Parkinson's Disease

Non-Motor and Non-Dopaminergic Features

Parkinson's Disease

Non-Motor and Non-Dopaminergic Features

EDITED BY

C. WARREN OLANOW MD, FRCPC
Henry P. and Georgette Goldschmidt Professor
Chairman Emeritus, Department of Neurology
Professor, Department of Neuroscience
Director, Robert and John M. Bendheim Parkinson's Disease Center
Mount Sinai School of Medicine
New York, NY, USA

FABRIZIO STOCCHI MD, PhD
Professor of Neurology
Director, Parkinson's Disease and Movement Disorders Research Centre
Institute for Research and Medical Care
IRCCS San Raffaele Pisana
Rome, Italy

ANTHONY E. LANG MD, FRCPC
Director, Division of Neurology, University of Toronto
Jack Clark Chair for Parkinson's Disease Research, University of Toronto
Director, Movement Disorder Centre, Toronto Western Hospital
Toronto, ON, Canada

WILEY-BLACKWELL
A John Wiley & Sons, Ltd., Publication

Blackwell Publishing was acquired by John Wiley & Sons in February 2007. Blackwell's publishing program has been merged with Wiley's global Scientific, Technical and Medical business to form Wiley-Blackwell.

Registered office: John Wiley & Sons, Ltd, The Atrium, Southern Gate, Chichester, West Sussex PO19 8SQ, UK

Editorial offices: 9600 Garsington Road, Oxford OX4 2DQ, UK
The Atrium, Southern Gate, Chichester, West Sussex PO19 8SQ, UK
111 River Street, Hoboken, NJ 07030-5774, USA

For details of our global editorial offices, for customer services and for information about how to apply for permission to reuse the copyright material in this book please see our website at www.wiley.com/wiley-blackwell

Library of Congress Cataloging-in-Publication Data
Parkinson's disease : non-motor and non-dopaminergic features / edited by C. Warren Olanow, Fabrizio Stocchi, Anthony E. Lang.
p. ; cm.
Includes bibliographical references and index.
ISBN 978-1-4051-9185-2 (hardcover : alk. paper) 1. Parkinson's disease–Diagnosis. 2. Parkinson's disease–Pathophysiology. I. Olanow, C. W. (Charles Warren), 1941- II. Stocchi, F. III. Lang, Anthony E.
[DNLM: 1. Parkinson Disease–complications. 2. Dopamine–physiology. 3. Parkinson Disease–physiopathology. WL 359]
RC382.P2657 2011
616.8′33–dc22

2010047397

A catalogue record for this book is available from the British Library.

This book is published in the following electronic formats: ePDF 9781444397956; Wiley Online Library 9781444397970; ePub 9781444397963

Set in 9.25/12pt Palatino by Aptara® Inc., New Delhi, India
Printed and bound in Malaysia by Vivar Printing Sdn Bhd

1 2011

Contents

Colour plate section can be found facing p. 182

List of Contributors

Garnik Akopian MD
Andrus Gerontology Center, University of Southern California, Los Angeles, CA, USA

Karen Anderson MD
Department of Neurology, University of Maryland Medical Center, Baltimore, MD, USA

Kailash P. Bhatia MD, FRCP
Sobell Department of Motor Neuroscience and Movement Disorders, Institute of Neurology, University College London, Queen Square, London, UK

Bastiaan R. Bloem MD
Department of Neurology and Parkinson Centre Nijmegen, Donders Institute for Brain Cognition and Behaviour, Radboud University Nijmegen Medical Centre. Nijmegen, The Netherlands

Heiko Braak MD
Clinical Neuroanatomy, Department of Neurology, Center for Clinical Research, University of Ulm, Ulm, Germany

Jonathan M. Brotchie PhD
Toronto Western Research Institute, Toronto Western Hospital, Toronto, ON, Canada

David J. Burn FRCP, MD, MA
Professor of Movement Disorders Neurology and Honorary Consultant Neurologist, Clinical Ageing Research Unit, Campus for Ageing and Vitality, Newcastle upon Tyne, UK

Antonio Carbone MD
Institute of Urology, University "La Sapienza", Rome, Italy

Cynthia L. Comella MD
Professor, Department of Neurological Sciences, Rush University Medical Center, Chicago, IL, USA

Michel A. Cramer Bornemann MD
Minnesota Regional Sleep Disorders Center and Hennepin County Medical Center, University of Minnesota Medical School, Minneapolis, MN, USA

Leonardo Cruz de Souza MD
Department of Neurology, Salpêtrière University Hospital, Paris, France

Virginie Czernecki PhD
Department of Neurology, Salpêtrière University Hospital, Paris, France

Kelly Del Tredici MD, PhD
Clinical Neuroanatomy, Department of Neurology, Center for Clinical Research, University of Ulm, Ulm, Germany

Dennis W. Dickson MD
Department of Neuroscience, Mayo Clinic, Jacksonville, FL, USA

Bruno Dubois MD
Professor of Neurology, Department of Neurology, Salpêtrière University Hospital, Paris, France

John E. Duda MD
Parkinson's Disease Research, Education and Clinical Center (PADRECC), Philadelphia Veterans Affairs Medical Center and Department of Neurology, University of Pennsylvania School of Medicine, Philadelphia, PA, USA

Mark J. Edwards PhD
Sobell Department of Motor Neuroscience and Movement Disorders, Institute of Neurology, University College London, Queen Square, London, UK

Murat Emre MD
Professor of Neurology, Istanbul Faculty of Medicine, Department of Neurology, Behavioral Neurology and Movement Disorders Unit, Istanbul University, Çapa Istanbul, Turkey

Andrew H. Evans MD, FRACP
Department of Neurology, Royal Melbourne Hospital, Parkville, Victoria, and Department of Medicine, University of Melbourne, Australia

Beth E. Fisher MD
Division of Biokinesiology and Physical Therapy, Department of Neurology, Keck School of Medicine, University of Southern California, Los Angeles, CA, USA

Cynthia M. Fox PhD, CCC-SLP
Research Associate, Department of Speech, Language and Hearing Science, University of Colorado–Boulder and the National Center for Voice and Speech–Denver, CO, USA

Susan H. Fox BSc, MB, ChB, MRCP (UK), PhD
Assistant Professor of Neurology, Movement Disorders Clinic, Division of Neurology, University of Toronto, Toronto, ON, Canada

Jospeph H. Friedman MD
Movement Disorders Program, Butler Hospital and Department of Neurology, Warren Alpert Medical School of Brown University, Providence, RI, USA

Christopher G. Goetz MD
Professor of Neurological Sciences and Professor of Pharmacology, Rush University Medical Center, Chicago, IL, USA

Anthony A. Grace PhD
Departments of Neuroscience, Psychiatry, and Psychology, University of Pittsburgh, Pittsburgh, PA, USA

Yvette Grimbergen MD
Department of Neurology, Leiden University Medical Centre, Leiden and Department of Neurology, Sint Franciscus Gasthuis, Rotterdam, The Netherlands

Staci Hoops BA
Department of Psychiatry, University of Pennsylvania, Philadelphia, PA, USA

Alex Iranzo MD
Neurology Service, Hospital Clinic and Institut d'Investigació Biomèdiques August Pi i Sunyer (IDIBAPS), Barcelona, Spain

Michael Jakowec MD
Department of Neurology, Keck School of Medicine and Division of Biokinesiology and Physical Therapy, University of Southern California, Los Angeles, CA, USA

Joseph Jankovic MD
Professor of Neurology, Director, Parkinson's Disease Center and Movement Disorders Clinic, Baylor College of Medicine, Houston, TX, USA

Carlos Juri MD
Clinica Universitaria and Medical School, Neuroscience Division, CIMA and Centro de Investigacion Biomedica en Red sobre Enfermedades Neurodegenerativas (CIBERNED), University of Navarra, Pamplona, Spain

Karl Kieburtz MD, MPH
Professor of Neurology and Community and Preventive Medicine, Department of Neurology, University of Rochester Medical Center, Rochester, NY, USA

Jeffrey H. Kordower PhD
Department of Neurological Sciences, Rush University Medical Center, Chicago, IL, USA

J. William Langston MD
Scientific Director and CEO, Parkinson's Institute, Sunnyvale, CA, USA

Andrew J. Lees FRCP
Director of Research, Reta Lila Weston Institute of Neurological Studies, Institute of Neurology, University College London, London, UK

Shen-Yang Lim MD, FRACP
Faculty of Medicine, University of Malaya, Kuala Lumpur, Malaysia

Andres W. Lozano MD, PhD, FRCSC, FRS
Professor and Dan Family Chairman of Neurosurgery, University of Toronto and Senior Scientist, Toronto Western Research Institute, Canada Research Chair in Neuroscience, Toronto, ON, Canada

Jun Lu MD, PhD
Department of Neurology, Program in Neuroscience and Division of Sleep Medicine, Harvard Medical School and Beth Israel Deaconess Medical Center, Boston, MA, USA

Mark W. Mahowald MD
Director, Minnesota Regional Sleep Disorders Center and Hennepin County Medical Center, University of Minnesota Medical School, Minneapolis, MN, USA

Christopher J. Mathias DPhil, DSc, FRCP, FMedSci
Autonomic and Neurovascular Medicine Unit, Imperial College London at St Mary's Hospital and Autonomic Unit, National Hospital for Neurology and Neurosurgery, Queen Square and Institute of Neurology, University College London, London, UK

Charlie K. Meshul MD
Department of Behavioral Neurosciences, Oregon Health Sciences University, Research Services, Portland VA Medical Center, Portland, OR, USA

Janis Miyasaki MD, FRCPC
Toronto Western Hospital (Movement Disorders Centre), University Health Network (UHN), University of Toronto, Toronto, ON, Canada

Uday Muthane DM, FNASc
Parkinson and Aging Research Foundation, Bangalore, India

Jose A. Obeso MD, PhD
Clinica Universitaria and Medical School, Neuroscience Division, CIMA and Centro de Investigacion Biomedica en Red sobre Enfermedades Neurodegenerativas (CIBERNED), University of Navarra, Pamplona, Spain

Carolyn F. Orr FRACP, PhD
Department of Neurology, Mayo Clinic, Rochester, NY, USA

Sean S. O'Sullivan MRCPI
Clincial Research Fellow, Reta Lila Weston Institute of Neurolgical Studies, Institute of Neurology, University College London, London, UK

Giovanni Palleschi MD
Institute of Urology, University "La Sapienza", Rome, Italy

Kimberly Pargeon MD
Department of Neurology, University of Maryland Medical Center, Baltimore, MD, USA

Daniel P. Perl MD
Professor of Pathology (Neuropathology), Uniformed Services University of the Health Sciences, Bethesda, MD, USA

Giselle Petzinger MD
Department of Neurology, Keck School of Medicine and Division of Biokinesiology and Physical Therapy, University of Southern California, Los Angeles, CA, USA

Ronald F. Pfeiffer MD
Department of Neurology, University of Tennessee Health Science Center, Memphis, TN, USA

Shilpa Ramaswamy PhD
Department of Neurological Sciences, Rush University Medical Center, Chicago, IL, USA

Lorraine Ramig PhD, CCC-SLP
Professor, University of Colorado–Boulder, Senior Scientist, National Center for Voice and Speech–Denver, CO, and Adjunct Professor, Columbia University, New York, NY, USA

Irene Hegeman Richard MD
Department of Neurology, University of Rochester School of Medicine and Dentistry, Rochester, NY, USA

Maria C. Rodriquez-Oroz MD, PhD
Clinica Universitaria and Medical School, Neuroscience Division, CIMA and Centro de Investigacion Biomedica en Red sobre Enfermedades Neurodegenerativas (CIBERNED), University of Navarra, Pamplona, Spain

Jospeh Rudolph MD
Department of Neurology, Mount Sinai School of Medicine, New York, NY, USA

Cristina Sampaio MD, PhD
Professor of Clinical Pharmacology and Therapeutics, Laboratory of Clinical Pharmacology and Therapeutics, Instituto de Medicina Molecular, Faculdade de Medicina de Lisboa, Lisbon, Portugal

Clifford B. Saper MD, PhD
Department of Neurology, Program in Neuroscience and Division of Sleep Medicine, Harvard Medical School and Beth Israel Deaconess Medical Center, Boston, MA, USA

Shimon Sapir PhD, CCC-SLP
Associate Professor, Communication Sciences and Disorders, Faculty of Social Welfare and Health Sciences, University of Haifa, Haifa, Israel

Carlos H. Schenck MD
Minnesota Regional Sleep Disorders Center and Hennepin County Medical Center, University of Minnesota Medical School, Minneapolis, MN, USA

Yvonne Schoon MD
Department of Geriatrics, Radboud University Nijmegen Medical Centre, Nijmegen, The Netherlands

Friederike Sixel-Döring MD
Paracelsus-Elena-Klinik, Center for Parkinsonism and Movement Disorders, Kassel and Philipps University, Marburg, Germany

Yoland Smith PhD
Professor of Neurology, Yerkes National Primate Research Center and Department of Neurology, Emory University, Atlanta, GA, USA

Brian J. Snyder MD
Division of Neurosurgery, Toronto Western Hospital, University of Toronto, Toronto, ON, Canada

Katherine E. Soderstrom BA
Department of Neurological Sciences, Rush University Medical Center, Chicago, IL, USA

Arlène D. Speelman MSc
Department of Neurology and Parkinson Centre Nijmegen, Donders Institute for Brain Cognition and Behaviour, Radboud University Nijmegen Medical Centre, Nijmegen, The Netherlands

Mark Stacy MD
Division of Neurology, Duke University Medical School, Durham, NC, USA

Thomas D.L. Steeves MD, FRCPC
Toronto Western Hospital (Movement Disorders Centre), University Health Network (UHN), University of Toronto, Toronto, ON, Canada

Matthew B. Stern MD
Parkinson's Disease Research, Education and Clinical Center (PADRECC), Philadelphia Veterans Affairs Medical Center, and Department of Neurology, University of Pennsylvania School of Medicine, Philadelphia, PA, USA

A. Jon Stoessl CM, MD, FRCPC
Pacific Parkinson's Research Centre, University of British Columbia, Vancouver, BC, Canada

Antonio P. Strafella MD, PhD, FRCPC
Associate Professor, Department of Medicine/Neurology, Movement Disorders Centre, Toronto Western Hospital and Senior Scientist, Division of Brain, Imaging and Behaviour–Systems Neuroscience, Toronto Western Research Institute and Associate Scientist, PET Imaging Center, Center for Addiction and Mental Health, University of Toronto, Toronto, ON, Canada

Michele Tagliati MD, FAAN
Vice Chairman, Department of Neurology, Director, Movement Disorders, Cedars-Sinai Medical Center, Los Angeles, CA, USA

Margherita Torti MD
Institute of Neurology, IRCCS San Raffaele Pisana, Rome, Italy

Claudia Trenkwalder MD
Paracelsus-Elena-Klinik, Center for Parkinsonism and Movement Disorders, Kassel and University of Göttingen, Göttingen, Germany

Marjolein A. van der Marck MSc
Department of Neurology and Parkinson Centre Nijmegen, Donders Institute for Brain Cognition and Behaviour, Radboud University Nijmegen Medical Centre, Nijmegen, The Netherlands

Tiffini Voss MD
Department of Neurology, University of Rochester School of Medicine and Dentistry, Rochester, NY, USA

John P. Walsh MD
Andrus Gerontology Center, University of Southern California, Los Angeles, CA, USA

William J. Weiner MD
Professor and Department Chairman, Department of Neurology, University of Maryland Medical Center, Baltimore, MD, USA

Daniel Weintraub MD
Assistant Professor of Psychiatry, University of Pennsylvania and Parkinson's Disease Research, Education and Clinical Center (PADRECC) and Mental Illness Research, Education and Clinical Center (MIRECC), Veterans Affairs Medical Center Philadelphia, PA, USA

Chapter 1
The Dopaminergic and Non-Dopaminergic Features of Parkinson's Disease

C. Warren Olanow[1], *Fabrizio Stocchi*[2], *& Anthony E. Lang*[3]
[1]Departments of Neurology and Neuroscience, Mount Sinai School of Medicine, New York, NY, USA
[2]Institute of Neurology, IRCCS San Raffaele Pisana, Rome, Italy
[3]Division of Neurology, University of Toronto, Toronto, ON, Canada

The dopamine story

Parkinson's disease (PD) is a common age-related neurodegenerative disorder, second only to Alzheimer's disease (AD). It is named in honor of James Parkinson, who provided a description of the disorder in his classic monograph written in 1817 [1]. Clinically, the disease is characterized by a series of cardinal motor features which include resting tremor, rigidity, bradykinesia, and gait impairment with postural instability. The hallmark pathologic features of the disease were described in the early twentieth century and are highlighted by degeneration of neurons in the substantia nigra pars compacta (SNc) coupled with proteinaceous Lewy bodies [2]. The presence of the brainstem dopaminergic system was first described by Dahlström and Fuxe [3]. The importance of dopamine depletion in the pathophysiology of PD was suggested in the late 1950s by Carlsson and colleagues, who showed that inhibition of dopamine uptake by reserpine led to a Parkinson-like syndrome in rabbits that could be reversed with the dopamine precursor levodopa [4]. Shortly afterwards, Ehringer and Hornykiewicz identified that there was a profound dopamine deficiency in the striatum of patients with PD [5]. It was subsequently established that dopamine is not simply a precursor in the norepinephrine pathway, but is itself a neurotransmitter that is manufactured in SNc neurons and transported to the striatum by way of the nigrostriatal tract.

Based on these observations, it was hypothesized that dopamine replacement might be an effective treatment strategy for PD. Dopamine itself does not cross the blood–brain barrier, so interest focused on the dopamine precursor levodopa, which can gain entry into the brain via the large neutral amino acid transport pathway and can then be decarboxylated to form dopamine. Initial studies in the early 1960s reported a dramatic benefit with small doses of levodopa [6], but these results were surprisingly difficult to confirm in early trials. It was not until the reports by Cotzias and co-workers in 1967 and 1969 that it was appreciated that consistent benefits could be obtained with relatively higher doses of levodopa [7,8]. These results were subsequently confirmed in double-blind trials [9], and the levodopa era had begun. Although levodopa provided benefit for the vast majority of PD patients, therapy was complicated by nausea and vomiting and could not be tolerated by as many as 50% of individuals. This problem was found to be due to the peripheral accumulation of dopamine and activation of dopamine receptors in the nausea and vomiting center of the brain (area postrema) that are not protected by the blood–brain barrier. This problem was resolved by administering levodopa in combination with a peripherally acting dopamine decarboxylase inhibitor [10], and levodopa today is routinely administered in combination with the decarboxylase inhibitor carbidopa (Sinemet®) or benserazide (Madopar®). Since its introduction, levodopa has been the standard of care for PD and has benefited millions of patients throughout the world. Virtually all patients improve, and benefits have been noted with respect to the classic motor features of the disease, quality of life, independence, employability, and mortality [11].

Levodopa-induced motor complications

Shortly after its introduction, it became appreciated that chronic levodopa therapy is associated with a series of motor complications, primarily comprised of fluctuations in motor response and involuntary movements or dyskinesias [12] (see Box 1.1). A review of the literature suggests that as many as 90% of patients who have received levodopa therapy for up to 10 years experience motor complications [13]. In severe cases, motor complications

Parkinson's Disease: Non-Motor and Non-Dopaminergic Features, First Edition. Edited by C. Warren Olanow, Fabrizio Stocchi, and Anthony E. Lang.

Box 1.1 Levodopa-induced motor complications

Motor fluctuations
- Wearing-off episodes
- Delayed on
- No "on"
- On/off phenomenon

Dyskinesia
- Peak dose dyskinesias
- Diphasic dyskinesia
- Dystonia

can be disabling and patients can cycle between "on" periods complicated by troublesome dyskinesias and "off" periods associated with severe parkinsonism and sometimes painful dystonia. This can result in severe disability for these patients and limit the utility of levodopa treatment.

The mechanism responsible for levodopa-induced motor complications in PD is not known. Levodopa does not cause motor complications in normal individuals, and the risk of their occurrence is increased with greater degrees of disease severity. Population studies and clinical trials indicate that motor complications are associated with the use of higher doses of levodopa [14,15], and they do not seem to be as troublesome today as they were a decade ago when physicians routinely employed higher doses. There is also evidence suggesting that the development of motor complications may relate to non-physiologic replacement of brain dopamine with standard formulations of levodopa [16]. In the normal state, SNc neurons fire continuously, striatal dopamine is maintained at a relatively constant level, and striatal dopamine receptors are continuously activated. With disease progression, as the striatum becomes progressively denervated, striatal dopamine levels become increasingly dependent on peripheral levodopa availability. Levodopa is typically administered to PD patients with a frequency of two to four times per day. As levodopa has a relatively short half-life (60–90 min), this intermittent administration of levodopa does not restore dopamine in a continuous and physiologic manner and leads to discontinuous or pulsatile stimulation of dopamine receptors. This in turn has been shown to result in molecular changes in striatal neurons, physiologic changes in pallidal neurons, and ultimately motor complications. It is now considered that the altered patterns of receptor stimulation by exogenously administered levodopa contribute to the development of motor complications in PD patients.

Over the past several decades, a number of interventions have been introduced to treat or prevent levodopa-induced motor complications by enhancing or prolonging the dopaminergic effect [17]. Dopamine agonists act directly on dopamine receptors and have longer half-lives than levodopa, MAO-B inhibitors block dopamine metabolism and increase synaptic dopamine concentrations, and COMT inhibitors block the peripheral metabolism of levodopa, thereby increasing brain availability of the drug. Each has been shown to reduce off-time in fluctuating patients. In addition, the early introduction of long-acting dopamine agonists reduces the risk of dyskinesia in comparison with levodopa and permits lower doses of levodopa to be employed. Surgical therapies that target nuclei within basal ganglia circuitry that have abnormal firing patterns associated with chronic levodopa treatment in PD have been shown to provide dramatic improvements for both motor fluctuations and dyskinesias [18]. Similar results have been reported with continuous infusion of dopaminergic agents such as levodopa and dopamine agonists [19,20], although these therapies have not yet been adequately evaluated in double-blind trials. It is noteworthy that no therapy has as yet been shown to provide anti-Parkinsonian benefits that are superior to what can be achieved with levodopa alone. Amazingly, 40 years after its introduction, levodopa remains the most effective symptomatic treatment for PD and the "gold standard" against which new therapies must be measured.

In the modern era, motor complications are not the problem they were a decade ago. This is related to the use of lower doses of levodopa, initiation of therapy with agents such as dopamine agonists that are less prone to induce motor complications, the availability of multiple medications that treat wearing-off effects, and surgical therapies that can control even severe motor complications. Research studies have examined the potential of dopamine cell transplantation or gene therapy strategies designed to restore the dopamine system in a physiologic manner, but benefits have not been observed in double-blind controlled studies and new research protocols continue to be explored. There is also an intensive effort to try to develop long-acting oral treatment strategies that can provide the benefits of levodopa without motor complications [21]. It is therefore realistic to consider that, in the not too distant future, we will be able to restore dopamine function to patients with PD and satisfactorily control the dopaminergic features of the disease for the vast majority of patients.

The non-motor and non-dopaminergic features of PD

Although treatment of the dopaminergic features has markedly changed the quality of life for most patients with PD, they continue to suffer from disability related to features that do not respond to levodopa. These are known as the non-dopaminergic features of PD because they likely relate to pathology that involves non-dopaminergic systems. It is now widely appreciated that pathology in PD involves more than just the nigrostriatal dopamine system. Neurodegeneration with Lewy bodies can be found in cholinergic neurons of the nucleus basalis of Meynert (NBM), epinephrine neurons of the locus coeruleus (LC), and serotonin neurons of the median raphe, in addition to neurons in the olfactory system, cerebral cortex, spinal cord, and peripheral autonomic nervous system [2,22]. Studies by Braak *et al.* based on α-synuclein immunostaining further suggest that in many PD patients pathologic changes occur in a progressive manner, beginning first in non-dopaminergic neurons of the dorsal motor nucleus of the vagus (DMV) and olfactory systems, involving dopamine neurons in the midbrain only in the mid-stage of the illness, and ultimately extending to involve the cerebral cortex in the later stages of the disease [23]. Although this precise sequence of Lewy pathology may not be found in all patients [24], and does not explain cases of dementia with Lewy bodies (DLB) where dementia is the presenting manifestation, it now seems likely that in most patients Lewy body pathology develops in non-dopaminergic regions of the nervous system before the dopamine system. Indeed, there is evidence of Lewy body pathology in autonomic neurons of the heart, gastrointestinal system, and cervical sympathetic ganglia in individuals with no clinical evidence of parkinsonism [25,26].

The non-dopaminergic clinical manifestations of PD are summarized in Box 1.2. These features, and particularly the non-motor manifestations, are frequently unrecognized and go untreated in as many as 50% or more of patients [27,28]. This is extremely relevant, as non-motor features have been shown to be a major determinant of the quality of life of PD patients and their caregivers [29–31]. In this respect, the 15 year follow-up from the prospective Sydney multicenter study is illuminating. Although 95% of patients experienced motor complications, it was the non-dopaminergic features of PD, such as falling, freezing, and dementia, that were the predominant causes of disability [32]. Indeed, 80% of surviving patients had experienced falls, with 23% suffering fractures, and 80% had dementia, with 50% being sufficiently severe to meet DSMIVR criteria. These non-dopaminergic features are also the main determinants of the need for nursing home placement [32–34] and survival [35,36] for PD patients.

Box 1.2 The non-dopaminergic features of PD

- *Motor disturbances*
  - Gait dysfunction, freezing and postural instability
  - Dysphagia
  - Drooling
- *Sensory disorders*
  - Pain and paresthesia
  - Anosmia
  - Visual discrimination defects
  - Ageusia
- *Autonomic dysfunction*
  - Orthostatic hypotension
  - Gastrointestinal disturbances – constipation, incontinence
  - Urinary impairment
  - Sexual dysfunction
  - Sweating
- *Sleep disturbances*
  - Sleep fragmentation
  - Excess daytime somnolence
  - Vivid dreaming
  - Insomnia
  - REM behavior disorder
  - RLS and periodic limb movements
  - Sleep apnea
- *Mood disturbances*
  - Depression
  - Anxiety and panic attacks
  - Apathy
- *Neuropsychiatric*
  - Hallucinations, illusions, delusions
  - Impulse control disorders
- *Cognitive impairment and dementia*
- *Others*
  - Seborrhea
  - Dry eyes
  - Fatigue
  - Diplopia
  - Blurred vision
  - Weight loss

The frequency with which non-motor features occur in PD is illustrated by recent studies which used newly developed questionnaires and scales to seek non-motor features in consecutive PD patients [37,38]. They illustrate that these symptoms occur far more frequently in PD patients than in age-matched controls, are present at the earliest stages of the illness, and gradually increase in number and severity over time in concert with the progression of the classical motor features of the illness. Different series show a broad range of prevalence of non-motor features in PD [35,37,39], probably due to the different methods used to assess and identify these features. It is estimated that between 50 and 100% of PD patients exhibit or are affected by non-motor features during the course of their disease [40]. In a cross-sectional population study, only 2.4% of PD patients reported not having non-motor symptoms, with milder PD patients reporting eight different types of symptoms compared with 12 in more severely affected patients [37]. Collectively, these studies illustrate the importance of non-dopaminergic and non-motor features in PD patients. The natural history of non-dopaminergic and non-motor features in PD is not well studied, and a large, longitudinal multicenter study is needed to assess formally the natural progression and risk factors for the development of these features in PD. The PRIAMO (PaRkInson And non Motor symptOms) study is ongoing and is expected to provide a better definition of the nature, extent, and relative importance of non-motor features in the PD population [41].

In keeping with the pathologic findings of Braak *et al.*, there is also evidence suggesting that many non-dopaminergic features, such as anosmia, constipation, and REM behavior disorder, may antedate the development of the classical dopaminergic motor features of PD [42–44]. Langston has suggested that patients who experience this triad of non-dopaminergic features are not just at risk for developing PD, but may actually have an early form of the disease [45]. Indeed, neuroimaging studies in at-risk populations have shown reduced dopaminergic activity [46], suggesting they may well be in an early phase of the disease consistent with this hypothesis. Originally, the term "preclinical" features was applied to these symptoms, but recognizing that they likely represent the earliest clinical manifestations of the disease, the term "premotor" PD is probably more accurate.

It should be appreciated that although non-motor features of PD may not be influenced by levodopa therapy, there can be fluctuations in association with doses of levodopa or dopamine agonists – this suggests that there may be a dopaminergic component to some of these non-motor features. For example, in some patients "off" periods are associated with pain, panic attacks, severe depression, confusion, sense of death, dysphagia, sweating, and/or difficulty with micturition and passing stool [47]. These symptoms can sometimes be improved, even dramatically, with levodopa or dopamine agonist therapy. Thus, non-motor features cannot be classified as being purely non-dopaminergic.

Importance of the non-dopaminergic features of PD

While the classical dopaminergic motor features continue to define PD, it is clear that we are entering a new era in which the non-dopaminergic features of the disease are being identified with increasing frequency and are an important source of disability for many individuals. In an age when PD patients had untreatable tremor, rigidity, and bradykinesia, the non-dopaminergic features of the illness were less evident and seemingly less important. Today, however, the classical motor features can usually be well controlled with dopaminergic therapies, and non-dopaminergic features have become increasingly problematic. Indeed, non-dopaminergic problems such as freezing, falling, and dementia, which cannot be adequately treated with dopaminergic therapies, are the major source of disability for patients with advanced PD. Research into their pathophysiology and the development of effective treatment strategies to control them are urgently required. Much of current research, particularly in areas such as cell-based and gene therapies, continues to be primarily focused on the dopamine system. Although this research is laudatory, it is currently not easy to conceive (although not inconceivable) how better restoration of the dopamine system will restore function to disabilities primarily related to degeneration of non-dopaminergic neurons. Clearly, more attention needs to be focused on the nature of non-dopaminergic pathology and the potentially disabling symptoms that ensue. Further, the evolution of the PD process to include these disabling problems emphasizes the need for neuroprotective therapies in PD that might be introduced early in the course of the disease to slow or stop disease progression and thereby potentially prevent their occurrence.

Non-dopaminergic features might also be important in facilitating the development of a neuroprotective therapy. In the laboratory, we routinely test promising agents in models of PD such as the MPTP monkey and the 6-OHDA lesioned rat, which primarily reflect dopamine depletion. They do not, however, replicate the pathologic or behavioral spectrum of the disorder. More importantly, there is no assurance that the etiopathogenesis of cell death in these models is in any way related to PD, or that agents that are protective in these models will prove beneficial in PD [48]. There is an intense effort to develop new models that more faithfully replicate the pathology of PD with involvement of the non-dopaminergic systems. Such a model might not only permit the development of therapies to treat non-dopaminergic features of PD, but might reflect a mechanism that more closely represents what is actually going on in PD than do current models. Unfortunately, the development of such models has not proven easy. It is hoped that the development of transgenic animals which carry gene mutations associated with PD might accomplish this goal, but to date this has proven to be difficult to achieve and further efforts are required.

Non-dopaminergic features of PD might also serve as primary endpoints in clinical trials seeking to identify a neuroprotective or disease-modifying therapy. Agents tested in studies performed to date cannot be definitively interpreted to have provided a neuroprotective effect even if the trial is positive, because a confounding symptomatic or pharmacologic effect of the study intervention cannot be excluded [49]. For example, it may not be possible to be sure whether positive results are due to the study agent slowing disease progression or to the agent having a symptomatic effect that merely masks ongoing neurodegeneration. Non-dopaminergic features of PD are defined by their lack of response to dopaminergic therapies, perhaps making them more suitable for endpoints than the classic motor features which have traditionally been employed to date. Even if neuroprotection cannot be definitively established, a determination that a given intervention slows or prevents the emergence of disability related to non-dopaminergic features for which there is currently no adequate therapy would be a welcome addition regardless of its mechanism of action. A composite endpoint that incorporates conventional UPDRS scores along with measures of non-dopaminergic features such as falling, freezing, and dementia is being employed as the primary outcome measure for an NIH-sponsored long-term simple study that aims to assess the effect of an intervention on cumulative disability. Although such studies are usually relatively long (approximately 5 years), the inclusion of non-dopaminergic features in the primary endpoint may provide greater insight into the effect of a new study drug on disease progression than current outcome measures.

Finally, if a neuroprotective therapy that slowed the rate of disease progression could be identified, early diagnosis would be extremely important. Non-dopaminergic features might permit the diagnosis of PD to be made prior to the emergence of the classical motor features of the disease, and thus permit a disease-modifying agent to be introduced at an earlier time point. Already, there is evidence suggesting that early treatment with a given agent might provide benefits that cannot be achieved by later treatment with the same agent, possibly by preserving beneficial compensatory mechanisms or preventing the development of maladaptive compensatory mechanisms [50,51,51a]. Early diagnosis, and the early introduction of therapy, have therefore become a major consideration in the current management of the early PD patient [52].

Conclusions

Interest in PD during the past half century has primarily focused on the dopamine system. However, it is evident that PD is a disorder with widespread pathology that involves more than just the nigrostriatal system. Clinical features of PD reflect this non-dopaminergic pathology and it is now appreciated that many disabling features of the disease do not respond to or are not adequately controlled by dopaminergic therapies. In a way, we are victims of our own success. Our ability to control the classical motor features of the illness with dopaminergic therapies has highlighted the importance of the non-dopaminergic features of the disease. Indeed, in the levodopa era, the non-dopaminergic features of PD constitute the major source of disability for advanced PD patients and their treatment constitutes an important unmet medical need. It is interesting to speculate on whether the same will hold true for other degenerative diseases such as AD and ALS once a satisfactory treatment for the primary cognitive and motor aspects of these illnesses has been developed.

Over the decades, there have been many textbooks that have addressed the clinical, pathologic, and etiopathologic features of PD, particularly as they relate to the dopamine system. We believe that there is now sufficient information and interest to warrant a full textbook dedicated to the non-dopaminergic features of PD. Here, we have gathered together a comprehensive series of chapters on the various clinical, pathologic, and scientific issues related to the non-dopaminergic aspects of PD written by a group of experts in their various fields. It is hoped that better recognition and understanding of the origin of these problems will lead to enhanced patient care and serve as a stimulus for the development of newer and more effective therapies for PD patients.

References

1. Parkinson J. *An Essay on the Shaking Palsy*. London: Whittingham and Rowland for Sherwood, Neely and Jones, 1817.
2. Forno LS. Neuropathology of Parkinson's disease. *J Neuropathol Exp Neurol* 1996;**55**(3):259–72.
3. Dahlström A, Fuxe K. Evidence for the existence of monoamine-containing neurons in the central nervous system. 1. Demonstration of monoamines in cell bodies of brainstem neurons. *Acta Physiol Scand Suppl* 1964;**232**:1–55.
4. Carlsson A, Lindqvist M, Magnusson T. 3,4-Dihydroxyphenylalanine and 5-hydroxytryptophan as reserpine antagonists. *Nature* 1957;**180**:1200.
5. Ehringer H, Hornykiewicz O. Distribution of noradrenaline and dopamine (3-hydroxytyramine) in the human brain and their behavior in diseases of the extrapyramidal system. *Klin Wochenschr* 1960;**38**:1236–9 (in German).
6. Birkmayer W, Hornykiewicz O. The L-3,4-dioxyphenylalanine (DOPA) effect in Parkinson-akinesia. *Wien Klin Wochenschr* 1961;**73**:787–8 (in German).
7. Cotzias GC, Van Woert MH, Schiffer LM. Aromatic amino acids and modification of parkinsonism. *N Engl J Med* 1967;**276**:374– 9.
8. Cotzias GC, Papavasiliou PS, Gellene R. Modification of parkinsonism – chronic treatment with L-dopa. *N Engl J Med* 1969;**280**:337–45.
9. Yahr MD, Duvoisin RC, Schear MJ, *et al*. Treatment of parkinsonism with levodopa. *Arch Neurol* 1969;**21**:343–54.
10. Papavasiliou PS, Cotzias GC, Duby SE, *et al*. Levodopa in parkinsonism: potentiation of central effects with a peripheral inhibitor. *N Engl J Med* 1972;**286**:8–14.
11. Olanow CW, Watts RL, Koller WC. An algorithm (decision tree) for the management of Parkinson's disease: treatment guidelines. *Neurology* 2001;**56**(Suppl 5):1–88.
12. Fox S, Lang AE. Levodopa-related motor complications – phenomenology. *Mov Disord* 2008;**23**(Suppl 3):S509–14.
13. Ahlskog JE, Muenter MD. Frequency of levodopa-related dyskinesias and motor fluctuations as estimated from the cumulative literature. *Mov Disord* 2001;**16**:448–58.
14. Schrag A, Quinn N. Dyskinesias and motor fluctuations in Parkinson's disease. A community-based study. *Brain* 2000;**123**:2297–305.
15. Fahn S, Oakes D, Shoulson I, *et al*. Levodopa and the progression of Parkinson's disease. *N Engl J Med* 2004;**351**:2498–508.

16. Olanow CW, Obeso JA, Stocchi F. Continuous dopamine receptor stimulation in the treatment of Parkinson's disease: scientific rationale and clinical implications. Lancet *Neurol* 2006;**5**:677–87.
17. Schapira AHV, Olanow CW. *Principles of Treatment for Parkinson's Disease*. Philadelphia, PA: Butterworth Heinemann, Elsevier, 2005.
18. The Deep-Brain Stimulation for Parkinson's Disease Study Group. Deep-brain stimulation of the subthalamic nucleus or the pars interna of the globus pallidus in Parkinson's disease. *N Engl J Med* 2001;**345**:956–63.
19. Nutt JG, Obeso JA, Stocchi F. Continuous dopamine-receptor stimulation in advanced Parkinson's disease. *Trends Neurosci* 2000;**23**(10 Suppl):S109–15
20. Stocchi F, Vacca L, Ruggieri S, Olanow CW. Infusion of levodopa methyl ester in patients with advanced PD: a clinical and pharmacokinetic study. *Arch Neurol* 2005;**62**:905–10.
21. Olanow CW. Levodopa – current use and future directions. *Mov Disord* 2008;**23**:S613–22.
22. Esiri M, Perl D. *Oppenheimer's Diagnostic Neuropathology; a Practice Manual*, 3rd edn. London: Hodder Arnold, 2008.
23. Braak H, Del Tredici K, Rub U, *et al*. Staging of brain pathology related to sporadic Parkinson's disease. *Neurobiol Aging* 2003;**24**:197–211.
24. Burke RE, Dauer WT, Vonsattel JP. A critical evaluation of the Braak staging scheme for Parkinson's disease. *Ann Neurol* 2008;**64**:485–91.
25. Wakabayashi K, Takahashi H, Takeda S, *et al*. Parkinson's disease: the presence of Lewy bodies in Auerbach's and Meissner's plexuses. *Acta Neuropathol* 1988;**76**:217–21.
26. Minguez-Castellanos A, Chamorro CE, Escamilla-Sevilla F, *et al*. Do alpha-synuclein aggregates in autonomic plexuses predate Lewy body disorders? A cohort study. *Neurology* 2007;**68**:2012–8.
27. Chaudhuri KR, Healy DG, Schapira AH, National Institute for Clinical Excellence. Non-motor symptoms of Parkinson's disease: diagnosis and management. *Lancet Neurol* 2006;**5**:235–45.
28. Shulman LM, Taback RL, Rabinstein AA, Weiner WJ. Nonrecognition of depression and other non-motor symptoms in Parkinson's disease. *Parkinsonism Relat Disord* 2002;**8**:193–7.
29. Forsaa EB, Larsen JP, Wentzel-Larsen T, *et al*. Predictors and course of health-related quality of life in Parkinson's disease. *Mov Disord* 2008;**23**:1420–7.
30. Rahman S, Griffin HJ, Quinn NP, Jahanshahi M. Quality of life in Parkinson's disease: the relative importance of the symptoms. *Mov Disord* 2008;**23**:1428–34.
31. Visser M, van Rooden SM, Verbaan D, *et al*. A comprehensive model of health-related quality of life in Parkinson's disease. *J Neurol* 2008;**255**:1580–7.
32. Hely MA, Morris JG, Reid WG, Trafficante R. Sydney Multicenter Study of Parkinson's Disease: non-L-dopa-responsive problems dominate at 15 years. *Mov Disord* 2005;**20**:190–9.
33. Aarsland D, Larsen JP, Tandberg E, Laake K. Predictors of nursing home placement in Parkinson's disease: a population-based, prospective study. *J Am Geriatr Soc* 2000;**48**:938–42.
34. Goetz CG, Stebbins GT. Risk factors for nursing home placement in advanced Parkinson's disease. *Neurology* 1993;**43**:2227–9.
35. Alves G, Forsaa EB, Pedersen KF, *et al*. Epidemiology of Parkinson's disease. *J Neurol* 2008;**255**(Suppl 5):18–32.
36. Chen H, Zhang SM, Schwarzschild MA, *et al*. Survival of Parkinson's disease patients in a large prospective cohort of male health professionals. *Mov Disord* 2006;**21**:1002–7.
37. Chaudhuri KR, Martinez-Martin P, Schapira AHV, *et al*. International multicentre pilot study of the first comprehensive self-completed nonmotor symptoms questionnaire for Parkinson's disease: The NMSQuest Study. *Mov Disord* 2006;**21**:916–23.
38. Chaudhuri KR, Martinez-Martin P, Brown RG, *et al*. The metric properties of a novel non-motor symptoms scale for Parkinson's disease: results from an international pilot study. *Mov Disord* 2007;**22**:1901–11.
39. Borek LL, Amick MM, Friedman JH. Non-motor aspects of Parkinson's disease. *CNS Spectrums* 2006;**11**:541–54.
40. Shulman LM, Taback RL, Bean J, Weiner WJ. Comorbidity of the nonmotor symptoms of Parkinson's disease. *Mov Disord* 2001;**16**:507–10.
41. Antonini A, Colosimo C, Marconi R, *et al*. The PRIAMO study: background, methods and recruitment. *Neurol Sci* 2008;**29**: 61–5.
42. Ponsen MM, Stoffers D, Booij J, *et al*. Idiopathic hyposmia as a preclinical sign of Parkinson's disease. *Ann Neurol* 2004;**56**:173–81.
43. Abbott RD, Petrovitch H, White LR, *et al*. Frequency of bowel movements and the future risk of Parkinson's disease. *Neurology* 2001;**57**:456–62.
44. Schenck CH, Bundlie SR, Mahowald MW. Delayed emergence of a parkinsonian disorder in 38% of 29 older men initially diagnosed with idiopathic rapid eye movement sleep behaviour disorder. *Neurology* 1996;**46**:388–93.
45. Langston JW. The Parkinson's complex: parkinsonism is just the tip of the iceberg. *Ann Neurol* 2006;**59**:591–6.
46. Horstink MW, Morrish PK. Preclinical diagnosis of Parkinson's disease. *Adv Neurol* 1999;**80**:327–33.
47. Stacy M, Bowron A, Guttman M, *et al*. Identification of motor and nonmotor wearing-off in Parkinson's disease: comparison of a patient questionnaire versus a clinician assessment. *Mov Disord* 2005;**20**:726–33.
48. Jenner P. Functional models of Parkinson's disease: a valuable tool in the development of novel therapies. *Ann Neurol* 2008;**64**(Suppl 2):S16–29.
49. Schapira AHV, Olanow CW. Neuroprotection in Parkinson's disease: myths, mysteries, and misconceptions. *JAMA* 2004;**291**:358–64.
50. Schapira AH, Obeso J. Timing of treatment initiation in Parkinson's disease: a need for reappraisal? *Ann Neurol* 2006;**59**:559–62.
51. Olanow CW. Hauser R, Jankovic J, *et al*. A randomized, double-blind, placebo-controlled, delayed start study to assess rasagiline as a disease modifying therapy in Parkinson's disease (The ADAGIO Study): rationale, design, and baseline characteristics. *Mov Disord* 2008;**23**:2194–201.

51a. Olanow CW, Rascol O, Hauser R. Double-blind delayed-start study of rasagiline in early Parkinson's disease. *N Engl J Med* 2009;**361**:1268–78.

52. Olanow CW, Stern MB, Sethi K. Scientific and clinical basis for the treatment of PD. *Neurology* 2009;**72**(21 Suppl 4): S1–136.

Chapter 2
Neuropathologic Involvement of the Dopaminergic Neuronal Systems in Parkinson's Disease

Daniel P. Perl
Uniformed Services University of the Health Sciences, Bethesda, MD, USA

Introduction: the neuroanatomy of the dopaminergic system

In 1964, based on their original work using histofluorescence, Dahlström and Fuxe [1] identified a number of monoaminergic neurons. Based on their findings, they proposed a nomenclature to identify these cell groups systematically. These monoamine (both dopamine and noradrenaline) neuronal groups were given an "A" designation and their order (A1, A2, A3, etc.) was arranged in a caudal to rostral orientation. The more caudal groups were predominantly noradrenergic and beginning in the mesencephalon the major dopaminergic neuronal populations of the brain were encountered. Three dopaminergic neuronal groups were identified in the mesencephalon and categorized as A8, A9, and A10. Since that original work in 1964, we have learned a great deal about these neuronal populations, their neuronal constituents, and their projections. Nevertheless, this nomenclature remains in wide use. However, the boundaries of these regions remain relatively imprecisely drawn and poorly defined. The Dahlström and Fuxe designations are still used in many publications, but the specifics of these designations may differ from one group of authors to another. This has caused some confusion in interpreting specific findings and, in particular, comparing results from different studies.

The substantia nigra pars compacta (SNc) is the grossly visible black substance in the midbrain located dorsal and medial to the cerebral peduncles. It is composed of prominently melanized neurons, the vast majority of which are tyrosine hydroxylase immunoreactive. Under the Dahlström and Fuxe classification, it is referred to as A9. Identifying this conspicuous nucleus is fairly straightforward; however, some of its boundaries have remained indistinct and distinction from its immediate neighbors is somewhat arbitrary. Within the SNc, a further subdivision of the neuronal populations has been proposed based on both neuroanatomic criteria and further neurochemical characterization. Based on tyrosine hydroxylase immunohistochemistry, the SNc forms two subcompartments or tiers, a dorsal tier and a roughly parallel ventral tier. In 1937, Hassler [2] provided perhaps the most comprehensive investigation of SNc anatomy and proceeded to divide this structure into 31 different subgroups. Although some of Hassler's subgroups are consistently recognizable, many appear to be rather arbitrarily drawn and are not sufficiently reproducible to make this a practical approach. Olszewski and Baxter, in their elegant atlas [3], subdivided the SNc into three parallel divisions, using the terms α, β, and γ. Using a somewhat similar approach, Gibbs and Lees [4] used this approach to create a simplified version of the Hassler classification. They described two parallel tiers, the ventrolateral group comparable to the α layer, and the dorsal group comparable to the β layer. The γ group is composed of a relatively small number of scattered cells that are mostly located in the region adjacent to the capsule of the red nucleus.

Damier *et al.* [5,6] employed a different approach to subdividing the SNc using calbindin D_{28K} immunohistochemistry. Using this approach, the SNc can be subdivided into calbindin-rich regions (matrix areas) and calbindin-poor regions (nigrosomes). In the calbindin-rich matrix areas, the neurons tend to be more diffusely oriented, whereas in the nigrosomes, they tend to be more densely packed. Within the SNc, there are a total of five nigrosomes (referred to as N1, N2, N3, N4, and N5), which can be consistently identified based on calbindin D_{28K} immunohistochemistry.

The A8 dopamine neurons represent a caudal and dorsal extension of the SNc (A9 neurons) and form a continuous band of cells without a clear distinction between

Parkinson's Disease: Non-Motor and Non-Dopaminergic Features, First Edition. Edited by C. Warren Olanow, Fabrizio Stocchi, and Anthony E. Lang.

the SNc and red nucleus. By and large, they comprise a retrorubral mesencephalic reticular extension and lie in a position that is dorsolateral to the SNc.

The A10 dopamine neurons are actually a combination of several populations of melanized neurons which are of variable size and found dorsomedial to the SNc. McRitchie, Hardman, and Halliday [7] characterized A10 in the human using detailed neuroanatomic preparations that rely on immunohistochemical markers. As they pointed out, when looked at in this fashion, the A10 region may be subdivided into seven separate and distinct subnuclei. To make the situation even more confusing, one of the seven regions they identified is referred to as the ventral tegmental area (VTA), a term that many others have employed to signify the entire A10 neuronal group.

The groups of dopaminergic neurons which are referred to as A11–A14 are relatively restricted small clusters of melanized cells which lie within the posterior aspect of the hypothalamus (A11), the arcuate nucleus (A12), and the periventricular nucleus (A13 and A14). With the exception of the A13 group characterized by Saper and colleagues [8,9], there has been relatively little study of these particular cell groups in the human.

Anatomic/functional considerations

For the past 20 years or more, there has been an increasing recognition that the mesencephalic dopaminergic system supports differing functions through its three separate pathways, namely the mesostriatal or nigrostriatal pathway, the mesolimbic projection, and the mesocortical pathway. The generally accepted concept has been that neurons of the SNc (A9) by way of the mesostriatal pathways provide dopaminergic innervation to the dorsal striatum. In the monkey, the more rostral portion of the SNc projects largely to the caudate (head) nucleus whereas the more posterior aspect of the nigra projects predominantly to the putamen. Further organization is provided with the more lateral portions of the SNc providing input to the dorsal portion of the head of the caudate. In this way, the A9 region is thought to be primarily involved in motor function through its modulating effects on the dorsal striatum.

The mesolimbic pathways involve the more medial tier of midbrain dopaminergic neurons, including the dorsomedial aspect of the SNc and the adjacent VTA (A10). The neurons of the VTA provide the major mesolimbic input and project primarily to the septal nuclei and nucleus accumbens. The retrorubral field neurons (A8) provide additional mesolimbic innervation. This mesolimbic input is involved in a wide range of motivation and goal-directed behaviors, in addition to pleasure-seeking activities. Further investigation has revealed rather diffuse and widespread dopaminergic input to the cerebral cortex, particularly the prefrontal regions, anterior olfactory nucleus and olfactory bulb, and hippocampus. The source of this mesocortical input has been considered to come primarily from VTA (A10) with some contribution also arising from A8 neurons. Such pathways are thought to involve the modulation of aspects of cognitive behavior, especially those concerning spatial working memory.

Although the concept of the three functionally and anatomically distinct ascending dopaminergic pathways, namely mesostriatal, mesolimbic, and mesocortical pathways, remains valid, ongoing research has cautioned that the origin of such projections from separate and discrete nuclear groups in the midbrain represents an oversimplification and will need to be revised and refined. It is clear that although the vast majority of SNc (A9) neurons do provide dopaminergic input to the dorsal striatum, this region also contains neurons that project to both cortical and limbic areas. Furthermore, striatal dopaminergic input derives, to some extent, from neurons in the VTA (A10) as well as from A8. In summary, the simplified notion of separate ventral and dorsal tiers in the midbrain tegmentum which serve to modulate discretely motor, motivational, and cognitive function has been useful but needs to be revised. There is clearly much overlap and integration of the innervations of the relevant structures and the specific functional role of these various neuroanatomic regions is more complex than was originally considered.

Morphometric quantitative studies of substantia nigra (A9) in normal aging

Over the past several decades, it has generally been accepted that there is a loss of dopaminergic neurons in the SNc in association with normal aging. This literature is complex, with rather differing approaches and results. Most point to the paper by McGeer, McGeer, and Suzuki [10] in 1977 as the original source of this concept. This study involved 13 normal controls (and four "parkinsonian" cases) and performed counts of pigmented neurons based on Cresyl Violet stains of every fifth section that had been cut serially through the entire SNc. How the SNc was delineated or the range of the dissection was not included in the Methods section of this rather brief paper, nor was there mention of how the cases were determined to be controls, on either a clinical or neuropathologic basis. The cases ranged in age from mid-teenage years to two cases in their early 80s. The cases had been obtained at autopsy from coroners and hospitals in the general Vancouver area. Although no specific neuronal counts are provided, from the correlation data graph that is included one may interpret that there was a 48% neuronal loss by age 60 years (about 7% per decade). Other somewhat similar studies [11–13] have reported a variable degree of loss. In each of these papers, what was counted, how neuronal counts were performed, and the nature of the case material were only briefly described or not mentioned at all. Interestingly, Fearnley and Lees [13] reported that SNc neuronal loss in controls was more prominent in the dorsal tier as opposed to the ventral tier, which is the predominant location of neuronal loss in association with Parkinson's disease (PD).

Kubis *et al.* [14] counted the numbers of tyrosine hydroxylase immunoreactive neurons in SNc (A9), VTA (A10), and the peri- and retrorubral areas (A8) of 21 brains derived from normal controls aged 44–110 years. These control specimens were derived from patients who had been without any significant neurologic symptomatology during life and who were also shown to be free of significant involvement by Lewy bodies, senile plaques, or neurofibrillary tangles on post-mortem examination. The entire rostal brainstem was cryoprotected, frozen, and serially sectioned with tyrosine hydroxylase staining of every 36th section for counting. Their approach to neuron counting, although exhaustive, was not strictly in adherence with the modern principles of non-biased serial sampling or stereology [15,16]. Nevertheless, this study failed to find any evidence of significant neuronal loss in any of the three dopaminergic neuronal compartments in their control cases.

More recently, there have been a series of studies in which stereologic principles have been employed for the counting SNc neurons in normal aging controls. These studies provided differing results and, for a number of reasons, are somewhat difficult to compare. As mentioned for the earlier studies, there were differences in how the controls were characterized and defined. There are also significant differences in which counting methods were used and what neuronal markers were employed. Cabello *et al.* [17] studied 28 brains derived from male controls, aged 19–92 years. The cases were described as being free of central nervous system disease yet the means by which that was determined is not specified. In this stereologically based study, melanized and non-melanized neurons that had been identified within the substantia nigra were counted in hematoxylin and eosin-stained plastic-embedded sections. How the boundaries of the substantia nigra were defined is not delineated in the paper. Nevertheless, they reported a significant decrease in the total number of melanin-containing neurons in the substantia nigra as a function of age. This correlation was not seen in the counts of non-melanized neurons within the substantia nigra. An additional finding was that advanced age was significantly associated with an increased in the size of the soma of the melanin-containing SNc neurons.

Using stereologically-based approaches, Chu, *et al.* [18] investigated the number of melanin-containing, tyrosine hydroxylase immunoreactive, and nuclear orphan receptor-related factor 1 (Nurr1) immunoreactive neurons of the SNc of 19 control subjects ranging in age from 18 to 102 years. The cases were subdivided into three subgroups, namely, young (aged 18–39 years, mean = 29.1 years), middle-aged (aged 44–68 years, mean = 56.5 years) and aged (aged 76–102 years, mean = 87.1 years) groups. The specimens were derived from patients who were stated to be without evidence of neurologic or psychiatric illness, although the means by which this was determined was not mentioned in the paper. Nurr1 is known to be essential for dopaminergic phenotype and motor function and was used as a surrogate marker for SNc dopamine neurons. This group found a significant reduction in Nurr1 immunoreactive neurons in the middle-aged (23.1% loss) and aged (46.3% loss) groups compared with the young group. The numbers of tyrosine hydroxylase immunoreactive neurons showed a very similar result. Of interest is the finding that the total melanized neuron counts were stable across all three age groups, suggesting the possibility of an age-related loss in these two dopamine-related neuronal markers but not in the actual number of cells.

Ma *et al.* [19] examined the number of melanin-containing neurons in the SNc of 26 controls with an age range of 17–90 years. The control cases had no signs or symptoms of PD or other neuropsychiatric diseases and were free of Lewy bodies (based on hematoxylin and eosin staining) and significant Alzheimer's disease-related changes. Using the physical dissector approach, they counted the number of pigmented neurons of the SNc in every 40th paraffin-embedded section stained with hematoxylin and eosin. In contrast to the previous study, they found a dramatic loss of pigmented neurons with aging ($r = -0.83$, $p < 0.001$); this decrease was equal to a 9.8% loss of SNc neurons per decade.

In a recent study, Rudow *et al.* [20] attempted to address many of these variables in the context of a stereologically based study of the substantia nigra in normal aging and PD. They examined seven young controls (aged 18–21 years) with no history of neurologic disease and who showed no neuropathologic abnormalities at autopsy, including being free of α-synuclein or tau-related lesions. Nine middle-aged controls (aged 43–59 years) met similar clinical and neuropathologic criteria. Finally, seven older controls (aged 76–96 years) were obtained from deceased enrollees in the Baltimore Longitudinal Study of Aging. These individuals had undergone extensive longitudinal neurologic, neuropsychological, and other clinical examinations with a mean last evaluation conducted within 8.6 months of death. Neuropathologic examination at autopsy revealed the absence of any underlying neurologic disease and no α-synuclein lesions, CERAD neuritic plaque scores of 0 or A (age-related normal) [21], and a Braak and Braak AD-related score of II or III [22]. Stereologically based neuronal counting was based on an examination of every 20th section of serially cut 50 μm paraffin-embedded sections through the entire extent of the substantia nigra. They used an optical fractionators approach to count total pigmented neurons and tyrosine hydroxylase immunoreactive neurons within the substantia nigra. The paper specifically mentions that they included both substantia nigra pars compacta and substantia nigra pars reticulata, despite the fact that the latter region is closely linked to the globus pallidus and is not part of the dopaminergic striatonigral projection system. The reason for this somewhat unusual approach is not explained. Dr Mark West is an author of this paper and, as one of the senior members of the group in Aarhus, Denmark, who developed and popularized the technique, one can assume that the orthodoxy of stereology was strictly adhered to. They found that the number and cell volume of melanin-containing neurons and tyrosine hydroxylase immunoreactive cells decreased significantly with respect to increasing age. There was a 28.3% pigmented neuronal loss when the young subjects were compared with the elderly group and a 36.2% loss of tyrosine hydroxylase immunoreactive neurons.

These important studies all report rather different results and some reach dramatically different conclusions. Each employs a somewhat different approach to defining what they consider to be a control, what region they include in their counting, and what type of cells they count. Further, many of the means by which these cell populations are counted vary considerably. Replication is a key to resolution of this problem, and additional work needs to be done with these factors in mind before these important questions can be considered to be properly answered. For the present, the majority of studies indicate that there is an age-related loss of dopamine markers and probably SNc neurons with aging.

Involvement of various dopaminergic neuronal groups in Parkinson's disease

Substantia nigra pars compacta (A9)

PD is defined for neuropathologists as neuronal loss of the dopaminergic neurons of the SNc accompanied by the appearance of Lewy bodies in some surviving neurons in this location (Plate 2.1). This definition has stood the test of time for almost 90 years, although the recent appearance of a very small number of familial parkinsonism cases which lack the diagnostic signature of the Lewy body have led to discussion of whether that definition remains viable [23,24]. In the context of this discussion, we will not venture into that debate but will point out that whether a sporadic case or a familial one, it is the neuronal loss within the nigrostriatal system that defines many, but certainly not all, of the motor features of PD and conceptually underlies virtually all of our currently available therapeutic approaches. The loss of pigmented neurons in the SNc is sufficiently complete that at autopsy of cases of PD the gross appearance on transverse section of the midbrain demonstrates obvious loss of black coloration. Some rare cases, particularly with relatively mild or early symptomatology, may only show blurring of the pigmentation at the edges of the SNc and require comparison with a normal specimen (see Plates 2.2–2.4).

In cases of PD, the neuronal loss is progressive and it is said that there is a significant lengthy presymptomatic phase and that clinical signs do not become apparent until at least 50% of nigral neurons are lost [25]. The actual data to support this often-quoted figure are rather scanty; however, it is clear that a significant degree of neuronal loss along with the dopaminergic projections they supply is needed for clinical symptomatology to ensue. For the most part, this is in accord with extrapolations of functional data supplied by PET scan studies of dopaminergic activity in early or presymptomatic patients [26].

The SNc is anatomically heterogeneous, with various components related to specific striatal projections. Based on a number of studies, there is evidence that in cases of PD, although involvement of the SNc may be encountered throughout the nucleus, it is not uniform in the degree of involvement and actually displays distinct regional specificities. Among the most detailed of such studies was the early work of Hassler [2,27], who categorized approximately 30 different neuronal subgroups within the SNc and then analyzed each with regard to involvement in cases of PD. In essence, Hassler's general conclusion was that involvement was most severe in the caudal and ventrolateral portions of the SNc.

The later study of Fearnley and Lees [13] looked at this issue using a less complicated parcellization of the SNc. They first divided the SNc into dorsal and ventral tiers. The dorsal tier was subdivided into three subregions, medial, lateral, and pars lateralis, while the ventral tier was divided in half into ventral and lateral portions. In the cases of PD that were examined, the most severe degree of neuronal loss was consistently found in the lateral portion of the ventral tier. This portion of the SNc is thought to project primarily to the dorsal portion of the putamen, the location in which the greatest degree of dopamine depletion is found in PD [28]. It should be noted that this finding essentially replicated that of Hassler, although he employed a much more complex approach to defining the distribution of cellular loss.

As mentioned above, Damier *et al.* [5,6] employed calbindin D_{28K} immunohistochemistry to subdivide the SNc into calbindin-rich (matrix areas) and calbindin-poor regions (nigrosomes). Using this approach to subdivide the SNc neuronal components (plus TH immunohistochemistry), five PD cases were examined and compared with five age-matched neurologically intact controls. In these cases they reported that neuronal loss was uneven in various dopaminergic cell groups, being greatest among neurons in the nigrosomes in comparison with those within the matrix area. Among the five nigrosome regions, the N1 nigrosome, the largest of these subregions that is located in the caudal and mediolateral aspect of the SNc, consistently showed the most significant degree of neuronal loss (98%, range 93–100%) in the PD cases when compared with the controls. Hence this region appears to show the greatest vulnerability to neurodegeneration in PD of any portion of the SNc. Of the other nigrosomes, there appeared to be a gradation of vulnerability to PD neurodegeneration extending caudal to rostral, lateral to medial, and ventral to dorsal with the progressive order of neuronal loss from nigrosome 1 to nigrosome 2, to 3, to 4, and then to 5, followed by greatest survival of neurons in the matrix area. Although this study is based on examination of only five PD cases, the authors suggested that their data supported the concept that this order of involvement could also be correlated with the clinical progression of the disease. This localization is, in general, in accord with the findings of extreme vulnerability of the ventrolateral neuronal clusters of the SNc of Hassler [27] and of Fearnley and Lees [13].

Medial and ventral tegmental region (A10)

These neurons are dorsomedial to the SNc and project to the nucleus acumbens and olfactory tubercle and, as such, are considered part of the mesolimbic dopamine system. They also project to the prefrontal and entorhinal cortex. van Domburg and ten Donkelaar [29] studied four cases of PD and four normal controls and showed that in the ventral tegmental area there was a 53% decrease in neuromelanin-containing neurons when compared with controls and a 35% loss of nonpigmented neurons. However, they also warned that these figures were based on a rather small numbers of cases. Rinne *et al.* [30] looked at neuronal loss in the SNc and the VTA in cases of PD, both with and without dementia and age-matched controls. Overall, they showed a 49% loss of VTA neurons in the PD cases, compared with controls. A negative correlation was found between the neuron number in the VTA and extent of dementia, as determined by the Global Deterioration Scale of Reisberg *et al.* [31]. In this study, neuron counts from other locations in the SNc did not correlate with measures of dementia severity. It should be pointed out that the common association of Alzheimer's disease (or at least Alzheimer's disease-related changes) with the presence of PD was not considered in this study and two of the six PD cases studied were said to show a significant degree of Alzheimer's disease-associated changes. Furthermore, the potential presence of cortical Lewy bodies was also not investigated in the PD cases, both with and without dementia. Finally, the neuronal counting was performed using a single 5 μm thick histologic section stained with hematoxylin and eosin that was taken within a histologic block at the level of the superior colliculus and the caudal red nucleus. The representativeness of this single section with respect to the remainder of the SNc cannot be determined, thus further reducing how much can be learned from the study.

Using a similar approach, McRitchie, Cartwright, and Halliday [32] compared the neuronal constituents within each of the seven subnuclei that comprise the A10 group in five normal controls and three PD-only cases, one case with progressive supranuclear palsy, one case of PD with Alzheimer's disease, and two cases with PD combined with significant small vessel cerebrovascular disease. Using nonbiased systematic sampling, they counted both tyrosine hydroxylase immunoreactive neurons and total Nissl-staining neurons in each of these seven subregions. They found that, although there was some variability, significant reductions in the total volume and the constituent dopaminergic and nondopaminergic neuron numbers were identified in the parabrachial pigmented nucleus and the parapeduncular nucleus of A10 in the PD cases. This change appeared to be selective since similar losses (in either dopaminergic or nondopaminergic neurons) were not seen in the other five subregions, including the selective region they referred to as the ventral tegmental area, itself (see Plate 2.5)

Peri- and retrorubral tegmental (lateral reticular formation) cell group (A8)

These neurons are encountered in the area of the mesencephalic reticular formation dorsolateral to the SNc. As noted above, these neurons project to striatal and limbic areas. This group of cells is also referred to as the retrorubral area (or A8), although their distribution also extends into the midbrain reticular fields. This is a relatively sparse region and these cells comprise only about 5% of the mesencephalic dopaminergic neurons. van Domburg and ten Donkelaar [29] reported a 65% decrease in neuromelanin-containing neurons in area A8 of cases of PD when compared with controls and a 20% loss of nonpigmented neurons in this location. On the other hand, McRitchie, Halliday, and Cartwright [33], using the nonbiased systematic sampling methods of stereology, reported no significant reduction in either tyrosine hydroxylase immunoreactive neurons or total Nissl-stained neurons within A8 when they compared PD cases and controls.

Hypothalamic dopaminergic neurons (A13)

In 1985, Spencer *et al.* [8] reported the presence of neurons in the human hypothalamus that by immunohistochemistry showed evidence of tyrosine hydroxylase and by histochemistry clearly contained neuromelanin. On the basis of these findings, these cells were considered to be dopaminergic neurons and they were localized to the arcuate and periventricular nuclei of the hypothalamus. These cells were considered to be part of the A13 dopaminergic cell group in rats [34], comparable to what had previously been found in non-human primates [35]. Matzuk and Saper [36] examined these melanized cells in seven cases of PD and five controls and found no significant loss on comparing the two groups. They considered that this indicated that although PD may cause severe dopaminergic cell loss in some regions, in other locations such cells could remain entirely intact.

Clinicopathologic correlations

It has long been the desire of neuropathologists studying PD to be able to develop an approach that will allow correlation of the distribution and degree of neurodegeneration in the brains of patients suffering from this disease with the specific clinical manifestations that they displayed during life. However, despite this important objective, few meaningful data have emerged to satisfy that goal. It must be recognized that PD is a chronic, slowly progressive disorder. Anatomic studies of cases of incidental Lewy body "disease" suggest that such asymptomatic patients actually represent preclinical examples of subjects who have yet to develop a sufficient degree of neurodegeneration to signal clinical evaluation and that for such cases the disease process has been undetected as it slowly evolved over many years. Furthermore, since patients do not die directly from PD, and with effective modern therapy available for their other medical conditions, it is not uncommon for such patients to survive for several decades following their initial neurologic diagnosis. Accordingly, neuropathologists typically encounter patients at the autopsy table who are in an extremely late stage of the disease. In such instances, the clinical picture has become rather stereotyped with overwhelming late-stage complications such as uncontrollable dyskinesias, autonomic disturbances, dementia, and other features. In our experience, unless one focuses on patients with an onset of PD at an extremely advanced age, where the inherent frailty of the extremely elderly comes into play, cases in early or even moderate stages of disease are relatively rarely encountered in the neuropathology laboratory.

Over the years, some studies have had the opportunity to examine relatively small numbers of PD patients who at death had been in only moderate stages of disease, at least as measured by their premortem Hoehn and Yahr stage [37]. In such instances, there has been the impression that, as might be anticipated, there was a lesser degree of neuronal loss in the SNc, when compared with later stages. Halliday *et al.* [38] published a neuropathologic study involving 13 levodopa-responsive PD cases, four patients dying in Hoehn and Yahr stages 2–3, and nine dying in stages 4–5. These cases were compared with the brains of 13 age-matched controls. This study showed that the earlier stage PD cases demonstrated a lesser degree of neuronal loss in the SNc (A9) than did the later stage patients (75% neuronal loss versus 87% loss, $p < 0.005$). As might be anticipated, there was also a significant correlation between neuronal loss in the SNc and the overall duration of disease ($r = 0.76$, $p = 0.002$). Similar data were produced by Ma *et al.* [39], who found a significant correlation between the numbers of pigmented neurons in the SNc and the stage of disease ($r = -0.58$, $p < 0.05$) and also the duration of disease ($r = 0.86$, $p < 0.01$).

Turning to the other mesencephalic dopaminergic sites, there has been consideration that in cases of PD, neurodegenerative involvement of mesolimbic and/or mesocortical pathways might underlie some of the non-motor manifestations of the disease. Rinne *et al.* [30] evaluated the brains of 12 cases of PD, some with dementia and others without, and also those of 18 controls. They examined a single transverse histologic section taken at the level of the superior colliculus and caudal red nucleus and divided the pigmented SNc neurons present into four portions ranging from most medial to the lateral portion. Pigmented neurons were counted and compared with the degree of dementia present, as measured by the six-point Global Dementia Rating Scale of Reisberg *et al.* [31]. Although the greatest degree of neuronal loss occurred in the most lateral portion of the SNc, there was a statistically significant negative correlation between the degree of dementia and the number of pigmented neurons seen in the most medial SNc compartment that they evaluated. Looking at the distribution map provided in the publication, this region might well correspond to the VTA (A10). Other studies of A10 in PD patients have achieved a variable degree of correlation with dementia levels. Hirsch, Graybiel, and Agid [40] found a 48% loss of tyrosine hydroxylase immunoreactive neurons in A10 in cases of PD (and 43% in A8). However, when an examination of A10 was subjected to the rigors of nonbiased serial sampling using the principles of stereology, no significant neuronal loss was detected in 13 PD cases when compared with 13 controls [38].

Recently, Torta and Castelli [41] reviewed the clinical/behavioral literature on PD with respect to possible evidence of dysfunction of reward-related behavior as one might expect to find with involvement of the mesolimbic and mesocortical dopaminergic pathways. Although this is an appealing theoretical possibility, there are no clinicopathologic studies which appear to support such a notion. However, it must be acknowledged that little scientific attention has yet been brought to bear on this subject.

Understanding selective vulnerability

Since the earliest work of Trétiakoff [42], Foix [43] and Hassler [27], there has been interest in understanding the basic nature of the selective neuronal vulnerability displayed by cases of PD. Although PD is considered to be the prototype dopaminergic neurodegenerative disorder, it is clear that the neurodegenerative process taking place in the disease is not selective for dopaminergic cells. It is widely acknowledged that in PD significant neurodegeneration involves multiple neuronal types, including adrenergic, serotoninergic, and cholinergic neuronal groups. Furthermore, as we have reviewed, there is ample evidence that neurodegeneration of dopaminergic cells is certainly not uniform and, even within particular neuroanatomic locations, neuronal loss follows a rather selective pattern, the basis for which has escaped scientific understanding to date. For example, within the SNc there is very severe neuronal loss in the N1 nigrosome whereas N5 remains relatively intact. What properties convey this unique sensitivity to the neurodegenerative process in PD and, conversely, what properties are associated with relative resistance to neuronal death of these nearby cell groups?

Hirsch, Graybiel, and Agid [40] noted that within the entire population of dopaminergic neurons in the midbrain, those containing a prominent neuromelanin content appear to be particularly prone to neurodegeneration in cases of PD. They also noted that non-melanized TH+ cells appeared to be relatively spared from the process of neuronal loss. Obviously, this does little to explain the fact that there is significant involvement of some non-pigmented neuronal groups in PD such as the nucleus basalis of Meynert. Further, as Gibb and Lees [4] have pointed out, the neurons of the ventral tier of the SNc have a lower content of neuromelanin than the neurons of the dorsal tier. A further line of research has suggested that increased levels of cellular calcium may mediate neuronal cell death in PD and that the presence of calcium-binding proteins such as calbindin D_{28K}, parvalbumin, calretinin, might have a protective effect for neuronal populations that contain significant concentrations of these calcium-buffering compounds. Most of the dopaminergic neurons in the SNc that undergo degeneration in association with PD do not contain immunoreactivity to such calcium-binding proteins; however, the neuronal distribution of such proteins within other mesencephalic dopaminergic regions fails to correlate well with their relative susceptibility to the neurodegenerative process. Clearly, with the current state of knowledge, the mystery of selective vulnerability in PD, as in any of the other forms of neurodegeneration, remains to be solved. When that occurs we will have made a major step forward in understanding the basic nature of these important disorders. The resolution of this problem could be of value in helping to define a neuroprotective therapy.

References

1. Dahlström A, Fuxe K. Evidence for the existence of monoamine-containing neurons in the central nervous system. 1. Demonstration of monoamines in cell bodies of brainstem neurons. *Acta Physiol Scand Suppl* 1964;**232**:3–55.
2. Hassler R. Zur Neuroanatomie de Substantia Nigra. *J Psychol Neurol* 1937;**48**:1–55.
3. Olszewski J, Baxter D. *Cytoarchitechture of the Human Brainstem*. Philadelphia, PA: JB Lippincott, 1954.
4. Gibb WR, Lees AJ. Anatomy, pigmentation, ventral and dorsal subpopulations of the substantia nigra, and differential cell death in Parkinson's disease. *J Neurol Neurosurg Psychiatry* 1991;**54**(5):388–96.
5. Damier P, Hirsch EC, Agid Y, Graybiel AM. The substantia nigra of the human brain. I. Nigrosomes and the nigral matrix, a compartmental organization based on calbindin D(28K) immunohistochemistry. *Brain* 1999;**122**(Pt 8):1421–36.
6. Damier P, Hirsch EC, Agid Y, Graybiel AM. The substantia nigra of the human brain. II. Patterns of loss of dopamine-containing neurons in Parkinson's disease. *Brain* 1999;**122**(Pt 8): 1437–48.
7. McRitchie DA, Hardman CD, Halliday GM. Cytoarchitectural distribution of calcium binding proteins in midbrain dopaminergic regions of rats and humans. *J Comp Neurol* 1996;**364**(1):121–50.
8. Spencer S, Saper CB, Joh T, *et al*. Distribution of catecholamine-containing neurons in the normal human hypothalamus. *Brain Res* 1985;**328**(1):73–80.
9. Saper CB, Petito CK. Correspondence of melanin-pigmented neurons in human brain with A1–A14 catecholamine cell groups. *Brain* 1982;**105**(Pt 1):87–101.
10. McGeer PL, McGeer EG, Suzuki JS. Aging and extrapyramidal function. *Arch Neurol* 1977;**34**(1):33–5.
11. Mann DM, Yates PO, Marcyniuk B. Monoaminergic neurotransmitter systems in presenile Alzheimer's disease and in senile dementia of Alzheimer type. *Clin Neuropathol* 1984;**3**(5): 199–205.
12. Thiessen B, Rajput AH, Laverty W, Desai H. Age, environments, and the number of substantia nigra neurons. *Adv Neurol* 1990;**53**:201–6.
13. Fearnley JM, Lees AJ. Ageing and Parkinson's disease: substantia nigra regional selectivity. *Brain* 1991;**114**(Pt 5):283–301.
14. Kubis N, Faucheux BA, Ransmayr G, *et al*. Preservation of midbrain catecholaminergic neurons in very old human subjects. *Brain* 2000;**123**(Pt 2):366–73.
15. West MJ. New stereological methods for counting neurons. *Neurobiol Aging* 1993;**14**:275–85.
16. Sterio DC. The unbiased estimation of number and size of arbitrary particles using the disector. *J Microsc* 1984;**134**:127–36.
17. Cabello CR, Thune JJ, Pakkenberg H, Pakkenberg B. Ageing of substantia nigra in humans: cell loss may be compensated by hypertrophy. *Neuropathol Appl Neurobiol* 2002;**28**(4):283–91.
18. Chu Y, Kompoliti K, Cochran EJ, *et al*. Age-related decreases in Nurr1 immunoreactivity in the human substantia nigra. *J Comp Neurol* 2002;**450**(3):203–14.

19. Ma SY, Roytt M, Collan Y, Rinne JO. Unbiased morphometrical measurements show loss of pigmented nigral neurones with ageing. *Neuropathol Appl Neurobiol* 1999;**25**(5):394–9.
20. Rudow G, O'Brien R, Savonenko AV, *et al*. Morphometry of the human substantia nigra in ageing and Parkinson's disease. *Acta Neuropathol* 2008;**115**(4):461–70.
21. Mirra SS, Heyman A, McKeel D, *et al*. The Consortium to Establish a Registry for Alzheimer's Disease (CERAD). Part II. Standardization of the neuropathologic assessment of Alzheimer's disease. *Neurology* 1991;**41**:479–86.
22. Braak H, Braak E. Neuropathological stageing of Alzheimer-related changes. *Acta Neuropathol (Berl)* 1991;**82**:239–59.
23. Calne DB, Mizuno Y. The neuromythology of Parkinson's disease. *Parkinsonism Relat Disord* 2004;**10**(5):319–22.
24. Weiner WJ. There is no Parkinson disease. *Arch Neurol* 2008; **65**(6):705–8.
25. Marsden CD. Parkinson's disease. *Lancet* 1990;**335**(8695): 948–52.
26. Snow BJ, Nygaard TG, Takahashi H, Calne DB. Positron emission tomographic studies of dopa-responsive dystonia and early-onset idiopathic parkinsonism. *Ann Neurol* 1993;**34**(5): 733–8.
27. Hassler R. Zur Pathologie der Paralysis Agitans und des postencephalitischen Parkinsonismus. *J Psychol Neurol* 1938; **48**:387–476.
28. Kish SJ, Shannak K, Hornykiewicz O. Uneven pattern of dopamine loss in the striatum of patients with idiopathic Parkinson's disease. Pathophysiologic and clinical implications. *N Engl J Med* 1988;**318**(14):876–80.
29. van Domburg PHMF, ten Donkelaar HJ. *The Human Substantia Nigra and Ventral Tegmental Area: a Neuroanatomical Study with Notes on Aging and Aging Diseases*. Berlin: Springer, 1991.
30. Rinne JO, Rummukainen J, Paljarvi L, Rinne UK. Dementia in Parkinson's disease is related to neuronal loss in the medial substantia nigra. *Ann Neurol* 1989;**26**(1):47–50.
31. Reisberg B, Ferris SH, de Leon MJ, Crook T. The Global Deterioration Scale for assessment of primary degenerative dementia. *Am J Psychiatry* 1982;**139**(9):1136–9.
32. McRitchie DA, Cartwright HR, Halliday GM. Specific A10 dopaminergic nuclei in the midbrain degenerate in Parkinson's disease. *Exp Neurol* 1997;**144**(1):202–13.
33. McRitchie DA, Halliday GM, Cartwright H. Quantitative analysis of the variability of substantia nigra pigmented cell clusters in the human. *Neuroscience* 1995;**68**(2):539–51.
34. Björklund A, Lindvall O, Nobin A. Evidence of an incerto-hypothalamic dopamine neurone system in the rat. *Brain Res* 1975;**89**(1):29–42.
35. Felten DL, Laties AM, Carpenter MB. Monoamine-containing cell bodies in the squirrel monkey brain. *Am J Anat* 1974; **139**(2):153–65.
36. Matzuk MM, Saper CB. Preservation of hypothalamic dopaminergic neurons in Parkinson's disease. *Ann Neurol* 1985;**18**(5):552–5.
37. Hoehn MM, Yahr MD. Parkinsonism: onset, progression and mortality. *Neurology* 1967;**17**:427–42.
38. Halliday GM, Ophof A, Broe M, *et al*. Alpha-synuclein redistributes to neuromelanin lipid in the substantia nigra early in Parkinson's disease. *Brain* 2005;**128**(Pt 11):2654–64.
39. Ma SY, Roytta M, Rinne JO, *et al*. Correlation between neuromorphometry in the substantia nigra and clinical features in Parkinson's disease using disector counts. *J Neurol Sci* 1997; **151**(1):83–7.
40. Hirsch E, Graybiel AM, Agid YA. Melanized dopaminergic neurons are differentially susceptible to degeneration in Parkinson's disease. *Nature* 1988;**334**(6180):345–8.
41. Torta DM, Castelli L. Reward pathways in Parkinson's disease: clinical and theoretical implications. *Psychiatry Clin Neurosci* 2008;**62**(2):203–13.
42. Trétiakoff MC. *Contribution a l'Étude de l'Anatomie Pathologique de Locus Niger de Soemmerling*. Université de Paris, 1919.
43. Foix C. Les lesions anatomiques de la maladie de Parkinson. *Rev Neurol* 1921;**37**:593–600.

Chapter 3
Non-Dopaminergic Pathology of Parkinson's Disease

Heiko Braak & Kelly Del Tredici
Department of Neurology, Center for Clinical Research, University of Ulm, Ulm, Germany

Introduction

Late-onset sporadic Parkinson's disease (sPD) is characterized by a progressive pathologic process that can last for decades. It affects neither nonhuman vertebrates [1] nor organs apart from the nervous system and is not known to go into remission.

There is a growing awareness that the definition of sPD as a monosystemic disorder with preferential obliteration of dopaminergic neurons in the nigrostriatal system is too narrow because increasing evidence shows that Lewy pathology is widely distributed throughout the nervous system, not only the central (CNS) but also the peripheral (PNS) and enteric nervous systems (ENS), and that not only dopaminergic neurons but also glutamatergic, GABAergic, noradrenergic, serotonergic, histaminergic, and cholinergic nerve cell types are vulnerable [2–6]. The neurotransmitters *per se* are not adequate criteria for predicting which neurons are predisposed or resistant to the pathologic process. Sensory regions of the nervous system mostly remain intact. Notable exceptions are olfactory structures and portions of the pain system. Whether cell loss, spine loss, or impaired axonal transport, the disease-related damage chiefly revolves around motor areas, and here, again, particularly around superordinate centers of the limbic, visceromotor, and somatomotor systems.

Lewy pathology

The ongoing formation of proteinaceous α-synuclein-containing intraneuronal inclusions (Lewy pathology, LP) is typical of sPD [7], and the presence of LP occupies a central role in the etiopathogenesis of sPD [8–11]. The pathologic process in its entirety is not confined to dopaminergic nerve cells but is marked by the development of the same forms of inclusion bodies (Lewy neurites/bodies, LNs/LBs) in the same neuronal types distributed at specific sites throughout the nervous system [12]. Individuals who lack LP but display parkinsonism suffer from disorders other than sPD [6]. Nor does the mere presence of LP justify the assumption that a given individual may have had clinically manifest sPD. Cases displaying incidental LP may have been in a premorbid, that is, presymptomatic or premotor, phase. Autopsy-controlled studies indicate that sPD is a disease entity with a broad spectrum of recognizable clinical, including non-motor, symptoms [13–18].

Selective vulnerability

Only a few of the many types of nerve cells within the human nervous system develop LP, and this selectivity is reflected in the regional distribution of the lesions. Other types directly in the vicinity of involved neurons maintain their morphologic and functional integrity for the duration of the disease [6,19–21]. Vulnerable nerve cells all have disproportionately long and thin axons that either lack a myelin sheath or are poorly myelinated [19–22]. Neurons with sturdily myelinated axons do not develop LP. The same can be said for short-axoned local circuit neurons or projection cells with short axons, such as those in the fourth neocortical layer. Susceptible cells also tend to have lipofuscin deposits or neuromelanin granules and all are capable of synthesizing α-synuclein [23–27]. Nerve cells that lack α-synuclein and pigment deposits may be innately capable of withstanding LP [27]. On the other hand, cells do exist that are plentifully supplied with α-synuclein but not especially susceptible to LP, such as the projection cells in the dorsal tegmental nucleus of Gudden. The lipofuscin-laden projection cells of the inferior olivary nucleus and the melanized dopaminergic neurons within the hypothalamic arcuate and periventricular nuclei are likewise among the cell types that generally resist the formation of LP [28].

Parkinson's Disease: Non-Motor and Non-Dopaminergic Features, First Edition. Edited by C. Warren Olanow, Fabrizio Stocchi, and Anthony E. Lang.

α-Synuclein

The natively unfolded protein α-synuclein is soluble in neuronal cytosol and is expressed in axons and presynaptic terminals. In sPD, monomeric α-synuclein is subject to misfolding and transition into a β-sheet conformation. Thereafter, possibly owing to this conformational defect, the protein is prone to aggregation and to the formation of insoluble inclusion bodies [7,29]. Many of the intrinsic and extrinsic factors that induce protein misfolding and aggregation are still unknown [30–33]. The resulting proteinaceous aggregates cannot be disposed of by physiologic clearance mechanisms [34–38] and persist as light microscopically visible spindle- or thread-like Lewy neurites (LNs) within cellular processes, and as punctate material or spherical pale bodies or Lewy bodies (LBs) in the somata of vulnerable nerve cells [12,39–43].

Of particular interest are the thread-like axonal LNs because, as a general rule, they precede LB formation [19,21,44–47]. One question is whether the α-synuclein that is physiologically present in axons suffices for protein aggregation or whether additional material has to be transported anterogradely from the soma to axonal aggregation sites. Because LNs may develop at the expense of the axonal cytoskeleton, it is to be anticipated that they disrupt somatopetal/somatofugal transport within the axon and, in so doing, become detrimental to other host nerve cell functions [48,49]. At present, there are no reports that aggregated α-synuclein causes "gridlock" at critical axonal junctures, for example, branching points. Nor can the transport gradient (i.e., somatopetal/somatofugal) be deduced from the shapes of LNs. If disrupted axonal transport were to result in the presence of abnormally high concentrations of α-synuclein within the cell body (inasmuch as the protein would be incapable of reaching its normally foreseen cellular locus), this might, in turn, trigger LB formation. Following the death of the host neuron, extraneuronal LBs are rapidly degraded by macrophages. Since a similar process for LNs is unknown, the axon membrane presumably remains intact for a long time despite the presence of the intra-axonal inclusions. Axons of some vulnerable nerve cells (e.g., dorsal motor projection neurons of the vagal nerve, projection neurons of the locus coeruleus, and magnocellular nuclei of the basal forebrain) can contain LNs in excess of 250 mm in length. However, there are other susceptible nerve cells, the axons of which do not develop LNs, among them nigral dopaminergic neurons and neocortical pyramidal cells in layers V–VI with corticostriatal or corticothalamic projections. Such exceptions indicate that it will not be easy to define universally applicable criteria for α-synuclein misfolding and aggregation because some cell types obviously are idiosyncratic.

It is unclear what leads to the formation of abnormal punctate material, pale bodies, and LBs, and what role is taken by lipofuscin and neuromelanin deposition in all of these processes. That some of the neurons involved – despite the presence of severe LP – apparently survive for decades has raised the issue of whether the inclusion bodies are deleterious at all for their host nerve cells. The aggregated material has also be viewed as (potentially) neuroprotective or neutral and the aggregation process as geared to isolating nonbiodegradable material, thereby preventing it from interfering with normal cellular metabolism [50–54]. Harmful or toxic effects are attributed chiefly to intermediate oligomeric byproducts [30,55]. Nevertheless, as pointed out above, the consequences of the protein aggregation process may be different for specific neuronal types, each of them with distinctly variable degrees of susceptibility. Dopaminergic nerve cells in the substantia nigra and noradrenergic neurons in the locus coeruleus [56], for example, probably react differently to the presence of stressors or LP than the motor neurons of the dorsal motor nucleus of the vagal nerve or cortical pyramidal cells.

Incidental Lewy disease

LP as an incidental finding has been observed in autopsy studies of individuals without clinical parkinsonism [57–67] and is sometimes regarded as a sequel to neuronal aging or as harmless epiphenomena accompanying other neurobiological processes [68]. However, because LP does not inevitably occur during aging, not even in the very old [1,59,63,69], incidental LNs/LBs also can be viewed as age associated rather than age dependent [6,22] and likely representative of early-phase sPD – when somatomotor symptoms are not detectable but a much larger (progressive) pathologic process is under way [3–5,16,17,70–72]. This view receives support from the fact that incidental lesions occur in the same types of nerve cells at the same topographical sites within the nervous system as those in clinically manifest sPD.

Progression of the pathologic process

sPD does not develop overnight. As in nearly every illness, some individuals cross the threshold from a presymptomatic disease state to symptomatic manifestation of the disorder [16,17,73]. By the time clinicians make the diagnosis based on typical motor signs, patients already are, relatively speaking, in an advanced phase of the pathologic process. The disease smolders, as it were, unnoticed in the nervous system, possibly for years [74], until it attains such dimensions that dysfunctions become evident.

Autopsy material from most patients with clinically diagnosed sPD can be assigned to one of four neuropathologic subgroups (stages 3–6) that differ from each other with respect to changes in the topographic distribution and extent of LP in the brain [6,19,22]. Each subgroup displays LP in increasing numbers of involved sites. Approximately 5–20% of individuals above the age of 60 years without motor symptoms display incidental LP [16,58,59,61,64,65,67,75]. Such cases usually can be assigned to one of three subgroups (stages 1–3) [19,22]. To the extent that the LP distribution pattern observable in stage 3 (often the last presymptomatic subgroup) closely resembles that of stage 4 (often the first symptomatic group), all six stages can be helpful in reconstructing the entire spectrum of the pathologic process associated with sPD (Figure 3.1) [6,19,21, 22,76–78]. This does not negate the possibility that in some individuals with stage 4 incidental brain pathology motor symptoms compatible with sPD might not be detectable.

Methodological limitations to this approach are that the theoretical progression of the pathologic process in sPD only can be reconstructed with the help of cross-sectional data gained from nonselected autopsy material. As such, the conclusions drawn from these data permit admissible but instructive assumptions [21,79]. Chief among these are that the pathologic process in sPD is progressive and does not begin simultaneously in all of the susceptible regions but at predisposed sites, advancing from there throughout additional portions of the nervous system. There is also evidence that cell-to-cell (transneuronal) contact may play a crucial role [36]. In the brain, the process follows an essentially caudo-rostral trajectory along the neuroaxis and progresses from the lower brainstem through basal portions of the mid- and forebrain until the cerebral cortex becomes involved (Figure 3.1) [6,19,20,80,81]. The LP process branches out in a manner resembling a dendrogram (Figure 3.2b). This concept has been confirmed in its essential accuracy in an interrater study [82]. Whereas our results achieved 88% convergence [19], other laboratories have obtained lower or higher convergence rates [14,42,50,51,62,72,76,77,83–88]. A number of cases are not stageable. These individuals often have more than one neurodegenerative disease [42,71,77,86–91]. The caudo-rostral advance in the lower brainstem does not achieve machine-like precision [72,77]; there is no evidence, however, to suggest that the pathologic process in sPD begins in all susceptible brain regions at once or that it progresses there and within the nervous system according to a hit-or-miss principle. It still is open whether the beginnings of the pathologic process are multicentric, for example, brain and spinal cord, brain and peripheral nervous system, spinal cord and peripheral nervous system [17,65,66,92–94], and whether the involvement of the sympathetic or parasympathetic system predominates. Very large autopsy-controlled prospective studies that include healthy "normals" are required to answer this question [11,72,81].

Stage 1

LP is seen in the dorsal motor nucleus of the vagal nerve, sometimes together with LP in the intermediate reticular zone, olfactory bulb, and anterior olfactory nucleus [19,95,96]. In the meantime, we have encountered cases displaying incidental LP confined to anterior olfactory structures, that is, "bulb only" cases (unpublished findings, presented September 2008, New York City).

Anterior olfactory structures

Nerve cells within the cellular islands of the anterior olfactory nucleus contain LNs and LBs [13,67,97–101]. Less conspicuous lesions occur in mitral and tufted cells of the olfactory bulb, and the olfactory epithelium remains free of LP [102]. Notably, the dopaminergic periglomerular cells of the olfactory bulb remain devoid of LP and, in sPD, they even increase in number [103]. From stage 3 onwards, additional secondary olfactory structures (piriform cortex, periamygdalar cortex, medial entorhinal region) become involved [19,104,105]. Evidence indicates that the gradient of the olfactory pathology in sPD is from more peripherally placed structures in the olfactory bulb to the anterior olfactory nucleus and the other olfactory structures rather than vice versa [67,106].

Pre- and postganglionic parasympathetic projection neurons

The lower brainstem dorsal motor nuclei of the vagal nerve display α-synuclein-immunoreactive inclusions in their somatodendritic compartment and also in central and peripheral portions of their long and unmyelinated axons that connect the CNS with postganglionic nerve cells of the ENS/PNS [19,22,97–99,107–109]. Other components of the dorsal vagal area, namely the gelatinosus nucleus, area postrema, the small-celled nuclei of the solitary tract, and the myelinated motor neurons of the ambiguus nucleus in the intermediate reticulate zone, remain uninvolved [95]. Catecholaminergic melanized nerve cells in the dorsal vagal area (A2 group) and intermediate reticular zone (A1 group) are not drawn into the disease process until stage 3 [19,25,110].

LP occurs in select postganglionic neuronal types of the gut, for example, vasoactive intestinal polypeptide (VIP) neurons of the Auerbach plexus [75,111–113; see also 114]. Lesions in these motor neurons are seen in both disease phases (presymptomatic and symptomatic), but it is unclear whether LP in the ENS develops prior to the CNS pathology (Plate 3.1a–d) [21,22,93]. Vagal preganglionic terminals synapse directly on inclusion-bearing motor neurons. In the esophagus and stomach, LNs can even extend into the mucosal lamina propria only micrometers away from the body's innermost environment [44,101].

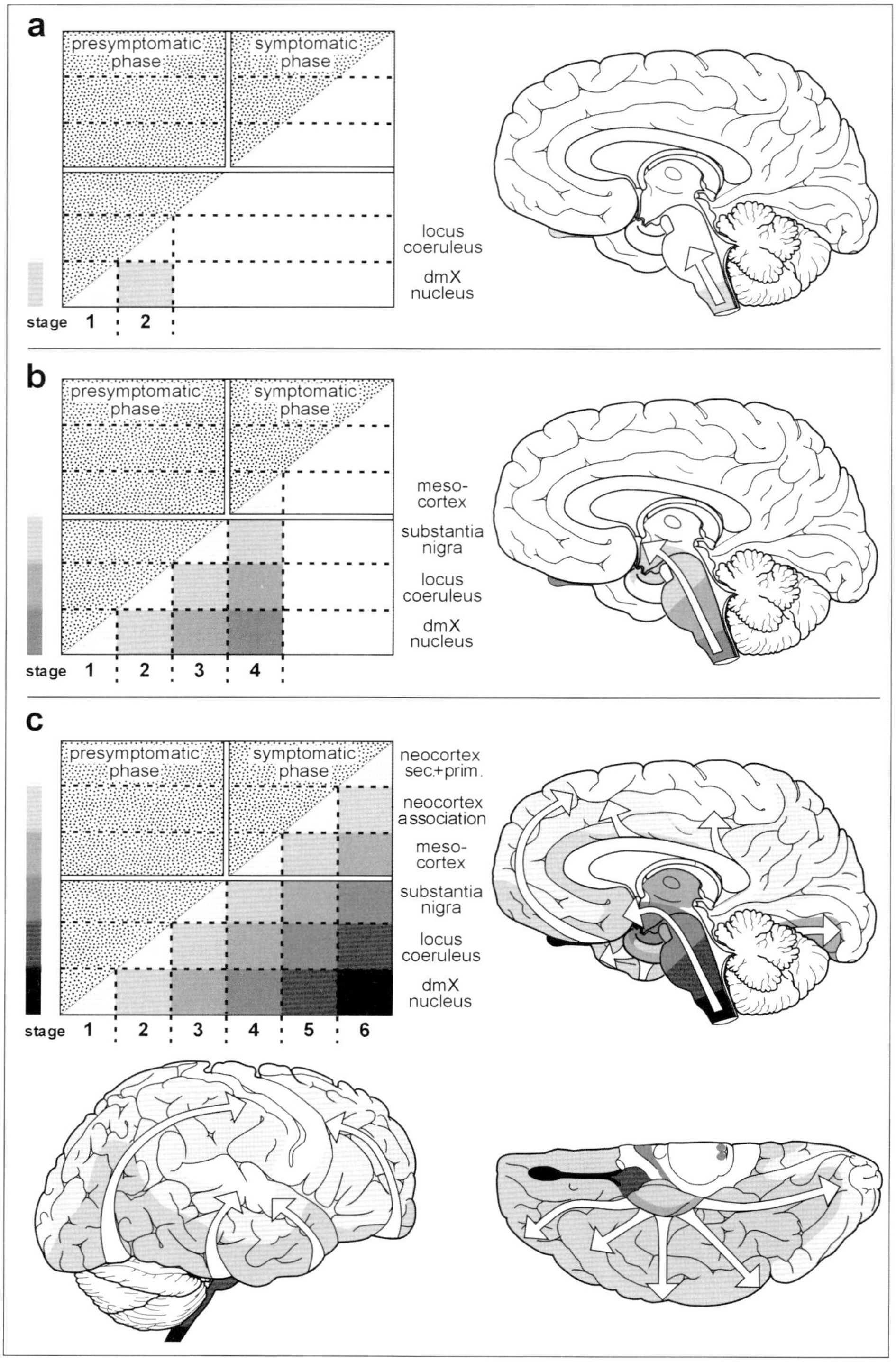

Figure 3.1 Six stages of brain pathology in sPD. (a) Initial lesions appear in stage 1 in the olfactory bulb, anterior olfactory nucleus, and dorsal motor nucleus of the vagal nerve. From there, the pathology follows a predominantly ascending path. In stage 2, lesions are seen for the first time in the level setting nuclei: the coeruleus–subcoeruleus complex, magnocellular nuclei of the reticular formation, and lower raphe nuclei. (b) The pathology in stage 3 continues its ascent and reaches the central subnucleus of the amygdala, pedunculopontine tegmental nucleus, the magnocellular nuclei of the basal forebrain, and pars compacta of the substantia nigra. The cerebral cortex becomes involved at stage 4, commencing with the anteromedial temporal mesocortex. At this juncture, the presymptomatic phase probably yields to the symptomatic phase of the disorder. (c) The higher order association areas of the neocortex become involved in stage 5, followed by the first-order association areas and primary fields in stage 6. Growing severity of the lesions is shown by increasing degrees of shading, as in Figure 3.2b.

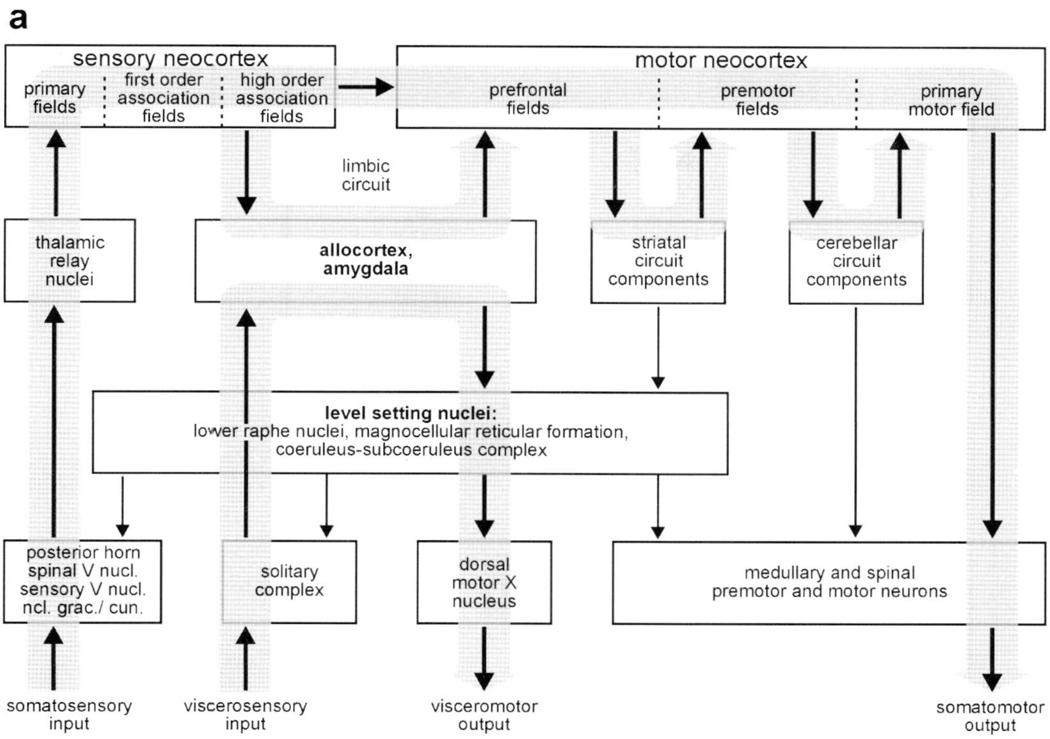

Figure 3.2 Simplified diagram of the limbic and somatomotor systems. (a) The neocortex is chiefly responsible for relationships with the world beyond the individual. It is the recipient of somatosensory, auditory, and visual input and regulates somatomotor activity that impinges on the organism's environment (see broad outer arrow in background). The allocortex is interconnected with the nuclear complex of the amygdala and, together, these structures receive not only exteroceptive information from the neocortex but also interoceptive data from the internal organs and influence endocrine and visceromotor functions (see broad inner arrow in background). As a result, they are optimally positioned to extract from the entire spectrum of incoming impulses the crucial information needed to produce an appropriate response to any given situation or set of circumstances. As custodians of memory and learning, limbic circuit centers serve as a neuronal bridge between the external and internal worlds. The neocortex consists of highly refined primary fields responsible for somatomotor activity and for initial processing of incoming data from sensory organs via specific thalamocortical projections. Each of the primary fields is flanked by somewhat less highly differentiated first-order sensory association areas and premotor fields. These, in turn, are interconnected with extensive but relatively simply organized high-order sensory association areas and the prefrontal cortex, which is the overriding executive instance of the human brain. Somatosensory, visual, and auditory data arriving at their respective primary sensory fields flow upstream via the first-order association areas to the high-order processing areas. From there, long and sparsely myelinated corticocortical projections convey the data to the prefrontal cortex terminating in layer IV of the target fields. Efferents from the prefrontal cortex are provided by corticocortical downstream projections that end in layer I of the premotor areas and primary motor field. The latter functions as a gateway for motor programs relayed to medullary and spinal premotor and motor neurons. However, the main routes for this return pathway are the striatal circuit and cerebellar circuit (see the two broad U-shaped arrows in background).
(*continued*)

Pre- and postganglionic sympathetic projection neurons

Gastrointestinal tract motility and functions are mainly driven by parasympathetic vagal output. These influences are constantly modified or inhibited by sympathetic antagonists (Figure 3.3) [115,116]. Sympathetic preganglionic centers that become involved during sPD include the intermediomedial and intermediolateral nuclei of the spinal cord and the postganglionic neurons in peripheral ganglia, such as the superior cervical and coeliac ganglia (Plate 3.1f,g) [65,66,75,92,94,117,118]. Lesions in preganglionic and postganglionic projection neurons of the sympathetic system have been observed at autopsy not only in the gastrointestinal tract and submandibular gland but also in the heart in both symptomatic individuals and cases with incidental LP [46,47,71,94,119,120].

Lamina I of the spinal cord

Unmyelinated or sparingly myelinated fibers that conduct thermal and nociceptive stimuli from the periphery to the CNS synapse almost exclusively on layer I neurons belonging to the pain system [121,122]. Layer I nerve cells almost completely filled with α-synuclein-immunoreactive material occur in both incidental and symptomatic sPD cases. The layer is decorated by a network of LNs (Plate 3.1e). The further caudally from

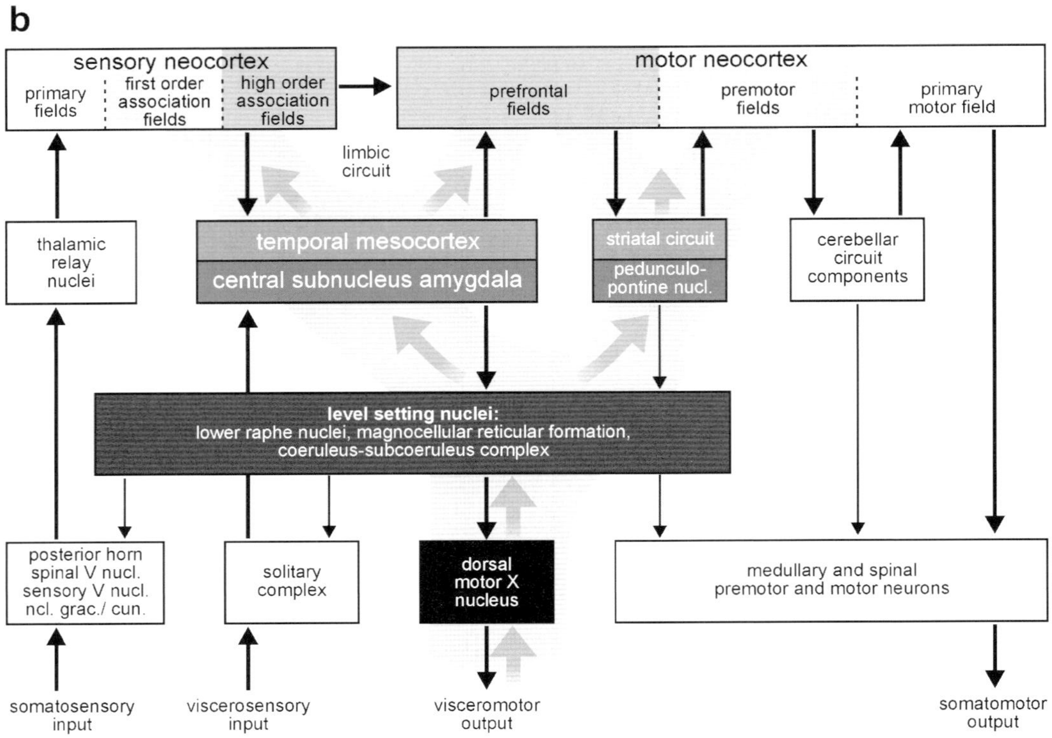

Figure 3.2 (*Contd.*) Simplified diagram of the limbic and somatomotor systems. (b) From stage 1 to stage 6, the pathologic process branches out in a manner resembling a dendrogram. The stem is given by the early involvement of the dorsal motor nucleus of the vagal nerve in stage 1 that broadens by affliction of the level setting nuclei as a unit in stage 2. A bifurcation of the pathologic process takes place in stage 3. Via one prong the process advances into centers of the central autonomic network (central subnucleus of the amygdala, components of the limbic circuit), via the other it progresses into centers of the somatomotor system (pedunculopontine tegmental nucleus, components of the striatal circuit). For shading, see Figures 3.1 and 3.4.

the cervical spinal cord, the denser the immunoreactive layer I neurons and associated network of LNs become, culminating in the lowermost thoracic, lumbar, and sacral segments [118]. The diagram in Figure 3.3 supplements the sympathetic and parasympathetic pathways that regulate the ENS by including portions of the pain system. Nerve cells in layer I receive modulatory supraspinal input from the lower raphe nuclei, reticular formation, and coeruleus/subcoeruleus complex – all of which sources also generate efferents to both sympathetic and parasympathetic preganglionic projection neurons (Figure 3.2a). Layer I axons provide excitatory input to sympathetic preganglionic neurons (Figure 3.3) and to the coeruleus–subcoeruleus complex before continuing their ascent within the spinothalamic tract. Hence nociceptive stimuli can activate sympathetic outflow [123]. Complaints of painful sensations are widespread in sPD and, combined with other clinical signs, can precede the classical motor symptoms [124–127].

Stage 2: Lewy pathology in the lower brainstem

In stage 2, LP is seen in additional nuclei of the lower brainstem, including the lower raphe system, magnocellular portions of the adjoining reticular formation, and noradrenergic neurons of the coeruleus–subcoeruleus complex (A6 and A7 groups) [19,20,44]. The nuclei that sustain damage during this stage all belong to a level setting system that is driven by supramedullary higher order centers of the limbic and somatomotor systems, such as the central subnucleus of the amygdala and pedunculopontine tegmental nucleus (Figure 3.2a). The level setting nuclei generate long and poorly myelinated descending axons. They inhibit relay nuclei that influence incoming somato- and viscerosensory input and also regulate the excitability levels of medullary and spinal premotor and motor neurons that receive data from the neocortex, the striatal and cerebellar circuits, and additional supramedullary sources (Figure 3.2a). An intact level setting system temporarily inhibits the conduction of incoming pain signals while placing the organism's motor neurons in a heightened state of preparedness in fight-or-flight situations [128–132].

During the first two neuropathologic stages, LP is usually found in olfactory areas, portions of the PNS and ENS, spinal cord, and lower brainstem. The pathologic process does not appear to have as its point of departure the substantia nigra [95]. On the contrary, nigral

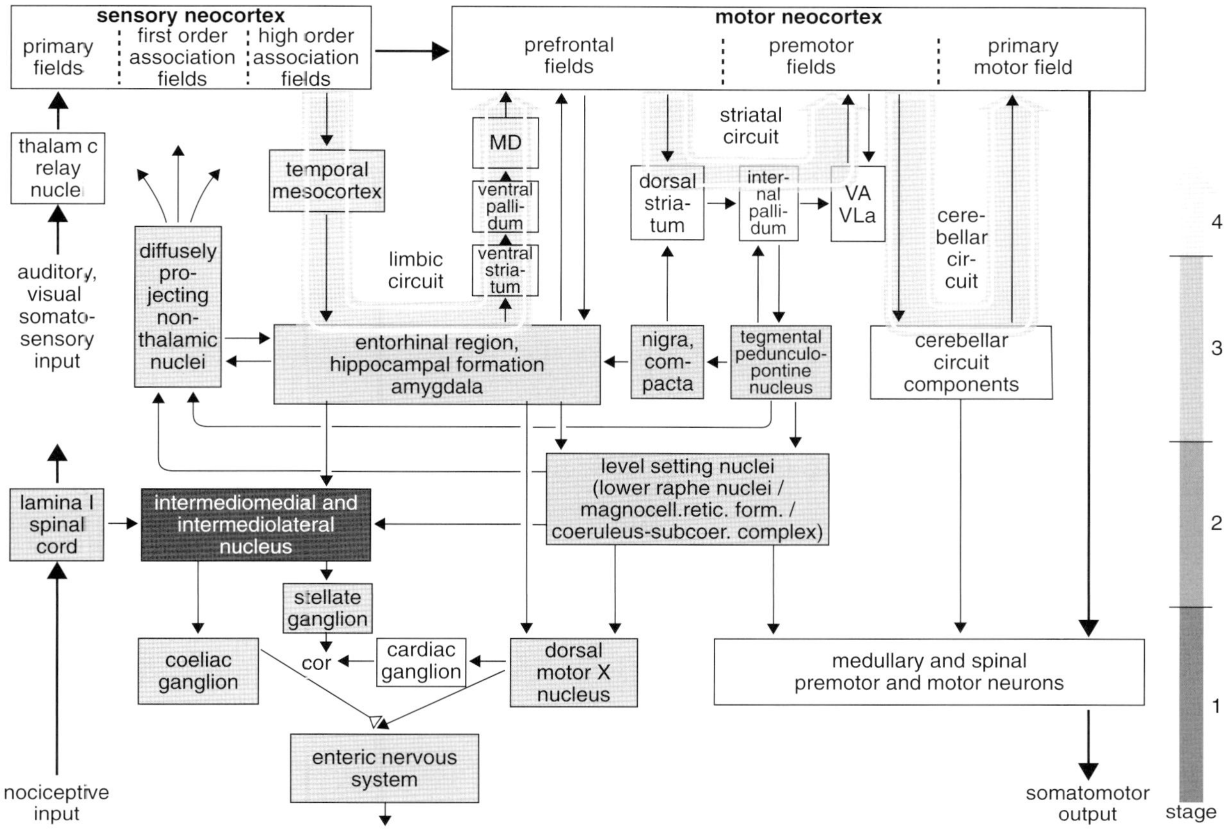

Figure 3.3 The diagram displays the progression of the pathologic process until stage 4 and a more detailed rendition of Figure 3.2a concerning the components of the limbic circuit. The greater the intensity of the shading, the more severe is the pathology. The entorhinal region, hippocampus, and amygdala participate in cortical data transfer at the nodal point where exteroceptive data are conveyed from neocortical high-order sensory association areas to the prefrontal cortex (limbic circuit). Data proceed via multiple neocortical areas to the anteromedial temporal mesocortex and, as if through a funnel, converge from there on both the entorhinal region and amygdala. The entorhinal region, hippocampal formation, and amygdala send projections that mainly terminate in the ventral striatum. From there, the data are conducted via the ventral pallidum and mediodorsal thalamus (MD) to the prefrontal cortex. The involvement of the anteromedial temporal mesocortex (from stage 4 onwards) leads to a marked reduction of the data transfer from the sensory neocortex to the prefrontal cortex and paves the way for cognitive impairment.

involvement presupposes the existence of LP in the lower medulla. Were it to become possible to diagnose sPD already in stage 1 or 2, and were a causal therapy to become available, the dopaminergic neuronal loss in the substantia nigra might be preventable [19].

Stage 3: Lewy pathology in the midbrain tegmentum and basal forebrain

The ascending disease process crosses the upper limit of the pontine tegmentum and encroaches upon basal portions of the mid- and forebrain in stage 3. Lesions occur in the central subnucleus of the amygdala and then in the pedunculopontine tegmental nucleus, the pars compacta of the substantia nigra, upper raphe nuclei, magnocellular nuclei of the basal forebrain (medial septal nucleus, interstitial nucleus of the diagonal band, basal nucleus of Meynert), and hypothalamic tuberomamillary nucleus. Involvement of all these sites is accompanied by the appearance of LP in the catecholaminergic melanized neurons of the medullary dorsal vagal area and intermediate reticular zone [19,22,113].

Whereas the level setting nuclei as a unit are the focal structures in stage 2, apparently a bifurcation of the pathologic process in the brain takes place during the third stage (Figure 3.2b). Via one prong it advances into high-order relay centers of the central autonomic network (central subnucleus of the amygdala, limbic circuit components), via another it progresses into superordinate centers of the somatomotor system, including the pedunculopontine nucleus and components of the striatal circuit. Both the central autonomic network and pedunculopontine nucleus regulate the level setting nuclei and both send projections to all diffusely projecting nonthalamic nuclei (Figures 3.3 and 3.4).

From the central subnucleus, the disease process encroaches on the basolateral subnuclei. Set off from

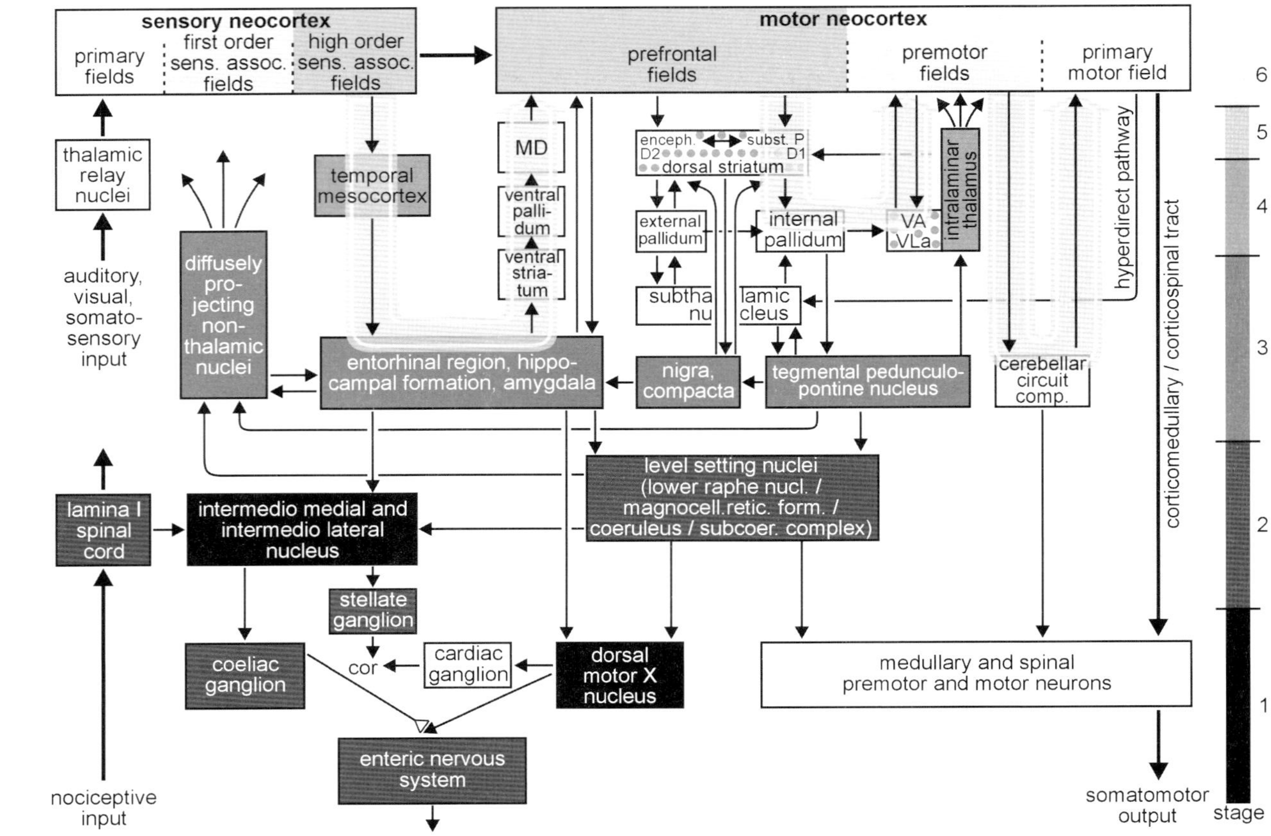

Figure 3.4 The diagram shows the progression of the pathologic process until stage 6 and displays the major components of the striatal circuit. Moving from left to right, the three broad gray arrows in the background are intended to facilitate recognition of the limbic, striatal, and cerebellar circuits. Damaged structures are marked by six degrees of shading: black (involved from stage 1 onwards), anthracite (from stage 2 onwards), dark gray (from stage 3 onwards), medium gray (from stage 4 onwards), gray (first affected in stage 5), and light gray (first involved in stage 6). White indicates noninvolvement or very minimal affection. Somatomotor functions are the result of activities in numerous smoothly interacting components that extend from the spinal cord to the telencephalon. The striatal circuit includes portions of the striatum, the external pallidum, subthalamic nucleus, internal pallidum, and associated relay nuclei of the thalamus (VA, VLa). The prefrontal cortex and additional portions of the neocortex activate the dorsal striatum via glutamatergic projections (see text for details). From there, data are transferred through the pallidum to the anteroventral thalamic nuclei, which relay the information back to the cortex. The pedunculopontine tegmental nucleus, dopaminergic nigral neurons, and intralaminar nuclei of the thalamus act upon the striatal circuit and modulate the data streaming through it. Speckled areas indicate nuclei with dot-like inclusions in stages 4–6.

the surrounding subnuclei by a mesh-like web of LNs, the central subnucleus sends descending, sparsely myelinated projections to the level setting nuclei and dorsal motor nucleus of the vagal nerve. In so doing, it exerts a "limbic" influence on each of these modulatory lower brainstem regions and regulates [104,105,133,134]. The central subnucleus receives afferents from the substantia nigra and basolateral complex of the amygdala; the latter group, in turn, is fed by projections from the cholinergic magnocellular nuclei of the basal forebrain and anteromedial temporal mesocortex (Figure 3.3).

The pedunculopontine tegmental nucleus provides a channel for the pathologic process into the striatal circuit. A dense network of LNs occurs within the nucleus followed by the appearance there of LBs in the somata of cholinergic projection cells [135–138]. The pedunculopontine nucleus consists of cholinergic and noncholinergic (GABA, glutamate) neurons [139]. Its main input originates from the internal pallidum (Figure 3.4). Thinly myelinated projections connect it with nigral dopaminergic neurons, the subthalamic nucleus, intralaminar nuclei of the thalamus, and nonthalamic nuclei with diffuse cortical projections (Figures 3.3 and 3.4). The ascending projections of the pedunculopontine tegmental nucleus outnumber by far its descending fiber tracts to the level setting nuclei and spinal cord [140,141; see also 142–146].

Nigral pathology begins, as a rule, in the posterolateral subnucleus of the pars compacta and then appears within the posterosuperior and posteromedial subnuclei, bypassing the magnocellular and anterior subnuclei or leaving behind mild LP [19,147–150]. As at previous sites, LNs occur first followed by punctate aggregations, pale bodies, and LBs in the somata of the melanized dopaminergic neurons (A9 group). There are no obvious signs of neuronal loss at this point. Nerve cell death occurs during the subsequent neuropathologic stages [19,20,22]. Lesions are not visible in the A10 group of melanized nerve cells (paranigral nucleus, parabrachial pigmented nucleus, perirubral formation) until stage 4 [22,110,151].

Although spaced widely apart, the noradrenergic coeruleus–subcoeruleus complex, serotonergic upper raphe nuclei, cholinergic magnocellular nuclei of the basal forebrain, and histaminergic tuberomamillary nucleus of the hypothalamus constitute a unit in that their long, thin, and sparsely myelinated fiber tracts project diffusely toward cortical areas, the striatum, and additional subcortical sites [150,152–154]. Whereas the coeruleus–subcoeruleus complex is involved at stage 2, each of the other nuclei is drawn into the disease process during stage 3 [19–22]. The magnocellular nuclei of the basal forebrain receive abundant data from the olfactory, insular, subgenual, and prefrontal cortex, the entorhinal region, amygdala, striatum, pallidum, and level-setting nuclei. These basal forebrain nuclei also project diffusely to the cortex and numerous subcortical sites, including the mediodorsal nuclei of the thalamus and the amygdala [145,154,155]. Most hypothalamic tuberomamillary neurons are GABAergic/histaminergic and generate diffuse projections of the same magnitude as those from the basal forebrain nuclei [142,156–158].

Clinical records of some stage 3 individuals and of most with stage 4 brain pathology mention sPD-related motor symptoms. This could be an indication that the presymptomatic (non-motor) phase gives way to the clinically recognizable phase of the disorder at about this time [6,19,22,78].

Stage 4: Lewy pathology in thalamus, meso- and allocortex, insular, subgenual, and anterior cingulate areas

In stage 4 the lesions are visible in the basolateral complex of the amygdala and interstitial nucleus of the terminal stria in addition to thalamic midline and intralaminar nuclei. The pathology also encroaches for the first time upon the cerebral cortex, that is, the anteromedial temporal mesocortex. During this stage, related areas of insular, subgenual, and anterior cingulate cortical regions become involved, and LP occurs in the entorhinal region and second sector of the Ammon's horn (CA2) [19,22,110]. The neocortical high-order association areas are intact. Remarkably, the small melanized dopaminergic neurons of the infundibular and periventricular nuclei (A12 group) belonging to the hypothalamus remain unaffected [28]. The axons of these nerve cells are short and lack connectivities with other nuclei that develop LP. Subtle abnormalities in the form of dot-like α-synuclein-immunoreactive inclusions show up in the temporal mesocortex, striatum, thalamic relay nuclei, claustrum, and amygdala [159].

An internal medullary layer divides the thalamus into lateral relay, mediodorsal relay, and anterior relay nuclei and harbors three groups of intralaminar nuclei (anterior nuclei, the centromediano–parafascicular complex, posterior nuclei). Midline thalamic nuclei fan out between the epithelial lining of the third ventricle and the mediodorsal relay nuclei. All thalamic relay nuclei are reciprocally connected with the cerebral cortex; their glutamatergic projection neurons generate sturdily myelinated axons that terminate in layer IV of defined cortical areas. By contrast, the glutamatergic neurons of the midline nuclei and intralaminar nuclei send poorly myelinated axons to layers I and VI of more than one cortical area. The intralaminar nuclei receive input from the pedunculopontine tegmental nucleus and generate, in addition to cortical connectivities, a powerful projection to the dorsal striatum (Figure 3.4) [160]. The midline nuclei furnish thalamo-allocortical circuits and pathways to the ventral striatum [161].

LP develops in the thalamus from stage 4 onwards. The midline nuclei and the intralaminar anterior and posterior groups are the most vulnerable [162,163]. In sPD, the severity of the LP that accumulates there contrasts sharply with the mild pathology seen in most of the thalamic relay nuclei. The centromedian nucleus, which also belongs to the intralaminar nuclei, is physiologically almost devoid of α-synuclein and, as such, LP does not develop there [22,27]. α-Synuclein-immunoreactive dot-like inclusions in thalamic relay nuclei and in astrocytes are described in greater detail below.

During the fourth stage, the pathologic process gains access to the cerebral cortex, where it reaches anteromedial portions of the temporal mesocortex (Figures 3.2b and 3.3). The mesocortex is a unique transitional zone wedged between the allocortex and neocortex. This region functions as an interface between the sensory neocortex and superordinate centers of the limbic system (entorhinal region, hippocampal formation, amygdala) (Figure 3.3). All vital data in transit from high-order sensory association areas to the prefrontal cortex must pass through the temporal mesocortex. From there, the data are relayed via the entorhinal region, hippocampal formation, and amygdala, and further, via the ventral striatum, ventral pallidum, and thalamic mediodorsal nuclei to the prefrontal cortex [155,164,165].

LNs are observable in all layers of the anteromedial temporal mesocortex. It is conceivable that the very dense network of LNs in layers II–III hampers the incoming data stream from neocortical high-order sensory association areas. LBs occur mainly in layers V–VI. Then, they appear in one of the deep layers of the entorhinal region, and a dense plexus of LNs develops in the second sector (CA2) of the hippocampal formation. In subsequent stages, the

CA2 lesions progress into adjoining portions of the CA1 and CA3 sectors [166]. LP also develops in the first sector (CA1) of the Ammon's horn and in the transitional region between the amygdala and hippocampal formation.

The insular, subgenual, and anterior cingulate cortex are located adjacent to cortical olfactory areas and represent the brain's preeminent organizational level for processing interoceptive data (internal organs) and also visceromotor and endocrine functions (blood pressure, heart rate, respiration, gastrointestinal motility). LP appears in these limbic regions directly following the lesions in the anteromedial temporal mesocortex, and the distribution pattern of LBs/LNs throughout the various cortical layers is very similar to that seen in the mesocortex.

The insular areas encompass gustatory fields and a topically organized representation of the internal organs and interior surface of the body. The region functions as a viscerosensory and limbic integration cortex because it is reciprocally connected with the subgenual and anterior cingulate areas, entorhinal region, amygdala, and intralaminar thalamic nuclei and sends projections to the magnocellular nuclei of the basal forebrain and ventral striatum [167–169]. The subgenual region represents a topically organized visceromotor center and acts as a visceromotor and limbic integration cortex. Reciprocal projections connect the subgenual region with adjoining prefrontal areas, the insular and anterior cingulate cortex, entorhinal region, hippocampal formation, amygdala, intralaminar and midline nuclei of the thalamus, lateral hypothalamus, and autonomic regions of the lower brainstem and spinal cord. The subgenual cortex also sends strong projections to the ventral striatum, ventral pallidum, and mediodorsal thalamus [168,170].

The limbic circuit

Eventually, the involvement of the anteromedial temporal mesocortex may seriously impede the data flow originating in neocortical high-order sensory association areas and heading to the prefrontal neocortex via the entorhinal region, hippocampal formation, ventral striatum, ventral pallidum, and mediodorsal thalamus [20–22]. Decreasing limbic input to the frontal lobe, in turn, may contribute to impaired executive functioning and pave the way for cognitive impairment [171–176]. Progressive deterioration of the nigrostriatal pathway not only causes greater impairment of somatomotor function but also interferes with the data flow coming from limbic centers – via the dopamine-deprived ventral striatum – to the ventral pallidum, mediodorsal thalamus, and prefrontal neocortex (Figure 3.3). At the same time, the direct dopaminergic innervation of the cerebral cortex is reduced [132].

Autonomic dysfunction begins during the preclinical phase of sPD [18,127,177], and early involvement of the final shared pathway in the autonomic system, for example, the preganglionic sympathetic and parasympathetic neurons of the brainstem and spinal cord, together with postganglionic cells of the PNS and ENS [116], is compounded by LP in the level setting nuclei and central nucleus of the amygdala. In stage 4, the superordinate cortical autonomic system relay centers (insular, subgenual, and anterior cingulate areas) also become involved. The functional integrity of these cortical areas is necessary for maintaining the sympathetically mediated increase in heart rate during physical exertion and emotional stress and the appropriate sudomotor response of the skin to emotional stimuli [168,178,179]. The progression of the lesions within the central autonomic network can serve to exacerbate already present dysautonomia [6,15,116,180].

Dot-like inclusions in cortex, striatum, and thalamus

Dot-like α-synuclein-immunoreactive inclusions appear during stage 4 in the anteromedial temporal mesocortex (layers II–III, V–VI) and continue from there into adjoining neocortical high-order association areas. Small dots correspond to pathologic aggregations in terminal axons. Somewhat larger punctate structures represent α-synuclein-immunoreactive accumulations in astrocytes. Apart from the cortical predilection sites, the dot-like inclusions also are visible in the striatum, thalamic relay nuclei, claustrum, and amygdala [181]. They only occur in these defined forebrain sites from stage 4 onwards and are not found in controls or between neuropathologic stages 1–3 [159].

The pace of the astrocytic inclusions matches the increasing degree of cortical involvement. The astrocytic reaction is most pronounced in layers V–VI, weaker in layers II–III, and nearly absent in layers I and IV. In involved areas, almost all astrocytes are immunolabeled and not only those in the vicinity of LB-bearing pyramidal cells. Immunoreactive astrocytes continue to maintain their normal intervals from each other. The intensity of the immunolabeling gradually tapers off at the limits of uninvolved sites, for example, layer IV or in deep portions of the white substance [159]. Nerve cells normally release traces of the soluble α-synuclein into the extracellular space. Thus, the protein can be detected in both cerebrospinal fluid and blood plasma [182–185]. Astrocytes are not known to synthesize α-synuclein in large quantities [186]. As such, it can be deduced that, in sPD, astrocytes take up already slightly altered α-synuclein as it leaks from terminal of diseased cortical pyramidal cells. Such abnormal material may then readily undergo transformation into astrocytic inclusions [159,183,184].

Because GABAergic projection neurons of the striatum and glutamatergic cells within the thalamic relay nuclei normally remain free of LP, it would be difficult to account for the astrocytic reaction in the thalamus and striatum were it not for the fact that dense connectivities exist between involved cortical areas and these nuclei

(Figure 3.4). The corticostriatal and corticothalamic projection neurons are small- to medium-sized pyramidal cells located primarily in layers V–VI [187,188]. This description closely fits that of the cortical neurons in which LBs develop. Moreover, the subthalamic nucleus also receives a projection from the cerebral cortex, although mainly from the primary motor field (Figure 3.4). These circumstances indicate that the immunoreactive material seen in cortical, striatal, and thalamic astrocytes originates from LB-bearing pyramidal cells having corticostriatal and corticothalamic projections. The absence of astrocytic immunoreactivity in the subthalamic nucleus lends credence to this explanation inasmuch as the projection cells of the corticosubthalamic tract in the primary motor field remain uninvolved [159].

Stages 5 and 6: Lewy pathology in neocortical prefrontal and high-order sensory association areas, premotor areas, first-order sensory association areas, and primary fields

In stage 5, LP is found in the high-order association areas of the neocortex. The inclusions are concentrated at the border of the mesocortex and gradually taper off the closer they are to the secondary and primary fields of the neocortex. Involved pyramidal cells are still predominantly those in layers V–VI [19,22]. In stage 6, cortical involvement gains additional momentum. LP occurs in the first-order sensory association areas and premotor fields, and eventually enters the neocortical primary sensory and motor fields. During stages 5 and 6, the dot-like immunoreactive inclusions observable in the cortex, striatum, and thalamic relay nuclei since stage 4 increase.

The striatal circuit

Within the striatal circuit, the dorsal striatum, external and internal pallidum, subthalamic nucleus, and ventrolateral thalamus begin to myelinate prenatally. As a result, they are exceptionally well myelinated in the adult human brain. With the exception of the substantia nigra and pedunculopontine nucleus (whose axons are thin and poorly myelinated), the projection neurons of the pallidum, subthalamic nucleus, and thalamic relay nuclei are resistant to the sPD-related pathologic process. The same applies to cerebellar circuit centers. They myelinate early and seldom become involved – and, if at all, during stages 5 and 6 [6,22].

The majority of striatal neurons are inhibitory medium-sized GABAergic projection cells with spiny dendrites and can be divided into two groups. One is characterized by enkephalin, expresses the D2 subtype of dopamine receptors, and projects chiefly to the external pallidum, whereas the second group contains substance P, expresses the D1 dopamine receptor subtype, and projects to the internal pallidum (Figure 3.4). Approximately 80% of all synapses within the striatum are derived from corticostriatal projections that terminate on the tips of spines belonging to medium-sized projection cells [189,190]. Dopaminergic projections from the substantia nigra form symmetric contacts on the stalks of the spines, whereas glutamatergic terminals from the intralaminar thalamic nuclei are found on the dendritic shafts. This means the dopaminergic fibers are optimally positioned to regulate excitatory input from the cortex and thalamus [190,191]. The main feature of the external pallidum is that it establishes, via the subthalamic nucleus, an "indirect" pathway to the main pallidal output structure, the internal pallidal segment (Figure 3.4) [132,160,192–196].

Under resting conditions, the activity of striatal spiny neurons is minimal. Temporary activation of the GABA/enkephalin neuronal subclass results in suppression of projection cells within the external pallidum and disinhibition or activation of the subthalamic nucleus, which, in turn, activates the internal segment of the pallidum (Figure 3.4). The inhibitory influence of this output structure suppresses thalamic activity (mainly the VA and VLa) and provides a negative feedback to the cerebral cortex (Figure 3.4). Increased activity of the skeletal musculature, on the other hand, requires predominance by striatal circuitry involved in the "direct" pathway. Activation of substance P neurons suppresses part of the activity in the internal pallidum and results in activation of related thalamic nuclei, thereby opening the way for positive feedback to the cortex (Figure 3.4). The dopaminergic projections from the substantia nigra exert opposing influences on the aforementioned striatal pathways by curbing the indirect and promoting the direct pathway [191,197].

Depletion of striatal dopamine in sPD probably induces postsynaptic changes in striatal projection neurons and causes an imbalance in the activity within both the direct pathway (insufficient activation) and the indirect pathway (insufficient inhibition). Hyperactivity of the subthalamic nucleus is the net effect. The resultant predominance of the internal pallidum leads to inhibition of thalamocortical activity and, clinically, to hypokinesia or akinesia [192,198–200]. The equilibrium between the indirect and direct pathways can be temporarily restored, to an extent, by pharmacologic alleviation of the striatal dopamine deficiency or by surgically induced reduction of the hyperactivity in the subthalamic nucleus (deep brain stimulation) [18,201–206].

Striatal dopamine deficiency leading to hyperactivity of striatal projection neurons is followed by loss of spines along their dendrites [207–209]. Striatal projection neurons may shed their spines as a protective response to dampen excessive corticostriatal drive and/or to ensure their own survival [210–212]. Moreover, the presence of axonal dot-like inclusions and α-synuclein-immunoreactive astrocytes in the striatum provides circumstantial evidence for a massive loss of cortical glutamatergic synapses that ultimately would render the spines useless. Destruction of the dominant cortical input to the striatum would interrupt the data stream directly at the "doorstep," so to speak, of the striatal circuit, and damage at this juncture would be accompanied by lesions of corticothalamic projections at the other end of the circuit (Figure 3.4) [132].

The hyperactivity in the subthalamic nucleus is not likely to result only from the disinhibitory influence of the external pallidum (Figure 3.4) [213], but is partially driven by the excitatory influence of corticosubthalamic connectivities (hyperdirect pathway) generated from the primary motor area. In sPD, the primary motor field remains almost fully intact and, as such, the corticosubthalamic pathway is functional even in the disorder (Figure 3.4). Whereas the corticostriatal projection forfeits its excitatory input, the subthalamic nucleus becomes increasingly subjected to the activating influence of the primary motor cortex [132].

Until recently, the striatal circuit has tended to be treated more or less in isolation. Figure 3.4, on the other hand, depicts striatal circuitry within the context of the limbic circuit, cerebellar circuit, lower brainstem, and spinal cord [132,214]. Moreover, this figure shows how the pathologic process may systematically progress within the nervous system and eventually involve regions that are vital for the regulation of somatomotor functions. Here, it should be emphasized that nuclei of the level setting system are drawn into the disease process in stage 2. Accumulation of LP within this system might suffice to induce mild but detectable somatomotor dysfunctions [215–217]. These could become exacerbated, and additional somatomotor symptoms become apparent following the involvement of the pedunculopontine tegmental nucleus and substantia nigra at stage 3. Affection of the thalamic intralaminar nuclei during stage 4 and deterioration of the corticostriatal and corticothalamic connectivities in stages 5–6 would seal the fate of the somatomotor system [127].

Acknowledgments

This work was supported by the German Research Council (Deutsche Forschungsgemeinschaft) and the Michael J. Fox Foundation for Parkinson's Research. We also wish to express our gratitude to Ms. I. Szász-Jacobi (graphics).

References

1. Chu Y, Kordower JH. Age-associated increases of α-synuclein in monkeys and humans are associated with nigrostriatal dopamine depletion: is this the target for Parkinson's disease? *Neurobiol Dis* 2007;**25**:134–49.
2. Jellinger KA. Pathology of Parkinson's disease. Changes other than the nigrostriatal pathway. *Mol Chem Neuropathol* 1991;**14**:153–97.
3. Lang AE, Obeso JA. Challenges in Parkinson's disease: restoration of the nigrostriatal dopamine system is not enough. *Lancet Neurol* 2004;**3**:309–16.
4. Langston JW. The Parkinson's complex: parkinsonism is just the tip of the iceberg. *Ann Neurol* 2006;**59**:591–6.
5. Ahlskog JE. Beating a dead horse: dopamine and Parkinson's disease. *Neurology* 2007;**69**:1701–11.
6. Braak H, Del Tredici K. Nervous system pathology in sporadic Parkinson's disease. *Neurology* 2008;**70**:1916–25.
7. Spillantini MG, Schmidt ML, Lee VMY, *et al.* α-Synuclein in Lewy bodies. *Nature* 1997;**388**:839–40.
8. Dickson DW. α-Synuclein and the Lewy body disorders. *Curr Opin Neurol* 2001;**14**:423–32.
9. Goedert M, Spillantini MG, Serpell LC, *et al.* From genetics to pathology: tau and α-synuclein assemblies in neurodegenerative diseases. *Philos Trans R Soc Lond B* 2001;**356**:213–7.
10. Norris EH, Giasson BI, Lee VM. α-Synuclein: normal function and role in neurodegenerative diseases. *Curr Top Dev Biol* 2004;**60**:17–54.
11. Litvan I, Halliday G, Hallett M, *et al.* The etiopathogenesis of Parkinson's disease and suggestions for further research. Part I. *J Neuropathol Exp Neurol* 2007;**66**:251–7.
12. Wakabayashi K, Tanji K, Mori F, Takahashi H. The Lewy body in Parkinson's disease: molecules implicated in the formation and degradation of alpha-synuclein aggregates. *Neuropathology* 2007;**27**:494–506.
13. Ross GW, Abbott RD, Petrovitch H, *et al.* Association of olfactory dysfunction with incidental Lewy bodies. *Mov Disord* 2006;**21**:2062–7.
14. Duda JE, Noorigian JV, Petrovitch H, White LR, Ross GW. Pattern of Lewy pathology progression suggested by Braak staging system is supported by analysis of a population-based cohort of patients. The Movement Disorders Society's 11th International Congress Late Breaking Abstracts A3, 2007.
15. Abbott RD, Ross GW, Petrovitch H, *et al.* Bowel movement frequency in late-life and incidental Lewy bodies. *Mov Disord* 2007;**22**:1581–6.
16. Beach TG, Adler CH, Sue LL, *et al.* Reduced striatal tyrosine hydroxylase in incidental Lewy body disease. *Acta Neuropathol* 2008;**115**:445–51.
17. Dickson DW, Fujishiro H, DelleDonne A, *et al.* Evidence that incidental Lewy body disease is presymptomatic Parkinson's disease. *Acta Neuropathol* 2008;**115**:437–44.
18. Olanow CW, Stern MB, Sethi K. The scientific and clinical basis for the treatment of Parkinson disease. *Neurology* 2009;**72**(Suppl 4):S1-136.
19. Braak H, Del Tredici K, Rüb U, *et al.* Staging of brain pathology related to sporadic Parkinson's disease. *Neurobiol Aging* 2003;**24**:197–210.
20. Braak H, Ghebremedhin E, Rüb U, *et al.* Stages in the development of Parkinson's disease-related pathology. *Cell Tiss Res* 2004;**318**:121–34.
21. Braak H, Müller CM, Bohl JR, *et al.* Stanley Fahn Lecture 2005: the staging procedure for the inclusion body pathology associated with sporadic Parkinson disease reconsidered. *Mov Disord* 2006;**21**:2042–51.

22. Braak H, Del Tredici K. Neuroanatomy and pathology of sporadic Parkinson's disease. *Adv Anat Embryol Cell Biol* 2009;**121**:1–119.
23. Hirsch E, Graybiel AM, Agid YA. Melanized dopaminergic neurons are differentially susceptible to degeneration in Parkinson's disease. *Nature* 1988;**334**:345–8.
24. Gray DA, Woulfe J. Lipofuscin and aging: a matter of toxic waste. *Sci Aging Knowl Environ* 2005;**5**:1–5.
25. Saper CB, Sorrentino DM, German DC, de Lacalle S. Medullary catecholaminergic neurons in the normal human brain and in Parkinson's disease. *Ann Neurol* 21991;**9**:577–84.
26. Terman A, Kurz T, Navratil M, *et al.* Mitochondrial turnover and aging of long-lived postmitotic cells: the mitochondrial-lysosomal axis theory of aging. *Antioxid Redox Signal* 2010;**12**, 503–35.
27. Braak H, Del Tredici K, Gai WP, Braak E. Alpha-synuclein is not a requisite component of synaptic boutons in the adult human central nervous system. *J Chem Neuroanat* 2001;**20**:245–52.
28. Matzuk MM, Saper CB. Preservation of hypothalamic dopaminergic neurons in Parkinson's disease. *Ann Neurol* 1985;**18**:552–5.
29. Tofaris GK, Spillantini MG. Physiological and pathological properties of α-synuclein. *Cell Mol Life Sci* 2007;**64**:2194–201.
30. Thomas PJ, Qu BH, Pedersen PL. Defective protein folding as a basis of human disease. *Trends Biochem Sci* 1995;**20**:456–9.
31. Dobson CM. Protein misfolding, evolution and disease. *Trends Biochem Sci* 1999;**24**:329–32.
32. Fortin DL, Nemani VM, Voglmaier SM, *et al.* Neural activity controls the synaptic accumulation of α-synuclein. *Neurobiol Dis* 2005;**25**:10913–21.
33. McAllister C, Karymov MA, Kawano Y, *et al.* Protein interactions and misfolding analyzed by AFM force spectroscopy. *J Mol Biol* 2005;**354**:1028–42.
34. Olanow CW, Perl DP, DeMartino GN, McNaught KSP. Lewy-body formation is an aggresome-related process: a hypothesis. *Lancet Neurol* 2004;**3**:496–503.
35. Olanow CW, McNaught KS. Ubiquitin–proteasome system and Parkinson's disease. *Mov Disord* 2006;**21**:1806–23.
36. Desplats P, Lee H-J, Bae E-J, *et al.* Inclusion formation and neuronal cell death through neuron-to-neuron transmission of α-synuclein. *PNAS* 2009;**106**:13010–5.
37. Terman A, Gustafsson B, Brunk UT. Autophagy, organelles and ageing. *J Pathol* 2007;**211**:134–43.
38. Pan T, Kondo S, Le W, Jankovic J. The role of autophagy-lysosome pathway in neurodegeneration associated with Parkinson's disease. *Brain* 2008;**131**:1969–78.
39. Gibb WR, Scott T, Lees AJ. Neuronal inclusions of Parkinson's disease. *Mov Disord* 1991;**6**:2–11.
40. Jellinger KA, Mizuno Y. Parkinson's disease. In: Dickson DW, ed. *Neurodegeneration: the Molecular Pathology of Dementia and Movement Disorders.* Basel: ISN Neuropathol Press, 2003 159–87.
41. Kuusisto E, Parkkinen L, Alafuzoff I. Morphogenesis of Lewy bodies: dissimilar incorporation of α-synuclein, ubiquitin, and p62. *J Neuropathol Exp Neurol* 2003;**62**:1241–53.
42. Saito Y, Kawashima A, Ruberu NN, *et al.* Accumulation of phosphorylated α-synuclein in aging human brain. *J Neuropathol Exp Neurol* 2003;**62**:644–54.
43. Wakabayashi K, Takahashi H, Obata K, Ikuta F. Immunocytochemical localization of synpatic vesicle-specific protein in Lewy body-containing neurons in Parkinson's disease. *Neurosci Lett* 1992;**138**:237–40.
44. Braak H, de Vos RAI, Bohl J, Del Tredici K. Gastric α-synuclein-immunoreactive inclusions in Meissner's and Auerbach's plexuses in cases staged for Parkinson's disease-related brain pathology. *Neurosci Lett* 2006;**396**: 67–72.
45. Orimo S, Amino T, Itoh Y, *et al.* Cardiac sympathetic denervation precedes neuronal loss in the sympathetic ganglia in Lewy body disease, *Acta Neuropathol* 2005;**109**:583–8.
46. Orimo S, Takahashi A, Uchihara T, *et al.* Degeneration of cardiac sympathetic nerve begins in the early disease process of Parkinson's disease. *Brain Pathol* 2007;**17**:24–30.
47. Orimo S, Uchihara T, Nakamura A, *et al.* Axonal alpha-synuclein aggregates herald centripetal degeneration of cardiac sympathetic nerve in Parkinson's disease. *Brain* 2008;**131**:642–50.
48. Saha AR, Hill J, Utton MA, *et al.* Parkinson's disease α-synuclein mutations exhibit defective axonal transport in cultured neurons. *J Cell Sci* 2004;**117**:1017–24.
49. Waxman EA, Duda JE, Giasson BI. Characterization of antibodies that selectively detect α-synuclein in pathological inclusions. *Acta Neuropathol* 2008;**116**:37–46.
50. Parkkinen L, Kauppinen T, Pirttila T, *et al.* Alpha-synuclein pathology does not predict extrapyramidal symptoms of dementia. *Ann Neurol* 2005;**57**:82–91.
51. Parkkinen L, Pirttilä T, Alafuzoff I. Applicability of current staging systems of α-synuclein pathology and their clinical relevance. *Acta Neuropathol* 2008;**115**:399–407.
52. Halliday GM, McCann H. Human-based studies on α-synuclein deposition and relationship to Parkinson's disease symptoms. *Exp Neurol* 2008;**209**:12–21.
53. Lee HG, Zhu X, Takeda A, *et al.* Emerging evidence for the neuroprotective role of α-synuclein. *Exp Neurol* 2006;**200**: 1–7.
54. Meredith G, Sonsalla P, Chesselet MF. Animal models of Parkinson's disease progression. *Acta Neuropathol* 2008;**115**:385–98.
55. Glabe CG, Kayed R. Common structure and toxic function of amyloid oligomers implies a common mechanism of pathogenesis. *Neurology* 2006;**66**(Suppl 1):74–8.
56. Dugger BN, Dickson DW. Cell type specific sequestration of choline acetyltransferase and tyrosine hydroxylase within Lewy bodies. *Acta Neuropathol* 2010;**120**:633–9.
57. Forno LS. Concentric hyaline intraneuronal inclusions of Lewy body type in the brain of elderly persons (50 incidental cases): relationship to parkinsonism. *J Am Geriatr Soc* 1969;**17**:557–75.
58. Gibb WRG, Lees AJ. The relevance of the Lewy body to the pathogenesis of idiopathic Parkinson's disease. *J Neurol Neurosurg Psychiatry* 1988;**51**:745–52.
59. Gibb WRG, Lees AJ. The significance of the Lewy body in the diagnosis of idiopathic Parkinson's disease. *Neuropathol Appl Neurobiol* 1989;**15**:27–44.
60. Smith PEM, Irving D, Perry RH. Density, distribution and prevalence of Lewy bodies in the elderly. *Neurosci Res Commun* 1991;**8**:127–35.

61. Forno LS, Langston JW. Lewy bodies and aging: relation to Alzheimer's and Parkinson's diseases. *Neurodegeneration* 1993;**2**:19–24.
62. Jellinger KA. Lewy body-related α-synucleinopathy in the aged human brain. *J Neural Transm* 2004;**111**:1219–35.
63. Saito Y, Ruberu NN, Sawabe M, *et al.* Lewy body-related α-synucleinopathy in aging. *J Neuropathol Exp Neurol* 2004;**63**:742–9.
64. Mikolaenko I, Pletnikova O, Kawas CH, *et al.* Alpha-synuclein lesions in normal aging, Parkinson disease, and Alzheimer disease: evidence from the Baltimore Longitudinal Study of Aging (BLSA). *J Neuropathol Exp Neurol* 2005;**64**:156–62.
65. Bloch A, Probst A, Bissig H, *et al.* α-Synuclein pathology of the spinal and peripheral autonomic nervous system in neurologically unimpaired elderly subjects. *Neuropathol Appl Neurobiol* 2006;**12**:284–95.
66. Klos KJ, Ahlskog JE, Josephs KA, *et al.* α-Synuclein pathology in the spinal cord of neurologically asymptomatic aged individuals. *Neurology* 2006;**66**:1100–2.
67. Hubbard PS, Esiri MM, Reading M, *et al.* Alpha-synuclein pathology in the olfactory pathways of dementia patients. *J Anat* 2007;**211**:117–24.
68. Tompkins MM, Hill WD. Contribution of somal Lewy bodies to neuronal death. *Brain Res* 1997;**775**:24–9.
69. Kubis N, Faucheux BA, Ransmayr G, *et al.* Preservation of midbrain catecholaminergic neurons in very old human subjects. *Brain* 2000;**123**:366–73.
70. Wolters EC, Braak H. Parkinson's disease: premotor clinico-pathological correlations. *J Neural Transm Suppl* 2006;**70**:309–19.
71. Fujishiro H, Frigerior R, Burnett M, *et al.* Cardiac sympathetic denervation correlates with clinical and pathologic stages of Parkinson's disease. *Mov Disord* 2008;**23**:1085–92.
72. Markesbery WR, Jicha GA, Liu H, Schmitt FA. Lewy body pathology in normal elderly subjects. *J Neuropathol Exp Neurol* 2009;**68**:816–22.
73. Thal DR, Del Tredici K, Braak H. Neurodegeneration in normal brain aging and disease. *Sci Aging Knowl Environ* 2004;**23**:1–13.
74. Hawkes CH. Parkinson's disease and aging: same or different process? *Mov Disord* 2008;**23**:47–53.
75. Wakabayashi K, Takahashi H. Neuropathology of autonomic nervous system in Parkinson's disease. *Eur Neurol* 1997;**38**(Suppl 2):2–7.
76. Halliday GM, Del Tredici K, Braak H. Critical appraisal of the Braak staging of brain pathology related to sporadic Parkinson's disease. *J Neural Transm Suppl* 2006;**70**:99–103.
77. Dickson DW, Uchikado H, Fujishiro H, Tsuboi Y. Evidence in favor of Braak staging of Parkinson's disease. *Mov Disord* 2010;**25**(Suppl 1):S78–82.
78. Kempster PA, O'Sullivan SS, Holton JL, *et al.* Relationships between age and late progression of Parkinson's disease: a clinico-pathological study. *Brain* 2010;**133**:1755–62.
79. Burke RE, Dauer WT, Vonsattel JP. A critical evaluation of the Braak staging scheme for Parkinson's disease. *Ann Neurol* 2008;**64**:485–91.
80. Dickson DW, Braak H, Duda JE, *et al.* Diagnostic criteria for the neuropathological assessment of Parkinson disease: Report of the Neuropathology and Genetics Working Group of the Second International Brainstorming Conference on Parkinson Disease. *Lancet Neurol* 2009;**8**:1150–7.
81. Beach, TG, Adler CH, Sue LI, *et al.* Multi-organ distribution of phophorylated α-synuclein histopathology in subjects with Lewy body disorders. *Acta Neuropathol* 2010;**119**:689–702.
82. Müller CM, de Vos RAI, Maurage CA, *et al.* Staging of sporadic Parkinson's disease-related alpha-synuclein pathology: inter- and intra-rater reliability. *J Neuropathol Exp Neurol* 2005;**64**:623–8.
83. Jellinger KA. Alpha-synuclein pathology in Parkinson's and Alzheimer's disease brain: incidence and topographic distribution – a pilot study. *Acta Neuropathol* 2003;**106**:191–201.
84. Kingsbury AE, Bandopadhyay R, Silveira-Moriyama L, *et al.* Brain stem pathology in Parkinson's disease: an evaluation of the Braak staging model. *Mov Disord* 2010;**25**:2508–15.
85. Neumann M, Müller V, Kretzschmar HA, *et al.* Regional distribution of proteinase-K-resistant α-synuclein correlates with Lewy body disease stage. *J Neuropathol Exp Neurol* 2004;**63**:1225–35.
86. Dickson DW, Uchikado H, Fujishoro H, Tsuboi Y. Evidence in favor of Braak staging of Parkinson's disease. *Mov Disord* 2010;**25**(Suppl 1):S78–S82.
87. Uchikado H, Lin WL, DeLucia MW, Dickson DW. Alzheimer disease with amygdala Lewy bodies: a distinct form of alpha-synucleinopathy. *J Neuropathol Exp Neurol* 2006;**65**:685–97.
88. Halliday GM, Hely M, Reid W, Morris J. The progression of pathology in longitudinally followed patients with Parkinson's disease. *Acta Neuropathol* 2008;**115**:409–15.
89. Parkkinen L, Soininen H, Alafuzoff I. Regional distribution of alpha-synuclein pathology in unimpaired aging and Alzheimer's disease. *J Neuropathol Exp Neurol* 2003;**62**:363–7.
90. Braak H, Müller CM, Rüb U, *et al.* Pathology associated with sporadic Parkinson's disease—where does it end? *J Neural Transm Suppl* 2006;**70**:89–97.
91. Hamilton RL. Lewy bodies in Alzheimer's disease: a neuropathological review of 145 cases using α-synuclein immunohistochemistry. *Brain Pathol* 2000;**10**:378–84.
92. Fumimura Y, Ikemura M, Saito Y, *et al.* Analysis of the adrenal gland is useful for evaluating pathology of the peripheral autonomic nervous system in Lewy body disease. *J Neuropathol Exp Neurol* 2007;**66**:354–62.
93. Minguez-Castellanos A, Chamorro CE, Escamilla-Sevilla F, *et al.* Do α-synuclein aggregates in autonomic plexuses predate Lewy body disorders? A cohort study. *Neurology* 2007;**68**:2012–8.
94. Del Tredici K, Hawkes CH, Ghebremedhin E, Braak H. Lewy pathology in the submandibular gland of individuals with incidental Lewy body disease and sporadic Parkinson's disease. *Acta Neuropathol* 2010;**119**:703–13.
95. Del Tredici K, Rüb U, de Vos RAI, *et al.* Where does Parkinson disease pathology begin in the brain? *J Neuropathol Exp Neurol* 2002;**61**:413–26.
96. Gai WP, Blumbergs PD, Geffen LB, Blessing WW. Age-related loss of dorsal vagal neurons in Parkinson's disease. *Neurology* 1992;**42**:2106–11.
97. Doty RL. Olfaction. *Annu Rev Psychol* 2001;**52**:423–52.
98. Doty RL. The olfactory vector hypothesis of neurogenerative disease: is it viable? *Ann Neurol* 2008;**63**:7–15.

99. Hawkes CH. Olfaction in neurodegenerative disorder. *Mov Disord* 2003 **18**:364–72.
100. Hawkes CH, Shephard BC, Daniel SE. Is Parkinson's disease a primary olfactory disorder? *Q J Med* 1999;**92**:473–80.
101. Hawkes CH, Del Tredici K, Braak H. Parkinson's disease: a dual-hit hypothesis. *Neuropathol Appl Neurobiol* 2007;**33**:599–614.
102. Duda JE, Shah U, Arnold SE, *et al*. The expression of alpha, beta-, and gamma-synucleins in olfactory mucosa. *Exp Neurol* 1999;**160**:515–22.
103. Huisman E, Uylings HB, Hoogland PV. A 100% increase of dopaminergic cells in the olfactory bulb may explain hyposmia in Parkinson's disease. *Mov Disord* 2004;**19**:687–92.
104. Harding AJ, Stimson E, Henderson JM, Halliday GM. Clinical correlates of selective pathology in the amygdala of patients with Parkinson's disease. *Brain* 2002;**125**:2431–45.
105. Braak H, Braak E, Yilmazer D, *et al*. Amygdala pathology in Parkinson's disease. *Acta Neuropathol* 1994;**88**:493–500.
106. Hubbard PS, Esiri NM, Reading M, *et al*. Alpha-synuclein pathology in the olfactory pathways of dementia patients. *J Anat* 2007;**211**:117–24.
107. Huang XF, Törk I, Paxinos G. Dorsal motor nucleus of the vagus nerve: a cyto- and chemoarchitectonic study in the human. *J Comp Neurol* 1993;**330**:158–82.
108. Hopkins DA, Bieger D, de Vente J, Steinbusch HWM. Vagal efferent projections: viscerotopy, neurochemistry and effects of vagotomy. *Prog Brain Res* 1996;**107**:79–96.
109. Blessing WW. Lower brain stem regulation of visceral, cardiovascular, and respiratory function. In: Paxinos G, Mai JK, eds. *The Human Nervous System*, 2nd edn. San Diego: Elsevier Academic Press, 2004:464–78.
110. Del Tredici K, Braak H. Idiopathic Parkinson's disease: staging an α-synucleinopathy with a predictable pathoanatomy. In: Kahle P, Haass C, eds. *Molecular Mechanisms in Parkinson's Disease*. Georgetown, TX: Landes Bioscience, 2004:1–32.
111. Wakabayashi K, Takahashi H, Ohama E, Ikuta F. Parkinson's disease: an immunohistochemical study of Lewy body-containing neurons in the enteric nervous system. *Acta Neuropathol* 1990;**79**:581–3.
112. Wakabayashi K, Takahashi H, Ohama E, *et al*. Lewy bodies in the visceral autonomic nervous system in Parkinson's disease. *Adv Neurol* 1993;**60**:609–12.
113. Benarroch EE. Enteric nervous system: functional organization and neurologic implications. *Neurology* 2007;**69**:1953–7.
114. Phillips RJ, Walter GC, Wilder SL, *et al*. Alpha-synuclein immunopositive myenteric neurons and vagal preganglionic terminals: autonomic pathway implicated in Parkinson's disease? *Neuroscience* 2008;**153**:733–50.
115. Loewy AD. Forebrain nuclei involved in autonomic control. *Prog Brain Res* 1991;**87**:253–68.
116. Cersósimo MG, Benarroch EE. Neural control of the gastrointestinal tract: implications for Parkinson disease. *Mov Disord* 2008;**23**:1065–75.
117. Wakabayashi K, Takahashi H. The intermediolateral nucleus and Clarke's column in Parkinson's disease. *Acta Neuropathol* 1997;**94**:287–9.
118. Braak H, Sastre M, Bohl JRE, *et al*. Parkinson's disease: lesions in dorsal horn layer I, involvement of parasympathetic and sympathetic pre- and postganglionic neurons. *Acta Neuropathol* 2007;**113**:421–9.
119. Iwanaga K, Wakabayashi K, Yoshimoto M, *et al*. Lewy body-type degeneration in cardiac plexus in Parkinson's and incidental Lewy body diseases. *Neurology* 1999;**52**:1269–71.
120. Ghebremedhin E, Del Tredici K, Langston JW, Braak H. Diminished tyrosine hydroxylase immunoreactivity in the cardiac conduction system and myocardium in Parkinson's disease: an anatomical study. *Acta Neuropathol* 2009;**118**:777–84.
121. Craig AD. Pain mechanisms: labeled lines versus convergence in central processing. *Annu Rev Neurosci* 2003;**26**:1–30.
122. Tracey I. Nociceptive processing in the human brain. *Curr Opin Neurobiol* 2005;**15**:478–87.
123. Samuels ER, Szabadi E. Functional neuroanatomy of the noradrenergic locus coeruleus: its roles in the regulation of arousal and autonomic function, part I: principles of functional organization. *Curr Neuropharmacol* 2009;**6**:235–53.
124. Quinn NP, Koller WC, Lang AE, Marsden CD. Painful Parkinson's disease. *Lancet* 1996;**i**:1366–9.
125. Buzas B, Max MB. Pain in Parkinson disease. *Neurology* 2004;**62**:2156–7.
126. Sage JI. Pain in Parkinson's disease. *Curr Treat Options Neurol* 2004;**6**:191–200.
127. Sethi K. Levodopa unresponsive symptoms in Parkinson's disease. *Mov Disord* 2008;**23**(Suppl 3):S521–33.
128. Holstege G. The somatic motor system. *Prog Brain Res* 1996;**107**:9–26.
129. Holstege G, Mouton LJ, Gerrits NM. Emotional motor system. In: Paxinos G, Mai JK, eds. *The Human Nervous System*, 2nd edn. San Diego: Elsevier Academic Press, 2004:1306–25.
130. Nieuwenhuys R. The greater limbic system, the emotional motor system and the brain. *Prog Brain Res* 1996;**107**:551–80.
131. Koutcherov Y, Huang XF, Halliday G, Paxinos G. Organisation of the human brain stem nuclei. In: Paxinos G, Mai KJ, eds. *The Human Nervous System*, 2nd edn. San Diego: Elsevier Academic Press, 2004:273–321.
132. Braak H, Del Tredici K. Cortico-basal ganglia-cortical circuitry in Parkinson's disease reconsidered. *Exp Neurol* 2008;**212**:129–31.
133. Sims KS, Williams RS. The human amygdaloid complex: a cytologic and histochemical atlas using Nissl, myelin, acetylcholinesterase and nicotinamide adenine dinucleotide phosphate diaphorase staining. *Neuroscience* 1990;**36**:449–72.
134. Bohus B, Koolhaas JM, Luiten PGM, *et al*. The neurobiology of the central nuleus of the amygdala in relation to neuroendocrine and autonomic outflow. *Prog Brain Res* 1996;**107**:447–60.
135. Hirsch EC, Graybiel AM, Duyckaerts C, Javoy-Agid F. Neuronal loss in the pedunculopontine tegmental nucleus in Parkinson disease and in progressive supranuclear palsy. *Proc Natl Acad Sci USA* 1987;**84**:5976–80.
136. Jellinger K. The pedunculopontine nucleus in Parkinson's disease, progressive supranuclear palsy and Alzheimer's disease. *J Neurol Neurosurg Psychiatry* 1988;**51**:540–3.
137. Zweig RM, Jankel WR, Hedreen JC, *et al*. The pedunculopontine nucleus in Parkinson's disease. *Ann Neurol* 1989;**26**:41–6.
138. Rinne JO, Ma SY, Lee MS, *et al*. Loss of cholinergic neurons in the pedunculopontne nucleus in Parkinson's disease is related to disability of the patients. *Parkinsonism Relat Disord* 2008;**14**:553–7.

139. Mesulam MM, Geula C, Bothwell MA, Hersh LB. Human reticular formation: cholinergic neurons of the pedunculopontine and laterodorsal tegmental nuclei and some cytochemical comparisons to forebrain cholinergic neurons. *J Comp Neurol* 1989;**283**:611–33.
140. Pahapill PA, Lozano AM. The pedunculopontine nucleus and Parkinson's disease. *Brain* 2000;**123**:1767–83.
141. Aravamuthan BR, Muthusamy KA, Stein JF, *et al.* Topography of cortical and subcortical connections of the human pedunculopontine and subthalamic nuclei. *NeuroImage* 2007;**37**:694–703.
142. Garcia-Rill E. The pedunculopontine nucleus. *Prog Neurobiol* 1991;**36**:363–89.
143. Steckler T, Inglis W, Winn P, Sahgal A. The pedunculopontine tegmental nucleus: a role in cognitive processes? *Brain Res Rev* 1994;**19**:298–318.
144. Inglis WL, Winn P. The pedunculopontine tegmental nucleus: where the striatum meets the reticular formation. *Prog Neurobiol* 1995;**47**:1–29.
145. Winn P, Brown VJ, Inglis WL. On the relationships between the striatum and the pedunculopontine tegmental nucleus. *Crit Rev Neurobiol* 1997;**11**:241–61.
146. Lee MS, Rinne JQ, Marsden CD. The pedunculopontine nucleus: its role in the genesis of movement disorders. *Yonsei Med J* 2000;**41**:167–84.
147. Braak H, Braak E. Nuclear configuration and neuronal types of the nucleus niger in the brain of the human adult. *Hum Neurobiol* 1986;**5**:71–82.
148. Fearnley JM, Lees AJ. Ageing and Parkinson's disease: substantia nigra regional selectivity. *Brain* 1991;**114**: 2283–301.
149. Gibb WRG, Lees AJ. Anatomy, pigmentation, ventral and dorsal subpopulations of the substantia nigra, and differential cell death in Parkinson's disease. *J Neurol Neurosurg Psychiatry* 1991;**54**:388–96.
150. Halliday GM. Substantia nigra and locus coeruleus. In: Paxinos G, Mai JK, eds. *The Human Nervous System*, 2nd edn. San Diego: Elsevier Academic Press, 2004:677–738.
151. McRitchie DA, Cartwright HR, Halliday GM. Specific A10 dopaminergic nuclei in the midbrain degenerate in Parkinson's disease. *Exp Neurol* 1997;**144**:202–13.
152. Saper CB. Cholinergic system. In: Paxinos G, ed. *The Human Nervous System*. San Diego: Academic Press, 1990: 1095–113.
153. Nieuwenhuys R. Structure and organisation of fibre systems. In: Nieuwenhuys R, Ten Donkelaar HJ, Nicholson C, eds. *The Central Nervous System of Vertebrates*, Vol. 1. Berlin: Springer, 1999:113–57.
154. Mesulam MM. The cholinergic innervation of the human cerebral cortex. *Prog Brain Res* 2004;**145**:67–78.
155. Heimer L, van Hoesen GW. The limbic lobe and its output channels: implications for emotional functions and adaptive behavior. *Neurosci Biobehav Rev* 2006;**30**:126–47.
156. Langston JW, Forno LS. The hypothalamus in Parkinson's disease. *Ann Neurol* 1978;**3**:129–33.
157. Panula P, Airaksinen MS, Pirvola U, Kotilainen E. A histamine-containing neuronal system in human brain. *Neuroscience* **3**1990;**4**:127–32.
158. Passani MB, Bacciottini L, Mannaioni F, Blandina P. Central histaminergic system and cognition. *Neurosci Biobehav Rev* 2000;**24**:107–13.
159. Braak H, Sastre M, Del Tredici K. Development of α-synuclein-immunoreactive astrocytes in the forebrain parallels stages of intraneuronal pathology in sporadic Parkinson's disease. *Acta Neuropathol* 2007;**114**:231–41.
160. Parent A, Hazrati LN. Functional anatomy of the basal ganglia. I. The cortico-basal ganglia–thalamo–cortical loop. *Brain Res Rev* 1995;**20**:91–127.
161. Groenewegen HJ, Berendse HW. The specificity of the "nonspecific" midline and intralaminar thalamic nuclei. *Trends Neurosci* 1994;**17**:52–7.
162. Henderson JM, Carpenter K, Cartwright H, Halliday GH. Loss of thalamic intralaminar nuclei in progressive supranuclear palsy and Parkinson's disease: clinical and therapeutic implications. *Brain* 2000;**123**:1410–21.
163. Rüb U, Del Tredici K, Schultz C, *et al.* Parkinson's disease: the thalamic components of the limbic loop are severely impaired by α-synuclein immunopositive inclusion body pathology. *Neurobiol Aging* 2002;**23**:245–54.
164. Heimer L, de Olmos J, Alheid GF, Zaborsky L. "Perestroika" in the basal forebrain: opening the border between neurology and psychiatry. *Prog Brain Res* 1991;**87**:109–65.
165. Groenewegen HJ, Trimble M. The ventral striatum as an interface between the limbic and motor systems. *CNS Spectr* 2007;**12**:887–92.
166. Dickson DW, Schmidt ML, Lee VMY, *et al.* Immunoreactivity profile of hippocampal CA2/3 neurites in diffuse Lewy body disease. *Acta Neuropathol* 1994;**87**:269–76.
167. Mesulam MM, Mufson EJ. The insula of Reil in man and monkey. In: Jones EG, Peters A, eds. *Cerebral Cortex. Association and Auditory Cortices*, Vol. 4. New York: Plenum Press, 1993:179–225.
168. van Hoesen GW, Morecraft RJ, Vogt BA. Connections of the monkey cingulate cortex. In: Vogt BA, Gabriel M, eds. *Neurobiology of Cingulate Cortex and Limbic Thalamus*. Boston: Birkhäuser, 1993:249–84.
169. Augustine JR. Circuitry and functional aspects of the insular lobe in primates including humans. *Brain Res Rev* 1996;**22**:229–44.
170. Cechetto DF, Saper CB. Role of the cerebral cortex in autonomic function. In: Loewy AD, Spyer KM, eds. *Central Regulation of Autonomic Function*. New York: Oxford University Press, 1990:208–23.
171. Hurtig HI, Trojanowski JQ, Galvin J, *et al.* Alpha-synuclein cortical Lewy bodies correlate with dementia in Parkinson's disease. *Neurology* 2000;**54**:1916–21.
172. Mattila PM, Rinne JO, Helenius H, *et al.* Alpha-synuclein-immunoreactive cortical Lewy bodies are associated with cognitive impairment in Parkinson's disease. *Acta Neuropathol* 2000;**100**:285–90.
173. Squire LR, Schacter DL. *Neuropsychology of Memory*. New York: Guilford Press, 2002.
174. Suzuki WA, Amaral DG. Functional neuroanatomy of the medial temporal lobe memory system. *Cortex* 2004;**40**:220–2.
175. Braak H, Rüb U, Jansen Steur ENH, *et al.* Cognitive status correlates with neuropathological stage in Parkinson disease. *Neurology* 2005;**64**:1404–10.
176. Emre M, Aarsland D, Brown R, *et al.* *Mov Disord* 2007;**22**: 1689–707.
177. Verbaan D, Marinus J, Visser M, *et al.* Patient-reported autonomic symptoms in Parkinson disease. *Neurology* 2007;**69**: 333–41.

178. Drevets WC, Price JL, Simpson JR, *et al.* Subgenual prefrontal cortex abnormalities in mood disorders. *Nature* 1997;**386**: 824–7.
179. Lane RD, Reiman EM, Ahern GL, *et al.* Neuroanatomical correlates of happiness, sadness, and disgust. *Am J Psychiatr* 1997;**154**:926–33.
180. Benarroch EE. The central autonomic network: functional organization, dysfunction, and perspective. *Mayo Clin Proc* 1993;**68**:988–1001.
181. Duda JE, Giasson BI, Mabon ME, *et al.* Novel antibodies to synuclein show abundant striatal pathology in Lewy body disease. *Ann Neurol* 2002;**52**:205–10.
182. El-Agnaf OM, Salem SA, Paleologou KE, *et al.* α-Synuclein implicated in Parkinson's disease is present in extracellular biological fluids, including human plasma. *FASEB J* 2003;**17**:1945–7.
183. Lee HJ, Patel S, Lee SJ. Intravesicular localization and exocytosis of α-synuclein and its aggregates. *J Neurosci* 2005;**25**:6016–24.
184. Lee SJ. Origins and effects of extracellular alpha synuclein: implications in Parkinson's disease. *J Mol Neurosci* 2008;**34**:17–22.
185. Mollenhauer B, Cullen V, Kahn I, *et al.* Direct quantification of CSF alpha-synuclein by ELISA and first cross-sectional study in patients with neurodegeneration. *Exp Neurol* 2008;**213**:315–25.
186. Mori F, Tanji K, Yoshimoto M, et al.. Demonstration of α-synuclein immunoreactivity in neuronal and glial cytoplasm in normal human brain tissue using proteinase K and formic acid pretreatment. *Exp Neurol* 2002;**176**:98–104.
187. Royce GJ. Laminar origin of cortical neurons which project upon the caudate nucleus: a horseradish peroxidase investigation in the cat. *J Comp Neurol* 1982;**205**:8–29.
188. Jones EG. Laminar distribution of cortical efferent cells. In: Peters A, Jones EG, eds. *Cerebral Cortex, Vol. 1: Cellular Components of the Cerebral Cortex.* New York: Plenum Press, 1984:521–53.
189. Pasik P, Pasik T, DiFiglia M. Quantitative aspects of neuronal organization in the neostriatum of the macaque monkey. In: Yahr MD, ed. *The Basal Ganglia.* New York: Raven Press, 1976:57–90.
190. Smith AD, Bolam JP. The neural network of the basal ganglia as revealed by the study of synaptic connections of identified neurones. *Trends Neurosci* 1990;**13**:259–65.
191. Gerfen CR. Molecular effects of dopamine on striatal-projection pathways. *Trends Neurosci* 2000;**23**(Suppl):64–70.
192. Alexander GE, Crutcher MD, DeLong MR. Basal ganglia-thalamocortical circuits: parallel substrates for motor, oculomotor, "prefrontal" and "limbic" functions. *Prog Brain Res* 1990;**85**:119–46.
193. Alheid GF, Heimer L, Switzer RC. Basal ganglia. In: Paxinos G, ed. *The Human Nervous System.* San Diego: Academic Press, 1990:483–582.
194. Parent A, Hazrati LN. Functional anatomy of the basal ganglia. II. The place of the subthalamic nucleus and external pallidum in basal ganglia circuitry. *Brain Res Rev* 1995;**20**: 128–54.
195. Haber SN, Gdowski MJ. The basal ganglia. In: Paxinos G, Mai JK, eds. *The Human Nervous System*, 2nd edn. San Diego: Elsevier Academic Press, 2004:677–738.
196. Tepper JM, Abercrombie ED, Bolam JP. Basal ganglia macrocircuits. *Prog Brain Res* 2007;**160**:3–7.
197. Starr MS. Glutamate/dopamine D1/D2 balance in the basal ganglia and its relevance to Parkinson's disease. *Synapse* 1995;**19**:264–93.
198. Obeso JA, Guridi J, Obeso JA, DeLong M. Surgery for Parkinson's disease. *J Neurol Neurosurg Psychiatry* 1997;**62**:2–8.
199. Wichmann T, DeLong MR. Functional neuroanatomy of the basal ganglia in Parkinson's disease. *Adv Neurol* 2003;**91**:9–18.
200. DeLong MR, Wichmann T. Circuits and circuit disorders of the basal ganglia. *Arch Neurol* 2007;**64**:20–4.
201. Benabid AL. Deep brain stimulation for Parkinson's disease. *Curr Opin Neurobiol* 2003;**13**:696–706.
202. Kopell BH, Rezai AR, Chang JW, Vitek JL. Anatomy and physiology of the basal ganglia: implications for deep brain stimulation for Parkinson's disease. *Mov Disord* 2006;**21**(Suppl 14):238–46.
203. Temel Y, Visser-Vandewalle V. Targets for deep brain stimulation in Parkinson's disease. *Expert Opin Ther Targets* 2006;**10**:1–8.
204. Wichmann T, DeLong M. Deep brain stimulation for neurologic and neuropsychiatric disorders. *Neuron* 2006;**52**:197–204.
205. Stefani A, Lozano AM, Peppe A, *et al.* Bilateral deep brain stimulation of the pedunculopontine and subthalamic nuclei in severe Parkinson's disease. *Brain* 2007;**130**:1596–607.
206. Volkmann J. Update on surgery for Parkinson's disease. *Curr Opin Neurol* 2007;**20**:465–9.
207. Stephens B, Mueller AJ, Shering AF, *et al.* Evidence of a breakdown of corticostriatal connections in Parkinson's disease. *Neuroscience* 2005;**132**:741–54.
208. Zaja-Milatovic S, Milatovic D, Schantz AM, *et al.* Dendritic degeneration in neostriatal medium spiny neurons in Parkinson's disease. *Neurology* 2005;**64**:545–7.
209. Kramer ML, Schulz-Schaeffer WJ. Presynaptic α-synuclein aggregates, not Lewy bodies, cause neurodegeneration in dementia with Lewy bodies. *J Neurosci* 2007;**27**:1405–10.
210. Deutch AY. Striatal plasticity in parkinsonism: dystrophic changes in medium spiny neurons and progression in Parkinson's disease. *J Neural Transm Suppl* 2006;**70**:67–70.
211. Gerfen CR. Indirect-pathway neurons lose their spines in Parkinson's disease. *Nature Neurosci* 2006;**9**:157–8.
212. Neely MD, Schmidt DE, Deutch AY. Cortical regulation of dopamine depletion-induced dendritic spine loss in striatal medium spiny neurons. *Neuroscience* 2007;**149**:457–64.
213. Blandini F, Nappi G, Tassorelli C, Martignioni E. Functional changes of the basal ganglia circuitry in Parkinson's disease. *Prog Neurobiol* 2000;**62**:63–88.
214. Jenkinson N, Nandi D, Muthusamy K, *et al.* Anatomy, physiology, and pathophysiology of the pedunculopontine nucleus. *Mov Disord* 2009;**23**:319–28.
215. Loza A, Pepin JL, Rapisarda G, *et al.* Functional changes of brainstem reflexes in Parkinson's disease. Conditioning of blink reflex R2 component by paired and index finger stimulation. *J Neural Transm* 1997;**104**:679–87.
216. Valls-Solé J. Neurophysiological characterization of parkinsonian syndromes. *Neurophysiol Clin* 2000;**30**:352–67.
217. Valls-Solé J, Valldeoriola F. Neurophysiological correlate of clinical signs in Parkinson's disease. *Clin Neurophysiol* 2002;**113**:792–805.

Chapter 4
Functional Anatomy of the Motor and Non-Motor Circuitry of the Basal Ganglia

Yoland Smith
Yerkes National Primate Research Center and Department of Neurology, Emory University, Atlanta, GA, USA

Introduction

The intricacy of the morphology and circuitry of the basal ganglia has long been of great interest for the neuroscience community. Since the first clear identification of the "corpus striatum" by Thomas Willis in the mid-1600s, our knowledge of the complex neural networks and microcircuits that integrate and process information through the basal ganglia has increased tremendously. The development of sophisticated tracing methods combined with high-resolution immunocytochemical techniques has set the stage for in-depth scrutiny of the cellular and subcellular substrates of neuronal communication within the basal ganglia system. These studies revealed complex features of the anatomy and synaptic connectivity of the basal ganglia that led to a reconsideration of various aspects of the pathophysiology of basal ganglia disorders and the potential role of basal ganglia in a variety of motor and non-motor functions. This chapter discusses the main features of the anatomic organization of the circuitry and synaptic organization of the primate basal ganglia with emphasis on most recent findings, which, we believe, must be considered in understanding the complex functions of basal ganglia in the normal and diseased states. Because of space constraints, this review does not aim to cover the whole literature on basal ganglia anatomy, and readers are referred to previous comprehensive reviews and compendiums for surveys of the early literature and a more general overview of this field [1–38].

Basal ganglia components and general circuitry

The basal ganglia comprise a group of tightly interconnected subcortical brain nuclei in the telencephalon, diencephalon, and midbrain that integrate and process complex sensorimotor, cognitive, and limbic information originating from the entire cortical mantle before it is conveyed to the thalamus and brainstem. The main basal ganglia structures comprise the striatum, made up of the caudate nucleus, putamen, nucleus accumbens, and olfactory tubercle in primates. The caudate nucleus and putamen are commonly referred to as the dorsal striatum, whereas the nucleus accumbens and olfactory tubercle form the ventral striatum. In rodents, the dorsal striatum is made up of a single mass of gray matter called the caudate–putamen complex. Other basal ganglia nuclei include the globus pallidus, which, in primates, is comprised of two parts, the internal and external segments, commonly referred to as the GPi and GPe, respectively. In rodents, the homolog of GPi is the entopeduncular nucleus and the structure corresponding to GPe is simply called globus pallidus (GP). These telencephalic structures are tightly linked with the subthalamic nucleus (STN), a small, almond-shaped nucleus located laterally just below the thalamus at the junction between the diencephalon and midbrain. Finally, another major component of the basal ganglia network is the substantia nigra that lies along the base of the mesencephalon up to the anterior part of the tegmentum. The substantia nigra is a complex meshwork of various populations of neurons divided into two major sub-nuclei; the dorsally located substantia nigra pars compacta (SNc), which is partly made up of dopaminergic neurons, and the substantia nigra pars reticulata (SNr), which is made up of GABAergic projection neurons. Other neighboring cellular groups related to the dopaminergic SNc include the ventral tegmental area (VTA) along the midline and the retrorubral field (RRF) located caudally along the ventrolateral edge of the upper brainstem. Information from the entire cerebral cortex and thalamus is sent to the basal ganglia, mainly via the striatum, which then processes, integrates and conveys this information back to frontal cortical regions or brainstem via functionally segregated

Parkinson's Disease: Non-Motor and Non-Dopaminergic Features, First Edition. Edited by C. Warren Olanow, Fabrizio Stocchi, and Anthony E. Lang.

channels of information that flow through GPi and SNr, commonly known as the basal ganglia output nuclei.

With the development of sensitive tracing methods, our view of the basal ganglia circuitry has changed considerably over time and become extremely complex. The discovery of new connections combined with the huge number of neurotransmitters and modulators known to be involved in the communication of basal ganglia networks provides a highly sophisticated and intricate framework that underlies basal ganglia function and dysfunction in normal and disease states. However, due to the limited amount of information on the functional role of many of these connections, and the lack of pharmacological tools to understand the mechanisms by which many of the molecules synthesized in basal ganglia neurons participate in neuronal communication, any attempt to incorporate this huge amount of information into basic models of the functional circuitry of the basal ganglia inevitably lead to incomprehensible maps of neural circuits and networks that are difficult to understand and to use efficiently for both research and clinical applications. Therefore, in this chapter, we will attempt to provide an accurate view of the complexity of the basal ganglia circuits, while trying to integrate this knowledge into working models that can be used to understand further the role of basal ganglia in various motor and non-motor functions.

Striatum: main entrance of extrinsic information to the basal circuits

The striatum is the largest and most complex integrative structure of the basal ganglia. As discussed above, it comprises two major components called the dorsal and ventral striatum named on the basis of their respective locations along the dorsoventral extent of the telencephalon. Most importantly, these striatal sub-regions process largely segregated information that originates from different regions of the cerebral cortex; the dorsal striatum receives its main cortical inputs from associative and sensorimotor areas, whereas the ventral striatum is predominantly innervated by limbic cortical regions. It is important to recognize that the relative size of the ventral striatum in comparison with the total striatal mass is significantly larger in rodents than in primates, but the structural, cellular, chemical, and hodological organization of ventral striatal regions in primates and nonprimates is very similar [27,28,38].

In addition to this functional organization, the striatum is also made up of two distinct compartments called the patch (or striosomes) and the extrastriosomal matrix. These two striatal compartments are characterized by distinct afferent and efferent projections and heterogeneous neurochemical phenotype (for reviews, see [2,39]). Although the functional significance of this compartmentalization remains poorly understood, recent findings showed that repeated exposure to motor or psychostimulants results in an imbalance of activity between patch and matrix compartments that correlate with repetitive behaviors known as motor stereotypies [40–43]. It has been proposed that the selective recruitment of patch (or striosome) neurons by chronic stimulant exposure may represent neural endpoints of the transmission from action–outcome associative behavior to conditioned habitual responses [43]. Selective neurodegeneration of patches occurs in X-linked progressive dystonia–parkinsonism [44,45], and differential dysregulation of the Ras/Rap/ERK MAP kinase signal transduction cascades between the patch and matrix compartments predicts the severity of motor side effects induced by chronic dopaminergic anti-parkinsonian therapy [46]. There is also evidence that variations in clinical symptomatology in Huntington's disease, mainly changes in mood, may be due to differential effects of GABA-A receptor subunits expression between the patch and matrix compartments [47].

The medium spiny neurons and striatum

At the cellular level, the striatum is largely made up of the so-called GABAergic medium spiny projection neurons, which can be divided into two major phenotypes based on their peptide and relative dopamine receptor expression (see below). There are about 2.8×10^6 medium spiny neurons in the rat striatum, which account for 95–97% of the total neuronal population [48]. These neurons are morphologically fairly homogeneous, being made up of a small- to medium-sized cell body that gives rise to smooth proximal dendrites from which emerges a heavily spiny dendritic tree that occupies a spherical radius of about 200 μm in the rat. Striatal projection neurons are divided into two main subtypes based on their preferential projection targets and their expression of dopamine receptors and neuropeptides. The so-called "direct pathway neurons" preferentially express D1 dopamine receptors, substance P, and dynorphin, and project directly to the basal ganglia output nuclei (GPi and SNr). The "indirect pathway neurons" preferentially express D2 dopamine receptors and enkephalin, and primarily project to the GPe. The degree of segregation between these two neuronal populations remains controversial (see the discussion below). There is a dichotomy in the extent of the dendritic tree of D1- and D2-containing striatal neurons in BAC-D1/EGFP versus BAC-D2/EGFP transgenic mice [49]. On average, the dendritic length of D1 projection neurons is significantly greater than D2 neurons, an anatomic feature that may underlie the increased excitability of D2 neurons in adult mice [49–51].

Another important criterion to consider when translating the morphologic differences to the physiologic dichotomy between the two populations of striatofugal neurons is the density and morphology of spines on D1 and D2 neurons. Although rigorous quantitative analysis must still be achieved, preliminary data suggest that in all species single striatal projection neurons of either pathway are covered by about 5000 spines distributed fairly homogeneously at about 1 spine per micrometer of distal dendritic length [52–55]. There is a severe loss of striatal spines in Parkinson's disease (PD), suggesting an important regulatory role of dopamine and glutamate in striatal spine plasticity and spinogenesis in normal and pathologic conditions (see below for more detail).

Axon collaterals of spiny neurons arborize profusely in the vicinity of their parent cell bodies, providing GABAergic innervation to neighboring projection neurons. Although this intrinsic inhibitory connectivity between medium spiny neurons has long been known as the substrate for lateral inhibition in the striatum [56], it seems that these connections are weak, distal, and likely mediate subtle modulatory influence on striatal projection neurons activity [57,58]. However, they are specifically organized and unidirectional between pairs of D1- or D2-containing neurons, or from D2- to D1-positive projection neurons [59]. In contrast, connections from D1- to D2-positive neurons are almost nonexistent. The strength of these intrinsic connections is significantly reduced in dopamine-depleted parkinsonian conditions [59]. Collaterals of substance P-containing medium spiny neurons of the direct pathway also provide strong GABAergic inputs to cholinergic interneurons (see below).

The striatal interneurons: main regulators of striatal integration and processing of extrinsic information

The striatal interneuron family is comprised of four chemically characterized populations. They represent only 2–3% of the total striatal neuronal population in rats, but as much as 23% of all striatal neurons in monkeys [15,60].

The *GABA/parvalbumin interneurons*, also referred to as "fast spiking interneurons," form multiple axosomatic synapses on projection neurons, are electrotonically coupled through gap junctions, and exert powerful control on spike timing in projection neurons, thereby providing the substrate for fastforward intrastriatal inhibition of projection neurons in response to cortical activation [61]. The *cholinergic interneurons*, of which more than 50% co-express calretinin in humans [62], likely correspond to the "tonically active" neurons (TANs) that can be physiologically identified in the rat and monkey striatum [63–65]. These neurons, which receive strong synaptic inputs from GABAergic axon collaterals of substance P-containing striatofugal neurons in rats [66], play a pivotal role in reward-related learning and motivated behaviors [67–72] that are also tightly linked to the dopaminergic nigrostriatal system, although the two populations of neurons encode task episodes differentially. The dopamine neurons encode mainly the cue and outcome delivery, whereas the TANs mainly encode outcome delivery and omission at termination of the behavioral trail episode [73,74]. In rats, cholinergic interneurons are connected to one another through GABAergic interneurons, which provide a mechanism whereby activation of cholinergic interneurons can induce widespread recurrent inhibition of these neurons via nicotinic excitation [75]. They are also key mediators of dopamine-dependent striatal plasticity and learning [76].

The *GABA/nitric oxide synthase/neuropeptide Y/somatostatin interneurons* are categorized physiologically as "persistent and low-threshold spike" neurons [61]. These cells induce large inhibitory currents in projection neurons and release nitric oxide that modulates plasticity at glutamatergic synapses [15]. On the other hand, somatostatin actions are responsible for the entrainment of projection neurons to the rhythms generated by other interneurons, and are thereby capable of modifying the processing and output of the striatum [77].

The *medium-sized GABA/calretinin interneurons* represent the largest population of striatal interneurons in humans [62]. They display physiologic characteristics similar to the persistent- and low-threshold spike neurons, and exert powerful monosynaptic inhibition on medium spiny projection neurons.

A small population of dopaminergic interneurons have also been described in the striatum of dopamine-depleted rats and monkeys, and in the caudate nucleus and putamen of human patients with PD [78–82]. These aspiny neurons co-express various markers of dopaminergic neurons, glutamic acid decarboxylase, and, for a small subset, calretinin [78,81]. They receive very scarce synaptic inputs and are preferentially expressed in the precommissural putamen and caudate nucleus [81]. Their density increases significantly following dopamine depletion and after administration of growth factors in the striatum [83], suggesting that they may serve a potential compensatory mechanism in PD.

The corticostriatal system: the main source of extrinsic information to the basal ganglia

The cerebral cortex is the main source of glutamatergic projections to the striatum. The corticostriatal projection originates from all cortical areas and displays a highly topographic and functionally organized pattern of distribution in the striatum. The sources of these projections impose functional maps upon the striatum which appear to be largely segregated throughout the basal ganglia–thalamocortical circuitry [84]. The anatomic organization of the corticostriatal system has been examined using a wide variety of neuroanatomic approaches in

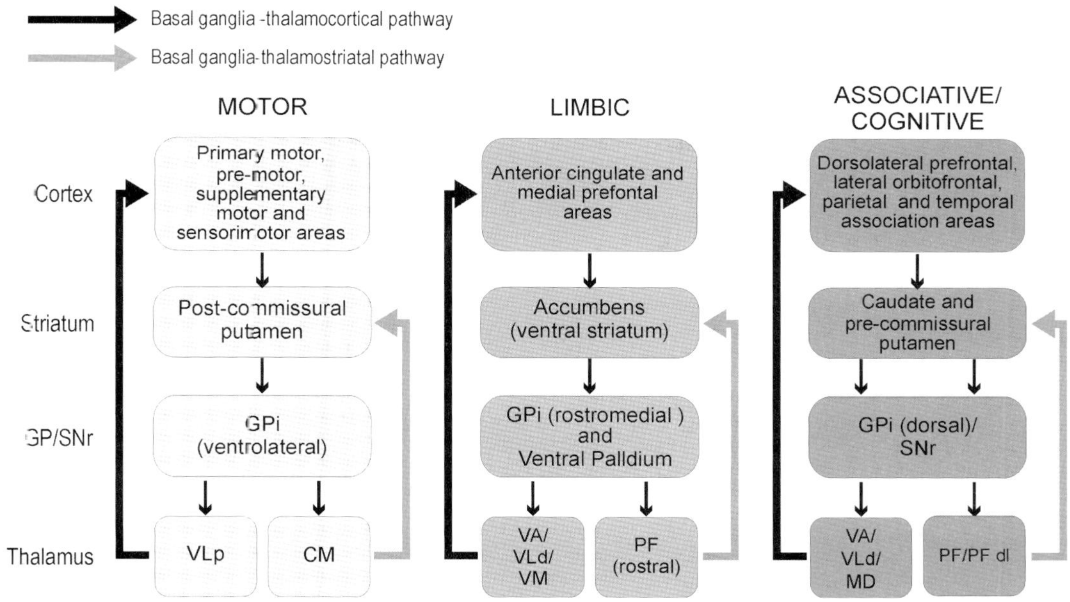

Figure 4.1 Segregated basal ganglia-thalamocortical (black arrows) and thalamostriatal (gray arrows) functional loops. Each functional modality is processed and travels through segregated regions of basal ganglia and thalamic nuclei (VA/VL and CM/PF) involved in motor, limbic and associative/cognitive functions.

rodents [85–93], carnivores [94–98], nonhuman primates (see below), and most recently humans using functional neuroimaging methods [99–106]. Because of the limited space, we will devote this section to a brief overview of the key features of the corticostriatal system in primates.

A large number of neuroanatomic studies have been published on the topographical and functional organization of the corticostriatal system in monkeys. This has led to a basic scheme outlining the functional connectivity between the cerebral cortex and striatum. The somatosensory, motor, and pre-motor cortices project somatotopically in a band-like pattern to the postcommissural region of the putamen, the associative cortical areas from frontal, parietal and temporal lobes project to the caudate nucleus, and the precommissural putamen, and the limbic cortices, the amygdala, and the hippocampus terminate preferentially in the ventral striatum [1,84,107,108] (Figure 4.1). The main source of cortical inputs to different striatal sub-regions in monkeys is shown in Table 4.1. There is also evidence for either convergence or segregation of functionally-related associative or sensorimotor cortical inputs in specific striatal territories [109–112].

In rats, the corticostriatal system originates from two distinct subsets of cortical pyramidal neurons; the so-called "intratelencephalic (IT)" neurons in superficial layers project solely to the striatum and the cerebral cortex, whereas the "pyramidal tract (PT)" neurons in deep cortical layers send their main axonal projections to the brainstem and spinal cord with collaterals to the striatum [113]. Although anatomic evidence suggests that cortical terminals from IT and PT neurons target preferentially "direct" or "indirect" pathway medium spiny projection neurons (see below) [114], recent electrophysiologic data demonstrate that IT neurons are the main source of excitatory inputs to both populations of striatal projection neurons [115], raising significant concerns about the functional significance of striatal projections from PT axon collaterals. The existence and functional significance of PT corticostriatal neurons thus remains controversial in primates [116–120].

Dendritic spines are, by far, the main targets of corticostriatal afferents [66, 119], although the GABA/PV-containing interneurons also receive significant cortical inputs in rats and monkeys [120]. Recent *in vivo* electrophysiologic data demonstrate that spike responses in GABA/PV interneurons occur earlier and can be induced by a lower intensity of cortical stimulation than that required for medium spiny projection neurons [121]. In general, increased cortical activity facilitates responses in GABA/PV interneurons, whereas opposite effects are found in projection neurons, which indicates that feedforward inhibition of GABA/PV interneurons filters cortical information effectively transmitted to striatal output neurons [121]. However, recent findings showing that fast spiking interneurons activity is not correlated with major task events suggest that these neurons play a more complex role than currently suggested based on theoretical models of striatal microcircuits [122]. Cortical inputs and feedforward inhibition from GABA/PV interneurons contribute to the imbalance of activity between the two

Table 4.1 Summary of major corticostriatal connections in nonhuman primates[a].

Cortical area	Head CD	Body CD	Tail CD	Pre-put	Post-put (dorsal)	Post-put (ventral)	Caudal put	Acc. shell	Acc. core
Prefrontal ass. areas									
Area 8a-FEF	+++	++							
SEF	+	+++							
Area 9 (dl PFC)	+++	+		+/–					
Area 24b, 32 (d ant. cing.)	++	+/–		+					+++
Area 24c	+/–	+/–		++	+				
Area 25, 14m (vm PFC)	++							+++	
Areas 11,12,13 (orbital ctx)	+++								++
Area 46r (dlPFC)	+++	+							
Area 46c (dlPFC)	+++	+		++					
PMdr	+++	+++		+/–					
Parietal ass. areas									
Rostral inf. parietal lobule						+	+		
Caudal inf. parietal lobule	+	++		+/–			++		
Rostral superior parietal lobule				+	+				
Caudal superior parietal lobule		+		+					
Lower IP sulcus		+					++		
Upper IP sulcus					+				
Caudal cingulate				+	+				
Medial parietal	+/–	+			+				
Rostral opercular						+			
Caudal opercular		+/–		+		+/–	+/–		
Temporal ass. areas									
Area 22	++		++						+
Rostral sup. temp. gyrus (TS1/TS2)	+		++	+		++			
Caudal sup. temp. gyrus (TS3)	+/–	+/–	+			+			
Prim. aud. ctx			+			+			
Sec. aud. ctx		+	+	++		+			
Visual areas									
Medial extrastriate	+	+			+/–				
DL extrastr.	+/–	++	+/–						
VL extrastr			++			+			
VM extrastr		+	++						
IT			++			++			
Area TE			++			++			
Motor areas									
M1					+++				
Pre-SMA		+		+	+				
SMA					+++				
PMd					+				
PMv					++				
CMA-rostral				++	+				
CMA-caudal				+	++		+		
Somato-sensory areas									
S1 (areas 1, 3a, 3b)					+++				

[a]Symbols and abbreviations: +/–, sparse, +, minor, ++, moderate, +++, strong; Acc, Nucleus accumbens; CD, Caudate nucleus; CMA, cingulate motor area; d ant. cing, dorsal anterior cingulate cortex; DL extrastr., dorsolateral extrastriate area; dl PFC, dorsolateral prefrontal cortex; FEF, frontal eye field; SEF, supplementary eye field; IP sulcus, intraparietal sulcus; IT, inferotemporal gyrus; PMd, dorsal pre-motor cortex; PM dr, dorsal and rostral pre-motor cortex; PMv, ventral pre-motor cortex; Pre-SMA, pre-supplementary area; Prim. aud. ctx, primary auditory cortex; Put, Putamen; Sec. aud. ctx, secondary auditory cortex; SMA, supplementary motor area; sup. temp. gyrus, superior temporal gyrus; VL extrastr., ventrolateral extrastriate area; VM extrastr., ventromedial extrastriate area; vm PFC, ventromedial prefrontal cortex [1,29,38,107–112,139].

Box 4.1 Dual thalamostriatal systems

CM/PF	Other thalamic nuclei
• Neurons have reticular dendrites	• Neurons have bushy-like dendrites
• Innervate preferentially the striatum with collaterals to cortex	• Innervate preferentially the cortex with collaterals to striatum
• Focal highly convergent sites of termination in the striatum	• Diffuse less convergent innervation of the striatum
• Form axo-dendritic synapses (75%)	• Form axo-spinous synapses (>95%)
• Do not display any relationships with dopaminergic afferents	• Converge with dopaminergic inputs on to common dendritic spines
• Discharge single spikes during cortical slow-wave activity	• Discharge low-threshold calcium bursts during cortical slow-wave activity
• Sensitive to attention-related multisensory information	• Respond to specific modalities (sensory, motor, limbic, etc.)
• Provide the striatum with attention-related information from brainstem	• Provide the striatum with context-dependent functionally related cortical information
• Key components of sub-cortical loops with basal ganglia and brainstem (superior colliculus, PPN, etc.)	• Key components of basal ganglia–thalamocorticothalamic loops
• Partly degenerate in PD	• Do not degenerate in PD

main populations of striatofugal neurons in the rat model of PD [121]. Cortical inputs to cholinergic interneurons are sparse and often located on distal dendrites [123,124]. Cortical inputs to other populations of interneurons have not been studied in great detail. There is anatomic evidence for differential cortical innervation of the two main populations of striatofugal neurons from motor cortical inputs in monkeys [125,126], but the functional significance of such possible segregation remains to be determined.

The dual thalamostriatal systems: two major extrinsic sources of striatal excitability

The thalamus has long been known as another source of glutamatergic projections to the striatum. However, because of limited information on the anatomic and physiologic organization of this system, very little is known about the functional integration of the thalamostriatal pathways in the basal ganglia network. Recent studies have suggested the existence of anatomically and functionally segregated dual thalamostriatal systems that originate from the caudal intralaminar thalamic nuclei versus other thalamic nuclei (Box 4.1). Significant interest in this system has recently been generated with evidence that deep brain stimulation of the caudal intralaminar nuclei, the main sources of thalamostriatal projections, alleviate some symptoms of PD and Tourette's syndrome (see below). This section will provide an overview of the main anatomic, physiologic, and pathologic features of the thalamostriatal systems in normal and diseased brains.

Thalamostriatal projections from the caudal intralaminar nuclei

The intralaminar thalamic nuclei are a major source of excitatory afferents to the striatum. In primates, the caudal intralaminar nuclear group, the centromedian (CM) and parafascicular (PF) nuclei, provide inputs that largely terminate in different functional territories in the striatum. The medial part of CM projects to the postcommissural sensorimotor putamen. The PF innervates predominantly the associative part of the caudate nucleus and the ventral striatum, while the dorsolateral PF projects selectively to the precommissural putamen (for reviews, see [14,33]) (Figure 4.1). Although CM/PF neurons send sparse projections to the cerebral cortex, their main termination target is the striatum [127], where they preferentially innervate the striatal matrix compartment [14]. At the ultrastructural level, CM and PF inputs innervate preferentially the dendritic shafts of striatal output neurons [128–131]. Striatal interneurons, immunoreactive for choline acetyltransferase, parvalbumin, and somatostatin, but not calretinin, also receive inputs from CM in monkeys [132]. In line with these electron microscopic data, there is evidence that projections from CM/PF tightly regulate the electrophysiologic activity of cholinergic interneurons [133,134] and are required for the sensory responses of TANs (likely cholinergic) that are acquired through sensorimotor learning in monkeys [135–137].

Thalamostriatal projections from other thalamic nuclei

The CM/PF complex is not the sole source of thalamostriatal projections. In fact, most thalamic nuclei contribute a varying degree of striatal innervation [14,37], but these projections display different anatomic and, most likely, functional features compared with striatal inputs from the CM/PF (Box 4.1). Albeit sparse compared with those from CM/PF, these projections are topographically and functionally organized in the rat and monkey striatum [14,37,131,138,139].

The synaptic connectivity of striatal projections from CM/PF is strikingly different from that of other thalamic nuclei. CM/PF terminals form synapses predominantly with dendritic shafts of medium spiny neurons, whereas projections from other nuclear groups, including the rostral intralaminar, midline, and relay thalamic nuclei, target almost exclusively dendritic spines [14,37,131,140]. Another main difference between striatal inputs from CM/PF and other thalamic nuclei relates to the degree of axon collateralization to the cerebral cortex; projections from CM/PF are mainly directed towards the striatum with minimal innervation of frontal cortical areas, whereas relay and rostral intralaminar nuclei project predominantly to the cerebral cortex with light to moderate striatal innervation [37,127]. In general, striatal projections from CM/PF are much more focused and give rise to a significantly larger number of terminals than individual corticostriatal axons [37,127,118]. The functional relevance of these differences in the striatal innervation pattern between thalamic and cortical inputs remains poorly understood (see below [134]).

The vesicular glutamate transporters 1 and 2 as segregated markers of cortical or thalamic inputs to the striatum

Vesicular glutamate transporter 1 and 2 (vGluT1 and vGluT2) immunostaining can be used as a selective marker of corticostriatal and thalamostriatal glutamatergic terminals, respectively [37,131,141]. More than 95% of vGluT1 terminals contact the heads of spines, whereas only 50–60% of vGluT2 terminals do so in monkeys, a pattern that does not change in parkinsonism [141]. In rats, there is a significant difference in the microcircuitry of vGluT2 terminals between the patch and matrix striatal compartments so that most axo-dendritic vGluT2 synapses are found in the matrix, consistent with the idea that the CM/PF complex is the main source of these synaptic inputs [14,37,131].

Functional roles of the thalamostriatal systems

The role(s) of the thalamostriatal system remain(s) poorly understood and likely differ(s) between projections that arise from CM/PF and those arising from other thalamic nuclei. In primates, the CM and PF supply striatal neurons with information that have attentional values, thus acting as detectors of behaviorally significant events occurring on the contralateral side [135,136]. In humans, changes in CM/PF activity are induced in response to attention-demanding reaction-time tasks [142]. Stimulation of the monkey CM induces complex excitatory and inhibitory electrophysiologic responses in striatal projection neurons and cholinergic interneurons [134]. On the other hand, stimulation of rostral intralaminar nuclei induces complex changes in cognitive processing, probably through regulation of cortical and striatal activity [143,144]. The function of other thalamostriatal systems might be to provide a positive reinforcer of specific populations of striatal neurons involved in performing a selected cortically driven behavior [14,37,139,145].

The CM/PF degenerates in Parkinson's disease

As many as 50% of CM/PF neurons degenerate in patients with progressive supranuclear palsy, Huntington's disease, and PD. In parkinsonian patients, subpopulations of parvalbumin-containing neurons are mainly affected in PF, whereas in CM non-parvalbumin/non-calbindin neurons are specifically targeted [14,37]. Asymmetries in the shape of thalami between patients with PD and healthy controls were recently reported [146]. Preclinical studies in rodents led to controversial data regarding cell loss in PF after nigrostriatal dopamine depletion; some studies showed significant loss of PF thalamostriatal neurons in 6-hydroxydopamine-treated rats and MPTP-treated mice, whereas others did not find any PF neuronal loss under similar conditions [14,37]. Although data from nonhuman primates are not available, electron microscopic data recently showed a significant reduction in the relative abundance of vGluT2-positive terminals forming axo-dendritic synapses in the putamen of MPTP-treated monkeys, suggesting a possible loss of CM-striatal neurons [141] in this animal model.

The striatal dopaminergic systems: major modulators of basal ganglia networks

The nigrostriatal system

The ventral midbrain dopaminergic neurons are subdivided into three main groups: the A8 (retrorubral field; RRF), A9 (substantia nigra pars compacta; SNc), and A10 (ventral tegmental area; VTA). Each of these regions is comprised predominantly of dopaminergic neurons with small groups of GABAergic interneurons, except in the VTA, where GABAergic projection neurons have also been documented [9]. Various neuropeptides have been identified in subsets of neurons in the medial SNc and VTA. In addition, calbindin D_{28K} (CB) is strongly expressed in neurons of the VTA and RRF and also dorsal tier neurons of the SNc (SNc-d), but is not found in ventral tier SNc neurons (SNc-v) [9,147,148]. This differential expression of CB may play a neuroprotective role in SNc-d and VTA neurons in PD, whereas its absence might account for the vulnerability of SNc-v neurons in PD [149–151]. SNc-v neurons express a higher level of dopamine transporter than other dopaminergic cell groups [152], which presumably accounts for the vulnerability of SNc-v neurons in MPTP-treated mice and monkeys [153,154].

The main groups of midbrain dopaminergic neurons differ in their projection patterns to the striatum: (1) the sensorimotor striatum in the postcommissural putamen is mainly innervated by dopaminergic cell columns in the SNc-v, (2) the limbic ventral striatum is targeted preferentially by VTA and SNc-d neurons, and (3) the associative striatum in the caudate nucleus is mainly targeted by dopaminergic neurons in the densocellular part of SNc-v [9,33]. The pattern is different in rats; where SNc-d neurons project predominantly to the dorsal striatum [155]. Two main types of nigrostriatal axons have been identified based on their origin and pattern of striatal innervation; thin, varicose, and widespread fibers that arise from neurons in the SNc-d, VTA and RRF and terminate preferentially in the matrix striatal compartment, and thick, more varicose fibers which originate from the SNc-v and terminate mostly in the patch striatal compartment [156]. The dichotomy between dopaminergic projections to patches or matrix, and the extent of striatal dopaminergic innervation, were recently challenged using a highly sensitive viral tracing method that resulted in much more extensive labeling of the axonal arbor of individual SNc dopaminergic neurons that did not show any preferential innervation of the patch or matrix compartments [157].

Although most midbrain dopaminergic neurons show a certain degree of degeneration in PD, the pattern of progressive cell loss is not homogeneous, but rather displays a complex topographic and regional organization. Two main features characterize the pattern of nigrostriatal degeneration in PD patients and MPTP-treated monkeys: (1) nigrostriatal projections to the sensorimotor striatal territory (postcommissural + lateral precommissural putamen) are more sensitive than those to the associative (caudate nucleus) and limbic (nucleus accumbens) striatal regions [158,159], and (2) VTA projections to the ventral striatum are selectively spared and show a far lesser degree of degeneration than other midbrain dopaminergic neurons [160,161]. There is also evidence for differential dopamine denervation of patches versus matrix compartments in MPTP-treated monkeys, but data remain controversial [151,162].

The pattern of nigrostriatal degeneration at the striatal and nigral levels correlates with the expression level of CB. At the striatal level, the most sensitive sensorimotor postcommissural putamen is devoid of CB-containing neurons [163]. In the substantia nigra, the relatively spared SNc-d and VTA neurons are enriched in CB, whereas the more sensitive SNc-v neurons express a low level of CB immunoreactivity [152,164]. Finally, SNc neurons in regions that receive strong CB innervation from the striatum are more resistant than those in CB-poor pockets called nigrosomes [160]. Together, these findings highlight the potential neuroprotective role of CB in PD pathogenesis.

Dopamine plays a critical role in regulating striatal activity through both pre- and post-synaptic mechanisms. The five dopamine receptor subtypes are expressed in projection neurons and interneurons of the striatum providing multiple targets whereby dopamine mediates its effects. Dopamine-mediated modulation of glutamatergic and cholinergic activity is severely affected in parkinsonian states, likely contributing to the abnormal basal ganglia network activity changes described in PD. The morphological and functional plasticity of dendritic spines is also tightly regulated by dopamine–glutamate interactions, providing a substrate for integration and processing of extrinsic information to the basal ganglia circuitry [6,9,33,55].

Other important modulatory systems that will not be discussed in this chapter include the serotonergic system from the raphe nuclei and the noradrenergic ascending projections from the locus coeruleus. Although not as much studied as the dopaminergic system, there is evidence that these two neurotransmitters regulate physiologic activity in various basal ganglia nuclei and possibly contribute to non-motor deficits and motor side effects of long-term dopaminergic therapy in PD [165–172].

Extrastriatal dopaminergic systems

Although the striatum is by far the main basal ganglia target of midbrain dopaminergic neurons, considerable evidence for extrastriatal dopamine function has been put forward to explain some of the paradoxical changes observed in basal ganglia circuitry in PD. Because of space limitations, we cannot expand much on this topic in this chapter, and readers are referred to recent publications and reviews that discuss evidence for nigropallidal, nigrosubthalamic, and nigrothalamic dopaminergic projections. The role of dendritic release of dopamine in the SNr has also been established as another major contributor of extrastriatal dopamine function in the basal ganglia [9,33].

The direct and indirect basal ganglia circuits: "a simplified model that brought us a long way"

A significant breakthrough in our understanding of the basal ganglia circuitry came in the early 1990s with the introduction of the model of "direct and indirect" pathways of the basal ganglia [173–175]. Although overly simplistic, this model has driven the field of basic and clinical basal ganglia research in recent decades. Obviously, since its introduction, our gain in knowledge of the basal ganglia circuitry has led to several revisions and updates that make it much more complex. However, it remains the most reliable working model that both physicians and basic scientists use to develop and refine functional hypotheses about the normal physiology and pathophysiology of basal ganglia in diseased states. In brief, the term "direct pathway" refers to the monosynaptic connection between the striatum and the basal ganglia output nuclei, the internal globus pallidus (GPi), and the substantia nigra pars reticulata (SNr), while the term "indirect pathway" refers to the polysynaptic pathway linking the striatum and GPi/SNr via the external globus pallidus (GPe) and the subthalamic nucleus (STN). Striatal neurons that give rise to either of these pathways are GABAergic, but can be segregated into two populations according to their peptide content (substance P-direct; enkephalin-indirect) and by the preferential expression of dopamine receptor subtypes (D1-direct; D2-indirect). By virtue of the neurotransmitters and basal activity in these neuronal networks, it has been proposed that activation of the direct and indirect pathways produces functionally opposite effects in GPi/SNr neurons. A balance between the activity of the two pathways is, therefore, essential for the normal functioning of basal ganglia. In PD, the loss of striatal dopamine leads to increased activity of indirect striatofugal neurons and decreased output from direct striatofugal neurons. Because of the polarity of connections in the direct/indirect pathways, this results in increased GABAergic basal ganglia outflow to the thalamus which, in turn, may reduce cortical excitability and decrease motor behaviors (Figure 4.2).

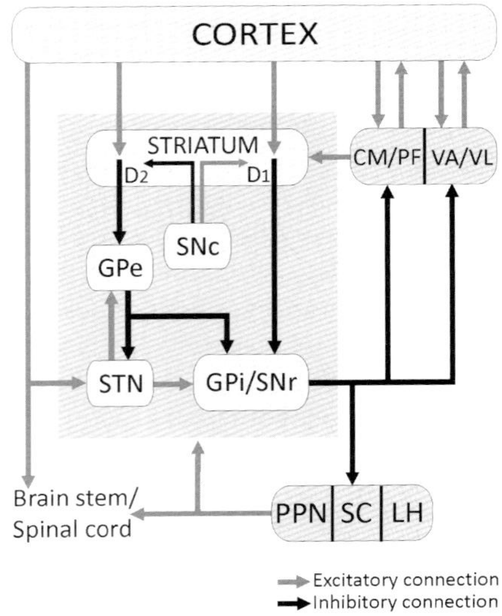

Figure 4.2 Direct and indirect pathway model of the basal ganglia. The gray box indicates tightly interconnected basal ganglia nuclei that receive extrinsic inputs from cortical, thalamic and brainstem regions. The black arrows indicate inhibitory connections, while the gray arrows illustrate excitatory connections. The extrastriatal SNc dopaminergic projections to GPe, STN and GPi/SNr have been omitted from this diagram. The connections between the basal ganglia and the PPN/SC/LH are depicted in more detail in Fig. 4.4. Abbreviations: CM, centromedian nucleus of the thalamus; D1 and D2, dopamine D1-type and D2-type receptors; GPe, globus pallidus external segment; GPi, globus pallidus internal segment; LH, lateral habenula; PF, parafascicular nucleus of thalamus; PPN, pedunculo pontine nucleus; SC, superior colliculus; SNc, substantia nigra pars compacta; SNr, substantia nigra pars reticulata; STN, subthalamic nucleus; VA/VL, ventral anterior and ventrolateral nuclei of thalamus.

The segregation of direct and indirect striatofugal pathway neurons: an ongoing dilemma?

This traditional scheme of the basal ganglia circuitry has been challenged in past decades based on some anatomic and molecular data suggesting that the two pathways may not be as segregated as previously thought. On the one hand, the use of single-cell filling studies has demonstrated that most striatofugal neurons of the direct pathway give off collaterals to the GPe [8,176–178]. However, it is noteworthy that many neurons in the primate striatum that innervate the GPe, GPi, and SNr often provide significantly more axon terminals to one of these structures than others, thereby maintaining a certain level of preferential targeting in their axonal projections [178]. The functional significance of these collateralized projections still remains poorly understood, but surely deserves consideration in the interpretation of functional changes in basal ganglia circuitry in normal and diseased states.

Another set of data that have generated strong interest and controversy about this model over the past 15 years come from molecular studies showing that D1 and D2 receptor mRNAs may not be as segregated as originally thought. Rather, they suggest that a significant proportion of striatal output neurons express mRNAs for both receptor subtypes [175,179–181]. This controversy originally came from the use of different techniques to examine the localization of D1 and D2 mRNA in striatal neurons. On the one hand, Gerfen and others, using the *in situ* hybridization approach, reported a clear and almost complete segregation of dopamine receptor mRNAs in striatonigral (D1-containing) and striatopallidal (D2-containing) neurons in rats and monkeys [175,179,182–184]. On the other hand, Surmeier and co-workers, using a more sensitive single-cell mRNA amplification technique, reported that most striatofugal neurons expressed a significant level of both dopamine receptors subtype mRNAs, shedding significant doubt on the segregation of the direct and indirect basal ganglia pathways originally proposed [180,181,185]. The hypothesis of co-expression was further supported by *in vitro* electrophysiologic data showing that a majority of striatal neurons are functionally responsive to both D1 and

D2 family receptor agonists [181]. Significant controversy about dopamine receptor segregation was also raised based on immunocytochemical studies, some reports showing that D1 and D2 receptor protein immunoreactivity was largely segregated in two distinct populations of striatal spines [114,186], whereas others demonstrated a high level of D1 and D2 receptor immunoreactivity at the single-cell level in the rat striatum [187].

More recently, bacterial artificial chromosome (BAC) transgenic mice in which striatal neurons express D1- or D2-enhanced green fluorescent protein (EGFP) have been engineered [188,189]. These mice have become a very useful tool to study the physiology, pharmacology, and anatomy of the two main populations of striatofugal neurons in normal and diseased states [25,49, 53,59,76, 190–192]. However, it is worth noting that there is a striking difference between the chemical phenotype of striatofugal neurons in these transgenic mice compared with data reported previously for normal rats (see above). The BAC-D1 and BAC-D2 mice indeed display a complete segregation of D1 and D2 receptor mRNA, even when measured with the highly sensitive single-cell mRNA amplification method, an approach that revealed significant D1/D2 co-localization in normal rats [25,53, 180,181,185]. Whether this strict segregation of the two dopamine receptor subtypes underlies distinct functional dopamine-mediated physiologic effects or variable mechanisms of synaptic plasticity between normal animals and these transgenic mice remains to be established.

Another important fact to keep in mind when interpreting dopamine-mediated effects in individual striatofugal neurons is the possible co-expression of other D1 or D2 receptor family subtypes (i e., D3, D4, and D5 receptors) in the two main populations of striatofugal neurons. In contrast to D1 and D2, the D3, D4, and D5 receptors are not as strictly segregated between the two striatofugal pathways, thereby providing a substrate for cross-talk and dual D1/D2-like dopamine-mediated effects on striatal projection neurons [6,185,193–198]. To our knowledge, there is no report on the relative expression level of D3, D4, or D5 receptors in striatofugal neurons of BAC-D1/EGFP or BAC-D2/EGFP transgenic mice. We believe that such information is absolutely essential to determine clearly the chemical phenotype of striatofugal neurons in these animals and ensure that functional data gathered from these mice can be translated to normal brains.

The hyperdirect corticosubthalamic system: anatomic and functional significance

In addition to the striatum, the STN represents another major entrance of extrinsic information to the basal ganglia circuitry. There is electrophysiologic evidence that information flowing along this tract is transmitted to the basal ganglia output nuclei, the SNr and GPi, at a faster pace than information flow along the direct and indirect corticostriatofugal systems [199]. A majority of SNr and GPi neurons, indeed, respond with a fast, likely monosynaptic, excitation following electrical stimulation of motor cortices. This excitation is abolished following STN lesion. In monkeys, the corticosubthalamic projection mainly originates from motor cortical areas and displays a strict somatotopic arrangement along the dorsolateral two-thirds of the STN. Inputs from M1 flow along the lateralmost part of the nucleus, while projections from the supplementary motor area (SMA), premotor cortices (PM), and the cingulate motor cortex (CM) terminate dorsomedially in an overlapping fashion. The somatotopy in the dorsolateral "M1 domain" and the dorsomedial "SMA/PM/CM domain" are reversed [199–201]. The ventrolateral half of the STN receives its main cortical inputs from the frontal and supplementary eye field areas, whereas the medial tip of the STN is related to the processing of limbic-related information (Figure 4.3).

A functional "center-surround model" has been proposed to explain the role of the hyperdirect pathway in the selection of motor programs. According to this hypothesis, the cortical information flowing along the hyperdirect pathway is transmitted to the GPi in a diffuse manner, thereby providing an overall excitation over a large pool of basal ganglia output neurons not related to the selected motor act (i.e., the "surround neurons"). In contrast, the corollary signal transmitted along the corticostriatal system is much more focused and conveyed to a restricted pool of GPi neurons (i.e., the "center neurons"). Despite its potential interest, this hypothesis relies on a questionable foundation, shedding doubt on its significance. First, the anatomic relationships between the STN and both pallidal segments are highly specific and topographic, opposing the assumption made by the model that the STN provides a diffuse projection to the GPi [202,203]. Second, most STN neurons increase their firing around the time of movement onset or after the movement during active step tracking movements in monkeys [204], thereby reducing the likelihood that the cortico-STN projection is involved in the preparation of movements as suggested by the center-surround hypothesis. However, most STN neurons are active before self-paced movements in human parkinsonians [205]. The relative importance of the corticosubthalamic versus corticostriatal projections in regulating motor behavior therefore necessitates further investigations.

The exact cellular origin of the hyperdirect corticosubthalamic projection remains poorly characterized. Although there is evidence that some of these axons might be collaterals of descending pyramidal tract axons in rats [206] and cats [207], recent single-cell filling of

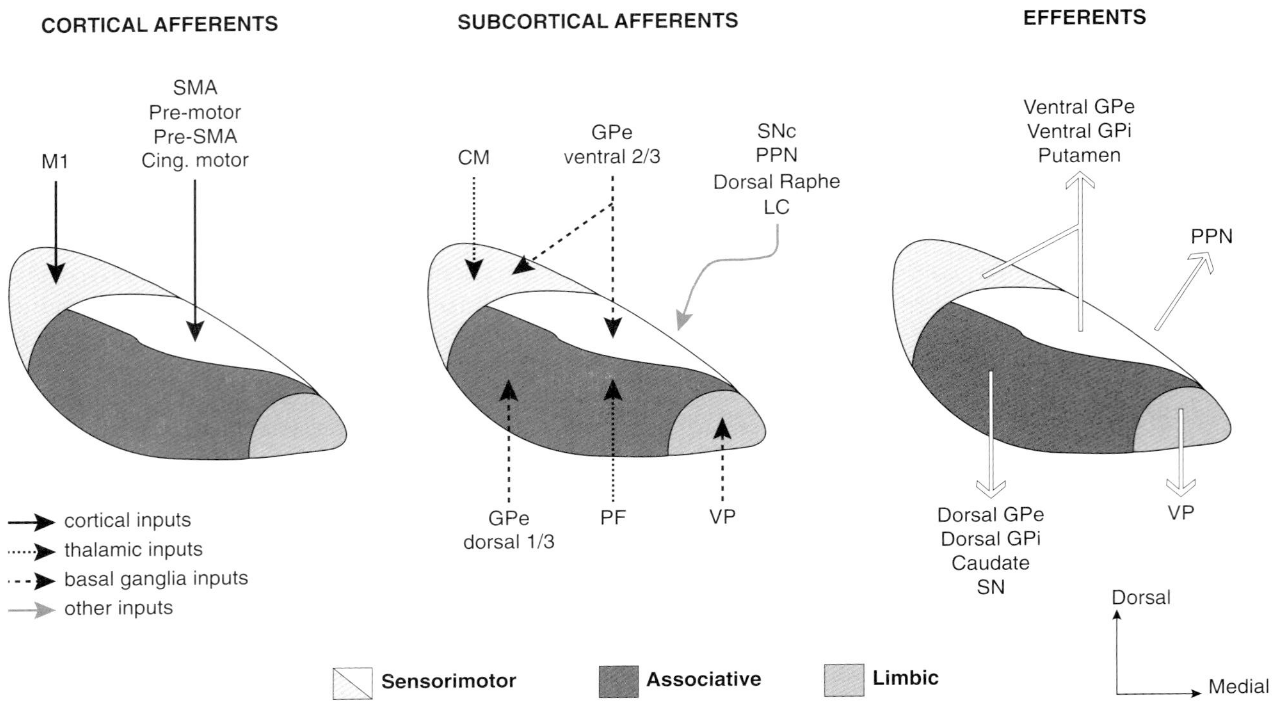

Figure 4.3 Afferent and efferent connections of functional subregions of the subthalamic nucleus. The sensorimotor region is further subdivided according to the source of primary motor (light gray) versus premotor, supplementary and cingulate motor cortical inputs (white). Abbreviations: Cing. mot., cingulate motor area of cortex; CM, centromedian nucleus of the thalamus; GPe, globus pallidus external segment; GPi, globus pallidus internal segment; LC, locus coeruleus M1, primary motor area of cortex; PF, parafascicular nucleus of thalamus; PPN, pedunculopontine nucleus; Pre-motor, pre-motor area of cortex; SMA, supplementary motor area of cortex; SN, substantia nigra; SNc, substantia nigra compacta.

pyramidal tract neurons in M1 resulted in only a few scarcely distributed fibers in the monkey STN [118], suggesting that this projection may have a more complex origin than previously thought in primates.

Non-motor components of the "hyperdirect" pathway

There is behavioral evidence that the corticosubthalamic projection from the prefrontal cortex plays a role in preparatory processes, attention, perseveration, and other important cognitive or limbic functions in rodents [208–213]. These behavioral effects are likely mediated by direct projections from the prefrontal cortex to the medial STN in rats [214–217]. Although the sources of associative and limbic cortical afferents to the STN remain poorly characterized in primates, recent diffusion-weighted magnetic resonance imaging methods have revealed connections between high-order associative areas of the frontal lobe and the STN in humans [218], providing a substrate for cognitive effects induced by bilateral STN DBS in some PD patients [219–226]. It is also important to keep in mind that areas in the ventromedial STN are tightly linked with the caudate nucleus and related associative regions of the GPe, providing another substrate for STN stimulation-mediated effects on complex cognitive functions [202,203,227,228]. In contrast to the striatum, the STN does not receive sensory cortical inputs [216,229]. The caudal intralaminar nuclei and the brainstem pedunculopontine nucleus are two additional sources of glutamatergic inputs to the STN [203] (Figure 4.3). In turn, the STN send glutamatergic projections back to the cortex and pedunculopontine nucleus [203,227,228,230].

The pedunculopontine nucleus: an intricate component of the basal ganglia circuitry

Intrinsic cellular organization of the PPN

The PPN comprises a chemically heterogeneous collection of neurons in the upper brainstem that lies around the superior cerebellar peduncle. It is bounded laterally by fibers of the medial lemniscus, medially by the decussation of the superior cerebellar peduncle, dorsally by the retrorubral field, rostrally by the dorsomedial sector of the caudalmost tip of the substantia nigra, and caudally by the cuneiform nuclei. It is made up of two major neuronal groups; the PPN compacta (PPNc), which is comprised of a densely packed population of cholinergic neurons located in the caudolateral half of the nucleus, and the PPN diffusa (PPNd), which is located more medially and is made up of sparsely distributed non-cholinergic neurons residing along the dorsoventral extent of the superior cerebellar peduncle. The human PPN contains about 10 000–15 000 cholinergic neurons [231,232], which make up more than 90% of cells in the PPNc [233]. In monkeys, as many as 40% of cholinergic neurons in the PPN express glutamate immunoreactivity. Smaller subsets of GABAergic, dopaminergic, and noradrenergic neurons have also been identified within the boundaries of the PPN. In addition, various neuropeptides are expressed in this region [234–239].

PPN connectivity

Many lines of anatomic and electrophysiologic evidence indicate that the PPN is reciprocally connected with the basal ganglia. The PPN receives substantial projections from the GPi and SNr (see below) and a more minor input from the STN. In turn, the PPN sends ascending projections to all basal ganglia nuclei. In rats and primates, the SNc and the STN are, by far, the most densely innervated basal ganglia structures by PPN efferents [240,241]. Both glutamate and acetylcholine are used as a neurotransmitter by these projections. The PPN innervation of the pallidal complex is not as dense as that of the STN and SNc, arborizes preferentially in the GPi, and uses both glutamate and acetylcholine as neurotransmitters. A light pedunculostriatal projection has also been described in rats and monkeys, but the chemical nature of this projection is still unknown. Taking into consideration these tight interconnections with basal ganglia structures combined with prominent descending projections to pontine, medullary, and spinal structures, the PPN is considered as a possible relay station where the striatum connects with neurons from the reticular formation and the spinal cord. Additional inputs to the PPN originate from the spinal cord, raphe nuclei, locus coeruleus, deep cerebellar nuclei, the superior colliculus, and the SNc [237–239]

The PPN sends massive cholinergic and non-cholinergic projections to various thalamic nuclei. These projections play a major role in mediating cortical desynchronization during waking and rapid eye movement (REM) sleep. Cholinergic and glutamatergic PPN inputs to thalamostriatal neurons have been demonstrated. A subpopulation of PPN neurons innervates simultaneously the basal ganglia and thalamic regions via axon collaterals. These findings suggest that the PPN conveys information to the basal ganglia not only directly, but also indirectly via thalamostriatal neurons. Therefore, the PPN occupies a strategic position that allows for modulation of neuronal activity in functional basal ganglia–thalamocortical and thalamostriatal loops [235,239,242]

The connectivity of the PPN described above using traditional tract-tracing methods in rats and nonhuman primates has recently been confirmed and extended in humans using diffusion tensor imaging. Despite the obvious shortcomings of this method to differentiate afferent versus efferent fiber pathways, and the likelihood that small fiber tracts may not be detected with tractography, this approach surely warrants attention because of its noninvasive nature and its possible use for tracing neural connections in the human brain [243–246].

PPN as a target for functional deep brain stimulation

Through this complex connection with basal ganglia, thalamus, and lower brainstem regions, the PPN is involved in the initiation and modulation of gait and other stereotyped movements in experimental animals [237,247–249], and there is evidence suggesting that the nucleus is involved in PD. Bilateral lesions of the PPN in normal nonhuman primates elicits bradykinesia [250,251]. Neuropathologic studies have shown as much as a 50% loss of cholinergic neurons in the PPN of human with PD [252,253]. In MPTP-treated parkinsonian monkeys, blockade of GABA-A receptors or low-frequency stimulation in the PPN reverses parkinsonian akinesia [254–256]. Based on this series of preclinical studies, the area of the PPN has been investigated as a possible target for DBS in parkinsonian patients who suffer from gait impairment, freezing, and poor balance that cannot be adequately controlled with dopaminergic therapy, and positive results have been reported in preliminary open-label studies [237,257–261]. However, the exact site to stimulate remains controversial. Some authors have argued that the peripeduncular nucleus, an aggregate of neurons located rostral and lateral to the PPN, is a main candidate target for DBS in patients with PD that warrants further exploration [262–266].

Basal ganglia outflow to the thalamus and brainstem

The GPi and SNr are the two main output nuclei of the basal ganglia. They receive functionally segregated inputs from the striatum and send this information through massive GABAergic projections that profusely innervate the thalamus, lateral habenula, superior colliculus, pedunculopontine tegmental nucleus, and reticular formation. These projections, which, in some cases originate from collaterals of the same axons, are highly specific and functionally compartmentalized in their respective targets (Figure 4.4). This section briefly reviews the anatomic organization of these various tracts and discusses their relevance in the transmission of basal ganglia information through cortical and subcortical loops that likely play a

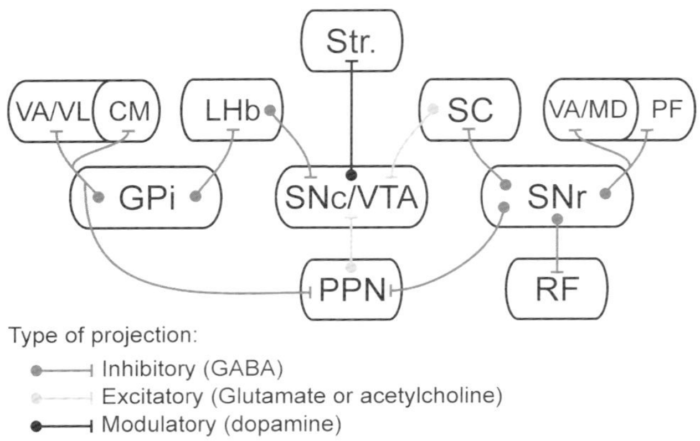

Figure 4.4 Main output projections of the GPi and SNr. This diagram also illustrates some of the subcortical inputs to SNc/VTA dopaminergic neurons that have been considered as sources of reward- or sensory-related influences to midbrain dopaminergic neurons. Abbreviations: CM: Centromedian nucleus; GPi: Globus pallidus, internal segment; LHb: Lateral habenular nucleus; MD: Mediodorsal nucleus; PF: Parafascicular nucleus; PPN: Pedunculopontine nucleus; RF: Reticular formation; SC: Superior colliculus; SNc: Substantia nigra compacta; SNr: Substantia nigra pars reticulata; Str: Striatum; VA: ventral anterior nucleus; VL: ventral lateral nucleus; VTA: ventral tegmental area.

major role in mediating changes in neural activity in normal and pathologic conditions.

Efferent projections of GPi

The pallidothalamic projection

The pallidothalamic projection travels via the ansa lenticularis and lenticular fasciculus to terminate in a topographic fashion in the ventral anterior/ventral lateral (VA/VL) nuclei of the thalamus [1,267,268]. The exact origin of the fibers that make up the two major pallidal outflow tracts remains controversial. According to recent anatomic data, pallidothalamic fibers originating from the caudal portion of the GPi, including the motor territory travel predominantly medially through the lenticular fasciculus en route to the thalamus, while fibers coursing below the ventral border of the pallidum in the so-called ansa lenticularis originate mostly from cells located in the rostral half of the GPi [269]. This scheme is much simpler than that published in other studies, which imply that fibers coursing through the ansa lenticularis frequently follow lengthy courses through the caudorostral extent of the GPi to reach the thalamus [270,271]. This apparent discrepancy may be the result of a higher degree of neuronal heterogeneity than previously thought in the primate GPi [271]. Understanding this delineation may be critical in optimizing the surgical treatment of various movement disorders [269].

Efferent projections from the sensorimotor GPi remain largely segregated from the associative and limbic projections at the level of the thalamus. In squirrel monkeys, the sensorimotor GPi outputs are directed towards the posterior VL (VLp), whereas the associative and limbic GPi innervate preferentially the parvocellular VA (VApc) and the dorsal VL (VLd). The ventromedial nucleus receives inputs from the limbic GPi only [268]. These findings, therefore, reveal that some associative and limbic cortical information, which is largely processed in segregated cortico-striatopallidal channels, converges to common thalamic nuclei in monkeys. These anatomic studies and many others provide clear evidence that the basal ganglia outflow from the GPi reaches cortical areas that extend far beyond motor-related cortices but also involve cognitive and associative regions of the prefrontal cortex [84, 272–275].

The pallidal-, nigral-, and cerebellar-receiving territories are largely segregated in the primate thalamus, whereas they slightly overlap in rodents [276–278]. It has long been thought that pallidothalamic outflow to the cerebral cortex was restricted to supplementary and premotor cortices, while information from the cerebellothalamic tract was solely directed to the primary motor cortex [279,280]. This simplistic view has now been replaced by a more sophisticated and complex view of thalamocortical projections which suggests that both pallidal and cerebellum information gains access to all motor-related cortices. However, the sources of GPi or cerebellar projections to specific motor cortical areas are quantitatively different and largely segregated. For instance, the GPi outflow to thalamic regions that innervate the supplementary and presupplementary motor is more massive than the dentate nucleus projections to these areas [275]. The high level of calbindin D_{28K} expression in the ventrolateral thalamus provides clear landmarks between GPi and cerebellar termination sites [267]. About 10–20% of pallidothalamic neurons in the monkey GPi project to the contralateral VA/VL [281].

Most pallidal neurons that project to thalamic motor nuclei send axon collaterals to the caudal intralaminar nuclei (Figures 4.1 and 4.4). These branched neurons are located in the central portion of GPi. Pallidal axons arising from the sensorimotor GPi terminate exclusively in CM, where they form synapses with thalamostriatal neurons projecting back to the sensorimotor territory of the striatum. In contrast, associative inputs from the GPi terminate massively in the dorsolateral extension of PF (PFdl), which does not project back to the caudate nucleus but rather innervates preferentially the precommissural region of the putamen. Finally, the limbic GPi innervates selectively the rostrodorsal part of PF, which, in turn, projects back to the nucleus accumbens. Therefore, it appears that CM/PF is part of closed and open functional loops with the striatopallidal complex [14,37,282] (Figure 4.1).

Recent single-cell filling studies have identified two major types of projection neurons in the monkey GPi: the type I neurons project to the ventral motor nuclei with collaterals to the pedunculopontine nucleus and/or the CM/Pf, whereas the type II neurons, located along the border of GPi, project to the lateral habenula with rare collaterals to the anterior thalamic nuclei [271].

The pallidotegmental projection

The pallidotegmental fibers terminate in the PPN. In monkeys, more than 80% of GPi neurons projecting to the PPN send axon collaterals to the ventral motor thalamus (Figure 4.4). Because the PPN gives rise to descending projections to the pons, medulla, and spinal cord, and also ascending projections to the thalamus and basal ganglia [237–239,241], the pallidotegmental projection may be a route by which cortical information processed in the basal ganglia can reach lower motor and autonomic centers. Another possibility could be that PPN acts as an important interface between different functional territories of the GPi and sends back the processed information to the basal ganglia. In contrast to the thalamus, there is significantly more overlap between projections from different functional regions of GPi in the PPN [283]. Pallidal fibers largely avoid cholinergic neurons in the pars compacta of the PPN, suggesting that the medial pars diffusa of the PPN is the potential site for the integration of information arising from different functional territories of the GPi in primates.

The pallidohabenular projection

In contrast to the pallidothalamic and pallidotegmental projections, which are largely collateralized, the pallidohabenular projection arises from a distinct population of neurons in the monkey GPi [271]. In rats, pallidohebenular neurons are located in the rostral part of the entopeduncular nucleus, whereas pallidothalamic and pallidotegmental projections arise preferentially from the caudal half of the nucleus. Interestingly, pallidohabenular cells receive afferents from striatofugal neurons in the patch compartment, whereas pallidothalamic and pallidotegmental neurons are innervated by striatal neurons in the matrix compartment. The ventral pallidum also contributes to the pallidohabenular projection in rats and cats.

In primates, retrograde labeling studies showed that pallidohabenular neurons are far less numerous than pallidothalamic cells and are mainly confined to a peri-GPi region which extends medially in the lateral hypothalamus. More recent studies in squirrel monkeys using sensitive anterograde labeling methods demonstrated that the pallidohabenular projection is functionally organized and more massive than previously thought [271]. The sensorimotor GPi innervates preferentially the centrolateral part of the lateral habenular nucleus whereas the limbic and associative GPi project massively to the medial part of the nucleus. The pallidohabenular projection is mainly GABAergic, although cholinergic neurons in the entopeduncular nucleus also contribute to this projection in rats. Because of its prominent connections with various limbic structures, the lateral habenula is considered as a functional interface between the limbic system and basal ganglia [284–290].

In addition, the lateral habenula is a major source of GABAergic inhibitory projections to midbrain dopaminergic neurons [284,291], although the details of the anatomic organization of this system remain to be characterized in primates (Figure 4.4). Recent studies have demonstrated that the pallidohabenular neurons located in the periphery of GPi change their activity in relation to expected rewards, thereby conveying reward-related signals to the lateral habenula. These in turn can influence the striatum and other basal ganglia nuclei through regulation of the dopaminergic and serotonergic systems [289] (Figure 4.4). There is also functional evidence that the lateral habenula plays important roles in learning, memory, and attention [292,293]. Because of its tight relationships with the different monoaminergic systems, the lateral habenula has been proposed as a potential target site for DBS in patients with severe depression [294].

Efferent projections of SNr

The nigrothalamic projection

In primates, the SNr and GPi inputs to the ventral thalamus are largely segregated from each other and from cerebellar afferents, but in nonprimates, the ventromedial nucleus receives convergent inputs from both basal ganglia output structures and the cerebellum. In monkeys, the nigrothalamic cells are distributed throughout the mediolateral extent of the SNr and form the largest population of nigrofugal neurons. Inputs from the medial part of the SNr terminate mostly in the medial magnocellular division of the VA (VAmc) and the mediodorsal nucleus (MDmc) that, in turn, innervate anterior regions of the frontal lobe including the principal sulcus and the orbital cortex. Neurons in the lateral part of the SNr project preferentially to the lateral posterior region of the VAmc and to different parts of MD mostly related to posterior regions of the frontal lobe including the frontal eye field areas of the pre-motor cortex (Figure 4.4). SNr outflow also gains access to thalamocortical neurons that project to the area TE in the inferotemporal cortex, providing a substrate whereby basal ganglia can influence higher order aspects of visual processing [273]. A dysfunction in this system may, therefore, contribute to alterations in visual perceptions, potentially accounting for the occurrence of visual hallucinations in basal ganglia disorders. In rats, a lamellar organization of nigrofugal neurons has been proposed as the main constituent for the parallel processing of information flow through the SNr. According to this model, functionally segregated striatal neurons project to different lamella of SNr neurons, which, in turn, convey the information to different thalamic nuclei. The dendrites of individual SNr neurons largely conform to the geometry of striatonigral projections, which strongly supports the concept of a parallel architecture of striatonigral circuits [295–297].

SNr neurons also project to rostral and caudal intralaminar thalamic nuclei. In monkeys, the nigro-intralaminar thalamic projection terminates exclusively in PF where nigral boutons form GABAergic synapses with thalamostriatal neurons that project to the caudate nucleus [14,37,282].

The nigrotegmental projection

The nigrotegmental projection displays a dorsoventral topography and terminates preferentially on non-cholinergic neurons in the medial two-thirds of the PPNd in rats. A much smaller number of nigral fibers innervate cholinergic neurons in the PPNc. In monkeys, the cells that give rise to the nigrotegmental projection are found throughout the mediolateral extent of the SNr and form the second largest population of SNr nigrofugal neurons. Most nigrotegmental cells send axon collaterals to the ventral anterior thalamic nucleus and receive direct inputs from the striatum. The pattern of distribution and postsynaptic targets of nigrotegmental neurons remain to be established in primates [1].

The nigrocollicular projection

The SNr sends a massive and topographically organized GABAergic projection to the intermediate layer of the superior colliculus. The nigral terminals form distinctive clusters in the deep and intermediate layers of the superior colliculus where they innervate neurons that project to the spinal cord, medulla, and periabducens area (Figure 4.4). This projection plays an important role in the control of saccadic eye movements orienting the eyes toward a stimulus in response to auditory of visual stimuli. This is consistent with the fact that SNr receiving neurons of the intermediate layer of the superior colliculus are targeted by visual inputs from the cortex and project to brainstem regions that control eye movements. In turn, the superior colliculus sends a significant projection to dopaminergic neurons in the SNc in rats and primates [298–303]. This projection is considered as a prime source of sensory-related events to dopaminergic nigrostriatal neurons, thereby suggesting that the phasic responses of midbrain dopaminergic neurons in complex tasks may be related to "sensory prediction errors" instead of "reward prediction errors" [304–312] (Figure 4.4).

The nigroreticular projection

The SNr also sends projections to the medullary reticular formation. In rats, this projection arises form a population of neurons in the dorsolateral SNr and terminates in the parvicellular reticular formation. Identified nigroreticular neurons receive GABAergic inputs from the striatum and the globus pallidus. This projection is thought to play a role in orofacial movements since the SNr receiving the neurons of the reticular formation are directly connected with orofacial motor nuclei [313,314].

Concluding remarks

Our knowledge of the functional anatomy of the basal ganglia has grown dramatically over recent decades. It has now become clear that the basal ganglia function extends far beyond the sensorimotor system, but also comprises major cognitive and limbic components. The complexity of the basal ganglia anatomy underlies some of the main symptomatic and pathophysiologic features of basal ganglia disorders which encompass multifarious motor and non-motor deficits which, in many cases, also include complex neuropsychiatric symptoms. We believe that continued growth of our understanding of the connections and cellular micro- and macrocircuits of the basal ganglia is the foundation for a deeper knowledge of normal basal ganglia function and further improvement of pharmacotherapeutic and neurosurgical approaches used to treat basal ganglia disorders.

Acknowledgments

I thank Adriana Galvan for her help in the preparation of figures and various members of my laboratory who have contributed to the original publication of some of the data discussed in this chapter. Thanks are also due the various funding agencies that have contributed to the support of research in my laboratory discussed in this chapter, including the National Institutes of Health (NINDS), National Parkinson Foundation, and Tourette Syndrome Association. I am also grateful for the continued support from a Yerkes National Primate Center NIH base grant.

References

1. Parent A, Hazrati LN. Functional anatomy of the basal ganglia. I. The cortico-basal ganglia-thalamo-cortical loop. *Brain Res Brain Res Rev* 1995;**20**:91–127.
2. Gerfen CR, Wilson CJ. The basal ganglia. In: Björklund A, Hökfeld T, Swanson L, eds. *Handbook of Chemical Neuroanatomy, Integrated Systems of the CNS, Part III*. Amsterdam: Elsevier, 1996: 369.
3. Middleton FA, Strick PL. New concepts about the organization of basal ganglia output. *Adv Neurol* 1997;**74**:57–68.
4. Middleton FA, Strick PL. Basal ganglia output and cognition: evidence from anatomical, behavioral, and clinical studies. *Brain Cogn* 2000;**42**:183–200.
5. Middleton FA, Strick PL. Basal ganglia and cerebellar loops: motor and cognitive circuits. *Brain Res Brain Res Rev* 2000;**31**:236–50.

6. Nicola SM, Surmeier J, Malenka RC. Dopaminergic modulation of neuronal excitability in the striatum and nucleus accumbens. *Annu Rev Neurosci* 2000;**23**:185–215.
7. Gerfen CR. Dopamine-mediated gene regulation in models of Parkinson's disease. *Ann Neurol* 2000;**47**:S42–50.
8. Parent A, Sato F, Wu Y, *et al.* Organization of the basal ganglia: the importance of axonal collateralization. *Trends Neurosci* 2000;**23**:S20–7.
9. Smith Y, Kieval JZ. Anatomy of the dopamine system in the basal ganglia. *Trends Neurosci* 2000;**23**:S28–33.
10. Bevan MD, Magill PJ, Terman D, *et al.* Move to the rhythm: oscillations in the subthalamic nucleus–external globus pallidus network. *Trends Neurosci*. 2002;**25**:525–31.
11. Afifi AK. The basal ganglia: a neural network with more than motor function. *Semin Pediatr Neurol* 2003;**10**:3–10.
12. Graybiel AM. Network-level neuroplasticity in cortico-basal ganglia pathways. *Parkinsonism Relat Disord* 2004;**10**:293–6.
13. Kelly RM, Strick PL. Macro-architecture of basal ganglia loops with the cerebral cortex: use of rabies virus to reveal multisynaptic circuits. *Prog Brain Res* 2004;**143**:449–59.
14. Smith Y, Raju DV, Pare JF, *et al.* The thalamostriatal system: a highly specific network of the basal ganglia circuitry. *Trends Neurosci* 2004;**27**:520–7.
15. Tepper JM, Bolam JP. Functional diversity and specificity of neostriatal interneurons. *Curr Opin Neurobiol* 2004;**14**:685–92.
16. Tepper JM, Koos T, *et al.* GABAergic microcircuits in the neostriatum. *Trends Neurosci* 2004;**27**:662–9.
17. Tepper JM, Abercrombie ED, *et al.* Basal ganglia macrocircuits. *Prog Brain Res* 2007;**160**:3–7.
18. McHaffie JG, Stanford TR, *et al.* Subcortical loops through the basal ganglia. *Trends Neurosci* 2005;**28**:401–7.
19. Boyes J, Bolam JP. Localization of GABA receptors in the basal ganglia. *Prog Brain Res* 2007;**160**:229–43.
20. Hammond C, Bergman H, *et al.* Pathological synchronization in Parkinson's disease: networks, models and treatments. *Trends Neurosci* 2007;**30**:357–64.
21. Wichmann T, Delong MR. Anatomy and physiology of the basal ganglia: relevance to Parkinson's disease and related disorders. *Handb Clin Neurol* 2007;**83**:1–18.
22. Graybiel AM. The basal ganglia: learning new tricks and loving it. *Curr Opin Neurobiol* 2005;**15**:638–44.
23. Graybiel AM. Habits, rituals, and the evaluative brain. *Annu Rev Neurosci* 2008;**31**:359–87.
24. Pisani A, Bernardi G, *et al.* Re-emergence of striatal cholinergic interneurons in movement disorders. *Trends Neurosci* 2007;**30**:545–53.
25. Surmeier DJ, Ding J, *et al.* D1 and D2 dopamine-receptor modulation of striatal glutamatergic signaling in striatal medium spiny neurons. *Trends Neurosci* 2007;**30**:228–35.
26. Wilson CJ. GABAergic inhibition in the neostriatum. *Prog Brain Res* 2007;**160**:91–110.
27. Haber SN. The primate basal ganglia: parallel and integrative networks. *J Chem Neuroanat* 2003;**26**:317–30.
28. Haber S. Parallel and integrative processing through the basal ganglia reward circuit: lessons from addiction. *Biol Psychiatry* 2008;**64**:173–4.
29. Braak H, Del Tredici K. Cortico-basal ganglia–cortical circuitry in Parkinson's disease reconsidered. *Exp Neurol* 2008;**212**:226–9.
30. Israel Z, Bergman H. Pathophysiology of the basal ganglia and movement disorders: from animal models to human clinical applications. *Neurosci Biobehav Rev* 2008;**32**:367–77.
31. Obeso JA, Rodriguez-Oroz MC, *et al.* Functional organization of the basal ganglia: therapeutic implications for Parkinson's disease. *Mov Disord* 2008;**23**(Suppl 3):S548–59.
32. Redgrave P, Gurney K, *et al.* What is reinforced by phasic dopamine signals? *Brain Res Rev* 2008;**58**:322–39.
33. Smith Y, Villalba R. Striatal and extrastriatal dopamine in the basal ganglia: an overview of its anatomical organization in normal and Parkinsonian brains. *Mov Disord* 2008;**23**(Suppl 3):S534–47.
34. Tepper JM, Wilson CJ, Koos T. Feedforward and feedback inhibition in neostriatal GABAergic spiny neurons. *Brain Res Rev* 2008;**58**:272–81.
35. Yelnik J. Modeling the organization of the basal ganglia. *Rev Neurol (Paris)* 2008;**164**:969–76.
36. Nambu A. Seven problems on the basal ganglia. *Curr Opin Neurobiol* 2009;**18**:251–8.
37. Smith Y, Raju D, *et al.* The thalamostriatal systems: anatomical and functional organization in normal and parkinsonian states. *Brain Res Bull* 2009;**78**:60–8.
38. Haber SN, Gdowski MJ. The basal ganglia. In: Paxinos G, Mai JK, eds. *The Human Nervous System*, 2nd edn. Amsterdam: Elsevier Academic Press, 2004: 677–738.
39. Graybiel AM. Neurotransmitters and neuromodulators in the basal ganglia. *Trends Neurosci* 1990;**13**:244–54.
40. Saka E, Graybiel AM. Pathophysiology of Tourette's syndrome: striatal pathways revisited. *Brain Dev* 2003;**25**(Suppl 1):S15–9.
41. Saka E, Goodrich C, Harlan P. Repetitive behaviors in monkeys are linked to specific striatal activation patterns. *J Neurosci* 2004;**24**:7557–65.
42. Canales JJ, Graybiel AM. A measure of striatal function predicts motor stereotypy. *Nat Neurosci* 2000;**3**:377–83.
43. Canales JJ. Stimulant-induced adaptations in neostriatal matrix and striosome systems: transiting from instrumental responding to habitual behavior in drug addiction. *Neurobiol Learn Mem* 2005;**83**:93–103.
44. Goto S, Lee LV, *et al.* Functional anatomy of the basal ganglia in X-linked recessive dystonia-parkinsonism. *Ann Neurol* 2005;**58**:7–17.
45. Sato K, Sumi-Ichinose C, *et al.* Differential involvement of striosome and matrix dopamine systems in a transgenic model of dopa-responsive dystonia. *Proc Natl Acad Sci USA* 2008;**105**:12551–6.
46. Crittenden JR, Cantuti-Castelvetri I, *et al.* Dysregulation of CalDAG-GEFI and CalDAG-GEFII predicts the severity of motor side-effects induced by anti-parkinsonian therapy. *Proc Natl Acad Sci USA* 2009;**106**:2892–6.
47. Tippett LJ, Waldvogel HJ, *et al.* Striosomes and mood dysfunction in Huntington's disease. *Brain* 2007;**130**:206–21.
48. Oorschot DE. Total number of neurons in the neostriatal, pallidal, subthalamic, and substantia nigral nuclei of the rat basal ganglia: a stereological study using the cavalieri and optical disector methods. *J Comp Neurol* 1996;**366**:580–99.
49. Gertler TS, Chan CS, *et al.* Dichotomous anatomical properties of adult striatal medium spiny neurons. *J Neurosci* 2008;**28**:10814–24.

50. Kreitzer AC, Malenka RC. Endocannabinoid-mediated rescue of striatal LTD and motor deficits in Parkinson's disease models. *Nature* 2007;**445**:643–7.
51. Cepeda C, Andre VM, *et al.* Differential electrophysiological properties of dopamine D1 and D2 receptor-containing striatal medium-sized spiny neurons. *Eur J Neurosci* 2008;**27**:671–82.
52. Ingham CA, Hood SH, *et al.* Spine density on neostriatal neurones changes with 6-hydroxydopamine lesions and with age. *Brain Res* 1989;**503**:334–8.
53. Day M, Wang Z, *et al.* Selective elimination of glutamatergic synapses on striatopallidal neurons in Parkinson disease models. *Nat Neurosci* 2006;**9**:251–9.
54. Wickens JR, Arbuthnott GW, *et al.* Simulation of GABA function in the basal ganglia: computational models of GABAergic mechanisms in basal ganglia function. *Prog Brain Res* 2007;**160**:313–29.
55. Villalba RM, Lee H, *et al.* Dopaminergic denervation and spine loss in the striatum of MPTP-treated monkeys. *Exp Neurol* 2009;**215**:220–7.
56. Wilson CJ, Groves PM. Fine structure and synaptic connections of the common spiny neuron of the rat neostriatum: a study employing intracellular inject of horseradish peroxidase. *J Comp Neurol* 1980;**194**:599–615.
57. Jaeger D, Kita H, *et al.* Surround inhibition among projection neurons is weak or nonexistent in the rat neostriatum. *J Neurophysiol* 1994;**72**:2555–8.
58. Koos T, Tepper JM, Wilson CJ. Comparison of IPSCs evoked by spiny and fast-spiking neurons in the neostriatum. *J Neurosci* 2004;**24**:7916–22.
59. Taverna S, Ilijic E, *et al.* Recurrent collateral connections of striatal medium spiny neurons are disrupted in models of Parkinson's disease. *J Neurosci* 2008;**28**:5504–12.
60. Graveland GA, DiFiglia M. The frequency and distribution of medium-sized neurons with indented nuclei in the primate and rodent neostriatum. *Brain Res* 1985;**327**:307–11.
61. Kawaguchi Y, Wilson CJ, *et al.* Striatal interneurones: chemical, physiological and morphological characterization. *Trends Neurosci* 1995;**18**:527–35.
62. Cicchetti F, Beach TG, *et al.* Chemical phenotype of calretinin interneurons in the human striatum. *Synapse* 1998;**30**:284–97.
63. Aosaki T, Graybiel AM, *et al.* Effect of the nigrostriatal dopamine system on acquired neural responses in the striatum of behaving monkeys. *Science* 1994;**265**:412–5.
64. Aosaki T, Tsubokawa H, *et al.* Responses of tonically active neurons in the primate's striatum undergo systematic changes during behavioral sensorimotor conditioning. *J Neurosci* 1994;**14**:3969–84.
65. Bennett BD, Wilson CJ. Spontaneous activity of neostriatal cholinergic interneurons in vitro. *J Neurosci* 1999;**19**:5586–96.
66. Smith AD, Bolam JP. The neural network of the basal ganglia as revealed by the study of synaptic connections of identified neurones. *Trends Neurosci* 1990;**13**:259–65.
67. Graybiel AM, Aosaki T, Flaherty AW. The basal ganglia and adaptive motor control. *Science* 1994;**265**:1826–31.
68. Kimura M, Yamada H, Matsumoto N. Tonically active neurons in the striatum encode motivational contexts of action. *Brain Dev* 2003;**25**(Suppl 1):S20–3.
69. Kimura M, Matsumoto N, Okahashi K. Goal-directed, serial and synchronous activation of neurons in the primate striatum. *Neuroreport* 2003;**14**:799–802.
70. Yamada H, Matsumoto N, Kimura M. Tonically active neurons in the primate caudate nucleus and putamen differentially encode instructed motivational outcomes of action. *J Neurosci* 22004;**4**:3500–10.
71. Apicella P. Leading tonically active neurons of the striatum from reward detection to context recognition. *Trends Neurosci* 2007;**30**:299–306.
72. Tan CO, Bullock D. A dopamine–acetylcholine cascade: simulating learned and lesion-induced behavior of striatal cholinergic interneurons. *J Neurophysiol* 2008;**100**:2409–21.
73. Joshua M, Adler A, Mitelman R. Midbrain dopaminergic neurons and striatal cholinergic interneurons encode the difference between reward and aversive events at different epochs of probabilistic classical conditioning trials. *J Neurosci* 2008;**28**:11673–84.
74. Joshua M, Adler A, Rosin B. Encoding of probabilistic rewarding and aversive events by pallidal and nigral neurons. *J Neurophysiol* 2009;**101**:758–72.
75. Sullivan MA, Chen H, *et al.* Recurrent inhibitory network among striatal cholinergic interneurons. *J Neurosci* 2008;**28**:8682–90.
76. Wang Z, Kai L, *et al.* Dopaminergic control of corticostriatal long-term synaptic depression in medium spiny neurons is mediated by cholinergic interneurons. *Neuron* 2006;**50**:443–52.
77. Galarraga E, Vilchis C, *et al.* Somatostatinergic modulation of firing pattern and calcium-activated potassium currents in medium spiny neostriatal neurons. *Neuroscience* 2007;**146**:537–54.
78. Betarbet R, Turner R, *et al.* Dopaminergic neurons intrinsic to the primate striatum. *J Neurosci* 1997;**17**:6761–8.
79. Cossette M, Levesque D, *et al.* Neurochemical characterization of dopaminergic neurons in human striatum. *Parkinsonism Relat Disord* 2005;**11**:277–86.
80. Cossette M, Lecomte F, *et al.* Morphology and distribution of dopaminergic neurons intrinsic to the human striatum. *J Chem Neuroanat* 2005;**29**:1–11.
81. Mazloom M, Smith Y. Synaptic microcircuitry of tyrosine hydroxylase-containing neurons and terminals in the striatum of 1-methyl-4-phenyl-1,2,3,6-tetrahydropyridine-treated monkeys. *J Comp Neurol* 2006;**495**:453–69.
82. Tande D, Hoglinger G, Debeir T, *et al.* New striatal dopamine neurons in MPTP-treated macaques result from a phenotypic shift and not neurogenesis. *Brain* 2006;**129**:1194–200.
83. Palfi S, Leventhal L, Chu Y, *et al.* Lentivirally delivered glial cell line-derived neurotrophic factor increases the number of striatal dopaminergic neurons in primate models of nigrostriatal degeneration. *J Neurosci* 2002;**22**:4942–54.
84. Alexander GE, DeLong MR, Strick PL. Parallel organization of functionally segregated circuits linking basal ganglia and cortex. *Annu Rev Neurosci* 1986;**9**:357–81.
85. Gerfen CR. The neostriatal mosaic: compartmentalization of corticostriatal input and striatonigral output systems. *Nature* 1984;**311**:461–4.
86. McGeorge AJ, Faull RL. The organization of the projection from the cerebral cortex to the striatum in the rat. *Neuroscience* 1989;**29**:503–37.

87. Wright AK, Norrie L, Ingham CA, *et al.* Double anterograde tracing of outputs from adjacent "barrel columns" of rat somatosensory cortex. Neostriatal projection patterns and terminal ultrastructure. *Neuroscience* 1999;**88**:119–33.
88. Alloway KD, Mutic JJ, Hoffer ZS, *et al.* Overlapping corticostriatal projections from the rodent vibrissal representations in primary and secondary somatosensory cortex. *J Comp Neurol* 42000;**28**:51–67.
89. Hoffer ZS, Alloway KD. Organization of corticostriatal projections from the vibrissal representations in the primary motor and somatosensory cortical areas of rodents. *J Comp Neurol* 2001;**439**:87–103.
90. Hoover JE, Hoffer ZS, Alloway KD. Projections from primary somatosensory cortex to the neostriatum: the role of somatotopic continuity in corticostriatal convergence. *J Neurophysiol* 2003;**89**:1576–87.
91. Reep RL, Cheatwood JL, Corwin JV. The associative striatum: organization of cortical projections to the dorsocentral striatum in rats. *J Comp Neurol* 2003;**467**:271–92.
92. Leergaard TB, Alloway KD, Pham TA, *et al.* Three-dimensional topography of corticopontine projections from rat sensorimotor cortex: comparisons with corticostriatal projections reveal diverse integrative organization. *J Comp Neurol* 2004;**478**:306–22.
93. Alloway KD, Lou L, Nwabueze-Ogbo F, *et al.* Topography of cortical projections to the dorsolateral neostriatum in rats: multiple overlapping sensorimotor pathways. *J Comp Neurol* 2006;**499**:33–48.
94. Royce GJ. Laminar origin of cortical neurons which project upon the caudate nucleus: a horseradish peroxidase investigation in the cat. *J Comp Neurol* 1982;**205**:8–29.
95. Updyke BV, Liles SL. The corticostriatal projection in cat: relation between axon terminals and evoked potentials. *Brain Res* 1987;**402**:365–9.
96. Norita M, McHaffie JG, Shimizu H, *et al.* The corticostriatal and corticotectal projections of the feline lateral suprasylvian cortex demonstrated with anterograde biocytin and retrograde fluorescent techniques. *Neurosci Res* 1991;**10**:149–55.
97. Updyke BV. Organization of visual corticostriatal projections in the cat, with observations on visual projections to claustrum and amygdala. *J Comp Neurol* 1993;**327**:159–93.
98. McHaffie JG, Thomson CM, Stein BE. Corticotectal and corticostriatal projections from the frontal eye fields of the cat: an anatomical examination using WGA-HRP. *Somatosens Mot Res* 2001;**18**:117–30.
99. Gerardin E, Lehericy S, Pochon JB, *et al.* Foot, hand, face and eye representation in the human striatum. *Cereb Cortex* 2003;**13**:162–9.
100. Lehericy S, Ducros M, Krainik A, *et al.* 3-D diffusion tensor axonal tracking shows distinct SMA and pre-SMA projections to the human striatum. *Cereb Cortex* 2004;**14**:1302–9.
101. Lehericy S, Ducros M, Van de Moortele PF, *et al.* Diffusion tensor fiber tracking shows distinct corticostriatal circuits in humans. *Ann Neurol* 2004;**55**:522–9.
102. Wiesendanger E, Clarke S, Kraftsik R, *et al.* Topography of cortico-striatal connections in man: anatomical evidence for parallel organization. *Eur J Neurosci* 2004;**20**:1915–22.
103. Postuma RB, Dagher A. Basal ganglia functional connectivity based on a meta-analysis of 126 positron emission tomography and functional magnetic resonance imaging publications. *Cereb Cortex* 2006;**16**:1508–21.
104. Dominey PF, Inui T, Hoen M. Neural network processing of natural language: II. Towards a unified model of corticostriatal function in learning sentence comprehension and non-linguistic sequencing. *Brain Lang* 2008;**109**:80–92.
105. Nagano-Saito A, Leyton M, Monchi O. Dopamine depletion impairs frontostriatal functional connectivity during a set-shifting task. *J Neurosci* 2008;**28**:3697–706.
106. Seger CA. How do the basal ganglia contribute to categorization? Their roles in generalization, response selection, and learning via feedback. *Neurosci Biobehav Rev* 2008;**32**:265–78.
107. Nakano K, Kayahara T, Tsutsumi T. Neural circuits and functional organization of the striatum. *J Neurol* 2000;**247**(Suppl 5):V1–15.
108. Nakano K. Neural circuits and topographic organization of the basal ganglia and related regions. *Brain Dev* 2000;**22**(Suppl 1):S5–16.
109. Yeterian EH, Van Hoesen GW. Cortico-striate projections in the rhesus monkey: the organization of certain cortico-caudate connections. *Brain Res* 1978;**139**:43–63.
110. Selemon LD, Goldman-Rakic PS. Longitudinal topography and interdigitation of corticostriatal projections in the rhesus monkey. *J Neurosci* 1985;**5**:776–94.
111. Parthasarathy HB, Schall JD, Graybiel AM. Distributed but convergent ordering of corticostriatal projections: analysis of the frontal eye field and the supplementary eye field in the macaque monkey. *J Neurosci* 1992;**12**:4468–88.
112. Flaherty AW, Graybiel AM. Two input systems for body representations in the primate striatal matrix: experimental evidence in the squirrel monkey. *J Neurosci* 1993;**13**:1120–37.
113. Reiner A, Jiao Y, Del Mar N, *et al.* Differential morphology of pyramidal tract-type and intratelencephalically projecting-type corticostriatal neurons and their intrastriatal terminals in rats. *J Comp Neurol* 2003;**457**:420–40.
114. Lei W, Jiao Y, Del Mar N, *et al.* Evidence for differential cortical input to direct pathway versus indirect pathway striatal projection neurons in rats. *J Neurosci* 2004;**24**:8289–99.
115. Ballion B, Mallet N, Bezard E, *et al.* Intratelencephalic corticostriatal neurons equally excite striatonigral and striatopallidal neurons and their discharge activity is selectively reduced in experimental parkinsonism. *Eur J Neurosci* 2008;**27**:2313–21.
116. Jones EG, Coulter JD, Burton H, *et al.* Cells of origin and terminal distribution of corticostriatal fibers arising in the sensory-motor cortex of monkeys. *J Comp Neurol* 1977;**173**:53–80.
117. Turner RS, DeLong MR. Corticostriatal activity in primary motor cortex of the macaque. *J Neurosci* 2000;**20**:7096–108.
118. Parent M, Parent A. Single-axon tracing study of corticostriatal projections arising from primary motor cortex in primates. *J Comp Neurol* 2006;**496**:202–13.
119. Kemp JM, Powell TP. The termination of fibres from the cerebral cortex and thalamus upon dendritic spines in the caudate nucleus: a study with the Golgi method. *Philos Trans R Soc Lond B Biol Sci* 1971;**262**:429–39.
120. Lapper SR, Smith Y, Sadikot AF, *et al.* Cortical input to parvalbumin-immunoreactive neurones in the putamen of the squirrel monkey. *Brain Res* 1992;**580**:215–24.
121. Mallet N, Le Moine C, Charpier S, *et al.* Feedforward inhibition of projection neurons by fast-spiking GABA

interneurons in the rat striatum *in vivo*. *J Neurosci* 2005;**25**: 3857–69.
122. Berke JD. Uncoordinated firing rate changes of striatal fast-spiking interneurons during behavioral task performance. *J Neurosci* 2008;**28**:10075–80.
123. Wilson CJ, Chang HT, Kitai ST. Firing patterns and synaptic potentials of identified giant aspiny interneurons in the rat neostriatum. *J Neurosci* 1990;**10**:508–19.
124. Thomas TM, Smith Y, Levey AI, *et al*. Cortical inputs to m2-immunoreactive striatal interneurons in rat and monkey. *Synapse* 2000;**37**:252–61.
125. Zemanick MC, Strick PL, Dix RD. Direction of transneuronal transport of herpes simplex virus 1 in the primate motor system is strain-dependent. *Proc Natl Acad Sci USA* 1991;**88**:8048–51.
126. Parthasarathy HB, Graybiel AM. Cortically driven immediate–early gene expression reflects modular influence of sensorimotor cortex on identified striatal neurons in the squirrel monkey. *J Neurosci* 1997;**17**:2477–91.
127. Parent M, Parent A. Single-axon tracing and three-dimensional reconstruction of centre median–parafascicular thalamic neurons in primates. *J Comp Neurol* 2005;**481**: 127–44.
128. Sadikot AF, Parent A, Smith Y, *et al*. Efferent connections of the centromedian and parafascicular thalamic nuclei in the squirrel monkey: a light and electron microscopic study of the thalamostriatal projection in relation to striatal heterogeneity. *J Comp Neurol* 1992;**320**:228–42.
129. Sadikot AF, Parent A, Francois C. Efferent connections of the centromedian and parafascicular thalamic nuclei in the squirrel monkey: a PHA-L study of subcortical projections. *J Comp Neurol* 1992;**315**:137–59.
130. Sidibe M, Smith Y. Differential synaptic innervation of striatofugal neurones projecting to the internal or external segments of the globus pallidus by thalamic afferents in the squirrel monkey. *J Comp Neurol* 1996;**365**:445–65.
131. Raju DV, Shah DJ, Wright TM, *et al*. Differential synaptology of vGluT2-containing thalamostriatal afferents between the patch and matrix compartments in rats. *J Comp Neurol* 2006;**499**:231–43.
132. Sidibe M, Smith Y. Thalamic inputs to striatal interneurons in monkeys: synaptic organization and co-localization of calcium binding proteins. *Neuroscience* 1999;**89**:1189–208.
133. Wilson CJ, Chang HT, Kitai ST. Origins of post synaptic potentials evoked in spiny neostriatal projection neurons by thalamic stimulation in the rat. *Exp Brain Res* 1983;**51**:217–26.
134. Nanda B, Galvan A, Smith Y, *et al*. Effects of stimulation of the centromedian nucleus of the thalamus on the activity of striatal cells in awake rhesus monkeys. *Eur J Neurosci*. 2009;**29**:588–98.
135. Minamimoto T, Kimura M. Participation of the thalamic CM-Pf complex in attentional orienting. *J Neurophysiol* 2002;**87**:3090–101.
136. Minamimoto T, Hori Y, Kimura M. Complementary process to response bias in the centromedian nucleus of the thalamus. *Science* 2005;**308**:1798–801.
137. Kimura M, Minamimoto T, Matsumoto N, *et al*. Monitoring and switching of cortico-basal ganglia loop functions by the thalamo-striatal system. *Neurosci Res* 2004;**48**:355–60.
138. McFarland NR, Haber SN. Convergent inputs from thalamic motor nuclei and frontal cortical areas to the dorsal striatum in the primate. *J Neurosci* 2000;**20**:3798–813.
139. Haber SN, Calzavara R. The cortico-basal ganglia integrative network: the role of the thalamus. *Brain Res Bull* 2009;**78**:69–74.
140. Lacey CJ, Bolam JP, Magill PJ. Novel and distinct operational principles of intralaminar thalamic neurons and their striatal projections. *J Neurosci* 2007;**27**:4374–84.
141. Raju DV, Ahern TH, Shah DJ, *et al*. Differential synaptic plasticity of the corticostriatal and thalamostriatal systems in an MPTP-treated monkey model of parkinsonism. *Eur J Neurosci* 2008;**27**:1647–58.
142. Kinomura S, Larsson J, Gulyas B, *et al*. Activation by attention of the human reticular formation and thalamic intralaminar nuclei. *Science* 1996;**271**:512–15.
143. Schiff ND, Giacino JT, Kalmar K A, *et al*. Behavioural improvements with thalamic stimulation after severe traumatic brain injury. *Nature* 2007;**448**:600–3.
144. Mair RG, Hembrook JR. Memory enhancement with event-related stimulation of the rostral intralaminar thalamic nuclei. *J Neurosci* 2008;**28**:14293–300.
145. Haber S, McFarland NR. The place of the thalamus in frontal cortical-basal ganglia circuits. *Neuroscientist* 2001;**7**:315–24.
146. McKeown MJ, Uthama A, Abugharbieh R, *et al*. Shape (but not volume) changes in the thalami in Parkinson disease. *BMC Neurol* 2008;**8**:8.
147. Gerfen CR, Baimbridge KG, Miller JJ. The neostriatal mosaic: compartmental distribution of calcium-binding protein and parvalbumin in the basal ganglia of the rat and monkey. *Proc Natl Acad Sci USA* 1985;**82**:8780–4.
148. Gerfen CR. The neostriatal mosaic. I. Compartmental organization of projections from the striatum to the substantia nigra in the rat. *J Comp Neurol* 1985;**236**:454–76.
149. Yamada T, McGeer PL, Baimbridge KG, *et al*. Relative sparing in Parkinson's disease of substantia nigra dopamine neurons containing calbindin-D28K. *Brain Res* 1990;**526**:303–7.
150. Damier P, Hirsch EC, Agid Y, *et al*. The substantia nigra of the human brain. II. Patterns of loss of dopamine-containing neurons in Parkinson's disease. *Brain* 1999;**122**(Pt 8):1437–48.
151. Iravani MM, Syed E, Jackson MJ, *et al*. A modified MPTP treatment regime produces reproducible partial nigrostriatal lesions in common marmosets. *Eur J Neurosci* 2005;**21**:841–54.
152. Haber SN, Ryoo H, Cox C, *et al*. Subsets of midbrain dopaminergic neurons in monkeys are distinguished by different levels of mRNA for the dopamine transporter: comparison with the mRNA for the D2 receptor, tyrosine hydroxylase and calbindin immunoreactivity. *J Comp Neurol* 1995;**362**:400–10.
153. Sanghera MK, Manaye K, McMahon A, *et al*. Dopamine transporter mRNA levels are high in midbrain neurons vulnerable to MPTP. *Neuroreport* 1997;**8**:3327–31.
154. Bezard E, Gross CE, Fournier MC, *et al*. Absence of MPTP-induced neuronal death in mice lacking the dopamine transporter. *Exp Neurol* 1999;**155**:268–73.
155. Gerfen CR, Herkenham M, Thibault J. The neostriatal mosaic: II. Patch- and matrix-directed mesostriatal dopaminergic and non-dopaminergic systems. *J Neurosci* 1987;**7**:3915–34.

156. Prensa L, Parent A. The nigrostriatal pathway in the rat: a single-axon study of the relationship between dorsal and ventral tier nigral neurons and the striosome/matrix striatal compartments. *J Neurosci* 2001;**21**:7247–60.
157. Matsuda W, Furuta T, Nakamura KC, *et al.* Single nigrostriatal dopaminergic neurons form widely spread and highly dense axonal arborizations in the neostriatum. *J Neurosci* 2009;**29**:444–53.
158. Kish SJ, Shannak K, Hornykiewicz O. Uneven pattern of dopamine loss in the striatum of patients with idiopathic Parkinson's disease. Pathophysiologic and clinical implications. *N Engl J Med* 1988;**318**:876–80.
159. Brooks DJ, Ibanez V, Sawle GV, *et al.* Differing patterns of striatal 18F-dopa uptake in Parkinson's disease, multiple system atrophy, and progressive supranuclear palsy. *Ann Neurol* 1990;**28**:547–55.
160. Damier P, Hirsch EC, Agid Y, *et al.* The substantia nigra of the human brain. I. Nigrosomes and the nigral matrix, a compartmental organization based on calbindin D(28K) immunohistochemistry. *Brain* 1999;**122**(Pt 8):1421–36.
161. Gibb WR, Lees AJ. Anatomy, pigmentation, ventral and dorsal subpopulations of the substantia nigra, and differential cell death in Parkinson's disease. *J Neurol Neurosurg Psychiatry* 1991;**54**:388–96.
162. Moratalla R, Quinn B, DeLanney LE, *et al.* Differential vulnerability of primate caudate–putamen and striosome–matrix dopamine systems to the neurotoxic effects of 1-methyl-4-phenyl-1,2,3,6-tetrahydropyridine. *Proc Natl Acad Sci USA* 1992;**89**:3859–63.
163. Karachi C, Francois C, Parain K, *et al.* Three-dimensional cartography of functional territories in the human striatopallidal complex by using calbindin immunoreactivity. *J Comp Neurol* 2002;**450**:122–34.
164. Iacopino A, Christakos S, German D, *et al.* Calbindin-D28K-containing neurons in animal models of neurodegeneration: possible protection from excitotoxicity. *Brain Res Mol Brain Res* 1992;**13**:251–61.
165. Fornai F, Ruffoli R, Soldani P, *et al.* The "Parkinsonian heart": from novel vistas to advanced therapeutic approaches in Parkinson's disease. *Curr Med Chem* 2007;**14**:2421–8.
166. Fornai F, di Poggio AB, Pellegrini A, *et al.* Noradrenaline in Parkinson's disease: from disease progression to current therapeutics. *Curr Med Chem* 2007;**14**:2330–4.
167. Rommelfanger KS, Edwards GL, Freeman KG, *et al.* Norepinephrine loss produces more profound motor deficits than MPTP treatment in mice. *Proc Natl Acad Sci USA* 2007;**104**:13804–9.
168. Rommelfanger KS, Weinshenker D. Norepinephrine: the redheaded stepchild of Parkinson's disease. *Biochem Pharmacol* 2007;**74**:177–90.
169. Carta M, Carlsson T, Munoz A, *et al.* Serotonin–dopamine interaction in the induction and maintenance of L-DOPA-induced dyskinesias. *Prog Brain Res* 2008;**172**:465–78.
170. Carta AR, Frau L, Pontis S, *et al.* Direct and indirect striatal efferent pathways are differentially influenced by low and high dyskinetic drugs: behavioural and biochemical evidence. *Parkinsonism Relat Disord* 2008;**14**(Suppl 2): S165–8.
171. Fox SH, Brotchie JM, Lang AE. Non-dopaminergic treatments in development for Parkinson's disease. *Lancet Neurol* 2008;**7**:927–38.
172. Fox SH, Chuang R, Brotchie JM. Parkinson's disease – opportunities for novel therapeutics to reduce the problems of levodopa therapy. *Prog Brain Res* 2008;**172**:479–94.
173. Albin RL, Young AB, Penney JB. The functional anatomy of basal ganglia disorders. *Trends Neurosci* 1989;**12**:366–75.
174. Bergman H, Wichmann T, DeLong MR. Reversal of experimental parkinsonism by lesions of the subthalamic nucleus. *Science* 1990;**249**:1436–8.
175. Gerfen CR, Engber TM, Mahan LC, *et al.* D1 and D2 dopamine receptor-regulated gene expression of striatonigral and striatopallidal neurons. *Science* 1990;**250**:1429–32.
176. Kawaguchi Y, Wilson CJ, Emson PC. Projection subtypes of rat neostriatal matrix cells revealed by intracellular injection of biocytin. *J Neurosci* 1990;**10**:3421–38.
177. Parent A, Charara A, Pinault D. Single striatofugal axons arborizing in both pallidal segments and in the substantia nigra in primates. *Brain Res* 1995;**698**:280–4.
178. Levesque M, Parent A. The striatofugal fiber system in primates: a reevaluation of its organization based on single-axon tracing studies. *Proc Natl Acad Sci USA* 2005;**102**:11888–93.
179. Le Moine C, Normand E, Bloch B. Phenotypical characterization of the rat striatal neurons expressing the D1 dopamine receptor gene. *Proc Natl Acad Sci USA* 1991;**88**:4205–9.
180. Surmeier DJ, Eberwine J, Wilson CJ, *et al.* Dopamine receptor subtypes colocalize in rat striatonigral neurons. *Proc Natl Acad Sci USA* 1992;**89**:10178–82.
181. Surmeier DJ, Reiner A, Levine MS, *et al.* Are neostriatal dopamine receptors co-localized? *Trends Neurosci* 1993;**16**: 299–305.
182. Gerfen CR, Keefe KA. Neostriatal dopamine receptors. *Trends Neurosci* 1994;**17**:2–3; author reply 4–5.
183. Le Moine C, Bloch B. D1 and D2 dopamine receptor gene expression in the rat striatum: sensitive cRNA probes demonstrate prominent segregation of D1 and D2 mRNAs in distinct neuronal populations of the dorsal and ventral striatum. *J Comp Neurol* 1995;**355**:418–26.
184. Svenningsson P, Le Moine C, Aubert I, *et al.* Cellular distribution of adenosine A2A receptor mRNA in the primate striatum. *J Comp Neurol* 1998;**399**:229–40.
185. Surmeier DJ, Song WJ, Yan Z. Coordinated expression of dopamine receptors in neostriatal medium spiny neurons. *J Neurosci* 1996;**16**:6579–91.
186. Hersch SM, Ciliax BJ, Gutekunst CA, *et al.* Electron microscopic analysis of D1 and D2 dopamine receptor proteins in the dorsal striatum and their synaptic relationships with motor corticostriatal afferents. *J Neurosci* 1995;**15**:5222–37.
187. Aizman O, Brismar H, Uhlen P, *et al.* Anatomical and physiological evidence for D1 and D2 dopamine receptor colocalization in neostriatal neurons. *Nat Neurosci* 2000;**3**:226–30.
188. Heintz N. BAC to the future: the use of bac transgenic mice for neuroscience research. *Nat Rev Neurosci* 2001;**2**:861–70.
189. Gong S, Zheng C, Doughty ML, *et al.* A gene expression atlas of the central nervous system based on bacterial artificial chromosomes. *Nature* 2003;**425**:917–25.
190. Shen W, Tian X, Day M, *et al.* Cholinergic modulation of Kir2 channels selectively elevates dendritic excitability in striatopallidal neurons. *Nat Neurosci* 2007;**10**:1458–66.

191. Shen W, Flajolet M, Greengard P, *et al.* Dichotomous dopaminergic control of striatal synaptic plasticity. *Science* 2008;**321**:848–51.
192. Ding J, Peterson JD, Surmeier DJ. Corticostriatal and thalamostriatal synapses have distinctive properties. *J Neurosci* 2008;**28**:6483–92.
193. Le Moine C, Bloch B. Expression of the D3 dopamine receptor in peptidergic neurons of the nucleus accumbens: comparison with the D1 and D2 dopamine receptors. *Neuroscience* 1996;**73**:131–43.
194. Gurevich EV, Joyce JN. Distribution of dopamine D3 receptor expressing neurons in the human forebrain: comparison with D2 receptor expressing neurons. *Neuropsychopharmacology* 1999;**20**:60–80.
195. Khan ZU, Gutierrez A, Martin R, *et al* Dopamine D5 receptors of rat and human brain. *Neuroscience* 2000;**100**:689–99.
196. Rivera A, Alberti I, Martin AB, *et al.* Molecular phenotype of rat striatal neurons expressing the dopamine D5 receptor subtype. *Eur J Neurosci* 2002;**16**:2049–58.
197. Noain D, Avale ME, Wedemeyer C, *et al.* Identification of brain neurons expressing the dopamine D4 receptor gene using BAC transgenic mice. *Eur J Neurosci* 2006;**24**:2429–38.
198. Araki KY, Sims JR, Bhide PG. Dopamine receptor mRNA and protein expression in the mouse corpus striatum and cerebral cortex during pre- and postnatal development. *Brain Res*, 2007;**1156**:31–45.
199. Nambu A, Tokuno H, Takada M. Functional significance of the cortico-subthalamo-pallidal "hyperdirect" pathway. *Neurosci Res* 2002;**43**:111–7.
200. Nambu A, Takada M, Inase M, *et al.* Dual somatotopical representations in the primate subthalamic nucleus: evidence for ordered but reversed body-map transformations from the primary motor cortex and the supplementary motor area. *J Neurosci* 1996;**16**:2671–83.
201. Strafella AP, Vanderwerf Y, Sadikot AF. Transcranial magnetic stimulation of the human motor cortex influences the neuronal activity of subthalamic nucleus. *Eur J Neurosci* 2004;**20**:2245–9.
202. Shink E, Bevan MD, Bolam JP, *et al.* The subthalamic nucleus and the external pallidum: two tightly interconnected structures that control the output of the basal ganglia in the monkey. *Neuroscience* 1996;**73**:335–57.
203. Smith Y, Bevan MD, Shink E, *et al.* Microcircuitry of the direct and indirect pathways of the basal ganglia. *Neuroscience* 1998;**86**:353–87.
204. Wichmann T, Bergman H, DeLong MR. The primate subthalamic nucleus. III. Changes in motor behavior and neuronal activity in the internal pallidum induced by subthalamic inactivation in the MPTP model of parkinsonism. *J Neurophysiol* 1994;**72**:521–30.
205. Paradiso G, Cunic D, Saint-Cyr JA, *et al.* Involvement of human thalamus in the preparation of self-paced movement. *Brain* 2004;**127**:2717–31.
206. Kitai ST, Deniau JM. Cortical inputs to the subthalamus: intracellular analysis. *Brain Res* 1981;**214**:411–5.
207. Giuffrida R, Li Volsi G, Maugeri G, *et al.* Influences of pyramidal tract on the subthalamic nucleus in the cat. *Neurosci Lett* 1985;**54**:231–5.
208. Baunez C, Humby T, Eagle DM, *et al.* Effects of STN lesions on simple vs choice reaction time tasks in the rat: preserved motor readiness, but impaired response selection. *Eur J Neurosci* 2001;**13**:1609–16.
209. Chudasama Y, Baunez C, Robbins TW. Functional disconnection of the medial prefrontal cortex and subthalamic nucleus in attentional performance: evidence for corticosubthalamic interaction. *J Neurosci* 2003;**23**:5477–85.
210. Winstanley CA, Baunez C, Theobald DE, *et al.* Lesions to the subthalamic nucleus decrease impulsive choice but impair autoshaping in rats: the importance of the basal ganglia in Pavlovian conditioning and impulse control. *Eur J Neurosci* 2005;**21**:3107–16.
211. Blandini F, Fancellu R, Armentero MT, *et al.* Unilateral lesion of the subthalamic nucleus enhances cortical fos expression associated with focally evoked seizures in the rat. *Brain Res* 2006;**1101**:145–50.
212. Eagle DM, Baunez C, Hutcheson DM, *et al.* Stop-signal reaction-time task performance: role of prefrontal cortex and subthalamic nucleus. *Cereb Cortex* 2008;**18**:178–88.
213. Le Jeune F, Peron J, Biseul I, *et al.* Subthalamic nucleus stimulation affects orbitofrontal cortex in facial emotion recognition: a PET study. *Brain* 2008;**131**:1599–608.
214. Tzagournissakis M, Dermon CR, Savaki HE. Functional metabolic mapping of the rat brain during unilateral electrical stimulation of the subthalamic nucleus. *J Cereb Blood Flow Metab* 1994;**14**:132–44.
215. Maurice N, Deniau JM, Glowinski J. Relationships between the prefrontal cortex and the basal ganglia in the rat: physiology of the corticosubthalamic circuits. *J Neurosci* 1998;**18**:9539–46.
216. Kolomiets BP, Deniau JM, Mailly P. Segregation and convergence of information flow through the cortico-subthalamic pathways. *J Neurosci* 2001;**21**:5764–72.
217. Kolomiets BP, Deniau JM, Glowinski J. Basal ganglia and processing of cortical information: functional interactions between trans-striatal and trans-subthalamic circuits in the substantia nigra pars reticulata. *Neuroscience* 2003;**117**:931–8.
218. Aron AR, Behrens TE, Smith S, *et al.* Triangulating a cognitive control network using diffusion-weighted magnetic resonance imaging (MRI) and functional MRI. *J Neurosci* 2007;**27**:3743–52.
219. Gerschlager W, Alesch F, Cunnington R. Bilateral subthalamic nucleus stimulation improves frontal cortex function in Parkinson's disease. An electrophysiological study of the contingent negative variation. *Brain* 1999;**122**(Pt 12):2365–73.
220. Schroeder U, Kuehler A, Haslinger B, *et al.* Subthalamic nucleus stimulation affects striato-anterior cingulate cortex circuit in a response conflict task: a PET study. *Brain* 2002;**125**:1995–2004.
221. Hershey T, Revilla FJ, Wernle A, *et al.* Stimulation of STN impairs aspects of cognitive control in PD. *Neurology* 2004;**62**:1110–4.
222. Haegelen C, Verin M, Broche BA. Does subthalamic nucleus stimulation affect the frontal limbic areas? A single-photon emission computed tomography study using a manual anatomical segmentation method. *Surg Radiol Anat* 2005;**27**:389–94.
223. Funkiewiez A, Ardouin C, Caputo E. Long term effects of bilateral subthalamic nucleus stimulation on cognitive

function, mood, and behaviour in Parkinson's disease. *J Neurol Neurosurg Psychiatry* 2004;**75**:834–9.

224. Funkiewiez A, Ardouin C, Cools R. Effects of levodopa and subthalamic nucleus stimulation on cognitive and affective functioning in Parkinson's disease. *Mov Disord* 2006;**21**:1656–62.
225. Campbell MC, Karimi M, Weaver PM, *et al.* Neural correlates of STN DBS-induced cognitive variability in Parkinson disease. *Neuropsychologia* 2008;**46**:3162–9.
226. Kalbe E, Voges J, Weber T. Frontal FDG-PET activity correlates with cognitive outcome after STN-DBS in Parkinson disease. *Neurology* 2009;**72**:42–9.
227. Parent A, Smith Y. Organization of efferent projections of the subthalamic nucleus in the squirrel monkey as revealed by retrograde labeling methods. *Brain Res* 1987;**436**:296–310.
228. Smith Y, Hazrati LN, Parent A. Efferent projections of the subthalamic nucleus in the squirrel monkey as studied by the PHA-L anterograde tracing method. *J Comp Neurol* 1990;**294**:306–23.
229. Afsharpour S. Topographical projections of the cerebral cortex to the subthalamic nucleus. *J Comp Neurol* 1985;**236**:14–28.
230. Degos B, Deniau JM, Le Cam J, *et al.* Evidence for a direct subthalamo-cortical loop circuit in the rat. *Eur J Neurosci* 2008;**27**:2599–610.
231. Garcia-Rill E, Biedermann JA, Chambers T, *et al.* Mesopontine neurons in schizophrenia. *Neuroscience* 1995;**66**:321–35.
232. Garcia-Rill E, Reese NB, Skinner RD. Arousal and locomotion: from schizophrenia to narcolepsy. *Prog Brain Res* 1996;**107**:417–34.
233. Mesulam MM, Geula C, Bothwell MA, *et al.* Human reticular formation: cholinergic neurons of the pedunculopontine and laterodorsal tegmental nuclei and some cytochemical comparisons to forebrain cholinergic neurons. *J Comp Neurol* 1989;**283**:611–33.
234. Inglis WL, Winn P. The pedunculopontine tegmental nucleus: where the striatum meets the reticular formation. *Prog Neurobiol* 1995;**47**:1–29.
235. Rye DB. Contributions of the pedunculopontine region to normal and altered REM sleep. *Sleep* 1997;**20**:757–88.
236. Winn P, Brown VJ, Inglis WL. On the relationships between the striatum and the pedunculopontine tegmental nucleus. *Crit Rev Neurobiol* 1997;**11**:241–61.
237. Pahapill PA, Lozano AM. The pedunculopontine nucleus and Parkinson's disease. *Brain* 2000;**123**(Pt 9):1767–83.
238. Winn P. Experimental studies of pedunculopontine functions: are they motor, sensory or integrative? *Parkinsonism Relat Disord* 2008;**14**(Suppl 2):S194–8.
239. Mena-Segovia J, Bolam JP, Magill PJ. Pedunculopontine nucleus and basal ganglia: distant relatives or part of the same family? *Trends Neurosci* 2004;**27**:585–8.
240. Charara A, Smith Y, Parent A. Glutamatergic inputs from the pedunculopontine nucleus to midbrain dopaminergic neurons in primates: *Phaseolus vulgaris*-leucoagglutionin anterograde labeling combined with postembedding glutamate and GABA immunohistochemistry. *J Comp Neurol* 1996;**364**:254–66.
241. Mena-Segovia J, Winn P, Bolam JP. Cholinergic modulation of midbrain dopaminergic systems. *Brain Res Rev* 2008;**58**:265–71.
242. Sidibe M, Pare JF, Raju DV, *et al.* Anatomical and functional relationships between intralaminar thalamic nuclei and basal ganglia in monkeys. In: Nicholson LFB, Faull RLM, eds. *The Basal Ganglia VII*. New York: Kluwer Academic/Plenum, 2002: 409–20.
243. Muthusamy KA, Aravamuthan BR, Kringelbach, *et al.* Connectivity of the human pedunculopontine nucleus region and diffusion tensor imaging in surgical targeting. *J Neurosurg* 2007;**107**:814–20.
244. Aravamuthan BR, Muthusamy KA, Stein JF, *et al.* Topography of cortical and subcortical connections of the human pedunculopontine and subthalamic nuclei. *Neuroimage* 2007;**37**:694–705.
245. Aravamuthan BR, Stein JF, Aziz TZ. The anatomy and localization of the pedunculopontine nucleus determined using probabilistic diffusion tractography. *Br J Neurosurg* 2008;**22**(Suppl 1):S25–32.
246. Aravamuthan BR, McNab JA, Miller KL, *et al.* Cortical and subcortical connections within the pedunculopontine nucleus of the primate *Macaca mulatta* determined using probabilistic diffusion tractography. *J Clin Neurosci* 2009;**16**:413–20.
247. Garcia-Rill E, Houser CR, Skinner RD, *et al.* Locomotion-inducing sites in the vicinity of the pedunculopontine nucleus. *Brain Res Bull* 1987;**18**:731–8.
248. Piallat B, Chabardes S, Torres N, *et al.* Gait is associated with an increase in tonic firing of the sub-cuneiform nucleus neurons. *Neuroscience* 2008;**158**:1201–5.
249. Weinberger M, Hamani C, Hutchison WD, *et al.* Pedunculopontine nucleus microelectrode recordings in movement disorder patients. *Exp Brain Res* 2008;**188**:165–74.
250. Kojima J, Yamaji Y, Matsumura M, *et al.* Excitotoxic lesions of the pedunculopontine tegmental nucleus produce contralateral hemiparkinsonism in the monkey. *Neurosci Lett* 1997;**226**:111–4.
251. Munro-Davies L, Winter J, Aziz TZ, *et al.* Kainate acid lesions of the pedunculopontine region in the normal behaving primate. *Mov Disord* 2001;**16**:150–1.
252. Hirsch EC, Graybiel AM, Duyckaerts C, *et al.* Neuronal loss in the pedunculopontine tegmental nucleus in Parkinson disease and in progressive supranuclear palsy. *Proc Natl Acad Sci USA* 1987;**84**:5976–80.
253. Jellinger KA. Neuropathology of movement disorders. *Neurosurg Clin N Am* 1998;**9**:237–62.
254. Jenkinson N, Nandi D, Muthusamy K, *et al.* Anatomy, physiology, and pathophysiology of the pedunculopontine nucleus. *Mov Disord* 2008;**24**:319–28.
255. Nandi D, Aziz TZ, Giladi N, *et al.* Reversal of akinesia in experimental parkinsonism by GABA antagonist microinjections in the pedunculopontine nucleus. *Brain* 2002;**125**:2418–30.
256. Jenkinson N, Nandi D, Miall RC, *et al.* Pedunculopontine nucleus stimulation improves akinesia in a Parkinsonian monkey. *Neuroreport* 2004;**15**:2621–4.
257. Pierantozzi M, Palmieri MG, Galati S. Pedunculopontine nucleus deep brain stimulation changes spinal cord excitability in Parkinson's disease patients. *J Neural Transm* 2008;**115**:731–5.
258. Ferraye MU, Debu B, Pollak P. Deep brain stimulation effect on freezing of gait. *Mov Disord* 2008;**23**(Suppl 2):S489–94.

259. Lozano AM, Snyder BJ. Deep brain stimulation for parkinsonian gait disorders. *J Neurol* 2008;**255**(Suppl 4):30–1.
260. Nandi D, Liu X, Winter JL, *et al*. Deep brain stimulation of the pedunculopontine region in the normal non-human primate. *J Clin Neurosci* 2002;**9**:170–4.
261. Nandi D, Jenkinson N, Stein J, *et al*. The pedunculopontinhe nucleus in Parkinson's disease: primate studies. *Br J Neurosurg* 2008;**22**(Suppl 1):S4–8.
262. Mazzone P, Lozano A, Stanzione P, *et al*. Implantation of human pedunculopontine nucleus: a safe and clinically relevant target in Parkinson's disease. *Neuroreport* 2005;**16**:1877–81.
263. Stefani A, Lozano AM, Peppe A, *et al*. Bilateral deep brain stimulation of the pedunculopontine and subthalamic nuclei in severe Parkinson's disease. *Brain* 2007;**130**:1596–607.
264. Yelnik J. PPN or PPD, what is the target for deep brain stimulation in Parkinson's disease? *Brain* 2007;**130**:e79; author reply e80.
265. Zrinzo L, Zrinzo LV, Hariz M. The peripeduncular nucleus: a novel target for deep brain stimulation? *Neuroreport* 2007;**18**:1301–2.
266. Zrinzo L, Zrinzo LV. Surgical anatomy of the pedunculopontine and peripeduncular nuclei. *Br J Neurosurg* 2008;**22**(Suppl 1):S19–24.
267. Percheron G, Francois C, Talbi B, *et al*. The primate motor thalamus. *Brain Res Brain Res Rev* 1996;**22**:93–181.
268. Sidibe M, Bevan MD, Bolam JP, *et al*. Efferent connections of the internal globus pallidus in the squirrel monkey: I. Topography and synaptic organization of the pallidothalamic projection. *J Comp Neurol* 1997;**382**:323–47.
269. Baron MS, Sidibe M, DeLong MR, *et al*. Course of motor and associative pallidothalamic projections in monkeys. *J Comp Neurol* 2001;**429**:490–501.
270. Kuo JS, Carpenter MB. Organization of pallidothalamic projections in the rhesus monkey. *J Comp Neurol* 1973;**151**:201–36.
271. Parent M, Levesque M, Parent A. Two types of projection neurons in the internal pallidum of primates: single-axon tracing and three-dimensional reconstruction. *J Comp Neurol* 2001;**439**:162–75.
272. Middleton FA, Strick PL. Anatomical evidence for cerebellar and basal ganglia involvement in higher cognitive function. *Science* 1994;**266**:458–61.
273. Middleton FA, Strick PL. The temporal lobe is a target of output from the basal ganglia. *Proc Natl Acad Sci USA* 1996;**93**:8683–7.
274. Middleton FA, Strick PL. Basal-ganglia "projections" to the prefrontal cortex of the primate. *Cereb Cortex* 2002;**12**:926–35.
275. Akkal D, Dum RP, Strick PL. Supplementary motor area and presupplementary motor area: targets of basal ganglia and cerebellar output. *J Neurosci* 2007;**27**:10659–73.
276. Ilinsky IA, Tourtellotte WG, Kultas-Ilinsky K. Anatomical distinctions between the two basal ganglia afferent territories in the primate motor thalamus. *Stereotact Funct Neurosurg* 1993;**60**:62–9.
277. Sakai ST, Stepniewska I, Qi HX, *et al*. Pallidal and cerebellar afferents to pre-supplementary motor area thalamocortical neurons in the owl monkey: a multiple labeling study. *J Comp Neurol* 2000;**417**:164–80.
278. Gallay MN, Jeanmonod D, Liu J. Human pallidothalamic and cerebellothalamic tracts: anatomical basis for functional stereotactic neurosurgery. *Brain Struct Funct* 2008;**212**:443–63.
279. Schell GR, Strick PL. The origin of thalamic inputs to the arcuate premotor and supplementary motor areas. *J Neurosci* 1984;**4**:539–60.
280. Strick PL. How do the basal ganglia and cerebellum gain access to the cortical motor areas? *Behav Brain Res* 1985;**18**:107–23.
281. Hazrati LN, Parent A. Contralateral pallidothalamic and pallidotegmental projections in primates: an anterograde and retrograde labeling study. *Brain Res* 1991;**567**:212–23.
282. Sidibe M, Pare JF, Smith Y. Nigral and pallidal inputs to functionally segregated thalamostriatal neurons in the centromedian/parafascicular nuclear compex in monkey. *J Comp Neurol* 2002;**447**:286–99.
283. Shink E, Sidibe M, Smith Y. Efferent connections of the internal globus pallidus in the squirrel monkey: II. Topography and synaptic organization of pallidal efferents to the pedunculopontine nucleus. *J Comp Neurol* 1997;**382**:348–63.
284. Matsumoto M, Hikosaka O. Lateral habenula as a source of negative reward signals in dopamine neurons. *Nature* 2007;**447**:1111–5.
285. Matsumoto M, Hikosaka O. Negative motivational control of saccadic eye movement by the lateral habenula. *Prog Brain Res* 2008;**171**:399–402.
286. Matsumoto M, Hikosaka O. Representation of negative motivational value in the primate lateral habenula. *Nat Neurosci* 2009;**12**:77–84.
287. Hikosaka O, Sesack SR, Lecourtier L, *et al*. Habenula: crossroad between the basal ganglia and the limbic system. *J Neurosci* 2008;**28**:11825–9.
288. Hikosaka O. Decision-making and learning by cortico-basal ganglia network. *Brain Nerve* 2008;**60**:799–813 (in Japanese).
289. Hong S, Hikosaka O. The globus pallidus sends reward-related signals to the lateral habenula. *Neuron* 2008;**60**:720–9.
290. Geisler S, Trimble M. The lateral habenula: no longer neglected. *CNS Spectr* 2008;**13**:484–9.
291. Ji H, Shepard PD. Lateral habenula stimulation inhibits rat midbrain dopamine neurons through a GABA(A) receptor-mediated mechanism. *J Neurosci* 2007;**27**:6923–30.
292. Klemm WR. Habenular and interpeduncularis nuclei: shared components in multiple-function networks. *Med Sci Monit* 2004;**10**:RA261–73.
293. Lecourtier L, Kelly PH. A conductor hidden in the orchestra? Role of the habenular complex in monoamine transmission and cognition. *Neurosci Biobehav Rev* 2007;**31**:658–72.
294. Sartorius A, Henn FA. Deep brain stimulation of the lateral habenula in treatment resistant major depression. *Med Hypotheses* 2007;**69**:1305–8.
295. Deniau JM, Menetrey A, Charpier S. The lamellar organization of the rat substantia nigra pars reticulata: segregated patterns of striatal afferents and relationship to the topography of corticostriatal projections. *Neuroscience* 1996;**73**:761–81.
296. Deniau JM, Mailly P, Maurice N, *et al*. The pars reticulata of the substantia nigra: a window to basal ganglia output. *Prog Brain Res* 2007;**160**:151–72.

297. Mailly P, Charpier S, Menetrey A, *et al.* Three-dimensional organization of the recurrent axon collateral network of the substantia nigra pars reticulata neurons in the rat. *J Neurosci* 2003;**23**:5247–57.
298. Coizet V, Comoli E, Westby GW, *et al.* Phasic activation of substantia nigra and the ventral tegmental area by chemical stimulation of the superior colliculus: an electrophysiological investigation in the rat. *Eur J Neurosci* 2003;**17**: 28–40.
299. Coizet V, Overton PG, Redgrave P. Collateralization of the tectonigral projection with other major output pathways of superior colliculus in the rat. *J Comp Neurol* 2007;**500**:1034–49.
300. Comoli E, Coizet V, Boyes J, *et al.* A direct projection from superior colliculus to substantia nigra for detecting salient visual events. *Nat Neurosci* 2003;**6**:974–80.
301. Dommett E, Coizet V, Blaha, *et al.* How visual stimuli activate dopaminergic neurons at short latency. *Science* 2005;**307**:1476–9.
302. May PJ, McHaffie JG, Stanford TR, *et al.* Tectonigral projections in the primate: a pathway for pre-attentive sensory input to midbrain dopaminergic neurons. *Eur J Neurosci.* 2009;**29**:575–87.
303. McHaffie JG, Jiang H, May PJ, *et al.* A direct projection from superior colliculus to substantia nigra pars compacta in the cat. *Neuroscience* 2006;**138**:221–34.
304. Redgrave P, Prescott TJ, Gurney K. Is the short-latency dopamine response too short to signal reward error? *Trends Neurosci* 1999;**22**:146–51.
305. Redgrave P, Gurney K. The short-latency dopamine signal: a role in discovering novel actions? *Nat Rev Neurosci* 2006;**7**:967–75.
306. Fiorillo CD, Newsome WT, Schultz W. The temporal precision of reward prediction in dopamine neurons. *Nat Neurosci.* 2008;**11**:966–73.
307. Redgrave P, Gurney K, Reynolds J. What is reinforced by phasic dopamine signals? *Brain Res Rev* 2008;**58**:322–39.
308. Laurent PA. The emergence of saliency and novelty responses from reinforcement learning principles. *Neural Networks* 2008;**21**:1493–9.
309. Kobayashi S, Schultz W. Influence of reward delays on responses of dopamine neurons. *J Neuroscience* 2008;**28**:7837–46.
310. Schultz W. Multiple dopamine functions at different time courses. *Annu Rev Neurosci* 2007;**30**:259–88.
311. Schultz W. Behavioral dopamine signals. *Trends Neurosci* 2007;**30**:203–10.
312. Schultz W, Preuschoff K, Camerer C. Explicit neural signals reflecting reward uncertainty. *Philos Trans R Soc Lond B Biol Sci* 2008;**363**:3801–11.
313. Mogoseanu D, Smith AD, Bolam JP. Monosynaptic innervation of trigeminal motor neurones involved in mastication by neurones of the parvicellular reticular formation. *J Comp Neurol* 1993;**336**:53–65.
314. Mogoseanu D, Smith AD, Bolam JP. Monosynaptic innervation of facial motoneurones by neurones of the parvicellular reticular formation. *Exp Brain Res* 1994;**101**:427–48.

Chapter 5
Functional Organization of the Basal Ganglia: Dopaminergic and Non-Dopaminergic Features

Carlos Juri, Maria C. Rodriguez-Oroz, & Jose A. Obeso
Clinica Universitaria and Medical School; Neuroscience Division, CIMA and Centro de Investigacion Biomedica en Red sobre Enfermedades Neurodegenerativas (CIBERNED), University of Navarra, Pamplona, Spain

Introduction

Parkinson's disease (PD) can be diagnosed clinically based on the presence of the cardinal motor manifestations of the disease (rest tremor, akinesia, rigidity) and a good response to dopaminergic therapy. However, the phenotype of PD has changed considerably due to the success of dopaminergic treatment, the increase in patients' life expectancy, which allows for features associated with the long-term course of the disease to emerge, and the recognition of non-motor and non-dopaminergic features of the illness. Accordingly, an attempt to understand the pathophysiologic basis of PD needs to take into account the following (Box 5.1):

1 Typical motor features which respond to levodopa.
2 The motor fluctuations and dyskinesias that complicate levodopa therapy.
3 Sensory symptoms such as pain, tingling, heat and cold, and numbness, which usually have a focal body distribution and are characteristically present in the "off" medication state but do not appear to be dopaminergic in origin.
4 Behavioral disorders and psychotic manifestations mediated by dopaminergic drugs and the underlying disease.
5 Non-motor manifestations (NMM) independent of treatment, such as cognitive impairment, mood disorders, and dysautonomia.
6 Motor abnormalities which respond poorly or not at all to dopaminergic drugs such as freezing of gait, disequilibrium, and postural abnormalities such as neck flexion, camptocormia, scoliosis, and hand and foot deformities, and are usually labeled "non-dopaminergic" features.

In this chapter, we shall mainly discuss the physiologic basis of the dopaminergic features and the sensory and non-dopaminergic motor manifestations of PD.

Functional organization of the basal ganglia

The organization of the basal ganglia in the normal and PD states has been extensively reviewed in Chapter 4 and elsewhere [1,2]. This chapter will focus on the role of the basal ganglia in the development of the non-motor features of PD, particularly with reference to sensory abnormalities and response fluctuations.

The basal ganglia are currently seen as a network, where different parts are activated depending on specific functions and circumstances [3,4]. The functional domains of the basal ganglia are not limited to movement control, but extend to involve learning, planning, working memory, and emotion [5–8] (Figure 5.1). It is now appreciated that these non-motor functions are also abnormal in PD.

Input–output of the basal ganglia

The motor circuit of the basal ganglia has two entry points [9], the striatum and the STN, and an efferent point, the globus pallidus (GPi)/substantia nigra pars reticulate (Snr), which send fibers to the cortex via the motor thalamus and to the brainstem (Figure 5.2). Cortical activity coding for movement and behavior access the basal ganglia by way of fast-conducting direct disynaptic projections to the GPi that synapse in the striatum or STN. The GPe modulates basal ganglia output (GPi) by means of connections to the striatum and by indirect tri-synaptic

Parkinson's Disease: Non-Motor and Non-Dopaminergic Features, First Edition. Edited by C. Warren Olanow, Fabrizio Stocchi, and Anthony E. Lang.

Box 5.1 Clinical spectrum of symptoms in Parkinson's disease

1 **Typical motor features** which respond well to levodopa

2 **Motor abnormalities which do not respond well or at all to dopaminergic drugs** (usually labeled "non-dopaminergic" features):
   Freezing of gait and disequilibrium
   Postural abnormalities such as neck flexion, camptocormia, scoliosis, hand and foot deformities

3 **Sensory symptoms** (usually have a focal body distribution and are characteristically present in the "off" medication state but disappear during the "on" state):
   Pain, tingling, heat and cold, numbness

4 **Behavioral disorders and psychotic manifestations mediated by dopaminergic drugs:**
   Psychosis, dopaminergic dysregulation syndrome, hallucinations

5 **Non-motor manifestations (NMM) independent of treatment:**
   Dementia
   Depression
   Autonomic dysfunction
   Sleep disorders

projections from the cortex (cortex–STN–GPe–GPi) (Figure 5.2). The GPe thus appears to be in a key position to regulate basal ganglia neuronal output and influences on thalamocortical projections within the motor loop [10,11].

Basal ganglia output modulates motor activity through variations of its inhibitory tone on the thalamus and brainstem projections, with enhanced motor function being associated with reduced inhibitor tone. Neuronal recordings in the SNr in monkeys that have been trained to generate saccadic eye movements showed that a cease or pause in GPi neuronal firing is associated with movement facilitation [12]. Similarly, movements of the arm

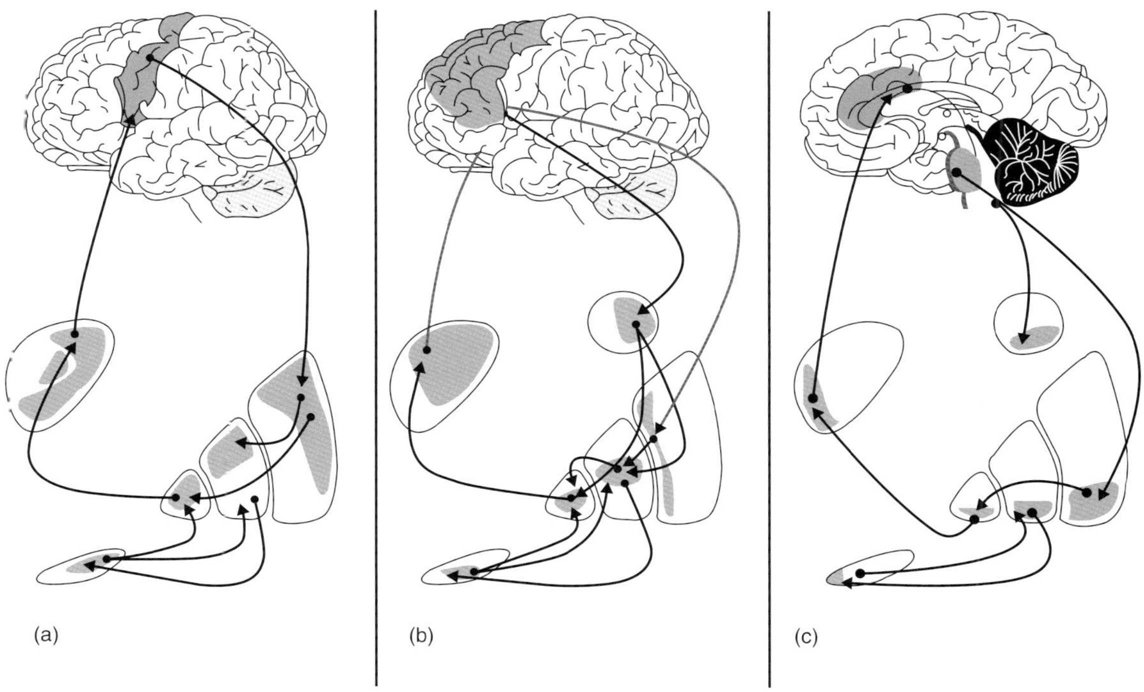

Figure 5.1 Functional division of the cortico-basal ganglia connections. (a) The motor loop, which involves the cortical motor areas (areas 4 and 6 and supplementary motor area), the posterolateral putamen, posterolateral globus pallidus pars externa and pars interna, the dorsolateral subthalamic nucleus, and the ventrolateral thalamus. The associative loop (b) and limbic loop (c) are also shown. Adapted from Cbeso *et al.* [1].

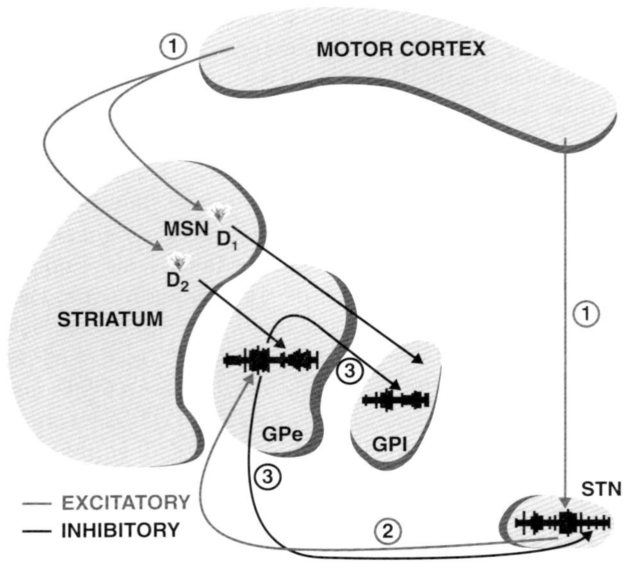

Figure 5.2 Summary of neurophysiologic events evoked by cortical activation. A cortical volley associated with movement initiation may presumably be dispatched simultaneously to the striatum and STN (step 1). One synapse later, the GPe and GPi are excited from the STN projection (step 2) and inhibited by the GABAergic–enkephalin projections from striatal medium spiny neurons in the "indirect pathway" and by the GABA striato-GPi projections in the "direct" pathway. A third synaptic connection (step 3) leads to inhibition of the STN and the GPi as a result of GPe firing in response to STN excitation. Minor changes in the excitability level of any one of these main nuclei may shift the predominant output of the basal ganglia to facilitation or inhibition. Dark arrows indicate GABAergic inhibition and light arrows glutamatergic excitation. Adapted from Obeso *et al.* [10].

are associated with decreased neuronal firing in the GPi prior to movement onset and a rebound in firing after movement initiation [13]. These observations led to the basic concept that reduced basal ganglia output leads to movement facilitation and increased activity to movement inhibition. According to this scheme, activation of corticostriatal–GPi activity (the direct pathway) facilitates a movement or an action, whereas activation of the cortico-STN–pallidal projection (the indirect pathway) is mainly inhibitory and restrains movements or actions.

The dopaminergic projection

DAergic mesencephalic neurons modulate basal ganglia excitability by two main systems: (1) the profuse DAergic nigrostriatal projection; and (2) extra-striatal fibers originating in the substantia nigra which project to the GPe, GPi, and STN. The ascending DAergic projections from ventral midbrain neurons are the only source of DA in the basal ganglia. These cells are located in the substantia nigra (A9 cell group), ventral tegmental area (A10), and retrorubral area (A8). The mesostriatal (or nigrostriatal) system is mainly composed of fibers originating from A9 cells. There are approximately 100 000 A9 neurons in the substantia nigra of each side in humans, each of which exhibits some 300 000 synaptic buttons, which densely innervate the striatum [14]. More than 90% of DA terminals form conventional synapses with the spines and dendrites of striatal projection neurons [15].

SNc neurons in the normal and awake monkey discharge continuously and sporadically at a low frequency (2–3 Hz) (tonic firing), but exhibit robust and highly synchronous burst firing in response to glutamate under special circumstances such as reward or anticipation of movement (phasic firing) [16]. Stable tonic firing is a fundamental characteristic of SNc neurons and is associated with continuous delivery of DA to the striatum. There is abundant experimental evidence indicating that DA exerts in the striatum both a neurotransmitter and a neuromodulatory function [15,16]. As a neurotransmitter, DA is released by action potentials, inducing a fast and short-lasting action restricted within the perisynaptic region [17]. As a neuromodulator, however, DA is released in the nonsynaptic extracellular space, inducing, after relatively lengthy diffusion, a slow, long-lasting, and widespread action that affects large striatal regions [18–20]. DAergic striatal activity, with either synaptic or extra-synaptic delivery, is finely tuned by pre-synaptic (i.e., SNc cell firing) and post-synaptic (i.e., re-uptake and metabolism) mechanisms [21–24] to provide relatively stable striatal dopamine levels. These ensure a continuous, albeit neither constant nor homogeneous, DAergic striatal effect. DA modulates the excitability of medium spiny striatal neurons primarily by exerting a filtering action and either enhancing or depressing specific subsets of cortico-striatal afferents [25,26]. Studies with organotypic cultures have shown that dopamine can facilitate or inhibit incoming striatal signals by activation of D-2 receptors located pre-synaptically on glutamatergic terminals [27].

DAergic neurons also innervate and modulate neuronal activity of other basal ganglia nuclei such as the GPe, STN, and GPi and also the thalamus and brainstem [28]. Changes in DA release on to these extra-striatal structures can modify the excitability and transmission of impulses through the different basal ganglia loops. For example, the importance of DAergic innervation of the GP and the reticularis nucleus of the thalamus [29] is illustrated by the fact that there is a direct projection from the GPe to the reticularis [30], a structure that can modify the excitability of specific thalamic nuclei which serve as a gating mechanism for afferent signals. Through this connection, DA and the GPe could modulate and sharpen the impact of the basal ganglia output on thalamocortical projections.

The parkinsonian state

The functional hallmarks of the parkinsonian state are striatal DA depletion and increased neuronal activity in the output nuclei of the basal ganglia. DA depletion leads to a series of functional changes that mediate the cardinal motor features of PD. The most important and characteristic feature is increased neuronal activity in the STN and GPi/SNr, leading to excessive inhibition of thalamocortical and brainstem motor nuclei [31,32]. There is a bulk of experimental and clinical evidence supporting this pathophysiologic feature of PD; indeed, the benefit achieved by lesions or DBS of the STN or GPi in PD patients provides strong support for the importance of this abnormality. On the other hand, a number of clinical features found in PD are not simply explained by increased neuronal activity in basal ganglia output nuclei. These range from the cardinal features of the disease such as tremor or rigidity, to the mechanisms responsible for fixed postures and the non-motor features of the disease such as pain and dementia.

The origin of sensory features in Parkinson's disease

Sensory symptoms in PD consist of pain, paresthesiae, itching, and burning sensations. These are typically focal and somatotopically distributed. For instance, pain is more common in the shoulder or in the foot. Burning more often affects the distal lower extremities. Sensory discomfort, associated with burning, pain, and other sensations, may be part of the restless leg syndrome, which is thought to occur with increased frequency in PD patients. Clinical examination of patients with these complaints typically fails to detect any defect of sensation, and peripheral nerve and central somatosensory conduction studies do not reveal any abnormality. Hence the origins of these manifestations are not believed to be a primary disorder of the somatosensory pathway.

The motor circuit through the basal ganglia is known to be somatotopically organized, and it is likely that the same is true with regard to the sensory system. The cortical motor areas (area 4, area 6, and supplementary motor area) and the primary somatosensory cortex project in a somatotopically organized fashion to the striatum (see Figure 5.3) [33]. The motor zone is situated in the dorsolateral region throughout the basal ganglia [34]. Conversely, no definite somatotopic arrangement has been found for the SNc and its nigrostriatal DAergic projection [14]. Less well appreciated or publicized is the existence of cortical projections from sensory areas, but this was the case for the motor system merely a decade ago, and it is certainly

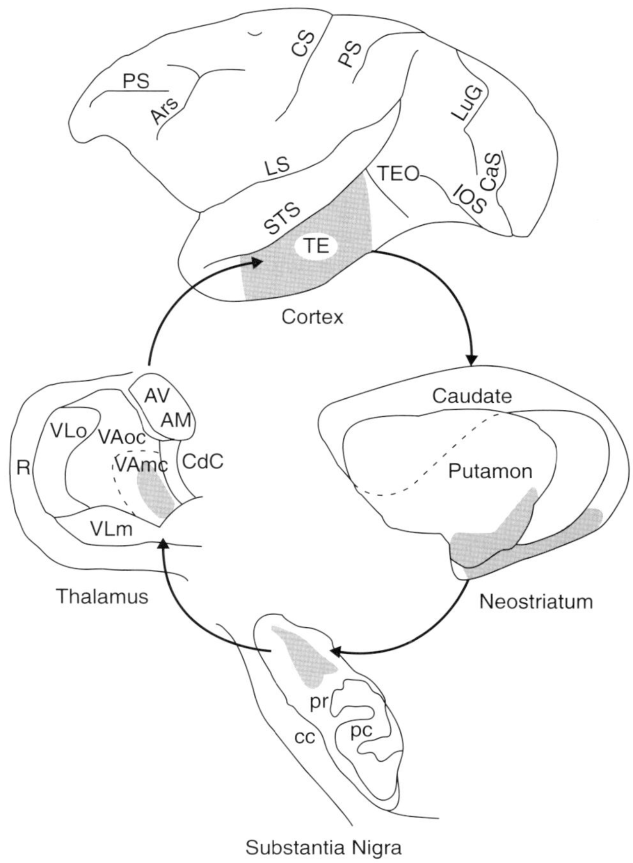

Figure 5.3 Visual loop: proposed loop for the processing of visual information by the basal ganglia. The circuit involves the cortical area TE (a higher visual association area), the posterior and ventral striatum, and the efferent substantia nigra pars reticulata that in turn projects to the thalamus and then back to the cortex. Note the similarities of this visual loop to the classical motor loop. Adapted from Middleton and Strick [34].

possible that there is somatotopic organization of sensory processing in the basal ganglia.

Somatosensory projections to the basal ganglia

Corticostriatal sensory pathways

Numerous studies in different mammalian species have demonstrated the presence of projections from the primary (SI) and secondary (SII) somatosensory cortices to the striatum. Neurophysiologic studies in both rats [36,37] and cats [38] have shown that there is activation of striatal neurons in response to somatosensory stimuli with different patterns depending on the nature of the stimulus. They found, for example, that some neurons discharged only in response to the stimulation of restricted corporal segments, whereas others responded to broader body segments, and yet others neurons were activated only when the stimulus was moving in a particular direction. A broad overlapping in the representation of the different corporal regions was observed [39].

Hoover, Hoffer, and Alloway [40], using anterograde tracers in the rat, demonstrated that there was overlap of somatosensory projections in the striatum from stimulation of different segments of the forelimb, but no overlap was found between different and distinct body parts such as the whiskers, forepaw, or hindpaw. Supported by these results, they proposed that the corticostriatal convergence in the neostriatum is based upon three principles: cortical proximity, somatotopic homology, and somatotopic continuity. According to these principles, the neurons originating in the somatosensory cortex in the rat are distributed to the neostriatum in an overlapping order. This arrangement could facilitate the functional integration at the striatal level of information proceeding from different cortical territories.

In the squirrel monkey, Flaherty and Graybiel [41], using electrophysiologic recording and anterograde tracer injections in the somatosensory cortex, evaluated the projections to the striatum. They demonstrated that neurons from different body regions send divergent projections which branch extensively and form patchy fields in the dorsal putamen. They found that there was no overlapping in those zones representing the foot, hand, or mouth, whereas overlapping was present in closely related areas such as the thumb and the fifth finger. This overlap was most predominant in the caudal putamen. They also found that regions from different zones of the somatosensory cortex representing distinct sensory modalities of the same regions of the body send convergent projections to the striatum, thereby facilitating multimodal sensory integration. On the basis of these findings, the authors suggested that convergence and transformation of the somatosensory cortical distribution could provide a basis for sensory modulation of motor output [41].

Studies using functional neuroimaging in humans and tracers in non-human primates have demonstrated that the sensory system is organized in the striatum is organized in a somatotopic arrangement [42–45], similar to what has been described for the motor system [46]. Thus, in both humans and monkeys, there is a foot–hand–face distribution along a dorsolateral to ventromedial gradient in which the foot is located dorsally, the face area ventrally and medially, and the hand area in between. This sensory representation is in marked proximity to the motor projections (frequently referred to as sensorimotor areas). There is considerable overlap between the somatotopic territories which may allow for interaction between information related to different body parts. In the putamen, the activated areas of the ipsi- and contralateral hand areas are not identical, suggesting a partial segregation of the ipsi- and contralateral striatal sensorimotor projections.

The interactions between the different striatal regions have also been explored. Haber, Fudge and McFarland [47] reviewed retrograde and anterograde tracing studies in non-human primates. They suggested that there was an interaction between the respective striatal regions that receive projections from the limbic, associative, and motor cortices by way of striatonigrostriatal (SNS) pathways. It is possible that a similar interaction could also occur for the sensory modalities represented in the striatum, which could explain the affective components of sensory perceptions.

In the cerebral cortex, a differential origin from the cortical layers is also a determinant of the destination of the pathways. Mercier, Clegg and Glickstein [48] have shown in the rat that the somatosensory (posteromedial barrel subfield) projections to basal ganglia arise in layer Va and consist of slow-conducting fibers, whereas projections to the cerebellum originate in layer Vb and are fast conducting.

Corticosubthalamic sensory pathways

Numerous studies have demonstrated that the STN in rodents and primates receives abundant projections from the pre-central, pre-motor, and pre-frontal cortices, [49–54]. However, there are few direct connections described between cortical non-motor areas and the STN [54]. Histologic studies indicate that projections arising from the visual and somatosensory cortices and directed to the STN are particularly sparse [55,56] and electrophysiological [57]. The role of the sensory cortico-subthalamic projections remains unclear [54]. Electrophysiologic studies in rats demonstrate convergence of information arising from stimulation of the motor, pre-frontal, and auditory cortices in the STN, suggesting an intermodal integrative role for this nucleus with respect to associative and limbic modalities [58].

Visual pathways

Middleton and Strick [34] have shown that in primates there is a connection between the substantia nigra pars reticulata and the inferotemporal cortex that extends through the thalamus. As the latter is a center for higher visual association, this suggests a role for the basal ganglia in the processing of visual information. This temporal cortical area also projects to the posterior striatum [59,60], which could give rise to a loop between the cortex, basal ganglia, thalamus, and cortex (Figure 5.3). This would provide an anatomic substrate for how the basal ganglia might process visual information. Another connection between SNpr and the anterior intraparietal cortex, an area devoted to seeing objects, has also been described in primates using modern radiotracer techniques with the rabies virus [61]. These findings emphasize that there are interconnections between visual circuits and the basal ganglia. A direct pathway from the retina though the superior colliculus to the substantia nigra pars compacta has also been described in the rat [62]. This projection synapses with both dopaminergic and non-dopaminergic neurons in the SNpc and could be involved in the fast detection and response to salient and unpredicted visual events.

Auditory pathways

Auditory connections with the basal ganglia have also been established in mammalians. Studies in cats have shown projections from the parieto-temporal cortices to the caudate nucleus and in particular to its ventral portion. However, in the monkey, studies have yielded conflicting results because only sparse connections have been demonstrated between the borders of the primary auditory cortices and the striatum, mainly the caudate nucleus [63]. Similar findings were reported by De la Mothe *et al.* [64] in marmosets. They found connections between the rostro-medial belt area and the tail of the caudate nucleus, but not between primary auditory cortices and striatum. Different results have been obtained in other mammalians. In the cat, Reale and Imig [65] showed the presence of cortical afferents from the cortical auditory cortices to the striatum in a topographical and tonotopical fashion. In humans, Prodoehl *et al.* [66], using fMRI techniques, found that visual and auditory feedback exert different influences over the activation of the basal ganglia. They found that the pattern of signal change measured by BOLD activation patterns in GPi and STN was altered by the type of feedback, being greater for auditory than visual feedback. These findings support the hypothesis that different kinds of sensory feedback can modify and in turn be processed within specific basal ganglia nuclei. This seems to be particularly relevant for both the GPi and STN. In rodents, neurophysiologic studies have demonstrated that auditory stimuli evoke responses in multisensory neurons [67]. These neurons are also activated by somatosensory stimulation in the caudate/putamen and GPi. The level of activation was higher when there was simultaneous stimulation with both modalities, supporting the likelihood that there is a multisensory integrative effect in the basal ganglia. In cats, Schneider [38] analyzed the activation of neurons in the dorsal lateral caudate nucleus of awake cats using different sensory modalities. They found that 22% of recorded neurons responded to tactile stimulation of the face, 7% had auditory responses, 6% had visual responses, and 6% were multimodal. In animals treated with MPTP, the results were similar if there were no motor features (asymptomatic group), but a marked decrease in the number of neurons responding to sensory stimuli was observed in those animals that experienced motor symptomatology (only 6% responded to somatosensory stimulation, 0.8% to auditory stimulation, and none to visual stimuli).

There is also evidence that auditory cortical fields project to the caudate and putamen in cats [65]. Anatomic connectivity studies are supported by several electrophysiologic studies which have recorded auditory-responsive neurons in the caudate, putamen, and globus pallidus [38,67]. Elegant work by Kolomiets *et al.* [58] on anesthetized rats showed that stimulating the auditory and motor cortex elicited converging responses on STN neurons, whereas different cells responded in the striatum. Other studies have reported that the regions functionally activated in the striatum with auditory stimuli represent only a partial component of the complete anatomic distribution of corticostriatal projections. These observations suggest that striatal activation following auditory stimuli is dependent on the behavioral context in which it occurs [68].

Pathophysiologic mechanisms and clinical relevance of sensory manifestations

The functional significance of sensory processing in the basal ganglia has not been clearly elucidated until now. It seems evident from the above anatomic summary that only a minority of the sensory modalities are processed independently, and most sensory processing seems to occur in a multimodal manner. Along these lines, Nagy *et al.* [69] have found evidence of multisensory function integration in caudate and substantia nigra neurons in the cat. They reported that activation of neurons in each of these nuclei occurs with visual, auditory, or tactile stimuli and the same neurons are affected in almost 50% of the cells. Similar interpretations have been observed in studies in the cat [38], monkey [41], and humans [66]. Accordingly, it has been proposed that the basal ganglia could exert a gating effect with integrative outputs based on sensory and motor input [70]. In PD, a dysfunction in the central processing of sensory information has been demonstrated [71,72]. It is plausible that the characteristic dopaminergic denervation in PD could alter sensory processing, inducing a disequilibrium in the parallel and convergent processing of the sensory information in the basal ganglia. This alteration could be responsible for the onset of abnormal perceptions, modification in the pain thresholds, alterations in temporal estimation, and the development of non-motor fluctuations related to dopaminergic stimulation. We shall review briefly the sensory fluctuations as an example of sensory disturbances in PD.

Non-motor fluctuations in Parkinson's disease

Fluctuations in non-motor features are a frequent complaint in PD, especially in those patients with advanced disease. Both pain and other non-painful sensory manifestations can fluctuate in PD, but pain is the aspect which has been best studied and most widely reported. Box 5.2 describes a classification of pain in PD based on its relationship to the dopaminergic status.

Witjas *et al.* [74] evaluated the presence of 54 non-motor manifestations in 50 PD patients, and found at least one symptom in all the subjects evaluated; the most frequent of these in their series were anxiety, drenching sweats, slowness of thinking, and fatigue. These fluctuations are mostly associated with the use of levodopa and dopaminergic agonists and they usually arise and progress in relationship to motor fluctuations. Racette *et al.* [75] evaluated the prevalence of mood fluctuations in 70 PD patients and found that 6.6% of this population said that they were affected by mood fluctuations. In comparison with those without fluctuations, this group had a significantly younger age at onset and longer disease duration and was significantly more likely to have dementia, psychosis, clinical depression, and fluctuations in motor symptoms.

The pathophysiology of non-motor fluctuations remains elusive. The variation observed in relation to dopaminergic treatment suggests that dopaminergic innervation may play some role in their physiopathology. In this respect, there is clinical evidence suggesting that non-motor fluctuations follow a similar pattern to typical motor fluctuations. Pursiainen *et al.* [76] evaluated sweating in 16 PD patients who experienced wearing-off effects as compared with 15 PD patients who did not have motor fluctuations. Using an evaporimeter on three different areas of the body, they found that maximum sweating coincided with the worst off-periods as measured by the motor UPDRS, suggesting a relationship to dopamine deficiency in the off state. However, patients without motor fluctuations had no change in sweating after a dose of levodopa. The authors suggested that differences in these groups could be accounted for by the possibility that thermoregulatory dysfunction could be related to impairment of both central and peripheral central nervous system structures. A similar result was recently reported by Lim *et al.* [77], who evaluated the response to a painful stimulus in PD subjects classified according to whether they were stable responders, fluctuators, or dyskinetic patients. They found that subjects with dyskinesia showed a large increase in pain threshold (48%) and tolerance (66%) following a levodopa dose that was absent in stable responders. These observations raise the possibility that pain and dyskinesia may share a common pathophysiologic mechanism.

The pharmacologic response of non-motor fluctuations has been reported previously. In 1995, Maricle *et al.* [78] reported a levodopa dose-related improvement in mood and anxiety in PD fluctuators. Fetoni *et al.* [79] also showed a significant improvement in symptoms of depression and anxiety in PD patients after a levodopa dose as compared with a poor response in patients with multiple system atrophy. Interestingly, recent studies have reported a reduction in non-motor fluctuations with continuous dopaminergic stimulation [80], which supports a role for discontinuous or pulsatile, non-physiologic replacement of dopamine in the origin of these complications, as has been suggested for the motor features of PD [81]. In their study, Eggert *et al.* [80] reported an improvement in motor and non-motor

Box 5.2 Classification of pain associated with Parkinson's disease.

A **Pain preceding diagnosis of Parkinson's disease**
1. Focal, i.e., shoulder or foot pain
2. Pseudo-radicular

B **Off-period pain (without dystonia) in patients with a fluctuating response to levodopa**
1. Morning pain
2. Wearing-off pain
3. Diphasic (beginning and end-of-dose) pain

C **Painful dystonic spasms**[a]
1. Early-morning dystonia
2. Off-period dystonia
3. Diphasic dystonia + pain

D **"On" medication "peak-dose" pain**

[a]Pain almost always coincides with body region affected by dystonia.
Source: Adapted from Quinn *et al.* [73].

fluctuations in 13 patients when they were switched to levodopa infusion as compared with standard oral treatments. These benefits were most noted with respect to anxiety and sleep disturbances, and a similar finding was reported by Isacson *et al.* in 12 patients following a continuous levodopa infusion for 6 months [82]. They found an improvement in quality of life and mood swings, but to a lesser extent than in motor symptoms and motor fluctuations.

There have been no published studies, to our knowledge, that report on neurophysiologic or molecular findings associated with non-motor fluctuations. All the structures supplied by dopaminergic innervation are possible candidates for the origin of the non-motor fluctuations in PD that appear to be improved with dopaminergic therapies. Dopaminergic neurotransmission is diffusely present in cortical and subcortical regions of the brain [83], and the importance of how dopamine is restored with respect to these systems has not been investigated. One of the limitations hindering our understanding of the physiologic origins of non-motor fluctuations is the lack of a reliable model for any of these manifestations.

Sensory dysfunction in other diseases of the basal ganglia

In addition to the sensory alterations observed in PD, other basal ganglia diseases are characterized by alterations in the processing of sensory information. In torsion dystonia, Bara-Jimenez *et al.* [84] showed that the pattern of sensory representation (homuncular organization) is altered in the primary somatosensory cortex of patients with focal dystonia of the hand. Similar results have been obtained with functional neuroimaging studies [85]. In Huntington's disease, Lawrence *et al.* [86] described alterations in visual processing, reinforcing the likelihood that the basal ganglia play an important role in visual processing, especially in context-dependent processing. Dysfunction of a temporo-basal ganglia loop could also be involved in the origin of peduncular hallucinosis, a condition observed in patients with lesions of the brainstem, thalamus, or thalamocapsular regions [87]. Dysfunction or hyperactivation of this circuit has also been proposed as an explanation for hallucinations that occur in other conditions such as Charles Bonnet syndrome and possibly PD itself [88].

Non-dopaminergic motor manifestations

Long-term evolution of PD is associated with a range of motor abnormalities which respond poorly or not at all to dopaminergic drugs and are therefore considered to be non-dopaminergic features. These include dysarthria, diplopia, gait disturbances, and postural abnormalities such as neck flexion, camptocormia, scoliosis, hand (Phakir's hand) and foot deformities. The pathophysiologic bases of these motor manifestations are not well understood and may vary for each of the different clinical signs. For instance, abnormal axial or distal limb postural abnormalities are probably associated with a reduction in or loss of necessary muscular tone in opposing back, neck, or intrinsic hand muscles, leading to skeletal deformities. These probably have a central origin and may even be directly related to basal ganglia dysfunction, as they can also be encountered after a focal lenticular lesion (i.e., stroke) [89], or bilateral striatal (i.e., Wilson's disease) or pallidal (i.e., anoxia, cyanide, and CO poisoning) lesions [90]. The precise pathophysiologic basis of these problems is not known, although it is noteworthy that these types of problems were much more frequent prior to the introduction of levodopa for PD treatment [90].

Gait impairment, freezing of gait (FOG), and disequilibrium deserve special attention. They can represent a major source of disability in PD, leading to frequent falls with associated skeletal injuries, and create a high caregiver burden and large economic cost. Clinically, FOG can include (1) start hesitation, which is a problem limited to initial stepping, (2) trepidation or freezing when turning or going through a doorway or another narrow space, and (3) actual freezing when walking, with a transient (seconds to minutes) inability to walk. These are probably all manifestations of the same problem, which in mild forms may seem to express independently. Either in partial or full form, an essential feature of FOG in PD is its remarkable capacity to improve with visual cues while at the same time having a high sensitivity to be triggered or worsened by visual input. FOG can also be induced by the subject attempting to undertake other movements with the upper limb or face, such as saluting or talking while walking. These features essentially underlie the marked difficulty that PD patients have in trying to undertake simultaneous or sequential tasks and are all thought to be intimately associated with basal ganglia dysfunction [91,92].

The mechanisms responsible for gait initiation and rhythmic stepping are complex and only starting to be understood (for a review, see [93]). The control of locomotion may be separated into three different steps. (1) *The initiation process*, which depends upon activation of the cerebral motor cortical areas which are required for the voluntary control of gait and limbic areas which are involved in the emotional components of walking (i.e., fear, escaping maneuvers, etc.). Gait also requires activation of the supplementary motor area (SMA). For example, reversible blockade of the SMA with the GABA agonist muscimol has been shown to disturb postural control during walking in monkeys [94]. In humans, lesion of pre-motor areas have also been reported to be associated with FOG and disequilibrium [95]. 2. *The regulation process*, whereby basal ganglia and cerebellar cortical loops regulate the parameters of locomotion. It is noteworthy that cerebellar lesions are not associated with FOG but with other features related to walking such as postural instability, impaired adjustment, and coordination problems. 3. *Basic locomotion execution*, which depends upon brainstem and spinal mechanisms regulating rhythm generation and muscle tone. Indeed, an overall analysis of the importance of the basal ganglia-brainstem connections in the control and automatic regulation of locomotion has led to the recognition that lesions of the pedunculopontine nucleus (PPN) and mesencephalic locomotor region (MLR) [93] likely play a key role in the development of gait problems in PD. The PPN is reciprocally connected with the basal ganglia [53]. There is a dense GABAergic projection from the globus pallidus and substantia nigra reticulata to the PPN, which in turn sends glutamatergic efferents to the STN and SNc [53]. In the cat, repetitive stimulation of the SNr modulates the rythmic activation of limb movements. This is mediated by the mesencephalic locomotor region and can be blocked by PPN-induced muscle tone suppression [96]. This suggests that increased activity in basal ganglia output directed towards these brainstem centers may underlie the termination of locomotion, which in animals is also associated with increased muscle tone. Recently, a case of failure of gait induced by a bilateral PPN stroke was described, supporting the central role of this structure in the control of gait [97].

The importance of the PPN in gait control was first suggested by the experimental demonstration that decerebrate cats were able to walk automatically following stimulation of the MLR (which includes both the PPN and the cuneiform nucleus) [98]. However, this function seems to be fully developed only in higher primates, as demonstrated by the fact that bilateral lesions of the PPN in rats has failed to induce spontaneous alterations in locomotor activity, though some changes can be detected in motor activity in response to pharmacologic stimuli [99]. The PPN has also been implicated in the control of the sleep–wake cycle [100], reward, and attention. However, the PPN is a complex and diffuse structure which is made up of many parts and surrounded by several other nuclei. It is therefore difficult to establish precise anatomico-functional correlations with individual signs and symptoms that occur in PD. Moreover, most functional studies regarding gait have been performed in quadruped animals, which may not share exactly the same anatomic and physiologic organization required for bipedal stance and gait.

Despite the limitations in our current knowledge and the implicit caution in making interpretations, the above-summarized data provide some hints towards understanding the interaction between the basal ganglia and brainstem in PD. Thus, it can be hypothesized that in the parkinsonian state the increased efferent (i.e., inhibitory) activity from the basal ganglia output nuclei [4] could lead to excessive inhibition of brainstem nuclei such as the PPN and MLR, with reduced facilitation of spinal cord pattern generators and a consequent impairment in gait initiation and locomotion. Admittedly, however, such a relationship has not been properly established and requires further testing. Studies in normal and parkinsonian non-human primates provide some support for this concept. Thus, a decrease of neuronal activity in the PPN has been demonstrated in MPTP monkeys, as evidenced by reductions in immunostaining for cytochrome oxidase and choline acetyltransferase and *in situ* hybridization measures of substance PD [101]. Further, in normal monkeys, selective PPN ablation, with preservation of fibers of passage, induced akinesia that resolved spontaneously over time with unilateral but not bilateral lesions [102]. Other studies have provided conflicting results. In the MPTP monkey, blockade of GABAergic neurotransmission in the PPN nuclei with biccuculine improved motor activity [103]. Physiologically, PPN neurons in PD patients, and also in patients with progressive supranuclear palsy, respond to contralateral active or passive limb movements in a proportion (about 30%) and there is also beta band activity (15–30 Hz) in close similarity with typical findings in the STN [104].

PPN neuronal loss has been reported in PD patients [105], in marked contrast to the absence of neuronal loss that has been reported with normal aging [106]. A relationship between the degree of PPN neuronal loss and gait dysfunction has been reported in PD [107], and cholinergic cell loss in the pedunculopontine tegmental nucleus has been reported to be related to disease severity [108], although the overall loss is comparatively mild and associated with the degree of SNc loss [109].

All of the above and the lack of effective treatments for a large number of patients with FOG and gait dysfunction in PD have led to consideration of DBS of the PPN region as a therapeutic option. In normal monkeys, PPN stimulation at 45–100 Hz induced akinesia and postural instability, whereas lower frequency stimulation induced slow arm tremor [110]. However, Mazzone *et al.* [111] reported the safety and short-term efficacy of PPN DBS in PD patients with gait impairment. Later, the same group compared the effects of STN and PPN DBS and reported improvements, particularly with respect to gait and axial symptoms, using PPN DBS with a stimulation rate of 25 Hz. This benefit was further enhanced when stimulation of the PPN was combined with dopaminergic therapy and was much greater than that observed with stimulation of the STN either alone or in combination with anti-parkinsonian medications [112]. Interestingly, spinal reflex excitability as assessed by the soleus–Hoffman reflex (HR) threshold can be normalized with PPN DBS alone or in combination with STN DBS, but not with levodopa therapy, suggesting that PPN affects spinal excitability [113].

In summary, whether or not FOG is really a non-DAergic motor problem is unanswered. This is not only a theoretical question but also a practical one. Because FOG is more often seen after long-term disease evolution, there is a tendency to associate it with spread of disease pathology. Clinical observation indicates that off-period FOG responds initially to levodopa and other DAergic drugs and also to deep brain stimulation of the subthalamic nucleus [114,115]. On the other hand, in a proportion of patients, FOG occurs during "on" periods and "off" period FOG is not resolved by tolerable amounts of DAergic drugs. In our experience, this often coincides with the development of postural instability and some degree of attention/cognitive impairment. Based on the above, we propose that FOG can have two different mechanisms/phases: (1) walking problems that are related to functional changes in the BG secondary to DA deficiency leading to hyper-inhibition of brainstem mechanisms mediating locomotion; and (2) spreading of neurodegeneration to affect directly brainstem nuclei and their efferents including descending reticulo-spinal projections and also ascending projections to the thalamus and cerebral cortex. This might explain the common association between FOG and attention/cognitive problems. The former is responsive to DAergic drugs and STN/GPi surgery and can be improved with visual cues whereas the latter is not. The association between FOG and disequilibrium likely relates to the fact that the initial phase of stepping is associated with changes in the center of gravity that are normally compensated for by anticipatory postural reflexes. Without adequate adjustment of equilibrium, the sequence of muscle synergies underlying step initiation is not possible and gait initiation is inevitably impaired.

Conclusions

Most interest in the physiology of PD has focused on the motor system. Here we have made great progress in understanding the basic mechanisms underlying the classic features of the disease and also those which underlie levodopa-induced dyskinesia. This understanding has in turn led to the introduction of more effective medical and surgical therapies which now benefit tens of thousands of PD patients. Only now are we beginning to appreciate the importance of the non-dopaminergic and non-motor features of PD, and the role that they play as a cause of disability in advanced patients. Neurophysiology now needs to focus its attention on these problems in an effort to understand better their pathophysiology and their relationship, if any, to the dopamine system. This has begun to occur with respect to the sensory system and it is anticipated that more information will quickly follow. It is hoped that this will lead to better insight into the organization of the basal ganglia and how it relates to these non-dopaminergic and non-motor features, how these systems become impaired in PD, and the development of novel therapeutic strategies. For the time being, we can summarize the state of our knowledge as follows:

1 Sensory pathways which extend from the primary or associative cortices to the basal ganglia are well characterized for the somatosensory, visual, and auditory systems. These pathways provide an anatomic basis for appreciating that the basal ganglia likely play an important role in the processing of sensory in addition to motor information.

2 Circuits duplicating the classical cortex–basal ganglia–thalamus–cortex motor loops are also present for sensory systems and presumably permit the processing of sensory information in the basal ganglia.

3 The convergence–divergence principle seems to be involved in the integration and regulation of sensory modalities in the basal ganglia. Context-guided processing appears to be a major component of how the basal ganglia analyze and relay sensory information. However, the precise mechanisms of how sensory information is processed in the basal ganglia and the role it plays in disease states remains elusive for the present.

4 The clinical pattern and evolution of non-motor features in PD and the corresponding pathologic changes are beginning to be delineated, but further work is required for them to be fully elucidated.

5 The origin of gait dysfunction and other motor manifestations of PD that do not respond or do not adequately respond to DAergic drugs is far from clear. Studies examining the role of brainstem nuclei such as the PPN in gait dysfunction and freezing of gait have attracted considerable attention and represent a framework for further studies.

References

1. Obeso JA, Rodriguez-Oroz MC, Benitez-Temino B, *et al.* Functional organization of the basal ganglia: therapeutic implications for Parkinson's disease. *Mov Disord* 2008;**23**(Suppl 3):S548–59.
2. Obeso JA, Marín C, Rodriguez-Oroz MC, *et al.* The basal ganglia in Parkinson's disease: current concepts and unexplained observations. *Ann Neurol* 2008;**64**:S30–46.
3. Marsden CD, Obeso JA. The functions of the basal ganglia and the paradox of stereotaxic surgery in Parkinson's disease. *Brain* 1994;**117**:877–97.

4. Obeso JA, Rodriguez-Oroz MC, Rodriguez M, *et al.* Pathophysiology of the basal ganglia in Parkinson's disease. *Trends Neurosci* 2000;**23**:S8–19.
5. Hikosaka O, Nakamura K, Sakai K, Nakahara H. Central mechanisms of motor skill learning. *Curr Opin Neurobiol* 2002;**12**:217–22.
6. Pasupathy A, Miller EK. Different time courses of learning-related activity in the prefrontal cortex and striatum. *Nature* 2005;**433**:873–6.
7. Seger CA. The basal ganglia in human learning. *Neuroscientist* 2006;**12**:285–90.
8. Yin HH, Knowlton BJ. The role of the basal ganglia in habit formation. *Nat Rev Neurosci* 2006;**7**:464–76.
9. Nambu A. A new dynamic model of the cortico-basal ganglia loop. *Prog Brain Res* 2004;**143**:461–6.
10. Obeso JA, Rodriguez-Oroz MC, Javier Blesa F, Guridi J. The globus pallidus pars externa and Parkinson's disease. ready for prime time? *Exp Neurol* 2006;**202**:1–7.
11. Kita H. Globus pallidus external segment. *Prog Brain Res* 2007;**160**:111–33.
12. Hikosaka O, Wurtz RH. Visual and oculomotor functions of monkey substantia nigra pars reticulata. III. memory-contingent visual and saccade responses. *J Neurophysiol* 1983;**49**:1268–84.
13. Turner RS, Anderson ME. Context-dependent modulation of movement-related discharge in the primate globus pallidus. *J Neurosci* 2005;**25**:2965–76.
14. . Bentivoglio M, Morelli M. Dopamine. In: Dunnett SB, Bentivoglio M, Björklund A, and Hökfelt T, eds. *Handbook of Chemical Neuroanatomy. Vol. 21. Dopamine*. Amsterdam: Elsevier, 2005: 1–107.
15. Smith Y, Bennett BD, Bolam JP, *et al.* Synaptic relationships between dopaminergic afferents and cortical or thalamic input in the sensorimotor territory of the striatum in monkey. *J Comp Neurol* 1994;**344**:1–19.
16. Schultz W. Predictive reward signal of dopamine neurons. *J Neurophysiol* 1998;**80**:1–27.
17. Abercrombie ED, DeBoer P, Heeringa MJ. Biochemistry of somatodendritic dopamine release in substantia nigra: an *in vivo* comparison with striatal dopamine release. *Adv Pharmacol* 1998;**42**:133–6.
18. Descarries L, Watkins KC, Garcia S, *et al.* Dual character, asynaptic and synaptic, of the dopamine innervation in adult rat neostriatum: a quantitative autoradiographic and immunocytochemical analysis. *J Comp Neurol* 1996;**375**: 167–86.
19. Gonon F. Prolonged and extrasynaptic excitatory action of dopamine mediated by D1 receptors in the rat striatum *in vivo*. *J Neurosci* 1997;**17**:5972–8.
20. Kawagoe KT, Garris PA, Wiedemann DJ, Wightman RM. Regulation of transient dopamine concentration gradients in the microenvironment surrounding nerve terminals in the rat striatum. *Neuroscience* 1992;**51**:55–64.
21. Hefti F, Enz A, Melamed E. Partial lesions of the nigrostriatal pathway in the rat. acceleration of transmitter synthesis and release of surviving dopaminergic neurones by drugs. *Neuropharmacology* 1985;**24**:19–23.
22. Rodriguez M, Gonzalez J, Sabate M, *et al.* Firing regulation in dopaminergic cells: effect of the partial degeneration of nigrostriatal system in surviving neurons. *Eur J Neurosci* 2003;**18**:53–60.
23. Rodriguez M, Pereda E, Gonzalez J, *et al.* How is firing activity of substantia nigra cells regulated? Relevance of pattern-code in the basal ganglia. *Synapse* 2003;**49**:216–25.
24. Rodriguez M, Morales I, Gonzalez-Mora JL, *et al.* Different levodopa actions on the extracellular dopamine pools in the rat striatum. *Synapse* 2007;**61**:61–71.
25. Bamford NS, Zhang H, Schmitz Y, *et al.* Heterosynaptic dopamine neurotransmission selects sets of corticostriatal terminals. *Neuron* 2004;**42**:653–63.
26. Onn SP, West AR, Grace AA. Dopamine-mediated regulation of striatal neuronal and network interactions. *Trends Neurosci* 2000;**23**:S48–56.
27. Bamford NS, Robinson S, Palmiter RD, *et al.* Dopamine modulates release from corticostriatal terminals. *J Neurosci* 2004;**24**:9541–52.
28. Sanchez-Gonzalez MA, Garcia-Cabezas MA, Rico B, Cavada C. The primate thalamus is a key target for brain dopamine. *J Neurosci* 2005;**25**:6076–83.
29. Anaya-Martinez V, Martinez-Marcos A, Martinez-Fong D, *et al.* Substantia nigra compacta neurons that innervate the reticular thalamic nucleus in the rat also project to striatum or globus pallidus: implications for abnormal motor behavior. *Neuroscience* 2006;**143**:477–86.
30. Hazrati LN, Parent A. Projection from the external pallidum to the reticular thalamic nucleus in the squirrel monkey. *Brain Res* 1991;**550**:142–6.
31. DeLong MR. Primate models of movement disorders of basal ganglia origin. *Trends Neurosci* 1990;**13**:281–5.
32. Hirsch EC, Perier C, Orieux G, *et al.* Metabolic effects of nigrostriatal denervation in basal ganglia. *Trends Neurosci* 2000;**23**:S78–85.
33. Takada M, Tokuno H, Nambu A, Inase M. Corticostriatal input zones from the supplementary motor area overlap those from the contra- rather than ipsilateral primary motor cortex. *Brain Res* 1998;**791**:335–40.
34. Middleton FA, Strick PL. The temporal lobe is a target of output from the basal ganglia. *Proc Natl Acad Sci USA* 1996;**93**:8683–7.
35. DeLong MR, Georgopoulos AP. Motor functions of the basal ganglia as revealed by studies of single cell activity in the behaving primate. *Adv Neurol* 1979;**24**:131–40.
36. Carelli RM, West MO. Representation of the body by single neurons in the dorsolateral striatum of the awake, unrestrained rat. *J Comp Neurol* 1991;**309**:231–49.
37. Chudler EH, Dong WK. The role of the basal ganglia in nociception and pain. *Pain* 1995;**60**:3–38.
38. Schneider JS. Responses of striatal neurons to peripheral sensory stimulation in symptomatic MPTP-exposed cats. *Brain Res* 1991;**544**:297–302.
39. Sedgwick EM, Williams TD. The response of single units in the caudate nucleus to peripheral stimulation. *J Physiol* 1967;**189**:281–98.
40. Hoover JE, Hoffer ZS, Alloway KD. Projections from primary somatosensory cortex to the neostriatum: The role of somatotopic continuity in corticostriatal convergence. *J Neurophysiol* 2003;**89**:1576–87.

41. Flaherty AW, Graybiel AM. Corticostriatal transformations in the primate somatosensory system. projections from physiologically mapped body-part representations. *J Neurophysiol* 1991;**66**:1249–63.
42. Flaherty AW, Graybiel AM. Two input systems for body representations in the primate striatal matrix: experimental evidence in the squirrel monkey. *J Neurosci* 1993;**13**:1120–37.
43. Alexander GE, DeLong MR. Microstimulation of the primate neostriatum. II. Somatotopic organization of striatal microexcitable zones and their relation to neuronal response properties. *J Neurophysiol* 1985;**53**:1417–30.
44. Kunzle H. Projections from the primary somatosensory cortex to basal ganglia and thalamus in the monkey. *Exp Brain Res* 1977;**30**:481–92.
45. Liles SL, Updyke BV. Projection of the digit and wrist area of precentral gyrus to the putamen: relation between topography and physiological properties of neurons in the putamen. *Brain Res* 1985;**339**:245–55.
46. Gerardin E, Lehericy S, Pochon JB, *et al.* Foot, hand, face and eye representation in the human striatum. *Cereb Cortex* 2003;**13**:162–9.
47. Haber SN, Fudge JL, McFarland NR. Striatonigrostriatal pathways in primates form an ascending spiral from the shell to the dorsolateral striatum. *J Neurosci* 2000;**20**:2369–82.
48. Mercier BE, Legg CR, Glickstein M. Basal ganglia and cerebellum receive different somatosensory information in rats. *Proc Natl Acad Sci USA* 1990;**87**:4388–92.
49. Brown LL. Somatotopic organization in rat striatum: Evidence for a combinational map. *Proc Natl Acad Sci USA* 1992; **89**:7403–7.
50. Hamani C, Saint-Cyr JA, Fraser J, *et al.* The subthalamic nucleus in the context of movement disorders. *Brain* 2004;**127**: 4–20.
51. Kunzle H. An autoradiographic analysis of the efferent connections from premotor and adjacent prefrontal regions (areas 6 and 9) in macaca fascicularis. *Brain Behav Evol* 1978;**15**:185–234.
52. Monakow KH, Akert K, Kunzle H. Projections of the precentral motor cortex and other cortical areas of the frontal lobe to the subthalamic nucleus in the monkey. *Exp Brain Res* 1978;**33**:395–403.
53. Parent A, Hazrati LN. Functional anatomy of the basal ganglia. I. The cortico-basal ganglia-thalamo-cortical loop. *Brain Res Brain Res Rev* 1995;**20**:91–127.
54. Romanelli P, Esposito V, Schaal DW, Heit G. Somatotopy in the basal ganglia: experimental and clinical evidence for segregated sensorimotor channels. *Brain Res Brain Res Rev* 2005;**48**:112–28.
55. Afsharpour S. Topographical projections of the cerebral cortex to the subthalamic nucleus. *J Comp Neurol* 1985;**236**:14–28.
56. Carpenter MB, Carleton SC, Keller JT, Conte P. Connections of the subthalamic nucleus in the monkey. *Brain Res* 1981;**224**:1–29.
57. DeLong MR, Crutcher MD, Georgopoulos AP. Primate globus pallidus and subthalamic nucleus: functional organization. *J Neurophysiol* 1985;**53**:530–43.
58. Kolomiets BP, Deniau JM, Mailly P, *et al.* Segregation and convergence of information flow through the cortico-subthalamic pathways. *J Neurosci* 2001;**21**:5764–72.
59. Francois C, Yelnik J, Percheron G, Fenelon G. Topographic distribution of the axonal endings from the sensorimotor and associative striatum in the macaque pallidum and substantia nigra. *Exp Brain Res* 1994;**102**:305–18.
60. Parent A, Bouchard C, Smith Y. The striatopallidal and striatonigral projections: two distinct fiber systems in primate. *Brain Res* 1984;**303**:385–90.
61. Clower DM, Dum RP, Strick PL. Basal ganglia and cerebellar inputs to "AIP". *Cereb Cortex* 2005;**15**:913–20.
62. Comoli E, Coizet V, Boyes J, *et al.* A direct projection from superior colliculus to substantia nigra for detecting salient visual events. *Nat Neurosci* 2003;**6**:974–80.
63. Borgmann S, Jurgens U. Lack of cortico-striatal projections from the primary auditory cortex in the squirrel monkey. *Brain Res* 1999;**836**:225–8.
64. de la Mothe LA, Blumell S, Kajikawa Y, Hackett TA. Cortical connections of the auditory cortex in marmoset monkeys: core and medial belt regions. *J Comp Neurol* 2006;**496**: 27–71.
65. Reale RA, Imig TJ. Auditory cortical field projections to the basal ganglia of the cat. *Neuroscience* 1983;**8**:67–86.
66. Prodoehl J, Yu H, Wasson P, *et al.* Effects of visual and auditory feedback on sensorimotor circuits in the basal ganglia. *J Neurophysiol* 2008;**99**:3042–51.
67. Chudler EH, Sugiyama K, Dong WK. Multisensory convergence and integration in the neostriatum and globus pallidus of the rat. *Brain Res* 1995;**674**:33–45.
68. Brown LL, Schneider JS, Lidsky TI. Sensory and cognitive functions of the basal ganglia . *Curr Opin Neurobiol* 1997;**7**:157–63.
69. Nagy A, Eordegh G, Paroczy Z, *et al.* Multisensory integration in the basal ganglia. *Eur J Neurosci* 2006;**24**:917–24.
70. Lidsky TI, Manetto C, Schneider JS. A consideration of sensory factors involved in motor functions of the basal ganglia. *Brain Res* 1985;**356**:133–46.
71. Boecker H, Ceballos-Baumann A, Bartenstein P, *et al.* Sensory processing in Parkinson's and Huntington's disease: investigations with 3D H(2)(15)O-PET. *Brain* 1999;**122**:1651–65.
72. Seiss E, Praamstra P, Hesse CW, Rickards H. Proprioceptive sensory function in Parkinson's disease and Huntington's disease: evidence from proprioception-related EEG potentials. *Exp Brain Res* 2003;**148**:308–19.
73. Quinn NP, Koller WC, Lang AE, Marsden CD. Painful Parkinson's disease. *Lancet* 1986;**i**:1366–9.
74. Witjas T, Kaphan E, Azulay JP, *et al.* Nonmotor fluctuations in Parkinson's disease: frequent and disabling. *Neurology* 2002;**59**:408–13.
75. Racette BA, Hartlein JM, Hershey T, *et al.* Clinical features and comorbidity of mood fluctuations in Parkinson's disease. *J Neuropsychiatry Clin Neurosci* 2002;**14**:438–42.
76. Pursiainen V, Haapaniemi TH, Korpelainen JT, *et al.* Sweating in parkinsonian patients with wearing-off. *Mov Disord* 2007;**22**:828–32.
77. Lim SY, Farrell MJ, Gibson SJ, *et al.* Do dyskinesia and pain share common pathophysiological mechanisms in Parkinson's disease? *Mov Disord* 2008;**23**:1689–95.
78. Maricle RA, Nutt JG, Valentine RJ, Carter JH. Dose–response relationship of levodopa with mood and anxiety in fluctuating

Parkinson's disease: a double-blind, placebo-controlled study. *Neurology* 1995;**45**:1757–60.
79. Fetoni V, Soliveri P, Monza D, *et al*. Affective symptoms in multiple system atrophy and Parkinson's disease: response to levodopa therapy. *J Neurol Neurosurg Psychiatry* 1999;**66**:541–4.
80. Eggert K, Schrader C, Hahn M, *et al*. Continuous jejunal levodopa infusion in patients with advanced Parkinson disease: practical aspects and outcome of motor and non-motor complications. *Clin Neuropharmacol* 2008;**31**:151–66.
81. Olanow CW, Obeso JA, Stocchi F. Continuous dopamine receptor stimulation in the treatment of Parkinson's disease: scientific rationale and clinical implications. *Lancet Neurol* 2006;**5**:677–87.
82. Isacson D, Bingefors K, Kristiansen IS, Nyholm D. Fluctuating functions related to quality of life in advanced Parkinson disease: effects of duodenal levodopa infusion. *Acta Neurol Scand* 2008;**118**:379–86.
83. Bjorklund A, Dunnett SB. Dopamine neuron systems in the brain: an update. *Trends Neurosci* 2007;**30**:194–202.
84. Bara-Jimenez W, Catalan MJ, Hallett M, Gerloff C. Abnormal somatosensory homunculus in dystonia of the hand. *Ann Neurol* 1998;**44**:828–31.
85. Butterworth S, Francis S, Kelly E, *et al*. Abnormal cortical sensory activation in dystonia: an fMRI study. *Mov Disord* 2003;**18**:673–82.
86. Lawrence AD, Watkins LH, Sahakian BJ, *et al*. Visual object and visuospatial cognition in Huntington's disease: implications for information processing in corticostriatal circuits. *Brain* 2000;**123**(Pt 7):1349–64.
87. Benke T. Peduncular hallucinosis: a syndrome of impaired reality monitoring. *J Neurol* 2006;**253**:1561–71.
88. Adachi N, Watanabe T, Matsuda H, Onuma T. Hyperperfusion in the lateral temporal cortex, the striatum and the thalamus during complex visual hallucinations: single photon emission computed tomography findings in patients with Charles Bonnet syndrome. *Psychiatry Clin Neurosci* 2000;**54**:157–62.
89. Marsden CD, Obeso JA, Zarranz JJ, Lang AE. The anatomical basis of symptomatic hemidystonia. *Brain* 1985;**108**:463–83.
90. Denny-Brown D, Yanagisawa N. The role of the basal ganglia in the initiation of movement. In: Yahr MD, ed. *The Basal Ganglia*. New York: Raven Press, 1976: 115–49.
91. Marsden CD. The mysterious motor function of the basal ganglia: The Robert Wartenberg Lecture. *Neurology* 1982;**32**:514–39.
92. Haaxma R, van Boxtel A, Brouwer WH, *et al*. Motor function in a patient with bilateral lesions of the globus pallidus. *Mov Disord* 1995;**6**:761–77.
93. Takakusaki K, Tomita N, Yano M. Substrates for normal gait and pathophysiology of gait disturbances with respect to the basal ganglia dysfunction. *J Neurol* 2008;**255**:19–29.
94. Mori F, Nakajima K, Tachibana A, *et al*. Cortical mechanisms for the control of bipedal locomotion in Japanese monkeys: II. Local inactivation of the supplementary motor area (SMA). *Neurosci Res* 2003;**46**:S157.
95. Freund HJ, Hummelsheim H. Lesions of premotor cortex in man. *Brain* 1985;**108**:697–733.
96. Jenkinson N, Nandi D, Muthusamy K, *et al*. Anatomy, physiology and pathophysiology of the –ine nucleus. *Mov Disord* 2009;**15**:319–28.
97. Kuo SH, Kenney C, Jankovic J. Bilateral pedunculopontine nuclei strokes presenting as freezing of gait. *Mov Disord* 2008;**4**:616–9.
98. Shik ML, Severin FV, Orlovsky GN. Control of walking and running by means of electrical stimulation of the mid-brain. *Biophysics* 1966;**11**:756–65.
99. Winn, P. How best to consider the structure and function of the pedunculopontine tegmental nucleus: evidence from animal studies. *J Neurol Sci* 2006;**248**:234–50.
100. Rye DB. Contributions of the pedunculopontine region to normal and altered REM sleep. *Sleep* 1997;**20**:757–88.
101. Gomez-Gallego M, Fernandez-Villalba E, Fernandez-Barreiro A, Herrero MT. Changes in the neuronal activity in the pedunculopontine nucleus in chronic MPTP-treated primates: an *in situ* hybridization study of cytochrome oxidase subunit I, choline acetyltransferase and substance P mRNA expression. *J Neural Transm* 2007;**3**:319–26.
102. Munro-Davies LE, Winter J, Aziz TJ, Stein JF. The role of the pedunculopontine region in basal-ganglia mechanisms of akinesia. *Exp Brain Res* 1999;**129**:511–17.
103. Nandi D, Aziz TZ, Giladi N, *et al*. Reversal of akinesia in experimental parkinsonism by GABA antagonist microinjections in the pedunculopontine nucleus. *Brain* 2002;**125**:2418–30.
104. Weinberger M, Hamani C, Hutchison WD, *et al*. Pedunculopontine nucleus microelectrode recordings in movement disorder patients. *Exp Brain Res* 2008;**188**:165–74.
105. Hirsch EC, Graybiel AM, Duyckaerts C, Javoy-Agid FJ. Neuronal loss in the pedunculopontine tegmental nucleus in Parkinson disease and in progressive supranuclear palsy. *Proc Natl Acad Sci USA* 1987;**84**:5976–80.
106. Manaye KF, Zweig R, Wu D, *et al*. Quantification of cholinergic and select non-cholinergic mesopontine neuronal populations in the human brain. *Neuroscience* 1999;**89**:759–70.
107. Jellinger K. The pedunculopontine nucleus in Parkinson's disease, progressive supranuclear palsy and Alzheimer's disease. *J Neurol Neurosurg Psychiatry* 1988;**51**:540–3.
108. Rinne JO, Maa SY, Leed MY, *et al*. Loss of cholinergic neurons in the pedunculopontine nucleus in Parkinson's disease is related to disability of the patients. *Parkinsonism Relat Disord* 2008;**14**:553–7.
109. Zweig RM, Jankel WR, Hedreen JC, *et al*. The pedunculopontine nucleus in Parkinson's disease. *Ann Neurol* 1989;**26**:41–6.
110. Nandi D, Liu X, Winter J, *et al*. Deep brain stimulation of the pedunculopontine region in the normal non-human primate. *J Clin Neurosci* 2002;**9**:170–4.
111. Mazzone P, Lozano A, Stanzione P, *et al*. Implantation of human pedunculopontine nucleus: a safe and clinically relevant target in Parkinson's disease. *Neuroreport* 2005;**16**:1877–81.

112. Stefani A, Lozano AM, Peppe A, *et al.* Bilateral deep brain stimulation of the pedunculopontine and subthalamic nuclei in severe Parkinson's disease. *Brain* 2007;**130**:1596–607.
113. Pierantozzi M, Palmieri MG, Galati1 S, *et al.* Pedunculopontine nucleus deep brain stimulation changes spinal cord excitability in Parkinson's disease patients. *J Neural Transm* 2008;**115**:731–5.
114. Sethi K. Levodopa unresponsive symptoms in Parkinson disease. *Mov Disord* 2008;**23**:S521–33.
115. Stolze H, Klebe S, Poepping M, *et al.* Effects of bilateral subthalamic nucleus stimulation on parkinsonian gait. *Neurology* 2001;**57**:144–6.

Chapter 6
Anatomy and Physiology of Limbic System Dysfunction in Parkinson's Disease

Anthony A. Grace
Departments of Neuroscience, Psychiatry, and Psychology, University of Pittsburgh, Pittsburgh, PA, USA

Introduction

Parkinson's disease (PD) is characterized by a degenerative loss of the dopamine innervation of motor areas of the striatum [1]; as such, PD is often considered to be a disorder exclusively of movement. However, there is growing recognition that the degeneration of the dopamine neurons is accompanied by mental disruptions. Moreover, treatment of the motor deficits with dopaminergic drugs can itself lead to a different set of psychiatric reactions. This is due to an involvement of the mesolimbic/mesocortical dopamine system and the propensity of dopaminergic drugs to affect multiple components of the dopamine system beyond those that regulate movement.

Anatomy of the dopamine system

There are four major dopamine pathways in the brain that are named according to their site of origin and termination. These are the nigrostriatal pathway that originates in the substantia nigra and projects to the caudate-putamen; this is the system that degenerates in PD [1]. The mesolimbic system originates in the mesencephalon and projects to limbic brain regions, including the ventral striatum/nucleus accumbens, septum, amygdala, hippocampus, and other regions. The mesocortical system also originates in the mesencephalon, and projects strongly to the frontal cortices and also other neocortical regions. Finally, the tuberoinfundibular system originates in the hypothalamus and projects to the pituitary; this system controls release of prolactin and growth hormone. This chapter focuses primarily on the nigrostriatal and mesolimbic/mesocortical dopamine systems, since these systems are most potently affected by drugs used in the treatment of PD.

Physiology of the dopamine system

Dopamine neurons located in the midbrain are medium-sized, non-spiny neurons with long dendrites extending from the multipolar somata. Spontaneous activity of dopamine neurons is driven by a pacemaker conductance that brings the neurons to spike firing threshold [2–4]. Because the spike threshold is comparatively depolarized, this pacemaker conductance plays an essential role in driving spike firing. As a result, inputs to the dopamine neuron appear to modulate activity from this spontaneously driven state.

In the intact rat, dopamine neuron activity can be divided into three states: inactive, spontaneously discharging single action potentials, or firing in bursts. At rest, it is estimated that at least 50% of the dopamine neurons in the substantia nigra are inactive [3], and this is believed to be maintained by a potent GABAergic inhibitory process [5] that likely arises from the pallidum [6–8]. The inactive neurons appear to be a population of neurons that can be recruited whenever a long-term demand is placed on the system, such as a dopamine antagonist [9] or loss of a portion of the neurons due to dopamine neuronal degeneration [10]. The presence of a reserve population appears to be critical in maintaining stability of the dopamine system, since a decrease in the reserve limits the dynamic range in which the dopamine system can respond. Thus, in animal models in which a portion of the dopamine neurons have been lesioned, although the animal may recover behaviorally by recruiting neuronal firing [10], it is much more susceptible to disruption when a demand is placed on the dopamine system. As a consequence, levels of dopamine blockade that do not affect locomotor activity in a normal animal will cause profound hyperexcitation and akinesia in the partially lesioned, but recovered animal [11,12]. Moreover, treatment with dopamine agonists such as

Parkinson's Disease: Non-Motor and Non-Dopaminergic Features, First Edition. Edited by C. Warren Olanow, Fabrizio Stocchi, and Anthony E. Lang.

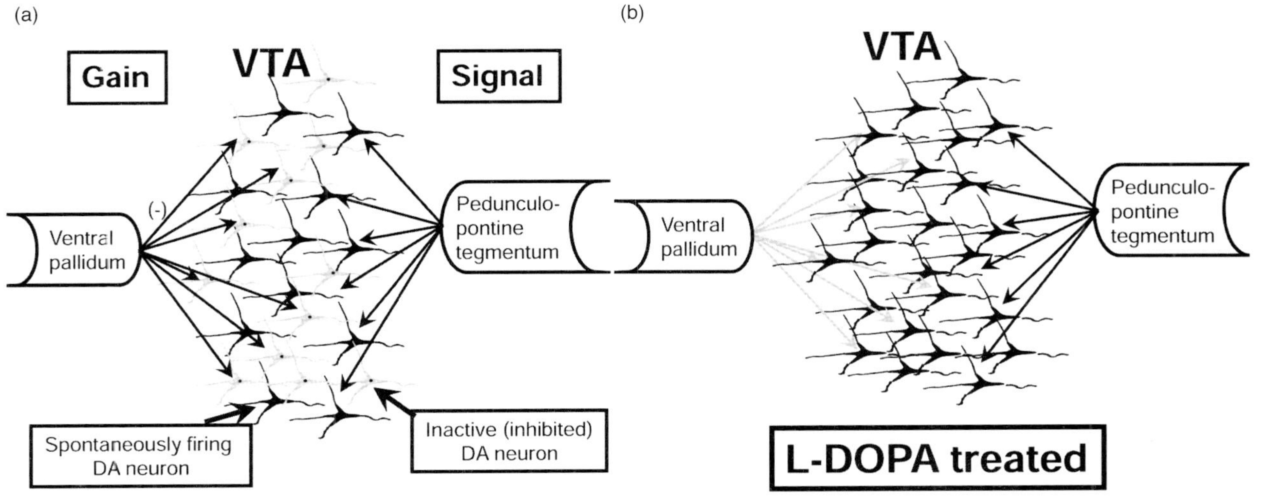

Figure 6.1 Dopamine neuronal activity states are regulated by distinct pathways. (a) In the normal organism, at least half of the dopamine neurons in the ventral tegmental area are not firing spontaneously. The number of spontaneously firing dopamine neurons is regulated via a powerful inhibitory influence originating in the ventral pallidum. In contrast, a glutamatergic input from the brainstem pedunculopontine tegmentum will drive dopamine neurons to fire in bursts, with burst firing proposed to be the behaviorally salient output of the dopamine system (the signal). In order for a dopamine neuron to fire in bursts, it must first be spontaneously firing. By regulating the number of dopamine neurons that are firing, the ventral pallidum sets the amplitude of the phasic response (i.e., the gain). (b) Following repeated treatment with dopaminergic drugs such as L-DOPA, there is proposed to be an increase in the number of dopamine neurons that fire spontaneously. As a result, all signals coming into the dopaminergic neurons will exert a maximum response. Although this may contribute to functional recovery in the nigrostriatal system, within the mesolimbic system it could lead to psychosis or abnormal perseverative behavior.

L-DOPA appears further to recruit spontaneously firing neurons [13]. Although this may be a factor in the effectiveness of L-DOPA treatment, it would also be expected to increase the instability of the system by decreasing its dynamic range. Such an unstable state could contribute to the on–off and freezing effects known to be associated with L-DOPA treatment.

The property of the DA neuron system to exhibit silent neurons held "in reserve" is also likely to play a role in some of the limbic properties of dopamine agonists. It is known that repeated treatment with indirect dopamine agonists such as psychostimulants will sensitize the dopamine system [14,15]. This appears to be a consequence of increasing the number of dopamine neurons that are firing, since the heightened response to psychostimulants correlates with the increase in the number of firing dopamine neurons [16]. Although the L-DOPA-induced increase in dopamine neuronal firing may contribute to its therapeutic actions within the damaged nigrostriatal system in PD [13], within the mesolimbic dopamine system it could have deleterious effects. Thus, with an increase in spontaneous firing, the dopamine system could demonstrate heightened responses to stimuli and to the psychological effects of L-DOPA [8,17]. As a result, stimuli might be expected to result in a heightened level of reward compared with that of the non-sensitized system, causing the patient to become locked into a highly self-rewarding but non-productive behavioral state [18,19]. This could manifest as a dependence on L-DOPA due to the rewarding properties of the drug itself [20]. Indeed, given that animal models of schizophrenia are found to exhibit an even greater increase in the number of firing dopamine neurons, the ability of L-DOPA to increase the firing activity of the dopamine neuronal population could underlie both its addictive properties and its propensity to induce psychosis (Figure 6.1).

In addition to modulation of the population of firing dopamine neurons, spontaneously firing dopamine neurons are known to exhibit two distinct patterns of activity: single-spike firing and burst firing. The single-spike firing appears to be the basal, non-activated state of spontaneously firing dopamine neurons. However, if an animal is exposed to an activating stimulus, the neurons can fire in bursts [21,22]. Burst firing is dependent on a glutamatergic drive acting on dopamine neurons [23–25]. The glutamatergic drive that initiates burst firing furthermore appears to depend on the specific dopamine neuronal population. Thus, burst firing in nigrostriatal dopamine neurons is potently regulated by subthalamic glutamatergic afferents [26], whereas mesolimbic burst firing is driven predominantly by the pedunculopontine tegmentum [7,8]. Since a dopamine neuron must be firing before it can be driven into a bursting mode, the amplitude of the response to a burst signal is regulated by the number of dopamine neurons that are active [8].

Dopamine actions on postsynaptic targets

The pattern of dopamine neuron activity determines the response elicited within postsynaptic targets. Thus, using local administration of dopamine antagonists, we found that stimulation of D2 receptors produces a potent inhibition of striatal neuron firing, whereas activation of D1 receptors facilitates striatal neuron responses to inputs [27]. Dopamine will also exert actions within the striatal system via its modulation of afferent inputs. The dorsal striatum receives convergent inputs from the motor and sensory cortex, and projects via the globus pallidus to the motor-related regions of the thalamus. Selective lesions of the dopamine innervation of the dorsal striatum result in disruption of voluntary movement [28,29]. Moreover, loss of the D1 bearing striatal neurons that are excited by dopamine, (i.e., direct pathway neurons [30,31]) results in an akinetic state. Finally, lesions of the output of this system at the level of the globus pallidus will relieve the akinesia associated with PD [32,33]. In summary, the nigrostriatal system, its targets within the striatum, and its output to the thalamus all form components of a system that regulates movements, and disruption of individual segments of this circuit will mimic many of the symptoms of PD.

Within the nucleus accumbens, the functional impact of dopamine may be even more complex, given the multitude of diverse inputs upon which dopamine may act. Thus, the nucleus accumbens receives powerful glutamatergic inputs from three primary structures: the amygdala, the hippocampus ventral subiculum, and the prefrontal cortex. Moreover, each of these systems provides a different functional modulation of the system. The amygdala is an area responsive to affective stimuli, and is proposed to gate affectively the nucleus accumbens [34,35]. The hippocampus subiculum has been proposed to be involved in context dependence [36–39], and therefore will serve to keep an organism focused on a specific task [17,40]. Finally, the medial prefrontal cortex is believed to be involved in behavioral flexibility [41]. Moreover, the impact that these systems have on the nucleus accumbens is potently modulated by dopamine. In studies examining the interaction of the ventral subicular and medial prefrontal cortical inputs, we found that activation of D2 receptors will provide a powerful and selective attenuation of the medial prefrontal cortical drive of the accumbens [42]. In contrast, the input from the ventral subiculum demonstrates potentiation in the presence of D1 receptor stimulation [43]. The receptor subtype stimulated is also dependent on the status of dopamine neuron activity. Thus, increases in the number of dopamine neurons firing will increase low-level tonic dopamine in the accumbens [7], which will selectively stimulate D2 receptors, whereas burst firing will result in a high-amplitude phasic dopamine release that preferentially activates D1 receptors [43] (Figure 6.2).

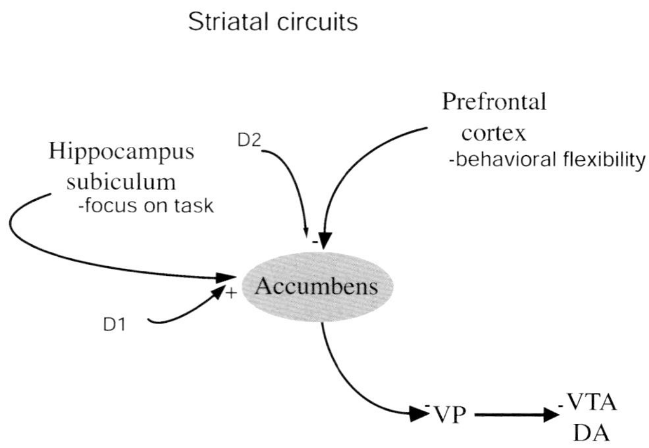

Figure 6.2 The nucleus accumbens receives afferent input from several structures involved in the control of motivated behavior. The ventral subiculum of the hippocampus is believed to regulate context-dependent actions; as such, this system will drive an organism to maintain focus on a current task. Moreover, the input from the ventral subiculum is potentiated via the actions of dopamine on D1 receptors. In contrast, the medial prefrontal cortex is believed to be involved in behavioral flexibility, or the ability to change response strategies when the current approach is ineffective. The prefrontal cortical input to the accumbens is potently inhibited by D2 receptor stimulation. If an organism is performing a task effectively, there is an activation of the dopamine system, which would potentiate subicular inputs and attenuate prefrontal cortical inputs, thereby favoring continuing the current strategy. This increase drive would also further maintain dopamine system activation via inhibition of the ventral pallidum (VP). In contrast, if a reward fails to occur, the resultant decrease in dopamine would now favor prefrontal cortical input and changing response strategies. This delicate balance can be disrupted by dopaminergic drugs, which would drive the system towards perseverative continuation of current behavioral strategies.

The ability of the dopamine system to modulate selectively nucleus accumbens afferents can also observed in behavioral studies in this system. For example, the prefrontal cortex can be functionally "disconnected" from the nucleus accumbens by inactivating the prefrontal cortex unilaterally and administering a D2 agonist contralaterally (to inhibit presynaptically prefrontal cortical afferents to the accumbens). Under this condition, the rat will exhibit perseveration, or the inability to change task performance in the face of altered reward contingencies. This is believed to be due to the loss of prefrontally driven behavioral flexibility. The ventral subiculum can also be disconnected from the accumbens, in this case by unilaterally inactivating the ventral subiculum while blocking D1-mediated potentiation of subicular afferents by administering a D1 agonist into the contralateral accumbens. In this case, the animal fails to learn effectively either component of the task [43]. Therefore, the dopamine system provides a potent balance between staying on task to achieve a goal, and the necessity to alter behavior flexibly if task contingencies fail (Figure 6.2).

The dopamine system is therefore positioned to modulate afferent drive in the nucleus accumbens. In the cases in which an organism is performing a task that leads to reward, the reward itself would lead to an activation of dopamine neuron firing, thereby increasing tonic and phasic dopamine release into the accumbens. This increase would shut down medial prefrontal cortical drive (via D2 receptor stimulation) and potentiate ventral subicular drive (via D1 receptor stimulation). The potentiation of ventral subicular drive would, in turn, maintain this increased dopamine neuron firing state and accumbens dopamine release. As a result, the organism would preferentially maintain its current activity (i.e., contextual focus on the current task via D1 potentiation of the ventral subicular input) while inhibiting competing behaviors (i.e., decreased behavioral flexibility via D2 inhibition of the medial prefrontal cortical input [40,44]). However, studies show that if the animal produces a behavior that it expects to result in a reward but no reward is forthcoming, there is an inhibition of dopamine neuron firing [45]. This decrease in dopamine would attenuate ventral subicular drive while potentiating medial prefrontal cortical drive. As a result, the organism would break from the current contextual focus (i.e., decreasing ventral subicular input) and flexibly shift to an alternative task (increased medial prefrontal cortical input).

Such a balance would therefore enable the organism to maintain optimal task performance and to shift strategies when the current response is no longer effective. On the other hand, if the dopamine system is disrupted, this process would be altered in a way that would interfere with optimal behavioral strategies. One way in which this delicate balance can be disrupted is by repeated cocaine administration. Thus, repeated cocaine administration mimics the condition of D1 activation, in that it induces a long-term potentiation [46] of the hippocampal subicular input while attenuating the ability of the medial prefrontal cortex to shift strategies [47]. This would lock the organism into a behavioral state that may not be an effective response strategy [40,44]. Furthermore, it appears that treatment of the Parkinson's patient with L-DOPA may be capable of producing a similar disruption in regulation.

Alteration of limbic system circuitry in Parkinson's disease: potential disruption by L-DOPA

The balance of limbic system drives is also likely to be altered in the Parkinson's patient. Thus, studies show that depletion of dopamine within the nucleus accumbens will prevent the hippocampus subiculum from influencing the subiculum nucleus–accumbens drive without affecting the actions of the medial prefrontal cortex [43]. Such a condition could contribute to the cognitive deficits observed in late PD [48,49]. On the other hand, repeated administration of L-DOPA would be expected to induce a different type of deficit. Thus, one of the consequences observed with repeated cocaine treatment is interference with simple behavioral tasks, such as reversal learning [47]. This is dependent on the ability of cocaine to induce sensitization, a phenomenon where cocaine will gradually have greater effects, provided that it is administered intermittently [50], and which correlates with the induction of subiculum-accumbens LTP as described above [46,47]. With L-DOPA administration, studies show that effective treatment with L-DOPA can affect the limbic system, such as in its ability to improve task-switching performance [51], a behavior that is dependent on a functional medial prefrontal cortical dopamine input [52]. However, repeated L-DOPA administration can also alter other types of deficits, such as reversal learning, which is present only during the "on" phase of the L-DOPA response [53]. Indeed, this impairment in reversal learning occurs in concert with activation of the nucleus accumbens during the "on" phase, but not the "off" phase of the response [54]. Such results would be consistent with what is observed with cocaine sensitization, that is, the failure of reversal learning due to ventral subicular overdrive of the nucleus accumbens [47].

Other potential alterations within limbic circuits in Parkinson's disease

In addition to disruption of movement, it is known that many patients with PD also exhibit signs that reach beyond the motor syndrome. Thus, more than 40% [55–59] of patients with PD demonstrate disorders related to mood, such as depression. Furthermore, depression has been most closely linked with poor quality of life [60,61]. The depression itself appears to arise independently of the Parkinson's symptoms, often occurring prior to onset of motor symptoms [62]. Moreover, the severity of Parkinson's symptoms accounts for only 9% of the variance in depression ratings [63]. Although the origins of the depressive syndrome have not been clearly characterized, it is known that the neurons that degenerate in PD in humans can encompass the entire midbrain dopamine system. Therefore, even though studies show that the nigrostriatal system is the first of the dopamine systems to degenerate, as the disease progresses there is a progressive involvement of more limbic regions [64]. Although a clear association has not been made between limbic degeneration and depression symptoms, the potential exists that this may correlate with mesolimbic dopamine neuron loss [65]. Indeed, postmortem studies suggest that degeneration of ventral tegmental area dopamine neurons may predict the severity of depression [66]. Animal model studies have shown that either lesions of the dopamine system [67] or dopamine antagonist administration [68] will lead to symptoms of anhedonia, or lack of pleasure from environmental stimuli. Restoration of dopamine transmission in these animal models will reverse the signs of anhedonia. Alternatively, early pathology in the serotonergic raphe and the noradrenergic locus coeruleus [69] in PD may be a factor, given the involvement of these two transmitter systems in the pathophysiology and treatment of depression [70]. Unlike classical depression, the depressive symptoms of PD have been reported to dissipate with dopamine agonist treatment of the motor symptomatology [71]. Moreover, dopamine agonists that preferentially activate the dopamine D3 receptor, such as pramipexole [72], a receptor that is preferentially localized to ventral striatal limbic circuits [73], are reported to be more effective in treating depression in PD [71,74].

There are also other dopamine-related disturbances in brain function other than those involved in movement and perseverative behaviors. Thus, Parkinson's patients exhibit lower levels of "novelty seeking" [75,76]. This is interesting given the link between risk-taking behavior and D4 receptors in the prefrontal cortex [77,78]. In addition, deficits in executive function are reported [79,80], a task which involves prefrontal cortical dopaminergic function [81,82]. Moreover, psychotic features have also been reported in up to one-third of Parkinson's patients [83,84]. The psychosis tends to appear later in the disorder. Given that these patients are typically on dopaminergic drugs, it is generally believed that the psychosis is a consequence of overstimulation of the dopamine system [85,86]. Indeed, the ability of L-DOPA administration to recruit dopamine neuron firing [13], which is similar to the manner in which amphetamine sensitizes the limbic dopamine system [16], suggests that a similar mechanism may be in place. Thus, dopamine receptor antagonists will relieve the psychotic symptoms [85]. Given the delayed degeneration of the limbic-projecting dopamine neurons, increasing dopaminergic agonist treatment could produce proportionately greater effects on the limbic dopamine system, leading to psychotic features. In order to treat the psychosis without exacerbating the Parkinson's symptoms, second-generation antipsychotic drugs (i.e., those that are not associated with motor side effects) are typically administered.

Parkinson's disease and impulse-control disorders

An increasing concern related to the use of anti-parkinson medication is the emergence of impulse-control disorders, such as compulsive gambling, eating, shopping, and other involvements [87]. This reflects an inability to resist a drive or over-involvement in normally pleasurable events that leads to harm to the individual or others. Unfortunately, the ability to attribute impulse-control disorders to PD or to dopamine replacement therapy has been confounded by the lack of an appropriate comparison group [87], although a recent study suggested that Parkinson's patients themselves are nearly 25 times more likely to exhibit impulse-control disorders [88], and 14% are reported to have a heightened interest in these activities [89]. In a number of cases, this has been associated with taking a direct-acting dopamine agonist, such as pramipexole [90,91]. This has been more often seen in patients treated for an extended period with dopamine agonists [89]. Typically, the patients who exhibit impulse-control disorders on dopamine agonist treatment are those who exhibited premorbid tendencies prior to the onset of PD or dopamine replacement therapy [92].

Animal studies have shed light on the neural substrates of impulse-control disorders. The orbitofrontal [93] and ventromedial prefrontal [94,95] cortices in particular have been implicated in impulsive behaviors. Both of these regions project to the limbic ventral striatum/nucleus accumbens, an area known to be involved in reward [96,97]. Given these data, a pathophysiology emerges that may account for impulse-control disorders and their exacerbation by dopaminergic agents. The premorbid tendency to exhibit impulsive behaviors may reflect an underlying disruption in orbital frontal cortical function that drives the need for increased impulsive behaviors related to reward. However, for the individual to experience reward, an intact mesolimbic dopamine circuit should be present. Indeed, diminished limbic dopamine system function has been associated with increased self-stimulation thresholds, suggesting a need for larger rewarding events to compensate for diminished dopaminergic capacity [98,99]. Thus, a decrease in ventral tegmental area dopamine in itself could be a facilitating factor. There is also the potential that this deficit could be magnified as a consequence of dopamine replacement drugs. Given the correlation between long-term administration of high doses of dopaminergic agonists and impulse-control disorders [87], one possibility is that the dopamine agonists may lead to a down-regulation of dopamine receptors within limbic structures, where the dopamine denervation is not as complete as in the more dorsal motor-related areas. One proposal is that a resultant decrease in the numbers of dopamine receptors may make stimuli less effective at producing a reward, and thereby require individuals to increase the "intensity" of their rewarding events to derive an equivalent amount of pleasure [100]. Indeed, it is known that animals with low levels of D2-like dopamine receptor availability are associated with impulsivity and cocaine administration

[101] and is thought to mediate vulnerability to addictive behaviors [100]. This may be particularly true for drugs which have a higher D3 agonist binding, due to the higher relative distribution of this receptor subtype within limbic structures [73]. Thus, although speculative, it may be that dopamine replacement therapy may be exacerbating an underlying impulsivity due to its actions on reward circuitry.

Conclusion

PD pathophysiology and treatment are dependent primarily on manipulation of the nigrostriatal motor system. However, there are other components of the dopamine system that can also be affected. When degeneration of the dopamine innervation extends to the limbic circuit, it could result in a loss of reward function, or anhedonia. Similarly, a loss of dopamine in the prefrontal cortex could interfere with novelty-seeking and task-switching behavior, both of which are described as being related to dopamine system function. The amygdala, an area involved in affective responses, is also potently modulated by dopamine [102,103]. Such alterations can also play a role in the pharmacotherapy of PD. Although dopamine replacement therapy is targeted to compensate for the loss of dopamine in nigrostriatal structures, one consequence of such treatments could be overstimulation of mesolimbic dopamine systems. Such a condition could underlie psychotic disturbances, cognitive dysfunctions, and addiction/impulse-control disruptions that have been observed in Parkinson's patients. A better knowledge of the subtle interplay of these parallel neurotransmitter systems may guide the development of more effective therapeutic approaches without the consequences of limbic system disruption.

References

1. Hornykiewicz O. Dopamine (3-hydroxytyramine) in the central nervous system and its relation to the Parkinson syndrome in man. *Dtsch Med Wochenschr* 1962;**87**:1807–10 (in German).
2. Grace AA, Bunney BS. Intracellular and extracellular electrophysiology of nigral dopaminergic neurons – 1. Identification and characterization. *Neuroscience* 1983;**10**(2):301–15.
3. Grace AA, Bunney BS. The control of firing pattern in nigral dopamine neurons: single spike firing. *J Neurosci* 1984;**4**(11):2866–76.
4. Grace AA, Onn SP. Morphology and electrophysiological properties of immunocytochemically identified rat dopamine neurons recorded *in vitro*. *J Neurosci* 1989;**9**(10):3463–81.
5. Grace AA, Bunney BS. Opposing effects of striatonigral feedback pathways on midbrain dopamine cell activity. *Brain Res* 1985;**333**(2):271–84.
6. Floresco SB, Todd CL, Grace AA. Glutamatergic afferents from the hippocampus to the nucleus accumbens regulate activity of ventral tegmental area dopamine neurons. *J Neurosci* 2001;**21**(13):4915–22.
7. Floresco SB, West AR, Ash B, *et al.* Afferent modulation of dopamine neuron firing differentially regulates tonic and phasic dopamine transmission. *Nat Neurosci* 2003;**6**(9):968–73.
8. Lodge DJ, Grace AA. The hippocampus modulates dopamine neuron responsivity by regulating the intensity of phasic neuron activation. *Neuropsychopharmacology* 2006;**31**:1356–61.
9. Bunney BS, Grace AA. Acute and chronic haloperidol treatment: comparison of effects on nigral dopaminergic cell activity. *Life Sci* 1978;**23**(16):1715–27.
10. Hollerman JR, Grace AA. The effects of dopamine-depleting brain lesions on the electrophysiological activity of rat substantia nigra dopamine neurons. *Brain Res* 1990;**533**(2):203–12.
11. Hollerman JR, Abercrombie ED, Grace AA. Electrophysiological, biochemical, and behavioral studies of acute haloperidol-induced depolarization block of nigral dopamine neurons. *Neuroscience* 1992;**47**(3):589–601.
12. Hollerman JR, Grace AA. Acute haloperidol administration induces depolarization block of nigral dopamine neurons in rats after partial dopamine lesions. *Neurosci Lett* 1989;**96**(1):82–8.
13. Harden DG, Grace AA. Activation of dopamine cell firing by repeated L-DOPA administration to dopamine-depleted rats: its potential role in mediating the therapeutic response to L-DOPA treatment. *J Neurosci* 1995;**15**(9):6157–66.
14. Segal DS, Mandell AJ. Long-term administration of *d*-amphetamine: progressive augmentation of motor activity and stereotypy. *Pharmacol Biochem Behav* 1974;**2**(2):249–55.
15. Post RM, Rose H. Increasing effects of repetitive cocaine administration in the rat. *Nature* 1976;**260**(5553):731–2.
16. Lodge DJ, Grace AA. Amphetamine activation of hippocampal drive of mesolimbic dopamine neurons: a mechanism of behavioral sensitization. *J Neurosci* 2008;**28**(31):7876–82.
17. Grace AA. Gating of information flow within the limbic system and the pathophysiology of schizophrenia. *Brain Res Brain Res Rev* 2000;**31**(2–3):330–41.
18. Merims D, Giladi N. Dopamine dysregulation syndrome, addiction and behavioral changes in Parkinson's disease. *Parkinsonism Rel Disord* 2008;**14**(4):273–80.
19. Fasano A, Elia AE, Soleti F, *et al.* Punding and computer addiction in Parkinson's disease. *Mov Disord* 2006;**21**(8):1217–8.
20. Spigset O, von Scheele C. Levodopa dependence and abuse in Parkinson's disease. *Pharmacotherapy* 1997;**17**(5):1027–30.
21. Freeman AS, Meltzer LT, Bunney BS. Firing properties of substantia nigra dopaminergic neurons in freely moving rats. *Life Sci* 1985;**36**(20):1983–94.
22. Schultz W. The phasic reward signal of primate dopamine neurons. *Adv Pharmacol* 1998;**42**:686–90.
23. Grace AA, Bunney BS. The control of firing pattern in nigral dopamine neurons: burst firing. *J Neurosci* 1984;**4**(11):2877–90.
24. Charlety PJ, Grenhoff J, Chergui K, *et al.* Burst firing of mesencephalic dopamine neuronsis inhibited by somatodendritic application of kynurenate. *Acta Physiol Scand* 1991;**142**:105–12.
25. Suaud-Chagny MF, Chergui K, Chouvet G, Gonon F. Relationship between dopamine release in the rat nucleus accumbens and the discharge activity of dopaminergic neurons during

local *in vivo* application of amino acids in the ventral tegmental area. *Neuroscience* 1992;**49**(1):63–72.
26. Smith ID, Grace AA. Role of the subthalamic nucleus in the regulation of nigral dopamine neuron activity. *Synapse* 1992;**12**(4):287–303.
27. West AR, Grace AA. Opposite influences of endogenous dopamine D1 and D2 receptor activation on activity states and electrophysiological properties of striatal neurons: studies combining *in vivo* intracellular recordings and reverse microdialysis. *J Neurosci* 2002;**22**(1):294–304.
28. Zigmond MJ, Berger TW, Grace AA, Stricker EM. Compensatory responses to nigrostriatal bundle injury. Studies with 6-hydroxydopamine in an animal model of parkinsonism. *Mol Chem Neuropathol* 1989;**10**(3):185–200.
29. Stachowiak MK, Bruno JP, Snyder AM, *et al.* Apparent sprouting of striatal serotonergic terminals after dopamine-depleting brain lesions in neonatal rats. *Brain Res* 1984;**291**(1):164–7.
30. Alexander GE, Crutcher MD, DeLong MR. Basal ganglia–thalamocortical circuits: parallel substrates for motor, oculomotor, "prefrontal" and "limbic" functions. *Prog Brain Res* 1990;**85**:119–46.
31. Alexander GE, DeLong MR, Strick PL. Parallel organization of functionally segregated circuits linking basal ganglia and cortex. *Annu Rev Neurosci* 1986;**9**:357–81.
32. Gross RE, Lozano AM, Lang AE, *et al.* The effects of pallidotomy on Parkinson's disease: study design and assessment techniques. *Acta Neurochir* 1997;**68**:24–8.
33. Schuurman PR, de Bie RM, Speelman JD, Bosch DA. Bilateral posteroventral pallidotomy in advanced Parkinson's disease in three patients. *Mov Disord* 1997;**12**(5):752–5.
34. O'Donnell P, Grace AA. Synaptic interactions among excitatory afferents to nucleus accumbens neurons: hippocampal gating of prefrontal cortical input. *J Neurosci* 1995;**15**(5 Pt 1):3622–39.
35. McGinty VB, Grace AA. Timing-dependent regulation of evoked spiking in nucleus accumbens neurons by integration of limbic and prefrontal cortical inputs. *J Neurophysiol* 2009;**101**(4):1823–35.
36. Jarrard LE. What does the hippocampus really do? *Behav Brain Res* 1995;**71**:1–10.
37. Maren S. Neurotoxic or electrolytic lesions of the ventral subiculum produce deficits in the acquisition and expression of Pavlovian fear conditioning in rats. *Behav Neurosci* 1999;**113**(2):283–90.
38. Sharp PE. Complimentary roles for hippocampal versus subicular/entorhinal place cells in coding place, context, and events. *Hippocampus* 1999;**9**(4):432–43.
39. Fanselow MS. Contextual fear, gestalt memories, and the hippocampus. *Behav Brain Res* 2000;**110**(1–2):73–81.
40. Grace AA, Floresco SB, Goto Y, Lodge DJ. Regulation of firing of dopaminergic neurons and control of goal-directed behaviors. *Trends Neurosci* 2007;**30**(5):220–7.
41. Ragozzino ME. The contribution of the medial prefrontal cortex, orbitofrontal cortex, and dorsomedial striatum to behavioral flexibility. *Ann N Y Acad Sci* 2007;**1121**:355–75.
42. O'Donnell P, Grace AA. Tonic D2-mediated attenuation of cortical excitation in nucleus accumbens neurons recorded *in vitro*. *Brain Res* 1994;**634**(1):105–12.
43. Goto Y, Grace AA. Dopaminergic modulation of limbic and cortical drive of nucleus accumbens in goal-directed behavior. *Nat Neurosci* 2005;**8**:805–12.
44. Goto Y, Grace AA. Limbic and cortical information processing in the nucleus accumbens. *Trends Neurosci* 2008;**31**(11):552–8.
45. Hollerman JR, Schultz W. Dopamine neurons report an error in the temporal prediction of reward during learning. *Nat Neurosci* 1998;**1**(4):304–9.
46. Conrad KL, Tseng KY, Uejima JL, *et al.* Formation of accumbens GluR2-lacking AMPA receptors mediates incubation of cocaine craving. *Nature* 2008;**454**(7200):118–21.
47. Goto Y, Grace AA. Dopamine-dependent interactions between limbic and prefrontal cortical plasticity in the nucleus accumbens: disruption by cocaine sensitization. *Neuron* 2005;**47**(2):255–66.
48. Owen AM, James M, Leigh PN, *et al.* Fronto-striatal cognitive deficits at different stages of Parkinson's disease. *Brain* 1992;**115**(Pt 6):1727–51.
49. Morrison CE, Borod JC, Brin MF, *et al.* Effects of levodopa on cognitive functioning in moderate-to-severe Parkinson's disease (MSPD). *J Neural Transm* 2004;**111**(10–11):1333–41.
50. Post RM. Intermittent versus continuous stimulation: effect of time interval on the development of sensitization or tolerance. *Life Sci* 1980;**26**(16):1275–82.
51. Mehta MA, Manes FF, Magnolfi G, *et al.* Impaired set-shifting and dissociable effects on tests of spatial working memory following the dopamine D2 receptor antagonist sulpiride in human volunteers. *Psychopharmacology* 2004;**176**(3–4):331–42.
52. Roberts AC, De Salvia MA, Wilkinson LS, *et al.* 6-Hydroxydopamine lesions of the prefrontal cortex in monkeys enhance performance on an analog of the Wisconsin Card Sort Test: possible interactions with subcortical dopamine. *J Neurosci* 1994;**14**(5 Pt 1):2531–44.
53. Cools R, Barker RA, Sahakian BJ, Robbins TW. Mechanisms of cognitive set flexibility in Parkinson's disease. *Brain* 2001;**124**(Pt 12):2503–12.
54. Cools R, Lewis SJG, Clark L, et al.. L-DOPA disrupts activity in the nucleus accumbens during reversal learning in Parkinson's disease. *Neuropsychopharmacology* 2007;**32**:180–9.
55. Tandberg E, Larsen JP, Aarsland D, Cummings JL. The occurrence of depression in Parkinson's disease. A community-based study. *Arch Neurol* 1996;**53**(2):175–9.
56. McDonald WM, Richard IH, DeLong MR. Prevalence, etiology, and treatment of depression in Parkinson's disease. *Biol Psychiatry* 2003;**54**(3):363–75.
57. Veazey C, Aki SO, Cook KF, *et al.* Prevalence and treatment of depression in Parkinson's disease. *J Neuropsychiatry Clin Neurosci* 2005;**17**(3):310–23.
58. Lemke MR, Brecht HM, Koester J, Reichmann H. Effects of the dopamine agonist pramipexole on depression, anhedonia and motor functioning in Parkinson's disease. *J Neurol Sci* 2006;**248**(1–2): 266–70.
59. Cummings JL, Masterman DL. Depression in patients with Parkinson's disease. *Int J Geriatr Psychiatry* 1999;**14**(9):711–8.
60. Kuopio AM, Marttila RJ, Helenius H, *et al.* The quality of life in Parkinson's disease. *Mov Disord* 2000;**15**(2):216–23.
61. Schrag A, Jahanshahi M, Quinn NP. What contributes to depression in Parkinson's disease? *Psychol Med* 2001;**31**(1):65–73.

62. Shiba M, Bower JH, Maraganore DM, *et al.* Anxiety disorders and depressive disorders preceding Parkinson's disease: a case–control study. *Mov Disord* 2000;**15**(4):669–77.
63. Menza MA, Mark MH. Parkinson's disease and depression: the relationship to disability and personality. *J Neuropsychiatry Clin Neurosci* 1994;**6**(2):165–9.
64. Manaye KF, Sonsalla PK, Barnett G, *et al.* 1-Methyl-4-(2′-methylphenyl)-1,2,3,6-tetrahydropyridine (2′CH_3-MPTP)-induced degeneration of mesostriatal dopaminergic neurons in the mouse: biochemical and neuroanatomical studies. *Brain Res* 1989;**491**(2):307–15.
65. Brown AS. Gershon S. Dopamine and depression. *J Neural Transm Gen Sect* 1993;**91**(2–3):75–109.
66. Torack RM, Morris JC. The association of ventral tegmental area histopathology with adult dementia. *Arch Neurol* 1988;**45**(5):497–501.
67. Carey RJ. An examination of parkinsonian versus anhedonia contributions to self-stimulation impairments induced by dopamine dysfunction. *Behav Brain Res* 1986;**22**(2):117–25.
68. Huang AC, Hsiao S. Haloperidol attenuates rewarding and aversively conditioned suppression of saccharin solution intake: reevaluation of the anhedonia hypothesis of dopamine blocking. *Behav Neurosci* 2002;**116**(4):646–50.
69. Braak H, Ghebremedhin E, Rub U, *et al.* Stages in the development of Parkinson's disease-related pathology. *Cell Tissue Res* 2004;**318**(1):121–34.
70. Nelson JC, Mazure CM, Jatlow PI, *et al.* Combining norepinephrine and serotonin reuptake inhibition mechanisms for treatment of depression: a double-blind, randomized study. *Biol Psychiatry* 2004;**55**(3):296–300.
71. Lemke MR. Dopamine agonists in the treatment of non-motor symptoms of Parkinson's disease: depression. *Eur J Neurol* 2008;**15**(Suppl 2):9–14.
72. Millan MJ, Maiofiss L, Cussac D, *et al.* Differential actions of antiparkinson agents at multiple classes of monoaminergic receptor. I. A multivariate analysis of the binding profiles of 14 drugs at 21 native and cloned human receptor subtypes. *J Pharmacol Exp Ther* 2002;**303**(2):791–804.
73. Sokoloff P, Giros B, Martres MP, *et al.* Molecular cloning and characterization of a novel dopamine receptor (D3) as a target for neuroleptics. *Nature* 1990;**347**(6289):146–51.
74. Rektorova I, Rektor I, Bares M, *et al.* Pramipexole and pergolide in the treatment of depression in Parkinson's disease: a national multicentre prospective randomized study. *Eur J Neurol* 2003;**10**(4):399–406.
75. Menza MA, Golbe LI, Cody RA, Forman NE. Dopamine-related personality traits in Parkinson's disease. *Neurology* 1993;**43**(3 Pt 1):505–8.
76. Fujii C, Harada S, Ohkoshi N, *et al.* Cross-cultural traits for personality of patients with Parkinson's disease in Japan. *Am J Med Genet* 2000;**96**(1):1–3.
77. Zuckerman M, Kuhlman DM. Personality and risk-taking: common biosocial factors. *J Personality* 2000;**68**(6):999–1029.
78. Comings DE, Gonzalez N, Wu S, *et al.* Studies of the 48 bp repeat polymorphism of the DRD4 gene in impulsive, compulsive, addictive behaviors: Tourette syndrome, ADHD, pathological gambling, and substance abuse. *Am J Med Genet* 1999;**88**(4):358–68.
79. Cooper JA, Sagar HJ, Jordan N, *et al.* Cognitive impairment in early, untreated Parkinson's disease and its relationship to motor disability. *Brain* 1991;**114**(Pt 5):2095–122.
80. Muslimovic D, Post B, Speelman JD, Schmand B. Cognitive profile of patients with newly diagnosed Parkinson disease. *Neurology* 2005;**65**(8):1239–45.
81. Weinberger DR. A connectionist approach to the prefrontal cortex. *J Neuropsychiatry Clin Neurosci* 1993;**5**(3):241–53.
82. Goldman-Rakic PS. The prefrontal landscape: implications of functional architecture for understanding human mentation and the central executive. *Philos Trans R Soc Lond B Biol Sci* 1996;**351**(1346): 1445–53.
83. Aarsland D, Larsen JP, Cummins JL, Laake K. Prevalence and clinical correlates of psychotic symptoms in Parkinson disease: a community-based study. *Arch Neurol* 1999;**56**(5):595–601.
84. Giladi N, Treves TA, Paleacu D, *et al.* Risk factors for dementia, depression and psychosis in long-standing Parkinson's disease. *J Neural Transm* 2000;**107**(1):59–71.
85. Friedman A, Sienkiewicz J. Psychotic complications of long-term levodopa treatment of Parkinson's disease. *Acta Neurol Scand* 1991;**84**(2):111–3.
86. Koller WC, Glatt SL, Hubble JP, *et al.* Apolipoprotein E genotypes in Parkinson's disease with and without dementia. *Ann Neurol* 1995;**37**(2):242–5.
87. Weintraub D. Dopamine and impulse-control disorders in Parkinson's disease. *Ann Neurol* 2008;**64**(Suppl 2):S93–100.
88. Avanzi M, Baratti M, Cabrini S, *et al.* Prevalence of pathological gambling in patients with Parkinson's disease. *Mov Disord* 2006;**21**(12):2068–72.
89. Giladi N, Weitzman N, Schreiber S, *et al.* New onset heightened interest or drive for gambling, shopping, eating or sexual activity in patients with Parkinson's disease: the role of dopamine agonist treatment and age at motor symptoms onset. *J Psychopharmacol* 2007;**21**(5):501–6.
90. Dodd ML, Klos KJ, Bower JH, *et al.* Pathological gambling caused by drugs used to treat Parkinson disease. *Arch Neurol* 2005;**62**(9):1377–81.
91. Driver-Dunckley E, Samanta J, Stacy M. Pathological gambling associated with dopamine agonist therapy in Parkinson's disease. *Neurology* 2003;**61**(3):422–3.
92. Weintraub D, Siderowf AD, Potenza MN, *et al.* Association of dopamine agonist use with impulse-control disorders in Parkinson disease. *Arch Neurol* 2006;**63**(7):969–73.
93. O'Doherty J, Kringelbach ML, Rolls ET, *et al.* Abstract reward and punishment representations in the human orbitofrontal cortex. *Nat Neurosci* 2001;**4**(1):95–102.
94. Potenza MN, Leung HC, Blumberg HP, *et al.* An FMRI Stroop task study of ventromedial prefrontal cortical function in pathological gamblers. *Am J Psychiatry* 2003;**160**(11): 1990–4.
95. Bechara A, Tranel D, Damasio H. Characterization of the decision-making deficit of patients with ventromedial prefrontal cortex lesions. *Brain* 2000;**123**(Pt 11):2189–202.
96. Fiorino DF, Coury A, Fibiger HC, Phillips AG. Electrical stimulation of reward sites in the ventral tegmental area increases dopamine transmission in the nucleus accumbens of the rat. *Behav Brain Res* 1993;**55**(2):131–41.

97. Wise RA. Drug-activation of brain reward pathways. *Drug Alcohol Depend* 1998;**51**(1–2): 13–22.
98. Koob GF. Neural mechanisms of drug reinforcement. *Ann N Y Acad Sci* 1992;**654**:171–91.
99. Baldo BA, Jain K, Veraldi L, *et al.* A dopamine D1 agonist elevates self-stimulation thresholds: comparison to other dopamine-selective drugs. *Pharmacol Biochem Behav* 1999; **62**(4):659–72.
100. Volkow ND, Wang GJ, Fowler JS, *et al.* Prediction of reinforcing responses to psychostimulants in humans by brain dopamine D2 receptor levels. *Am J Psychiatry* 1999;**156**(9): 1440–3.
101. Dalley JW, Fryer TD, Brichard L, *et al.* Nucleus accumbens D2/3 receptors predict trait impulsivity and cocaine reinforcement. *Science* 2007;**315**(5816):1267–70.
102. LeDoux JE. Emotion circuits in the brain. *Annu Rev Neurosci* 2000;**23**:155–84.
103. Rosenkranz JA, Grace AA. Dopamine-mediated modulation of odour-evoked amygdala potentials during pavlovian conditioning. *Nature* 2002;**417**(6886):282–7.

Chapter 7
Animal Models of Parkinson's Disease: the Non-Motor and Non-Dopaminergic Features

Katherine E. Soderstrom[1], *Shilpa Ramaswamy*[1], *C. Warren Olanow*[2], *& Jeffrey H. Kordower*[1]
[1]Department of Neurological Sciences, Rush University Medical Center, Chicago, IL, USA
[2]Department of Neurology and Neuroscience, Mount Sinai School of Medicine, New York, NY, USA

Parkinson's disease

Parkinson's disease (PD) has historically been diagnosed based on the cardinal motor symptoms of resting tremor, rigidity, bradykinesia, and gait disturbance [1,2]. The characteristic pathologic feature of the disease is a loss of neurons in the substantia nigra pars compacta (SNc) coupled with intracytoplasmic inclusions or Lewy bodies (LBs). LBs are comprised of a central core containing protein aggregates surrounded by a filamentous halo made up primarily of neurofilament and α-synuclein [3,4]. The cardinal motor symptoms of PD are believed to arise primarily as a result of the progressive degeneration of dopaminergic neurons in the SNc. These neurons project to the striatum (putamen and caudate nucleus), where they synapse on to the resident GABAergic medium spiny neurons. Dopaminergic innervation modulates the glutamatergic input from the cortex and thalamus and stabilizes the basal ganglia network. In PD, when nigral cells degenerate, there is a loss of the dopaminergic innervation of the striatum leading to dysfunction of basal ganglia circuitry and the development of the classic motor features [5,6].

Pathology in PD is now known to extend well beyond the nigrostriatal dopamine system. Indeed, neurodegeneration with LBs is found in cholinergic neurons of the nucleus basalis of Meyneret, epinephrine neurons of the locus coeruleus, and serotonin neurons of the raphe, and also in neurons in the olfactory system, cerebral hemisphere, dorsal motor nucleus, spinal cord, and peripheral autonomic nervous system [7]. This non-dopaminergic pathology is thought to be responsible for the development of clinical features that are not adequately controlled with dopaminergic therapies such as sleep disturbances, mood disorders, autonomic dysfunction, sensory impairment, gait and balance difficulties, and dementia. These are known as non-dopaminergic features and can comprise some of the earliest complaints associated with the development of PD, including anosmia, constipation, fatigue, depression, and sleep disturbances [8]. They can also represent an important source of disability in advanced patients. Aarsland, Beyer, and Kurz showed that dementia is an important co-morbidity in late-stage PD patients [9], and long-term studies have demonstrated that features which do not respond to dopaminergic therapies, such as falling, freezing, and dementia, are the primary source of disability and nursing home placement in advanced patients [10].

In a seminal series of papers, Braak and colleagues looked at the distribution pattern of α-synuclein pathology in the aging control and PD brain [11–14]. They confirmed that synucleinopathy is not limited to the nigrostriatal system, and extends to involve neurons in the upper and lower brain stem, olfactory system, cerebral hemispheres, spinal cord, and peripheral autonomic system. By observing the α-synuclein immunohistochemistry of patients in various stages of normal aging and disease, they observed that synucleinopathy actually begins in the olfactory bulb and lower brainstem, and progresses through the brain in a rostral–caudal fashion, affecting the SNc in mid-stages of the illness, and eventually reaching the cerebral hemispheres [14]. These findings have led some to suggest that PD is in fact a disease *complex* with traditional motor parkinsonism due to dopamine neuronal degeneration in the SNc representing only a middle stage of the disease process. Patients with anosmia, constipation, and RBD who do not have motor features at all might nonetheless have an early form of PD [15].

Although the cause of nigral cell loss is unknown, several clues have been used to develop animal models of PD. The presence of proteinaceous LBs, and also the accumulation of oxidized proteins [16], findings of alterations

Parkinson's Disease: Non-Motor and Non-Dopaminergic Features, First Edition. Edited by C. Warren Olanow, Fabrizio Stocchi, and Anthony E. Lang.

in proteasomal structure and function [17,18], and the discovery that some gene mutations associated with familial PD have the potential to increase protein formation or interfere with their clearance [19], have focused attention on the importance of proteolytic stress in the pathogenesis of PD. Similarly, findings of mitochondrial defects in patients with sporadic PD [20] and the appreciation that several mutant proteins in PD are linked to mitochondria [21] have also implicated this structure as a potential cause of PD. Postmortem studies also provide evidence that oxidative stress, inflammation, and excitotoxicity potentially play a role in the pathogenesis of SNc nigral cell death in PD, which is thought to occur by way of a signal-mediated apoptotic process [22]. Each of these factors thought to be associated with the etiopathogenesis of PD can be used to try to generate an animal model of the disease.

Classic PD models

The classic animal models that have traditionally been used to study PD have focused on the nigrostriatal dopamine system and the motor deficits associated with dopamine depletion. This has served the PD community well in understanding the pathophysiology of the classic motor features of PD and developing medical and surgical interventions that treat the dopaminergic symptoms and their associated motor complications. However, these dopaminergic models do not model the non-dopaminergic pathology and non-motor features of PD, and have not reliably predicted agents that have neuroprotective or disease modifying effects in the clinic. As awareness of the importance of the non-motor features of PD has grown, researchers have begun to clamor for models that more closely replicate the pathology and the etiopathogenesis of PD. In addition, there has been an attempt to re-evaluate the traditional models of PD to determine to what extent, if any, they induce non-motor and non-dopaminergic deficits. This chapter considers the classic models and begins to review progress that has been made with newer models that might address the non-dopaminergic and non-motor features of PD.

Classic models of PD

6-Hydroxydopamine

6-Hydroxydopamine (6-OHDA) is a dopamine analog that is selectively taken up by dopamine neurons via the dopamine transporter [23]. Once in the cell, its metabolism results in the production of toxic molecules such as free radicals and hydrogen peroxide [23], which induce oxidative stress and damage critical biomolecules, leading to cell death. 6-OHDA does not cross the blood–brain barrier and must be delivered to the brain via stereotaxic surgery. Dependent on the location (typically striatum, SNc, or medium forebrain bundle), dose, and number of injection sites, the severity of the lesion can vary greatly [24]. This variation has allowed researchers to achieve relatively successful models of early-, mid- and late-stage PD. Unilateral lesions, if severe, can induce circling behaviors (ipsilateral with amphetamine and contralateral with dopamine agonists), which can be counted in order to provide a measure of the severity of the dopamine lesion and the efficacy of a dopaminergic therapy. Direct infusion of 6-OHDA into the nigra, striatum, or median forebrain bundle results in a relatively selective loss of dopaminergic cells, making it a good model for evaluating the pathologic and physiologic effects of a dopamine lesion, the benefits and side effects of a dopaminergic therapy, and the influence of a dopamine lesion on the development of non-motor symptoms.

1-Methyl-4-phenyl-1,2,3,6-tetrahydropyridine (MPTP)

Arguably one of the best animal models of PD, 1-methyl-4-phenyl-1,2,3,6-tetrahydropyridine (MPTP) was first discovered when it was self-administered by drug users who went on to develop the classic motor features of PD [25]. MPTP can cross the blood–brain barrier, where it is taken up primarily by astrocytes and converted to the toxic metabolite MPP+ by monoamine oxidase type B. Dopaminergic cells take up MPP+ via the dopamine transporter, and its interaction with cytosolic proteins, dopamine storage vesicles, and the mitochondrial electron transport chain (particularly complex I) results in cell toxicity and death [26,27]. MPP+ is preferentially toxic to dopaminergic neurons, but it does not exclusively affect these cells. MPTP can be delivered systemically to induce a model of generalized parkinsonism, or it can be injected into the carotid artery unilaterally to create a model of dopamine depletion where the affected side can be compared with the "normal" side. Limitations of the MPTP model include the fact that it is an acute toxin which selectively damages the SNc and locus coeruleus but not other areas affected in PD, and is not associated with the formation of LBs. However, recent studies demonstrate that chronic infusion of MPTP can induce a dopaminergic lesion that is coupled with inclusion bodies [28]. This may reflect the possibility that LBs represent an aggresome-like inclusion that forms as a protective measure in response to excess levels of misfolded proteins [29], and acute administration of MPTP prevents this compensation from occurring. MPTP can also be used to provide a model to determine the influence of primary dopamine dysfunction on non-dopaminergic neurons and other neurotransmitter systems. Paraquat is an environmental pesticide that can be reduced to form MPTP, but does not itself cross the blood–brain barrier.

Rotenone

Rotenone is a pesticide that has also been shown to be toxic to complex I of the mitochondrial respiratory chain, and reported to induce a model of PD with nigral degeneration and inclusion bodies [30]. However, the toxin is associated with variable results, widespread CNS degeneration with involvement of structures that are not affected in PD, and systemic toxicity with fatality in relatively large numbers of animals [31]. For these reasons, this model is not routinely employed in assessing new therapies for PD. Some of these problems may have been overcome with new treatment protocols and the model may have increased importance in the future [32].

A review of the classic models of Parkinson's disease illustrates that although they have proven to be excellent models of dopamine deficiency and its sequelae, they are sadly inadequate with respect to reproducing the non-dopaminergic and non-motor features of PD. They do not replicate the full spectrum of pathology found in PD, they do not induce the formation of LBs which are the pathological hallmark of the disease, and they do not induce a progressive and gradual loss of function. Further, they do not necessarily reflect the etiology or pathogenesis of the cell death that occurs in PD. Hence positive results in these models with candidate neuroprotective agents have not been shown to translate into comparable effects in PD patients [33]; similarly, negative results in these models do not necessarily mean that the agent being investigated would not prove to be effective in PD. Remedying these deficiencies and developing novel models that take into account our evolving knowledge of the disease are essential if we are to develop more effective therapies for PD.

Novel models of PD

Genetic models of PD

With the discovery of genetic mutations known to result in familial forms of PD, researchers have developed a number of transgenic mouse and fly models that carry these mutations, in an attempt to try to replicate the pathological pattern of PD with an etiologic agent that is known to be associated with the development of at least some forms of PD. In principle, these genetic models provide an excellent opportunity to replicate the non-dopaminergic pathology and non-motor/non-dopaminergic deficits that occur in PD, and to use these for high-throughput screening in an attempt to develop more effective symptomatic and protective therapies for PD. This, however, has proven difficult to accomplish and none of the transgenic models developed to date precisely replicates either the dopaminergic or non-dopaminergic pathology of PD. This may reflect the fact that mutant proteins which are pathogenic in PD may be metabolized differently and have different physiologic functions in animal models, and lead to no pathology or a different pathologic syndrome to what occurs in humans. Nonetheless, this approach remains of considerable interest, and efforts to utilize information derived from gene mutations associated with PD in order to create a faithful transgenic model of the disease continue to be actively pursued.

Among these approaches, overexpression of α-synuclein has so far attracted the most attention. This is based on the fact that familial forms of PD have been associated with mutations in the α-synuclein protein [34], and because α-synuclein is the dominant protein in LBs in patients with sporadic PD [3]. Perhaps even more interestingly, it has also been shown that duplication or triplication of the wild-type α-synuclein protein can lead to a form of PD [35,36]. Overexpression of both mutant and wild-type α-synuclein has been shown to induce dopamine neuronal degeneration with inclusions and motor abnormalities in *Drosophila* [37]. Interestingly, transgenic mice that express these mutations do not develop a PD phenotype, but do develop neuronal degeneration with α-synuclein pathology [38,39]. Although these models may not represent PD *per se*, they likely represent a form of neurodegeneration that occurs via a similar pathogenic mechanism to what occurs in PD and might prove more valuable than traditional models for testing putative neuroprotective agents. Another approach has been to use viral vectors to deliver wild-type or mutant α-synuclein to rodents or primates by direct injection. This approach induces neurodegeneration with LB-like inclusions and has been used to mirror the dopaminergic features of PD [40]. It remains to be seen if this approach can be used to mirror the non-dopaminergic pathology of PD.

There has also been great interest in developing models of PD based on LRRK2, as mutations in this protein are associated with both familial and sporadic forms of PD, and make up a large proportion of PD cases in some subgroups such as Ashkenazy Jews and North African Arabs. Recently, a transgenic model of PD has been generated in *Drosophila* using both wild-type and mutant LRRK2 [41]. The flies had selective loss of dopamine cells and a levodopa-responsive locomotor abnormality. This is thought to represent the first transgenic model that recapitulates key features of PD based on a gain of function gene mutation. On the other hand, dopamine cell loss with impaired locomotor activity has also been described in transgenic LRRK2 knockout *Drosophila* [42]. The development of LRRK2 transgenic mice is awaited.

Aphakia mouse model of PD

The transgenic aphakia mouse lacks Pitx3, a transcription factor necessary for dopamine neuron development, which results in a 90% loss of A9 dopamine neurons while leaving neighboring populations virtually intact [43]. The aphakia mouse model has been used in an attempt to replicate dopaminergic cell loss while preventing severe motor impairments that would prevent evaluation of non-motor symptoms such as cognitive decline [44]. The aphakia mouse may prove very useful in the evaluation of dopamine's role in the expression of some non-motor symptoms of PD.

Lipopolysaccaride model of PD

The emerging understanding of the critical role of inflammation in the progression of PD has led researchers to model this feature in the lipopolysaccharide (LPS) model of PD. Recent studies have shown that LPS injections into α-synuclein transgenic mice can lead to dopamine neuronal degeneration with α-synuclein-positive inclusions [45]. Like other systemic models, the LPS model is not limited to being used to cause dopaminergic dysfunction and may therefore prove useful in the study of non-dopaminergic mechanisms in the non-motor deficits observed in PD patients. Additionally, its ability to replicate the progressive nature of PD may allow for the evaluation of early- and late-stage dysfunction within the same animal.

Proteasome inhibition model of PD

Based on the observation that there is protein accumulation and proteasomal dysfunction in PD, attempts have been made to generate a model based on the use of proteasome inhibitors. Direct injections of proteasome inhibitors have been shown to induce dopamine neuronal degeneration with inclusion bodies in rats [46]. There has also been a report indicating that systemic administration of a proteasome inhibitor induces neurodegeneration coupled with LB-like inclusions in the SNc and also in the non-dopaminergic brain stem sites that are affected in PD [47]. Although some aspects of these studies have been confirmed [48–51], several groups have been unable to replicate any of these findings [52–54]. The basis for these conflicting results remains unknown, but the potential of a model of PD that impairs protein clearance remains of interest. Interest has been rekindled in this approach by the recent report that transgenic mice lacking essential subunits of the 26S proteasome experience dopamine cell loss with inclusion bodies in the SNc and in other brain regions [55].

Aged animal model of PD

Although controversial, some hypothesize that PD represents an extreme end on the continuum of aging [56]. It is well established that aging is the single most important risk factor for the development of PD [57]. With normal aging there is a loss of tyrosine hydroxylase-positive (TH+) nigral cells and an increase in α-synuclein accumulation and also increased protein accumulation and impaired proteasomal function [56]. Indeed, approximately 10% of individuals aged 60 years or older who did not have neurological abnormalities during life have LBs in the SNc [58]. These are referred to as incidental LBs, and are thought to represent a preclinical form of PD. Additionally, nuclei that are also affected in PD such as the locus coeruleus have been shown to demonstrate cell loss in the aged brain [59]. Because of the systemic and progressive nature of age-related deficits, these animals may prove to be useful models for evaluating the non-motor and non-dopaminergic features of PD and for testing putative neuroprotective agents.

Use of animal models to assess the non-motor and non-dopaminergic features of PD

Autonomic dysfunction

One of the more prevalent and potentially troubling features of autonomic dysfunction in PD patients is orthostatic hypotension (OH), a condition defined as at least a 20 mmHg decrease in systolic blood pressure [60]. OH was historically believed to be a side effect of pharmacological therapy; however, it is now considered to be a primary symptom of PD that may be exacerbated by treatment. Additionally, many PD patients experience hypotension following exercise and meals [61]. This cardiovascular dysfunction may be due to a loss of noradrenergic cardiac innervation that is typically seen in PD patients. However, it is important to note that in many patients this denervation exists in the absence of OH. In a study comparing individuals with familial genetic cases of PD, patients with increased α-synuclein expression showed a loss of cardiac innervation that was not seen in those with a parkin-related form of PD [62]. This finding suggests a role for synucleinopathy in cardiac dysfunction [60]. Indeed, α-synuclein-positive inclusions have been detected in cardiac sympathetic neurons in both PD patients and in some without clinical features of the disorder, suggesting that it may be an early pre-motor feature of the disease [63].

Treating OH in PD patients can be difficult as it is exacerbated by the use of dopaminergic agonists that are regularly used to treat the motor symptoms of PD. Non-pharmacological therapies can be employed, such as compression socks, elevation of the head of the bed to avoid naturesis, and dietary changes with increased salt load [64]. In the event that these are not effective, traditional blood pressure medications such as fluorohydrocortisone and midodrine can be used.

One measure that has been used to assess autonomic dysfunction in animal models is piloerection (erection of the hair). When the autonomic nervous system is intact, piloerection occurs in animals in response to cold temperature and/or fear. When an animal is suffering from autonomic dysfunction there is an overall increase in spontaneous piloerection. Researchers have reported an increase in piloerection in rats receiving 6-OHDA lesions to the medium forebrain bundle [65], suggesting that this model may mimic some features of the autonomic dysfunction observed in PD patients.

Digestive dysfunction with slowing of gastrointestinal (GI) transit time and constipation is another prominent and troublesome autonomic symptom that is frequently observed in PD patients. GI disturbances are often an early symptom in patients which may predate the onset of motor symptoms, and increase in severity with disease progression. These dysfunctions include dysphagia and related drooling, gastroparesis, anorectal dysfunction, and colonic dysmobility [61]. Although the etiology of GI dysfunction remains uncertain, a loss of sympathetic innervation of the gut coupled with musculature impairments due to dopamine loss have been suggested [66].

Constipation is the commonest GI problem and can be very difficult to treat. Aside from diet and laxatives, treatment of constipation in PD patients can include agents that enhance GI motility. This may be accomplished with 5-hydroxytryptamine type 4 (5-HT$_4$) agonists such as mosapride [67]. The activation of these serotonergic receptors results in the release of acetylcholine, and positive effects for constipation in PD patients has been reported in two open-label trials [68,69].

Potentially, some of the classic motor models of PD may exhibit GI dysfunction that researchers have failed to record. This would appear to be the case with the MPTP mouse model of PD. In a recent study [70], researchers found a 40% decrease in enteric TH+ cells in mice that had received an acute dose of MPTP (total dose = 60 mg over four injections). However, in mice this cell loss resulted in an increase in colonic emptying, whereas in human PD colonic emptying is delayed. Genetic models of PD that overexpress the α-synuclein gene have also shown some success in replicating GI dysfunction. One group has reported abnormal GI activity in transgenic mice overexpressing human α-synuclein via the Thy1 promoter (Thy1–αSyn) [71]. These mice showed significantly slower colonic motility when compared with wild-type littermates.

Other autonomic dysfunctions in PD patients include urological symptoms, thermoregulatory dysfunction, and sexual dysfunction [61]. Like the symptoms mentioned above, these dysfunctions can be important problems for the PD patient and are often overlooked by the Parkinson's community of scientists despite the enormous challenge and disturbance that they may present to PD patients. A more detailed evaluation of autonomic functions in the various models of PD is warranted.

Sleep dysfunction

Sleep disturbance has recently attracted attention as a symptom of PD that can be problematic for PD patients and may precede the development of motor dysfunction by as much as a decade. Sleep disturbances in PD patients can include insomnia, difficulty in falling asleep, fragmented sleep, sleep apnea, and daytime fatigue [72]. Rapid eye movement (REM) sleep behavior disorder (RBD) is an important problem for some PD patients and is characterized by having REM cycle sleep without atonia. This results in patients "acting out" their dreams, often in a violent and dangerous manner [73]. The pathophysiology of sleep disturbances in PD is not known, although studies in the cat have suggested that atonia in sleep is controlled by the pedunculopontine nucleus [74], a brainstem region that may be involved even in the early stages of PD [14]. Clinically, RBD has also been shown to precede the development of the classic motor features of PD. In one study, RBD symptoms preceded the development of parkinsonism by years in 38% of PD patients [75].

Although dopamine deficiency has been implicated as a possible factor in sleep disturbances, dopamine replacement with levodopa or dopamine agonists may actually aggravate sleep and increase daytime sleepiness. Indeed, high doses of dopamine agonists have been implicated in PD patients experiencing sudden episodes of falling asleep while driving [76]. Another study found no significant effect of the dopamine agonist pramipexole on RBD-associated behaviors despite improving parkinsonian symptoms [77]. Alternatively, non-dopaminergic therapies such as clonazepam and melatonin have been used in PD patients suffering from RBD with relative success [78]. Although these findings argue against dopamine deficiency as a primary factor in PD-associated sleep disturbances and specifically RBD, it should be noted that by the time patients present with the classic motor symptoms of the disease, they may have had sleep disorders such as RBD for decades. The delivery of dopaminergic agonists to a mid-stage PD patient may just be a case of too little, too late. In fact, a study using pramipexole in idiopathic RBD patients, a condition many argue truly represents a preclinical stage of PD [79], found significant improvements in RBD symptoms [77]. Taken together, these findings highlight the necessity for further study of the pathogenesis and therapeutic options for patients with sleep disorders and particularly RBD in PD patients.

Analyzing sleep dysfunction in the 6-OHDA model of PD has been largely neglected. This may in part be due to the lack of appropriate animal models of RBD and other sleep-related disorders. One means of detecting sleep disturbances in animal models has been through activity monitoring, observing both the overall amount of activity displayed by animals and the times in which activities are demonstrated (in relation to the animal's light–dark cycle). In one study, rats that received unilateral 6-OHDA nigral lesions showed an overall decrease in total activity, as would be expected, but no disturbance in the circadian rhythm of their activity [80]. Further investigation is necessary to determine if nigrostriatal dysfunction is a causative factor of sleep disturbance in PD.

Abnormal sleep patterns have been noted in MPTP-treated animals. One study, looking at sleep structure in MPTP-treated monkeys, found that animals exhibiting severe parkinsonism displayed lighter sleep and had significantly less REM sleep than a similar monkey that failed to develop motor dysfunction [81]. Similarly, studies have determined that MPTP-treated mice also show increased occurrence and length of paradoxical sleep episodes compared with untreated controls [82]. Although these findings seem to support a role for dopamine in PD-associated sleep disturbances, a more recent study suggests that the paradoxical sleep observed in MPTP-treated mice may be transient, despite the permanent loss of dopaminergic cells [83].

Sensory dysfunction

Braak *et al.* observed that one of the first brain areas affected by Lewy pathology in the parkinsonian brain was the olfactory bulb [14]. It is not surprising, therefore, that one of the first complaints of many PD patients is anosmia, the loss of smell. Although the predominance of olfactory dysfunction varies depending on study parameters, one group recently reported close to a 75% loss of olfactory function in PD patients compared with age-matched controls [84].

As might be expected, research has focused primarily on using anosmia as an early detector for PD rather than investigating therapies for its reversal. Despite this apparent neglect, a few reports have looked at the effects of various therapies on olfactory dysfunction. Interestingly, dopaminergic agonists and levodopa fail to elicit improvements in olfaction despite having antiparkinsonian effects [85]. In fact, studies have shown that there is an increase in TH+ cells in the olfactory bulbs of PD patients [86]. As olfactory dopamine neurons act as inhibitors in this system, this finding makes sense physiologically but does not correlate with what would be expected in PD. What has been reported to be successful in improving olfactory deficits in PD patients is deep brain stimulation (DBS) of the subthalamic nucleus (STN) [87]. STN-DBS results in the prevention of excitation of the internal segment of the globus pallidus (GPi) by the STN, resulting in less inhibition of the thalamus by the GPi and greater activation of the cortex by the thalamus. It is important to note that STN-DBS resulted in improved odor discrimination (a function of cortical function) but not the threshold of odor detection (a function of the olfactory bulb).

Analysis of olfactory dysfunction in animal models has been extremely limited. One study investigating olfactory function found impairments in the MPTP-treated non-human primate model of PD [88]. This finding is surprising as human patients with MPTP-induced parkinsonism do not display the olfactory dysfunction seen in patients with idiopathic PD [89]. Less surprising is the finding that olfactory deficits have been noted in a genetic model of PD. In a study using mice expressing a mutated form of α-synuclein via the Thy 1 promoter (Thy1–h[A30P]αSyn), transgenic animals displayed olfactory deficits and also significant synucleinopathy of the olfactory bulb [90]).

Visual dysfunction has also been observed in PD patients. Visual disturbances in PD can include decreased visual acuity, color vision, and contrast sensitivity [87]. Although these symptoms have been noted in early-stage PD, they are often not discernible by regular eye tests and increase in severity with disease progression. Many of these visual disturbances are believed to be associated with decreased retinal dopamine, although their responsiveness to dopamine agonists has not been definitively shown [61]. A search for visual alterations has not been performed in animal models of PD.

Another very serious and understudied aspect of PD is dysfunction in pain sensation. Studies have reported that many PD patients suffer from an increased prevalence of musculoskeletal, radicular, and central pain [91]. Musculoskeletal pain is often attributed to the alterations in posture and gait that occur in PD patients. One of the earliest symptoms that lead patients to report to the clinic can be shoulder pain that is often misdiagnosed as bursitis. An increased frequency of radicular or nerve pain is also reported in PD patients. Both musculoskeletal and radicular pain can usually be successfully treated with pain medication and exercise regimes. Much more difficult to treat is central or primary pain which may also be increased in PD patients, although thankfully it is much less common. Unlike the aforementioned varieties, central pain is believed to be a primary symptom of the disease, not the result of altered movement, and is therefore treated with varying success with dopaminergic agonists [61].

There is very little literature evaluating the ability of the 6-OHDA model of PD to mimic the sensory dysfunction observed in PD patients. The exception has been in the area of pain perception. In a recent study, rodents receiving intrastriatal 6-OHDA lesions showed a delayed response (as measured by the tail flick test), but an excessive response (as measured by the formalin test), to pain stimulation [92]. These findings support the hypothesis that an intact nigrostriatal system is required for appropriate responses to pain. Similar findings in mice receiving MPTP investigating pain perception have found that mice receiving both acute and chronic injections of MPTP ($80\ \text{mg kg}^{-1}$ total) show an increased sensitivity to pain as determined by the tail flick and hot plate tests [93].

Neuropsychiatric dysfunction

Depression is believed to be one of the commonest comorbidities associated with PD [94], with the number of sufferers varying depending on the diagnostic criteria employed [95]. Although sharing many of the features of primary depression, the PD-associated disorder is believed to be a distinct entity. Although its etiology is uncertain, and could develop secondary to a patient knowing that they having a chronic progressive neurodegenerative disease, PD-associated depression is believed to result from decreases in mood-altering monoamines including serotonin, noradrenalin, and dopamine associated with degeneration in the raphe nucleus, locus coeruleus, and SNc respectively. Additionally frontal cortical dysfunction known to exist in PD has also been suggested as a factor in the development of depression [95].

Anxiety has been shown to be more prevalent in PD patients than in the unaffected population. According to some reports, as many as 40% of patients may experience anxiety-related disorders [96], primarily expressed as general anxiety disorder, panic disorder, and social anxiety disorder [97]. Anxiety is often manifested in combination with depression in PD patients and determining a unique causation for anxiety has proven to be difficult. Like PD-associated depression, anxiety in PD patients is often manifest prior to the onset of motor symptoms and represents a distinct disorder from non-PD associated anxiety.

One of the most frequently utilized animal models of depression is the learned helplessness model. First developed by psychologists Martin Seligman and Steve Maier, the learned helplessness theory proposes that depression is a response to continual failed attempts at achieving a goal [98]. In this model, animals receive an inescapable stimulus, such as a repeated shock. The animals fail to be able to escape from the stimulus, demonstrating a "learned helplessness" [99]. Anxiety and depression-like symptoms can also be measured in animals by using the social interaction test, which measures the amount of social behavior between two previously unacquainted animals. Animals experiencing depression will typically display less social interaction than normal controls. Another popular animal model of depression is the forced swim task [100]. In this paradigm, animals are placed in water at a depth which necessitates swimming. Initially animals will swim attempting to find a platform or means of escape, but as the task continues the animals will demonstrate an immobile posture, floating on the water. In subsequent trials the amount of time spent swimming will decrease and the time spent immobile will increase. These and other methods have been used reliably as models in the evaluation of classic depression and increasingly in the evaluation of PD-associated depression.

6-OHDA lesions have also been used to assess whether the location of cell loss (i.e., SNc, ventral tegmental area, or a combination of loss to these areas) plays a role in the development of depression in PD patients. A recent study used 6-OHDA lesions placed in the SNc or in the ventral tegmental area to determine if there was a comorbidity between depression or psychiatric symptoms and parkinsonism in this model. They found that both lesions resulted in increased depression-like symptoms in rats, as measured by the learned helplessness task [101]. These findings suggest that dopamine cell loss is intimately related to the development of depression. Interestingly, the delivery of a selective serotonin uptake inhibitor class of anti-depressant resulted in the alleviation of the depression-like symptoms. Whether this suggests an as yet unidentified involvement of the serotonergic neurons in this model, or that the drug elicits its effects through modulating the dopaminergic system, is unclear.

Researchers have also used less severely affected early PD models to study some the psychiatric symptoms that can precede or coincide with the motor symptoms of PD. In a recent study, investigators looked at the cognitive and emotional deficits elicited in rats receiving low-dose 6-OHDA lesions (10.5 μg) bilaterally into the striatum [102]. In this relatively mild model, where striatal dopamine levels were decreased by only about 36%, rats showed significant emotional deficits, as measured by social interaction tests and the forced swim test, but no significant deficit in cognitive function when compared to rats receiving vehicle injections despite the absence of motor impairment [102]. Interestingly, in contrast to what is found in PD, rats receiving mild lesions showed a decrease in anxiety-related behaviors. A further analysis of this model may provide insight into the possible role of dopamine in the development of the non-motor psychiatric symptoms that are manifest in early in PD. For instance, an assay of monoamine and monoamine metabolite levels in the brains of these rats determined that whereas dopamine was reduced in 6-OHDA-treated rats, serotonin was not, a finding that differs from what is found in PD patients who typically have more extensive neurodegeneration. It will be interesting to discover if this biochemical discrepancy is responsible for the behavioral discrepancies noted, particularly the decreased anxiety observed in experimental animals.

Another study administered a low dose of 6-OHDA (12 μg) bilaterally into the striatum to try to characterize the cognitive and emotional deficits in a rat with mild to moderate striatal dopamine depletion [103]. The researchers found a significant increase in depression-like behaviors similar to what was reported in the previous study, but saw an increase in anxiety-like behaviors, more in keeping with what is found in PD. The authors reported a progressive loss of dopamine in the prefrontal cortex, which they proposed as a possible explanation for the increased anxiety observed. It may be that the increased dose of 6-OHDA from 10 to 12 μg, although small, may have resulted in a large enough loss of striatal dopamine to cross a threshold eliciting prefrontal cortical dopamine level alterations and anxiety-like behaviors.

Cognitive dysfunction

Cognitive dysfunction is arguably one of the most debilitating non-motor symptoms associated with PD patients and the major reason for nursing home placement for patients with advanced PD. Cognitive dysfunction can include a broad spectrum of functions, including executive function, learning and memory, and language [104,105]. The striatum, in addition to the motor cortex–striatal loop, also extends and receives projections from many other cortical areas, including the prefrontal cortex [106]. Dysfunction to this prefrontal–striatal circuitry may be responsible for some of the cognitive deficits seen in PD patients. Executive dysfunction in PD patients can include impairments in working memory [107], attention [108], and the initiation of goal-directed behaviors [109]. PD-associated cognitive dysfunction is distinct from the dementia that is seen in Alzheimer's disease (AD) [110] For instance, memory impairment is a more prominent feature of AD, whereas executive dysfunction is a more characteristic feature of PD. Further, whereas PD patients do show deficits in information recall (frontal lobe-dependent, responsive to cues), AD patients show deficits primarily in the encoding of information (hippocampal-dependent, unresponsive to cues) [111].

Sadly, in many PD patients cognitive dysfunction can progress to a frank dementia (PDD). Whereas information encoding is spared in PD patients without dementia, it begins to be lost as patients progress to a frank dementia. Likewise, many of the cognitive dysfunctions discussed above begin to worsen in severity. Additionally, patients suffering from PDD experience hallucinations at a much greater frequency than PD patients without dementia [112]. Unlike hallucinations in other forms of psychosis that are typically auditory, hallucinations in PDD are primarily visual. Additionally, PDD patients show a higher frequency of mood-related disorders than non-demented PD patients [113]. Although similarities do exist between PD- and AD-associated dementia, including the existence of β-amyloid plaques, LB pathology in the limbic and cerebral cortices is the principle pathology of PDD [113].

To date, the most effective treatment for cognitive dysfunction in PD and PDD has been cholinesterase inhibitors, particularly rivastigmine. In a large double-blind placebo-controlled clinical trial, rivastigmine was found to improve performance significantly in a battery of cognitive tests with few side effects and little to no worsening of parkinsonism (an exception was tremor, which worsened by 6% in rivastigmine-treated patients compared with placebo) in patients diagnosed with PDD [114].

Dysfunction of the cholinergic basal forebrain system has been implicated in the dementia of both AD and PD. This has been modeled in animals using excitotoxic lesions to the cholinergic neurons of the nucleus basalis. Interestingly, this nucleus shows LB pathology in the brains of PD patients, making this animal model potentially relevant to PDD. Animals with nucleus basalis lesions, produced with ibotenic acid or other excitotoxins, show deficits in learning and memory tasks. A similar approach to creating an animal model of cholinergic dysfunction has been to block the activity of the neural growth factor (NGF) on cholinergic neurons by using the immunotoxin 192 IgG-saporin (SAP). This antibody binds p75 receptors blocking the activity of NGF and creating learning and memory deficits in SAP-treated animals. Finally, dementia has been modeled in animals using fornix transections. This physical interruption of hippocampal efferents results in cognitive deficits in animals; however, this model is not particularly useful in determining the restorative effects of therapeutic interventions as they might apply to PD.

Cognitive dysfunction has also been relatively well studied in the classical models of PD. Interestingly, cognitive deficits have been studied in the MPTP-treated rat. Generally, rats are believed to be resistant to MPTP-induced toxicity, in part due to their high expression of monoamine oxidase B (MAO-B). However, bilateral delivery of MPTP (100 μg) to the SNc of rats can result in a very mild lesion that may model the very early pre-motor phase of PD [115]. Using this model, it has been shown that mild nigral lesions can lead to deficits in the Morris water maze test even in the absence of motor deficit [116]. Cognitive dysfunction has also been noted in the MPTP-treated monkey. In one study, monkeys treated with MPTP showed deficits in spatial memory that persisted for up to 10 years following toxin administration [117]. It remains uncertain whether pre-motor cognitive dysfunction and long-term deficits that worsen with disease progression occur via the same mechanisms.

Genetic models of PD have also been used to study cognitive deficits in PD. In Thy1–h[A30P]αSyn transgenic mice, progressive cognitive decline was noted when compared with wild-type controls as measured by the Morris water maze test [118]. In keeping with observations in human PD, Thy1–h[A20P]αSyn mice did not exhibit deficits until a relatively late age (12 months), and at sacrifice were found to show significant synucleinopathy throughout the central nervous system.

Some of the newer PD models have also been used to investigate cognitive decline. A recent study using the aphakia mouse model found that in addition to performing significantly worse in motor tasks (as measured by the rotorod task), affected mice showed significant deficits in the swimming T-maze task, the dry T-maze task, and passive avoidance learning when compared with wild-type controls, all behaviors dependent on intact prefrontal–striatal circuitry [44]. Aphakia mice are responsive to levodopa [119]; however, it is not yet known if this drug or other dopaminergic agents are able to reverse the cognitive deficits observed in these mice.

The LPS model of PD has also been used to study cognitive decline. In one study, acute administration of LPS (200 μg) to adult male rats resulted in subsequent suppression of gaping behavior, a learned conditioned response to toxic stimuli [120]. This finding is in keeping with other studies that have suggested that LPS-induced neuroinflammation can result in cognitive deficits [121,122]. How deficits in these and other models relate to the cognitive impairment that occurs in PD is not yet known.

Gait disturbances in PD

Gait dysfunction with postural instability is another of the major sources of disability in patients with advanced PD. These features may be improved with dopaminergic therapies in the early stages of the disease, but with disease progression cannot be controlled with available therapies and can force patients to be confined to bed or a wheelchair. Some patient with the akinetic rigid form of PD will have relatively early impairment of gait and balance, but the possibility of an atypical parkinsonism should be considered in these cases. Gait impairment is frequently associated with transient freezing at the onset or during the course of movement, particularly walking. Freezing of gait that occurs in off periods can often be improved with dopaminergic therapies, suggesting that dopamine degeneration somehow contributes to the development of this problem. On the other hand, freezing that occurs during off periods tends not to be helped with levodopa, suggesting that degeneration of other components of the motor system is primarily responsible for these problems.

Most assessments of gait dysfunction in PD have been descriptive, noting reduced automatic movements, decreased arm swing, small steps, and periods of retropulsion and festination. More recently, gait in PD has been assessed and mathematically modeled using a state-of-the-art OPTOTAK motion detection system. PD patients were found to have relatively normal swing and stance phases, but an inability automatically to dorsiflex the foot during the swing phase of gait [123]. There is no effective therapy for those aspects of gait impairment that do not respond to dopaminergic therapies, although it has been noted that freezing episodes can sometimes be improved by visual or auditory cueing.

Gait has not been adequately assessed in animal models, and it is not at all clear that the slowness of locomotion that occurs in the 6-OHDA or MPTP models are due to anything more than a dopamine lesion, and thus do not accurately replicate the gait disorder of PD. Studies in cats have shown that lesions in the region around the PPN can slow gait and reproduce some features of parkinsonism, and stimulation of this region can stimulate movement and improve gait [124]. For this reason, the area is often referred to as the mesencephalic locomotor region (MLR). The PPN is known to be affected in PD, and it is possible that degeneration in this region contributes to the gait dysfunction that occurs in PD. Attempts to generate a model of PD based on lesions in the PPN are currently being made. It is noteworthy that DBS of the PPN has been reported to improve gait dysfunction that cannot be improved with levodopa or DBS-STN in open-label studies in a small number of patients with advanced PD [125]. A recent report noted that stimulation of the dorsal columns in the spinal cord improved the gait disorder associated with 6-OHDA and dopamine depletion [126]. The authors postulated that this type of stimulation might break up a synchronization pattern that was responsible for gait dysfunction in this model but, as mentioned, it is not at all clear that this benefit was not due to simple excitation and perhaps dopamine release associated with stimulation. Further work to try to model the PD gait disorder in order to understand better the underlying anatomico-physiologic mechanisms and to develop more effective therapies is urgently required.

Therapy-induced non-motor features of PD

In addition to the use of animal models of PD to gain knowledge regarding the pathogenesis of cell death, the pathophysiology of disease symptoms, candidate targets for symptomatic and protective therapies, and as a model for testing new therapies, they have also been used to define and understand better the causation and treatment of the motor side effects of dopaminergic therapy. In addition to the motor complications of levodopa therapy, which are discussed in detail elsewhere [127], these include a series of non-motor problems such as impulse control disorders, dopamine dysregulation syndrome, and hallucinations.

Impulse control disorder and dopaminergic dysregulation syndrome can be debilitating non-motor side effects that typically result following high-dose therapy with dopaminergic agents. Impulse control disorders consist of pathological gambling, hypersexuality, and compulsive disorders such as eating and shopping. They have primarily been described in association with dopamine agonists. Dopamine dysregulation syndrome is more commonly seen with levodopa, and consists of an addiction-like syndrome where patients take increasing quantities of levodopa even though there is no obvious motor deficit. This can also be associated with punding, a repetitive series of purposeless activities that are performed for no apparent reason. These behaviors can be the most devastating to patients as they result in profound behavioral and personality changes [128]. Depending on the diagnosis criteria and on whether the patients themselves or loved ones are reporting, incidences of impulse control disorders can be as high as 14% [129]. One possible explanation for this high prevalence in treated PD patients is that dopaminergic therapies may be acting on the dopamine-sensitive mesolimbic reward system. Whereas dopamine therapies are designed to replace dopamine deficiency in nigrostriatal system, they also provide dopamine to the relatively intact mesolimbic system, which may cause it to become hyperactivated [128]. Indeed, functional neuroimaging studies demonstrate alterations in the ventral striatum of patients with pathological gambling tendencies.

The effective management of impulse control disorders in PD patients has not been extensively studied. However, current treatment includes the reduction or withdrawal of dopamine agonists and behavioral–cognitive therapy [130]. Because of its indirect effects on dopaminergic systems, many researchers hoped that STN-DBS would provide a possible therapy for PD that would not induce this debilitating side effect. Although inconclusive, two recent case studies in which PD patients developed hypersexuality following STN-DBS argue against this hypothesis [131]. Indeed, recent studies suggest that DBS-STN is more likely to induce an impulse control disorder than are dopamine agonists [132].

There are few animal experiments trying to model these features. Recently, a fascinating series of experiments were carried out by Frank *et al.* in animals and PD patients receiving DBS-STN [133]. These studies showed that stimulation of the STN was associated with a reduced capacity to inhibit making wrong selections. This important study indicates that although most attention has focused on the dopamine system as the basis for these disorders, alterations in non-dopaminergic components of the basal ganglia may be a factor. Further experiments testing the nature of these disorders and how the dopamine system, VTA–ventral striatum, and STN systems interrelate are required.

Visual hallucinations are another debilitating side effect of dopamine replacement that may occur in as many as 40% of late-stage PD patients [134]. Although these tend to be not threatening and patients are typically aware that their visual hallucinations are not real, they can become associated with delusions and paranoia, and are a risk factor for developing PDD. The first course of treatment is typically a reduction in dopamine agonists followed by cholinesterase inhibitors if the hallucinations persist [2].

Conclusion

It is becoming increasingly clear that the behavioral and pathological features of PD extend far beyond the classical motor symptoms associated with nigrostriatal dopamine deficiency. As this realization spreads, so to do the needs of researchers for new models in which to study the prevalent and potentially disabling non-motor and non-dopamine symptoms of PD. To date, the models that have been used to study PD have been nearly exclusively ones that concentrate on disruption of the dopamine system. These have proven extremely helpful in developing new symptomatic therapies for PD. They have also proven useful in understanding the pathophysiology of the motor complications associated with dopaminergic therapies and for designing new therapeutic strategies. However, it is now clear that there is involvement of the serotonergic, noradrenergic, and acetylcholinergic systems and also neuronal degeneration in the cerebral cortex, upper and lower brain stem, spinal cord, and peripheral autonomic nervous system in PD. Further, it is highly likely that this pathology underlies the various motor and non-motor features that do not respond to or are not adequately controlled by dopaminergic therapies. Indeed, these now represent the major source of disability for advanced PD patients. While the explosion of clinical interest focusing attention on these problems is encouraging, it is clear that these problems have not been adequately addressed or are not replicated in current models. A review of current PD models, such as in this chapter, makes it clear how much more work is necessary.

References

1. Chou K, Hurtig H. Classical motor features of Parkinson's disease. In: Ebadi M, Pfeiffer R, eds. *Parkinson's Disease.* Boca Raton, FL: CRC Press, 2005: 403–6.
2. Olanow CW, Stern MB, Sethi K. Scientific and clinical basis for the treatment of Parkinson disease. *Neurology* 2009;**72**(21 Suppl 4):S1–136
3. Spillantini MG, Crowther RA, Jakes R, *et al.* Alpha-synuclein in filamentous inclusions of Lewy bodies from Parkinson's disease and dementia with Lewy bodies. *Proc Natl Acad Sci USA* 1998;**95**:6469–73.
4. Golbe LI. Alpha-synuclein and Parkinson's disease. *Adv Neurol* 2003;**91**:165–74.
5. Blandini F, Nappi G, Tassorelli C, Martignoni E. Functional changes of the basal ganglia circuitry in Parkinson's disease. *Prog Neurobiol* 2000;**62**(1):63–88.
6. Obeso JA, Marin C, Rodriguez-Oroz MC, *et al.* The basal ganglia in Parkinson's disease: current concepts and unexplained observations. *Ann Neurol* 2008;**64**:S30–46.
7. Forno LS. Neuropathology of Parkinson's disease. *J Neuropathol Exp Neurol* 1996;**55**:259–72.
8. Chaudhuri KR, Healy DG, Schapira AHV. Non-motor symptoms of Parkinson's disease: diagnosis and management. *Lancet Neurol* 2006;**5**(3):235–45.
9. Aarsland D, Beyer MK, Kurz MW. Dementia in Parkinson's disease. *Curr Opin Neurol* 2008;**21**(6):676–82.

10. Hely MA, Morris JG, Reid WG, Trafficante R. Sydney Multicenter Study of Parkinson's disease: non-L-dopa-responsive problems dominate at 15 years. *Mov Disord* 2005;**20**:190–9.
11. Braak H, Braak E. Pathoanatomy of Parkinson's disease. *J Neurol* 2000;**247**(Suppl 2):459–69.
12. Braak H, Del Tredici K, Bratzke H, *et al.* Staging of the intracerebral inclusion body pathology associated with idiopathic Parkinson's disease (preclinical and clinical stages). *J Neurol* 2002;**249**(Suppl 3:III):1–5.
13. Braak H, Ghebremedhin E, Rub U, *et al.* Stages in the development of Parkinson's disease-related pathology. *Cell Tissue Res* 2004;**318**(1):121–34.
14. Braak H, Bohl JR, Muller CM, *et al.* Stanley Fahn Lecture 2005. The staging procedure for the inclusion body pathology associated with sporadic Parkinson's disease reconsidered. *Mov Disord* 2006;**21**(12):2042–51.
15. Langston JW. The Parkinson's complex: parkinsonism is just the tip of the iceberg. *Ann Neurol* 2006;**59**(4):591–6.
16. Jenner, P. Oxidative stress and Parkinson's disease. *Handb Clin Neurol* 2007;**83**:507–20.
17. McNaught KSP, Olanow CW, Halliwell B, *et al.* Failure of the ubiquitin–proteasome system in Parkinson's disease. *Nat Rev Neurosci* 2001;**2**:589–94.
18. Lim KL. Ubiquitin–proteasome system dysfunction in Parkinson's disease: current evidence and controversies. *Expert Rev Proteomics* 2007;**4**(6):769–81.
19. Olanow CW, McNaught K. The ubiquitin–proteasome system in Parkinson's disease. *Mov Disord* 2006;**21**:1806–23.
20. Schapira AHV, Cooper JM, Dexter D, *et al.* Mitochondrial complex I deficiency in Parkinson's disease. *J Neurochem* 1990;**54**:823–7.
21. Gupta A, Dawson VL, Dawson TM. What causes cell death in Parkinson's disease? *Ann Neurol* 2008;**64**(Suppl 2):S3–15.
22. Olanow CW. Pathogenesis of cell death in Parkinson's disease. *Mov Disord* 2007;**22**:S335–342.
23. Sachs C, Jonsson G. Mechanisms of action of 6-hydroxydopamine. *Biochem Pharmacol* 1975;**24**:1–8.
24. Soderstrom KE, Baum G, Kordower JH. Animal models of Parkinson's disease. In: Squire LR, ed. Encyclopedia of Neuroscience, Vol. 1. Oxford: Academic Press, 2009: 455–63.
25. Langston JW, Ballard P, Tetrud JW, Irwin I. Chronic parkinsonism in humans due to a product of meperidine-analog synthesis. *Science* 1983;**219**:979–80.
26. Przedborski S, Vila M. The 1-methyl-4-phenyl-1,2,3,6-tetrahydropyridine mouse model: a tool to explore the pathogenesis of Parkinson's disease. *Ann N Y Acad Sci* 2003;**991**:189–98.
27. Schultz, W. MPTP-induced parkinsonism in monkeys: mechanism of action, selectivity and pathophysiology. *Gen Pharmacol* 1988;**19**:153–61.
28. Fornai F, Schlüter OM, Lenzi P, *et al.* Parkinson-like syndrome induced by continuous MPTP infusion: convergent roles of the ubiquitin–proteasome system and alpha-synuclein. *Proc Natl Acad Sci USA* 2005;**102**:3413–8.
29. Olanow CW, Perl DP, DeMartino GN, McNaught K. Lewy-body formation is an aggresome-related process: a hypothesis. *Lancet Neurol* 2004;**3**:496–503.
30. Betarbet R, Sherer TB, MacKenzie G, *et al.* Chronic systemic pesticide exposure reproduces features of Parkinson's disease. *Nat Neurosci* 2000;**3**:1301–6.
31. Lapointe N, St-Hilaire M, Martinoli MG, *et al.* Rotenone induces non-specific central nervous system and systemic toxicity. *FASEB J* 2004;**18**:717–9.
32. Cannon JR, Tapias V, Na HM, *et al.* A highly reproducible rotenone model of Parkinson's disease. *Neurobiol Dis* 2009;**34**:279–90.
33. Schapira AHV, Olanow CW. Neuroprotection in Parkinson's disease: myths, mysteries, and misconceptions. *JAMA* 2004;**291**:358–64.
34. Polymeropoulos MH, Lavedan C, Leroy E, *et al.* Mutation in the alpha-synuclein gene identified in families with Parkinson's disease. *Science* 1997;**276**:2045–7.
35. Singleton AB, Farrer M, Johnson J. Alpha-synuclein locus triplication causes Parkinson's disease. *Science* 2003;**302**:841.
36. Chartier-Harlin MC, Kachergus J, Roumier C, *et al.* Alpha-synuclein locus duplication as a cause of familial Parkinson's disease. *Lancet* 2004;**364**:1167–9.
37. Feany MB, Bender WW. A *Drosophila* model of Parkinson's disease. *Nature* 2000;**404**:394–8.
38. van der Putten H, Wiederhold KH, Probst A, *et al.* Neuropathology in mice expressing human alpha-synuclein. *J Neurosci* 2000;**20**:6021–9.
39. Masliah E, Rockenstein E, Veinbergs I, *et al.* Dopaminergic loss and inclusion body formation in alpha-synuclein mice: implications for neurodegenerative disorders. *Science* 2000;**287**(5456):1265–9.
40. Kirik D, Björklund A. Modeling CNS neurodegeneration by overexpression of disease-causing proteins using viral vectors. *Trends Neurosci* 2003;**26**:386–92.
41. Liu Z, Wang X, Yu Y, et al. A *Drosophila* model for LRRK2-linked parkinsonism. *Proc Natl Acad Sci USA* 2008;**105**: 2693–8.
42. Lee SB, Kim W, Lee S, Chung J. Loss of LRRK2/PARK8 induces degeneration of dopaminergic neurons in *Drosophila*. *Biochem Biophys Res Commun* 2007;**358**:534–9.
43. Hwang DY, Ardayfio P, Kang UJ, *et al.* Selective loss of dopaminergic neurons in the substantia nigra of Pitx3- deficient aphakia mice. *Brain Res Mol Brain Res* 2003;**114**(2): 123–31.
44. Ardayfio P, Moon J, Leung KK, *et al.* Impaired learning and memory in Pitx3 deficient aphakia mice: a genetic model for striatum-dependent cognitive symptoms in Parkinson's disease. *Neurobiol Dis* 2008;**31**(3):406–12.
45. Gao HM, Kotzbauer PT, Uryu K, *et al.* Neuroinflammation and oxidation/nitration of alpha-synuclein linked to dopaminergic neurodegeneration. *J Neurosci* 2008;**28**: 7687–98.
46. McNaught KS, Björklund LM, Belizaire R, *et al.* Proteasome inhibition causes nigral degeneration with inclusion bodies in rats. *Neuroreport* 2002;**13**:1437–41.
47. McNaught KSP, Perl DP, Brownell AL, Olanow CW. Systemic exposure to proteasome inhibitors causes a progressive model of Parkinson's disease. *Ann Neurol* 2004;**56**:149–62.
48. Zeng BY, Bukhatwa S, Hikima A, *et al.* Reproducible nigral cell loss after systemic proteasomal inhibitor administration to rats. *Ann Neurol* 2006;**60**:248–52.
49. Schapira AH, Cleeter MW, Muddle JR, *et al.* Proteasomal inhibition causes loss of nigral tyrosine hydroxylase neurons. *Ann Neurol* 2006;**60**:253–5.

50. Nair VD, McNaught KS, González-Maeso J, *et al.* p53 mediates nontranscriptional cell death in dopaminergic cells in response to proteasome inhibition. *J Biol Chem* 2006;**281**:39550–60.
51. Bukhatwa S, Iravani MM, Zeng BY, *et al.* An immunohistochemical and stereological analysis of PSI-induced nigral neuronal degeneration in the rat. *J Neurochem* 2009;**109**: 52–9.
52. Bové J, Zhou C, Jackson-Lewis V, *et al.* Proteasome inhibition and Parkinson's disease modeling. *Ann Neurol* 2006;**60**: 260–4.
53. Kordower JH, Kanaan NM, Chu Y, *et al.* Failure of proteasome inhibitor administration to provide a model of Parkinson's disease in rats and monkeys. *Ann Neurol* 2006;**60**: 264–8.
54. Manning-Boğ AB, Reaney SH, Chou VP, *et al.* Lack of nigrostriatal pathology in a rat model of proteasome inhibition. *Ann Neurol* 2006;**60**:256–60.
55. Bedford L, Hay D, Devoy A, *et al.* Depletion of 26S proteasomes in mouse brain neurons causes neurodegeneration and Lewy-like inclusions resembling human pale bodies. *J Neurosci* 2008;**28**:8189–98.
56. Chu Y, Kordower JH. Age-associated increases of alpha-synuclein in monkeys and humans are associated with nigrostriatal dopamine depletion: is this the target for Parkinson's disease? *Neurobiol Dis* 2007;**25**(1):134–49.
57. Lang AE, Lozano AM. Parkinson's disease – first of two parts. *Med Prog* 1998;**339**:1044–53.
58. Gibb WR, Lees AJ. The relevance of the Lewy body to the pathogenesis of idiopathic Parkinson's disease. *J Neurol Neurosurg Psychiatry* 1988;**51**(6):745–52.
59. Manaye K, McIntire D, Mann D, German D. Locus coeruleus cell loss in the aging human brain: a non-random process. *J Comp Neurol* 2004;**358**(1):79.
60. Goldstein DS. Cardiac denervation in patients with Parkinson's disease. *Cleveland Clin J Med* 2007;**74**(Suppl 1):S91–4.
61. Pfeiffer RF. Non-motor parkinsonism. *Parkinsonism Relat Disord* 2007;**13**(Suppl 3):S211–20.
62. Suzuki M, Hattori N, Orimo S, *et al.* Preserved myocardial [^{123}]metaiodobenzylguanidine uptake in autosomal recessive juvenile parkinsonism: first case report. *Mov Disord* 2005;**20**(5):634–6.
63. Iwanaga K, Wakabayashi K, Yoshimoto M, *et al.* Lewy body-type degeneration in cardiac plexus in Parkinson's and incidental Lewy body diseases. *Neurology* 1999;**52**:1269.
64. Walter BL. Cardiovascular autonomic dysfunction in patients with movement disorders. *Cleveland Clin J Med* 2008;**75**(Suppl 2):S54–8.
65. Henderson JM, Schleimer SB, Allbutt H, *et al.* Behavioral effects of parafascicular thalamic lesions in an animal model of parkinsonism. *Behav Brain Res* 2005;**162**:222–32.
66. Natale G, Pasquali L, Ruggieri S, *et al.* Parkinson's disease and the gut: a well known clinical association in need of an effective cure and explanation. *Neurogastroenterol Motil* 2008;**20**:741–9.
67. Fox SH, Brotchie JM, Lang AE. Non-dopaminergic treatments in development for Parkinson's disease. *Lancet Neurol* 2008;**7**(10):927–38.
68. Liu Z, Sakakibara R, Odaka T, *et al.* Mosapride citrate, a novel 5-HT4 agonist and partial 5-HT3 antagonist, ameliorates constipation in parkinsonian patients. *Mov Disord* 2005;**20**(6):680–6.
69. Asai H, Udaka F, Hirano M, *et al.* Increased gastric motility during 5-HT4 agonist therapy reduces response fluctuations in Parkinson's disease. *Parkinsonism Relat Disord* 2005;**11**(8): 499–502.
70. Anderson G, Noorian AR, Taylor G, *et al.* Loss of enteric dopaminergic neurons and associated changes in colon motility in an MPTP mouse model of Parkinson's disease. *Exp Neurol* 2007;**207**(1):4–12.
71. Wang L, Fleming SM, Chesselet MF, Tache Y. Abnormal colonic motility in mice overexpressing human wild-type alpha-synuclein. *Neuroreport* 2008;**19**(8):873–6.
72. Comella CL. Sleep disorders in Parkinson's disease: an overview. *Mov Disord* 2007;**22**(Suppl 17):S367–73.
73. Boeve BF, Silber MH, Saper CB, *et al.* Pathophysiology of REM sleep behavior disorder and relevance to neurodegenerative disease. *Brain* 2007;**130**:2770–88.
74. Rye D. Contributions of the pedunculopontine region to normal and altered REM sleep. *Sleep* 1997;**20**:757–88.
75. Schenck CH, Bundlie SR, Mahowald MW. Delayed emergence of a parkinsonian disorder in 38% of 29 older men initially diagnosed with idiopathic rapid eye movement sleep behavioral disorder. *Neurology* 1996;**46**(2):388–93.
76. Homann CN, Wenzel K, Suppan K, *et al.* Sleep attacks in patients taking dopamine agonists: review. *BMJ* 2002;**324** (7352):1483–7.
77. Schmidt MH, Koshal VB, Schmidt HS. Use of prmipexole in REM sleep behavior disorder: results from a case series. *Sleep Med* 2006;**7**(5):418–23.
78. Gagnon JF, Postuma RB, Montplaisir J. Update on the pharmacology of REM sleep behavior disorder. *Neurology* 2006;**67**(5):742–7.
79. Schenck C, Bundlie S, Mahowald M. REM behavior disorder (RBD): delayed emergence of parkinsonism and/or dementia in 65% of older men initially diagnosed with idiopathic RBD, and an analysis of the minimum and maximum tonic and/or phasic electromyographic abnormalities found during REM sleep. *Sleep* 2003;**26**:A3316.
80. Baier P, Branisa P, Kock R, *et al.* Circadian distribution of motor activity in unilaterally 6-hydroxy-dopamine lesioned rats. *Exp Brain Res* 2006;**169**:283–8.
81. Almirall H, Pigarev I, de la Clazada MD, *et al.* Nocturnal sleep structure and temperature slope in MPTP treated monkeys. *J Neural Transm* 1999;**106**(11–12): 1125–34.
82. Monaca C, Laloux C, Jacquesson JM, *et al.* Vigilance states in a parkinsonian model, the MPTP mouse. *Eur J Neurosci* 2004;**20**(9):2472–8.
83. Laloux C, Derambure P, Kreisler A, *et al.* MPTP-treated mice: long-lasting loss of nigral TH-ir neurons but not paradoxical sleep alteration. *Exp Brain Res* 2008;**186**:635–42.
84. Johnston AN, Mellick GD, Herting B, *et al.* Prevalence of smell loss in Parkinson's disease – a multicenter study. *Parkinsonism Relat Disord* 2009;**15**(7):490–4.
85. Doty RL, Singh A, Tetrud J, Langston JW. Lack of major olfactory dysfunction in MPTP-induced parkinsonism. *Ann Neurol* 1992;**32**(1):97–100.
86. Huisman E, Uylings HBM, Hoogland PV. A 100% increase of dopaminergic cells in the olfactory bulb may explain hyposmia in Parkinson's disease. *Mov Disord* 2004;**19**(6):687–92.

87. Guo, X, Guo G, Wang X, *et al.* Effects of bilateral deep brain stimulation of the subthalamic nucleus on olfactory function in Parkinson's disease patients. *Stereotactic Funct Neurosurg* 2008;**86**:237–44.
88. Miwa T, Watanabe A, Mitsumoto Y, *et al.* Olfactory impairment and Parkinson's disease-like symptoms observed in the common marmoset following administration of 1-methyl-4-phenyl-1,2,3,6-tetrahyddropyridine. *Acta Oto-laryngol* 2004; **124**(Suppl 553):80–4.
89. Doty RL, Stern MB, Pfeiffer C, *et al.* Bilateral olfactory dysfunction in early stage treated and untreated idiopathic Parkinson's disease. *J Neurol Neurosurg Psychiatry* 1992;**55**(2):138–42.
90. Fleming SM, Tetreault NA, Mulligan CK, *et al.* Olfactory deficits in mice overexpressing human wildtype α-synuclein. *Eur J Neurosci* 2008;**28**:247–56.
91. Ford B. Pain in Parkinson's disease. *Clin Neurosci* 1998;**5**(2): 63–72.
92. Tassorelli C, Armetero M, Greco R, *et al.* Behavioral response and Fos activation following painful stimuli in a rodent model of Parkinson's disease. *Brain Res* 2007;**1176**:53–61.
93. Rosland JH, Hunskaar S, Brock OJ, Hole K. Acute and long term effects of 1-methyl-4-phenyl-1,2,3,6-tetrahydorpyridine (MPTP) in tests of nociception in mice. *Pharmacol Toxicol* 1992;**70**(1):31–7.
94. Cummings JL, Masterman DL. Depression in patients with Parkinson's disease. *Int J Geriatr Psychiatry* 1999;**14**:711–8.
95. Lemke MR, Fuchs G, Gemende I, *et al.* Depression and Parkinson's disease. *J Neurol* 2004;**251**(Suppl 6: VI):24–7.
96. Richard IH, Schiffer RB, Kurlan R. Anxiety and Parkinson's disease. *J Neuropsychiatry Clin Neurosci* 1996;**8**(4):383–92.
97. Richard IH. Anxiety disorders in Parkinson's disease. *Adv Neurol* 2005;**96**:42–55.
98. Maier SF. Learned helplessness and animal models of depression. *Prog Neuro-psychopharmacol Biol Psychiatry* 1984;**8**(3):435–46.
99. Seligman ME, Beagley G. Learned helplessness in the rat. *J Comp Physiol Psychol* 1975;**88**(2):534–41.
100. Porsolt RD, Brossard G, Hautbois C, Roux S. Rodent models of depression: forced swimming and tail suspension behavioral despair tests in rats and mice. *Curr Protocols Neurosci* 2001;Unit 8.10A.
101. Winter C, von Rumohr A, Mundt A, *et al.* Lesions of dopaminergic neurons in the substantia nigra pars compacta and in the ventral tegmental area enhance depressive-like behaviors in rats. *Behav Brain Res* 2007;**184**:133–41.
102. Branchi I, D'Andrea I, Armida M, *et al.* Nonmotor symptoms in Parkinson's disease: investigating early-phase onset of behavioral dysfunction in the 6-hydroxydopamine-lesioned rat model. *J Neurosci Res* 2008;**86**:2050–61.
103. Tadaiesky MT, Dombrowski PA, Figueiredo CP, *et al.* Emotional, cognitive and neurochemical alterations in a premotor stage model of Parkinson's disease. *Neuroscience* 2008;**156**:830–40.
104. Caballol N, Marti MJ, Tolosa E. Cognitive dysfunction and dementia in Parkinson's disease. *Mov Disord* 2007;**22**(Suppl 17):S358–66.
105. Emre M, Aarsland D, Brown R, *et al.* Clinical diagnostic criteria for dementia associated with Parkinson's disease. *Mov Disord* 2007;**22**:1689–707.
106. Alexander GE, DeLong MR, Strick PL. Parallel organization of functionally segregated circuits linking basal ganglia and cortex. *Annu Rev Neurosci* 1986;**9**:357–81.
107. Owen AM, Iddon JL, Hodges JR, *et al.* Spatial and non-spatial working memory at different stages of Parkinson's disease. *Neuropsychologia* 1997;**35**(4):519–32.
108. Bloxham CA, Dick DJ, Moore M. Reaction times and attention in Parkinson's disease. *J Neurol Neurosurg Psychiatry* 1987;**50**: 1178–83.
109. Hanna-Pladdy B. Dysexecutive syndromes in neurologic disease. *J Neurol Phys Ther* 2007;**31**(3):119–27.
110. Huber SJ, Shuttleworth EC, Freidenberg DL. Neuropsychological differences between the dementias of Alzheimer's and Parkinson's disease. *Arch Neurol* 1989;**46**(12):1287–91.
111. Zgaljardic DJ, Borod JC, Foldi NS, Mattis P. A review of cognitive and behavioral sequelae of Parkinson's disease: relationship to frontostriatal circuitry. *Cogn Behav Neurol* 2003;**16**(4): 193–210.
112. Aarsland D, Larsen JP, Lim NG, *et al.* Range of neuropsychiatric disturbances in patients with Parkinson's disease. *J Neurol Neurosurg Psychiatry* 1999;**67**(4):492–6.
113. Goetz CG, Emre M, Dubois B. Parkinson's disease dementia: definitions, guidelines, and research perspectives in diagnosis. *Ann Neurol* 2008;**64**(Suppl 2):S81–92.
114. Emre M, Aarsland D, Albanese A, *et al.* Rivastigmine for dementia associated with Parkinson's disease. *N Engl J Med* 2004;**351**:2509–18.
115. Da Cunha C, Gevaerd MS, Vital M, *et al.* Memory disruption in rats with nigral lesions induced by MPTP: a model for early Parkinson's disease amnesia. *Behav Brain Res* 2001;**124**:9–18.
116. Ferro M, Bellissimo M, Anselmo-Franci, J, *et al.* Comparison of bilaterally 6-OHDA- and MPTP-lesioned rats as models of the early phase of Parkinson's disease: histological, neurochemical, motor and memory alterations. *J Neurosci Methods* 2005;**148**:78–87.
117. Fernandez-Ruiz J, Douden DJ, Aigner TG. Long-term cognitive impairment in MPTP-treated rhesus monkeys. *Neuroreport* 1995;**7**(1):102–4.
118. Freichel C, Neumann M, Ballard T, *et al.* Age-dependent cognitive decline and amygdala pathology in alpha-synuclein transgeneic mice. *Neurobiol Aging* 2007;**28**(9):1421–35.
119. Hwang DY, Fleming SM, Ardayfio P, *et al.* 3,4-Dihydoxyphenyalanine reverses the motor deficits in Pitx3-deficient aphakia mice: behavioral characterization of a novel genetic model of Parkinson's disease. *J Neurosci* 2005;**25**(8): 2132–7.
120. Chan M, Cross-Mellor S, Kavaliers M, Pssenkopp KP. Lipopolysaccharide (LPS) blocks the acquisition of LiCl-induced gaping in a rodent model of anticipatory nausea. *Neurosci Lett* 2009;**450**:301–305.
121. Hennigan A, Trotter C, Kelly A. Lipopolysaccharide impairs long-term potentiation and recognition memory and increases p75NTR expression in the rat dentate gyrus. *Brain Res* 12007;**130**:158–66.
122. Kelly A, Vereker E, Nolan Y, *et al.* Activation of p38 plays a pivotal role in the inhibitory effect of lipopolysaccharide and interleukin-1 beta on long term potentiation in rat dentate gyrus. *J Biol Chem* 2003;**278**:19453–62.
123. Cho C, Osaki Y, Kunin M, *et al.* A model-based approach for assessing parkinsonian gait and effects of levodopa and

deep brain stimulation. *IEEE Eng Med Biol Soc* 2006;**1**:1228–31.

124. Pahapill PA, Lozano AM. The pedunculopontine nucleus and Parkinson's disease. *Brain* 2000;**123**:1767–83.
125. Stefani A, Lozano AM, Peppe A, *et al.* Bilateral deep brain stimulation of the pedunculopontine and subthalamic nuclei in severe Parkinson's disease. *Brain* 2007;**130**:1596–607.
126. Fuentes R, Petersson P, Siesser WB, *et al.* Spinal cord stimulation restores locomotion in animal models of Parkinson's disease. *Science* 2009;**323**:1578–82.
127. Olanow CW, Obeso JA, Stocchi F. Continuous dopamine receptor stimulation in the treatment of Parkinson's disease: scientific rationale and clinical implications. *Lancet Neurol* 2006;**5**:677–87.
128. Lim SY, Evans AH, Miyasaki JM. Impulse control and related disorders in Parkinson's disease: review. *Ann N Y Acad Sci* 2008;**1142**:85–107.
129. Merims D, Giladi N. Dopamine dysregulation syndrome, addiction and behavioral changes in Parkinson's disease. *Parkinsonism Relat Disord* 2008;**14**(4):273–80.
130. Galpern WR, Stacy M. Management of impulse control disorders in Parkinson's disease. *Curr Treat Options Neurol* 2007;**9**(3):189–97.
131. Doshi P, Bhargava P. Hypersexuality following subthalamic nucleus stimulation for Parkinson's disease. *Neurol India* 2008;**56**(4):474–6.
132. Hälbig TD, Tse W, Frisina PG, *et al.* Subthalamic deep brain stimulation and impulsivity in Parkinson's disease. *Eur J Neurol* 2009;**16**:493–7.
133. Frank MJ, Samanta J, Moustafa AA, Sherman SJ. Hold your horses: impulsivity, deep brain stimulation, and medication in parkinsonism. *Science* 2007;**318**:1309–12.
134. Poewe W. When a Parkinson's disease patient starts to hallucinate. *Pract Neurol* 2008;**8**(4):238–41.

Chapter 8
The Emerging Entity of Pre-Motor Parkinson's Disease

J. William Langston
Parkinson's Institute, Sunnyvale, CA, USA

Prologue

Although this chapter will focus on the "pre-motor" features of Parkinson's disease (PD), it must be set in the frame of a larger picture of our evolving concept of what the disease actually is. At the current time, PD is not diagnosed unless typical motor features are present. Indeed, most clinicians will consider the diagnosis only when at least two of the classical motor features of rest tremor, rigidity, and bradykinesia are present. These features are so well ensconced in the neurologic lexicon that they have been given birth to the more generic term "parkinsonism," a constellation of clinical signs rather than a disease. However, we are now in a somewhat historic time in which researchers and clinicians are re-evaluating the scope and nature of PD. During the last 10 years, the breadth of the disorder has become much more obvious and it is now clear that the pathologic process, at least as measured by the presence of α-synuclein containing Lewy bodies and Lewy neurites, is widely distributed throughout the brain, spinal cord, and peripheral autonomic nervous system, with parkinsonism representing only the tip of the iceberg [1]. While clues to this have been accumulating for three-quarters of a century, these changes have become dramatically apparent with the advent of immunohistochemical stains for the protein α-synuclein, a major component of Lewy bodies and neurites [2] (see also Chapter 2) and have led to an entirely new staging system [3]. As the clincopathologic correlates of non-parkinsonian features of the disease are becoming better defined, it is increasingly apparent that the motor features of PD are part of a much broader spectrum of signs and symptoms [1,4,5]

Does this mean that we should change the diagnostic criteria for PD? The answer is – not yet. On a practical basis, the field is still at a point where few if any would make a diagnosis of Parkinson's disease in the absence of the classic motor features. Ironically, many neuropathologists will not make a diagnosis of PD without a history of parkinsonism during life, no matter how typical the pathologic findings are (a fact that has skewed the literature as cases without parkinsonism in life are not included in pathologic reports of what otherwise might have been diagnosed as PD). This puts the field into something of a vicious cycle, as we have become trapped in our own definitions. However, it seems increasingly plausible that certain combinations of non-motor signs and symptoms [5] will prove to be just as accurate at predicting the presence of a chronic, progressive synucleinopathy of the brain and peripheral nervous system as are the classical PD features that meets the British brain bank research criteria [6].

This broader view of pre-motor PD has several conceptual implications. First, if one accepts that all of the pre-motor features of the PD are a part of the disease, then they are not risk factors or biomarkers, but actually manifestations of the disease itself. This is a concept that takes some time getting used to, because the concept of PD so strongly implies motor dysfunction. Second, as will be discussed later, if Lewy body diseases are part of a continuum, then in some instances dementia could be a pre-motor feature of PD, even though by certain consensus criteria when dementia precedes parkinsonism, or occurs within 1 year of the onset of parkinsonism, it is called dementia with Lewy bodies (DLB) [7] rather than PD or Parkinson's disease dementia (PDD). Complicating matters even more is that fact that some classical pre-motor features of PD, such as REM sleep behavior disorder (RBD) or depression, may never be followed by clinically diagnosable PD, even though postmortem examination reveals full-blown pathologic features of typical Lewy body PD [8,9]. Alternatively, other "pre-motor" features may not occur until the post-motor phase, or may never occur at all [10]. Hence putting the pieces of the parkinsonian puzzle into a clear-cut continuum is likely to be challenging, and the major burden

Parkinson's Disease: Non-Motor and Non-Dopaminergic Features, First Edition. Edited by C. Warren Olanow, Fabrizio Stocchi, and Anthony E. Lang.

of nomenclature will probably be borne by the clinicians. It is against this challenge in redefining our concepts PD and related Lewy body disorders that this chapter tackles what we know about the "pre-motor" features of PD.

Introduction

Until recently, what are generally becoming known as the pre-motor features of PD have been largely neglected in PD. There are many historical reasons for the lack of focus on these features. First and foremost is the legacy from the pre-L-dopa days. When the neurodegenerative process that underlies classical PD strikes the dopaminergic substantia nigra with enough force, in the absence of effective dopaminergic therapies, the physical symptoms are catastrophic. Indeed, because of the profound motor deficits, disability was severe and the average life-span of patients was significantly shortened. Little wonder, then, that the motor features gained such prominence. This changed with the discovery that these motor symptoms were largely due to the degeneration of nigrostriatal neurons [11,12] and the corresponding striatal dopamine deficiency [13]. Even more remarkable was the dramatic discovery that this motor deficit could be overcome by administering the dopamine precursor levodopa [14]. It is not surprising, then, that for the past 50 years the field has largely focused, some would say obsessively, on the motor symptoms of PD. Interestingly, the success that we have achieved with dopaminergic therapies has led to the unmasking of the non-motor features of the disease, many of which had been overshadowed by the parkinsonism when left in an untreated state [15]. Indeed, it would not be an overstatement to say that the last 10 years has led to a profound awakening regarding the significance of the non-motor features of PD. This is illustrated by the longitudinal Sydney Multicenter Study, which showed that disability at 15 years was predominantly due to the non-motor features of the disease [16]. This historic evolution has provided insights into the importance of the many non-dopaminergic systems that are affected in the disease.

As the non-motor features of PD have become increasingly well characterized, another, related, question has begun to emerge, namely how many of these non-motor features can precede the onset of classic parkinsonism, and for those that can, when and how often does this occur? That the disease begins well before motor features become manifest has long been assumed based on the fact that a substantial depletion of striatal dopamine is required before symptoms emerge. Indeed, imaging studies employing ligands that assess the dopaminergic nigrostriatal system suggest that the process of nigrostriatal degeneration has been ongoing for at least 5–6 years prior to motor symptoms (see Chapter 9). However, these imaging studies typically do not measure other aspects of the disease. It is now becoming increasingly clear that some of these other features may precede the onset of parkinsonism by many years or even decades, and represent not pre-symptomatic disease, but pre-motor symptoms of the disease.

There is little doubt that one of the factors that triggered interest in this evolving concept is the work of Braak *et al.* [3], who hypothesized that the evolution of PD follows a relatively orderly process after it begins in the central nervous system (CNS), first appearing in the dorso-motor nucleus of the vagus and the olfactory bulb (stage 1), then ascending up the brainstem and eventually involving the cortices (Braak stage 6 – see Chapter 3). While Braak's staging system is based on the static pictures of postmortem brain, the hypothesis that the disease begins in the brainstem and/or olfactory bulb drew even more interest in the possibility that Braak's stages 1 and 2 might not be "pre-symptomatic" stages as suggested in their illustrations [3], but rather could be associated with their own clinical manifestations, albeit not those of classical PD. Since in Braak's staging the involvement of the substantia nigra comes midway in disease evolution (stage 3), it did not take long for both clinicians and basic scientists to search in earnest for signs and symptoms that predate the motor features of these disease. Although many of these clues have been in front of us for nearly as long as the disease has been recognized, the pieces of the puzzle really did not come together forcefully until recently. Nowhere was this more obvious than with the recognition of the importance of RBD and its relationship to PD and related Lewy body disorders.

REM sleep behavioral disorder (RBD) – the concept of pre-motor PD comes of age

One of the major blocks to investigating the pre-motor signs and symptoms of PD is that, until recently, there has been no known way to identify a meaningful cohort of individuals who are going to develop diagnosable PD prospectively and then study them objectively for signs and symptoms that occur before the actual motor features PD become manifest. RBD appears to be one of the few opportunities to do this (LRRK2 mutations [17] and hyposmia may represent others). RBD is extensively reviewed elsewhere in this volume (see Chapter 23), so the focus here will on the role that the discovery of this syndrome has had in shaping interest in pre-motor features of the disease. First described by Schenk *et al.* [18], this disorder was largely limited to the sleep literature until the same group reported that, after 13 years, nearly 40% of affected patients developed PD [19]. Not surprisingly, the last few years have witnessed a dramatic increase in interest in RBD because of the accumulating evidence that RBD is a manifestation of a Lewy body disease in the brainstem that can progress to PD or related Lewy body disorders. For example, Posthuma *et al.* [20] reported that the 5 year risk of developing a neurodegenerative disease in patients diagnosed with RBD is approximately 18%, with a 12 year risk of 52%. Similarly, Hickey *et al.* [21] found that 45% of patients with RBD developed PD or Lewy body dementia at 11.5 years. By far the most parsimonious explanation for these findings is that RBD is a manifestation of a brainstem synucleinopathy that has not yet progressed to the point that it affects brain structures leading to parkinsonism or dementia.

Adding credence to this hypothesis are the three autopsy studies of pure RBD that have been reported to date. One patient had a 20 year history of RBD without parkinsonian features, and yet exhibited all of they typical neuropathologic findings of PD at autopsy [8], including nigral cell loss and α-synuclein-positive Lewy bodies and neurites. A second patient had a 15 year history of RBD without a history of any other neurologic disorder. Autopsy findings revealed pathologic findings consistent with Braak stage 3 PD [22]. The third case, which predated α-synuclein immunohistochemistry, was found to have cortical Lewy bodies using ubiquitin staining, in addition to changes typical of Alzheimer's disease [23]. If all the cases with RBD that have been examined neuropathologically are considered, the majority appear to have Lewy body disease, and virtually all do if MSA is included [24].

What is all the more remarkable about this story is that RBD now stands alone as the most effective predictor of developing typical PD or a related synucleinopathy. Not even LRRK2 mutations are as predictive of developing PD and/or a DLB-like condition. On the other hand, not all patients with PD will express clinical manifestations of RBD. Approximately 20–40% of patients with PD give a history compatible with RBD. However, if patients who fail to demonstrate an absence of muscle tone during REM sleep as assessed during polysomnography are included, even though there is no history of dream-enacting behavior (so-called subclinical RBD), this figure reaches around 60% [10]. So, while a brainstem synucleinopathy (Braak stage 1–3) seems capable of causing RBD, it is equally clear that not all such cases manifest RBD, even when the process has reached its most advance stages. It is also important to note that some patients go on to develop a dementia with Lewy bodies (DLB) picture rather than PD [24]. This harks back to the Prologue of this chapter, where the point was made that Lewy body diseases may all be a part of a continuum, and that the real problem may be using parkinsonism as the anchor for diagnosing what is in essence a chronic progressive synucleinopathy of the brain, spinal cord, and peripheral autonomic nervous systems.

In summary, there are several important lessons to be learned from RBD. The first is that the progressive synucleinopathy that seems to be an integral part of PD can clearly cause brainstem symptoms before sufficient damage in the substantia nigra leads to parkinsonism; as a result, these symptoms can precede the classical features of PD. This echoes a theme that will be encountered throughout this chapter, namely that parkinsonism is just one manifestation of a much wider spread disorder. Second, of course, is that patients with pure (or idiopathic RBD) provide an opportunity to investigate the pre-motor features of the disease. Since there are no population-based studies of RBD, we really do not know how common it is, and even if we did, cases are difficult to ascertain in the general population, as it is not clear how many ever come to medical attention. Therefore, it is unlikely to provide a way to screen the general population for pre-motor PD, something that is becoming increasingly important as there are more and more clinical trials aimed disease modification. What is very clear, however, is that we now have a tool to develop a research cohort of individuals with pre-motor PD (Braak stage 2 or early stage 3) that could be invaluable for investigating other pre-motor features of the disease. This remarkable parasomnia offers us an exceptional window to identify patients with a progressive synucleinopathy of the brainstem that is very likely to be part of the continuum that includes PD and DLB.

Olfactory dysfunction

First reported as a feature of PD by Anasri and Johnson in 1975 [25], this novel aspect of PD was for a long time disregarded as an odd curiosity. However, it is now becoming recognized as an important feature of the disease for a variety of reasons. First, there is a compelling body of literature indicating that it is one of the most consistent features of PD. It is present in 60–100% of patients with motor features of PD, particularly when formally tested [26–33], and detection can be improved by extending testing across different tasks [26]. This frequency of hyposmia cannot be explained by aging alone [34]. Second, from a pathologic standpoint, the olfactory bulb appears to be one of the most consistently involved areas of the brain [3,35]. Indeed, the presence of Lewy bodies in the olfactory bulb is highly predictive of Lewy bodies elsewhere in the brain [36]. In a recent study highlighting the importance of olfaction in PD, Bohen *et al.* [37] compared the accuracy of various clinical motor and non-motor tests for the diagnosis of PD and found that the hyposmia was the single most accurate predictive factor of PD among all of motor and non-motor features tested. In another remarkable observation, Goldstein and Sewell [38] actually found a correlation between hyposmia and cardiac sympathetic innervation of the heart as measured by

[6-^{18}F]fluorodopamine positron emission tomography (PET) imaging. As will be discussed later, loss of autonomic innervation of the heart appears to be one of the most fundamental findings not only in motor PD, but also in the pre-motor stage of the disease.

Once again, the emerging interest in olfactory dysfunction as a pre-motor and perhaps sentinel feature of PD was inspired, at least in part, by the work of Braak *et al.*, who pointed to pathologic involvement of the olfactory bulb as one of the earliest pathologic features of the disease (stage 1) [3]. As a result, there is now a wealth of studies indicating that olfactory dysfunction can precede the onset of motor features. Perhaps the most compelling of these was carried out by Ross *et al.* [39], who took advantage of the Honolulu–Asian Aging Study (HAAS) cohort to study 2267 subjects without PD (aged 71–95 years) who had undergone testing for olfactory function. and assessed incident PD over the subsequent 8 years. They found a 5.2-fold increase in the risk of developing PD for subjects in the lowest quartile of olfactory function compared with those in the top two quartiles, and concluded that impaired olfaction can precede the onset of PD by at least 4 years. In another study that involved 30 patients with idiopathic olfactory loss [40], 11 were found to have increased echogenicity of the substantia nigra with transcranial sonography, which is thought to be a marker of nigral degeneration. Ten of these 11 patients underwent SPECT scans with [^{123}I]FP-CIT, and five had abnormal scans suggesting preclinical degeneration of the nigrostriatal system (another two had borderline changes). After 4 years, 7% had developed PD and another 13% had developed at least some motor features of the disease [41].

Berendse *et al.* [42] took another approach to this question by evaluating 250 relatives of patients with PD. From this group, 25 hyposmic and 23 normosmic individuals were chosen for [^{123}I]beta-CIT SPECT scanning. Four of the hyposmic individuals had abnormal scans, and two of these eventually developed PD, thus providing evidence that anosmia can precede the onset of the motor features of PD; importantly, none of the normosmic individuals had abnormal scans or developed PD. In another study of 361 normal first-degree relatives of PD patients, those with olfactory dysfunction were found to have a significantly increased risk of developing PD in a 5-year period [43]. These studies have been compelling enough that a large multicenter study has been launched to assess 3000 first-degree relatives of patients with PD. Those with hyposmia and also a subset of normosmic controls are being enrolled in a long-term follow-up study to determine the risk for developing PD. This study, known as the Parkinson's Associated Risk Syndrome (PARS) study, includes an assessment of a variety of non-motor features in addition to SPECT imaging, and represents the largest study of this nature to date.

As pointed out in the previous section, RBD patients present a unique opportunity to search for other signs and symptoms of pre-motor PD. With this in mind, Stiasny-Kolster *et al.* [44] examined a group of 30 patients with pure RBD for hyposmia. Remarkably, they found that 97% had an abnormal sense of smell. They observed that the combination of hyposmia and RBD is highly compatible with Braak stage 2 disease, and is supportive of the hypothesis that hyposmia can precede the onset of PD. Adding additional evidence to this hypothesis was the fact that on neurologic examination, five patients had newly discovered signs of PD. In four of these the findings actually met British Brain Bank criteria for a diagnosis of PD, again providing compelling evidence that in some patients there is a constellation of clinical features that suggest early per-motor PD. Finally, two of the pure RBD patients showed evidence of preclinical nigrostriatal degeneration on [^{123}I]FP-CIT SPECT scanning.

Because olfactory testing is dependent on patient responses, there is interest in finding ways to measure olfaction objectively. In one study, a deficit in olfactory arousal was detected in nine of 10 of PD patients using EEG recordings [45]; however, EEGs are unlikely to be used as a screening procedure. Sakuma, Nakashima, and Takahashi reported that the olfactory deficit in PD can be assessed by using evoked potentials [46], and several studies have attempted to image the olfactory system. Mueller *et al.* found that olfactory bulb volume is not changed in PD patients [47]. However, Westerman *et al.* [48] used fMRI to assess brain activity during olfactory processing and reported that activity was reduced in hippocampus and amygdala under certain conditions.

Finally, it is difficult to discuss the olfactory bulb in PD without pointing out its possible relationship to the cause of the disease, as the bulb could presumably represent a portal of entry of a parkinsonogenic pathogen. Indeed, olfactory bulb involvement is so sensitive to the disease process that it is an important area for future study of mechanisms of disease development. Ultimately, it will be important to screen a large population of normal individuals in mid-life to obtain an unbiased cohort of individuals with "idiopathic hyposmia" to determine how great a risk factor it is for PD. At the moment there are no populations where such data have already been collected, with the exception of the HAAS study cited above, which was limited to Asian American males. It should also be noted that selectivity may be limited in using olfaction as a screening tool for pre-motor PD, as a similar deficit has been reported in Alzheimer's disease [49,50], although the defect may be more marked in PD [51]. Since the nasal mucosa is accessible and could be biopsied, this approach could be very attractive to establish a diagnosis in PD. However, to date no differences have been found on histological or biochemical assessment of olfactory mucosa in PD patients compared with controls, including staining for α-synuclein deposition [52,53].

Constipation

Widely recognized as a common and often very bothersome symptom of PD, constipation was recognized as an important feature of the disease by James Parkinson himself [54]. There is little doubt that this non-motor feature of the disease is due, at least in part, to direct involvement of the innervation of the intestinal tract, as a number of investigators have reported Lewy bodies and Lewy neuritic pathology in nerve fibers in the colon, stomach, and esophagus [55–60]. It is not surprising, then, that abnormalities of intestinal motility have been well documented, including abnormalities of colonic contractility and anal sphincter dysfunction [61,62], suggesting that bowel dysfunction is a primary feature of the disease rather than the effects of immobility or poor hydration. These features are reviewed elsewhere in this volume (Chapter 24).

There is now increasing evidence that constipation is also a pre-motor feature of the disease. The seminal study in this regard came once again from the HAAS cohort. In 2003, Abbott *et al.* [63] reported that midlife constipation in this group bestowed approximately a fourfold risk for PD later in life, suggesting that changes in the gut could be a very early pre-motor feature of the disease. This prospective study was complemented by a retrospective study which found that 33 of 74 PD patients reported that constipation preceded the onset of parkinsonism, by an average of 18 years [64], an interval not dissimilar to that reported in the HAAS study. The problem is that constipation is a common problem in the general population, and, although an important pre-motor feature, it is unlikely to be a very specific diagnostic indicator of the disease. On the other hand, as will be discussed later, in combination with other pre-motor features it could be a important component of a pre-motor diagnostic battery.

Cardiac autonomic denervation

There is a compelling body of evidence that autonomic denervation of the heart is a nearly universal feature of PD, a phenomenon that has been documented in over 40 imaging studies [65]. It can be seen fairly early in the disease [66] and appears to progress over time [67]. Evidence of a decline in autonomic innervation has also been documented electrophysiologically by assessing heart rate variability, which declines as autonomic innervation is lost [68,69]. These clinical studies have been complemented by a number of pathologic studies. For example, Iwanaga *et al.* [70] observed Lewy bodies and α-synuclein-positive neurites in the hearts from nine of 11 patients with PD but, equally important in the search for pre-motor features of PD, they observed similar changes in seven of seven individuals with so-called incidental Lewy bodies, which is thought by many to represent pre-motor PD; others have made similar observations [71]. In another study, in virtually all patients with PD ($N = 11$) and DLB ($N = 7$), tyrosine hydroxylase (TH) nerve fiber staining had nearly disappeared in the heart [72]. These investigators also found that Lewy bodies were present in both TH-positive and TH-negative nerve processes, which are nerves of extrinsic sympathetic and intrinsic origin, respectively. In a later study, Orimo *et al.* found complete or moderate loss of TH fibers in the heart of 10 of 20 incidental Lewy body cases [73], again suggesting that cardiac changes can precede clinical manifestation PD. Using [^{123}I]-*m*-iodobenzylguanidine (MIBG), the primary ligand used for imaging cardiac sympathetic innervation, at least one group has reported that loss of cardiac sympathetic innervation correlates with disease status [74]. However others have failed to observe such a correlation with cardiac imaging [71] or a striatal dopamine depletion as measured by PET [75]. Interestingly, at least one study has shown that MIBG and olfaction are highly correlated, whereas loss of MIBG uptake did not correlate with disease status or duration [76]. Finally, at least one autopsy case has been reported in a PD patient who had an abnormal MIBG scan during life. At postmortem examination, this patient was found to have marked pathologic involvement of the cardiac sympathetic nerve plexus that was more pronounced than that seen in the sympathetic ganglion [77].

Given how important cardiac autonomic denervation (CAD) is likely to be for understanding mechanisms that underlie PD and its evolution, it is surprising that it still not clear what symptoms this abnormality causes. Therefore, it is difficult to include CAD among the pre-motor symptoms of PD. However, it clearly appears to be a physical sign that can be measured by imaging and possibly electrophysiologic techniques. In a theme that is becoming recurrent in this chapter, to determine if CAD is a pre-motor sign, several groups have turned to RBD. Perhaps the most impressive study to date was reported by Miyamoto *et al.* [78], who carried out cardiac MIBG scintigraphy in 13 patients with RBD, and found abnormal uptake in all 13. The same group also reported that these changes are no different than those observed in PD and DLB, thereby providing even more compelling evidence that RBD is part of a continuum that includes PD and DLB [79]. However, MIBG scanning of the heart is far from a routine procedure, and is unlikely to be used as a screening procedure. On the other hand, heart rate variability (HRV) also occurs in PD, presumably as a result of decreased autonomic input, raising the question as to whether or not these changes may also precede the onset of PD.

To explore this question, we recently carried out the spectral analysis of 3–5 min segments of waking EKGs from 11 patients with RBD and 11 control subjects [80]. Tracings were analyzed for three different domains of HRV; time domain, frequency domain, and geographic and non-linear measures. Ten of the 14 parameters measured were statistically different in the RBD patients. Of particular interest was the fact that, using a discriminant analysis, the EKG spectral analysis correctly identified all 11 RBD patients and incorrectly identified only one control as having RBD (specificity of 95%). Although this study needs to be replicated in a larger and different population, it raises the intriguing possibility that EKG can be used as a simple, non-invasive, and inexpensive tool to identify pre-motor PD. If so, routine EKGs could also be used to screen the general population for an early synucleinopathy well before PD or dementia becomes clinically manifest. This could be an attractive approach because data from modern digital EKGs can now be downloaded into software programs that automatically calculate all domains of HRV.

Pure autonomic failure

While autonomic dysfunction is a well known feature of typical PD, there is increasing evidence that pure autonomic failure (PAF) may be an early manifestation of a synucleinopathy, and therefore should be considered as a possible pre-motor feature of PD. As pointed out earlier in this chapter, hyposmia is likely one of the earliest pre-motor features of PD (Braak stage 1). Therefore, Silveira-Moriyama *et al.* [81] tested odor identification in 16 patients with PAF and found that mean UPSIT scores were lower than in controls (although not as much as in PD). On the other hand, Goldstein and Sewell [38] found that the hyposmia in PAF is very similar to that seen in PD. Carrying this approach a step further, the same group [82] imaged cardiac sympathetic function in three PAF patients with [6-^{18}F]fluorodopamine and found a complete loss of uptake, indicating marked CAD in each. This combination of hyposmia and CAD would appear to provide strong evidence for an early synucleinpathy of the brain and peripheral autonomic nervous. Adding even more evidence to the hypothesis that these patients may have pre-motor PD is a report by Compta *et al.* [83], who carried out DAT imaging in a patient with PAF and found that it was decreased, suggesting early nigrostriatal involvement, consistent with pre-motor PD.

The most extensive study on the pathology of this disorder comes from Hishikawa *et al.* [84], who reported on the neuropathology of 30 Lewy body disorders, PD DLB, and PAF and found no pathologic distinctions among them. They concluded that PD, DLB, and PAF share a common pathologic phenotype. In addition, several case reports suggest the peripheral autonomic nervous system and brainstem may be involved first. Hague *et al.* [85] reported a patient with PAF who had had orthostatic hypotension and urinary symptoms for 15 years prior to death at age 63 years, but who never manifested PD. Neuropathologic findings included the presence of Lewy bodies in the substantia nigra, locus coeruleus, and substantia innominata. There was also mild neuronal loss with extraneuronal pigment in the substantia nigra. Lewy bodies were also seen in the sympathetic ganglia, and also in autonomic axons in a variety of areas, including epicardial fat, periadrenal adipose tissue, and muscle layer of the urinary bladder. In a second autopsied case of PAF [86], the primary findings were a loss of intermediolateral column cells in the spinal cord and sympathetic ganglionic neurons and Lewy bodies in sympathetic ganglia neurons. The pigmented brainstem nuclei were completely normal although the olfactory bulb was not mentioned as having been examined. Although the authors concluded that the case showed that patients with PAF did not always have pre-motor PD, this patient could be very important, indicating that the very earliest appearance of LB may occur in peripheral sympathetic neurons and spinal cord.

In summary, there is a growing body of evidence that PAF may be joining the ranks as a pre-motor feature of PD based on pathologic findings and an association with other pre-motor signs and symptoms of PD, although cases in which the disorder clearly advances to motor PD are lacking. At the very least, we can say that this disorder is due to a synucleinopathy of the peripheral autonomic nervous system, spinal cord, and brainstem and CAD may be a core feature. A longitudinal study of individuals with PAF including idiopathic orthostatic hypotension would certainly be of interest, but the disorder is not common and so far no such study has been carried out.

Before closing this section on autonomic dysfunction, one additional study is worth mentioning. Minguez-Castellanos *et al.* [87] assessed the prevalence of α-synuclein pathology in the abdominal and pelvic autonomic plexuses in the general population. An additional goal was to determine if individuals with a peripheral synucleinopathy would go on to develop a neurodegenerative disease. They employed a novel approach of examining surgical specimens from 100 patients (aged 44–84 years) who had undergone resections of an abdominal organs and found α-synuclein deposits in the autonomic nervous system of nine patients. These were most common in the vesicoprostatic (26%) tissues. By comparison, synuclein pathology was present in 4% in the digestive tract tissues. Of particular interest was the fact that MIGB uptake was significantly reduced in the α-synuclein-positive group compared with a group of subjects who had no evidence of synuclein pathology. Although no patient had developed an obvious neurodegenerative process within 16 months, striatal [^{123}I]ioflupane uptake was abnormally low in one synuclein positive subject. At 30 months after the biopsy, lower cardiac and striatal uptake values tended to correlate with mild parkinsonian features as measured by UPDRS part III scores ($p = 0.07$). The authors concluded that α-synuclein pathology in peripheral autonomic neurons could represent pre-motor PD or the early stages of a related Lewy body disorder.

Depression

Although depression is common in PD and makes almost everyone's list as a pre-motor symptom of PD [5,88–91], there is a little prospective evidence showing that it precedes the onset of PD in a predictable fashion. However, there are a number of retrospective case–control studies supporting this possibility. For example, Leentjens *et al.* [92] used data from a general practice-based registry and found that at the time of diagnosis, 9.2% of PD patients had a history of depression compared with 4% of controls (odds ratio of 2.4). In a similar study, Schuurman *et al.* [93] found an odds ratio of 3 for developing PD in a retrospective cohort study of patients, and Nilsson, Kessing and Bolwig [94] found a similar odds in a retrospective study using linked public hospital registers. Using the Rochester Epidemiology Project in Olmsted County, Shiba *et al.* [95] employed a case–control design and found an odds ratio of 1.9 for developing PD; however, this association disappeared when the analysis was restricted to a history of depression of 5 years or more. In a case–control study of Indian patients with PD, a 10 year or greater history of depression was found to be a risk factor for PD [96]. A hospital-based retrospective case–control has also shown that depression bestowed a threefold increase risk for PD [97]. Another group examined the use of antidepressants from a large computerized database from the General Practice Research Database cohort, and assessed 999 PD cases and 6261 controls [98]. Initiation of antidepressants was associated with an increased risk of PD (rate ratio of 1.85), which was stronger if they had been initiated within 2 years of diagnosis (rate ratio of 2.19). However, not all groups have found such a relationship [99] and the HAAS study, which utilized prospective data, failed to detect depression as a risk factor for PD [63]. At the moment, there are no ongoing prospective studies similar to the PARS study to tackle this potentially important question, but it is a study that should be done.

Before closing this section on depression, it is worth summarizing an interesting autopsy proven case that is relevant to this discussion. Iritani *et al.* [9] reported an 84-year-old woman who developed a later-life major depression without parkinsonism, cognitive changes, or hallucinations. At autopsy she had Lewy bodies in the substantia nigra, locus ceruleus, and dorsal raphae and also in the hippocampus and cerebral cortex (Braak stage 6).

Dementia

Dementia is rarely listed as pre-motor feature of PD. Rather, most consider it a post-motor feature that comes later in the illness, when it is typically referred to as PDD. In fact, by one definition, if the dementia precedes PD or occurs within 1 year after the diagnosis, it should be designated as DLB [100]. However, if one considers DLB part of the Lewy body continuum of disease, then it could be argued that dementia can just as easily be a pre-motor feature of Lewy body disease, as many cases have little if any parkinsonism when the dementia is first evident. While it is beyond the scope of this chapter to take on the longstanding debate as to whether or not PD and DLB are the same entity, the important point here is that in most cases of pathologically proven DLB, the dementia not a "prenigral" event when viewed from a neuropathologic standpoint. Indeed, a number of reports have suggested that PDD is indistinguishable from DLB when viewed under the microscope [84,101], although others have found subtle differences in the neuropathologic substrate of DLB [102]. Lippa *et al.* argued that Lewy body pathology is a unifying basis for PDD, PD, and DLB (they suggested the term Lewy body disorders), but recommended that three categories should be maintained based on clinical differences [103]. On the other hand, at least some reports have suggested that pure DLB and PDD can be virtually identical at the clinical level also [104].

Regardless of one's views on PDD versus DLB, one of the most interesting aspects of the study of the pre-motor features of the PD is that they are increasingly providing unifying features between the two disorders. For example, it is now becoming apparent that CAD is major feature of DLB, just as for PD and RBD. In fact, this feature of DLB has become so well documented that it is now being advocated as a means of separating DLB from Alzheimer's disease [105–109]. In one study, it was superior to [^{99m}Tc]ethyl cysteinate dimer SPECT in differentiating the two [110]. In a highly relevant study, Miyamoto *et al.* found that cardiac MIGB SPECT scanning was similar among RBD, PD, and DLB [79]. It is also interesting to note that many of the pre-motor features of PD, such as RBD and depression, are also considered supportive of a diagnosis of DLB [100]. Furthermore, a decrease in DAT binding on SPECT or PET scanning [111] and neuroleptic sensitivity [112] are also considered as supportive evidence of a diagnosis of DLB. Of course, both of these features would also be supportive of pre-motor PD.

Where do we go from here? The need for prospective cohorts

A major problem that has plagued the investigation of pre-motor PD is the lack of identifiable cohorts in which to study these features. As is evident, RBD may be one vehicle to enable this, but most investigators do not have enough patients with pure RBD to carry out meaningful studies. Identifying larger cohorts will be essential if we are to pursue this line of research. A second approach is the search for LRRK2 carriers, with the goal of assembling a large enough cohort to carry out meaningful research. The LRRK2 G2019S mutation accounts for about 1.5% of all PD in some European populations and in the United States [113], and there may be equivalents of this mutation in other populations throughout the world. The numbers rise to around 18% in Ashkenazi Jews [114], and approximately 40% in Berber Arabs in North Africa [115]. Currently there are efforts to ascertain asymptomatic carriers, as this mutation significantly increases the risk for developing PD (penetrance is estimated at around 30% by age 75–85 years [116–119]). Long-term follow-up of LRRK2 carriers could therefore provide a population in which to study pre-motor features of the disease. Interestingly, at least two groups have already attempted to use LRRK2 G2019S mutation carriers as a way to study hyposmia as a pre-motor feature of PD [120,121]. Both groups found a deficit in olfaction similar to that in PD in patients who had developed a parkinsonian phenotype, but asymptomatic carriers could not be distinguished from non-carrier controls. The likely explanation for these results relates to the variable penetrance of the disorder and the relatively older onset of LRRK2 parkinsonism. Hence these studies point out the need for long-term follow-up of such cohorts. It is hoped that we will see such cohorts assembled and enrolled in longitudinal follow-up studies in the not too distant future.

Another approach is to follow an elderly cohort of non-parkinsonian individuals, examining them annually for all of the suspected pre-motor features of PD, and then obtain whole-body autopsies at death to evaluate both the central and peripheral autonomic nervous system for α-synuclein pathology. Such a study is currently in progress in Sun City, AZ, USA, and has already yielded some important results. The research group observed the high specificity and sensitivity of an olfactory bulb synucleinopathy in Lewy body disorders [36]. They also made the important and novel observation that patients with so-called incidental Lewy bodies actually have reduced striatal tyrosine hydroxylase [122], representing one of the strongest pieces of evidence to date that such cases actually have pre-motor PD.

Ultimately, it will necessary to assemble large cohorts of individuals in their 50s or 60s with one or more pre-motor features of pre-motor PD (e.g., idiopathic hyposmia, depression, and PAF) from the general population. Although such populations would be of great value for the prospective study of pre-motor PD, investigations of this nature are labor and time intensive and costly. However, if a decrease in HRV as measured by a routine EKG can be validated as an instrument to measure CAD, it would change the landscape dramatically. This is because it would be much easier to identify large population-based cohorts by simply piggy-backing on routine EKGs. This approach would be particularly attractive as CAD has the potential to be a unifying and early feature of the different Lewy body diseases.

Conclusion

Investigating and understanding better pre-motor PD are becoming a major focus of research, for many reasons. First, elucidating the earliest features of PD could reshape our understanding of the nature and extent of the disease process. Second, since pre-motor features are signs of very early disease processes, they could give us clues as to the cause of PD [123]. For example, the fact that the olfactory bulb is almost always (if not always) one of the first structures in the CNS to manifest a synucleinopathy raises the intriguing question as to whether not the nose could be a portal of entry for a parkinsonogenic pathogen. One can speculate in a similar manner about the gut, as it is not difficult to imagine a pathogen crossing the mucus membranes of the gastrointestinal tract and gaining entry into the neuronal structures that innervate the intestinal tract [124]. Indeed, this might explain the early involvement of the dorsomedial nucleus of the vagus, with its direct connection to the gastrointestinal tract. Recently, Hawkes, Del Tredici, and Braak [125] have suggested a double hit hypothesis that suggests that both portals of entry might be involved. Finally, and perhaps most importantly, recognition of the early pre-motor features could lead to much earlier intervention in the disease. At the moment, we are still lacking proven ways to halt or slow the progression of the disease, but a great deal of research is currently directed towards this goal, and proven success with a disease-modifying therapy would make pre-motor identification hugely important, as there is a general consensus that one of the reasons for lack of success to date is that we are starting disease-modifying trials too late in the disease process.

Although we are not yet at the stage where we can easily screen for pre-motor PD, this possibility could come quickly. For example, if a combination of decreased HRV and hyposmia were to prove highly indicative of an early Lewy body disorder such as PD, one could design a multi-tiered approach, starting with annual assessment of HRV on routine annual EKGs starting at age 50 years. Individuals reaching a certain threshold of HRV decline could then undergo testing for hyposmia (something that could be done in any physician's office) as a tier two, and referred for further testing if olfaction was abnormal. If successful, and disease-modifying agents become available, we may have within our reach secondary prevention, as such agents could be instituted at a very early pre-motor stage, and the catastrophic motor syndrome that James Parkinson so ably describe in 1817 [54] might then become a thing of the past.

Epilogue

As should become evident from reading this chapter, there is an evolving body of diseases characterized by α-synuclein-positive Lewy bodies and Lewy neurites that affect the peripheral autonomic nervous system and CNS, often in a fairly well-defined order. Named diseases include PD, DLB, PAF, and RBD, all of which have a synuclein-based pathology as the most common neuropathologic phenotype. What is becoming evident is that there seem to be several core features that are common to all of these disorders which probably deserve attention since they seem to be cross-roads for all of these disorders. The first is CAD, which has been identified and studied extensively over the last 15 years. It is becoming obvious that CAD is a nearly universal feature of these diseases. Unfortunately, this feature is not yet readily accessible to the clinician unless appropriate SPECT or PET scanning with ligands such as MIGB is readily available. The other is hyposomia, a feature that is readily accessible for clinical testing. It is suggested that these features could be important in the investigation and diagnosis of PD and other Lewy body disorders, and may hold critical keys to solving the puzzle of synucleinopathies of the brain, spinal cord, and peripheral autonomic nervous system.

References

1. Langston JW. The Parkinson's complex: parkinsonism is just the tip of the iceberg. *Ann Neurol* 2006;**59**(4):591–6.
2. Braak H, Braak E. Pathoanatomy of Parkinson's disease. *J Neurol* 2000;**247**(Suppl 2):II3–10.
3. Braak H, Del Tredici K, Bratzke H, *et al*. Staging of the intracerebral inclusion body pathology associated with idiopathic Parkinson's disease (preclinical and clinical stages). *J Neurol* 2002;**249**(Suppl 3):III/1–5.
4. Fox SH, Brotchie JM, Lang AE. Non-dopaminergic treatments in development for Parkinson's disease. *Lancet Neurol* 2008;**7**(10):927–38.
5. Tolosa E, Gaig C, Santamaria J, Compta Y. Diagnosis and the premotor phase of Parkinson disease. *Neurology* 2009;**72**(7 Suppl):S12–20.
6. Hughes AJ, Daniel SE, Lees AJ. Improved accuracy of clinical diagnosis of Lewy body Parkinson's disease. *Neurology* 2001;**57**(8):1497–9.
7. McKeith IG, Dickson DW, Lowe J, *et al*. Diagnosis and management of dementia with Lewy bodies: third report of the DLB Consortium. *Neurology* 2005;**65**(12):1863–72.
8. Uchiyama M, Isse K, Tanaka K, *et al*. Incidental Lewy body disease in a patient with REM sleep behavior disorder. *Neurology* 1995;**45**(4):709–12.
9. Iritani S, Tsuchiya K, Arai T, *et al*. An atypical autopsy case of Lewy body disease with clinically diagnosed major depression: a clinical, radiological and pathological study. *Neuropathology* 2008;**28**(6):652–9.
10. Gagnon JF, Bedard MA, Fantini ML, *et al*. REM sleep behavior disorder and REM sleep without atonia in Parkinson's disease. *Neurology* 2002;**59**(4):585–9.
11. Greenfield JG, Bosanquet FD. The brain-stem lesions in Parkinsonism. *J Neurol Neurosurg Psychiatry* 1953;**16**(4):213–26.
12. Carlsson A. The occurrence, distribution and physiological role of catecholamines in the nervous system. *Pharmacol Rev* 1959;**11**(2, Pt 2):490–3.
13. Ehringer H, Hornykiewicz O. Distribution of noradrenaline and dopamine (3-hydroxytyramine) in the human brain and their behavior in diseases of the extrapyramidal system. *Klin Wochenschr* 1960;**38**:1236–9 (in German).
14. Cotzias GC. L-Dopa for Parkinsonism. *N Engl J Med* 1968;**278**(11):630.
15. Lang AE, Obeso JA. Time to move beyond nigrostriatal dopamine deficiency in Parkinson's disease. *Ann Neurol* 2004;**55**(6):761–5.
16. Hely MA, Morris JG, Reid WG, Trafficante R. Sydney Multicenter Study of Parkinson's disease: non-L-dopa-responsive problems dominate at 15 years. *Mov Disord* 2005;**20**(2):190–9.
17. Lees AJ, Hardy J, Revesz T. Parkinson's disease. *Lancet* 2009;**373**(9680):2055–66.
18. Schenck CH, Bundlie SR, Ettinger MG, Mahowald MW. Chronic behavioral disorders of human REM sleep: a new category of parasomnia. *Sleep* 1986;**9**(2):293–308.
19. Schenck CH, Bundlie SR, Mahowald MW. Delayed emergence of a parkinsonian disorder in 38% of 29 older men initially diagnosed with idiopathic rapid eye movement sleep behaviour disorder. *Neurology* 1996;**46**(2):388–93.
20. Postuma RB, Gagnon JF, Vendette M, *et al*. Quantifying the risk of neurodegenerative disease in idiopathic REM sleep behavior disorder. *Neurology* 2009;**72**(15):1296–300.
21. Hickey MG, Demaerschalk BM, Caselli RJ, *et al*. "Idiopathic" rapid-eye-movement (REM) sleep behavior disorder is associated with future development of neurodegenerative diseases. *Neurologist* 2007;**13**(2):98–101.
22. Boeve BF, Dickson DW, Olson EJ, *et al*. Insights into REM sleep behavior disorder pathophysiology in brainstem-predominant Lewy body disease. *Sleep Med* 2007;**8**(1):60–4.
23. Schenck CH, Mahowald MW, Anderson ML, *et al*. Lewy body variant of Alzheimer's disease (AD) identified by postmortem ubiquitin staining in a previously reported case of AD associated with REM sleep behavior disorder. *Biol Psychiatry* 1997;**42**(6):527–8.
24. Boeve BF, Silber MH, Ferman TJ. REM sleep behavior disorder in Parkinson's disease and dementia with Lewy bodies. *J Geriatr Psychiatry Neurol* 2004;**17**(3):146–57.
25. Ansari KA, Johnson A. Olfactory function in patients with Parkinson's disease. *J Chronic Dis* 1975;**28**(9):493–7.
26. Boesveldt S, de Muinck Keizer RJ, Knol DL, *et al*. Extended testing across, not within, tasks raises diagnostic accuracy

of smell testing in Parkinson's disease. *Mov Disord* 2009;**24**(1): 85–90.

27. Iijima M, Kobayakawa T, Saito S, *et al.* Smell identification in Japanese Parkinson's disease patients: using the odor stick identification test for Japanese subjects. *Intern Med* 2008;**47**(21):1887–92.
28. Quagliato LB, Viana MA, Quagliato EM, Simis S. Olfactory dysfunction in Parkinson's disease. *Arq Neuropsiquiatr* 2007;**65**(3A):647–52 (in Portuguese).
29. Bohnen NI, Gedela S, Kuwabara H, *et al.* Selective hyposmia and nigrostriatal dopaminergic denervation in Parkinson's disease. *J Neurol* 2007;**254**(1):84–90.
30. Muller A, Reichmann H, Livermore A, Hummel T. Olfactory function in idiopathic Parkinson's disease (IPD): results from cross-sectional studies in IPD patients and long-term follow-up of de-novo IPD patients. *J Neural Transm* 2002;**109**(5–6):805–11.
31. Hawkes CH, Shephard BC, Daniel SE. Olfactory dysfunction in Parkinson's disease. *J Neurol Neurosurg Psychiatry* 1997;**62**(5):436–46.
32. Doty RL, Bromley SM, Stern MB. Olfactory testing as an aid in the diagnosis of Parkinson's disease: development of optimal discrimination criteria. *Neurodegeneration* 1995;**4**(1):93–7.
33. Ward CD, Hess WA, Calne DB. Olfactory impairment in Parkinson's disease. *Neurology* 1983;**33**(7):943–6.
34. Hawkes CH. Parkinson's disease and aging: same or different process? *Mov Disord* 2008;**23**(1):47–53.
35. Beach TG, Adler CH, Lue L, *et al.* Unified staging system for Lewy body disorders: correlation with nigrostriatal degeneration, cognitive impairment and motor dysfunction. *Acta Neuropathol* 2009;**117**(6):613–34.
36. Beach TG, White CL III, Hladik CL, *et al.* Olfactory bulb alpha-synucleinopathy has high specificity and sensitivity for Lewy body disorders. *Acta Neuropathol* 2009;**117**(2):169–74.
37. Bohnen NI, Studenski SA, Constantine GM, Moore RY. Diagnostic performance of clinical motor and non-motor tests of Parkinson disease: a matched case–control study. *Eur J Neurol* 2008;**15**(7):685–91.
38. Goldstein DS, Sewell L. Olfactory dysfunction in pure autonomic failure: implications for the pathogenesis of Lewy body diseases. *Parkinsonism Relat Disord* 2009;**15**(7):516–20.
39. Ross GW, Petrovitch H, Abbott RD, *et al.* Association of olfactory dysfunction with risk for future Parkinson's disease. *Ann Neurol* 2008;**63**(2):167–73.
40. Sommer U, Hummel T, Cormann K, *et al.* Detection of presymptomatic Parkinson's disease: combining smell tests, transcranial sonography, and SPECT. *Mov Disord* 2004;**19**(10):1196–202.
41. Haehner A, Hummel T, Hummel C, *et al.* Olfactory loss may be a first sign of idiopathic Parkinson's disease. *Mov Disord* 2007;**22**(6):839–42.
42. Berendse HW, Booij J, Francot CM, *et al.* Subclinical dopaminergic dysfunction in asymptomatic Parkinson's disease patients' relatives with a decreased sense of smell. *Ann Neurol* 2001;**50**(1):34–41.
43. Ponsen MM, Stoffers D, Twisk JW, *et al.* Hyposmia and executive dysfunction as predictors of future Parkinson's disease: a prospective study. *Mov Disord* 2009;**24**(7):1060–5.
44. Stiasny-Kolster K, Doerr Y, Moller JC, *et al.* Combination of 'idiopathic' REM sleep behaviour disorder and olfactory dysfunction as possible indicator for alpha-synucleinopathy demonstrated by dopamine transporter FP-CIT-SPECT. *Brain* 2005;**128**(Pt 1):126–37.
45. Gori S, Massetani R, Murri L. Evaluation of olfactory function by topographic EEG analysis in patients with Parkinson's disease. *Ital J Neurol* Sci 1995;**16**(9):595–601.
46. Sakuma K, Nakashima K, Takahashi K. Olfactory evoked potentials in Parkinson's disease, Alzheimer's disease and anosmic patients. *Psychiatry Clin Neurosci* 1996;**50**(1):35–40.
47. Mueller A, Abolmaali ND, Hakimi AR, *et al.* Olfactory bulb volumes in patients with idiopathic Parkinson's disease a pilot study. *J Neural Transm* 2005;**112**(10):1363–70.
48. Westermann B, Wattendorf E, Schwerdtfeger U, *et al.* Functional imaging of the cerebral olfactory system in patients with Parkinson's disease. *J Neurol Neurosurg Psychiatry* 2008;**79**(1):19–24.
49. Mesholam RI, Moberg PJ, Mahr RN, Doty RL. Olfaction in neurodegenerative disease: a meta-analysis of olfactory functioning in Alzheimer's and Parkinson's diseases. *Arch Neurol* 1998;**55**(1):84–90.
50. Lehrner JP, Brucke T, Dal-Bianco P, *et al.* Olfactory functions in Parkinson's disease and Alzheimer's disease. *Chem Senses* 1997;**22**(1):105–10.
51. Williams SS, Williams J, Combrinck M, *et al.* Olfactory impairment is more marked in patients with mild dementia with Lewy bodies than those with mild Alzheimer disease. *J Neurol Neurosurg Psychiatry* 2009;**80**(6):667–70.
52. Hawkes C. Olfaction in neurodegenerative disorder. *Adv Otorhinolaryngol* 2006;**63**:133–51.
53. Witt M, Bormann K, Gudziol V, *et al.* Biopsies of olfactory epithelium in patients with Parkinson's disease. *Mov Disord* 2009;**24**(6):906–14.
54. Parkinson J. *An Essay on the Shaking Palsy*. London: Whittingham and Rowland: 1817.
55. Qualman SJ, Haupt HM, Yang P, Hamilton SR. Esophageal Lewy bodies associated with ganglion cell loss in achalasia. Similarity to Parkinson's disease. *Gastroenterology* 1984;**87**(4):848–56.
56. Kupsky WJ, Grimes MM, Sweeting J, *et al.* Parkinson's disease and megacolon: concentric hyaline inclusions (Lewy bodies) in enteric ganglion cells. *Neurology* 1987;**37**(7):1253–5.
57. Wakabayashi K, Takahashi H, Takeda S, *et al.* Parkinson's disease: the presence of Lewy bodies in Auerbach's and Meissner's plexuses. *Acta Neuropathol (Berl)* 1988;**76**(3):217–21.
58. Wakabayashi K, Takahashi H, Ohama E, Ikuta F. Parkinson's disease: an immunohistochemical study of Lewy body-containing neurons in the enteric nervous system. *Acta Neuropathol (Berl)* 1990;**79**(6):581–3.
59. Wakabayashi K, Takahashi H, Ohama E, *et al.* Lewy bodies in the visceral autonomic nervous system in Parkinson's disease. *Adv Neurol* 1993;**60**:609–12.
60. Takeda S, Yamazaki K, Miyakawa T, Arai H. Parkinson's disease with involvement of the parasympathetic ganglia. *Acta Neuropathol (Berl)* 1993;**86**(4):397–8.
61. Ashraf W, Pfeiffer RF, Quigley EM. Anorectal manometry in the assessment of anorectal function in Parkinson's disease: a

comparison with chronic idiopathic constipation. *Mov Disord* 1994;**9**(6):655–63.

62. Ashraf W, Wszolek ZK, Pfeiffer RF, *et al.* Anorectal function in fluctuating (on–off) Parkinson's disease: evaluation by combined anorectal manometry and electromyography. *Mov Disord* 1995;**10**(5):650–7.
63. Abbott RD, Ross GW, White LR, *et al.* Environmental, lifestyle, and physical precursors of clinical Parkinson's disease: recent findings from the Honolulu–Asia Aging Study. *J Neurol* 2003;**250**(Suppl 3):III30–9.
64. Ueki A, Otsuka M. Life style risks of Parkinson's disease: association between decreased water intake and constipation. *J Neurol* 2004;**251**(Suppl 7):vII18–23.
65. Goldstein DS. Cardiac denervation in patients with Parkinson disease. *Cleve Clin J Med* 2007;**74**(Suppl 1):S91–4.
66. Takatsu H, Nishida H, Matsuo H, *et al.* Cardiac sympathetic denervation from the early stage of Parkinson's disease: clinical and experimental studies with radiolabeled MIBG. *J Nucl Med* 2000;**41**(1):71–7.
67. Li ST, Dendi R, Holmes C, Goldstein DS. Progressive loss of cardiac sympathetic innervation in Parkinson's disease. *Ann Neurol* 2002;**52**(2):220–3.
68. Akincioglu C, Unlu M, Tunc T. Cardiac innervation and clinical correlates in idiopathic Parkinson's disease. *Nucl Med Commun* 2003;**24**(3):267–71.
69. Kallio M, Suominen K, Haapaniemi T, *et al.* Nocturnal cardiac autonomic regulation in Parkinson's disease. *Clin Auton Res* 2004;**14**(2):119–24.
70. Iwanaga K, Wakabayashi K, Yoshimoto M, *et al.* Lewy body-type degeneration in cardiac plexus in Parkinson's and incidental Lewy body diseases. *Neurology* 1999;**52**(6):1269–71.
71. Fujishiro H, Frigerio R, Burnett M, *et al.* Cardiac sympathetic denervation correlates with clinical and pathologic stages of Parkinson's disease. *Mov Disord* 2008;**23**(8):1085–92.
72. Orimo S, Amino T, Itoh Y, *et al.* Cardiac sympathetic denervation precedes neuronal loss in the sympathetic ganglia in Lewy body disease. *Acta Neuropathol (Berl)* 2005;**109**(6): 583–8.
73. Orimo S, Takahashi A, Uchihara T, *et al.* Degeneration of cardiac sympathetic nerve begins in the early disease process of Parkinson's disease. *Brain Pathol* 2007;**17**(1):24–30.
74. Spiegel J, Hellwig D, Farmakis G, *et al.* Myocardial sympathetic degeneration correlates with clinical phenotype of Parkinson's disease. *Mov Disord* 2007;**22**(7):1004–8.
75. Raffel DM, Koeppe RA, Little R, *et al.* PET measurement of cardiac and nigrostriatal denervation in Parkinsonian syndromes. *J Nucl Med* 2006;**47**(11):1769–77.
76. Lee PH, Yeo SH, Kim HJ, Youm HY. Correlation between cardiac 123I-MIBG and odor identification in patients with Parkinson's disease and multiple system atrophy. *Mov Disord* 2006;**21**(11):1975–7.
77. Mitsui J, Saito Y, Momose T, *et al.* Pathology of the sympathetic nervous system corresponding to the decreased cardiac uptake in ^{123}I-metaiodobenzylguanidine (MIBG) scintigraphy in a patient with Parkinson disease. *J Neurol Sci* 2006 Apr 15;**243**(1–2): 101–4.
78. Miyamoto T, Miyamoto M, Inoue Y, *et al.* Reduced cardiac ^{123}I-MIBG scintigraphy in idiopathic REM sleep behavior disorder. *Neurology* 2006;**67**(12):2236–8.
79. Miyamoto T, Miyamoto M, Suzuki K, *et al.* ^{123}I-MIBG cardiac scintigraphy provides clues to the underlying neurodegenerative disorder in idiopathic REM sleep behavior disorder. *Sleep* 2008;**31**(5):717–23.
80. Valappil RA J, Black J, Broderick MJ, *et al.* Exploring the electrocardiogram as a potential tool to screen for premotor Parkinson's disease. *Mov Disord* 2010;**25**:2296–303.
81. Silveira-Moriyama L, Mathias C, Mason L, *et al.* Hyposmia in pure autonomic failure. *Neurology* 2009;**72**(19):1677–81.
82. Goldstein DS, Holmes C, Cannon RO III, *et al.* Sympathetic cardioneuropathy in dysautonomias. *N Engl J Med* 1997;**336**(10):696–702.
83. Compta Y, Marti MJ, Paredes P, Tolosa E. Pure autonomic failure with altered dopamine transporter imaging. *Arch Neurol* 2006;**63**(4):604–5.
84. Hishikawa N, Hashizume Y, Yoshida M, Sobue G. Clinical and neuropathological correlates of Lewy body disease. *Acta Neuropathol (Berl)* 2003;**105**(4):341–50.
85. Hague K, Lento P, Morgello S, *et al.* The distribution of Lewy bodies in pure autonomic failure: autopsy findings and review of the literature. *Acta Neuropathol (Berl)* 1997;**94**(2):192–6.
86. van Ingelghem E, van Zandijcke M, Lammens M. Pure autonomic failure: a new case with clinical, biochemical, and necropsy data. *J Neurol Neurosurg Psychiatry* 1994;**57**(6):745–7.
87. Minguez-Castellanos A, Chamorro CE, Escamilla-Sevilla F, *et al.* Do alpha-synuclein aggregates in autonomic plexuses predate Lewy body disorders?: a cohort study. *Neurology* 2007;**68**(23):2012–8.
88. Berg D. Biomarkers for the early detection of Parkinson's and Alzheimer's disease. *Neurodegener Dis* 2008;**5**(3–4):133–6.
89. Lim SY, Fox SH, Lang AE. Overview of the extranigral aspects of Parkinson disease. *Arch Neurol* 2009;**66**(2):167–72.
90. Tolosa E, Compta Y, Gaig C. The premotor phase of Parkinson's disease. *Parkinsonism Relat Disord* 2007;**13**(Suppl):S2–7.
91. Wolters E, Braak H. Parkinson's disease: premotor clinico-pathological correlations. *J Neural Transm Suppl* 2006;(70):309–19.
92. Leentjens AF, van den Akker M, Metsemakers JF, *et al.* Higher incidence of depression preceding the onset of Parkinson's disease: a register study. *Mov Disord* 2003;**18**(4):414–8.
93. Schuurman AG, van den Akker M, Ensinck KT, *et al.* Increased risk of Parkinson's disease after depression: a retrospective cohort study. *Neurology* 2002;**58**(10):1501–4.
94. Nilsson FM, Kessing LV, Bolwig TG. Increased risk of developing Parkinson's disease for patients with major affective disorder: a register study. *Acta Psychiatr Scand* 2001;**104**(5):380–6.
95. Shiba M, Bower JH, Maraganore DM, *et al.* Anxiety disorders and depressive disorders preceding Parkinson's disease: a case–control study. *Mov Disord* 2000;**15**(4):669–77.
96. Behari M, Srivastava AK, Das RR, Pandey RM. Risk factors of Parkinson's disease in Indian patients. *J Neurol Sci* 2001;**190**(1–2):49–55.
97. Taylor CA, Saint-Hilaire MH, Cupples LA, *et al.* Environmental, medical, and family history risk factors for Parkinson's disease: a New England-based case–control study. *Am J Med Genet* 1999;**88**(6):742–9.
98. Alonso A, Rodriguez LA, Logroscino G, Hernan MA. Use of antidepressants and the risk of Parkinson's disease: a

prospective study. *J Neurol Neurosurg Psychiatry* 2009;**80**(6): 671–4.

99. McCann SJ, LeCouteur DG, Green AC, *et al.* The epidemiology of Parkinson's disease in an Australian population. *Neuroepidemiology* 1998;**17**(6):310–7.
100. McKeith IG, Perry EK, Perry RH. Report of the second dementia with Lewy body international workshop: diagnosis and treatment. Consortium on Dementia with Lewy Bodies. *Neurology* 1999;**53**(5):902–5.
101. Colosimo C, Hughes AJ, Kilford L, Lees AJ. Lewy body cortical involvement may not always predict dementia in Parkinson's disease. *J Neurol Neurosurg Psychiatry* 2003;**74**(7):852–6.
102. Gomez-Tortosa E, Newell K, Irizarry MC, Albert M, *et al.* Clinical and quantitative pathologic correlates of dementia with Lewy bodies. *Neurology* 1999;**53**(6):1284–91.
103. Lippa CF, Duda JE, Grossman M, *et al.* DLB and PDD boundary issues: diagnosis, treatment, molecular pathology, and biomarkers. *Neurology* 2007;**68**(11):812–9.
104. Galvin JE, Pollack J, Morris JC. Clinical phenotype of Parkinson disease dementia. *Neurology* 2006;**67**(9):1605–11.
105. Estorch M, Camacho V, Paredes P, *et al.* Cardiac (123)I-metaiodobenzylguanidine imaging allows early identification of dementia with Lewy bodies during life. *Eur J Nucl Med Mol Imaging* 2008;**35**(9):1636–41.
106. Oide T, Tokuda T, Momose M, *et al.* Usefulness of [^{123}I]metaiodobenzylguanidine ([^{123}I]MIBG) myocardial scintigraphy in differentiating between Alzheimer's disease and dementia with Lewy bodies. *Intern Med* 2003;**42**(8):686–90.
107. Schmidt SL, Correa PL, Tolentino JC, *et al.* Value of combining activated brain FDG-PET and cardiac MIBG for the differential diagnosis of dementia: differentiation of dementia with Lewy bodies and Alzheimer disease when the diagnoses based on clinical and neuroimaging criteria are difficult. *Clin Nucl Med* 2008;**33**(6):398–401.
108. Taki J, Yoshita M, Yamada M, Tonami N. Significance of ^{123}I-MIBG scintigraphy as a pathophysiological indicator in the assessment of Parkinson's disease and related disorders: it can be a specific marker for Lewy body disease. *Ann Nucl Med* 2004;**18**(6):453–61.
109. Yoshita M, Taki J, Yamada M. A clinical role for [(123)I]MIBG myocardial scintigraphy in the distinction between dementia of the Alzheimer's-type and dementia with Lewy bodies. *J Neurol Neurosurg Psychiatry* 2001;**71**(5):583–8.
110. Tateno M, Kobayashi S, Shirasaka T, *et al.* Comparison of the usefulness of brain perfusion SPECT and MIBG myocardial scintigraphy for the diagnosis of dementia with Lewy bodies. *Dement Geriatr Cogn Disord* 2008;**26**(5):453–7.
111. McKeith I, O'Brien J, Walker Z, *et al.* Sensitivity and specificity of dopamine transporter imaging with ^{123}I-FP-CIT SPECT in dementia with Lewy bodies: a phase III, multicentre study. Lancet Neurol 2007;**6**(4):305–13.
112. Aarsland D, Perry R, Larsen JP, *et al.* Neuroleptic sensitivity in Parkinson's disease and parkinsonian dementias. *J Clin Psychiatry* 2005;**66**(5):633–7.
113. Brice A. Genetics of Parkinson's disease: LRRK2 on the rise. *Brain* 2005;**128**(Pt 12):2760–2.
114. Ozelius LJ, Senthil G, Saunders-Pullman R, *et al.* LRRK2 G2019S as a cause of Parkinson's disease in Ashkenazi Jews. *N Engl J Med* 2006;**354**(4):424–5.
115. Lesage S, Durr A, Tazir M, *et al.* LRRK2 G2019S as a cause of Parkinson's disease in North African Arabs. *N Engl J Med* 2006;**354**(4):422–3.
116. Clark LN, Wang Y, Karlins E, *et al.* Frequency of LRRK2 mutations in early- and late-onset Parkinson disease. *Neurology* 2006;**67**(10):1786–91.
117. Goldwurm S, Zini M, Mariani L, *et al.* Evaluation of LRRK2 G2019S penetrance: relevance for genetic counseling in Parkinson disease. *Neurology* 2007;**68**(14):1141–3.
118. Ozelius LJ, Foroud T, May S, *et al.* G2019S mutation in the leucine-rich repeat kinase 2 gene is not associated with multiple system atrophy. *Mov Disord* 2007;**22**(4):546–9.
119. Kachergus J, Mata IF, Hulihan M, *et al.* Identification of a novel LRRK2 mutation linked to autosomal dominant parkinsonism: evidence of a common founder across European populations. *Am J Hum Genet* 2005;**76**(4):672–80.
120. Lohmann E, Leclere L, De Anna F, *et al.* A clinical, neuropsychological and olfactory evaluation of a large family with LRRK2 mutations. *Parkinsonism Relat Disord* 2009;**15**(4):273–6.
121. Silveira-Moriyama L, Guedes LC, Kingsbury A, *et al.* Hyposmia in G2019S LRRK2-related parkinsonism: clinical and pathologic data. *Neurology* 2008;**71**(13):1021–6.
122. Beach TG, Adler CH, Sue LI, *et al.* Reduced striatal tyrosine hydroxylase in incidental Lewy body disease. *Acta Neuropathol* 2008;**115**(4):445–51.
123. Del Tredici K, Rub U, De Vos RA, *et al.* Where does parkinson disease pathology begin in the brain? *J Neuropathol Exp Neurol* 2002;**61**(5):413–26.
124. Braak H, Rub U, Gai WP, Del Tredici K. Idiopathic Parkinson's disease: possible routes by which vulnerable neuronal types may be subject to neuroinvasion by an unknown pathogen. *J Neural Transm* 2003;**110**(5):517–36.
125. Hawkes CH, Del Tredici K, Braak H. Parkinson's disease: a dual-hit hypothesis. *Neuropathol Appl Neurobiol* 2007;**33**(6): 599–614.

Chapter 9
Functional Imaging Studies in Parkinson's Disease: the Non-Dopaminergic Systems

A. Jon Stoessl
Pacific Parkinson's Research Centre, University of British Columbia, Vancouver, BC, Canada

Introduction

Although imaging techniques such as magnetic resonance imaging (MRI), functional MRI (fMRI), diffusion tensor imaging, and magnetic resonance spectroscopy (MRS) can provide useful information, changes observed in Parkinson's disease (PD) with these techniques are often limited. In contrast, it is the ability of positron emission tomography (PET) to provide specific neurochemical information that has led to its particular utility in the diagnosis and investigation of PD. Naturally, the major focus has been on studies of the dopamine (DA) system, which will be reviewed only briefly here. It should not be forgotten, however, that PET can also be used in PD to study not only DA function, but also the function of other monoamine systems, non-monoaminergic neurotransmitter systems, and general function and connectivity. Additionally, PET may provide insights into autonomic innervation of other organs such as the heart which may be involved early in the disease, and into non-neuronal factors that may contribute to the etiology and/or progression of PD (see Table 9.1).

Changes in the DA system in PD

Changes in the DA system have been extensively reviewed in numerous publications and will be addressed only briefly here. There are three major approaches to studying the integrity of presynaptic DA function: (i) the density of the vesicular monoamine transporter type 2 (VMAT2), assessed with [^{11}C]dihydrotetrabenazine, (ii) binding to the plasmalemmal dopamine transporter (DAT), assessed using a large variety of ^{11}C- and ^{18}F-labeled tropane (cocaine-like) derivatives or with [^{11}C]-*d-threo*-methylphenidate (MP) [and also a number of γ-emitting analogs that can be analyzed using single photon emission computed tomography (SPECT)], and (iii) [6-^{18}F]fluoro-L-dopa (FD), which is sensitive to and provides a measure of the rate of aromatic acid decarboxylation and also storage of fluorodopamine in synaptic vesicles. A limited number of centers use [6-^{18}F]-*m*-tyrosine, which is decarboxylated in a fashion similar to FD, but which is trapped and therefore not useful for measuring DA turnover.

As expected, all of these tracers show analogous changes in PD. These consist of a substantial loss of striatal DA innervation that is asymmetric with a characteristic rostral–caudal gradient, such that the posterior putamen is most severely affected, whereas the caudate is relatively spared. Such changes are seen in the clinically unaffected striatum in patients with early unilateral disease and may also be seen in subjects who are clinically unaffected but who have a high risk of going on to develop PD based on genetic mutations [1,2] or exposure to DA neurotoxins [3]. Although there is a loose relationship between the severity of DA denervation as assessed by PET (or SPECT) and clinical measures of disease severity, there is sufficient discordance that imaging cannot be used as a biomarker [4,5].

DA function can also be assessed by using ligands that bind to post-synaptic DA receptors. There are few if any changes in D1 receptor binding associated with PD or its complications [6,7]. Small increases in D2 binding have been described in early, untreated disease, but these vanish with dopaminergic replacement therapy [7–10]. In addition, competition for binding of ligands with relatively low affinity for DA receptors such as [^{11}C]raclopride can be used to assess changes in the levels of synaptic DA. Thus, in response to an oral dose of levodopa, it can be demonstrated that subjects prone to the future development of motor fluctuations [11], and also subjects with levodopa-induced dyskinesias [12], have relatively greater but shorter duration changes in synaptic DA levels compared with those with a stable response to medication. The degree of improvement

Parkinson's Disease: Non-Motor and Non-Dopaminergic Features, First Edition. Edited by C. Warren Olanow, Fabrizio Stocchi, and Anthony E. Lang.

Table 9.1 Changes associated with PD and its complications.

Complication	Measure	Findings	Ref.
PD	Dopamine innervation (DAT, VMAT2, FD)	Asymmetric reduction with rostral–caudal gradient	53–58
	Dopamine turnover	Increased, related to DAT	59,60
	5HT innervations ([^{11}C]DASB)	Widespread reductions	25,27
	Glucose metabolism	Altered metabolic network with decreases in SMA, parietal cortex, increases in striatum, pallidum and cerebellum	40,61
	Microglial activation	Increases, widespread or localized, related or unrelated to disease severity	45,46
Motor complications			
Fluctuations	Dopamine release following levodopa	Short duration, predates development of fluctuations	11
	DA receptors	No relationship	10
Dyskinesias	Dopamine release following levodopa	Increased magnitude, short duration	12
	DAT binding	Decreased expression, corrected for DA nerve terminal density	62
	DA receptors	No relationship	7,9
	Opioid receptors	Decreased in striatum of dyskinetic PD patients	33
Other			
Depression	DA/NE innervation	Decreased in VS, thalamus, amygdala	29
	5HT innervation	Increased in cortex of depressed PD patients	26
Dementia	Glucose metabolism	Widespread decreases, especially occipital cortex	63
	Cholinergic innervation	Widespread decreases	30,31
	Amyloid deposition	Increased in DLB, not PDD	50–52

in bradykinesia and rigidity (but interestingly not tremor) also correlates with levodopa-induced DA release as assessed by this method [13].

More recently, a similar approach has been used to study non-motor complications in PD. Thus, PD patients with the dopamine dysregulation syndrome demonstrate sensitized DA release in the ventral striatum in response to a dose of levodopa compared with those with similar disease severity but without this complication, although the degree of dopamine release is similar between both groups in the motor striatum [14]. This is consistent with the role of ventral striatal DA release in signaling expectation of reward and is in keeping with ventral striatal DA release in response to amphetamine [15], pleasurable food [16], and indeed placebos [17,18] and sham transcranial magnetic stimulation [19].

Displacement of [^{11}C]raclopride binding can also be used to detect endogenous DA release during performance of a set shift in a card-sorting task [20] and during performance of a spatial working memory task. In the latter study, whereas PD subjects demonstrated reduced DA release in the caudate during performance of this task, DA release in medial prefrontal cortex was comparable to controls [21]. These findings are compatible with earlier studies in which alterations in FD uptake in caudate nucleus and frontal cortex were associated with cognitive dysfunction in patients with PD [22].

Changes in monoamine transmitters other than DA

There is an extremely limited number of studies on the status of serotonergic innervation in PD. Using the $5HT_{1A}$ ligand [^{11}C]WAY 100635, which binds to presynaptic serotonin autoreceptors as well as post-synaptic receptors, Doder *et al.* [23] demonstrated that tremor in PD, which does not correlate with measures of DA innervation [24], is related to serotonin binding in the midbrain raphe (therefore presumably reflecting the density of surviving serotonergic neurons in this region). A more specific approach to the study of 5HT innervation is the use of a ligand selective for the 5HT reuptake transporter. Using [^{11}C]DASB, Guttman *et al.* have shown widespread reductions in 5HT nerve terminal density in PD patients compared with healthy controls [25]. Contrary to expectations, there is no evidence of a more profound reduction in serotonin innervation in depressed PD patients compared with those without depression, and indeed increases are seen in some extra-striatal sites, particularly the dorsolateral and prefrontal cortex [26]. Recently, Albin *et al.* confirmed the loss of serotonergic innervation in PD using [^{11}C]DASB. They reported that forebrain serotonergic innervation was more severely affected than hindbrain innervation [27], a finding that would appear to be in conflict with the Braak hypothesis [28] of caudal to rostral progression of PD.

The noradrenergic system is even less well studied in PD, in large part owing to the lack of specific tracers. A number of the agents used to label the dopamine transporter are relatively non-specific and may also bind to the noradrenalin reuptake site. Although there is no easy way to distinguish *in vivo* the relative proportion of binding to a particular site, differences in anatomic distribution allow one to make a reasonable inference. Using the combined dopamine–noradrenaline transporter ligand [^{11}C]RTI-32, Remy *et al.* [29] compared PD subjects with anxiety and/or depression with PD subjects without these features. In the depressed PD subjects, there were reductions in tracer uptake in the locus coeruleus, thalamus, amygdala, and ventral striatum compared with PD subjects without depression. In the locus coeruleus, this reduction presumably reflects a relative loss of noradrenergic neurons, whereas in the amygdala and ventral striatum, the findings likely suggest a loss of dopamine innervation. In the thalamus, the changes may point to changes in the function of either or both neurotransmitters.

Other neurotransmitters

Acetylcholine

In keeping with postmortem neurochemical and immunocytochemical findings, dementia in PD is associated with a profound loss of cholinergic innervation as measured by PET with the cholinesterase substrates PMP [30] and MP4A [31]. The cholinergic deficit is widespread in PD, greater in those with dementia than in those who are congnitively intact, and greater in PD subjects with dementia than in patients with Alzheimer's disease [30].

Neuropeptides

Opioid binding is normal in PD subjects compared with controls [32]. However, PD patients with levodopa-induced dyskinesias have reduced striatal [^{11}C]diprenorphine binding compared with those without motor complications [33]. This presumably reflects increased occupancy of opioid receptors resulting from increased expression of dynorphin in the direct striatal pathway and/or enkephalin in the indirect pathway.

There are even fewer studies on non-opioid peptides in PD. Analogous to the situation for the opioid peptides, one preliminary study demonstrated reduced levels of striatal NK1 neurokinin/tachykinin receptor binding in PD subjects with dyskinesias [34]. This might reflect increased receptor occupancy due to increased synaptic levels of substance P associated with dyskinesias, but the interpretation is difficult, as the tracer used has a high affinity for the neurokinin receptor (and may therefore not be subject to competition from endogenous ligand), and the source of substance P input to the striatum is not clear.

Amino acid transmission

Although PD is associated with important changes in the expression of both inhibitory and excitatory amino acids, there are to date no imaging studies using specific markers for these compounds to study either the disease or its complications. However, these changes undoubtedly contribute to altered synaptic activity and the consequent perturbations of metabolic networks that are seen in PD (see below).

Neurotransmitter expression in the peripheral nervous system

The monoamines [6-^{18}F]-fluorodopamine and [^{11}C]hydroxyephedrine (or the SPECT analog [^{123}I]-*m*-iodobenzylguanidine (MIBG)) are taken up by post-ganglionic sympathetic neurons and their density can be readily assessed in the heart (after correcting for myocardial blood flow). Autonomic dysfunction in PD arises from degeneration of these post-ganglionic sympathetic neurons and is therefore associated with decreased cardiac uptake of these tracers. This contrasts with multiple system atrophy, where the degeneration is predominantly preganglionic and cardiac uptake is consequently normal in most reports [35,36]. As differentiation between PD and multiple system atrophy can be an enormous diagnostic challenge in some patients, there has been considerable interest in the potential clinical utility of this approach. However, some caution is necessary, as at least one report has called into question the specificity of decreased cardiac tracer uptake for PD [37] and further investigations are warranted.

Network activity in Parkinson's disease

PET can also be used to study regional cerebral blood flow (rCBF) and glucose metabolism (rCMRGlc) at rest or in response to a variety of physiologic, pharmacologic or cognitive stimuli. Regional glucose metabolism is generally held to be a measure of synaptic activity, and could therefore theoretically be increased in response to either excitation or inhibition. Blood flow is generally tightly coupled to cellular metabolism, although certain interventions may alter the two measures differently

[38]. In PD, the expected movement-induced increases in both rCBF and rCMRGlc in the motor regions are attenuated, but can be restored with a variety of dopaminergic medications or with deep brain stimulation, as can in fact altered patterns of glucose metabolism in the resting state [39,40]. Altered metabolic networks in PD include changes in corticostriatal– pallido– thalamocortical (CSPTC) loops, which may in turn arise from reduced dopamine innervation. These networks can be normalized with dopaminergic therapies. Therapeutic interventions downstream to striatal dopamine receptors such as subthalamic nucleus stimulation [40] or conversion of excitatory glutamatergic subthalamic activity to inhibitory GABAergic activity [41] can also modify the expression of the abnormal metabolic network independent of dopamine.

Alterations in metabolic or cerebral blood flow networks may also reflect compensatory changes that are essentially independent of dopaminergic modulation of CSPTC loops. For example, impaired activation of CSPTC loops during performance of voluntary movements may result in *increased* activity in parietal and premotor cortices [42,43]. In a planning task (Tower of London) that is thought to assess procedural memory, PD patients shift from normal activation of the caudate nucleus to activation of the hippocampus, suggesting a shift to circuitry that usually subserves declarative memory [44].

Clues from functional imaging into etiology of PD and pathogenesis of complications

While the majority of functional imaging studies have focused on either measurement of neurotransmitters and their receptors or on the analysis of patterns of cerebral activation and metabolic networks, PET can also be used to study the pathological mechanisms that underlie PD. Thus, inflammation, thought possibly to contribute to the progression if not the primary neural degeneration of PD, can be imaged using the peripheral benzodiazepine receptor ligand [^{11}C]PK11195, which binds to activated microglia. However, although one group of investigators have reported binding largely restricted to the midbrain which correlates with disease severity as measured by UPDRS motor scores and dopamine transporter binding (but not with disease duration) [45], other investigators have found widespread microglial activation that does not correlate with other measures of disease severity [46]. The interesting and provocative suggestion that PD might be associated with impaired blood–brain barrier *P*-glycoprotein-mediated extrusion of potential toxins in the midbrain (as assessed by binding of the L-type calcium channel ligand [^{11}C]verapamil) [47] could not be reproduced in a subsequent report by the original authors, conducted in patients with early PD [48].

Dementia in PD may be associated with numerous changes, including cortical Lewy body deposition with or without concurrent Alzheimer's disease. In recent years, many investigators have felt that for the majority of cases, the distinction between PD dementia and dementia with Lewy bodies is mainly semantic, based on the temporal evolution of cognitive decline relative to the timing of the appearance of motor manifestations. The thioflavin compound Pittsburgh B labeled with C-11 ([^{11}C]PIB) binds to widespread regions of brain in Alzheimer's disease in a fashion presumed to reflect amyloid deposition [49]. Very little information is available in PD. In one recent study, PIB binding was seen in only two out of 10 demented PD patients [50]. In two other recent studies, PIB binding was seen in patients with DLB, but not in the majority of those with PDD [51,52]. A search for compounds that bind α-synuclein and could permit imaging of this protein is under way and will surely provide important clues as to the nature and distribution of pathology in the course of PD. This has proven difficult, however, as α-synuclein is primarily an intracellular protein, making the development of such tracers considerably more difficult.

Conclusion

Functional imaging with PET (and SPECT) has provided significant insights into the dopaminergic basis for the manifestations of PD and complications of therapy, and also alterations in patterns of cerebral activation. To date, the information on non-dopaminergic mechanisms is only just beginning to receive the attention it deserves. As there is increased recognition of the importance of the non-dopaminergic features of PD and, importantly, as new tracers are developed that allow the quantitative assessment of relevant functions, we are likely to see a steady growth in publications over the next few years. It is anticipated that this will provide useful information for purposes of diagnosis, assessment of new interventions, and studies related to better understanding of the etiopathogenesis and pathophysiology of PD.

References

1. Piccini P, Burn DJ, Ceravolo R, *et al.* The role of inheritance in sporadic Parkinson's disease: evidence from a longitudinal study of dopaminergic function in twins. *Ann Neurol* 1999;**45**:577–82.
2. Adams JR, van Netten H, Schulzer M, *et al.* PET in LRRK2 mutations: comparison to sporadic Parkinson's disease and evidence for presymptomatic compensation. *Brain* 2005;**128**(Pt 12):2777–85.

3. Calne DB, Langston JW, Martin WR, *et al.* Positron emission tomography after MPTP: observations relating to the cause of Parkinson's disease. *Nature* 1985;**317**(6034):246–8.
4. Brooks DJ, Frey KA, Marek KL, *et al.* Assessment of neuroimaging techniques as biomarkers of the progression of Parkinson's disease. *Exp Neurol* 2003;**184**(Suppl 1):S68–79.
5. Ravina B, Eidelberg D, Ahlskog JE, *et al.* The role of radiotracer imaging in Parkinson disease. *Neurology* 2005;**64**(2):208–15.
6. Shinotoh H, Inoue O, Hirayama K, *et al.* Dopamine D1 receptors in Parkinson's disease and striatonigral degeneration: a positron emission tomogrphy study. *J Neurol Neurosurg Psychiatry* 1993;**56**:467–72.
7. Turjanski N, Lees AJ, Brooks DJ. In vivo studies on striatal dopamine D1 and D2 site binding in L-dopa-treated Parkinson's disease patients with and without dyskinesias. *Neurology* 1997;**49**(3):717–23.
8. Antonini A, Schwarz J, Oertel WH, *et al.* Long-term changes of striatal dopamine D2 receptors in patients with Parkinson's disease: a study with positron emission tomography and [^{11}C]raclopride. *Mov Disord* 1997;**12**:33–8.
9. Kishore A, de la Fuente-Fernandez R, Snow BJ, *et al.* Levodopa-induced dyskinesias in idiopathic parkinsonism (IP): a simultaneous PET study of dopamine D1 and D2 receptors. *Neurology* 1997;**48**(Suppl 2):A327 [Abstract].
10. de la Fuente-Fernandez R, Kishore A, Snow BJ, *et al.* Dopamine D1 and D2 receptors and motor fluctuations in idiopathic Parkinsonism (IP): a simultaneous PET study. *Neurology* 1997;**48**(Suppl 2):A208 [Abstract].
11. de la Fuente-Fernandez R, Lu JQ, Sossi V, *et al.* Biochemical variations in the synaptic level of dopamine precede motor fluctuations in Parkinson's disease: PET evidence of increased dopamine turnover. *Ann Neurol* 2001;**49**(3):298–303.
12. de la Fuente-Fernandez R, Sossi V, *et al.* Levodopa-induced changes in synaptic dopamine levels increase with progression of Parkinson's disease: implications for dyskinesias. *Brain* 2004;**127**(Pt 12):2747–54.
13. Pavese N, Evans AH, Tai YF, *et al.* Clinical correlates of levodopa-induced dopamine release in Parkinson disease: a PET study. *Neurology* 2006;**67**(9):1612–7.
14. Evans AH, Pavese N, Lawrence AD, *et al.* Compulsive drug use linked to sensitized ventral striatal dopamine transmission. *Ann Neurol* 2006;**59**(5):852–8.
15. Leyton M, Boileau I, Benkelfat C, *et al.* Amphetamine-induced increases in extracellular dopamine, drug wanting, and novelty seeking: a PET/[^{11}C]raclopride study in healthy men. *Neuropsychopharmacology* 2002;**27**(6):1027–35.
16. Small DM, Jones-Gotman M, Dagher A. Feeding-induced dopamine release in dorsal striatum correlates with meal pleasantness ratings in healthy human volunteers. *Neuroimage* 2003;**19**(4):1709–15.
17. de la Fuente-Fernandez R, Ruth TJ, Sossi V, *et al.* Expectation and dopamine release: mechanism of the placebo effect in Parkinson's disease. *Science* 2001;**293**(5532):1164–6.
18. de la Fuente-Fernandez R, Schulzer M, Stoessl AJ. Placebo mechanisms and reward circuitry: clues from Parkinson's disease. *Biol Psychiatry* 2004;**56**(2):67–71.
19. Strafella AP, Ko JH, Monchi O. Therapeutic application of transcranial magnetic stimulation in Parkinson's disease: the contribution of expectation. *Neuroimage* 2006;**31**(4):1666–72.
20. Monchi O, Ko JH, Strafella AP. Striatal dopamine release during performance of executive functions: a [(11)C] raclopride PET study. *Neuroimage* 2006;**33**(3):907–12.
21. Sawamoto N, Piccini P, Hotton G, *et al.* Cognitive deficits and striato-frontal dopamine release in Parkinson's disease. *Brain* 2008;**131**(Pt 5):1294–302.
22. Rinne JO, Portin R, Ruottinen H, *et al.* Cognitive impairment and the brain dopaminergic system in Parkinson disease: [^{18}F]fluorodopa positron emission tomographic study. *Arch Neurol* 2000;**57**:470–5.
23. Doder M, Rabiner EA, Turjanski N, *et al.* Tremor in Parkinson's disease and serotonergic dysfunction: an ^{11}C-WAY 100635 PET study. *Neurology* 2003;**60**(4):601–5.
24. Vingerhoets FJG, Schulzer M, Calne DB, Snow BJ. Which clinical sign of Parkinson's disease best reflects the nigrostriatal lesion? *Ann Neurol* 1997;**41**:58–64.
25. Guttman M, Boileau I, Warsh J, *et al.* Brain serotonin transporter binding in non-depressed patients with Parkinson's disease. *Eur J Neurol* 2007;**14**(5):523–8.
26. Boileau I, Warsh JJ, Guttman M, *et al.* Elevated serotonin transporter binding in depressed patients with Parkinson's disease: a preliminary PET study with [(11)C]DASB. *Mov Disord* 2008;**23**:1776–80.
27. Albin RL, Koeppe RA, Bohnen NI, *et al.* Spared caudal brainstem SERT binding in early Parkinson's disease. *J Cereb Blood Flow Metab* 2008;**28**(3):441–4.
28. Braak H, Del Tredici K, Rub U, *et al.* Staging of brain pathology related to sporadic Parkinson's disease. *Neurobiol Aging* 2003;**24**(2):197–211.
29. Remy P, Doder M, Lees A, *et al.* Depression in Parkinson's disease: loss of dopamine and noradrenaline innervation in the limbic system. *Brain* 2005;**128**(Pt 6):1314–22.
30. Bohnen NI, Kaufer DI, Ivanco LS, *et al.* Cortical cholinergic function is more severely affected in parkinsonian dementia than in Alzheimer disease: an *in vivo* positron emission tomographic study. *Arch Neurol* 2003;**60**(12):1745–8.
31. Hilker R, Thomas AV, Klein JC, *et al.* Dementia in Parkinson disease: functional imaging of cholinergic and dopaminergic pathways. *Neurology* 2005;**65**(11):1716–22.
32. Burn DJ, Rinne JO, Quinn NP, *et al.* Striatal opioid receptor binding in Parkinson's disease, striatonigral degneration and Steele–Richardson–Olszewski syndrome, a [^{11}C]diprenorphine PET study. *Brain* 1995;**118**:951–8.
33. Piccini P, Weeks RA, Brooks DJ. Alterations in opioid receptor binding in Parkinson's disease patients with levodopa-induced dyskinesias. *Ann Neurol* 1997;**42**:720–6.
34. Whone AL, Rabiner EA, Arahata Y, *et al.* Reduced substance P binding in Parkinson's disease complicated by dyskinesias: an ^{18}F-L829165 PET study. *Neurology* 2002;**58**(Suppl 3):A488–9 [Abstract].
35. Goldstein DS, Holmes CS, Dendi R, *et al.* Orthostatic hypotension from sympathetic denervation in Parkinson's disease. *Neurology* 2002;**58**(8):1247–55.
36. Berding G, Schrader CH, Peschel T, *et al.* [*N*-Methyl-^{11}C]*meta*-hydroxyephedrine positron emission tomography in Parkinson's disease and multiple system atrophy. *Eur J Nucl Med Mol Imaging* 2003;**30**(1):127–31.

37. Raffel DM, Koeppe RA, Little R, *et al*. PET measurement of cardiac and nigrostriatal denervation in Parkinsonian syndromes. *J Nucl Med* 2006;**47**(11):1769–77.
38. Hirano S, Asanuma K, Ma Y, *et al*. Dissociation of metabolic and neurovascular responses to levodopa in the treatment of Parkinson's disease. *J Neurosci* 2008;**28**(16):4201–9.
39. Jenkins IH, Fernandez W, Playford ED, *et al*. Impaired activation of the supplementary motor area in Parkinson's disease is reversed when akinesia is treated with apomorphine. *Ann Neurol* 1992;**32**:749–57.
40. Asanuma K, Tang C, Ma Y, *et al*. Network modulation in the treatment of Parkinson's disease. *Brain* 2006;**129**(Pt 10):2667–78.
41. Feigin A, Kaplitt MG, Tang C, *et al*. Modulation of metabolic brain networks after subthalamic gene therapy for Parkinson's disease. *Proc Natl Acad Sci USA* 2007;**104**:19559–64.
42. Samuel M, Ceballos-Baumann AO, Blin J, *et al*. Evidence for lateral premotor and parietal overactivity in Parkinson's disease during sequential and bimanual movements. A PET study. *Brain* 1997;**120**(Pt 6):963–76.
43. Haslinger B, Erhard P, Kampfe N, *et al*. Event-related functional magnetic resonance imaging in Parkinson's disease before and after levodopa. *Brain* 2001;**124**(Pt 3):558–70.
44. Dagher A, Owen AM, Boecker H, Brooks DJ. The role of the striatum and hippocampus in planning: a PET activation study in Parkinson's disease. *Brain* 2001;**124**(Pt 5):1020–32.
45. Ouchi Y, Yoshikawa E, Sekine Y, *et al*. Microglial activation and dopamine terminal loss in early Parkinson's disease. *Ann Neurol* 2005;**57**(2):168–75.
46. Gerhard A, Pavese N, Hotton G, *et al*. *In vivo* imaging of microglial activation with [^{11}C](*R*)-PK11195 PET in idiopathic Parkinson's disease. *Neurobiol Dis* 2006;**21**(2):404–12.
47. Kortekaas R, Leenders KL, van Oostrom JC, *et al*. Blood–brain barrier dysfunction in parkinsonian midbrain *in vivo*. *Ann Neurol* 2005;**57**(2):176–9.
48. Bartels AL, van Berckel BN, Lubberink M, *et al*. Blood–brain barrier P-glycoprotein function is not impaired in early Parkinson's disease. *Parkinsonism Relat Disord* 2008;**14**:505–8.
49. Klunk WE, Engler H, Nordberg A, *et al*. Imaging brain amyloid in Alzheimer's disease with Pittsburgh Compound-B. *Ann Neurol* 2004;**55**(3):306–19.
50. Maetzler W, Reimold M, Liepelt I, *et al*. [^{11}C]PIB binding in Parkinson's disease dementia. *Neuroimage* 2008;**39**(3):1027–33.
51. Edison P, Rowe CC, Rinne JO, *et al*. Amyloid load in Parkinson's disease dementia and Lewy body dementia measured with [^{11}C]PIB-PET. *J Neurol Neurosurg Psychiatry* 2008;**79**:1331–8.
52. Gomperts SN, Rentz DM, Moran E, *et al*. Imaging amyloid deposition in Lewy body diseases. *Neurology* 2008;**71**(12):903–10.
53. Leenders KL, Palmer AJ, Quinn N, *et al*. Brain dopamine metabolism in patients with Parkinson's disease measured with positron emission tomography. *J Neurol Neurosurg Psychiatry* 1986;**49**:853–60.
54. Brooks DJ, Salmon EP, Mathias CJ, *et al*. The relationship between locomotor disability, autonomic dysfunction, and the integrity of the striatal dopaminergic system in patients with multiple system atrophy, pure autonomic failure, and Parkinson's disease, studied with PET. *Brain* 1990;**113**:1539–52.
55. Frost JJ, Rosier AJ, Reich SG, *et al*. Positron emission tomographic imaging of the dopamine transporter with ^{11}C-WIN 35,428 reveals marked declines in mild Parkinson's disease. *Ann Neurol* 1993;**34**:423–31.
56. Marek KL, Seibyl JP, Zoghbi SS, *et al*. [^{123}I]beta-CIT/SPECT imaging demonstrates bilateral loss of dopamine transporters in hemi-Parkinson's disease. *Neurology* 1996;**46**:231–7.
57. Lee CS, Samii A, Sossi V, *et al*. *In vivo* positron emission tomographic evidence for compensatory changes in presynaptic dopaminergic nerve terminals in Parkinson's disease. *Ann Neurol* 2000;**47**(4):493–503.
58. Frey KA, Koeppe RA, Kilbourn MR, *et al*. Presynaptic monoaminergic vesicles in Parkinson's disease and normal aging. *Ann Neurol* 1996;**40**:873–84.
59. Sossi V, de la Fuente-Fernandez R, Holden JE, *et al*. Increase in dopamine turnover occurs early in Parkinson's disease: evidence from a new modeling approach to PET ^{1}8F-fluorodopa data. *J Cereb Blood Flow Metab* 2002;**22**:232–9.
60. Sossi V, Fuente-Fernandez R, Schulzer M, *et al*. Dopamine transporter relation to dopamine turnover in Parkinson's disease: a positron emission tomography study. *Ann Neurol* 2007;**62**(5):468–74.
61. Moeller JR, Eidelberg D. Divergent expression of regional metabolic topographies in Parkinson's disease and normal ageing. *Brain* 1997;**120**(Pt 12):2197–206.
62. Troiano AR, de la Fuente-Fernandez R, Sossi V, *et al*. Positron emission tomography demonstrates reduced dopamine transporter expression in PD patients with dyskinesia. *Mov Disord* 2006;**21**(Suppl 15):S634 [Abstract].
63. Minoshima S, Foster NL, Sima AA, *et al*. Alzheimer's disease versus dementia with Lewy bodies: cerebral metabolic distinction with autopsy confirmation. *Ann Neurol* 2001;**50**(3):358–65.

Chapter 10
Assessment of Non-Motor Features of Parkinson's Disease: Scales and Rating Tools

Christopher G. Goetz[1] *& Cristina Sampaio*[2]
[1]Rush University Medical Center, Chicago, IL, USA
[2]Laboratory of Clinical Pharmacology and Therapeutics, Instituto de Medicina Molecular Faculdade de Medicina de Lisboa, Lisbon, Portugal

Introduction: principles of scale development and usage

The care of patients and research efforts related to non-motor aspects of PD demand the availability of reliable and valid clinical rating instruments. Measurement tools allow the documentation of the presence and severity of characteristics of behaviors over time and permit a uniform comparability of outcomes.

Measurement is the assignment of numerals to symptoms, behaviors, or clinical signs according to pre-agreed rules [1]. Most scales used in clinical medicine can be classified as nominal, ordinal, or interval scales. In *Nominal* or categorical scales, the basic relationship described is equality or difference, and therefore signs are rated as present or absent. In an *Ordinal* scale, an attribute is classified according to its rank order, but the steps in the scale are not necessarily presumed to be equal. The basic relationship described in an ordinal scale is greater or less. Most of the rating scales used in Parkinson's disease (PD) are ordinal, in that patients rated 4 are more disabled than patients rated 3, but the difference between 3 and 4 may not be of the same magnitude as that between 2 and 3. *Interval* scales, like ordinal scales, order behaviors, but in this case all steps in the scale are presumed to be equal. Other than measures of number of hours spent in the on or off state, true interval scales are not commonly used in PD or other neurological assessments.

The ability of scales to produce consistent results and therefore to be useful instruments in monitoring patients and conducting research depends on their clinimetric properties. Several terms are used in this chapter in comparing the relative merits of different scales. *Reliability* is the extent to which a measurement tool yields the same results on repeated trials. Reliability conceptually captures the proportion of variation in any given measurement that is due to true variation in the behavior and not to error. Reliability can be classified as intra-rater and inter-rater reliability, the former referring to the reproducibility of a single examiner's rating over time (test–retest) and the latter to the reproducibility of ratings when multiple examiners examine the same behavior in the same patient. *Dimensionality* refers to the ability of a rating instrument to measure appropriate subdomains of a particular construct. *Internal consistency* is the extent to which the items making up a composite score are measuring the same concept or latent factor. Dimensionality and internal consistency are important in forming both composite measures of severity and in developing subscale scores of clinical pertinence. *Validity* is the core feature of clinimetric interest, because it measures the extent to which an instrument measures what it is designed to assess. Finally, *responsivity* assesses whether a scale can detect change whether it is related to disease progression (presumed worsening) or to a treatment intervention (presumed improvement).

Rating scales assessing non-motor aspects of PD focus on two primary concepts of dysfunction, impairment and disability. Whereas impairment relates to objective deficits (cognitive testing batteries or tilt table testing for blood pressure), disability refers to the impact of disease on patient function. As such, items usually rated by the investigator and based solely on the neurologic examination assess impairment, whereas interviews that involve the patient's or caregiver's assessment measure disability. Some scales are uniquely impairment ratings, whereas others are uniquely disability assessments. Many others combine the two, allowing a total score to estimate a global level of disease severity as it relates to the behavior being studied.

This chapter focuses on three approaches to measuring non-motor aspects of PD. The first section discusses

Parkinson's Disease: Non-Motor and Non-Dopaminergic Features, First Edition. Edited by C. Warren Olanow, Fabrizio Stocchi, and Anthony E. Lang.

global PD scales that have some embedded items that address non-motor problems. The prototype of this type of measurement tool is the Unified Parkinson's Disease Rating Scale (UPDRS) and its official Movement Disorder Society-sponsored revised version, the MDS-UPDRS. The second section focuses on scales that target specifically the breadth of non-motor elements of PD rather than motor elements of the disease. The third section reviews scales focusing on individual non-motor impairments or disabilities. In the latter group, such scales have sometimes been developed specifically for PD, but in most instances they have been applied to PD after development for a wider patient population. The Movement Disorder Society has developed a Task Force on PD Rating Scales, and this group is in the process of reviewing scales that assess all non-motor behaviors covered by single screening questions in the MDS-UPDRS. This group effort and related programs sponsored by the MDS anchor the summary of this third section.

Global PD scales

Unified Parkinson's Disease Rating Scale (UPDRS)

The UPDRS is the international "gold standard" of clinical rating scales for PD [2]. It combines assessments of impairment and disability derived from several earlier scales and currently is the most widely applied scale in clinical trials. The UPDRS is a four-part scale, but the predominant areas of clinical focus are Part II (Activities of Daily Living) and Part III (Objective Motor Examination). Non-motor elements are not extensively assessed. Part I, termed Mentation, Behavior, and Mood, has four questions, covering screening assessments of Intellectual impairment, Thought disorder (fused with dreaming), Depression, and Motivation/Initiative. In Part II, there is a question on Sensory Complaints. Each item is rated using a five-point system, where 0 is normal and 4 represents severe abnormality. Finally, a series of present versus absent questions cover sleep abnormalities, orthostatic hypotension, and anorexia/nausea/vomiting. In spite of excellent clinimetric properties for the two primary sections of the scale (Parts II and III), no careful study has assessed the clinimetric properties of the non-motor items spread throughout the scale. The official MDS-sponsored critique of the UPDRS identified the relatively poor coverage of non-motor aspects of PD as one of the critical weaknesses of the original scale [3]. The critique considered the scale insufficient to allow a fair assessment of the breadth or severity of non-motor involvement. Based largely on the inadequacy of the original scale to assess non-motor features of PD, the final conclusion by the Panel was to develop a new version of the UPDRS (see below).

Movement Disorder Society revision of the UPDRS (MDS-UPDRS)

The MDS-UPDRS is a modification of the original UPDRS and has been developed to replace the earlier scale [4,5]. It is a 65-item assessment, divided into four parts, one of them specifically designated "Non-Motor Experiences of Daily Living." This section covers 13 items (Box 10.1), seven related to behavior, two to sleep patterns, one to pain, and three to autonomic nervous system symptoms. All questions follow a standard format with five possible responses anchored in the clinical concept that 0 = normal, 1 = slight, 2 = mild, 3 = moderate, and 4 = severe disability.

The clinimetric profile of the MDS-UPDRS includes high reliability, internal consistency, concurrent validity, and high correlations with the original UPDRS [4]. Specifically related to non-motor assessments, internal consistency is high for Part I ($\alpha = 0.78$). Further, MDS-UPDRS Part I scores correlate well with the shorter Part I of the original UPDRS ($r = 0.76$). As a measure of internal validity, inter-correlations have measured how Part I relates to the three others parts of the MDS-UPDRS (Part II Motor Experiences of Daily Living, Part III Objective Motor Examination, and Part IV Motor Complications). These analyses confirm that Part I assesses a very different aspect of PD than the other parts, such that low correlations are found between Part I and all other parts: Parts I and II $r = 0.66$, Parts I and III $r = 0.41$, and Parts and I and IV $r = 0.40$.

Box 10.1 MDS-UPDRS

Part I: Non-Motor Aspects of Experiences of Daily Living

- Cognitive impairment
- Hallucinations and psychosis
- Depressed mood
- Anxious mood*
- Apathy
- Features of dopamine dysregulation syndrome*
- Sleep problems*+
- Daytime sleepiness*+
- Pain and other sensations+
- Urinary problems*+
- Constipation problems*+
- Lightheadedness on standing*+
- Fatigue*+

Items marked with an asterisk (*) are domains not previously assessed with 0–5 ratings. The unmarked items are newly written, but covered in some capacity in the original UPDRS. Items marked with a plus (+) are covered by the patient/caregiver questionnaire without direct input from the investigator.

Table 10.1 Factor structures of Part I of the MDS-UPDRS.

Factor No.	Factor/item	Item factor loading
Part I: Non-Motor Aspects of Experiences of Daily Living (Section CFI = 0.94, RSMEA = 0.06, WRMR = 1.10)		
Factor 1	Daytime sleepiness	0.57
	Sleep problems	0.40
	Cognitive impairment	0.48
	Pain and other sensations	0.48
	Hallucinations and psychosis	0.40
	Urinary problems	0.59
	Constipation problems	0.49
	Features of DDS	0.49
	Light headedness on standing	0.45
	Fatigue	0.54
Factor 2	Depressed mood	0.83
	Anxious mood	0.66
	Apathy	0.53

Factor structure analysis identified two robust factors for Part I, one focusing on general non-motor symptoms and one on mood disturbance (CFI = 0.94). (Table 10.1). Differential item function analysis identified that the question on dopamine dysregulation may be clinimetrically problematic and may need revision. In the large clinimetric testing program of over 800 PD patients, few patients endorsed any response other than normal to this socially delicate question. Further, Caucasians and minorities responded to this question differently relative to their response patterns on the rest of Part I. Further testing of this question in cross-cultural and treatment trials of the MDS-UPDRS are planned, in addition to wording modifications and considerations of dropping it from the scale altogether. Admittedly the delicate nature of the question's content, covering sexual urges and anti-social compulsions, poses implicit challenges to data acquisition on this behavioral domain and has not been previously approached in global scales for PD.

Part I of the MDS-UPDRS was developed to provide screening questions on non-motor aspects of PD and its treatment, but the section was not envisioned to be comprehensive for in-depth examination of any single item. To guide researchers and clinicians to scales that can be used for more extensive monitoring of each non-motor item, the MDS-UPDRS is accompanied by an Appendix to Additional Scales. This Appendix is considered an ongoing list that will evolve and be updated as new clinimetric analyses and new scales are developed. The Appendix is anchored in the reports prepared by the MDS Task Force on PD Rating Scales (see below).

Multi-dimensional assessment tools

The identification, characterization, and evaluation of the non-motor features of PD are still a field in evolution. In the context of current scientific knowledge, it is not yet possible to establish accurately which non-motor features are core manifestations of the disease itself, which are common co-morbidities, and which are adverse reactions to treatment. This lack of firm knowledge impacts negatively on the ability to interpret data generated by prospective all-inclusive assessment tools.

Nonetheless, a few multi-dimensional assessment tools for non-motor signs and symptoms have been developed and tested clinimetrically. The Non-Motor Symptom Questionnaire (NMSQuest) comprises 30 common symptoms scored yes or no, and is designed to provide a rapid screen for problematic non-motor symptoms as an aid to clinical management [6]. This version was not a rating scale to be used as a measure of treatment response. A subsequent revised version of the NMSQuest reorganized the symptoms into nine domains: cardiovascular (two items); sleep/fatigue (four items); mood/cognition (six items); perceptual problems/hallucinations (three items); attention/memory (three items); gastrointestinal tract (three items); urinary (three items); sexual function (two items); and miscellaneous (four items). This scale was formally validated and data are available for scaling, reliability, internal consistency, construct validity, and factor analysis. This new scale is known as the Non-Motor Symptoms Scale (NNMS) [7].

The SCOPA program was established in The Netherlands as an attempt to develop a complete array of tools to evaluate all dimensions of PD. The SCOPA project is driven by the aim of developing tools that are practical and quick to apply. They target the practicing physician over the researcher. So far, this program has produced a number of independent scales tackling different topics, but there is no single SCOPA instrument to cover all non-motor elements. Several of the individual SCOPA scales are discussed in the next section.

Focal non-motor scales

Overview

This section reviews a process developed by the Movement Disorder Society to evaluate systematically rating scales applicable to non-motor aspects of PD. For each question in Part I of the MDS-UPDRS, the Steering Committee of the MDS Task Force on PD Rating Scales invited a program Chairperson to form a team of experts to critique existing rating scales for that non-motor problem in PD and to place the critique in a clinical and clinimetric context. Scales were selected through literature searchers and assessed following a format utilized across the different programs. The results of the reviews and conclusions were then summarized by the Chair and the draft report revised following feedback and discussion with all Task Force members. Each report was reviewed and altered according to suggestions by the members of the Steering Committee and submitted and approved by the Scientific Issues Committee of the MDS before submission for publication in the journal *Movement Disorders*.

For all these reports, pre-specified definitions were utilized. A scale is considered *Recommended* if it has been applied to PD populations, there are data on its use in studies beyond the group that developed the scale, and it has been studied clinimetrically and found valid, reliable, and sensitive to change. A scale is considered *Suggested* if it has been applied to PD populations, but only one of the other criteria applies. A scale is described as *Listed* if it meets only one of the three criteria defined for recommended scales. These qualifications may pertain to specific properties of the scale, such as screening for the presence or absence of the behavior and measuring severity and change in severity during treatment.

This overall effort is fully integrated with the MDS-UPDRS program and the Appendix for Additional Scales from the MDS-UPDRS is based on these conclusions (Table 10.2). Where the Task Force report is not yet complete, the Appendix Committee from the MDS-UPDRS Task Force has provided provisional conclusions (Table 10.3).

Scales with official reports by the MDS Task Force on PD Rating Scales

Depressed mood

A systematic literature review was conducted to explore the use of depression scales in PD and determine which scales should be selected as Recommended or Suggested (Table 10.2) [8]. The scales reviewed were the Beck Depression Inventory (BDI), Hamilton Depression Scale (Ham-D), Hospital Anxiety and Depression Scale (HADS), Zung Self-Rating Depression Scale (SDS), Geriatric Depression Scale (GDS), Montgomery–Asberg Depression Rating Scale (MADRS), Unified Parkinson's Disease Rating Scale (UPDRS) Part I, Cornell Scale for the Assessment of Depression in Dementia (CSDD), and Center for Epidemiologic Studies Depression Scale (CES-D). Seven clinical researchers with clinical and research experience in the assessment of PD depression were assigned to review the scales using a structured format. From the onset of the review process, the group considered that the determination of appropriate scales is dependent on the clinical or research goal for its application. As a rule, observer-rated scales were considered preferred. Based on the Task Force document and input from the UPDRS

Table 10.2 Scale evaluations from the reports by the MDS Task Force on PD Rating Scales.

A. Depression

Scale[a]	Goal: diagnostic screening or rating severity	Grading[b]	General comments
HAM-D	Screening	R	1. Scales selection (criteria): scales analyzed have either been used previously to assess depression in PD in more than one study or, based on literature review and expert evaluation, have potential utility in PD based on their content, their widespread use, and clinimetric evidence from studies in depressed patients without PD. The latter criterion was just applicable to CES-D and CSDD. Only depression-specific scales were considered. Multi-dimensional scales were excluded
	Severity	R	
MADRS	Screening	S	
	Severity	R	
BDI	Screening	R	
	Severity	S	
HADS	Screening	S	
	Severity	L	
SDS	Screening	S	2. Temporal window: up to June 2005
	Severity	S	
GDS	Screening	R	3. Based on Schrag *et al.*[8] with input from the MDS-UPDRS Appendix Committee (C. Sampaio, Chair)
	Severity	L	
UPDRS I	Screening	S	
	Severity	L	4. The Task Force considered that it was not appropriate to invest efforts in developing a new scale of PD depression rather one of the recommended should be systematically studied and characterized clinimetrically
CES-D	Screening	L	
	Severity	L	
CSDD	Screening	L	
	Severity	L	

[a]Beck Depression Inventory (BDI), Hamilton Depression Scale (Ham-D), Hospital Anxiety and Depression Scale (HADS), Zung Self-Rating Depression Scale (SDS), Geriatric Depression Scale (GDS), Montgomery–Asberg Depression Rating Scale (MADRS), Unified Parkinson's Disease Rating Scale (UPDRS) Part I, Cornell Scale for the Assessment of Depression in Dementia (CSDD), and Center for Epidemiologic Studies Depression Scale (CES-D).
[b]R, Recommended; S, Suggested; L, Listed.

Table 10.2 (*Cont.*)

B. Psychosis

Scale[a]	Goal: diagnostic screening or rating severity	Grading[b]	General comments
PPRS	Not specified	S	1. Scales selection (criteria): scales analyzed were used in published, peer-reviewed PD psychosis studies
PPQ	Not specified	S	
RHI	Not specified	L	
BHQ	Not specified	L	2. Temporal window: up to September 2005
NPI	Not specified	R	
BEHAVE-AD	Not specified	S	3. Based on Fernandez *et al.*[9]
BPRS	Not specified	R	
PNSS	Not specified	R	4. The Task Force considered that none of the scales evaluated captures the full phenomenology of PD psychosis and therefore recommends the investment in the development of a dedicated scale
SAPS	Not specified	R	
NOSIE	Not specified	L	
CGIS	Not specified	S	
UPDRS Part I	Not specified	L	

[a]Parkinson Psychosis Rating Scale (PPRS), Parkinson Psychosis Questionnaire (PPQ), Rush Hallucination Inventory (RHI), Baylor Hallucinations Questionnaire (BHQ), Neuropsychiatric Inventory (NPI), Behavioral Pathology in Alzheimer's Disease Rating Scale (BEHAVE-AD), Brief Psychiatric Rating Scale (BPRS), Positive and Negative Syndrome Scale (PANSS), Schedule for Assessment of Positive Symptoms (SAPS), Nurses' Observation Scale for Inpatient Evaluation (NOSIE-30), Clinical Global Impression Scale (CGIS), Unified Parkinson's Disease Rating Scale (UPDRS) Part I.
[b]R, Recommended; S, Suggested; L, Listed.

C. Anxious mood

Scale[a]	Goal: diagnostic screening or rating severity	Grading[b]	General comments
BAI	Screening *Only for panic attacks*	S	1. Scales selection (criteria): scales analyzed have been designed to assess anxiety and that have been either validated or used in studies with PD patients. Multi-dimensional scales were excluded. An exception was made for the anxiety subscale of the Neuropsychiatric Inventory (NPI), because of the frequency with which this instrument is used to assess psychiatric symptoms in PD. Although obsessive compulsive disorder is considered an anxiety disorder in the DSM classification (but not in the ICD classification), scales assessing obsessive-compulsive symptoms were not considered here
	Severity	S	
HADS	Screening	S	
	Severity	L	
Zung SAS	Screening	S	
	Severity	S	
Zung ASI	Screening	S	
	Severity	S	
STAI	Screening	S	2. Temporal window: up to February 2007
	Severity	S	
HARS	Screening	S	3. Based on Leentjens *et al.*[10]
	Severity	S	
NPI Item 5	Screening	S	4. The Task Force considered it is not clear if efforts to develop a new scale for Anxiety in PD will be cost effective. They recommended further investment in characterizing and validating the available scales
	Severity	S	

[a]Beck Anxiety Inventory (BAI), Hospital Anxiety and Depression Scale (HADS), Zung Self-rating Anxiety Scale (Zung SAS), Zung Anxiety Status Inventory (Zung ASI), Spielberger State Trait Anxiety Inventory (STAI), Hamilton Anxiety Rating Scale (HARS), Neuropsychiatric Inventory (NPI).
[b]S, Suggested; L, Listed.

(*continued*)

Table 10.2 (*Cont.*)

D. Apathy/anhedonia

Scale[a]	Goal: diagnostic screening or rating severity	Grading[b]	General comments
AES	Screening	S	1. Scales selection (criteria): scales analyzed have been designed to assess apathy or anhedonia and that have been either validated or used in studies
	Severity	S	with PD patients. Multi-dimensional scales were excluded. Scales
AS	Screening	R	assessing momentary mood states, such as the Profile of Moods States
	Severity	R	Questionnaire (POMS), were also excluded. Because of its special status in
AI	Screening	L	the assessment of PD patients, and also its wide use, an exception was
	Severity	L	made for item 4 (motivation) of Part I of the Unified Parkinson's Disease
LARS	Screening	S	Rating Scale (UPDRS)
	Severity	L	
UPDRS Item 4	Screening	R	2. Temporal window: up to February 2007
	Severity	L	
NPI Item 7	Screening	S	3. Based on Leentjens *et al.*[11]
	Severity	L	
SHAPS	Screening	S	4. The Task Force considered that there is a need to characterize better the
	Severity	S	definitions of apathy and anhedonia before engaging in further validation
Chapman	Screening	L	studies for the existing scales that are considered necessary
	Severity	L	

[a]Apathy Evaluation Scale (AES), the Apathy Scale (AS), the Apathy Inventory (AI), and the Lille Apathy Rating Scale (LARS). In addition, item 4 (motivation/initiative) of the Unified Parkinson's Disease Rating Scale (UPDRS) and item 7 (apathy) of the Neuropsychiatric Inventory (NPI) were included. Anhedonia scales identified for review were the Snaith–Hamilton Pleasure Scale (SHAPS) and the Chapman scales for physical and social anhedonia.
[b]R, Recommended; S, Suggested; L, Listed.

E. Dysautonomia. Upper and lower gastrointestinal dysautonomia symptoms (GIDS)

Item	Scale[a]	Goal: diagnostic screening or rating severity	Grading[b]	General comments
Sialorrhea	DSFS-S	Not specified	S	1. Scale selection (criteria): scales analyzed were used in the
	DRL	Not specified	S	assessment of sialorrhea, dysphagia and constipation.
	SCS-PD-S	Not Specified	S	Scales previously used as outcome measures in studies
Dysphagia	SDQ	Not specified	S	of patients with PD were selected for evaluation. If no
	SWAL	Not specified	S	such scales were identified, scales used in other
	QOL-S			populations were selected for evaluation
Constipation	No scales identified			
	ROME III module			2. Temporal window: up to June 2007
Generic scales	SCOPA	Screening	R	
	AUT	Follow-up	L	3. Based on Evatt *et al.*[12]
	NMS	Screening	R	
		Follow-up	L	
	NMSS	Screening	S	
		Follow-up	L	

[a]Drooling Severity and Frequency Scale (DSFS), Drooling Rating Scale (DRS), Sialorrhea Clinical Scale for Parkinson's Disease (SCS-PD), Swallowing Disturbance Questionnaire (SDQ), Generic Scale for Dysphagia-Related Outcomes (Quality of Life) – SWALQOL, The Scales for Outcomes in Parkinson's Disease – Autonomic, or SCOPAAUT, Nonmotor Symptoms Questionnaire for Parkinson's Disease (NMSQuest), Nonmotor Symptoms Scale (NMSS).
[b]R, Recommended; S, Suggested; L, Listed.

Table 10.3 Recommendations from the Appendix Committee of the MDS-UPDRS[a]

Domain	Scale[b]	Goal: diagnostic screening or rating severity	Grading[c]	General comments
Pain[5]	VAS	Screening	R	1. Scales selection (criteria): scales considered in the EFNS systematic review on the assessment of neuropathic pain were considered. Pain associated with PD is considered central in origin, which makes it a type of neuropathic pain. However, it is also admitted that there are cases where peripheral stimuli are the pain trigger; this pain is probably nociceptive. Pain in PD is not fully understood but for the purpose of this table we consider that primary pain associated with PD is neuropathic
		Severity	R	
	NRS	Screening	S	
		Severity	S	
	VRS	Screening	S	
		Severity	S	
	11-Likert	Screening	S	
		Severity	S	2. Temporal window: up to June 2007
	PRS	Screening	NA	
		Severity	L	3. Based on Cruccu *et al.*[13]
	GPS	Screening	L	
		Severity	L	4. Grading was inferred by the MDS-UPDRS Appendix Committee Chair from the quoted paper plus the specific references on pain and PD retrieved from PubMed
	MPQ	Screening	L	
		Severity	L	
	SF-MPQ	Screening	R	5. A full report from the Task Force is still in preparation but it seems import to invest in characterizing the pain phenomenology in PD before taking the decision about developing a specific scale or not
		Severity	S	
	SSS	Screening	L	
		Severity	L	
	NPS	Screening	L	
		Severity	L	
	NPSI	Screening	S	
		Severity	S	
	CGI	Screening	NA	
		Severity	L	

[a]Subject to modification when full evaluations by the MDS Task Force on PD Rating Scales are complete.
[b]Visual Analog Scale (VAS), Numeric Rating Scale (NRS), Verbal Rating Scale (VRS), 11-point Likert Scale (11-Likert), Parin Relief Scale (PRS), Global Pain Scale (GPS), McGill Pain Questionnaire (MPQ), Short Form of McGill Pain Questionnaire (SF-MPQ), Symptom Severity Scale (SSS), Neuropathic Pain Scale (NPS), Neuropathic Pain Scale Inventory (NPSI), Clinical Global Impression (CGI).
[b]R, Recommended; S, Suggested; L, Listed; NA, not applicable.

Domain	Scale selection (criteria)	Temporal window	Scale[a]	Goal: diagnostic screening or rating severity	Grading[b]	General comments
Cognition (not dementia)	Relative to age-matched normal controls, most non-demented patients with PD are impaired in several cognitive tasks. Poor performance even occurs in early stages. Only scales specifically develop for cognitive impairment in PD were considered	Up to April 2004	MMP	Not specified	L	Based on the Appendices Committee original report
			SCOPA-Cog	Not specified	S	
			BAECD	Not specified	S	
			FAB	Not specified	L	

[a]Mini Mental Parkinson (MMP), Scales for Outcomes of Parkinson's Disease – Cognition (SCOPA-Cog), Brief Assessment of Executive Control Dysfunction (BAECD), Frontal Battery Dysfunction (FAB).
[b]S, Suggested; L, Listed.

Domain	Scale selection (criteria)	Temporal window	Scale[a]	Goal: diagnostic screening or rating severity	Grading[b]	General comments
Parkinson's disease dementia	Scales analyzed were used in published, peer-reviewed PD dementia studies	Up to April 2004	MMSE	Not specified	L	Based on the Appendices Committee original report and the MDS PDD Task Force second paper, in press
			ADAS-Cog	Not specified	S	
			MDRS	Not specified	R	
			NPI	Not specified	L	

[a]Mini Mental Score (MMSE), The Alzheimer's Disease Assessment Scale – Cognitive Subscale (ADAS-Cog), The Mattis' Dementia Ratings Scale (MDRS), The Neuropsychiatric Inventory (NPI).
[b]R, Recommended; S, Suggested; L, Listed.

(*continued*)

Table 10.3 (*Cont.*)

Domain	Scale selection (criteria)	Temporal window	Scale[a]	Goal: diagnostic screening or rating severity	Grading[b]	General comments
Fatigue	Scales analyzed were used in published, peer-reviewed PD studies	Up to March 2008	FSS	Not specified	R	Based on the Appendices Committee original report and a new search of PubMed made in March 2008. Analysis was only preliminary, made by CS
			MFI	Not specified	S	
			PFS	Not specified	R	

[a]Fatigue Severity Scale (FSS), Multidimensional Fatigue Inventory (MFI), Parkinson Fatigue Scale (PFS).
[b]R, Recommended; S, Suggested.

Domain	Scale selection (criteria)	Temporal window	Scale[a]	Goal: diagnostic screening or rating severity	Grading[b]	General comments
Nocturnal sleep	Scales analyzed have been designed to assess insomnia and/or quality of sleep in PD studies	Up to March 2008	PSQI	Screening	R	Based on the Appendices Committee original report and a new search of PubMed made in March 2008
				Severity	R	
			SCOPA-SLEEP	Screening	S	
				Severity	S	
			SDQ	Screening	L	
				Severity	NA	
			NSFSS	Screening	L	
				Severity	NA	
			PDSS	Screening	R	
				Severity	R	
			MPDSS	Screening	L	
				Severity	L	

[a]The Pittsburgh Sleep Quality Index (PSQI), SCOPA-SLEEP night-time sleep sub-scale (SCOPA-SLEEP), Sleep Disorders Questionnaire (SDQ), National Sleep Foundation Sleep Survey (NSFSS), Parkinson's Disease Sleep Scale (PDSS), Modified Parkinson's Disease Sleep Scale (MPDSS).
[b]R, Recommended; S, Suggested; L, Listed.

Domain	Scale selection (criteria)	Temporal window	Scale[a]	Goal: diagnostic screening or rating severity	Grading[b]	General comments
Daytime sleepiness	Scales analyzed have been designed to assess daytime sleepiness or "sleep attacks" in PD studies	Up to March 2008	ESS	Screening	R	Based on the Appendices Committee original report and a new search of PubMed made in March 2008
				Severity	R	
			SCOPA-SLEEP Day	Screening	S	
				Severity	S	
			PDSS Item 15	Screening	L	
				Severity	L	
			SSS	Screening	L	
				Severity	L	
			KSS	Screening	L	
				Severity	L	

[a]Epworth Sleepiness Scale (ESS), SCOPA-SLEEP daytime sleepiness sub-scale (SCOPA-SLEEP Day), Parkinson's Disease Sleep Scale (PDS), The Stanford Sleepiness Scale (SSS) The Karolinska Sleepiness Scale (KSS).
[b]R, Recommended; S, Suggested; L, Listed.

(*continued*)

Table 10.3 (*Cont.*)

Domain	Scale selection (criteria)	Temporal window	Scale[a]	Goal: diagnostic screening or rating severity	Grading[b]	General comments
Orthostatic hypotension	Scales analyzed included a number of generic scales assessing autonomic related symptoms, including OH. Some of these scales are specific for PD. There are also generic autonomic scales with OH subdomains not specific for PD, but used in studies of PD. Additionally, there are scales developed to evaluate symptoms associated with orthostatic intolerance (not exclusively related to OH, but they have not been applied to PD cohorts (see text)	Up to March 2008	SCOPA-AUT	Screening	L	Based on the Appendices Committee original report and a new search of PubMed made in March 2008
				Severity	L	
			NMS Quest	Screening	L	
				Severity	L	
			NMSS	Screening	L	
				Severity	L	
			COMPASS	Screening	L	
				Severity	L	
			OGS	Screening	L	
				Severity	L	
			OHSA	Screening	L	
				Severity	L	

[a]Autonomic Subscale of the SCOPA program (SCOPA-AUT), Non-Motor Symptom Questionnaire (NMSQuest), Non-Motor Symptoms Scale (NMSS), Composite Autonomic Symptom Scale (COMPASS), Orthostatic Grading Scale (OGS), Orthostatic Hypotension Symptoms Assessment (OHSA).
[b]L, Listed.

Domain	Scale selection (criteria)	Temporal window	Scale[a]	Goal: diagnostic screening or rating severity	Grading[b]	General comments
Erectile dysfunction	See text	Up to March 2008	IIEF	Not specified	S	Based on the Appendices Committee original report and a new search of PubMed made in March 2008
			IIEF-5	Not specified	S	
			SHIM			

[a]International Index of Erectile Function (IIEF), International Index of Erectile Function 5 Item (short version) (IIEF-5), also known as Sexual Health Inventory for Men (SHIM).
[b]S, Suggested.

Domain	Scale selection (criteria)	Temporal window	Scale[a]	Goal: diagnostic screening or rating severity	Grading[b]	General comments
Urinary tract symptoms	Scales analyzed included standard urinary symptom scoring methods, but for men these scales do not differentiate symptoms due to neurological dysfunction from benign prostatic hypertrophy. Other scales deal with overall pelvic organ dysfunction (see text)	Up to March 2008	AUASI (men)	Screening	S	Based on the Appendices Committee original report and a new search of PubMed made in March 2008
				Severity	L	
			UDI-6 (women)	Screening	S	
				Severity	L	
			Sakakibara	Screening	L	
				Severity	L	
			IPSS	Screening	S	
				Severity	L	

[a]American Urological Association Symptom Index (AUASI), Urogenital Distress Inventory-6 (UDS-6), International Prostate Symptoms Score (IPSS).
[b]S, Suggested; L, Listed.

Appendix Committee rating group, Recommended scales for diagnostic screening of PD-related depression are HAM-D, BDI, and GDS. Suggested scales are MADRS, HADS, Zung SDS, and UPDRS I. The CES-D and CSDD are alternative instruments that were considered promising, but fall short of both the Recommended and Suggested categories because they still need validation studies in PD depression. For measurement of the *severity* of depressive symptoms, the HAM-D and MADRS are Recommended whereas the BDI and Zung are Suggested. Further studies are needed to validate the CSDD which could be potentially useful for the assessment of the severity of PD-related depression in patients with coexisting dementia.

The report considered the problem of overlapping symptoms between depression and parkinsonism (weight loss, slowness, sleep disruption). To account for overlapping motor and non-motor symptoms of depression, adjusted instrument cut-off scores were considered necessary for PD-related depression, and scales to assess the severity of motor symptoms, such as the UPDRS or MDS-UPDRS, should also be included to help adjust for confounding factors. The HADS and the GDS include limited motor symptom assessment and may therefore be potentially useful in rating depression severity across a range of PD severity; however, these scales appear insensitive in severe depression and therefore could not be rated as either Recommended or Suggested. In the document summary, the Task Force considered that the available scales were overall useful for studying depression and that the complex and time-consuming task of developing a new scale to measure depression specifically for patients with PD was currently not warranted.

Hallucinations and psychosis

Following the same procedure as applied to the assessment of depression, a new group was assembled to assess scales focusing on the problem of hallucinations and psychotic behavior in PD [9]. Twelve psychosis scales/questionnaires were reviewed: Parkinson's Psychosis Rating Scale, Parkinson Psychosis Questionnaire, Rush Hallucination Inventory, Baylor Hallucination Questionnaire, Neuropsychiatric Inventory (NPI), Behavioral Pathology in Alzheimer's Disease Rating Scale (BEHAVE-AD), Brief Psychiatric Rating Scale (BPRS), Positive and Negative Syndrome Scale (PANSS), Schedule for Assessment of Positive Symptoms (SAPS), Nurses' Observation Scale for Inpatient Evaluation, Clinical Global Impression Scale (CGIS), and Unified Parkinson's Disease Rating Scale Part I. Each had different advantages and disadvantages in terms of time requirements, training demands on raters, and clinimetric application in PD (Table 10.2). This evaluation did not separate the scales' utility separately for diagnostic screening versus severity rating. The Task Force labeled the NPI, BPRS, PNSS, and SAPS as Recommended and the PPRS, PPQ, BEHAVE-AD, and the CGIS as Suggested. Although these ratings were based on the defined criteria listed above, the Task Force report emphasized that none of the scales was comprehensive and all were lacking in some respects in terms of basic content, mechanistic, or psychometric properties. Different scales were considered most suited for some settings and others for different situations. Because one scale was unable to serve all needs, a scale used to measure clinical response and change over time such as the CGIS was considered important to combine with other selected scales as a means of cataloging rater or patient-based considerations of the impact on function. This type of global impression was felt to be an important adjunct especially to scales such as the NPI or SAPS. Based on the clinimetric analysis, the Task Force considered that in clinical trials on PD psychosis, the primary outcome scales should be NPI (for the cognitively impaired PD population or when a caregiver is required), and the SAPS, PANSS, or BPRS (for the cognitively intact PD population or when the patient is the sole informant). The CGIS was considered to be an important accompanied secondary outcome scale to measure change and response to treatment over time.

The Task Force was cognizant that even with these Recommended scales, elements of PD-related hallucinations and psychosis were inadequately captured. In this light, the final recommendation of the group was the development of a new scale specifically designed for the assessment of psychotic symptoms in PD. This effort is in the first phases of organization.

Anxious mood

As discussed in other chapters of this book, anxiety syndromes are considered to be common in patients with PD, with some patients meeting criteria for generalized anxiety disorder, others experiencing episodes of non-specific anxiety, and still others developing panic disorders. The systematic review of available scales to assess anxiety in PD focused on six anxiety rating scales: the Beck Anxiety Inventory (BAI), the Hospital Anxiety and Depression Scale (HADS), the Zung Self-Rating Anxiety Scale (SAS) and Anxiety Status Inventory (ASI), the Spielberger State Trait Anxiety Inventory (STAI), and the Hamilton Anxiety Rating Scale (HARS). In addition, item 5 (anxiety) of the Neuropsychiatric Inventory (NPI) was included in the review [10]. Although all scales met at least some of the Task Force predetermined criteria for ranking, no scale met all criteria and therefore none was Recommended. In this report, the utility of scales for diagnostic screening of anxiety and for rating severity of anxiety symptoms was evaluated. For diagnostic screening, all were Suggested. For the evaluation of severity, similarly, most could be Suggested (BAI, Zung SAS, Zung ASI, STAI, HARS, and NPI), but again none met the criteria for Recommended (Table 10.2). Because of the number of scales already in the literature, most of them appearing clinically applicable to the issues faced by PD patients but still inadequately utilized and studied, the Task Force recommended further studies of these instruments and did not recommend developing a new scale for assessing anxiety in PD.

Apathy and anhedonia

Apathy is generally defined as a lack of interest or a state of emotional neutrality, whereas anhedonia involves the inability to experience pleasure. The systematic literature review of scales addressing these symptoms identified the following scales: Apathy Evaluation Scale (AES), Apathy Scale (AS), Apathy Inventory (AI), and Lille Apathy Rating Scale (LARS). In addition, item 4 (motivation/initiative) of the Unified Parkinson's Disease Rating Scale (UPDRS), and item 7 (apathy) of the Neuropsychiatric Inventory (NPI) were reviewed [11]. Anhedonia scales identified for review were the Snaith–Hamilton Pleasure Scale (SHAPS) and the Chapman scales for physical and social anhedonia. As with the reports on depression and anxiety, the evaluation examined the utility of scales for diagnostic screening and for severity of apathy/anhedonia. Only the AS qualified as Recommended for both diagnostic screening and for severity (Table 10.2). Item 4 on the UPDRS Part I met the specified criteria to be Recommended for diagnosis, but because it is a single-item inventory, it cannot be considered for in-depth assessment of severity. For apathy, Suggested diagnostic screening scales were AES, LARS, and NPI. For the diagnosis of anhedonia, the SHAPS was Suggested. For severity assessment, the AES was Suggested for apathy and the SHAPS for anhedonia. Information on the validity of apathy and anhedonia scales in PD is limited largely because of the lack of consensus on precise diagnostic criteria for these conditions. One of the goals of the MDS-UPDRS will be a clearer definition of apathetic mood in PD once the scale is utilized across large populations and in different cultural settings.

Gastrointestinal dysautonomia

The Task Force on Rating Scales considered autonomic symptoms in two categories, the first concerning several problems related to gastrointestinal function. Upper and lower gastrointestinal dysautonomia symptoms (GIDS) included for this review were sialorrhea, dysphagia, and constipation. In contrast to the behavioral assessments discussed above, for dysautonomia there are extensive, invasive quantitative measurement tools for assessing symptoms and responses to therapy; however, these tests are time consuming, require specialized equipment, can cause patient discomfort, and present patients with some medical risk. For this review of scales, the Task Force restricted its critique to symptom-based scales that could be administered in an office setting without the need for specialized equipment. Based on the systematic review, scales for individual symptoms of sialorrhea, dysphagia, and constipation were identified along with three global scales that include these symptoms in the context of assessing wider forms of dysautonomia or non-motor symptoms [12]. Although no sialorrhea scales met criteria for Recommended, three fulfilled criteria for Suggested: Drooling Severity and Frequency Scale (DSFS), Drooling Rating Scale, and Sialorrhea Clinical Scale for PD (SCS-PD). Likewise, two dysphagia scales, the Swallowing Disturbance Questionnaire (SDQ) and Dysphagia-Specific Quality of Life (SWAL-QOL), met criteria for Suggested. Although Rome III constipation module is widely accepted in the gastroenterology community and the earlier version from the Rome II criteria has been used in a single study of PD patients, neither met the criteria for Suggested or Recommended.

This Task Force team also evaluated global scales that assessed larger areas of dysautonomia, but concentrated for their review on the adequacy of the gastrointestinal evaluations. In this category they examined, the Scales for Outcomes in Parkinson's Disease – Autonomic (SCOPA-AUT) and the Non-Motor Symptoms Questionnaire for Parkinson's Disease (NMSQuest), finding that both met criteria for Recommended scales for diagnostic screening purposes of gastrointestinal dysautonomia. They also evaluated the Nonmotor Symptoms Scale (NMSS) and rated it as Suggested in terms of the diagnosis of gastrointestinal symptoms. None was Recommended or Suggested for evaluating severity of symptoms. The group concluded that further application of available scales should be encouraged and no new scales were specifically needed until the available scales were fully tested clinimetrically.

Other non-motor evaluations in progress by Task Force: recommendations of the MDS-UPDRS Appendix Committee

In the near future, the MDS-sponsored Task Force program will provide reports on available scales of Pain, Cognition and Dementia, Fatigue, Nocturnal Sleep Disturbance and Daytime Sleepiness, and Non-Gastrointestinal Dysautonomia (orthostatic hypotension, urinary and sexual dysfunction). Because final critiques are not yet published, the Appendix Committee of the MDS-UPDRS Task Force has provided provisional guides for non-motor elements that are included in the MDS-UPDRS. These recommendations are listed in Table 10.3. When the full Task Force Reports are prepared, the Appendix to the MDS-UPDRS will incorporate those recommendations.

Pain

Under the auspices of The European Federation of Neurological Societies (EFNS), Cruccu *et al.* developed a systematic review of the assessment tools available for evaluating neuropathic pain [13]. Pain associated with PD is often considered central in origin, but has multiple likely causes including compressive neuropathies and local musculoskeletal pains. PD lowers the pain threshold, making PD patients more prone to experience pain whatever the origin [14]. Given its multi-factorial nature, pain in PD is likely to be best assessed by a dedicated pain scale that can capture the different features of the syndrome in this disease. Currently, such a tool does not exist. The MDS-UPDRS Appendix Committee considered that the Cruccu assessment for neuropathic pain is an appropriate starting point for pain assessment in PD, but accepted that direct extrapolation of recommendations on neuropathic pain to PD-related pain was limited. Quantitative sensory testing (QST) is not a scale but rather a laboratory measurement. It is not considered appropriate for screening but it may be useful for quantification of treatment effects. It has been the method most frequently used in papers dedicated to pain in PD. The Leeds Assessment of Neuropathic Symptoms and Signs (LANSS scale) and Neuropathic Pain Questionnaire (NPQ) were developed to differentiate neuropathic from nociceptive pain patients, but they are not tools for quantitative assessment of pain perception or interference in daily life. The Brief Pain Inventory (BPI) was developed to measure pain in cancer patients. It was not analyzed in the Cruccu *et al.* systematic review, but it was used once in a study of pain in PD. The scales considered as potentially useful in neuropathic pain are Visual Analog Scale (VAS), Numerical Rating Scale (NRS), Verbal Rating Scale (VRS), 11-Likert Scale, Gracely Pain Scale (GPS), McGill Pain Questionnaire (MPQ), short form, Symptom Score Scale (SSS), Neuropathic Pain Scale (NPS), Neuropathic Pain Symptom Inventory (NPSI), Pain Relief Scale (PRS), and Clinical Global Impression (CGI). The short form of the McGill Pain Questionnaire (SF-MPQ) has been used in a controlled clinical trial with duloxetine in PD patients and it proved to be sensitive to change [15]. The MDS-UPDRS Appendix Committee considered that, for screening purposes for the presence of pain, the SF-MPQ and the VAS are Recommended. Scales to screen patients for the diagnosis of PD-related pain that met the criteria for Suggested were NRS, VRS, 11-Likert and NPSI. For the assessment of pain severity or intensity, the VAS was Recommended. The NRS, VRS, and 11-Likert Scale are validated scales, but so far have not been used in PD studies. They are therefore classified as Suggested. Also Suggested are the SF-MPQ and NPSI, which go beyond measuring just intensity and attempt to qualify and quantify the different components of the pain sensation.

Cognition

There are two categories of cognition impairment in PD, a full dementia syndrome and cognitive impairment without dementia. The diagnosis and characterization of dementia in PD is a complex process, difficult to capture in a single instrument. A detailed algorithm to accomplish the accurate description of that process has been proposed utilizing standard cognitive tests that do not require special neuropsychological expertise. This algorithm has not yet been validated, but it serves as the first major definition of PD dementia [16]. The Mattis Dementia Rating Scale has been validated in assessing PD dementia, and it is the only instrument for which an adequate set of clinimetric data derived from PD cohorts is available [17,18]. The MDS-UPDRS Appendix Committee considered the Mattis Scale as Recommended for the assessment of PD dementia. The largest clinical trial ever conducted in the field of PD dementia used a scale developed for Alzheimer's Disease – ADAS-Cog [19]. This instrument was able to detect a modest treatment effect of rivastigmine [20]. In the absence of a formal validation of ADAS-Cog for PD dementia, its empirical use, in therapeutic trials, has been legitimized by the EXPRESS trial database. However, it is considered a non-optimal instrument, and its face validity has been questioned, particularly because its content does not cover executive function. Accordingly, the MDS-UPDRS Appendix Committee rated the ADAS-Cog as Suggested. Although the Mini-Mental Status Examination and Neuropsychiatric Inventory have sometimes been applied to the assessment of dementing illnesses, for PD neither scale was rated as Recommended or Suggested.

Cognitive impairment without dementia, sometimes referred to as minimal cognitive impairment (MCI) in PD, calls for assessment tools different from those used in dementia. Only two rating scales specifically developed for cognitive impairment assessments in PD were identified. The Mini-Mental Parkinson is a brief screening test derived from the Mini-Mental State Examination of Folstein [21]. It has not been fully validated, and there are no other known studies beyond the original report. The SCOPA-Cog is intended for comparing groups in research situations and for assessing change in cognitive functioning over time. In the validation process, the items that emerged as the most relevant were selected for the final composition of the scale. These functions suggest that the scale is an instrument that assesses "subcortical" functions in PD, including executive function and attention [22]. Additionally, the Brief Assessment of Executive Control Dysfunction (BAECD) [23] was specifically designed to evaluate relatively subtle impairment of executive function and compared normal controls and patients with schizophrenia, Huntington's disease, and PD. The SCOPA-Cog and the BAECD are considered Suggested by the MDS-UPDRS Appendix Committee.

Fatigue

Fatigue is a symptom frequently associated with chronic neurological disorders, and sometimes is a relevant determinant of disability. Fatigue is likely a multi-factorial symptom that can be part of weakness, apathy, depression, and bradykinesia. There are a number of scales that attempt to capture and quantify fatigue across all medical illnesses, and one scale has been specifically designed to assess fatigue in PD. Despite the small number of studies of fatigue in PD, the Appendix Committee considered two scales that fit the criteria for Recommended: the Fatigue Severity Scale (FSS) and Parkinson Fatigue Scale (PFS) [24,25].

Nocturnal sleep

Nocturnal sleep disruption is a common and disabling feature of PD with multiple origins, ranging from akinesia and tremor to sleep architectural alternations implicit to PD, to medication side effects. Scales identified as potentially relevant to nocturnal sleep assessment in PD are the Pittsburgh Sleep Quality Index (PSQI), SCOPA-SLEEP night-time sleep sub-scale (SCOPA-Sleep), Sleep Disorders Questionnaire (SDQ), National Sleep Foundation Sleep Survey (NSFSS), Parkinson's Disease Sleep Scale (PDSS) and the Modified Parkinson's Disease Sleep Scale (MPDSS) [26]. The SCOPA-SLEEP night-time sub-scale and the MPDSS were specifically developed to target PD patients [27]. Among the disease-specific scales, only the PDSS has undergone a full validation process and therefore only the PDSS is considered Recommended by the MDS-UPDRS Appendix Committee for assessing the presence and severity of nocturnal sleep disruption. Among the other non-disease specific scales, the PSQI is a frequently applied scale in PD studies, and, given its wide usage and good validation in other disease categories, the MDS-UPDRS Appendix Committee graded the PSQI as Recommended. The SCOPA-SLEEP scale was rated as Suggested for assessing the presence and severity of nocturnal sleep problems.

Daytime sleepiness

Daytime sleepiness related to PD itself or medication effects has a strong impact on daily function [28–30]. The scales identified as possibly relevant to evaluated daytime sleepiness in PD patients are the Epworth Sleepiness Scale (ESS), SCOPA-SLEEP daytime sleepiness sub-scale, Parkinson's Disease Sleep Scale (PDSS), Stanford Sleepiness Scale (SSS), and Karolinska Sleepiness Scale (KSS). The ESS is the most widely applied scale in PD studies; it is a self-administered questionnaire with eight items, asking subjects to rate on a four-point scale their chances of falling asleep in eight different daily life situations. The ESS score is the sum of the eight item-scores and can vary from 0 to 24. Acceptable validity, test–retest reliability, and internal consistency reliability of the ESS have been reported.

The SCOPA-SLEEP daytime sleepiness sub-scale was validated in one postal survey against the PSQI in 143 PD patients and 104 controls. The PDSS has been evaluated in relation to nocturnal sleep only. For the SSS and KSS, there are no data in PD. The MDS-UPDRS Appendix Committee rated the ESS as the only Recommended scale for evaluating of daytime sleepiness, both presence and severity. The SCOPA-SLEEP was rated as Suggested [27].

Orthostatic hypotension

Orthostatic hypotension (OH) is a frequent occurrence in PD. The gold standard for diagnosis and severity is the objective measurement of the drop in systolic and diastolic blood pressures using a tilt table. However, it is well established that there is no direct correspondence between the objective severity of OH and patient complaints of lightheadedness. There are a number of generic scales assessing autonomic related symptoms, including items associated with OH, and some of these scales are specific for PD (SCOPA-AUT, NMSQuest, NMSS). There are also generic autonomic scales with OH subdomains, such as the Composite Autonomic Symptom Scale (COMPASS). Although these are not specific for PD, they nonetheless have been used in studies of PD cohorts. The MDS-UPDRS Appendix Committee found that none of these scales met the criteria for Recommended or Suggested for the purpose of evaluating symptoms associated with OH. Additionally there are scales developed to evaluate symptoms associated with orthostatic intolerance (not exclusively related to orthostatic hypotension). These are the Orthostatic Grading scale (OGS) and the Orthostatic Hypotension Symptoms Assessment (OHSA), but they have never been applied to PD cohorts [31].

Erectile dysfunction

Erectile dysfunction has usually been evaluated by laboratory methods based on plistimography and manometry. The need to conduct large double-blind clinical trials to develop sidenafil fostered the development of the International Index of Erectile Function (IIEF), a scale of 15 items covering five domains [32]. This scale has been fully validated in non-PD subjects, but validation studies have not been extended to PD cohorts. An abridged five-item version of the IIEF [IIEF-5 or the Sexual Health Inventory for Men (SHIM)] was developed and validated as a brief, easily administered, patient-reported diagnostic tool [33]. IIEF has been the primary outcome measure in at least two open trials that evaluated the efficacy of sidenafil and pergolide in PD patients with erectile dysfunction, but in the sidenafil trial the population included patients with MSA [34,35]. The SHIM has also been used in a trial of sidenafil in PD patients [36]. Based on these data, the MDS-UPDRS Appendix Committed graded the IIEF and SHIM as Suggested for PD studies.

Urinary dysfunction

Nocturia is the most prevalent of the lower urinary tract symptoms (LUTS) reported by patients with PD (>60%). Patients complain of urgency (33–54%) and frequency (16–36%), which may be severe. Urgency incontinence can become problematic particularly if poor mobility compounds bladder disorders. Although co-existing benign prostatic hypertrophy (BPH) may occur in men with PD and be confused with PD-related urinary symptoms, urinary problems in PD are otherwise similar in men and women [37]. Standard urinary symptom scoring methods have been applied to patients with PD, but these scales do not differentiate symptoms due to neurological dysfunction from BPH. Such scales include the American Urological Association Symptom Index (AUASI) for men and the Urogenital Distress Inventory-6 (UDI-6) for women [38]. Sakakibara *et al.* developed a dedicated questionnaire for pelvic organ dysfunction that covers bladder, bowel, and sexual function in PD [39]. This questionnaire has not been formally validated despite having been applied to a cohort of PD patients. In another study of PD patients (men and women), the International Prostate Symptoms Score (IPSS) was used [40]. All the questionnaires mentioned above were used for screening purposes in diagnosing the presence of urinary complaints. The non-PD specific questionnaires were validated outside the context of PD, and therefore the MDS-UPDRS Appendix Committee judged that they could be considered as Suggested scales for diagnostic screening purposes. The Sakakibara P-specific questionnaire has been insufficiently validated and therefore is not rated as either Suggested or Recommended. There are no controlled trials of therapeutic interventions in PD patients with urinary symptoms and therefore there is no scale to rate severity and sensitivity of change available for assessment in this context.

Dopamine dysregulation syndrome

A range of impulse control and repetitive behaviors, termed "dopamine dysregulation syndrome" (DDS), are presumed to be related to dopaminergic medications. They have long been recognized in PD, but more recently highlighted in relation to the use of dopamine agonists [41]. These behaviors include pathological gambling, hypersexuality, compulsive shopping, and compulsive eating. They may also be related to the phenomenon of "punding" or incessant repetitive unnecessary behaviors, and, in the view of several researchers, also include compulsive medication use or abuse. Estimates of DDS in PD typically exceed those in the general population, affecting about 5% of patients at any given time and between 5 and 10% at some point during the course of their disease [42].

There is still controversy on the best way to classify these behaviors. Specific criteria for the most prevalent categories have been derived from DSM-IV or proposed by different authors following the DSM-IV model (gambling, hypersexuality, compulsive shopping, compulsive eating, punding, compulsive medication use) [43].

A dedicated rating scale to screen and/or measure the severity of these behaviors in PD has not yet been published. Each of the above-mentioned behaviors has been studied using methods imported from the psychiatric literature and not specifically developed for PD. In most instances, the method used was a structured clinical interview including the modified Minnesota Impulse Disorder Interview. Because this field is in the developmental phase only, the MDS-UPDRS Appendix Committee could not list any scale as Suggested or Recommended. No table is shown for this behavior in Table 10.3.

Future perspectives: other specific scale critiques in development

A unified set of Recommended scales to assess non-motor elements of PD will complement the MDS-UPDRS and allow for a greater likelihood that researchers world-wide will use similar measures when developing research protocols and assessing new interventions. As new clinimetric studies are conducted, as new scales are tested, and as new statistical analyses are provided, the ranking of Recommended and Suggested for scales may change and the authors are committed to encouraging the MDS to maintain these reports and categorizations as fluid and evolving. Reference to the Movement Disorder Society website (Movementdisorders.org) will assure up-to-date recommendations.

References

1. Rocca NG. Statistical and methodologic considerations in scale construction. In: Munsat TL, ed. *Quantification of Neurologic Deficit*. Boston: Butterworth, 1989: 49–67.
2. Fahn S, Elton RL, the UPDRS Development Committee. Unified Parkinson's Disease Rating Scale. In: Fahn S, Marsden CD, Calne D, Goldstein M, eds. *Recent Developments in Parkinson's Disease*. Florham Park, NJ: Macmillan Healthcare Information, 1987: 153–63.
3. Movement Disorder Society Task Force on Rating Scales for Parkinson's Disease: Goetz CG, Poewe W, Rascol O, *et al.* UPDRS: Status and Recommendations. *Mov Disord* 2003;**18**: 738–50.
4. Goetz CG, Fahn S, Martinez-Martin P, *et al.* Movement Disorder Society-sponsored revision of the Unified Parkinson's Disease Rating Scale (MDS-UPDRS): process, format, and clinimetric testing plan. *Mov Disord* 2007;**22**:41–7.
5. Goetz CG, Tilley BC, Shaftman S, *et al.* Movement Disorder Society-sponsored revision of the Unified Parkinson's Disease Rating Scale (MDS-UPDRS): scale presentation and clinimetric profile. *Mov Disord*. 2008;**23**:2129–70.
6. Chaudhuri KR, Martinez-Martin P, Schapira AHV. An international multicenter pilot study of the first comprehensive self-completed non motor symptoms questionnaire for Parkinson's disease: the NMSQuest study. *Mov Disord* 2006;**21**:916–23.
7. Chaudhuri KR, Martinez-Martin P, Brown RG, *et al.* The metric properties of a novel non-motor symptoms scale for Parkinson's disease: results from an international pilot study. *Mov Disord* 2007;**22**:1901–11.

8. Schrag A, Barone P, Brown RG, *et al.* Depression rating scales in Parkinson's disease: critique and recommendations. *Mov Disord* 2007;**22**:1077–92.
9. Fernandez HH, Aarsland D, Fénelon G, *et al.* Scales to assess psychosis in Parkinson's disease: critique and recommendations. *Mov Disord* 2008;**23**:484–500.
10. Leentjens AFG, Dujardin K, Marsh L, *et al.* Anxiety rating scales in Parkinson's disease: critique and recommendations. *Mov Disord* 2008;**23**(14):2015–25.
11. Leentjens AFG, Dujardin K, Marsh L, *et al.* Apathy and anhedonia rating scales in Parkinson's disease: critique and recommendations. *Mov Disord* 2008;**23**(14):2004–14.
12. Evatt ML, Chaudhuri KR, Chou KL, *et al.* Dysautonomia rating scales in Parkinson's disease: sialorrhea, dysphagia, and constipation: critique and recommendations to Movement Disorders Task Force on Rating Scales for Parkinson's Disease. *Mov Disord* 2008;**24**(5):635–46.
13. Cruccu G, Anand P, Attal N, *et al.* Guidelines on assessment of neuropathic pain and response to treatment. In: *European Handbook of Neurological Management Official EFNS Guidelines*, Hughes R, Brainin M, Gilhus NE, eds, 1st edn. Blackwell: Oxford, 2006: 234–47.
14. Djaldetti R, Shifrin A, Rogowski Z, *et al.* Quantitative measurement of pain sensation in patients with Parkinson disease. *Neurology* 2004;**62**:2171–5.
15. Djaldetti R, Yust-Katz S, Kolianov V, *et al.* The effect of duloxetine on primary pain symptoms in Parkinson disease. *Clin Neuropharmacol* 2007;**30**:201–5.
16. Dubois B, Burn D, Goetz C, *et al.* Diagnostic procedures for Parkinson's disease dementia: recommendations from the Movement Disorder Society Task Force. *Mov Disord* 2007;**22**:2314–24.
17. Brown GG, Rahill AA, Gorell JM, *et al.* Validity of the Dementia Rating Scale in assessing cognitive function in Parkinson's disease. *J Geriatr Psychiatry Neurol* 1999;**12**:180–188.
18. Llebaria G, Pagonabarraga J, Kulisevsky J, *et al.* Cut-off score of the Mattis Dementia Rating Scale for screening dementia in Parkinson's disease. *Mov Disord* 2008;**23**(11):1546–50.
19. Mohs RC, Rosen WG, Davis KL The Alzheimer's Disease Assessment Scale: an instrument for assessing treatment efficacy. *Psychopharmacol Bull* 1983;**19**:448–50.
20. Emre M, Aarsland D, Albanese A, *et al.* Rivastigmine for dementia associated with Parkinson's disease. *N Engl J Med* 2004;**351**:2509–18.
21. Mahieux F, Michelet D, Manifacier MJ, *et al.* Mini-Mental Parkinson: first validation study of a new bedside test constructed for Parkinson's disease. *Behav Neurol* 1995;**8**:15–22.
22. Marinus J, Visser M, Verwey NA, *et al.* Assessment of cognition in Parkinson's disease. *Neurology* 2003;**61**:1222–8.
23. Hanes KR, Andrewes DG, Deidre JS, Pantelis C. A brief assessment of executive control dysfunction: discriminant validity and homogeneity of planning, set shift, and fluency measures. *Arch Clin Neuropsychol* 1996;**11**:185–91.
24. Herlofson K, Larsen JP. Measuring fatigue in patients with Parkinson's disease: the Fatigue Severity Scale. *Eur J Neurol* 2002;**9**:595–600.
25. Brown RG, Dittner A, Findley L, Wessely SC. The Parkinson Fatigue Scale. *Parkinsonism Relat Disord* 2005;**11**:49–55.
26. Chaudhuri KR, Pal S, DiMarco A, *et al.* The Parkinson's Disease Sleep Scale: a new instrument for assessing sleep and nocturnal disability in Parkinson's disease. *J Neurol Neurosurg Psychiatry* 2002;**73**:629–35.
27. Marinus J, Visser M, van Hilten JJ, *et al.* Assessment of sleep and sleepiness in Parkinson disease. *Sleep* 2003;**26**:1049–54.
28. Fabbrini G, Barbanti P, Aurilia C, *et al.* Excessive daytime sleepiness in *de novo* and treated Parkinson's disease. *Mov Disord* 2002;**17**:1026–30.
29. Shulman LM, Taback RL, Rabinstein AA, Weiner WJ. Non-recognition of depression and other non-motor symptoms in Parkinson's disease. *Parkinsonism Relat Disord* 2002;**8**:193–7.
30. Iranzo A, Valldeoriola F, Santamaria J, *et al.* Sleep symptoms and polysomnographic architecture in advanced Parkinson's disease after chronic bilateral subthalamic stimulation. *J Neurol Neurosurg Psychiatry* 2002;**72**:661–4.
31. Winker R, Barth A, Dorner W, *et al.* Diagnostic management of orthostatic intolerance in the workplace. *Int Arch Occup Environ Health* 2003;**76**:143–50.
32. Rosen RC, Riley A, Wagner G, *et al.* The international index of erectile function (IIEF): a multidimensional scale for assessment of erectile dysfunction. *Urology* 1997;**49**:822–30.
33. Rosen RC, Cappelleri JC, Smith MD, *et al.* Development and evaluation of an abridged, 5-item version of the International Index of Erectile Function (IIEF) as a diagnostic tool for erectile dysfunction. *Int J Impot Res* 1999;**11**:319–26.
34. Hussain IF, Brady CM, Swinn MJ, *et al.* Treatment of erectile dysfunction with sildenafil citrate (Viagra) in parkinsonism due to Parkinson's disease or multiple system atrophy with observations on orthostatic hypotension. *J Neurol Neurosurg Psychiatry* 2006;**77**:822–5.
35. Pohanka M, Kanovský P, Bares M, *et al.* Pergolide mesylate can improve sexual dysfunction in patients with Parkinson's disease: the results of an open, prospective, 6-month follow-up. *Eur J Neurol* 2004;**11**:483–8.
36. Zesiewicz TA, Helal M, Hauser RA. Sildenafil citrate (Viagra) for the treatment of erectile dysfunction in men with Parkinson's disease. *Mov Disord* 2000;**15**:305–8.
37. Winge K, Fowler CJ. Bladder dysfunction in Parkinsonism: mechanisms, prevalence, symptoms, and management. *Mov Disord* 2006;**21**; 737–45.
38. Lemack GE, Dewey RB Jr, Roehrborn CG, *et al.* Questionnaire-based assessment of bladder dysfunction in patients with mild to moderate Parkinson's disease. *Urology* 2000;**56**:250–4.
39. Sakakibara R, Shinotoh H, Uchiyama T, *et al.* Questionnaire-based assessment of pelvic organ dysfunction in Parkinson's disease. *Auton Neurosci* 2001;**92**:76–85.
40. Araki I, Kuno S. Assessment of voiding dysfunction in Parkinson's disease by the international prostate symptom score. *J Neurol Neurosurg Psychiatry* 2000;**68**:429–33.
41. Voon V, Potenza MN, Thomsen T. Medication-related impulse control and repetitive behaviors in Parkinson's disease. *Curr Opin Neurol* 2007;**20**:484–92.
42. Mamikonyan E, Siderowf AD, Duda JE, *et al.* Long-term follow-up of impulse control disorders in Parkinson's disease. *Mov Disord* 2008;**23**:75–80.
43. Voon V, Fox S. Medication-related impulse control and repetitive behaviors in Parkinson disease. *Arch Neurol* 2007;**64**:1089–96.

Chapter 11
Clinical Trial Measures of the Non-Motor Features of Parkinson's Disease

Karl Kieburtz
Department of Neurology, University of Rochester Medical Center, Rochester, NY, USA

Introduction

The majority of therapeutic clinical trials that have been performed in Parkinson's disease (PD) to date have primarily focused on the motor features of the disease, generally using change in the Unified Parkinson's Disease Rating Scale (UPDRS) and "on" and "off" times as the primary endpoints. "On" and "off" times refer to the amount of time anti-parkinsonian drugs are working well or not working, respectively, and are typically assessed by patient-completed home diaries. The motor and activities of daily living (ADL) subscales of the UPDRS and quality-of-life measures have frequently been used as secondary outcome measures. In early disease, the emphasis has been on change from baseline in UPDRS score. Indeed, European and North American regulatory agency guidelines for pivotal trials cite the use of the UPDRS and its motor and ADL subscales as preferred outcome measures. Time to the development of dyskinesia, a motor complication of levodopa therapy, has also been employed as a primary endpoint in several studies, although no drug has yet received approval for this indication. It should be noted that all of these measures, including the ADL subsection of the classic UPDRS, primarily focus on motor disability. Motor features are again emphasized in later stage clinical trials where the outcome measures that are most often employed are change in UPDRS score, and the amount of self-reported "on" or "off" time and time with troublesome dyskinesia, using home diaries. These clinical trial measures reflect the traditional clinical and research emphasis on the motor aspects of Parkinson's disease. Indeed, the triad of rigidity, rest tremor, and bradykinesia have historically served as the basis for making the diagnosis of PD. However, this is only part of the story of the clinical spectrum of PD. It is now evident that there can also be functional impairments in mood, cognitive performance, gait and balance, motor freezing, sleep and daytime sleepiness, sensory phenomena, autonomic dysfunction, and other non-motor and non-dopamine areas, as discussed extensively in various chapters of this book. Indeed, non-motor features of the disease are commonly seen in the early stages of the disease [1], and may even precede the onset of the classical motor triad of parkinsonism [2].

The progressive disability in PD can be attributed as much, if not more so, to the non-motor symptoms and non-dopaminergic features of the illness as to the classic levodopa-responsive motor symptoms. For example, Dooneief *et al.* [3] found that roughly half of PD patients across a broad clinical spectrum had experienced depression. The Sydney Multicenter Study [4] followed an initial cohort of 149 people for 15 years. Although the study was designed to compare the effect of initial levodopa versus bromocriptine treatment on motor complications, the long term follow-up of the subjects provides a window into the progression of PD. Only one-third of subjects survived to 15 years and the large majority in both groups had motor complications, although interestingly these were not a significant contributor to disability. However, of the initial cohort, only four patients were living alone and none were working. The remainder were in nursing homes or assisted living facilities. About 80% of the subjects had fallen, and 25% had sustained fractures. Roughly 80% had cognitive impairment, 50% had dementia sufficient to meet DSMIVR criteria, and approximately 50% had experienced visual hallucinations. Over half of the patients also had depression. These were the symptoms that were primarily responsible for disability and nursing home placement. In another study, a questionnaire which focused on non-motor symptoms was administered to 525 patients in North America, Europe, Japan and Israel. This relatively simple questionnaire incorporated 30 yes/no questions, and patients with over 5 years of disease duration endorsed, on average, more than 10 non-motor symptoms, with a progressive increase associated with disease progression [5]. Overall, non-motor

Parkinson's Disease: Non-Motor and Non-Dopaminergic Features, First Edition. Edited by C. Warren Olanow, Fabrizio Stocchi, and Anthony E. Lang.

and non-dopaminergic complaints occurred with a significantly higher frequency than in age-matched controls. These findings point to the high prevalence of non-motor and non-dopaminergic symptoms and signs in patients with advanced PD. Indeed, in a cross-sectional study performed by Muslimovic *et al.* [6] it was found that axial impairment (postural instability and gait difficulty) and self-reported mood status were the main determinants of quality-of-life in patients who had PD for an average of 3 years. In a longitudinal secondary analysis of the DATATOP data, Marras *et al.* [7] similarly found that approximately 5–6 years after early PD patients had been enrolled in the trial, the Hamilton Depression Scales scores and self-rating of cognitive function were predictors of decline in health-related quality-of-life, and postural instability/gait disorder was found to decline concurrently with deterioration in health-related quality-of-life. Together these studies suggest that non-motor and non-dopaminergic features such as depression, cognitive impairment, and ambulatory dysfunction are the most important predictors of decreasing function and quality-of-life in patients with PD. These features are to some extent defined by the inability of dopaminergic therapies to provide benefit, and the development of alternative and effective therapies for these problems is a major goal of PD research. To accomplish this, it will be necessary to develop standardized measures of these domains (see Chapter 10), an understanding of the natural history of the emergence of these symptoms in PD, and a determination of if, and how, these might be used as primary outcome measures in clinical trials designed to capture the potential benefits of therapeutic interventions introduced at various stages of the disease.

Parkinson's disease pathology and clinical features

The study of PD pathology has also largely focused on motor features, and indeed there is a correlation between the degree of nigrostriatal pathology, dopamine deficiency, and severity of motor impairment. Recent attention has now begun to focus on non-dopaminergic pathology which extends throughout the nervous system [8], which likely accounts for the emergence of features that do not respond to levodopa therapy (see Chapters 2 and 3). Early pathological abnormalities can be detected in olfactory structures, preganglionic parasympathetic projection neurons, the enteric nervous system, and the lower brainstem. In more advanced PD, in concert with the progression of the motor manifestations of the disease, there are also pathologic changes in temporal mesocortex, hippocampus, pre-frontal neocortex, and eventually in primary sensory and motor cortical fields. This extensive pathology may help to explain the broad range of clinical manifestations that eventually develop in PD. Involvement of parasympathetic and sympathetic projection neurons and also the loss of enteric nervous system neurons may explain autonomic symptoms, such as constipation and orthostatic hypotension, which are often seen in the earliest stages of PD. There are not yet good data to correlate the degree of pathology in these areas with the magnitude of symptoms, and this process is partly hampered by our lack of good measurement tools in the non-motor domains of PD.

The World Health Organization initially developed a schema for classifying impairments, disabilities, and handicaps (ICIDH), which was revised into an international classification of functioning, disability, and health, commonly abbreviated as "ICF." Although there are debates about the specific use of the language, for clinicians and clinical researchers more or less common-sense definitions may be used. Scales of "impairment" measure an individual's ability to perform tasks, usually in a given domain such as motor, cognitive, or autonomic functions. The UPDRS is an example of a scale that measures "impairment." Different types of scales would capture the functional implication of these impairments and are frequently called "measures of function." An examples of this kind of scale in PD is the Schwab and England Activities of Daily Living scale. How functional limitation shapes a person's view of their illness and their life is captured in "health-related quality-of-life" instruments. We will review some of the instruments that have been developed to capture impairments in several non-motor domains (cognitive, mood, hallucinations and psychiatric function, autonomic function, sleep, and fatigue) and then review some of the scales of disability and health-related quality-of-life that have been used in PD. This review is not exhaustive as there are hundreds of such instruments available. The Movement Disorders Society is currently carrying out a review of scales in several domains in an effort to help identify those which can be used by researchers to permit different studies to be compared and contrasted. Where these reviews have been completed and published they are cited below. Examples of measures of impairment and disability that are available for testing various non-motor features of PD and that have been used in specific clinical trials are also described. In addition, we will consider some new study designs that can be used to try to assess the effect of interventions on the cumulative motor and non-motor disability associated with PD.

Measures of impairment (see Table 11.1)

Cognition

Cognitive impairment has been recognized as an important aspect of PD for many years, affecting as many as 80%

Table 11.1 Impairment scales in PD.

Domain	Scale
Motor	UPDRS
Cognition	SCOPA-Cog [14] MMSE ADAS-Cog
Depression	Beck Depression Scale Zung Montgomery–Asberg Depression Rating Scale Hamilton Depression Scale
Hallucinations	Brief Psychiatric Rating Scale Schedule for Assessment of Positive Symptoms Neuropsychiatric Inventor
Sleep	Pittsburg Sleep Quality Index Epworth Daytime Sleepiness Scale

of PD patients, although until recently there have not been PD-specific measures of cognitive impairment. Aarsland and colleagues [9] followed a longitudinal population-based cohort in Norway for 12 years. Following an initial assessment of PD prevalence, they assessed dementia using DSMIII-R criteria based on a semi-structured caregiver interview, the Mattis Dementia Rating Scale, and the Mini Mental State Examination (MMSE). For those without severe impairment, a neuropsychological test battery assessing visual memory, visual/spatial ability, and executive functions was also used. This is a fairly typical pattern whereby an extensive and complex use of formal neuropsychologic testing along with patient and caregiver interviews are used to reach a formal diagnosis of dementia. Marder *et al.* [10] pursued a similar strategy, evaluating PD patients for dementia in a defined community in upper Manhattan using a neuropsychologic test battery and subject evaluation to diagnose dementia based on DSMIII-R criteria. In the Rotterdam population-based study of dementia [11], a two-step process was used. Participants were screened with the MMSE and the Geriatric Mental State Schedule. If the screening was positive, subjects were further examined with the Cambridge Examination of Mental Disorders in the Elderly, and if necessary a further examination was done by neuropsychologists, again yielding a diagnosis based on DSMIII-R criteria. These studies all demonstrated an increased frequency of dementia in PD patients compared with age-matched controls, but these techniques used for diagnosing dementia on a research basis are excessively cumbersome for routine use in practice or in clinical trials. In the DATATOP study, cognition was assessed by a battery of neuropsychologic retests including Digit Span, Symbol Digit, Selective Reminding, Odd Man Out, Spot-the-Dot, Verbal Fluency, and MMSE [12].

In the EXCEL trial [13], which tested the potential of rivastigmine to improve or slow progression of dementia associated with PD, the primary measure of cognitive performance was the Alzheimer's Disease Assessment Scale Cognitive Subscale (ADAS-Cog) which is the most widely used outcome measure in AD trials. An Alzheimer's-based clinical global impression scale and an ADL scale were also used along with the MMSE and additional neuropsychologic tests. Again, this is a relatively intensive battery and the primary outcome measure is not specific to PD. Nonetheless, the inclusion criteria employed and the positive results obtained in this trial were sufficient to convince the regulatory authorities to accept Parkinson's disease with dementia (PD-D) as a specific entity distinct from AD and to authorize approval of the drug. Although the study showed positive results in favor of ravistigmine, it is interesting to speculate on the likelihood that more specific measures of executive functions which are preferentially impaired in PD dementia would have shown even more positive results. Alternatively, the use of endpoints that primarily assess cognitive function in AD might have been negative in PD dementia and failed to detect benefits of the drug.

van Hilten and colleagues [14] have developed a scale specific for assessing cognition in PD called the SCOPA-COG as part of a project to develop scales for outcomes in PD. SCOPA-COG is relatively brief, containing 10 items that cover memory, attention, executive functioning, and visual/spatial functioning. The maximum score is 43. Four hundred PD patients were evaluated and demonstrated to have significantly worse performance in comparison with 150 controls. Across disease severity, as judged by the Hoehn and Yahr scale, cognitive impairment increased. The SCOPA-COG appears to be a well-validated instrument designed to assess cognition in PD, and is similar to the MMSE in terms of simplicity of administration.

More recently, the Movement Disorder Society (MDS) commissioned a panel to provide an operational definition of dementia in PD [15], and to provide a battery of tests that could be used as endpoints for research studies and clinical trials [16]. While these include a relatively exhaustive series of evaluations, it is anticipated that this will facilitate defining PD-D patients and conducting research in this area.

Depression

Depression is a common problem in PD, occurring in as many as 50% of patients. Once again, clinical research in PD has primarily been performed using depression rating scales that have been developed in psychiatry. Perhaps the most commonly used scales are the Hamilton Depression Scale [17], the Beck Depression Scale [18], and the Montgomery–Asberg Depression Scale (MADRS) [19]. The Hamilton Scale is an interviewer-rated scale and the MADRS is an observer-rated scale requiring some experience in depression. In contrast, the Beck is a self-rating instrument. Other rating scales that have been used in PD research including the Hospital Anxiety and Depression Scale, the Zung Self-Rating Depression Scale, the Geriatric Depression Scale, the Cornell Scale for the Assessment of Depression in Dementia, and the Center for Epidemiologic Studies Depression Scale. These were reviewed by Schrag *et al.* on behalf of the MDS [20]. Their conclusions were that as screening tools the Hamilton Depression Scale, the Beck, the Hospital Anxiety and Depression Scale, the MADRS and the GDS were recommended and have been validated in PD. In contrast, for measurement of the severity of depressive symptoms, which is perhaps more relevant to clinical trials, the Hamilton, MADRS, Beck, and Zung Self-Rating scales were recommended. Based on the recommendations of the MDS Task Force, both the Hamilton and MADRS seem appropriate as examiner-completed evaluations and the Beck and Zung scales are appropriate as self-reported measures of depression in PD. In a recent clinical trial of desipramine and citalopram in depression in PD [21], the primary outcome measure was the MADRS. Despite a strong placebo effect, both interventions demonstrated a significant improvement at 30 days. This suggests that the scale is responsive to the treatment effects of drugs in PD depression.

Hallucinations

Schrag [22] reviewed the psychiatric aspects of PD, which include depression, cognitive impairment (as discussed above), apathy, and psychosis, which is most commonly treatment related. Fernandez *et al.* [23] reviewed the scales for psychosis in PD for the MDS. Although several scales have been developed to assess psychosis in PD, they have not been widely used. In the general population, a variety of scales have been developed, including the Neuropsychiatric Inventory (NPI), the Brief Psychiatric Rating Scale (BPRS), the Positive and Negative Symptom Scale, and the Schedule for Assessment for Positive Symptoms (SAPS). The authors concluded that there were no validated tools that capture adequately the phenomenology of PD psychosis. However, they found that the Brief Psychiatric Rating Scale and the Schedule for the Assessment for Positive Symptoms appear to be sensitive to change. The NPI is probable a good scale in cataloging the presence of psychotic phenomenon, but is a highly descriptive scale. The group concluded that the NPI, the SAPS, the Positive and Negative Syndrome Scale, and the BPRS were all appropriate for use as primary outcome measures for clinical trials of PD psychosis. In a clinical trial of clozapine [24] for the treatment of drug-induced psychosis in PD, the Clinical Global Impression Scale, the BPRS, and the SAPS were all used as outcome measures. Each of these demonstrated improvement on active treatment, demonstrating their responsiveness as outcome measures in a clinical trial.

Autonomic Dysfunction

Autonomic dysfunction can have a variety of manifestations in PD, including difficulty with swallowing, orthostatic hypotension with positional lightheadedness, bowel and bladder impairment, and sexual dysfunction. Evaluations used to date have relied primarily on clinical assessments, including blood pressure changes when standing and lying, and historical questions about urinary frequency and constipation. No multi-system scales to evaluate these autonomic features have been developed until recently. The non-motor questionnaire asks for symptoms in several of these domains [1], and has proven useful in determining if problems exist (as patients frequently will not mention these unless directly probed). The PRO-PARK project led by van Hilten and colleagues [25] has also developed an instrument designed to assess autonomic symptoms in PD patients, the SCOPA-AUT. This was evaluated in 420 PD patients and compared with 150 controls, similarly to the SCOPA-COG. They found an increasing prevalence of autonomic symptoms in older patients and in those with more severe disease and with greater medication usage. There are no other validated scales that have been used to assess multiple areas of autonomic function. Autonomic outcome scales for use as a primary outcome measure in clinical trials are not well developed and have historically relied on historical measures (see above). The SCOPA-AUT remains to be used as a major outcome measure in a clinical trial.

Sleep

Sleep disorders including fragmentation of sleep architecture, insomnia, REM behavior disorder, sleep apnea, restless leg syndrome, and difficulties with excess daytime sleepiness have all been described in PD. Most clinical research on sleep dysfunction has relied on formal polysomnography and multiple sleep latency studies. There are no PD-specific instruments for assessing sleep quality or excessive daytime sleepiness. The Pittsburgh Sleep Quality Index [26] has been used in assessment of non-PD populations and was specifically devised to assess sleep quality among psychiatric patients. Its utility in PD is not well established. The Epworth Daytime Sleepiness Scale (EDSS) [27] has been developed for assessment of patients with sleep apnea, and has been used successfully to assess the extent of sleepiness in PD populations [28]. Small trials of modafinil [29] have used the EDSS as an outcome measure. In one small study of 40 subjects, modafinil failed to improve Epworth sleepiness scores; this was confirmed by a more formal assessment using the multi-sleep latency test.

Measures of function and health-related quality-of-life

Measures of function focus on individuals' ability to care for themselves and to interact with others. The Schwab and England ADL Scale [30] is probably the best established PD disability scale and has been used extensively in clinical trials, but rarely as a primary outcome measure. There are not many other pure disability scales, as most PD-specific scales have focused on subjects' perception of how their disability impacts their life, and are better described as health-related quality-of-life scales. Several of these have been developed for PD, specifically including the PDQ-39 [31] and PD-QUAL [32]. In addition, generic health-related quality-of-life instruments have been evaluated in PD, including the EQ-5D [33] and the Medical Outcome Survey 36-Item Short Form (SF-36) [34]. More recently, the SCOPA-PS has been developed for testing psycho-social functions in PD patients [35]. This is a short psycho-social questionnaire assessing psycho-social functioning in PD patients that behaves similarly to other PD and generic health-related quality-of-life instruments. Despite concerns that these instruments might be insensitive to change in PD patients, they have been used with success in clinical trials. The CALM-PD study demonstrated changes in the EQ-5D [36] that paralleled changes in UPDRS score. In contrast, there was little association between new onset motor complications and changes in health-related quality-of-life. In studies of the COMT inhibitors entacapone [37] and tolcapone [38], conducted in stable treated PD patients, improvements were seen in health-related quality-of-life instruments, including the PDQ-39 and the SF-36. These changes in health-related quality-of-life were seen despite no significant change in motor functioning, as assessed by UPDRS scores in another trial [37]. These types of studies suggest that in early PD patients there are benefits in non-motor features associated with study interventions which are not captured by the UPDRS. To try to address this problem and to capture subtle change in both motor and non-motor features in PD, the MDS formulated a new UPDRS scale known as the MDS-UPDRS [39,40]. This is more extensive than the original and is not suited for routine office assessment, but should be useful in clinical research, particularly in trials testing putative neuroprotective therapies that are aiming to detect subtle changes in patients with early disease.

Lastly, it is worth noting that much of the impact of PD in its advanced state falls on the caregivers. Instruments have been developed by Carter *et al.* [41] and Schrag *et al.* [42] to assess caregivers' strain or burden. These studies found that caregiver strain is experienced across all stages of PD, but that it accumulates significantly as the disease progresses. Schrag *et al.* found that non-motor symptoms of psychiatric disturbance and falls were most closely associated with increases in caregiver burden.

New Study Designs (see Table 11.2)

Treatments that can favorably influence the progression of PD are clearly needed. Most trials of such agents have focused on early PD, usually before the start of dopaminergic therapy. The clinical milestone of need for dopaminergic therapy has been one of the most common outcomes in such trials and probably integrates some non-motor aspects of PD. More recently, there has been a focus on the change in UPDRS scores (Parts I–III) in early disease. Parts I and II of the UPDRS incorporate mental and ADL aspects of PD, but the "total" UPDRS score is still largely driven by motor aspects of PD. There have been fewer studies that examined the progression of "treated PD," and these have usually focused on the evolution of motor complications, namely dyskinesias and motor fluctuations. As outlined throughout this book, such a focus on motor features misses important clinical aspects of PD. How can clinical trials be designed differently?

The National Institute of Neurological Disorders and Stroke (NINDS) is currently funding a PD clinical research program designed to identify treatments that could help slow PD progression. The NINDS Exploratory Trials in PD (NET-PD) program included pilot studies to assess

Table 11.2 Outcomes in clinical trials in PD.

Stage of illness	Motor outcome	Non-motor outcomes of interest
Pre-manifest	Onset of motor signs	Olfaction Autonomic dysfunction (e.g., constipation) Sleep
Early, untreated	UPDRS	Cognition Mood Sleep
Early, treated	UPDRS Ambulation	Cognition Mood Function Health-related quality-of-life Sleep
Advanced treated	On/off diaries Postural stability UPDRS on/off	Dementia Depression Health-related quality-of-life Hallucinations

potential interventions. Based, in part, on those studies, creatine (10 g per day) was chosen as the intervention for a large clinical trial of individuals with PD concurrently treated with a dopaminergic agent. The study plan calls for approximately 1700 individuals to be followed for a minimum of 5 years. Subjects are randomized to receive creatine or placebo in combination with the best medical and surgical therapy available. The outcome measures were selected in an effort to assess a broad range of both motor and non-motor PD features. The measures of impairment assess complex motor function (ambulatory ability) and cognition. Ambulatory ability is assessed using five questions from the UPDRS, three from the ADL section (Part II, falls, freezing, and walking) and two from the motor section (Part III, gait and postural stability). Cognition is screened by the Symbol Digit Modality test [41], which requires the participant to match numbers with geometric figures. This task is administered orally. The two measures of function are the Schwab and England and the Modified Rankin scale. The Schwab and England scale was developed for PD and is widely used, as described earlier. It rates function from 0 to 100%, with anchor descriptions at 10% intervals. The Rankin scale [42] is widely used as a functional outcome (0–4 scale) primarily in stroke studies. Lastly, the PDQ-39 is used as a measure of health-related quality of life. It is a 39-item self-administered questionnaire that covers a broad array of domains, and is scored from 0 to 100. Secondary measures included in the study are the UPDRS Parts I–IV, SCOPA-COG, Beck Depression Inventory, health care utilization and EQ-5D.

The primary outcome consists of all five primary measures, equally weighted, because each is thought to measure an important aspect of PD. The method of analysis is a Global Statistical Test. This test essentially ranks all the participants on each scale and then calculates a mean rank across all five tests. The mean rank is then compared between the groups. A similar analysis was used in the NINDS *t*PA trial. This study design assesses the cumulative development of disability over the course of the illness that are most important to the patient and the treating physician and has the advantage of avoiding issues of mechanism.

Another approach to disease-modifying trials may be to use non-motor features not as outcome measures, but as inclusion criteria. Loss of olfactory discrimination, constipation, REM sleep behavior disorder, and depression have all been identified as single or combined signs of a state that may precede the classic motor features of PD. The pathology identified by Braak provides an insight into these possible early features. Some investigators have found that individuals with these signs and a family history of PD have an increased risk of dopamine transporter imaging abnormalities, suggestive of very early PD. A possible trial design would be to identify individuals with signs such as diminished olfaction, constipation, and dopamine transporter imaging abnormalities who do not have the motor features of PD, and to randomize them to potential disease-modifying agents. A relevant outcome would be the onset of motor signs and symptoms sufficient for a diagnosis of PD. In such a trial, non-motor features would play a role as some of the earliest features of PD, rather than as later features as they are used in the NET-PD trial.

Conclusion

Despite the high prevalence of non-motor symptoms across a range of PD severity, there is still a paucity of well-designed and validated instruments. Scales for cognition and mood are perhaps the most advanced. There is more limited experience with scales for psychosis in PD. Scales for autonomic dysfunction and sleep are even less well developed. There is a pressing need for standardization and validation of these instruments to assess the impact of treatments on these domains. Initial experience with scales not directed at specific domains of impairment (e.g., mood, cognition) but focused on disability and health-related quality-of-life can be responsive to treatment effects and have utility in clinical trials. The data collected to date suggest that non-motor symptoms contribute heavily to the worsening of health-related quality-of-life in PD patients. A major challenge for the near future is to define the natural rate of progression of these features and to develop reliable, validated instruments to assess these features that are generally accepted and used across multiple centers for evaluating the potential value of new study interventions. New long-term study designs which capture cumulative disability related to both motor and non-motor features are likely to be increasingly more widely employed.

References

1. Chaudhuri KR, Martinez-Martin P, Schapira AH, *et al.* International multicenter pilot study of the first comprehensive self-completed nonmotor symptoms questionnaire for Parkinson's disease: The NMSQuest study. *Mov Disord* 2006;**21**:916–23.
2. Langston JW. The Parkinson's complex: parkinsonism is just the tip of the iceberg. *Ann Neurol* 2006;**59**:591–6.
3. Dooneief G, Mirabello E, Bell K, *et al.* An estimate of the incidence of depression in idiopathic Parkinson's disease. *Arch Neurol* 1992;**49**:305–7.
4. Hely MA, Morris JGL, Reid WGJ, Trafficante R. Sydney multicenter study of Parkinson's disease: non-L-dopa-responsive problems dominate at 15 years. *Mov Disord* 2005;**20**(2): 190–199.

5. Martinez-Martin P, Schapira AHV, Stocchi F, *et al.* Prevalence of nonmotor symptoms in Parkinson's disease in an international setting; study using nonmotor symptoms questionnaire in 545 patients. *Mov Disord* 2007;**22**(11):1623–9.
6. Muslimovic D, Post B, Speelman JD, *et al.*, for the CARPA Study Group. Determinants of disability and quality of life in mild to moderate Parkinson disease. *Neurology* 2008;**70**: 2241–7.
7. Marras C, McDermott MP, Rochon PA, *et al.*, and the Parkinson Study Group DATATOP Investigators. Predictors of deterioration in health-related quality of life in Parkinson's disease: results from the DATATOP trial. *Mov Disord* 2008;**23**(5): 653–9.
8. Braak H and Del Tredici K. Invited article: nervous system pathology in sporadic Parkinson disease. *Neurology* 2008;**70**:1916–25.
9. Buter TC, van den Hout A, Matthews FE, *et al.* Dementia and survival in Parkinson disease. A 12-year population study. *Neurology* 2008;**70**:1017–22.
10. Marder K, Tang MX, Cote L, *et al.* The frequency and associated risk factors for dementia in patients with Parkinson's disease. *Arch Neurol* 1995;**52**:695–701.
11. de Lau LML, Schipper MA, Hofman A, *et al.* Prognosis of Parkinson disease. Risk of dementia and mortality: The Rotterdam Study. *Arch Neurol* 2005;**62**:1265–9.
12. Kieburtz K, McDermott M, Como P, *et al.* The effect of deprenyl and tocopherol on cognitive performance in early untreated Parkinson's disease. *Neurology* 1994;**44**:1756–9.
13. Emre M, Aarsland D, Albanese A, *et al.* Rivastigmine for dementia associated with Parkinson's disease. *N Engl J Med* 2004;**351**:2509–18.
14. Verbaan D, Marinus J, Visser M, *et al.* Cognitive impairment in Parkinson's disease. *J Neurol Neurosurg Psychiatry* 2007;**78**:1182–7.
15. Emre M, Aarsland D, Brown R, *et al.* Clinical diagnostic criteria for dementia associated with Parkinson's disease. *Mov Disord.* 2007;**22**:1689–707.
16. Dubois B, Burn D, Goetz C, *et al.* Movement Disorder Society Task Force: diagnostic procedures for Parkinson's disease dementia. *Mov Disord* 2007;**22**:2314–24.
17. Hamilton M. A rating scale for depression. *J Neurol Neurosurg Psychiatry* 1960;**23**:56–62.
18. Beck AT, Ward CH, Mendelson M, *et al.* An inventory for measuring depression. *Arch Gen Psychiatry* 1960;**4**:53–63.
19. Montgomery ST, Asberg M. A new depression scale designed to be sensitive to change. *Br J Psychiatry* 1979;**134**: 382–9.
20. Schrag A, Barone P, Brown RG, *et al.* Depression rating scales in Parkinson's disease: critique and recommendations. *Mov Disord* 2007;**22**(8):1077–92.
21. Devos D, Dujardin K, Poirot I, *et al.* Comparison of desipramine and citalopram treatments for depression in Parkinson's disease: a double-blind, randomized, placebo-controlled study. *Mov Disord* 2008;**23**(6):850–7.
22. Schrag A. Psychiatric aspects of Parkinson's disease. An update. *J Neurol* 2004;**251**:795–804.
23. Fernandez HH, Aarsland D, Fenelon G, *et al.* Task Force Report. Scales to assess psychosis in Parkinson's disease: critique and recommendations. *Mov Disord* 2008;**23**(4):484–500.
24. The Parkinson Study Group. Low-dose clozapine for the treatment of drug induced psychosis in Parkinson's disease. *N Engl J Med* 1999;**340**:747–63.
25. Verbaan D, Marinus J, Visser M, *et al.* Patient-reported autonomic symptoms in Parkinson disease. *Neurology* 2007;**69**: 333–41.
26. Buyssee DJ, Reynolds CF, Monk TH, *et al.* The Pittsburgh Sleep Quality Index: a new instrument for psychiatric practice and research. *Psychiatry Res* 1989;**28**:193–213.
27. Johns MW. A new method for measuring daytime sleepiness: The Epworth Sleepiness Scale. *Sleep* 1991;**14**(6):540–54.
28. Brodsky MA, Godbold J, Roth T, Olanow CW. Sleepiness in Parkinson's disease: a controlled study. *Mov Disord* 2003;**18**: 668–72.
29. Ondo WG, Fayle R, Atassi F, Jankovic J. Modafinil for daytime somnolence in Parkinson's disease: double blind, placebo controlled parallel trial. *J Neurol Neurosurg Psychiatry* 2005;**76**(12):1636–9.
30. Schwab RS, England AC Jr. Projection techniques for evaluating surgery in Parkinson's disease. In: *Third Symposium on Parkinson's Disease, Royal College of Surgeons in Edinburgh, May 20–22, 1968*. Edinburgh: Livingstone, 1969: 152–7 (153, Table 1).
31. Peto V, Jenkinson C, Fitzpatrick R, Greenhall R. The development and validation of a short measure of functioning and well being for individuals with Parkinson's disease. *Qual Life Res* 1995;**4**(3):241–8.
32. Welsch M, McDermott MP, Holloway RG, *et al.*, and The Parkinson Study Group. Development and testing of the Parkinson's disease quality of life scale. *Mov Disord* 2003;**18**(6): 637–45.
33. Schrag A, Selai C, Jahanshahi M, Quinn NP. The EQ-5D – a generic quality of life measure – is a useful instrument to measure quality of life in patients with Parkinson's disease. *J Neurol Neurosurg Psychiatry* 2000;**69**:67–73.
34. Ware JE Jr, Sherbourne CD. The MOS 36-item short-form health survey (SF-36). I. Conceptual framework and item selection. *Med Care* 1992;**30**(6):473–83.
35. Marinus J, Visser M, Martinez-Martin P, *et al.* A short psychosocial questionnaire for patients with Parkinson's disease: the SCOPA-PS. *J Clin Epidemiol* 2003;**56**:61–7.
36. Marras C, Lang A, Krahn M, *et al.*, and The Parkinson Study Group. Quality of life in early Parkinson's disease: impact of dyskinesias and motor fluctuations. *Mov Disord* 2004;**19**(1): 22–8.
37. Olanow CW, Kieburtz K, Stern M, *et al.*, for the US01 Study Team. Double-blind, placebo-controlled study of entacapone in levodopa-treated patients with stable Parkinson disease. *Arch Neurol* 2004;**61**:1563–8.
38. Waters CH, Kurth M, Bailey P, *et al.*, and the Tolcapone Stable Study Group. Tolcapone in stable Parkinson's disease: efficacy and safety of long-term treatment. *Neurology* 1998;**59**(5): 665–671.
39. Goetz CG, Fahn S, Martinez-Martin P, *et al.* Movement Disorder Society-sponsored revision of the Unified Parkinson Disease Rating Scale (MDS-UPDRS): process, format and clinimetric testing plan. *Mov Disord* 2007;**22**:41–7.
40. Goetz CG, Tilley BC, Shaftman SR, *et al.*, for the Movement Disorder Society UPDRS Revision Task Force. Movement

Disorder Society-sponsored revision of the Unified Parkinson's Disease Rating Scale (MDS-UPDRS): scale presentation and clinimetric testing results. *Mov Disord* 2008;**23**:2129–70.

41. Carter JH, Stewart BJ, Archbold PG, *et al.* Living with a person who has Parkinson's disease: the spouse's perspective by stage of disease. *Mov Disord* 1998;**13**(1):20–8.

42. Schrag A, Hovris A, Morley D, *et al.* Caregiver-burden in Parkinson's disease is closely associated with psychiatric symptoms, falls and disability. *Parkinsonism Relat Disord* 2006;**12**:35–41.

43. Schapira AHV, Olanow CW. Neuroprotection in Parkinson's disease: myths, mysteries, and misconceptions. *JAMA* 2004;**291**:358–34.

Chapter 12
Clinical Features of Dementia Associated with Parkinson's Disease and Dementia with Lewy Bodies

David J. Burn
Institute for Ageing and Health, Newcastle University, Newcastle upon Tyne, UK

Introduction

Dementia with Lewy bodies (LBD) and Parkinson's disease with dementia (PDD) are typically differentiated by the "1 year rule." Dementia that develops prior to the onset of PD symptoms, or within 1 year after diagnosis, is referred to as DLB, whereas dementia developing more than 1 year after the onset of PD features is diagnosed as PDD. In writing a chapter on the clinical features of dementia associated with PDD and DLB, one imagines a dog walking out at night in between two lamp-posts. The lamp-post on the left is most frequently visited by the Movement Disorder specialist, a vicious beast who fiercely guards his territory, while the post on the right is the domain of the Old Age Psychiatrist, a lean animal who has had to become increasingly streetwise in order to survive. Looking at the two near-identical lamp-posts, we ask ourselves, do these territories really matter? The answer is probably not. In a recent review on the subject, McKeith wrote: "Other than age of onset, temporal course, and possibly levodopa-responsiveness, no major differences between DLB and PDD have been found in any variable examined thus far, including cognitive profile, attentional performance, neuropsychiatric features, sleep disorder, autonomic dysfunction, type and severity of parkinsonism, neuroleptic sensitivity, and responsiveness to cholinesterase inhibitors" [1]. Indeed, it is not unreasonable to consider that they represent different spectra of the same disease.

Of course, patients with PDD are generally under the care of movement disorders specialists at the time their dementia develops, whereas patients with DLB are usually first referred to geriatric psychiatrists, often with suspected Alzheimer's disease (AD) as dementia frequently precedes the onset of parkinsonian features. Hence, despite the fact that the two conditions may be part of a single disorder, entry into the health care system frequently differs, and patient support organizations add another element of "identity" to the disorders. Unambiguous diagnostic labels are clearly important. This chapter will concentrate on PDD and DLB as two very similar conditions and part of a disease spectrum. It will consider the clinical features that typify these dementias. Where differences exist, or study data are only available for one or the other diagnosis, this will be specified.

The interface between PDD and DLB

PDD refers to dementia developing in the context of established PD. For DLB, dementia is frequently (but not invariably) the first feature to develop and parkinsonism usually develops (but not always) at a later stage. The clinical interface between the two is arbitrary and the infamous "1 year rule" is frequently invoked for an operational definition [2]. This "rule" states that if extrapyramidal motor features have been present for 12 months or more before the onset of dementia, the diagnosis should be PDD, but if dementia precedes the motor features or occurs within 12 months of the onset of the motor features, the diagnosis should be DLB. This polarization based upon the temporal evolution of clinical features is reasonable in one sense, but ignores the fact that biology does not work in "straight lines" or "cut-offs" and there is no reason to think that dementia that begins 11 months after the onset of motor features is different to the dementia that begins after a latency of 13 months. Most clinicians and researchers therefore regard PDD and DLB as a continuum on a spectrum of disorders characterized by neuronal loss, Lewy-related pathology and synuclein deposition [3]. A useful unifying term for the dementia associated with PD and DLB is "Lewy body dementia."

Parkinson's Disease: Non-Motor and Non-Dopaminergic Features, First Edition. Edited by C. Warren Olanow, Fabrizio Stocchi, and Anthony E. Lang.

Unfortunately, "DLB" and "Lewy body dementia" are frequently interchanged, leading to further confusion.

Descriptive epidemiology

Prevalence estimates for DLB, depending on case criteria, range from 0 to 5% with regard to the general population, and from 0 to 30.5% of all dementia cases [4]. The only estimate for DLB incidence is 0.1% per year for the general population and 3.2% per year for all new dementia cases [4].

Cognitive deficits are evident even in early PD. Depending upon the neuropsychologic tests used and the criteria applied, impairments have been reported in 24–36% of newly diagnosed PD cases [5,6]. People with PD have an increased risk of full-blown dementia of up to six times that of age-matched controls [7]. In a systematic review of prevalence studies of PDD, 24–31% of PD patients have dementia and 3–4% of dementia burden in the population is due to PDD [8]. The prevalence of PDD in the general population aged over 65 years has been estimated as 0.2–0.5%. Studies providing data for dementia incidence in PD have yielded figures of between 30 and 112 per 1000 person-years [9].

A majority of people with PD will develop dementia if followed up for long enough. The cumulative incidence of dementia steadily increases with age and duration of PD and, conditional on survival, increases to 80–90% by age 90 years [10]. At 20 years of follow-up in a cohort of patients recruited in Sydney, Australia, 100 of 136 (74%) had died, and 83% of the surviving patients were demented [11]. This high cumulative incidence was also suggested by a clinicopathologic study in which 80% of PD cases had been reported with dementia antemortem [12].

Predicting dementia in PD

Current age, rather than age at onset, is the most important determinant of dementia risk in PD [13]. Increasing motor disability is also predictive of dementia and is synergistic with current age [14]. Non-demented PD patients with a "postural instability–gait difficulty" motor phenotype show more rapid cognitive decline [15] and this phenotype is associated with a fourfold increased risk of dementia [9]. One may speculate that these observations relate to increasing cholinergic neuronal loss and/or dysfunction, particularly within the pedunculopontine nucleus, "modulating" the clinical phenotype and simultaneously producing a range of non-motor problems, including cognitive impairment.

Longer disease duration and male gender have also been associated with increased risk of PDD. Less well-established risk factors include low educational attainment, depression, excessive daytime somnolence, REM sleep behavior disorder, and orthostatic hypotension (OH). A recent study suggested that cerebrovascular risk factors may not be associated with incident dementia in PD [16]. This finding is somewhat counterintuitive and, despite this, cigarette smoking prior to disease onset has been associated with worse cognitive function in PD [17]. Dementia *may* be associated with weight loss in PD, together with worsening of parkinsonism, age at diagnosis, and emergence of visual hallucinations, but the predictive value of antecedent weight loss is not known.

Regarding drug effects, anti-cholinergic agents may be a risk factor for PDD, and prolonged use of these agents has been associated with an increased frequency of cortical plaques and tangles in non-demented PD patients [18]. This is biologically plausible since muscarinic M1 receptors have been linked with amyloid precursor protein secretion. Poor response to L-dopa and hallucinations on dopaminergic treatment also predict dementia, while there is limited evidence from an observational study that amantadine may delay and attenuate dementia [19]. L-Dopa-induced elevation in plasma homocysteine levels could contribute towards cognitive failure, although this has not been confirmed in prospective studies. Visual hallucinations in PD predict more rapid cognitive deterioration [20].

Psychosis requiring anti-psychotic therapy has been associated with development and progression of dementia, while the use of atypical anti-psychotics may have adverse effects upon disease progression. Deficits in auditory verbal learning and non-verbal reasoning, picture completion, Stroop interference, and verbal fluency have all been independently associated with an increased risk of cognitive failure in PD. Two simple bedside tests, pentagon copying and semantic fluency, may also be predictive of cognitive decline and dementia. There is an association between apathy and cognitive dysfunction, particularly executive impairment, but it is unknown whether apathy is independently predictive of dementia.

Cognitive features

The neuropsychologic profile of PDD is covered in detail in Chapter 13, so this aspect will therefore be covered only briefly here. Suffice it to say that the dementia syndrome associated with PD is clinically heterogeneous, presumably reflecting a variable underlying pathologic and neurochemical substrate. Executive deficits are, however, common and typical of PDD [6]. These deficits may be "subclinical" from an early stage in the disease process and only revealed by formal neuropsychologic testing. Subsequently, they become more disruptive, may be associated with "word finding" problems, and begin to impact upon activities of daily living. Impairment in tasks requiring initiation, planning, concept formation, rule finding, set shifting, or set maintenance, together with impaired mental processing speed (bradyphrenia), constitutes executive dysfunction. Such an apparent lack of mental flexibility, inability to multitask or complete simple or previously familiar tasks, and mental slowness are frustrating to both patients and carers, yet may be overlooked by the unwary physician and not captured by performing a Mini-Mental State Examination (MMSE). The dysexecutive syndrome of PDD may be so severe as to dominate neuropsychologic testing at this stage, making the interpretation of other tests difficult (for example, by impacting upon memory retrieval strategies and the patient's approach to pentagon copying) [21]. Notwithstanding the executive impairment, memory and visuoperceptual deficits also typify many cases of PDD [22]. Memory problems may arise via disturbance of retrieval rather than storage (in contrast with AD), although not all studies have confirmed this distinction. In the former case, the memory deficit is classically improved by cueing. Impairment in spontaneous and focused attention and poor performance on attentional tasks constitute another typical component in the dementia syndrome associated with PD. This may be recognized clinically by brief or more prolonged "absences," with the patient staring into space, or appearing to become distracted. Attentional performance may fluctuate during the day and from day to day, leading to frustratingly variable levels of function and a significant impact upon activities of daily living [23,24].

Less commonly, the pattern of dementia in PD is similar to that encountered in AD. The exact frequency of such a phenotype has not been established, although in an incident community-based PD cohort, 8% of cases had deficits on a pattern recognition task at first assessment, believed to be sensitive to temporal lobe dysfunction [5]. It may be speculated that this clinical phenotype is determined by a greater burden of Alzheimer-type pathology in the medial temporal lobe. In a study of PD to characterize dementia and its relationship to visual hallucinations, this "AD" dementia phenotype was encountered in only 5% of prevalent PDD cases [25].

Regarding DLB, the cognitive profile is also typified by marked impairments in visuospatial, attentional, and executive function, with relative sparing of memory in comparison with AD [26]. Several studies have compared the cognitive profiles of DLB and PDD. No significant differences were found, although DLB cases may have greater executive dysfunction [27]. When assessed using the Mattis Dementia Rating Scale, 56 and 55% of patients with PDD and DLB, respectively, were classified as having a so-called "subcortical" cognitive profile compared with only 33% of patients with AD [28]. Conversely, 30% of patients with PDD and 26% of those with DLB had a "cortical" profile.

In summary, both PDD and DLB are typified by a dysexecutive–visuoperceptual dementia syndrome, although there may be heterogeneity. There is no significant difference in the dementia profile between the two Lewy body dementias, and where differences exist they are more likely to represent temporal effects rather than fundamental biological differences.

Neuropsychiatric features

Neuropsychiatric disturbances are extremely common in PDD and DLB. In a study of 537 PDD patients, 89% presented with at least one neuropsychiatric symptom when assessed using the Neuropsychiatric Inventory, and 77% had two or more symptoms [29]. Hallucinations occur in 45–65% of PDD patients and 60–70% of DLB patients, considerably more commonly than in AD (where typically fewer than 10% are affected). One study has suggested that the frequency of visual hallucinations in PDD may be as high as 87% [25], although this requires confirmation. Visual hallucinations in the Lewy body dementias are at least twice as frequent as auditory hallucinations, the majority being complex formed hallucinations. The characteristics of recurrent visual hallucinations are similar in PDD and DLB, with phenomenology suggesting involvement of dorsal and ventral visual pathways in their generation [30]. Tactile hallucinations are uncommon. Visual hallucinations, which are commonly preceded by illusionary phenomena (that is, the misinterpretation of visual stimuli) may be simple and ill-defined – a feeling that someone is behind the patient ("presence"), or that someone has passed across their visual field ("passage"). Subsequently, the hallucinations become more formed and detailed, often in color, static, and centrally located. Both anonymous people and family members (living or dead) are common, as are animals. As insight is lost, delusional misinterpretation of the hallucinations may occur. Delusions have a frequency in PDD of 25–30% and 55–70% in DLB [27]. Paranoid ideation, such as spousal infidelity and "phantom boarder" (believing strangers are living in the house) are common themes. Capras syndrome, characterized by a delusional belief that a person has been replaced by an imposter, is also common in the Lewy body dementias, and frequently accompanied by visual hallucinations [31]. In a prospective study of 30 PDD cases, delusional misinterpretation was found in 16.7% of patients [32]. In common with the previous study, all of these cases also experienced visual hallucinations that were significantly more severe than in PDD cases without delusional misinterpretation. There is some evidence that PDD patients with Capras and related syndromes have more severe memory and language deficits, possibly implicating greater temporal lobe involvement [32].

The frequency of major depression in PDD has been found to be 13%, compared with 9% for non-demented PD patients [33]. Major depression occurs in 19% of DLB cases at presentation, with nearly 50% of patients experiencing depressive symptoms at some stage of their illness [34]. Both severity of depressed mood and prevalence of major depression may be higher in PDD and DLB than in AD. Anxiety is also common in the Lewy body dementias (30–50%) and tends to cluster with depressed mood. Irritability and aggression, common in AD, are not prominent features in PDD or DLB. Apathy affects over 50% of people with PDD, and in 70% this may be severe [29]. This contrasts with a previously reported frequency of 17% for non-demented PD. Demented PD patients are significantly more likely to underestimate their apathy compared with non-demented cases, so an informant assessment is important [35].

Motor, sleep, and other neurologic features

Given the predisposition of patients with a "postural instability–gait disorder" phenotype to go on and develop dementia in PD, it is not surprising that this phenotype is over-represented in PDD and DLB compared with more standard forms of PD [36]. Although parkinsonism is common in DLB, it is not invariable, occurring in 70–92% of cases during the disease course [37,38]. Although some reports have suggested reduced L-dopa responsiveness in PDD patients, this has not been formally established, particularly after controlling for confounders such as subcortical small vessel disease. No significant difference in mean improvement on UPDRS motor score to a single-dose 200 mg L-dopa challenge was recorded in one study, although more non-demented patients experienced greater than 20% improvement compared with those with PDD (90% versus 65%) [39]. Another study included patients with DLB, PD, and PDD and failed to detect differences in L-dopa responsiveness between PD and PDD groups [40]. Approximately one-third of the DLB patients were found to respond to L-dopa, and these tended to be younger than the non-responders. The use of L-dopa did not appear to have adverse cognitive or neuropsychiatric effects in the DLB cases over 3 months of follow-up [41]. There are insufficient data to infer differences in the occurrence of L-dopa-induced motor complications in PDD and DLB patients compared with PD, but they might be expected to be less as PDD patients tend to be older.

Falls are common in the Lewy body dementias and are likely to be multi-factorial in nature, resulting from not only cognitive and neuropsychiatric factors, but also motor and autonomic impairments. Over one-third of DLB patients suffer more than 20 falls per year [42]. The risk of gait and balance disorder is higher in non-Alzheimer's dementia [vascular dementia (VaD), PDD, and DLB] than in an AD (odds ratio = 15, 95% confidence interval 6–37) [43]. Moreover, if a gait disorder is present in mild dementia, this may be diagnostic of non-Alzheimer's dementia, with sensitivity of 78% and specificity of 100%.

Electro-oculography has demonstrated that PDD and DLB patients have impairment in both reflexive and complex saccades, compared with AD patients who show deficits only in complex saccades, although such distinctions cannot be made on bedside testing [44]. Using the Epworth Sleepiness Scale, 57% of PDD, 50% of DLB, and 41% of PD subjects were classified as having excessive daytime somnolence, compared with only 18% of AD patients and 10% of controls [45]. Furthermore, sleep quality was poorer in PDD, PD, and DLB patients compared with AD and normal controls.

Rapid eye movement (REM) sleep behavior disorder (RBD), a common sleep disturbance in neurodegenerative disorders, is characterized by loss of normal skeletal muscle atonia during REM sleep with resultant motor activity and "acting out of dreams" [46]. Behaviors range from verbal outbursts to pugilistic movements and even more dramatic motor activity. Injuries to bed partners and the patients themselves are common. Estimates from specialist centers place the frequency of RBD in DLB at 50–80% [47]. Prospective population-based studies are needed to assess the true incidence and prevalence of RBD in DLB. A recent cross-sectional study of 65 PD patients using the Mayo Sleep Questionnaire for RBD determined that 24 met the criteria for a clinical diagnosis of RBD. Of the 24 patients with RBD, 10 (42%) also met Diagnostic and Statistical Manual (4th edition) (DSM-IV) criteria for PDD. The frequency of RBD was significantly higher in the PDD group (77%) compared with the non-demented PD cases (27%) [48]. Cognitive impairment in non-demented PD patients may also be closely related to the presence of RBD [49]. Patients with PD and concomitant RBD show significantly poorer performance on standardized tests measuring episodic verbal memory, executive functions, and visuospatial and visuoperceptual processing as compared with PD patients without RBD and control subjects. Although suggestive, therefore, prospective studies are required to confirm whether the occurrence of RBD in PD is an independent risk factor for incident dementia. A higher frequency of symptomatic orthostasis has been reported in association with cognitive impairment in PD [50]. In a cross-sectional study of cardiovascular autonomic function in PDD, DLB, AD, and VaD, compared with elderly controls, significant differences were found in severity of cardiovascular autonomic dysfunction between the four dementias [51]. PDD and DLB groups had considerable impairment, whereas the VaD group showed limited evidence of autonomic dysfunction and in AD, apart from orthostatic hypotension, autonomic function was relatively normal. The PDD patients showed consistent impairment of both parasympathetic and sympathetic function tests in comparison with controls and AD. Moreover, higher autonomic symptom scores in PDD are associated with poorer outcomes in all measures of physical activity, activities of daily living, depression, and quality-of-life [52].

Urologic symptoms and urodynamic abnormalities are very common in DLB and result not only from dementia and immobility but also from central and peripheral somato-autonomic dysfunction [53]. Urgency and urge incontinence, suggesting detrusor overactivity, are more frequent in DLB cases compared with AD, with up to 90% of DLB patients being affected [54]. This may relate to greater subcortical pathology in DLB, leading to disinhibition of pontine micturition centers. In common with PD, anosmia is frequent in DLB [55]. Adding anosmia as a core feature to diagnostic criteria improved sensitivity for detecting DLB, but did not improve discrimination between AD and DLB owing to a concomitant increase in false positives.

Diagnosis of PDD and DLB

Usually, when dementia develops in the context of well-established PD, there is no doubt about the diagnosis. In certain situations, for example a new referral where the temporal sequence of events is unclear, there is significant co-morbid illness, or when the clinical course is atypical (e.g., a rapid onset of confusion), the differential may include DLB (since a distinction is usually expected in the clinic), vascular parkinsonism, AD with or without drug-induced parkinsonism, delirium, and depressive pseudodementia or other coincidental causes of dementia. Many of these conditions are excluded by taking a careful collateral history, blood tests, structural (e.g., computed tomography) and functional (e.g., dopamine transporter) imaging. In one recent clinicopathologic study, features that distinguished PDD from AD included cognitive fluctuations, but also several neuropsychiatric features, including visual and auditory hallucinations, depression, and sleep disturbance [12]. Mild depression or dysthymia has little, if any, impact on cognition in PD, whereas significant depression appears to impair executive functions and memory [56].

Diagnostic criteria for PDD

Until recently, there were no disease-specific diagnostic criteria for PDD. As mentioned above, reliance upon a single MMSE score less than the traditional value of 24 out of 30 is insensitive because this instrument is heavily biased towards mnemonic deficits and does not include robust measures of executive function. Hence PD patients may still be demented with scores above this cut-off. Furthermore, as described above, variability in spontaneous and focused attention may mean that at the time of assessment, "spuriously" high or low scores may be obtained that are not representative of day-to-day impairment. DSM-IV criteria subsume PDD under "dementia due to other medical conditions," and the section fails to capture the spectrum of cognitive and neuropsychiatric problems associated with this disorder.

New diagnostic criteria for PDD, produced by a Task Force commissioned by the Movement Disorder Society, have recently been proposed [21] (Boxes 12.1 and 12.2). These criteria were developed through a comprehensive literature review in which the characteristic cognitive, behavioral, motor and other features of PDD were defined. On the basis of this review, four groups of features were derived (Box 12.1). Two levels of certainty (probable or possible PDD) were then suggested, based upon the presence and/or absence of these features (Box 12.2). The diagnosis of PD, according to Queen Square Brain Bank criteria, before the development of dementia symptoms is an essential first step in the process. The diagnosis of dementia must be based on the presence of deficits in two or more of the four core cognitive domains (attention, memory, executive, and visuospatial functions) and should be severe enough to impact upon normal daily activities, independent of the influence of motor and other impairments. Neuropsychiatric and behavioral symptoms are frequent in PDD, but are not invariable, and this is reflected in the criteria.

In a second paper, also commissioned by the Movement Disorder Society, practical guidelines were provided as to how the diagnostic criteria might be operationalized [57]. These guidelines offer two diagnostic levels, depending upon the clinical scenario and the expertise of the evaluator. The level I assessment is aimed primarily at the clinician with no particular expertise in neuropsychologic methods, but who requires a simple, pragmatic set of tests that are not excessively time consuming (Box 12.3). Thus, in addition to a clinical history and caregiver account, the MMSE [58], supplemented by a clock drawing test and the four-item Neuropsychiatric Inventory [59], are sufficient to complete a level I assessment. Fluctuating attention, which, as described above, is a dominant factor in determining disability in PDD, is examined by asking the patient to give the months of the year backwards, starting from December, or by repeatedly subtracting 7, starting at 100. It remains to be determined whether these tests are sufficiently sensitive to detect this feature, or whether additional instruments such as the "Ferman four-item test," which has been shown to be highly sensitive for discriminating DLB from AD, may also be necessary [60].

Box 12.1 Features of dementia associated with Parkinson's disease [21]

I. Core features

1) Diagnosis of PD according to Queen Square Brain Bank criteria
2) A dementia syndrome with insidious onset and slow progression, developing within the context of established PD and diagnosed by history, clinical and mental examination, defined as:
   - Impairment in more than one cognitive domain
   - Representing a decline from pre-morbid level
   - Deficits severe enough to impair daily life (social, occupational or personal care), independent of the impairment ascribable to motor or autonomic symptoms

II. Associated clinical features

1) **Cognitive features:**
   - Attention: Impaired. Impairment in spontaneous and focused attention, poor performance in attentional tasks; performance may fluctuate during the day and from day to day
   - Executive functions: Impaired. Impairment in tasks requiring initiation, planning, concept formation, rule finding, set shifting or set maintenance; impaired mental speed (bradyphrenia)
   - Visuospatial functions: Impaired. Impairment in tasks requiring visual-spatial orientation, perception or construction
   - Memory: Impaired. Impairment in free recall of recent events or in tasks requiring learning new material, memory usually improves with cueing, recognition is usually better than free recall
   - Language: Core functions largely preserved. Word finding difficulties and impaired comprehension of complex sentences may be present
2) **Behavioral features:**
   - Apathy: decreased spontaneity; loss of motivation, interest and effortful behavior
   - Changes in personality and mood including depressive features and anxiety
   - Hallucinations: mostly visual, usually complex, formed visions of people, animals or objects
   - Delusions: usually paranoid, such as infidelity, or phantom boarder (unwelcome guests living in the home) delusions
   - Excessive daytime sleepiness

III. Features which do not exclude PD-D, but make the diagnosis uncertain

1) Co-existence of any other abnormality, which may by itself cause cognitive impairment, but judged not to be the cause of dementia. e.g., presence of relevant vascular disease in imaging
2) Time interval between the development of motor and cognitive symptoms not known

IV. Features suggesting other diseases as cause of mental impairment, which when present make it impossible to diagnose PD-D reliably

1) Cognitive and behavioral symptoms appearing *solely* in the context of other conditions such as acute confusion due to:
   - systemic diseases or abnormalities
   - drug intoxication
   - major depression according to DSM IV
2) Features compatible with "probable vascular dementia" criteria according to NINDS-AIREN (dementia in the context of cerebrovascular disease as indicated by focal signs in neurologic examination such as hemiparesis, sensory deficits, and evidence of relevant cerebrovascular disease by brain imaging *and* a relationship between the two as indicated by the presence of one or more of the following: onset of dementia within 3 months after a recognized stroke, abrupt deterioration in cognitive functions, and fluctuating, stepwise progression of cognitive deficits)

The four questions in the Ferman instrument are administered to the caregiver and comprise: Does the patient experience excessive daytime sleepiness? Does the patient sleep for more than 2 hours during the day? Are there times when his/her words occasionally come out jumbled up? Does the patient sometimes stare into space for periods of time? Informant endorsement of three out of four of these items has been shown to have a positive predictive value of 83% for diagnosis of DLB versus AD [60], but the sensitivity of the instrument in detecting fluctuating attention in PDD is not yet known.

The level I assessment can be used alone or in combination with level II, which is better suited to the case when there is the need to specify the pattern and the severity of dementia associated with PD [57]. The level II assessment is appropriate for detailed clinical monitoring, research

Box 12.2 Criteria for the diagnosis of probable and possible PD-D [21]

Probable PDD

A Core features: both must be present

B Associated clinical features:
Typical profile of cognitive deficits including impairment in at least two of the four core cognitive domains (impaired attention which may fluctuate, impaired executive functions, impairment in visuospatial functions and impaired free recall memory which usually improves with cueing).
The presence of at least one behavioral symptom (apathy, depressed or anxious mood, hallucinations, delusions, excessive daytime sleepiness) supports the diagnosis of Probable PDD; the lack of behavioral symptoms, however, does not exclude the diagnosis

C None of the group III criteria present

D None of the group IV criteria present

Possible PDD

A Core features: both must be present

B Associated clinical features:
Atypical profile of cognitive impairment in one or more domains, such as prominent or receptive-type (fluent) aphasia, or pure storage-failure type amnesia (memory does not improve with cueing or in recognition tasks) with preserved attention.
Behavioral symptoms may or may not be present
OR

C One or more of the group III criteria present

D None of the group IV criteria present

Box 12.3 Guidelines for diagnosis of PDD at level I [57]

1 A diagnosis of PD based on the Queen's Square Brain Bank criteria

2 PD developed prior to the onset of dementia

3 MMSE score below 26

4 Cognitive deficits severe enough to impact upon daily living (elicited via caregiver interview or "Pill Questionnaire"[a])

5 Impairment in at least two of the following cognitive domains:
- months reversed or subtract seven backwards
- lexical fluency or clock drawing
- MMSE pentagons
- MMSE three-word recall
- The presence of one of the following behavioral symptoms: apathy or depressed mood or delusions or excessive daytime sleepiness supports the diagnosis of probable PDD[b]
- The presence of major depression or delirium or any other abnormality which may by itself cause significant cognitive impairment makes the diagnosis uncertain[c]

[a] This item, described in an Appendix in reference 50, requires validation. In brief, the patient is asked to describe verbally their treatment and its time schedule. Even if the patient does not manage their own treatment, it is suggested that they have lost at least a part of their autonomy if they can no longer describe their treatment. The criterion of impairment is met if the patient is no longer able to explain their daily PD medication, or if errors are made that are considered clinically significant.
[b] These can be assessed with the four-item Neuropsychiatric Inventory [52], which includes hallucinations, depression, delusions, and apathy. A cut-off score of ≥3 for each item is proposed. Excessive daytime sleepiness may be assessed by specific questions.
[c] Should be absent to permit diagnosis of "Probable" PDD.

studies, or pharmacologic trials. It requires neuropsychologic expertise and is much more time consuming than level I assessment.

Both the diagnostic criteria and the accompanying diagnostic procedures need to be validated in carefully conducted, prospective studies, preferably with pathologic confirmation of diagnosis. It is almost inevitable that they will require refinement, but at least represent a solid attempt at deriving "disease-specific" criteria for defining the dementia syndrome associated with PD, with practical suggestions for their application in routine clinical use.

Diagnostic criteria for DLB

Consensus clinical diagnostic criteria were first published in 1996 and were updated in 1999 and, most recently, in 2005 (Box 12.4). The central feature of DLB is characterized as a progressive dementia in which episodic memory impairment is often minimal in the early stages, whereas attentional, executive, and visuospatial deficits may be disproportionately prominent [2,61,62]. The presence of two or more of three core clinical features (fluctuating attention and alertness, recurrent visual hallucinations, parkinsonism), together with the variable presence of suggestive or supportive features, indicates probable DLB. This, of course, means that the presence of parkinsonism is not necessary for the diagnosis of DLB. In addition, the criteria refer to "spontaneous features" of parkinsonism to differentiate drug-induced (most commonly the use of neuroleptics) from degenerative parkinsonism.

Box 12.4 Revised criteria for the clinical diagnosis of DLB [2]

1 *Central feature (essential for a diagnosis of possible or probable DLB)*
Dementia defined as progressive cognitive decline of sufficient magnitude to interfere with normal social or occupational function. Prominent or persistent memory impairment may not necessarily occur in the early stages but is usually evident with progression. Deficits on tests of attention, executive function, and visuospatial ability may be especially prominent.

2 *Core features (two core features are sufficient for a diagnosis of probable DLB, one for possible DLB)*
Fluctuating cognition with pronounced variations in attention and alertness
Recurrent visual hallucinations that are typically well formed and detailed
Spontaneous features of parkinsonism

3 *Suggestive features (if one or more of these is present in the presence of one or more core features, a diagnosis of probable DLB can be made. In the absence of any core features, one or more suggestive features is sufficient for possible DLB. Probable DLB should not be diagnosed on the basis of suggestive features alone)*
REM sleep behavior disorder
Severe neuroleptic sensitivity
Low dopamine transporter uptake in basal ganglia demonstrated by SPECT or PET imaging

4 *Supportive features (commonly present but not proven to have diagnostic specificity)*
Repeated falls and syncope
Transient, unexplained loss of consciousness
Severe autonomic dysfunction, e.g., orthostatic hypotension, urinary incontinence
Hallucinations in other modalities
Systematized delusions
Depression
Relative preservation of medial temporal lobe structures on CT/MRI scan
Generalized low uptake on SPECT/PET perfusion scan with reduced occipital activity
Abnormal (low uptake) MIBG myocardial scintigraphy
Prominent slow wave activity on EEG with temporal lobe transient sharp waves

5 *A diagnosis of DLB is less likely*
In the presence of cerebrovascular disease evident as focal neurologic signs or on brain imaging
In the presence of any other physical illness or brain disorder sufficient to account in part or in total for the clinical picture
If parkinsonism only appears for the first time at a stage of severe dementia

6 *Temporal sequence of symptoms*
DLB should be diagnosed when dementia occurs before or concurrently with parkinsonism (if it is present). The term Parkinson's disease dementia (PDD) should be used to describe dementia that occurs in the context of well-established parkinsonian disease. In a practice setting, the term that is most appropriate to the clinical situation should be used and generic terms such as LB disease are often helpful. In research studies in which a distinction needs to be made between DLB and PDD, the existing 1 year rule between the onset of dementia and parkinsonism DLB continues to be recommended. Adoption of other time periods will simply confound data pooling or comparison between studies. In other research settings that may include clinicopathologic studies and clinical trials, both clinical phenotypes may be considered collectively under categories such as LB disease or α-synucleinopathy.

"Suggestive features" now included in the criteria are RBD, severe neuroleptic sensitivity, and abnormal dopamine uptake on single photon emission computed tomography (SPECT) or positron emission tomography (PET) imaging. These have a similar diagnostic weighting as the core features but require further validation before being considered sufficient for a diagnosis of probable DLB without the presence of core features. Features listed in Box 12.4 and considered as supportive of a diagnosis of DLB lack specificity because they may also occur in a variety of other disorders.

When DLB presents as a primary dementia syndrome, the main differential diagnoses are AD, VaD, delirium secondary to systemic or pharmacologic toxicity, prion disease, or other neurodegenerative syndromes. When applied correctly, consensus guidelines for the clinical diagnosis of DLB have prospective diagnostic accuracy at least as good as those for AD. One of the main reasons for reduced sensitivity in the diagnosis of DLB is the failure to enquire about, or elicit, fluctuations in attention. The discriminating value of the diagnostic criteria is greatest in the early stages, suggesting that DLB should be considered in any new dementia presentation [63]. The inability of moderately impaired DLB patients to copy pentagons accurately has been reported to have a sensitivity of 88% and a specificity of 59% compared with AD, suggesting this as a useful screening test [64]. The best model for differentiating DLB from AD in the earliest disease stages may include visual hallucinations and visuospatial/constructional dysfunction, but not spontaneous extrapyramidal signs, as predictors [65].

The degree of concomitant Alzheimer tangle pathology has a major influence upon diagnostic accuracy for DLB. Thus, the greater the "Alzheimerization" of the DLB case, the less likely it is that the final clinical diagnosis will be correct [66]. In DLB patients with a low neurofibrillary tangle burden, visual hallucinations occurred in 65% of cases, compared with only 33% of those cases with high tangle counts in one study [66]. Not surprisingly, diagnostic accuracy was therefore greater in the low tangle burden cases (75%) compared with high neurofibrillary tangle load cases (39%).

Natural history and determinants of prognosis

Overall, women live with PD longer than men and spend more years with dementia [10]. In a recent register-based study of 10 347 PD subjects with a mean age of 77 years receiving dopaminergic agents, 35% had required an antipsychotic drug by 7 years into their disease [67]. In turn, psychosis (and visual hallucinations in particular) frequently progresses to dementia over a 2 year period [68]. Using data from a population-based study in Norway and 12 years of follow-up, progression from PD to PDD and death has been modeled, using a three-state irreversible Markov model [10]. From this model, for example, it may be predicted that at age 70 years, a man with PD but no dementia has a life expectancy of 8 years, of which 5 years would be expected to be dementia free and 3 years would be expected to be with dementia. A mean annual rate of decline of 2.3 MMSE points has been reported for PDD once it has developed [69]. Visual hallucinations in PDD predict more rapid cognitive deterioration [20].

Rate of progression for DLB, as evidenced by change in global cognitive measures such as the MMSE or Cambridge Cognitive Examination (CAMCOG), is equivalent to or faster than that seen in AD and VaD, with a decline of 4–5 MMSE points per year [70–72]. The neuropsychologic changes as DLB progresses are not well characterized, although differences from AD are more pronounced in the early stages and lessen as the dementia progresses.

A retrospective study of 243 autopsy-confirmed Lewy body (predominantly DLB) dementia cases found a median survival of 5 years from symptom onset [73]. Older age at disease onset, fluctuating cognition, and visual hallucinations predicted shorter survival. Interestingly, after adjusting for the presence of age, gender, and Alzheimer-type pathology, fluctuating cognition at symptom onset was identified as the best predictor of a poor outcome.

Future directions

The Lewy body dementias represent a vigorous research area at present, particularly as we strive to discover better symptomatic treatments and, ultimately, disease-modifying strategies. There is more work to be done to validate clinical diagnostic criteria for PDD, preferably through longitudinal clinicopathologic studies. Such studies will also help to determine the pathologic and neurochemical basis for phenotypic variability in PDD and DLB. The development of functional imaging techniques utilizing ligands such as PIB which binds β-amyloid with high affinity, also offers the possibility of determining *in vivo* the correlates of clinical features with the burden and topography of pathologic protein aggregation. Fluctuating attention, which is such a key symptom in determining the patient's ability to perform activities of daily living, yet which is often overlooked in the clinical assessment, requires further study, especially in validating simple clinical instruments for its detection. Although current age is probably a dominant factor in determining risk for dementia in PD, it should be possible to derive better predictive models for this complication, thus identifying patient groups at high risk and suitable for putative dementia-modifying approaches at an early stage.

Conclusion

Both PDD and DLB have come to the attention of the medical community in recent years. With regard to PDD, the frequency of dementia in PD is far higher than was previously imagined. In part, this relates to the secular trend for an increasingly aged society, but also the fact that dementia is now being systematically considered in the context of PD and not being dismissed as "co-existing AD." For DLB, the main battleground has been differentiating the syndrome from AD, and it is now accepted that there are major clinical differences, largely dependent upon underlying α-synuclein pathology and strategic cell loss. Furthermore, as the worlds of the geriatric psychiatrist and neurologist have collided, the clinical similarities between the two Lewy body dementias have become apparent. It is no longer helpful to defend jealously our respective lampposts, as collaborative working and patient management will pay far greater dividends. It is therefore time to share the same kennel!

References

1. McKeith I. Dementia with Lewy bodies and Parkinson's disease with dementia: where two worlds collide. *Pract. Neurol.* 2007;**7**:374–82.
2. McKeith I, Dickson D, Lowe J, *et al.* Diagnosis and management of dementia with Lewy bodies: third report of the DLB Consortium. *Neurology* 2005;**65**:1863–72.
3. Lippa CF, Duda JE, Grossman M, *et al.* DLB and PDD boundary issues: diagnosis, treatment, molecular pathology and biomarkers. *Neurology* 2007;**68**:812–9.
4. Zaccai J, McCracken C, Brayne C. A systematic review of prevalence and incidence studies of dementia with Lewy bodies. *Age Ageing* 2005;**34**:561–6.
5. Foltynie T, Brayne CEG, Robbins TW, Barker RA. The cognitive ability of an incident cohort of Parkinson's disease patients in the UK. The CamPaIGN study. *Brain* 2004;**127**:550–60.
6. Muslimovic D. Post B, Speelman JD, Schmand B. Cognitive profile of patients with newly diagnosed Parkinson disease. *Neurology* 2005:**65**:1239–45.
7. Hobson P, Meara J. Risk and incidence of dementia in a cohort of older subjects with Parkinson's disease in the United Kingdom. *Mov Disord* 2004;**19**:1043–9.
8. Aarsland D, Zaccai J, Brayne C. A systematic review of prevalence studies of dementia in Parkinson's disease. *Mov Disord* 2005;**10**:1255–63.
9. Williams-Gray CH, Foltynie T, Brayne CEG, *et al.* Evolution of cognitive dysfunction in an incident Parkinson's disease cohort. *Brain* 2007;**130**:1787–98.
10. Buter TC, van den Hout A, Matthews FE, *et al.* Dementia and survival in Parkinson disease: a 12-year population study. *Neurology* 2008;**70**:1017–22.
11. Hely MA, Reid WG, Adena MA, *et al.* The Sydney multicenter study of Parkinson's disease: the inevitability of dementia at 20 years. *Mov Disord* 2008;**23**:837–44.
12. Galvin JE, Pollack J, Morris JC. Clinical phenotype of Parkinson disease dementia. *Neurology* 2006;**67**:1605–11.
13. Aarsland D, Kvaløy JT, Andersen K, *et al.* The effect of age of onset of PD on risk of dementia. *J Neurol* 2007;**254**:38–45.
14. Levy G, Schupf N, Tang MX, *et al.* Combined effect of age and severity on the risk of dementia in Parkinson's disease. *Ann Neurol* 2002;**51**:722–9.
15. Burn D, Rowan E, Allan L, *et al.* Motor subtype and cognitive decline in Parkinson's disease, Parkinson's disease with dementia, and dementia with Lewy bodies. *J Neurol Neurosurg Psychiatry* 2006;**77**:585–9.
16. Haugarvoll K, Aarsland D, Wentzel-Larsen T, Larsen J. The influence of cerebrovascular risk factors on incident dementia in patients with Parkinson's disease. *Acta Neurol Scand* 2005;**112**:386–90.
17. Weisskopf MG, Grodstein F, Ascherio A. Smoking and cognitive function in Parkinson's disease. *Mov Disord* 2007;**22**: 660–5.
18. Perry EK, Kilford L, Lees AJ, *et al.* Increased Alzheimer pathology in Parkinson's disease related to antimuscarinic drugs. *Ann Neurol* 2003;**54**:235–8.
19. Inzelberg R, Bonuccelli U, Schechtman E, *et al.* Association between amantadine and the onset of dementia in Parkinson's disease. *Mov Disord* 2006;**21**:1375–9.
20. Burn D, Emre M, McKeith I, *et al.* Effects of rivastigmine in patients with and without visual hallucinations in dementia associated with Parkinson's disease. *Mov Disord* 2006;**21**:1899–907.
21. Emre M, Aarsland D, Brown R, *et al.* Clinical diagnostic criteria for dementia associated with Parkinson disease. *Mov Disord* 2007;**22**:1689–707.
22. Noe E, Marder K, Bell KL, *et al.* Comparison of dementia with Lewy bodies to Alzheimer's disease and Parkinson's disease with dementia. *Mov Disord* 2004;**19**:60–7.
23. Bradshaw JSM, Hopwood M, Anderson V, Brodtmann A. Fluctuating cognition in dementia with Lewy bodies and Alzheimer's disease is qualitatively distinct. *J Neurol Neurosurg Psychiatry* 2004;**75**:382–7.
24. Bronnick K, Ehrt U, Emre M, *et al.* Attentional deficits affect activities of daily living in dementia-associated with Parkinson's disease. *J Neurol Neurosurg Psychiatry* 2006;**77**:1136–42.
25. Kitayama M, Wada-Isoe K, Nakaso K, *et al.* Clinical evaluation of Parkinson's disease dementia: association with aging and visual hallucination. *Acta Neurol Scand* 2007;**116**:190–5.
26. Collerton D, Burn D, McKeith I, O'Brien J. Systematic review and meta-analysis show dementia with Lewy bodies is a visual perceptual and attentional-executive dementia. *Dement Geriat Cog Disord* 2003;**16**:229–37.
27. Aarsland D, Ballard CG, Halliday G. Are Parkinson's disease with dementia and dementia with Lewy bodies the same entity? *J Geriatr Psychiatry Neurol* 2004;**17**:137–45.
28. Janvin C, Larsen J, Salmon D, *et al.* Cognitive profiles of individual patients with Parkinson's disease and dementia: comparison with dementia with Lewy bodies and Alzheimer's disease. *Mov Disord* 2006;**21**:337–42.
29. Aarsland D, Brønnick K, Ehrt U, *et al.* Neuropsychiatric symptoms in patients with Parkinson's disease and dementia: frequency, profile and associated care giver stress. *J Neurol Neurosurg Psychiatry* 2007;**78**:36–42.
30. Mosimann U, Rowan E, Partington C, *et al.* Characteristics of visual hallucinations in Parkinson disease dementia and dementia with Lewy bodies. *Am J Geriatr Psychiatry* 2006;**14**:153–60.
31. Josephs KA. Capgras syndrome and its relationship to neurodegenerative disease. *Arch Neurol* 2007;**64**:1762–6.
32. Pagonabarraga J, Llebaria G, García-Sánchez C, *et al.* A prospective study of delusional misidentification syndromes in Parkinson's disease with dementia. *Mov Disord* 2008;**23**:443–8.
33. Aarsland D, Ballard CG, Larsen JP, McKeith IG. A comparative study of psychiatric symptoms in dementia with Lewy bodies and Parkinson's disease with and without dementia. *Int J Geriatr Psychiatry* 2001;**16**:528–36.
34. Ballard CG, Holmes C, McKeith IG, *et al.* Psychiatric morbidity in dementia with Lewy bodies: a prospective clinical and neuropathological comparative study with Alzheimer's disease. *Am J Psychiatry* 1999;**156**:1039–45.
35. Dujardin K, Sockeel P, Delliaux M, *et al.* The Lille Apathy Rating Scale: validation of a caregiver-based version. *Mov Disord* 2008;**23**:845–9.
36. Burn DJ, Rowan EN, Minnett T, *et al.* Extrapyramidal features in Parkinson's disease with and without dementia and dementia with Lewy bodies: a cross-sectional comparative study. *Mov Disord* 2003;**18**:884–9.

37. Del Ser T, McKeith I, Anand R, *et al.* Dementia with Lewy bodies: findings from an international multicentre study. *Int J Geriatr Psychiatry* 2000;**15**:1034–45.
38. Aarsland D, Ballard C, McKeith I, *et al.* Comparison of extrapyramidal signs in dementia with Lewy bodies and Parkinson's disease. *J Neuropsychiatry Clin Neurosci* 2001;**13**:374–9.
39. Bonelli SB, Ransmayr G, Steffelbauer M, *et al.* L-Dopa responsiveness in dementia with Lewy bodies, Parkinson's disease with and without dementia. *Neurology* 2004;**63**:376–8.
40. Molloy S, McKeith IG, O'Brien JT, Burn DJ. The role of levodopa in the management of dementia with Lewy bodies. *J Neurol Neurosurg Psychiatry* 2005;**76**:1200–3.
41. Molloy S, Rowan EN, McKeith IG, *et al.* The effect of levodopa on cognitive function in Parkinson's disease with and without dementia and dementia with Lewy bodies. *J Neurol Neurosurg Psychiatry* 2006;**77**:1323–8.
42. Ballard CG, Shaw F, Lowery K, *et al.* The prevalence, assessment and associations of falls in dementia with Lewy bodies and Alzheimer's disease. *Dement Geriatr Cogn Disord* 1999;**10**:97–103.
43. Allan L, Ballard C, Burn D, Kenny R. Prevalence and severity of gait disorders in Alzheimer's and non-Alzheimer's dementias. *J Am Geriatr Soc* 2005;**53**:1681–7.
44. Mosimann UP, Müri RM, Burn DJ, *et al,* Saccadic eye movement changes in Parkinson's disease dementia and dementia with Lewy bodies. *Brain* 2005;**128**:1267–76.
45. Boddy F, Rowan EN, Lett D, *et al,* Sleep quality and excessive daytime somnolence in Parkinson's disease with and without dementia, dementia with Lewy bodies and Alzheimer's disease: a comparative, cross-sectional study. *Int J Geriatr Psychiatry* 2007;**22**:529–35.
46. Schenck CH, Hurwitz TD, Mahowald MW. Symposium: normal and abnormal REM sleep regulation: REM sleep behaviour disorder: an update on a series of 96 patients and a review of the world literature. *J Sleep Res* 1993;**2**:224–31.
47. Boeve BF, Silber MH, Ferman TJ. REM sleep behavior disorder in Parkinson's disease and dementia with Lewy bodies. *J Geriatr Psychiatry Neurol* 2004;**17**:146–57.
48. Marion MH, Qurashi M, Marshall G, Foster O. Is REM sleep behaviour disorder (RBD) a risk factor of dementia in idiopathic Parkinson's disease? *J Neurol* 2008;**255**:192–6.
49. Vendette M, Gagnon JF, Décary A, *et al.* REM sleep behavior disorder predicts cognitive impairment in Parkinson disease without dementia. *Neurology* 2007;**69**:1843–9.
50. Graham JM, Sagar HJ. A data-driven approach to the study of heterogeneity in idiopathic Parkinson's disease: identification of three distinct subtypes. *Mov Disord* 1999;**14**:10–20.
51. Allan LM, Ballard CG, Allen J, *et al.* Autonomic dysfunction in dementia. *J Neurol Neurosurg Psychiatry* 2007;**78**:671–7.
52. Allan L, McKeith I, Ballard C, Kenny RA. The prevalence of autonomic symptoms in dementia and their association with physical activity, activities of daily living and quality of life. *Dement Geriatr Cogn Disord* 2006;**22**:230–7.
53. Sakakibara R, Ito T, Uchiyama T, *et al.* Lower urinary tract function in dementia of Lewy body type. *J Neurol Neurosurg Psychiatry* 2005;**76**:729–32.
54. Ransmayr GN, Holliger S, Schletterer K, *et al.* Lower urinary tract symptoms in dementia with Lewy bodies, Parkinson disease, and Alzheimer disease. *Neurology* 2008;**70**:299–303.
55. Olichney JM, Murphy C, Hofstetter CR, *et al.* Anosmia is very common in the Lewy body variant of Alzheimer's disease. *J Neurol Neurosurg Psychiatry* 2005;**76**:1342–7.
56. Tröster AI, Stalp LD, Paolo AM, *et al.* Neuropsychological impairment in Parkinson's disease with and without depression. *Arch Neurol* 1995;**52**:1164–9.
57. Dubois B, Burn D, Goetz C, *et al.* Diagnostic procedures for Parkinson's disease dementia. *Mov Disord* 2007;**22**:2314–24.
58. Folstein MF, Folstein SE, McHugh PR. "Mini-mental state." A practical method for grading the cognitive state of patients for the clinician. *J Psychiatr Res* 1975;**12**:189–98.
59. Bronnick K, Aarsland D, Larsen JP. Neuropsychiatric disturbances in Parkinson's disease clusters in five groups with different prevalence of dementia. *Acta Psychiatr Scand* 2005;**112**:201–7.
60. Ferman TJ, Smith GE, Boeve BF, *et al.* DLB fluctuations: specific features that reliably differentiate DLB from AD and normal aging. *Neurology* 2004;**62**:181–7.
61. McKeith IG, Galasko D, Kosaka K, *et al.* Consensus guidelines for the clinical and pathological diagnosis of dementia with Lewy bodies (DLB): report of the consortium on DLB international workshop. *Neurology* 1996;**47**:1113–24.
62. McKeith IG, Perry EK, Perry RH. Report of the second dementia with Lewy body international workshop: diagnosis and treatment. Consortium on Dementia with Lewy Bodies. *Neurology* 1999;**53**:902–5.
63. McKeith IG, Ballard CG, Perry RH, *et al.* Prospective validation of consensus criteria for the diagnosis of dementia with Lewy bodies. *Neurology* 2000;**54**:1050–8.
64. Ala TA, Hughes LF, Kyrouac GA, *et al.* Pentagon copying is more impaired in dementia with Lewy bodies than in Alzheimer's disease. *J Neurol Neurosurg Psychiatry* 2001;**70**:483–8.
65. Tiraboschi P, Salmon D, Hansen L, *et al.* What best differentiates Lewy body from Alzheimer's disease in early-stage dementia? *Brain* 2006;**129**:729–35.
66. Merdes AR, Hansen LA, Jeste DV, *et al.* Influence of Alzheimer pathology on clinical diagnostic accuracy in dementia with Lewy bodies. *Neurology* 2003;**60**:1586–90.
67. Marras C, Kopp A, Qiu F, *et al.* Antipsychotic use in older adults with Parkinson's disease. *Mov Disord* **1**2007;**5**:319–23.
68. Factor SA, Feustel PJ, Friedman JH, *et al.* Longitudinal outcome of Parkinson's disease patients with psychosis. *Neurology* 2003;**60**:1756–61.
69. Aarsland D, Andersen K, Larsen JP, *et al.* The rate of cognitive decline in Parkinson's disease. *Arch Neurol* 2004;**61**:1906–11.
70. Simard M, van Reekum R, Cohen T. A review of the cognitive and behavioural symptoms in dementia with Lewy bodies. *J Neuropsychiatry Clin Neurosci* 2000;**12**:425–50.
71. Ballard CG, O'Brien J, Morris CM, *et al.* The progression of cognitive impairment in dementia with Lewy bodies, vascular dementia and Alzheimer's disease. *Int J Geriatr Psychiatry* 2001;**16**:499–503.
72. Johnson D, Morris J, Galvin J. Verbal and visuospatial deficits in dementia with Lewy bodies. *Neurology* 2005;**65**:1232–8.
73. Jellinger KA, Wenning GK, Seppi K. Predictors of survival in dementia with Lewy bodies and Parkinson dementia. *Neurodegener Dis* 2007;**4**:428–30.

Chapter 13
Neuropsychologic Features of Parkinson's Dementias

Leonardo Cruz de Souza, Virginie Czernecki, & Bruno Dubois
Department of Neurology, Salpêtrière University Hospital, Paris, France

Introduction

The cognitive impairments in Parkinson's disease (PD) patients have received attention since the first description of the illness, even though James Parkinson stated in his initial study of six patients that there was not a mental dysfunction in PD. It was not until Charcot's publications in 1861–1862 that cognitive impairment began to be recognized as a feature of this disorder [1]. Nowadays, even if PD is mainly considered to be a movement disorder, it has been increasingly acknowledged that it is frequently accompanied by cognitive deficits and that approximately 30% of PD patients develop the so-called Parkinson's disease dementia (PDD). The main risk factors for PDD are old age, severity of motor impairment, and compromised cognitive functions at the time of baseline assessment. In a longitudinal follow-up study of 149 patients with PD (Sydney Multicenter Study of Parkinson's disease), Hely *et al.* [2] have shown that the predominant problems after 15 years of disease duration are non-motor and mainly concern cognitive decline (84%) and dementia (48%).

Parkinson's disease dementia

Neuropsychologic profile

Dementia in PD can be recognized on the basis of a severe dysexecutive syndrome with memory deficit in the absence of aphasia, apraxia, or agnosia. Several factors can make it difficult to recognize or assess the dementia of PD. In the levodopa "off" state, patients can be severely akinetic, with slowing of movement and hypophonic and slurred speech. Together with the anxiety that frequently accompanies these features, these can interfere with performance in tests of motor and verbal cognitive function. In the levodopa "on" state, patients may be inattentive and hampered by uncontrolled dyskinesias which can also interfere with cognitive testing. Further, depression, which is observed in about 40% of patients with PD, can be associated with a significant decrease in frontal metabolism on PET scan studies and with attention and memory disorders which impair cognitive function, especially in the executive system [3,4]. Another confounding factor is the frequent presence of medications such as anti-cholinergic drugs which can specifically impair cognitive performance in PD patients because of the underlying loss of cholinergic neurons of the nucleus basalis of Meynert [5,6]. The neuropsychologic pattern of PDD is thus less clearly established than one would except, because in many studies the diagnosis has relied primarily on clinical judgment or on informal tests. The recent DSM-IV criteria allow for a more accurate detection of PDD than previous versions because they include the presence of a dysexecutive syndrome.

Recent papers have described the neuropsychologic profile of PD dementia (see review in reference 7). It is characterized by a rather homogeneous profile with a predominant executive dysfunction associated with attentional disorders and episodic memory retrieval deficits. Attention is preferentially affected in PDD and is more severe than is found in AD patients, with fluctuations in attention observed in approximately 29% of the patients [8]. Accordingly, PDD has been classified as a "dysexecutive dementia" [9], thought to be related to predominant subcortico-frontal dysfunction.

Fluctuating memory complaints are common among PDD patients: up to 67% of the patients report it as the presenting symptom [10], and an objective memory deficit is regularly demonstrated in PDD patients. This is characterized by impaired immediate and delayed recall performance in both verbal and visual memory tests. The mechanism of this episodic memory impairment is interesting to consider. Generally, a recall deficit can result from three different causes: (1) *an impaired registration*, due to an attention disorder or executive dysfunction as are frequently found in PDD, or to depression, drugs

Parkinson's Disease: Non-Motor and Non-Dopaminergic Features, First Edition. Edited by C. Warren Olanow, Fabrizio Stocchi, and Anthony E. Lang.

(benzodiazepines), or sleep disorders; for that reason, there is a need to use tests that assess whether information has been truly registered; (2) *a storage deficit*, for example, due to damage of medio-temporal lobe structures as is found in Alzheimer's disease (AD); and (3) *a retrieval deficit*, due to an impaired ability to activate strategies necessary for retrieving stored information as is seen with frontal lobe damage or in patients with subcortico-frontal dysfunction. In PDD, the recall deficit is thought to result from registration and/or retrieval deficits, rather than from a storage problem. This is the reason why the recall performance is generally improved, or even normalized, with the use of semantic cueing and/or recognition procedures. However, some reports have shown that cued recall [11] and recognition for both verbal and non-verbal material [10] can also be impaired in PDD.

Executive functions, including concept formation, planning, cognitive control, initiation, and inhibition control, have been shown to be impaired in PDD [12,13]. In addition, short-term and working memory are disturbed in PDD, as assessed either by the digit span test [14] or by the digit ordering test [15]. PDD patients also perform badly in lexical fluency. This test provides an excellent means for determining how well subjects activate pathways to retrieve specific information, and it is sensitive to cognitive changes of Parkinson's disease [16]. Clinically evident aphasia is rare in PDD patients. However, linguistic problems with word-finding difficulties, decreased information content of spontaneous speech, diminished word list generation, and impaired strategies in sentence comprehension are commonly seen [17,18]. In general, patients with PDD have less impairment in core language functions than patients with AD. Visuospatial construction is impaired in PDD, probably to a greater extent than that seen in AD [19]. Praxis disorders may also be observed, although their nature is still a matter of debate [20]. As a rule, these instrumental deficits are less severe than in AD, but similar to those found in patients with dementia with Lewy bodies (DLB) [20].

In summary, the subcortico-frontal involvement in PDD is considered to be the cause of the clinical features, especially executive dysfunction (impaired working memory, attention, conceptualization, and shifting aptitude), and also behavioral changes (apathy) and memory retrieval deficit. Visuospatial functions may also be impaired, but core language functions are relatively preserved. Although some overlap can be demonstrated with AD and DLB with respect to lesions of cortical and subcortical cholinergic neuronal system, the cognitive profile of PDD seems to be relatively specific.

Criteria for PDD diagnosis

In the absence of accepted guidelines for the diagnosis of PDD, the Movement Disorders Society (MDS) set up a Task Force aimed at proposing new criteria [21] and practical guidelines [9] for PDD. Box 13.1 summarizes the criteria for the diagnosis of probable and possible PDD.

Box 13.1 Criteria for the diagnosis of probable and possible PDD [21]

Probable PDD

A Core features: a dementia syndrome developing within the context of established PD

B Associated clinical features:
- Typical profile of cognitive deficits including impairment in at least two of the four core cognitive domains (impaired attention which may fluctuate, impaired executive functions, impairment in visuospatial functions, and impaired free recall memory which usually improves with cueing)
- The presence of at least one behavioral symptom (apathy, depressed or anxious mood, hallucinations, delusions, excessive daytime sleepiness) supports the diagnosis of Probable PDD; lack of behavioral symptoms, however, does not exclude the diagnosis

C Absence of any other abnormality which may by itself cause cognitive impairment

D None of the group IV features present

Possible PDD

A Core features: both must be present

B Associated clinical features:
- Atypical profile of cognitive impairment in one or more domains, such as prominent or receptive-type (fluent) aphasia, or pure storage-failure type amnesia (memory does not improve with cueing or in recognition tasks) with preserved attention
- Behavioral symptoms may or may not be present

OR

C One or more of the group III features present

D None of the group IV features present

MDS guidelines for the diagnosis of PDD

In parallel, the MDS Task Force has operationalized the diagnosis of PDD and has proposed practical guidelines based on a two-level algorithm depending on the clinical scenario and the expertise of the examiner involved in the assessment [9]. Level I is the diagnostic level. It should be done by the neurologist in an office setting or at the beside. It does not require particular expertise in neuropsychologic methods, and employs a simple, pragmatic set of tests that are not excessively time consuming. Level II is more qualitative and is recommended for more specific purposes such as clinical monitoring, research studies, and pharmacologic trials.

Level I testing

The proposed guidelines for the diagnosis of PDD rely on the following set of considerations. (1) The diagnosis of dementia is a *clinical diagnosis* that should be made by a clinician. It should not be based on neuropsychologic test scores alone, whatever battery or set of neuropsychologic evaluations is employed (i.e., Mattis DRS [22], Montreal Cognitive Assessment – MoCA [23], MMS [24], FAB [25], or composite battery of memory, executive and instrumental functions). (2) The clinician who will have to make the diagnosis of dementia is primarily a specialist in movement disorders, generally with a limited knowledge in neuropsychology. (3) The major criterion of dementia is the evidence of a loss of autonomy: a person who is no longer able to manage and take care of himself/herself and who needs assistance such that they are dependent on others. Accordingly, an evaluation of activities of daily living is an important step in the process of making the diagnosis of dementia. This impact must be significantly relevant and not related solely to the severity of the motor deficit such that the cognitive problems themselves compromise the autonomy of the patient. We have proposed a simple measure for assessing the impact of cognitive dysfunction on patient autonomy, called the "Pill Questionnaire": if the patient still independently manages a his/her treatment lone or if the patient is still able to describe explicitly his/her anti-parkinsonian treatment regimen without significant errors, we consider that the patient maintained his/her autonomy. (4) A derivative point from the above is that the diagnosis of PDD is a clinical decision that should be made by an experienced clinician who has full knowledge of the patient's anti-parkinsonian treatment and PD status. (5) If an impact on ADL is the keystone for the diagnosis of PDD, the additional cognitive requirements should be easy and fast to obtain. This is why the MMSE [24] was proposed: the test can provide a global score of general intellectual efficiency, the evidence of an attention (serial 7s), memory (missing word), and visuo-constructive (pentagons) impairment. An additional test that can be simply performed is verbal fluency (number of words with letter S in 1 min).

Accordingly, the diagnosis of PDD relies on an algorithm of five criteria (see Box 13.2):

1 *A diagnosis of idiopathic Parkinson's disease.*

The diagnosis should be based on: (i) the diagnostic criteria for PD proposed by the Queen Square Brain Bank; and (ii) the occurrence of PD prior for at least 1 year prior to the onset of dementia. The information is gathered by the clinician from the patient/caregiver history or from ancillary records. If dementia develops in the context of established PD, a diagnosis of PDD is warranted. Dementia in a PD patient that develops prior to this time point would be diagnosed as dementia with Lewy bodies. It remains uncertain whether there is any advantage in making this somewhat arbitrary distinction.

Box 13.2 Algorithm for diagnosing PDD [9]

1 A diagnosis of idiopathic PD based on the Queen's Square Brain Bank criteria for PD
2 PD developed prior to the onset of dementia
3 MMSE below 26
4 Cognitive deficits severe enough to impact daily living (caregiver interview or Pill Questionnaire)
5 Impairment in at least two of the following tests:
- months reversed or subtract seven backwards
- lexical fluency or clock drawing
- MMSE pentagons
- Three-word recall

The presence of one of the following behavioral symptoms: apathy or depressed mood or delusions or excessive daytime sleepiness may support the diagnosis of probable PDD
The presence of major depression or delirium or any other abnormality which may by itself cause significant cognitive impairment makes the diagnosis uncertain.

2 *PD is associated with a decreased global cognitive efficiency.*
The MMSE [24] is the proposed test for assessing cognitive efficiency because it is universal, and can be assessed in the clinician's office or at the beside in a relatively brief period of time. A score of 25 or below is proposed for identifying cognitively impaired patients. This cutoff is adequate in patients below the age of 80 years and in those with at least 10 years of formal education.

3 *The cognitive deficiency is severe enough to impair daily life.*
The diagnosis of dementia requires evidence of an impact on daily living activities that cannot be attributed to motor or autonomic symptoms. The examiner should ask questions about daily functioning, such as the patient's ability to manage finances, use pieces of equipment, organize independently the daily distribution of anti-parkinsonian medication (the Pill Questionnaire, see Box 13.3), and cope in social situations.

4 *Impairment in more than one of the following cognitive domains.*

The proposed diagnostic criteria require a profile of cognitive deficits, typical of those described for PDD, in two or more of four cognitive domains:

(i) *Attention.* The proposed tests are: serial 7s of the MMSE [24] (cutoff: at least two uncorrected responses) and months reversed (cutoff: omission of two or more months, uncorrected sequencing of the months, or failure to complete the test within 90 s).

(ii) *Executive functions.* The proposed tests are lexical fluency (considering the number of words beginning with the letter S in 1 min, with a score below 10 being

Box 13.3 The Pill Questionnaire [9]

Instructions:
Ask the patient to describe verbally his/her treatment and its time schedule

Scoring:

1 There is no impact:
- if the patient is able to describe spontaneously and clearly the drugs, doses (mg or color or tablet) and timing of treatment;
- if the patient needs some help from the examiner (what time do you take your medication?; which drugs and which doses?) but he/she is successful without clinically pertinent errors;
- if the caregiver certifies that the patient can (or could) safely and reliably take the pills without supervision in daily life

2 There is an impact on daily living:
- if the patient is not able to describe, even with the help of the examiner, the time and nature (drugs and doses) of his/her treatment;
- if the caregiver certifies that the patient can (or could) no longer safely and reliably take the pills without supervision in daily life

acknowledged as an impairment) and the clock drawing test (the cutoff is the inability to insert the correct clock face numbers and/or the clock hands pointing to the correct time).

(iii) *Visuo-constructive ability*. The proposed test is: drawing of the MMSE [24] pentagons (the copy should include two pentagons that overlap).

(iv) *Memory impairment*. The proposed test is three-word recall of the MMSE [24] (at least one missing word in the free recall is considered sufficient to suggest the existence of a memory/retrieval problem).

5 *The absence of major depression or delirium.*

An absence of depression is generally required for the diagnosis of a dementia. In PD, depression is frequent and should not be *a priori* an exclusionary criterion for the diagnosis of dementia. However, as it may aggravate cognitive changes, it should be documented and it is recommended that, in case of major depression, anti-depressant treatment should be tried before determining the existence of a dementia.

To summarize, the diagnosis of PD dementia is made by the neurologist. It is fairly easy to make, simply requiring the physician to diagnose idiopathic Parkinson's disease; to use the MMSE [24] and Verbal Fluency Test, and to question the patient or the family on the function in activities of daily living such as with the Pill Questionnaire (Box 13.3).

Level II testing

In most cases, the level I algorithm is sufficient to make a diagnosis of PDD and for initiation of appropriate treatment. However, it may happen that an additional evaluation is required, either for a better characterization of the neuropsychologic pattern or for research purposes. In such cases, complementary investigations are required that should ideally be performed by trained neuropsychologists. In this eventuality, no cutoff scores are necessary because the studies are not performed for diagnostic purposes.

1 For assessing global efficiency, we have recommended the MATTIS Dementia Rating Scale (DRS) [22] because the subtests of this scale (attention, initiation and perseveration, conceptualization, and memory) are more sensitive to the subcortico-frontal dysfunction of PDD, compared with the MMSE, which is probably more sensitive to the dementia of AD. The global score (maximum of 144) can be useful to follow the severity of dementia in patients over time.

2 Executive functions can be assessed with specific tests that are listed in Table 13.1. Generally, executive functions refer to the processes that are needed for elaboration of goal-directed behaviors: the ability to analyze the situation correctly, to select pertinent information, to manipulate this information within working memory, to elaborate and execute the response program, to evaluate its appropriateness according to the requirements of the environment, or to change the response if needed. Different tests are proposed to evaluate these different processes (test for finding rule, mental set shifting, solving problems, attention resource allocation) in a more or less specific manner.

3 Apathy is frequently observed in disorders of the basal ganglia, even in the absence of a depressed mood. It is thought to be related to dysfunction of the ventral striatum/orbital anterior-cingulate loop and can be evaluated with the Apathy Scale or with the NeuroPsychiatric Inventory (NPI) [26].

4 Episodic long-term memory is currently assessed with the recall of a word list after a time delay. However, a recall deficit may result from different causes:

(a) Decreased registration: as can be observed in attention disorders that can occur in a variety of situations, for example, depression, anxiety, drug side effects (benzodiazepines, anti-cholinergics), and sleep disorders. Interestingly, all of these factors can be present in patients with PD or PDD. Here, the items to be remembered are not – or are poorly – encoded, and it is not surprising, therefore, that the recall is low. In other words, a recall deficit in patients with PDD may not result from a true memory deficit but from a low registration of the items to be remembered. This is the reason why it is important to establish whether a true registration has been performed with

Table 13.1 Recommended tests for level II (data from Dubois *et al.* [9]).

Global efficiency	Mattis DRS
Executive functions	
Working memory	Digit Span Spatial Span (CANTAB) Digit Ordering Test
Conceptualization	Similarities (WAIS-III) Wisconsin CST
Set activation	Verbal Fluency (C, F, L)
Set shifting	TMT
Set maintenance	Stroop Test Odd Man Out Test
Behavioral control	Prehension Behavior
Memory	RAVLT Free and Cued Recall Test
Instrumental functions	
Language	Boston Naming Test
Visuo-constructive	Copy of the Clock
Visuo-spatial	Benton Line Orientation Test Cube Analysis (VOSP)
Visuo-perceptive	Benton Face Recognition Test Fragmented Letters (VOSP)
Neuropsychiatric functions	
Apathy	Apathy Scale
Depression	MADRS Hamilton Beck Depression Inventory GDS-15
Visual hallucination	PPQ
Psychosis	NPI

tests that evaluate encoding before studying memory *per se*.

(b) A storage deficit: as is seen in cases with damage to the hippocampo–mamillo–thalamic circuit (e.g., Korsakoff's syndrome and AD). In this situation, information is not stored in the brain even if it has been well encoded. Accordingly, there is a recall deficit due to a true memory disorder.

(c) Decreased retrieval: as typically seen in patients with subcortico-frontal dysfunction. In this condition, there is not a genuine memory deficit but only difficulty in internally activating appropriate retrieval strategies that guide the memory search, as required, for example, in the Rey Auditory Verbal Learning Test [27]. The use of semantic cues may improve the performance of patients with a dysexecutive syndrome by facilitating the retrieval of information. This is the case with the Free and Cued Recall Test [28]. With this test, patients with PDD have a specific pattern of performance: a very low recall deficit (as in a typical dementia) with significant improvement – and even normalization – with cueing. Therefore, it may be possible to define precisely the nature of an episodic memory deficit: impaired mediotemporal component with a storage deficit as in AD; impaired subcortico-frontal component with predominant retrieval deficit as in PDD.

5 Instrumental functions. PDD should be considered mainly a dysexecutive dementia, as opposed to AD, where instrumental functions are severely impaired (e.g., aphasia, apraxia, and agnosia). These latter functions have also been shown to be mildly impaired in PDD, reflecting possible cortical involvement in this condition. Therefore, these functions should be assessed by specific tests (see Table 13.1).

6 Neuropsychiatric symptoms are common in PDD, and have important clinical implications. The most characteristic features are apathy and visual hallucinations, with depression and psychosis occurring in more severely affected patients.

Dementia with Lewy bodies

Neuropsychologic profile

The profile of neuropsychologic impairments in patients with DLB differs from that of AD and other dementia syndromes, reflecting the combined involvement of cortical and subcortical pathways with relative sparing of the hippocampus. Patients with DLB perform better than those with AD on tests of verbal memory [29] but worse on tests of visual perception [30,31], tests that require drawing and copying [32], and tests of attention and executive functions [33]. Fifty patients with autopsy-verified DLB performed significantly worse than 95 patients with autopsy-verified AD on tests of visuospatial ability, verbal fluency, psychomotor speed, and abstract reasoning. A logistic regression model designed to distinguish between DLB and AD patients showed that performance on tests of verbal fluency (i.e., the Phonemic Fluency Test), visuospatial ability (i.e., the WISC-R Block Design Test, the Clock Drawing Test), psychomotor speed (i.e., Part A of the Trail-Making Test), and general semantic knowledge (i.e., the Number Information Test) was highly significant and correctly classified approximately 60% of patients with DLB and 88% of patients with AD [34].

In an extension to these studies, the COGDRAS computer-based test system has been used to record attentional performance (speed and accuracy) [35] and to measure cognitive fluctuations which are the core feature of DLB (which until very recently have proven difficult to quantify by other means) [36,37]. DLB and PDD patients show similar attentional slowing on the COGRAS choice reaction time test compared with AD and non-demented PD subjects, and also show greater between-test

Box 13.4 Revised criteria for the clinical diagnosis of dementia with Lewy bodies (DLB) [44]

1 **Central feature** (*essential for a diagnosis of possible or probable DLB*)
Dementia defined as progressive cognitive decline of sufficient magnitude to interfere with normal social or occupational function
Prominent or persistent memory impairment may not necessarily occur in the early stages but is usually evident with progression
Deficits on tests of attention, executive function, and visuospatial ability may be especially prominent

2 **Core features** (*two core features are sufficient for a diagnosis of probable DLB, one for possible DLB*)
Fluctuating cognition with pronounced variations in attention and alertness
Recurrent visual hallucinations that are typically well formed and detailed
Spontaneous features of parkinsonism

3 **Suggestive features** (*If one or more of these is present in the presence of one or more core features, a diagnosis of probable DLB can be made. In the absence of any core features, one or more suggestive features is sufficient for possible DLB. Probable DLB should not be diagnosed on the basis of suggestive features alone*)
REM sleep behavior disorder
Severe neuroleptic sensitivity
Low dopamine transporter uptake in basal ganglia demonstrated by SPECT or PET imaging

4 **Supportive features** (*commonly present but not proven to have diagnostic specificity*)
Repeated falls and syncope
Transient, unexplained loss of consciousness
Severe autonomic dysfunction, e.g., orthostatic hypotension, urinary incontinence
Hallucinations in other modalities
Systematized delusions
Depression
Relative preservation of medial temporal lobe structures on CT/MRI scan
Generalized low uptake on SPECT/PET perfusion scan with reduced occipital activity
Abnormal (low-uptake) MIBG myocardial scintigraphy.
Prominent slow wave activity on EEG with temporal lobe transient sharp waves

5 **A diagnosis of DLB is less likely**
In the presence of cerebrovascular disease evident as focal neurologic signs or on brain imaging
In the presence of any other physical illness or brain disorder sufficient to account in part or in total for the clinical picture
If parkinsonism only appears for the first time at a stage of severe dementia

6 **Temporal sequence of symptoms**
DLB should be diagnosed when dementia occurs before or concurrently with parkinsonism (if it is present). The term Parkinson disease dementia (PDD) should be used to describe dementia that occurs in the context of well-established PD. In a practice setting the term that is most appropriate to the clinical situation should be used and generic terms such as LB disease are often helpful. In research studies in which distinction needs to be made between DLB and PDD, the existing 1-year rule between the onset of dementia and parkinsonism DLB continues to be recommended. Adoption of other time periods will simply confound data pooling or comparison between studies. In other research settings that may include clinicopathologic studies and clinical trials, both clinical phenotypes may be considered collectively under categories such as LB disease or a-synucleinopathy

variability (a measure of fluctuation) when the choice reaction time paradigm is repeatedly presented at 3 s intervals. There is a debate about whether or not there are distinct neuropsychologic patterns in patients with DLB and PDD. Whereas the cognitive patterns have been reported to differ in the relatively mild stages of the disease [38,39], they were similar in the more severe stages [39,40], leading to the conclusion that the two diseases might be a spectrum of the same disorder. Before making a definitive determination on this point, it should be reminded that (1) from a neuropsychologic point of view, differences might be blunted by the severity of the dementia and by the sensitivity of tests that might not be high enough to detect subtle differences, (2) psychiatric symptoms are significantly more frequent in patients with DLB [41,42], and (3) PIB retention in the brain on imaging studies is significantly higher in patients with DLB (similar to that of patients with AD) than in patients with PDD [43].

Diagnosis

In 2005, the Third Report of the DLB Consortium was published [44], in which new consensus criteria for the clinical and pathologic diagnosis of DLB were proposed (Box 13.4). The clinical diagnosis of DLB should be considered when there is a dementia that is associated with fluctuating cognition, hallucinations, and parkinsonism. As established by the Consortium, the dementia should occur before or concurrently with parkinsonism.

Neuropsychologic evaluation is a valuable tool for differential diagnosis and should be routinely performed. Neuropsychologic tests can characterize the profile of cognitive impairment, which can be used for improving the specificity of the diagnosis. In a given patient with parkinsonism and cognitive fluctuations, the confirmation of a "amnestic syndrome of the medial temporal type" in tests of episodic memory may favor the diagnosis of DLB rather than of PDD. These are reviewed in more detail in Chapter 12.

References

1. Goetz C. The historical background of behavioral studies in Parkinson's disease. In: Huber SJ, Cummings JL, eds. *Parkinson's Disease – Neurobehavioral Aspects*. New York: Oxford University Press, 1992: 3–9.
2. Hely MA, Morris JG, Reid WG, Trafficante R. Sydney Multicenter Study of Parkinson's disease: non-L-dopa-responsive problems dominate at 15 years. *Mov Disord* 2005;**20**(2):190–9.
3. Starkstein SE, Bolduc PL, Mayberg HS, *et al.* Cognitive impairments and depression in Parkinson's disease: a follow up study. *J Neurol Neurosurg Psychiatry* 1990;**53**(7):597–602.
4. Kuzis G, Sabe L, Tiberti C, *et al.* Cognitive functions in major depression and Parkinson disease. *Arch Neurol* 1997;**54**(8): 982–6.
5. Candy JM, Perry RH, Perry EK, *et al.* Pathological changes in the nucleus of Meynert in Alzheimer's and Parkinson's diseases. *J Neurol Sci* 1983;**59**(2):277–89.
6. Dubois B, Ruberg M, Javoy-Agid F, *et al.* A subcortico-cortical cholinergic system is affected in Parkinson's disease. *Brain Res* 1983;**288**(1–2):213–8.
7. Pillon B, Boller F, Levy R, Dubois B. Cognitive deficits and dementia in Parkinson's disease. In: Boller F, Cappa SF, eds. *Handbook of Neuropsychology*, 2nd edn, Vol. 6, 2001: 307–67.
8. Bronnick K, Emre M, Lane R, *et al.* Profile of cognitive impairment in dementia associated with Parkinson's disease compared with Alzheimer's disease. *J Neurol Neurosurg Psychiatry* 2007;**78**(10):1064–8.
9. Dubois B, Burn D, Goetz C, *et al.* Diagnostic procedures for Parkinson's disease dementia: recommendations from the movement disorder society task force. *Mov Disord* 2007;**22**(16):2314–24.
10. Noe E, Marder K, Bell KL, *et al.* Comparison of dementia with Lewy bodies to Alzheimer's disease and Parkinson's disease with dementia. *Mov Disord* 2004;**19**(1):60–7.
11. Higginson CI, Wheelock VL, Carroll KE, Sigvardt KA Recognition memory in Parkinson's disease with and without dementia: evidence inconsistent with the retrieval deficit hypothesis. *J Clin Exp Neuropsychol* 2005;**27**(4):516–28.
12. Pillon B, Deweer B, Agid Y, Dubois B. Explicit memory in Alzheimer's, Huntington's, and Parkinson's diseases. *Arch Neurol* 1993;**50**(4):374–9.
13. Zgaljardic DJ, Borod JC, Foldi NS, Mattis P. A review of the cognitive and behavioral sequelae of Parkinson's disease: relationship to frontostriatal circuitry. *Cogn Behav Neurol* 2003;**16**(4):193–210.
14. Woods SP, Tröster AI. Prodromal frontal/executive dysfunction predicts incident dementia in Parkinson's disease. *J Int Neuropsychol Soc* 2003;**9**(1):17–24.
15. Hoppe CD, Müller UD, Werheid KD, *et al.* Digit Ordering Test: clinical, psychometric, and experimental evaluation of a verbal working memory test. *Clin Neuropsychol* 2000;**14**(1):38–55.
16. Levy G, Jacobs DM, Tang MX, *et al.* Memory and executive function impairment predict dementia in Parkinson's disease. *Mov Disord* 2002;**17**(6):1221–6.
17. Piatt AL, Fields JA, Paolo AM, *et al.* Lexical, semantic, and action verbal fluency in Parkinson's disease with and without dementia. *J Clin Exp Neuropsychol* 1999;**21**(4):435–43.
18. Grossman M, Zurif E, Lee C, *et al.* Information processing speed and sentence comprehension in Parkinson's disease. *Neuropsychology* 2002;**16**(2):174–81.
19. Mosimann UP, Mather G, Wesnes KA, *et al.* Visual perception in Parkinson disease dementia and dementia with Lewy bodies. *Neurology* 2004;**63**(11):2091–6.
20. Zadikoff C, Lang AE. Apraxia in movement disorders. *Brain* 2005;**128**(Pt 7):1480–97.
21. Emre M, Aarsland D, Brown R, *et al.* Clinical diagnostic criteria for dementia associated with Parkinson's disease. *Mov Disord* 2007;**22**(12):1689–707.
22. Mattis S. *Dementia Rating Scale: Professional Manual*. Odessa, FL: Psychological Assessment Resources, 1988.
23. Nasreddine ZS, Phillips NA, Bédirian V, *et al.* The Montreal Cognitive Assessment, MoCA: a brief screening tool for mild cognitive impairment. *J Am Geriatr Soc* 2005;**53**(4):695–9.
24. Folstein M, Folstein SE, McHugh,PR. 'Mini-mental state'. A practical method for grading the cognitive state of patients for the clinician. *J Psychiatr Res* 1975;**12**:189–98.
25. Dubois B, Slachevsky A, Litvan I, Pillon B. The FAB: a Frontal Assessment Battery at bedside. *Neurology* 2000;**55**:1621–6.
26. Cummings JL, Mega M, Gray K, *et al.* The Neuropsychiatric Inventory: comprehensive assessment of psychopathology in dementia. *Neurology* 1994;**44**(12):2308–14.
27. Schmidt, M. *Rey Auditory and Verbal Learning Test: A Handbook*. Los Angeles, CA: Western Psychological Services, 1996.
28. Grober E, Buschke H: Genuine memory deficits in dementia. *Dev Neuropsychol* 1987;**3**:13–36.
29. McKeith IG, Perry RH, Fairbairn AF, *et al.* Operational criteria for senile dementia of Lewy body type (SDLT). *Psychol Med* 1992;**22**(4):911–22.
30. Mori E, Shimomura T, Fujimori M, *et al.* Visuoperceptual impairment in dementia with Lewy bodies. *Arch Neurol* 2000;**57**(4):489–93.
31. Calderon J, Perry RJ, Erzinclioglu SW, *et al.* Perception, attention, and working memory are disproportionately impaired in dementia with Lewy bodies compared with Alzheimer's disease. *J Neurol Neurosurg Psychiatry* 2001;**70**(2):157–64.
32. Gnanalingham KK, Byrne EJ, Thornton A, *et al.* Motor and cognitive function in Lewy body dementia: comparison with Alzheimer's and Parkinson's diseases. *J Neurol Neurosurg Psychiatry* 1997;**62**(3):243–52.

33. Ballard C, O'Brien J, Gray A, *et al.* Attention and fluctuating attention in patients with dementia with Lewy bodies and Alzheimer disease. *Arch Neurol* 2001;**58**(6):977–82.
34. Dubois B, Pillon B, McKeith IG. Parkinson's disease with and without dementia and Lewy body dementia. In: Miller B, Cummings JL, eds. *The Human Frontal Lobes – Functions and Disorders*, 2nd edn. New York: Guilford Press, 2007: 472–504.
35. Wesnes KA, McKeith IG, Ferrara R, *et al.* Effects of rivastigmine on cognitive function in dementia with Lewy bodies: a randomised placebo-controlled international study using the cognitive drug research computerised assessment system. *Dement Geriatr Cogn Disord* 2002;**13**(3):183–92.
36. Walker MP, Ayre GA, Cummings JL, *et al.* The Clinician Assessment of Fluctuation and the One Day Fluctuation Assessment Scale. Two methods to assess fluctuating confusion in dementia. *Br J Psychiatry* 2000;**177**:252–6.
37. Ferman TJ, Smith GE, Boeve BF, *et al.* DLB fluctuations: specific features that reliably differentiate DLB from AD and normal aging. *Neurology* 2004;**62**(2):181–7
38. Downes JJ, Priestley NM, Doran M, *et al.* Intellectual, mnemonic, and frontal functions in dementia with Lewy bodies: a comparison with early and advanced Parkinson's disease. *Behav Neurol* 1998;**11**(3):173–83.
39. Aarsland D, Litvan I, Salmon D, *et al.* Performance on the dementia rating scale in Parkinson's disease with dementia and dementia with Lewy bodies: comparison with progressive supranuclear palsy and Alzheimer's disease. *J Neurol Neurosurg Psychiatry* 2003;**74**(9):1215–20.
40. Horimoto Y, Matsumoto M, Nakazawa H, *et al.* Cognitive conditions of pathologically confirmed dementia with Lewy bodies and Parkinson's disease with dementia. *J Neurol Sci* 2003;**216**(1):105–8.
41. Aarsland D, Ballard C, Larsen JP, McKeith I. A comparative study of psychiatric symptoms in dementia with Lewy bodies and Parkinson's disease with and without dementia. *Int J Geriatr Psychiatry* 2001;**16**(5):528–36
42. Noe E, Marder K, Bell KL, *et al.* Comparison of dementia with Lewy bodies to Alzheimer's disease and Parkinson's disease with dementia. *Mov Disord* 2004;**19**(1):60–7.
43. Gomperts SN, Rentz DM, Moran E, *et al.* Imaging amyloid deposition in Lewy body diseases. *Neurology* 2008;**71**(12): 903–10.
44. McKeith IG, Dickson DW, Lowe J, et al.; Consortium on DLB. Diagnosis and management of dementia with Lewy bodies: third report of the DLB Consortium. *Neurology* 2005;**65**(12): 1863–72.

Chapter 14
Neuropathology of Dementia in Parkinson's Disease

Dennis W. Dickson[1] *& Carolyn F. Orr*[2]
[1]Department of Neuroscience, Mayo Clinic, Jacksonville, FL, USA
[2]Department of Neurology, Mayo Clinic, Rochester, MN, USA

Introduction

Parkinson's disease (PD) is the most common, age-associated neurodegenerative movement disorder and is characterized by bradykinesia, rigidity, tremor, and postural instability [1]. Many of these patients eventually develop cognitive problems or even dementia, referred to as Parkinson's disease dementia (PDD). Clinical criteria for PDD have only recently been formulated [2] and recommendations for systematic clinical evaluation of PDD proposed [3]. Clinical aspects of PDD are discussed elsewhere in this book; this chapter deals with the neuropathology of PDD. Neuropathologic criteria for PD based upon consensus of experts [4] have not been rigorously tested, but are widely used and in line with other accepted criteria [5,6]. At present there are no neuropathologic criteria for PDD, but there are neuropathologic criteria for the related clinical disorder, dementia with Lewy bodies (DLB) [7], that have been validated in prospectively diagnosed individuals [8]. Both DLB [7] and PDD [2] are distinct clinical entities in terms of temporal aspects and relative severity of various clinical features, but they have few significant differences in terms of neuropathology based upon currently available information, and none that are sufficiently robust to allow their differentiation to be made without access to clinical information [9–11]. Additional studies are needed to determine if there are any pathologic features that differentiate PDD from DLB. In the meantime, it has been suggested that since the two cannot be differentiated, the neuropathologic diagnosis should be expressed as a description of the objective findings, with respect to Alzheimer-type pathology and Lewy-related pathology, and a comment on the probability that the observed pathology would be consistent with a Lewy-related cognitive disorder, to encompass both PDD and DLB. The probability that the Alzheimer- and Lewy-related pathological findings would be associated with a dementia syndrome with parkinsonism is directly related to the severity of the Lewy-related pathology and inversely related to the Alzheimer-type pathology [7]. The basis for this is thought to be that when Alzheimer-type pathology is severe, the clinical presentation is usually that of Alzheimer's disease (AD), regardless of the severity of Lewy-related pathology [12]. This latter hypothesis has been tested in DLB [8], but not yet in PDD.

The neuropathologic substrate for PDD has been reviewed recently, and this chapter builds upon that description [2]. Some PD patients may have cognitive problems related to cerebrovascular disease or other concurrent neurodegenerative disease processes [13], but this is not the focus of the current description. This chapter is based upon a review of the literature and also perspective from personal evaluation of cases of PD and PDD who have come to autopsy, mostly from retrospective studies [9,14–17].

Neuropathology of PD

Dementia in PD evolves in the context of pre-existing PD. While most cases of PD that come to autopsy have Lewy body disease, in all reported autopsy series there are also cases thought to have PD or PDD who in fact have other pathologic processes [18–20]. In a personal consecutive series of 149 autopsy cases of PD and PDD from a diverse referral base, including patients evaluated in life by movement disorder specialists and also patients who were not seen by specialists, about 25% of the PD and PDD cases have other pathologies. In the PD group, cases considered to have PD included equal numbers of multiple system atrophy, progressive supranuclear palsy, corticobasal degeneration, and vascular parkinsonism, whereas AD, progressive supranuclear palsy, and corticobasal

Parkinson's Disease: Non-Motor and Non-Dopaminergic Features, First Edition. Edited by C. Warren Olanow, Fabrizio Stocchi, and Anthony E. Lang.

Table 14.1 Comparison of neuropathology in PD and PDD[a].

Parameter	PD ($N = 58$)	PDD ($N = 52$)	p-Value
Age at death (years; mean ± standard deviation)	75 ± 10	77 ± 7	n.s.
Sex (% men)	78	67	n.s.
Family history (% positive)	19	33	n.s.
APOE ε4 (% positive)	33	40	n.s.
MAPT H1H1 (% positive)	61	67	n.s.
Vascular pathology (% positive)	14	15	n.s.
Brain weight (g) (mean ± standard deviation)	1250 ± 150	1210 ± 130	n.s.
Senile plaque score (median: 25%-, 75%-tile)	0 (0, 0)	2 (0, 2)	<0.001
Braak NFT stage (median: 25%-, 75%-tile)	II (I, III)	III (II, IV)	<0.001
DLB type (median: 25%-, 75%-tile)	T (B, D)	D (T, D)	<0.001

[a]Comparison of autopsy-confirmed cases of PD and PDD that have Lewy body pathology as the substrate of parkinsonism. There are no significant differences between PD and PDD for age at death; male to female ratio; presence of family history of parkinsonism or dementia; or carrier frequency of apolipoprotein E ε4 or tau gene (*MAPT*) H1H1 genotype. Brain weight and presence of cerebrovascular pathology (i.e., infarcts or leukoencephalopathy) were also not different. On the other hand, there were significantly more senile plaques (senile plaque score: 0 = none, 1 = sparse cortical plaques; 2 = moderate to frequent diffuse amyloid plaques; 3 = moderate to frequent neuritic plaques); a higher Braak neurofibrillary tangle stage [145] (ranging from 0 to VI, with stages V and VI associated with a diagnosis of high likelihood AD); and more cortical Lewy bodies (Lewy body type [146]: B = brainstem predominant, T = transitional or limbic Lewy bodies; D = diffuse cortical Lewy bodies). Statistical analysis: SigmaStat ver. 3.0 9 (Systat Software, Point Richmond, CA, USA); *t*-tests for age and brain weight; Mann–Whitney rank sum test for senile plaque score, Braak stage, Lewy body type; chi-squared for sex, family history vascular pathology; and Fisher exact test for *APOE* and *MAPT*.

degeneration were over-represented in the PDD group. Of those that had Lewy bodies, there was no significant difference in the age at death or the male-to-female ratio between PD ($N = 58$) and PDD ($N = 52$), although PDD tended to be in slightly older patients and more frequent in women (Table 14.1). Family history of dementia or parkinsonism and apolipoprotein E ε4 carrier state, which is a risk factor for Alzheimer-type pathology in the setting of neurodegenerative disorders [21], tended to be higher in PDD than PD, but the differences were not statistically significant.

The external appearance of the brain in PD is usually relatively unremarkable, with a brain weight that is within normal limits (Table 14.1). The degree of cortical atrophy is minimal and not more than expected for the age of the individual. In PDD, the atrophy is not significantly greater than in PD and age-matched controls (Plate 14.1a). The most consistent macroscopic finding is a decrease in visible pigmentation of monoaminergic brainstem nuclei, namely the substantia nigra and locus coeruleus (Plate 14.1b). This pallor reflects loss of neurons containing neuromelanin pigment. The degree of depigmentation has been shown to correlate with the extent of neuronal loss [22].

Loss of dopaminergic neurons in the substantia nigra in the midbrain leads to loss of striatal dopamine [23]. Ventrolateral neurons in the pars compacta of the substantia nigra are preferentially affected, and it is estimated that more than half of the substantia nigra pars compacta neurons must be lost before the onset of parkinsonian symptoms [24]. Neuronal loss in the ventrolateral substantia nigra pars compacta correlates with disease duration [25]. Neuronal loss is also present in the noradrenergic neurons in the locus coeruleus [26,27], cholinergic neurons in the basal nucleus of Meynert [28,29], cholinergic neurons of the mesopontine nuclei (i.e., pedunculopontine tegmental and laterodorsal tegmental nuclei) [30], and serotonergic neurons in median raphe nuclei [30]. In the medulla, neuronal loss occurs in adrenergic neurons in the ventrolateral tegmentum, serotonin neurons in the raphe obscurus nucleus, substance P-containing neurons in the lateral reticular formation, and dorsal motor nucleus of the vagus [30]. There is neuronal loss in intralaminar thalamic nuclei [31] and hypocretin and melanin concentrating hormone neurons in the hypothalamus [32,33]. There is also loss of neurons in the olfactory bulb [34].

The histopathologic hallmark of PD is the Lewy body. Lewy bodies are granulofilamentous intraneuronal inclusions composed of α-synuclein and other proteins [35,36]. Typical Lewy bodies are easily recognized, consisting of round cytoplasmic inclusions (Plate 14.2a), but more subtle lesions are also found, so-called cortical Lewy bodies (Plate 14.2c). Inclusions similar to Lewy bodies are also found within neuronal processes as intra-neuritic Lewy bodies (Plate 14.3c). In addition to these lesions, which are readily detected with routine histologic methods, there are also aggregates of α-synuclein in neuronal processes referred to as Lewy neurites (Plate 14.3). Although originally described in the hippocampus [37] and later the amygdala [38], Lewy neurites are now known to be more widely distributed than originally suspected and may be the most abundant type of pathologic lesion in any given region that is affected by the disease process. Their detection can be enhanced by proteolytic treatment of tissue sections [39–41]. They may also be the earliest cytologic alteration in affected neurons [42,43], and they may precede Lewy body formation in perikarya or axons. The combination of abnormal α-synuclein immunoreactive inclusions in neuronal cell bodies and neurites is referred to as Lewy-related pathology.

Distribution of Lewy-related pathology

Lewy-related pathology is found consistently in the substantia nigra, locus coeruleus, dorsal motor nucleus of the vagus, and most regions in the brainstem that show neuronal loss. Lewy bodies and Lewy neurites also are found in the olfactory bulb in most cases, and it is increasingly recognized that olfactory bulb pathology can occur early in the disease process [34,44–48]. Cortical and subcortical areas associated with the olfactory system, including the amygdala [38], are often severely affected. The density of Lewy-related pathology in the olfactory bulb correlates with density of cortical and amygdala Lewy bodies and concurrent Alzheimer-type pathology [49,50]. Lewy-related pathology is also common in the hypothalamus and basal forebrain, including the basal nucleus of Meynert. Cortical areas that are most vulnerable include limbic structures (e.g., cingulate gyrus, in addition to perirhinal and entorhinal cortices), insular cortex, temporal pole, and frontal cortex. Lewy-related pathology is usually less dense in parietal and occipital lobes, and it largely spares primary motor, somatosensory, and visual cortices. Amongst subcortical structures that are affected, the striatum often has fine curvilinear or dot-like α-synuclein immunoreactive neurites [51]. Neuraxonal spheroids, which are relatively common in the globus pallidus and the pars reticularis of the substantia nigra, also frequently have α-synuclein immunoreactivity [52]. Lewy-related pathology is also detected in the intralaminar thalamic nuclei [31]. Brainstem nuclei that are vulnerable, in addition to those noted above for neuronal loss, include periaqueductal gray and the pontine and medullary tegmentum, but not the pontine base or inferior olivary nucleus.

Accompanying neuronal loss in the substantia nigra are activated microglia expressing class II major histocompatibility antigens [53–55]. Microglia may also contain neuromelanin or even Lewy bodies consistent with neuronal phagocytosis. A subset of astrocytes in PD display abnormal α-synuclein immunoreactivity, and these have been noted to occur in the amygdala, thalamus, basal ganglia, and cerebral cortex [56]. Oligodendroglia immunoreactive for α-synuclein have also been described in PD, especially in vulnerable brainstem nuclei and the basal ganglia [57,58].

Staging Lewy-related pathology

Based upon evaluation of a large number of normal brains and PD brains, Braak and co-workers proposed a staging scheme for PD [48,59–61]. According to this pathologic staging scheme, substantia nigra dopaminergic neurodegeneration develops at the mid-stage of the illness, whereas involvement of olfactory bulb, medulla, and pontine tegmentum occurs at an earlier time point [59,60]. The final stages are characterized by widespread cortical Lewy bodies [61], similar to those found in diffuse Lewy body disease [62]. Diffuse cortical Lewy body pathology is the most common finding in patients with an antemortem clinical presentation of DLB [7]. In addition, it is the type of Lewy-related pathology detected in many studies of PDD [14,16,25,63,64] (see Table 14.1).

The general principles of the proposed staging system have been confirmed in several studies of PD, but there are some caveats [65]. Large cross-sectional studies by Parkkinen and co-workers [66–68] and Jellinger [69] largely concurred with the Braak staging scheme; however, they also described cases in which Lewy bodies are found in the substantia nigra without involvement of the medulla. It is increasingly recognized that Lewy bodies are frequent in the setting of advanced AD [70] and that the most common location for Lewy bodies in AD is the amygdala [71–73], with Lewy body formation almost completely limited to the amygdala in about 15–20% of the cases [71]. Most of these cases did not have brainstem pathology, including the dorsal motor nucleus of the vagus and surrounding areas, which is the earliest stage in the scheme proposed by Braak and co-workers. Thus, Lewy bodies in advanced AD do not fit the PD staging scheme [74].

Neuropathologic correlates of dementia in PD: a historical perspective

The interpretation of the pathologic basis of dementia in PD has changed as neuropathologic methods have evolved. When routine histologic methods, including silver impregnation techniques, were the only means available for evaluation of brains, dementia was most often attributed to Alzheimer-type pathology [75,76]. It is true that the majority of PDD cases, in part because of their advanced age, have some degree of Alzheimer-type pathology, most often in the form of neocortical amyloid plaques with few or no neocortical neurofibrillary tangles. As the nature of Alzheimer-type pathology has been investigated in prospective longitudinal cohorts of normal and demented subjects, it has become clear that there is heterogeneity in Alzheimer-type lesions, with some neurologically normal elderly individuals displaying many cortical amyloid plaques [77–81], but few or no neurofibrillary tangles, a process we refer to as "pathological aging" [77,82]. Amyloid plaques in neurologically normal individuals are composed of diffuse amyloid deposits without significant neuritic elements (Plate 14.4c), in contrast to plaques in AD where neuritic plaques (Plate 14.4b) are common and of diagnostic significance [83]. The clinical significance of cortical amyloid plaques has come into question with the advent of positron emission tomographic (PET) methods and imaging tracers for amyloid, which have shown many neurologically normal individuals with cerebral amyloid [84–87]. Multifactorial analyses indicate that cognitive deficits associated with amyloid plaques are mediated by neurofibrillary degeneration [88,89] or other pathologic processes. Review of demented individuals previously considered to have "plaque-only AD" [90] has revealed other pathology rather than amyloid that likely contributed to dementia, with a major factor being Lewy body disease [91]. In our consecutive autopsy series of PD and PDD, senile plaque score was significantly greater in PDD than in PD (Table 14.1), but the effect of the senile plaque score is lost in a multiple logistic regression analysis, while both neurofibrillary tangles (Braak NFT stage) and Lewy bodies (Lewy body disease type) remain significant correlates of dementia in PD (Table 14.2).

In the late 1970s and early 1980s, there was increasing interest in the role of the cholinergic system in dementia, as deficits in cortical cholinergic innervation due to neuronal loss in the basal nucleus of Meynert had been reported in AD [92] and other disorders, particularly PD and Lewy body dementia [93–96]. These studies indicated that dementia in PD was likely heterogeneous – some had concurrent AD, but others had dementia due to severe neuronal loss in the basal nucleus of Meynert and other nuclei that had wide cortical projections (i.e., the isodendritic core [97]), such as mesolimbic dopaminergic fibers originating in the ventral tegmental region (A10 dopaminergic neurons) and noradrenergic fibers from the locus coeruleus [27,28,62,98–102].

Table 14.2 Multiple logistic regression analysis of neuropathologic variables for dementia in PD ($N = 110$)[a].

Parameter	Odds ratio	5% confidence interval	95% confidence interval	*p*-Value
Senile plaque score	1.1	0.65	1.7	n.s.
DLB type	2.3	1.1	4.6	0.019
Braak NFT stage	2.2	1.3	3.8	0.004

[a]Multiple logistic regression of pathologic variables that were significantly different between PD and PDD (Table 14.1). Effects of senile plaque on dementia are negated, whereas both Lewy bodies and neurofibrillary tangles remain significant.

In the late 1980s, Lewy bodies were discovered to have ubiquitin immunoreactivity [103], which soon became the method of choice for detecting Lewy bodies. With the advent of this new technique, it was much easier to detect cortical Lewy bodies, in addition to neuritic pathology that prior to that time had gone unnoticed [37]. Increasingly, cortical Lewy bodies and Lewy neurites were recognized as contributing to dementia in PD [19,104]. Application of more sensitive and specific measures for tau protein, which had by then been discovered to be the major protein within Alzheimer-type neurofibrillary tangles [105], drew attention to tau pathology in PDD also [106]. It was also recognized that neurofibrillary tangles were ubiquitinated [107] and that the use of ubiquitin to study brains with Lewy bodies was fraught with difficulties if there was any degree of Alzheimer-type pathology, since there was no good way of differentiating Lewy bodies from small neurofibrillary tangles. Only double immunostaining for tau and ubiquitin permitted unequivocal differentiation of Lewy bodies from neurofibrillary tangles [37], but this method was never widely used by most laboratories. More recently, interest has shifted to tau pathology that may not be visible as a structural lesion in the brain, with evidence to suggest that abnormal phospho-tau in synaptic structures may be increased in PDD [108].

A major breakthrough in the pathologic investigation of PD and PDD was the discovery that Lewy bodies were composed of α-synuclein [109] and that immunohistochemistry for α-synuclein could unequivocally differentiate Lewy bodies and Lewy neurites from neurofibrillary tangles and neuropil threads. Immunohistochemistry for α-synuclein clearly showed more cortical α-synuclein pathology than previously recognized, even with ubiquitin immunohistochemistry [110]. Subsequent studies indicated that the density of cortical Lewy bodies correlated with dementia in PD [16,63,64,111–117]. Braak and coworkers are credited with the conceptual breakthrough in putting cortical and subcortical α-synuclein pathology into a relentlessly progressive continuum [43,59,60], with the last stage associated with widespread cortical pathology [61] and associated with dementia in PD [118–121]. While the Braak staging scheme is valuable from a conceptual framework for PD and PDD, as noted previously, it may not fit well for all types of Lewy-related pathologies, particularly Lewy bodies in individuals with AD [49,65]. Particularly troubling are more recent reports that cortical Lewy bodies can be detected in PD patients who are not demented [68,114,122,123] or even in individuals with no evidence of either parkinsonism or dementia [66,67,122]. These reports have refocused attention to other types of pathology that are usually present in PD patients with dementia, such as amyloid plaques in cortex [123] or striatum [124,125] and neuritic α-synuclein pathology in cortex and striatum, which has been found to be greater in PDD than PD [17,51].

Significance of cortical Lewy-related pathology in PDD

Lewy-related pathology is considered by many to be the main substrate driving cognitive impairment in PD [16,63,64,112,117]. In PDD, Lewy body counts in the limbic cortex, amygdala, and neocortex are increased nearly 10-fold compared with PD [25]. The density of cortical Lewy bodies, especially in the limbic cortex, has been shown to correlate with cognitive impairment [104,111]. Cognitive decline in PD has also been shown to correlate with Braak PD stage, with one-third having cognitive decline at stage 3, two-thirds at stage 4, more than 90% at stage 5, and all patents at stage 6 [61,118]. In our consecutive autopsy series of PD and PDD cases, PDD was significantly more likely to have diffuse cortical Lewy bodies, whereas transitional/limbic Lewy bodies were most common in PD (Table 14.1).

As noted above, several studies have shown that cortical Lewy bodies can be detected in non-demented individuals [68,122], which raises the question of whether the α-synuclein pathology that is visible with immunohistochemistry is functionally relevant to cognitive impairment. The analogous situation has plagued correlations of cortical amyloid plaques and cognition. While amyloid is felt to be fundamental to the pathogenesis of AD, it is increasingly clear that some neurologically normal individuals have extensive amyloid at autopsy [77] which can be detected during life with PET using amyloid-biding ligands [84]. Thus, the challenge is to determine the relationship between the observed pathology and its functional consequences. Increasingly, for amyloid and other protein aggregation disorders, the toxic species is felt to represent oligomers rather than the fibrillar deposits that are observed with the microscope (or PET scan) [126]. Similarly, the toxic species of α-synuclein may not be that which is observed, but rather a soluble oligomer that may contribute to cellular dysfunction and death [127–130]. While much discussion has focused on intracytoplasmic Lewy bodies, neuritic α-synuclein pathology may be more significant. Descriptions of cortical Lewy bodies in normal individuals rarely indicate the extent of Lewy-related neuritic pathology, which may be a better correlate of cognitive dysfunction since it is usually more widespread and denser than the Lewy bodies in patients with PDD and DLB (Plate 14.3)

Significance of Alzheimer-type pathology in PDD

Some degree of Alzheimer-type pathology, namely amyloid plaques and neurofibrillary tangles, is common in most cases of PDD (Plate 14.4), but usually not sufficient to diagnose AD by current neuropathologic criteria [131], in which neocortical tangles are required to consider the pathology highly likely to contribute to dementia. In our consecutive autopsy series of PD and PDD, the median Braak neurofibrillary tangle stage was II in PD and only III in PDD. Even with a high density of cortical plaques, this degree of neurofibrillary degeneration would not likely be clinically significant [132], and would warrant no more than a low-to-intermediate likelihood of this pathology contributing to dementia using the NIA–Reagan criteria for AD [131]. In retrospective studies of PDD, amyloid plaques may be numerous. This fits with recent PET imaging studies that have shown cortical amyloid deposits in many patients with PDD [133,134]. In our consecutive autopsy series of PD and PDD, the median plaque score for PD was 0, whereas it was 2 for PDD, indicative of moderate to frequent cortical amyloid deposits for patients with this condition (Table 14.1). Alzheimer-type pathology in PDD is usually characterized by diffuse amyloid plaques (Plate 14.4c) rather than neuritic plaques, which are characteristic of AD. When neurofibrillary tangles are detected they are often confined to medial temporal lobe structures (e.g., entorhinal cortex (Plate 14.4a), but not the neocortex. Rather, evidence suggests that the effect of amyloid deposits on cognitive dysfunction in PDD is mediated by α-synuclein and tau pathology. In addition to cortical amyloid deposits, amyloid deposits are not uncommon in the striatum in AD [135], and they have been reported to be a characteristic finding in PDD [124] (Plate 14.4d). The significance of this observation has been debated [125].

There is evidence to suggest that amyloid influences the burden of both α-synuclein and tau pathology [50,123], but the mechanism whereby this might occur is uncertain. In transgenic mice, α-synuclein pathology is increased if α-synuclein transgenic mice are crossed with mice that overproduce amyloid [136]. Similarly, tau pathology is enhanced in tau transgenic mice crossed with transgenic mice that overproduce amyloid [137]. The availability of animal models that recapitulate the modulating effects of amyloid on α-synuclein and tau suggests that an explanation for the interaction might be discovered in the future.

Subcortical pathology in PDD

Loss of ascending inputs from brainstem nuclei that project diffusely to cortical areas has been implicated in dementia in PD [97]. The nuclei that consistently show neuronal loss and Lewy-related pathology in PD and PDD include noradrenergic neurons of the locus coeruleus, dopaminergic neurons of the mesolimbic projecting ventral tegmental area, and cholinergic neurons of the basal nucleus of Meynert, in addition to serotonergic neurons of the raphe nuclei [58,101,138,139]. This pathology is predicted to be associated with functional disturbances that may not be tightly linked to cortical α-synuclein or Alzheimer-type pathology and may account for the less than perfect correlations between structural lesions and cognitive dysfunction in PD.

Cortical synaptic pathology in PDD

It has been argued that synaptic loss is the common denominator of cognitive dysfunction in a wide range of neurodegenerative disorders, and also the cognitive deficits that accompany aging [140,141]. There are relatively few studies that have addressed synaptic pathology in PDD, despite the fact that α-synuclein is a major presynaptic protein felt to be involved in synaptic vesicle release [142]. Quantitative assessment of presynaptic proteins, such as synaptophysin, has shown decreases in cortical synaptic proteins in PDD compared with neurologically normal controls, but less consistently than in AD [143,144]. Further studies are warranted in this area. Synaptic loss and neurotransmitter deficiencies are not easily appreciated with routine neuropathologic methods. Both may contribute to the imperfect fit for correlations between structural lesions (e.g., Alzheimer- and Lewy-related pathologies) and cognition in PD. How Alzheimer- and Lewy-related pathologies contribute to synaptic dysfunction and loss is currently unclear.

Acknowledgment

DWD is supported by NIH grants P01-AG03949, P50-AG16574, P01-AG17216, P50-AG25711, and P50-NS40256.

References

1. Jellinger KA, Mizuno Y. Parkinson's disease. In: Dickson DW, ed. *Neurodegeneration: the Molecular Pathology of Dementia and Movement Disorders*. Basel: ISN Neuropath Press, 2003: 159–87.
2. Emre M, Aarsland D, Brown R, *et al.* Clinical diagnostic criteria for dementia associated with Parkinson's disease. *Mov Disord* 2007;**22**:1689–707.
3. Dubois B, Burn D, Goetz C, *et al.* Diagnostic procedures for Parkinson's disease dementia: recommendations from the Movement Disorder Society Task Force. *Mov Disord* 2007;**22**:2314–24.
4. Gelb DJ, Oliver E, Gilman S. Diagnostic criteria for Parkinson disease. *Arch Neurol* 1999;**56**:33–9.
5. Daniel SE, Lees AJ. Parkinson's Disease Society Brain Bank, London: overview and research. *J Neural Transm Suppl* 1993;**39**:165–72.
6. Hughes AJ, Daniel SE, Kilford L, Lees AJ. Accuracy of clinical diagnosis of idiopathic Parkinson's disease: a clinico-pathological study of 100 cases. *J Neurol Neurosurg Psychiatry* 1992;**55**:181–4.
7. McKeith IG, Dickson DW, Lowe J, *et al.* Diagnosis and management of dementia with Lewy bodies: third report of the DLB Consortium. *Neurology* 2005;**65**:1863–72.
8. Fujishiro H, Ferman TJ, Boeve BF, *et al.* Validation of the neuropathologic criteria of the third consortium for dementia with Lewy bodies for prospectively diagnosed cases. *J Neuropathol Exp Neurol* 2008;**67**:649–56.
9. Tsuboi Y, Dickson DW. Dementia with Lewy bodies and Parkinson's disease with dementia: are they different? *Parkinsonism Relat Disord*. 2005;**11**(Suppl 1):47–51.
10. Aarsland D, Ballard CG, Halliday G. Are Parkinson's disease with dementia and dementia with Lewy bodies the same entity? *J Geriatr Psychiatry Neurol* 2004;**17**:137–45.
11. Guo L, Itaya M, Takanashi M, *et al.* Relationship between Parkinson disease with dementia and dementia with Lewy bodies. *Parkinsonism Relat Disord* 2005;**11**:305–9.
12. Lopez OL, Becker JT, Kaufer DI, *et al.* Research evaluation and prospective diagnosis of dementia with Lewy bodies. *Arch Neurol* 2002;**59**:43–6.
13. Jellinger KA. Prevalence of vascular lesions in dementia with Lewy bodies. A postmortem study. *J Neural Transm* 2003;**110**:771–8.
14. Algom AA, Dickson DW. Parkinson's disease dementia (PDD) and Alzheimer dementia (AD): a retrospective clinical comparison and quantitative neuropathologic study. *Neurology* 2008;**70**:A276.
15. Bower JH, Dickson DW, Taylor L, *et al.* Clinical correlates of the pathology underlying parkinsonism: a population perspective. *Mov Disord* 2002;**17**:910–6.
16. Apaydin H, Ahlskog JE, Parisi JE, *et al.* Parkinson disease neuropathology: later-developing dementia and loss of the levodopa response. *Arch Neurol* 2002;**59**:102–12.
17. Tsuboi Y, Uchikado H, Dickson DW. Neuropathology of Parkinson's disease dementia and dementia with Lewy bodies with reference to striatal pathology. *Parkinsonism Relat Disord*. 2007;**13**(Suppl 3):221–224.
18. Jellinger KA. Morphological substrates of parkinsonism with and without dementia: a retrospective clinico-pathological study. *J Neural Transm Suppl* 2007;91–104.
19. Hughes AJ, Daniel SE, Blankson S, Lees AJ. A clinicopathologic study of 100 cases of Parkinson's disease. *Arch Neurol* 1993;**50**:140–8.
20. Hughes AJ, Daniel SE, Lees AJ. Improved accuracy of clinical diagnosis of Lewy body Parkinson's disease. *Neurology* 2001;**57**:1497–9.
21. Josephs KA, Tsuboi Y, Cookson N, *et al.* Apolipoprotein E epsilon 4 is a determinant for Alzheimer-type pathologic features in tauopathies, synucleinopathies, and frontotemporal degeneration. *Arch Neurol* 2004;**61**:1579–84.
22. Greffard S, Verny M, Bonnet AM, *et al.* A stable proportion of Lewy body bearing neurons in the substantia nigra suggests a model in which the Lewy body causes neuronal death. *Neurobiol Aging* 2008;**31**:99–103.
23. DelleDonne A, Klos KJ, Fujishiro H, *et al.* Incidental Lewy body disease and preclinical Parkinson disease. *Arch Neurol* 2008;**65**:1074–80.

24. Fearnley JM, Lees AJ. Ageing and Parkinson's disease: substantia nigra regional selectivity. *Brain* 1991;**114**:2283–301.
25. Harding AJ, Halliday GM. Cortical Lewy body pathology in the diagnosis of dementia. *Acta Neuropathol (Berl)* 2001;**102**:355–63.
26. Mann DM, Yates PO, Hawkes J. The pathology of the human locus coeruleus. *Clin Neuropathol* 1983;**2**:1–7.
27. Zweig RM, Cardillo JE, Cohen M, *et al.* The locus coeruleus and dementia in Parkinson's disease. *Neurology* 1993;**43**:986–91.
28. Nakano I, Hirano A. Parkinson's disease: neuron loss in the nucleus basalis without concomitant Alzheimer's disease. *Ann Neurol* 1984;**15**:415–8.
29. Whitehouse PJ, Hedreen JC, White CL III, Price DL. Basal forebrain neurons in the dementia of Parkinson disease. *Ann Neurol* 1983;**13**:243–8.
30. Halliday GM, Blumbergs PC, Cotton RG, *et al.* Loss of brainstem serotonin- and substance P-containing neurons in Parkinson's disease. *Brain Res* 1990;**510**:104–7.
31. Brooks D, Halliday GM. Intralaminar nuclei of the thalamus in Lewy body diseases. *Brain Res Bull* 2009;**78**:97–104.
32. Fronczek R, Overeem S, Lee SY, *et al.* Hypocretin (orexin) loss in Parkinson's disease. *Brain* 2007;**130**:1577–85.
33. Thannickal TC, Lai YY, Siegel JM. Hypocretin (orexin) cell loss in Parkinson's disease. *Brain* 2007;**130**:1586–95.
34. Beach TG, White CL III, Hladik CL, *et al.* Olfactory bulb alpha-synucleinopathy has high specificity and sensitivity for Lewy body disorders. *Acta Neuropathol* 2009;**117**:169–74.
35. Pollanen MS, Dickson DW, Bergeron C. Pathology and biology of the Lewy body. *J Neuropathol Exp Neurol* 1993;**52**:183–91.
36. Shults CW. Lewy bodies. *Proc Natl Acad Sci USA* 2006;**103**:1661–8.
37. Dickson DW, Ruan D, Crystal H, *et al.* Hippocampal degeneration differentiates diffuse Lewy body disease (DLBD) from Alzheimer's disease: light and electron microscopic immunocytochemistry of CA2-3 neurites specific to DLBD. *Neurology* 1991;**41**:1402–9.
38. Braak H, Braak E, Yilmazer D, *et al.* Amygdala pathology in Parkinson's disease. *Acta Neuropathol* 1994;**88**:493–500.
39. Dickson DW. Misfolded, protease-resistant proteins in animal models and human neurodegenerative disease. *J Clin Invest* 2002;**110**:1403–5.
40. Neumann M, Kahle PJ, Giasson BI, *et al.* Misfolded proteinase K-resistant hyperphosphorylated alpha-synuclein in aged transgenic mice with locomotor deterioration and in human alpha-synucleinopathies. *J Clin Invest* 2002;**110**:1429–39.
41. Beach TG, White CL, Hamilton RL, *et al.* Evaluation of alpha-synuclein immunohistochemical methods used by invited experts. *Acta Neuropathol* 2008;**116**:277–88.
42. Braak E, Sandmann-Keil D, Rub U, *et al.* Alpha-synuclein immunopositive Parkinson's disease-related inclusion bodies in lower brain stem nuclei. *Acta Neuropathol* 2001;**101**:195–201.
43. Braak H, Del Tredici K, Bratzke H, *et al.* Staging of the intracerebral inclusion body pathology associated with idiopathic Parkinson's disease (preclinical and clinical stages). *J Neurol.* 2002;**249**(Suppl 3):III/1–5.
44. Bloch A, Probst A, Bissig H, *et al.* Alpha-synuclein pathology of the spinal and peripheral autonomic nervous system in neurologically unimpaired elderly subjects. *Neuropathol Appl Neurobiol* 2006;**32**:284–95.
45. Hubbard PS, Esiri MM, Reading M, *et al.* Alpha-synuclein pathology in the olfactory pathways of dementia patients. *J Anat* 2007;**211**:117–24.
46. Sengoku R, Saito Y, Ikemura M, *et al.* Incidence and extent of Lewy body-related alpha-synucleinopathy in aging human olfactory bulb. *J Neuropathol Exp Neurol* 2008;**67**:1072–83.
47. Daniel SE, Hawkes CH. Preliminary diagnosis of Parkinson's disease by olfactory bulb pathology. *Lancet* 1992;**340**:186.
48. Del Tredici K, Rub U, De Vos RA, *et al.* Where does Parkinson disease pathology begin in the brain? *J Neuropathol Exp Neurol* 2002;**61**:413–26.
49. Fujishiro H, Tsuboi Y, Lin WL, *et al.* Co-localization of tau and alpha-synuclein in the olfactory bulb in Alzheimer's disease with amygdala Lewy bodies. *Acta Neuropathol* 2008;**116**:17–24.
50. Tsuboi Y, Wszolek ZK, Graff-Radford NR, *et al.* Tau pathology in the olfactory bulb correlates with Braak stage, Lewy body pathology and apolipoprotein epsilon4. *Neuropathol Appl Neurobiol* 2003;**29**:503–10.
51. Duda JE, Giasson BI, Mabon ME, *et al.* Novel antibodies to synuclein show abundant striatal pathology in Lewy body diseases. *Ann Neurol* 2002;**52**:205–10.
52. Newell KL, Boyer P, Gomez-Tortosa E, *et al.* Alpha-synuclein immunoreactivity is present in axonal swellings in neuroaxonal dystrophy and acute traumatic brain injury. *J Neuropathol Exp Neurol.* 1999;**58**, 1263–8.
53. McGeer PL, McGeer EG. Glial reactions in Parkinson's disease. *Mov Disord* 2008;**23**:474–83.
54. McGeer PL, Itagaki S, Boyes BE, McGeer EG. Reactive microglia are positive for HLA-DR in the substantia nigra of Parkinson's and Alzheimer's disease brains. *Neurology* 1988;**38**:1285–91.
55. McGeer PL, Itagaki S, Akiyama H, McGeer EG. Rate of cell death in parkinsonism indicates active neuropathological process. *Ann Neurol* 1988;**24**:574–6.
56. Braak H, Sastre M, Del Tredici K. Development of alpha-synuclein immunoreactive astrocytes in the forebrain parallels stages of intraneuronal pathology in sporadic Parkinson's disease. *Acta Neuropathol* 2007;**114**:231–41.
57. Wakabayashi K, Hayashi S, Yoshimoto M, *et al.* NACP/alpha-synuclein-positive filamentous inclusions in astrocytes and oligodendrocytes of Parkinson's disease brains. *Acta Neuropathol* 2000;**99**:14–20.
58. Bohnen NI, Kaufer DI, Hendrickson R, *et al.* Cognitive correlates of cortical cholinergic denervation in Parkinson's disease and parkinsonian dementia. *J Neurol* 2006;**253**:242–7.
59. Braak H, Del Tredici K, Rub U, *et al.* Staging of brain pathology related to sporadic Parkinson's disease. *Neurobiol Aging* 2003;**24**:197–211.
60. Braak H, Ghebremedhin E, Rub U, *et al.* Stages in the development of Parkinson's disease-related pathology. *Cell Tissue Res* 2004;**318**:121–34.
61. Braak H, Muller CM, Rub U, *et al.* Pathology associated with sporadic Parkinson's disease – where does it end? *J Neural Transm Suppl* 2006;89–97.
62. Kosaka K, Tsuchiya K, Yoshimura M. Lewy body disease with and without dementia: a clinicopathological study of 35 cases. *Clin Neuropathol* 1988;**7**:299–305.

63. Hurtig HI, Trojanowski JQ, Galvin J, *et al.* Alpha-synuclein cortical Lewy bodies correlate with dementia in Parkinson's disease. *Neurology* 2000;**54**:1916–21.
64. Mattila PM, Rinne JO, Helenius H, *et al.* Alpha-synuclein-immunoreactive cortical Lewy bodies are associated with cognitive impairment in Parkinson's disease. *Acta Neuropathol (Berl)* 2000;**100**:285–90.
65. Burke RE, Dauer WT, Vonsattel JP. A critical evaluation of the Braak staging scheme for Parkinson's disease. *Ann Neurol* 2008;**64**:485–91.
66. Parkkinen L, Soininen H, Alafuzoff I. Regional distribution of alpha-synuclein pathology in unimpaired aging and Alzheimer disease. *J Neuropathol Exp Neurol* 2003;**62**:363–7.
67. Parkkinen L, Kauppinen T, Pirttila T, *et al.* Alpha-synuclein pathology does not predict extrapyramidal symptoms or dementia. *Ann Neurol* 2005;**57**:82–91.
68. Parkkinen L, Pirttila T, Alafuzoff I. Applicability of current staging/categorization of alpha-synuclein pathology and their clinical relevance. *Acta Neuropathol* 2008;**115**:399–407.
69. Jellinger KA. Lewy body-related alpha-synucleinopathy in the aged human brain. *J Neural Transm* 2004;**111**:1219–35.
70. Hamilton RL. Lewy bodies in Alzheimer's disease: a neuropathological review of 145 cases using alpha-synuclein immunohistochemistry. *Brain Pathol* 2000;**10**:378–84.
71. Uchikado H, Lin WL, DeLucia MW, Dickson DW. Alzheimer disease with amygdala Lewy bodies: a distinct form of alpha-synucleinopathy. *J Neuropathol Exp Neurol* 2006;**65**:685–97.
72. Leverenz JB, Fishel MA, Peskind ER, *et al.* Lewy body pathology in familial Alzheimer disease: evidence for disease- and mutation-specific pathologic phenotype. *Arch Neurol* 2006;**63**:370–6.
73. Lippa CF, Pulaski-Salo D, Dickson DW, Smith TW. Alzheimer's disease, Lewy body disease and aging: a comparative study of the perforant pathway. *J Neurol Sci* 1997;**147**:161–6.
74. Dickson DW, Uchikado H, Fujishiro H, Tsuboi Y. Evidence in favor of Braak staging of Parkinson's disease. *Mov Disord*. 2009;**25**(Suppl 1):S78–82.
75. Hakim AM, Mathieson G. Dementia in Parkinson disease: a neuropathologic study. *Neurology* 1979;**29**:1209–14.
76. Boller F, Mizutani T, Roessmann U, Gambetti P. Parkinson disease, dementia, and Alzheimer disease: clinicopathological correlations. *Ann Neurol* 1980;**7**:329–35.
77. Dickson DW, Crystal HA, Mattiace LA, *et al.* Identification of normal and pathological aging in prospectively studied non-demented elderly humans. *Neurobiol Aging* 1992;**13**:179–89.
78. Mufson EJ, Chen EY, Cochran EJ, *et al.* Entorhinal cortex beta-amyloid load in individuals with mild cognitive impairment. *Exp Neurol* 1999;**158**:469–90.
79. Naslund J, Haroutunian V, Mohs R, *et al.* Correlation between elevated levels of amyloid beta-peptide in the brain and cognitive decline. *JAMA* 2000;**283**:1571–7.
80. Wang DS, Lipton RB, Katz MJ, *et al.* Decreased neprilysin immunoreactivity in Alzheimer disease, but not in pathological aging. *J Neuropathol Exp Neurol* 2005;**64**:378–85.
81. Wang J, Dickson DW, Trojanowski JQ, Lee VM. The levels of soluble versus insoluble brain Abeta distinguish Alzheimer's disease from normal and pathologic aging. *Exp Neurol* 1999;**158**:328–37.
82. Dickson DW. The pathogenesis of senile plaques. *J Neuropathol Exp Neurol* 1997;**56**:321–39.
83. Mirra SS, Heyman A, McKeel D, *et al.* The Consortium to Establish a Registry for Alzheimer's Disease (CERAD). Part II. Standardization of the neuropathologic assessment of Alzheimer's disease. *Neurology* 1991;**41**:479–86.
84. Aizenstein HJ, Nebes RD, Saxton JA, *et al.* Frequent amyloid deposition without significant cognitive impairment among the elderly. *Arch Neurol* 2008;**65**:1509–17.
85. Jack CR Jr, Lowe VJ, Weigand SD, *et al.* Serial PIB and MRI in normal, mild cognitive impairment and Alzheimer's disease: implications for sequence of pathological events in Alzheimer's disease. *Brain* 2009;**132**:1355–65.
86. Reiman EM, Chen K, Liu X, *et al.* Fibrillar amyloid-β burden in cognitively normal people at 3 levels of genetic risk for Alzheimer's disease. *Proc Natl Acad Sci USA* 2009;**106**:6820–5.
87. Villemagne VL, Pike KE, Darby D, *et al.* Abeta deposits in older non-demented individuals with cognitive decline are indicative of preclinical Alzheimer's disease. *Neuropsychologia* 2008;**46**:1688–97.
88. Bennett DA, Schneider JA, Wilson RS, *et al.* Neurofibrillary tangles mediate the association of amyloid load with clinical Alzheimer disease and level of cognitive function. *Arch Neurol* 2004;**61**:378–84.
89. Wang DS, Uchikado H, Bennett DA, *et al.* Cognitive performance correlates with cortical isopeptide immunoreactivity as well as Alzheimer-type pathology. *J Alzheimers Dis* 2008;**13**:53–66.
90. Terry RD, Hansen LA, DeTeresa R, *et al.* Senile dementia of the Alzheimer type without neocortical neurofibrillary tangles. *J Neuropathol Exp Neurol* 1987;**46**:262–8.
91. Hansen LA, Masliah E, Galasko D, Terry RD. Plaque-only Alzheimer disease is usually the lewy body variant, and vice versa. *J Neuropathol Exp Neurol* 1993;**52**:648–54.
92. Davies P, Maloney AJ. Selective loss of central cholinergic neurons in Alzheimer's disease. *Lancet* 1976;**ii**:1403.
93. Perry EK, Tomlinson BE, Blessed G, *et al.* Correlation of cholinergic abnormalities with senile plaques and mental test scores in senile dementia. *Br Med J* 1978;**ii**:1457–9.
94. Candy JM, Perry RH, Perry EK, *et al.* Pathological changes in the nucleus of Meynert in Alzheimer's and Parkinson's diseases. *J Neurol Sci* 1983;**59**:277–89.
95. Perry RH, Perry EK, Smith CJ, *et al.* Cortical neuropathological and neurochemical substrates of Alzheimer's and Parkinson's diseases. *J Neural Transm Suppl* 1987;**24**:131–6.
96. Perry EK, Marshall E, Perry RH, *et al.* Cholinergic and dopaminergic activities in senile dementia of Lewy body type. *Alzheimer Dis Assoc Disord* 1990;**4**:87–95.
97. Rossor MN. Parkinson's disease and Alzheimer's disease as disorders of the isodendritic core. *Br Med J* 1981;**283**:1588–90.
98. Gaspar P, Gray F. Dementia in idiopathic Parkinson's disease. A neuropathological study of 32 cases. *Acta Neuropathol (Berl)* 1984;**64**:43–52.
99. Sudarsky L, Morris J, Romero J, Walshe TM. Dementia in Parkinson's disease: the problem of clinicopathological correlation. *J Neuropsychiatry Clin Neurosci* 1989;**1**:159–66.
100. Rinne JO, Rummukainen J, Paljarvi L, Rinne UK. Dementia in Parkinson's disease is related to neuronal loss in the medial substantia nigra. *Ann Neurol* 1989;**26**:47–50.

101. Yoshimura M. Pathological basis for dementia in elderly patients with idiopathic Parkinson's disease. *Eur Neurol* 1988;**28**(Suppl 1):29–35.
102. Jellinger K, Grisold W. Cerebral atrophy in Parkinson syndrome. *Exp Brain Res*. 1982;Suppl 5:26–35.
103. Kuzuhara S, Mori H, Izumiyama N, *et al.* Lewy bodies are ubiquitinated. A light and electron microscopic immunocytochemical study. *Acta Neuropathol (Berl)* 1988;**75**:345–53.
104. Churchyard A, Lees AJ. The relationship between dementia and direct involvement of the hippocampus and amygdala in Parkinson's disease. *Neurology* 1997;**49**:1570–6.
105. Goedert M, Wischik CM, Crowther RA, *et al.* Cloning and sequencing of the cDNA encoding a core protein of the paired helical filament of Alzheimer disease: identification as the microtubule-associated protein tau. *Proc Natl Acad Sci USA* 1988;**85**:4051–5.
106. Vermersch P, Delacourte A, Javoy-Agid F, *et al.* Dementia in Parkinson's disease: biochemical evidence for cortical involvement using the immunodetection of abnormal tau proteins. *Ann Neurol* 1993;**33**:445–50.
107. Mori H, Kondo J, Ihara Y. Ubiquitin is a component of paired helical filaments in Alzheimer's disease. *Science* 1987;**235**:1641–4.
108. Muntane G, Dalfo E, Martinez A, Ferrer I. Phosphorylation of tau and alpha-synuclein in synaptic-enriched fractions of the frontal cortex in Alzheimer's disease, and in Parkinson's disease and related alpha-synucleinopathies. *Neuroscience* 2008;**152**:913–23.
109. Spillantini MG, Schmidt ML, Lee VM, *et al.* Alpha-synuclein in Lewy bodies. *Nature* 1997;**388**:839–40.
110. Irizarry MC, Growdon W, Gomez-Isla T, *et al.* Nigral and cortical Lewy bodies and dystrophic nigral neurites in Parkinson's disease and cortical Lewy body disease contain alpha-synuclein immunoreactivity. *J Neuropathol Exp Neurol* 1998;**57**:334–7.
111. Kovari E, Gold G, Herrmann FR, *et al.* Lewy body densities in the entorhinal and anterior cingulate cortex predict cognitive deficits in Parkinson's disease. *Acta Neuropathol (Berl)* 2003;**106**:83–8.
112. Aarsland D, Perry R, Brown A, *et al.* Neuropathology of dementia in Parkinson's disease: a prospective, community-based study. *Ann Neurol* 2005;**58**:773–6.
113. Bertrand E, Lechowicz W, Szpak GM, *et al.* Limbic neuropathology in idiopathic Parkinson's disease with concomitant dementia. *Folia Neuropathol* 2004;**42**:141–50.
114. Colosimo C, Hughes AJ, Kilford L, Lees AJ. Lewy body cortical involvement may not always predict dementia in Parkinson's disease. *J Neurol Neurosurg Psychiatry* 2003;**74**:852–6.
115. Brown DF, Dababo MA, Bigio EH, *et al.* Neuropathologic evidence that the Lewy body variant of Alzheimer disease represents coexistence of Alzheimer disease and idiopathic Parkinson disease. *J Neuropathol Exp Neurol* 1998;**57**:39–46.
116. Wakabayashi K, Kakita A, Hayashi S, *et al.* Apolipoprotein E epsilon4 allele and progression of cortical Lewy body pathology in Parkinson's disease. *Acta Neuropathol (Berl)* 1998;**95**:450–4.
117. Mattila PM, Roytta M, Torikka H, *et al.* Cortical Lewy bodies and Alzheimer-type changes in patients with Parkinson's disease. *Acta Neuropathol (Berl)* 1998;**95**:576–582.
118. Braak H, Rub U, Jansen Steur EN, *et al.* Cognitive status correlates with neuropathologic stage in Parkinson disease. *Neurology* 2005;**64**:1404–10.
119. Galvin JE, Pollack J, Morris JC. Clinical phenotype of Parkinson disease dementia. *Neurology* 2006;**67**:1605–11.
120. Halliday G, Hely M, Reid W, Morris J. The progression of pathology in longitudinally followed patients with Parkinson's disease. *Acta Neuropathol* 2008;**115**:409–15.
121. Ballard C, Ziabreva I, Perry R, Larsen JP, *et al.* Differences in neuropathologic characteristics across the Lewy body dementia spectrum. *Neurology* 2006;**67**:1931–4.
122. Zaccai J, Brayne C, McKeith I, *et al.* Patterns and stages of alpha-synucleinopathy: relevance in a population-based cohort. *Neurology* 2008;**70**:1042–8.
123. Pletnikova O, West N, Lee MK, *et al.* Abeta deposition is associated with enhanced cortical alpha-synuclein lesions in Lewy body diseases. *Neurobiol Aging* 2005;**26**:1183–92.
124. Kalaitzakis ME, Graeber MB, Gentleman SM, Pearce RK. Striatal beta-amyloid deposition in Parkinson disease with dementia. *J Neuropathol Exp Neurol* 2008;**67**:155–61.
125. Jellinger KA, Attems J. Does striatal pathology distinguish Parkinson disease with dementia and dementia with Lewy bodies? *Acta Neuropathol* 2006;**112**:253–60.
126. Selkoe DJ. Soluble oligomers of the amyloid beta-protein impair synaptic plasticity and behavior. *Behav Brain Res* 2008;**192**:106–13.
127. Danzer KM, Haasen D, Karow AR, *et al.* Different species of alpha-synuclein oligomers induce calcium influx and seeding. *J Neurosci* 2007;**27**:9220–32.
128. Outeiro TF, Putcha P, Tetzlaff JE, *et al.* Formation of toxic oligomeric alpha-synuclein species in living cells. *PLoS ONE* 2008;**3**:e1867.
129. Volles MJ, Lansbury PT Jr. Zeroing in on the pathogenic form of alpha-synuclein and its mechanism of neurotoxicity in Parkinson's disease. *Biochemistry* 2003;**42**:7871–8.
130. Waxman EA, Giasson BI. Molecular mechanisms of alpha-synuclein neurodegeneration. *Biochim Biophys Acta*. 2008;**1792**:616–24.
131. Hyman BT, Trojanowski JQ. Consensus recommendations for the postmortem diagnosis of Alzheimer disease from the National Institute on Aging and the Reagan Institute Working Group on diagnostic criteria for the neuropathological assessment of Alzheimer disease. *J Neuropathol Exp Neurol* 1997;**56**:1095–7.
132. Braak H, Braak E. Frequency of stages of Alzheimer-related lesions in different age categories. *Neurobiol Aging* 1997;**18**:351–7.
133. Edison P, Rowe CC, Rinne JO, *et al.* Amyloid load in Parkinson's disease dementia and Lewy body dementia measured with [^{11}C]PIB positron emission tomography. *J Neurol Neurosurg Psychiatry* 2008;**79**:1331–8.
134. Gomperts SN, Rentz DM, Moran E, *et al.* Imaging amyloid deposition in Lewy body diseases. *Neurology* 2008;**71**:903–10.
135. Gearing M, Levey AI, Mirra SS. Diffuse plaques in the striatum in Alzheimer disease (AD): relationship to the striatal mosaic and selected neuropeptide markers. *J Neuropathol Exp Neurol* 1997;**56**:1363–70.
136. Masliah E, Rockenstein E, Veinbergs I, *et al.* Beta-amyloid peptides enhance alpha-synuclein accumulation and neuronal

deficits in a transgenic mouse model linking Alzheimer's disease and Parkinson's disease. *Proc Natl Acad Sci USA* 2001;**98**:12245–50.

137. Lewis J, Dickson DW, Lin WL, *et al*. Enhanced neurofibrillary degeneration in transgenic mice expressing mutant tau and APP. *Science* 2001;**293**:1487–91.

138. Jellinger KA. Morphological substrates of dementia in parkinsonism. A critical update. *J Neural Transm Suppl* 1997;**51**:57–82.

139. Perry EK, McKeith I, Thompson P, *et al*. Topography, extent, and clinical relevance of neurochemical deficits in dementia of Lewy body type, Parkinson's disease, and Alzheimer's disease. *Ann N Y Acad Sci* 1991;**640**:197–202.

140. Masliah E, Terry R. The role of synaptic proteins in the pathogenesis of disorders of the central nervous system. *Brain Pathol* 1993;**3**:77–85.

141. Terry RD, Katzman R. Life span and synapses: will there be a primary senile dementia? *Neurobiol Aging* 2001;**22**:347–8.

142. Clayton DF, George JM. The synucleins: a family of proteins involved in synaptic function, plasticity, neurodegeneration and disease. *Trends Neurosci* 1998;**21**:249–54.

143. Wakabayashi K, Honer WG, Masliah E. Synapse alterations in the hippocampal-entorhinal formation in Alzheimer's disease with and without Lewy body disease. *Brain Res* 1994;**667**:24–32.

144. Hansen LA, Daniel SE, Wilcock GK, Love S. Frontal cortical synaptophysin in Lewy body diseases: relation to Alzheimer's disease and dementia. *J Neurol Neurosurg Psychiatry* 1998;**64**:653–6.

145. Braak H, Braak E. Neuropathological stageing of Alzheimer-related changes. *Acta Neuropathol (Berl)* 1991;**82**:239–59.

146. Kosaka K, Yoshimura M, Ikeda K, Budka H. Diffuse type of Lewy body disease: progressive dementia with abundant cortical Lewy bodies and senile changes of varying degree – a new disease? *Clin Neuropathol* 1984;**3**:185–92.

Chapter 15
Treatment of Dementia Associated with Parkinson's Disease

Murat Emre
Istanbul Faculty of Medicine, Department of Neurology, Behavioral Neurology and Movement Disorders Unit, Istanbul University, Çapa Istanbul, Turkey

Introduction

Until recently, treatment of cognitive dysfunction and dementia was not an issue on the agenda of clinicians treating patients with Parkinson's disease (PD). This has changed, however, as both cross-sectional and prospective epidemiological studies revealed the high prevalence and functional significance of mental dysfunction [1,2]. Cognitive impairment and dementia are among the most frequent problems in the later course of the disease and this becomes more relevant as more patients survive to older ages due to more effective treatment of motor symptoms. Cognitive dysfunction is now recognized to be an integral part of PD: in the prospectively followed-up Sydney cohort, 85% of patients were reported to develop cognitive impairment of various degrees 15 years after diagnosis [2]. The realization that PD is not simply a motor disorder prompted searches for the treatment of mental dysfunction. It also resulted in a paradigm shift in the conception of future treatment strategies, demanding a more holistic approach to disease pathology rather than simply rescuing or restoring dopaminergic cells. Although such strategies have not yet borne fruit, we have witnessed several important developments in the past few years with regard to dementia in PD, including the description of clinical diagnostic criteria for this condition [3] and the introduction of the first specific treatment for dementia associated with PD (PDD).

General considerations on the treatment of PDD

It is customary to divide the treatment approaches to neurodegenerative diseases into two sub-categories, disease-modifying and symptomatic treatments. The first approach includes strategies to delay, halt, or reverse the cellular loss, commonly defined as neuroprotective or neurorestorative therapies, whereas the second approach basically encompasses interventions which deal with the consequences of cellular loss. The latter includes treatment of symptoms which are considered to be directly related to cellular–synaptic loss (deficit symptoms such as impaired attention or memory) and those related to malfunctioning of remaining cells due to erratic signal processing, such as psychotic symptoms. Rational drug design strategies to halt the neurodegenerative process require an understanding of pathophysiological events that lead to cell death. Downstream events may be generic to many disorders, whereas understanding of and interfering with more upstream processes may result in more specific interventions. A popular starting point for neurodegenerative diseases characterized by accumulation of intra- or extracellular proteins is to understand the nature, mechanisms, and consequences of abnormal protein aggregation.

Although Alzheimer-type pathology, in particular amyloid plaques, is frequently coexistent, the main pathology associated with PDD is Lewy bodies (LBs) in limbic and cerebral cortical areas [4]. The main constituent of LBs is α-synuclein, which abnormally misfolds and accumulates in these intracellular inclusion bodies. As yet, there is no treatment method in clinical testing to inhibit or reverse the accumulation of α-synuclein. Furthermore, it is also unknown if this would favorably affect the disease progression as the causative role of α-synuclein aggregation in the disease process is still not certain.

Hence, with the lack of any disease-modifying agents directed against the disease pathology, the current therapeutic approaches consist of symptomatic treatment. This can also be divided into two main groups: specific or neurotransmitter-based substitution therapy based on the neurochemical deficits associated with PDD, and

Parkinson's Disease: Non-Motor and Non-Dopaminergic Features, First Edition. Edited by C. Warren Olanow, Fabrizio Stocchi, and Anthony E. Lang.

non-specific treatment targeted at behavioral symptoms frequently present in this disorder.

Specific treatment

Biochemical deficits in PDD

Biochemically, impairments in practically all ascending monoaminergic pathways have been suggested to be associated with PDD. The presence and magnitude of such deficits, however, have not been consistent, as deficits reported in some studies for one or the other system have not been confirmed in other studies [4,5]. These deficits are likely to exist to variable extents across patients. It has been suggested that each of them may contribute to certain aspects of the disease, for example, serotoninergic deficits to mood disorder, noradrenergic deficits to impaired attention and mood, and cholinergic deficits to impaired memory, attention, and executive functions [6].

Overall, the most consistent findings have been those demonstrating cholinergic deficits. Morphologically, a prominent loss of cholinergic neurones in the nucleus basalis of Meynert (nbM) was reported in 1983 [7]. This cellular loss was subsequently found to be associated with the loss of cholinergic markers, as demonstrated by reduced cholinacetyltransferase (ChAT) and acetylcholinesterase (AChE) activity in nbM and in the cerebral cortex, the severity of which positively correlated with the severity of dementia [8,9]. Comparative studies, both *in vitro* and *in vivo*, revealed the relative magnitude of these deficits across common forms of dementia. In a postmortem study, mean midfrontal ChAT activity was found to be markedly reduced in patients with PD and dementia with Lewy bodies (DLB) as compared with normal controls; interestingly, this reduction was more extensive than that seen in patients with Alzheimer's disease (AD), which is the prototypical disorder with cholinergic deficits [10]. Functional imaging studies with PET revealed similar findings: compared with controls, mean cortical AChE activity was lowest in patients with PDD, followed by patients with PD without dementia and AD patients with equal severity of dementia [11]. In a subsequent study, the same researchers were able to show that the degree of cortical cholinergic deficits correlated particularly well with typical cognitive deficits found in PDD, such as impaired performance on tests of attention and executive functions [12].

Clinical studies with cholinesterase inhibitors

As the evidence suggesting cholinergic deficits to be the main biochemical substrate of cognitive dysfunction in PD mounted, the obvious therapeutic consequence was the investigation of cholinergic substitution therapy in these patients. Previous attempts with other cholinergic strategies such as the acetylcholine precursors lecithin and choline, and nicotinergic or muscarinergic receptor agonists, had failed in AD trials. Cholinesterase inhibitors (ChE-I) emerged as the sole method of enhancing cholinergic neurotransmission with proven clinical efficacy in AD. These substances inhibit the enzyme acetylcholinesterase, which breaks down acetylcholine in the synaptic cleft, terminating its post-synaptic effects. Through this inhibition, the synaptic half-life of acetylcholine is prolonged. Following the establishment of ChE-I as standard therapy in AD, they were also investigated in PDD, despite initial worries that enhanced cholinergic activity might worsen motor symptoms. Following a small, open-label study with the first clinically available ChE-I, tacrine [13], which reported favorable effects on mental symptoms without worsening of motor functions, all available ChE-I, including donepezil, rivastigmine, and galantamine, have been tested in PDD, mostly in the form of open-label and, in a few, randomized, placebo–controlled studies in small samples. Despite their methodological limitations with regard to open-label design or small sample size, a consistent pattern emerged in these studies suggesting favorable effects on cognitive and behavioral symptoms; worsening of motor symptoms such as increased tremor was observed in only a small proportion of cases. An overall analysis of these earlier studies concluded that treatment with ChE-I may provide improvements in cognitive and behavioral symptoms without having detrimental effects on motor functions in the majority of patients [14]. These preliminary findings prompted the initiation of large-scale studies, one with rivastigmine and the other with donepezil.

The first large, randomized, placebo-controlled, double-blind study in patients with PDD was conducted with rivastigmine, which inhibits both acetyl- and butyrylcholinesterase [15]. In this multicenter study, denoted EXPRESS and performed in 12 countries, 541 patients with mild to moderate PDD were assigned to receive rivastigmine or placebo over 24 weeks, with an unequal randomization ratio of 2:1. Rivastigmine was slowly titrated with monthly increments of 3 mg per day over the first 16 weeks up to 12 mg per day and then maintained at the highest tolerated dose for a further 8 weeks. Primary efficacy parameters included Alzheimer's Disease Assessment Scale – Cognitive Subscale (ADAS-cog) for the assessment of cognitive functions and Alzheimer's Disease Collaborative Study – Clinical Global Impression of Change (ADCS-CGIC) for the assessment of overall changes from baseline. There were a number of secondary efficacy parameters which assessed different aspects of dementia. These included Mini Mental State Examination (MMSE) for screening and staging, an activities of daily living (ADL) scale to assess activities of daily living (ADCS-ADL), Neuropsychiatric Inventory (NPI) to capture behavioral symptoms, a computerized test battery for the assessment of attention (CDR battery), and two tests for the assessment of executive functions, namely verbal fluency and Ten Point Clock Drawing test. In addition to standard safety measures, Part III (motor section) of the Unified Parkinson's Disease Rating Scale (UPDRS) was used in order to evaluate motor functions objectively.

Of the 541 randomized patients, 410 completed the study as per protocol. Premature discontinuations, 131 in total, were more frequent in the rivastigmine group (27.3% versus 17.9% under placebo), and this was also the case for discontinuations due to adverse events (17.1% versus 7.8% under placebo). Both primary endpoints showed statistically significant improvements in favor of rivastigmine. On the composite cognitive scale, ADAS-cog, patients on rivastigmine showed a 2.1 point improvement at week 24. whereas patients on placebo deteriorated by 0.7 points ($p < 0.001$). The mean score for the 7-point ADCS-CGIC at week 24 was 3.8 in the rivastigmine group and 4.3 in the placebo group (score 4 indicating no change, lower scores indicating improvement, and higher scores indicating worsening from baseline). More patients on rivastigmine showed any degree of improvement (40.8% versus 29.7% on placebo) and more patients on placebo had deteriorated (42.5% on placebo versus 33.7% on rivastigmine) ($p = 0.007$). Similarly, all secondary efficacy measures revealed statistically significant differences in favor of rivastigmine: neuropsychiatric symptoms as assessed by NPI showed an improvement on rivastigmine and no change from baseline on placebo, and there were improvements in Ten Point Clock Drawing test, verbal fluency, attention tests, and MMSE scores on rivastigmine, whereas patients on placebo worsened compared with baseline. The ADL scores showed a minimal worsening in patients on rivastigmine, whereas those on placebo showed significantly greater worsening. Adverse events were significantly more frequent on rivastigmine; the main adverse events were gastrointestinal led by nausea and vomiting (29.0% versus 11.2% nausea, and 16.6% versus 1.7% vomiting on rivastigmine and placebo, respectively). In general, worsening of parkinsonian symptoms was reported more frequently as an adverse event on rivastigmine (27.3% versus 15.6% on placebo), basically driven by worsening of tremor (10.2% on rivastigmine versus 3.9% on placebo). The objective measures of motor symptoms, however, as assessed by UPDRS Part III, did not reveal any significant differences between the two treatments. Interestingly, orthostatic hypotension, syncope, and deaths were slightly more frequent in the placebo group [16]. Vital signs, body weight, ECG, and laboratory assessments did not reveal any clinically relevant changes.

In order to assess the long-term effects of rivastigmine, the EXPRESS study was extended for an additional 6 months, where all patients (including those who were assigned to placebo during the double-blind phase) received rivastigmine. All patients were re-titrated in order to maintain the original treatment assignment blinded. The results demonstrated that the beneficial effects seen during the first 6 months were by and large maintained, although there was some decline from the initial improvement. Patients who initially received placebo and then switched to rivastigmine showed a comparable benefit to those who had been on rivastigmine for the whole duration of the study, but not in all parameters, suggesting potential benefits of earlier treatment initiation [17]. The analysis of adverse events during the extension phase, with particular emphasis on motor symptoms, revealed that worsening tremor as an adverse event occurred more frequently on previously placebo-treated patients, and the frequency was lower in those who were treated with rivastigmine from the beginning. Importantly, there was no evidence of worsening motor function over the course of 1 year of treatment [18]. A subsequent study in PDD patients, with quantified assessments of tremor, confirmed that there may be a slight worsening of tremor under rivastigmine treatment [19].

The EXPRESS study provided a large database on which several sub-analyses were subsequently performed. One of these analyses was based on the hypothesis that visual hallucinations may be associated with more severe cholinergic deficits, and such patients may benefit more from cholinergic treatment. A comparison of patients who had visual hallucinations at baseline with those who did not, showed that hallucinators drew more benefits in cognitive outcomes, and this was mainly driven by a more rapid decline from baseline in the hallucinating group [20]. Impairment in attentional functions is one of the main deficits in patients with PDD. Hence a more in-depth analysis of rivastigmine's effects on various aspects of attention was performed, as assessed by a computerized test battery during the study. This analysis revealed that all tested aspects of attention (including focused attention, sustained attention, consistency of responding, and central processing speed) improved significantly under rivastigmine treatment [21]. Another sub-analysis using the baseline data from EXPRESS assessed the correlation between various cognitive domains and activities of daily living, The results demonstrated that impaired attention is an important determinant of ADL in patients with PDD, putting the improvement in attentional functions in a clinical perspective [22].

On the basis of the EXPRESS study, rivastigmine was granted a marketing approval for treatment of patients with mild to moderate PDD, both in the European Union and the United States, becoming the first specific treatment for this condition. In the meantime, a patch form of rivastigmine has also become available, which has been approved for PDD in a number of countries.

Previously, two small randomized, placebo-controlled studies in PD patients with cognitive impairment [23,24] and one small placebo-controlled, cross-over study in patients with PDD [25] demonstrated beneficial effects of donepezil on mental functions. Subsequently, a large randomized, double-blind, placebo-controlled study in PDD was conducted with donepezil. The results have not yet been published, but reported in abstract form [26]. This was also a 24-week study, in which 550 patients with mild to moderate PDD (MMSE range 10–26) were randomized into three groups to receive either placebo, donepezil 5 mg, or donepezil 10 mg. The primary efficacy parameters were ADAS-cog and an overall measure of change from baseline, Clinician Interview Based Impression of Change-plus (CIBIC-plus); secondary measures included tests for attention, working memory, executive and visuo-spatial functions, Disability Assessment for Dementia (DAD) scale to assess activities of daily living, NPI for behavioral symptoms, and MMSE as a general measure. UPDRS Part III was included to assess the effects of donepezil on motor function.

At week 24, there was a 0.3 score improvement in ADAS-cog under placebo, a 2.45 score improvement under 5 mg, and a 3.72 score improvement under 10 mg donepezil. The difference between placebo and the donepezil groups, however, did not reach statistical significance in the primary analysis of efficacy; type II weighted analysis and omission of country interaction resulted in significance ($p < 0.001$). The second primary endpoint CIBIC-plus showed statistically significant superiority for 10 mg, but not for 5 mg donepezil. Statistically significant differences in favor of donepezil were also found on MMSE, Brief Test of Attention and Verbal Fluency Test, whereas there were no statistically significant differences from placebo on the activities of daily living scale DAD and the behavioral scale NPI. UPDRS Part III scores did not reveal any significant worsening of motor functions under donepezil.

Effects of donepezil on central processing speed and other attentional measures were evaluated using computerized tests in an open-label study over 20 weeks of treatment. Compared with baseline, power of attention, continuity of attention, and reaction time variability were found to have improved after donepezil treatment [27].

Other neurotransmitter-based treatment approaches

Dopaminergic, noradrenergic, and serotoninergic deficits have all been suggested to be associated with PDD, or at least to underlie some of the symptoms seen in demented PD patients.

The effects of dopaminergic treatment on mental functions have hardly been studied in patients with PDD; most formal studies have been performed in non-demented patients. The results have been equivocal, describing either no effects, or improvement in some and worsening in other functions. In one of the few studies which specifically included demented patients, 22 subjects with PD, 27 with PDD, and 11 with DLB were tested for cognitive functions and behavioral symptoms after acute L-dopa challenge and following 3 months of treatment. After acute challenge, patients reported improvement in subjective alertness, but fluctuations increased; reaction time and accuracy remained unchanged in those with PDD. After 3 months of treatment, neuropsychiatric scores improved in both PD and PDD, mean global cognitive score was better, but attention and memory scores were worse in PD patients without dementia. Reaction time became slower in those with PDD; there were, however, no patients with marked deterioration. The authors concluded that L-dopa does not adversely affect cognitive function in PDD [28].

There have been no studies investigating the effect of serotoninergic or noradrenergic substitution therapy in patients with PDD, partly because of a lack of appropriate substances such as selective noradrenergic agents.

The other treatment modality approved for AD, the NMDA antagonist memantine, has not yet been tested in large, randomized, controlled studies in PDD. Conflicting results have been described in a small number of case reports or case series in patients with DLB, reporting both worsening and improvement [29,30]. In a small case series, good tolerability and possible benefits have been suggested in patients with PDD [31]. A large randomized, controlled trial with memantine in patients with PDD and DLB is currently under way.

Another substance with antagonistic effects at NMDA receptors, amantadine, which is being used increasingly to treat levodopa-induced dyskinesias, was evaluated in a retrospective study. A total of 593 PD patients were included in this analysis, 263 of whom had received amantadine treatment. In the total of 116 patients who developed dementia, the time to onset of dementia was 9.1 years in the amantadine group versus 5.9 years in those who had never received amantadine. Duration of amantadine exposure positively correlated with time to dementia; in the survival analysis, mental decline was slower in the group which was ever exposed to amantadine and the MMSE scores were also significantly higher. The authors concluded that amantadine use may delay the onset of dementia in PD and may attenuate its severity [32]. Given the retrospective nature of the study, however, these results should be interpreted with caution until they are confirmed in prospective studies.

Safinamide, a new, selective, and reversible monoamine oxidase type B (MAO-B) inhibitor that also inhibits glutamate release, is currently under development for treatment of PD. In a recent placebo-controlled trial in which safinamide or placebo were added to treatment in patients with early PD stabilized on a single dopamine agonist, cognitive functions were evaluated using a cognitive test battery. A preliminary analysis in 123 patients revealed that there were trends or significant improvements in tests of spatial working memory, verbal working memory, and executive functions in patients treated with safinamide [33]. Although this study was not in patients with PDD, the results are encouraging and merit further study of safinamide in this population.

Non-specific treatment

Treatment of behavioral symptoms

Neuropsychiatric and behavioral symptoms such as psychosis, depressive features, apathy, and sleep–wake cycle disturbances are frequently encountered problems in patients with PDD [34]. Their management is described in detail in other chapters. The principles of pharmacological treatment will be briefly mentioned here, emphasizing particular aspects relevant for demented patients.

Psychotic symptoms such as visual hallucinations may improve under treatment with ChE-I. Hence treatment with a ChE-I should be considered first in PDD patients with hallucinations before reverting to anti-psychotics. Neuroleptic treatment, however, may sometimes become unavoidable, especially in patients with overt psychosis or psychotic agitation. Classical neuroleptics are prohibited as they worsen motor function and may result in life-threatening neuroleptic hypersensitivity. Although most new generation or "atypical" neuroleptics have been tried to treat psychosis in patients with PD in some form, specific studies in PDD populations are scarce; those mentioned below were basically performed in PD patients with hallucinations or psychosis, not selected for the presence or absence of dementia. Randomized, placebo-controlled studies showing significant improvement of psychosis in PD without worsening of motor symptoms exist only for clozapine [35,36]. In controlled trials, olanzapine did not significantly improve psychosis, but worsened motor function [37,38]; risperidone also is associated with a high risk of worsening motor symptoms [39,40]. In two small randomized, placebo-controlled studies, quetiapine up to 200 mg was not found to be more effective than placebo against hallucinations or psychosis, but it did not worsen motor symptoms [41,42]. Two small comparative trials against clozapine revealed that it may improve psychosis, less so than clozapine, without worsening parkinsonism [43,44]. In a retrospective analysis of all PD patients receiving quetiapine in a single center, more quetiapine non-responders were found in those who had dementia and motor worsening also tended to occur more frequently in demented patients [45]. Finally, in one open-label [46] and one randomized, placebo-controlled study [47], both of which included patients with PDD, quetiapine did not show significant benefits for treating agitation or psychosis; motor symptoms did not worsen. In a systematic review of atypical neuroleptics for the treatment of psychosis in PD, clozapine was concluded to be the only drug with proven efficacy and acceptable tolerability provided that appropriate safety monitoring is performed [48].

Although disorders of affective and depressive features are amongst the most frequent behavioral symptoms in PD and PDD, surprisingly there have been no randomized, controlled studies of anti-depressants in these populations. A meta-analysis of all available studies conducted in PD patients with depression revealed large effect sizes, under both active treatment and placebo; however, there were no statistically significant differences between them. Increasing age and major depression predicted better response [49]. In another systematic review performed by the American Academy of Neurology Quality Standards Sub-committee, amitriptyline was found to be the only compound with evidence of efficacy in PD depression [50]. Tricyclic antidepressants such as amitriptyline, however, should be avoided in patients with PDD because of their anti-cholinergic effects and their potential to worsen cognition. Selective serotonin and selective serotonin and noradrenaline re-uptake inhibitors (SSRIs and SNRIs) should be preferred, taking into account their adverse effects and other concomitant medication such as MAO-B inhibitors.

Treatment of excessive daytime sleepiness

Excessive daytime sleepiness is a frequent problem in PDD, and it probably occurs more often in demented patients than those without dementia. Although not specifically tested in PDD, modafinil, an agent which promotes wakefulness, can be considered to treat excessive daytime sleepiness. In studies performed in non-demented PD patients, modafinil was found to be significantly better than placebo in two small randomized, placebo-controlled and one open-label study [51–53], although no difference was found in another small placebo-controlled trial [54]. The drug was well tolerated in all patients.

Conclusion

Dementia is an integral part of the disease spectrum in PD, affecting approximately one-third of patients in cross-sectional studies. Cognitive impairment of variable degrees develops in 85% of patients 15 years following the diagnosis. Currently, there is no treatment which halts or reverses the disease pathology to avoid development of dementia. Symptomatic treatment approaches are based on substituting accompanying neurotransmitter deficits or ameliorating associated behavioral symptoms. The most prominent biochemical deficits are cholinergic; treatment with ChE-I has been shown to provide mild to moderate benefits in cognitive and behavioral symptoms without undue worsening in motor functions. Based on a large randomized, placebo-controlled trial, the ChE-I rivastigmine has been approved for the treatment of PDD, becoming the first specific therapy registered for this condition. Patients with PDD should be offered treatment with ChE-I, taking into account expected therapeutic benefits and any potential tolerability issues. Rivastigmine should be started with 1.5 mg b.i.d., and the dose should be increased by 3 mg per day at monthly intervals up to 12 mg per day. Although no significant deterioration of motor symptoms was reported in clinical trials, motor functions should be monitored in order not to overlook individual sensitivities, in particular worsening of tremor, which may occur in a small proportion of patients.

References

1. Aarsland D, Zaccai J, Brayne C. A systematic review of prevalence studies of dementia in Parkinson's disease. *Mov Disord* 2005;**20**:1255–63.
2. Hely MA, Morris JG, Reid WG, Trafficante R. Sydney Multicenter Study of Parkinson's disease: non-L-dopa-responsive problems dominate at 15 years. *Mov Disord* 2005;**20**(2):190–9.
3. Emre M, Aarsland D, Brown R, *et al.* Clinical diagnostic criteria for dementia associated with Parkinson's disease. *Mov Disord* 2007;**22**:1689–707.
4. Emre M. What causes mental dysfunction in Parkinson's disease? *Mov Disord* 2003;**18**(Suppl 6):S63–71.
5. Emre M. Dementia associated with Parkinson's disease. *Lancet Neurol* 2003;**2**:229–37.
6. Pillon B, Boller F, Levy R, Dubois B. Cognitive deficits and dementia in Parkinson's disease. In: Boller F, Cappa S, eds. *Handbook of Neuropsychology*, 2nd edn. Amsterdam: Elsevier Sciences, 2001: 311–71.
7. Whitehouse PJ, Hedreen JC, White CL III, Price DL. Basal forebrain neurons in the dementia of Parkinson disease. *Ann Neurol* 1983;**13**:243–8.
8. Perry EK, Curtis M, Dick DJ, Candy JM, *et al.* Cholinergic correlates of cognitive impairment in Parkinson's disease: comparisons with Alzheimer's disease. *J Neurol Neurosurg Psychiatry* 1985;**48**:413–21.
9. Perry RH, Perry EK, Smith CJ, *et al.* Cortical neuropathological and neurochemical substrates of Alzheimer's and Parkinson's diseases. *J Neural Transm Suppl* 1987;**24**:131–6.
10. Tiraboschi P, Hansen LA, Alford M, *et al.* Cholinergic dysfunction in diseases with Lewy bodies. *Neurology* 2000;**54**:407–11.
11. Bohnen NI, Kaufer DI, Ivanco LS, *et al.* Cortical cholinergic function is more severely affected in parkinsonian dementia than in Alzheimer disease: an *in vivo* positron emission tomographic study. *Arch Neurol* 2003;**60**:1745–8.
12. Bohnen NI, Kaufer DI, Hendrickson R, *et al.* Cognitive correlates of cortical cholinergic denervation in Parkinson's disease and parkinsonian dementia. *J Neurol* 2006;**253**(2):242–7.
13. Hutchinson M, Fazzini E. Cholinesterase inhibition in Parkinson's disease. *J Neurol Neurosurg Psychiatry* 1996;**61**(3):324–5.
14. Aarsland D, Mosimann UP, McKeith IG. Role of cholinesterase inhibitors in Parkinson's disease and dementia with Lewy bodies. *J Geriatr Psychiatry Neurol* 2004;**17**:164–71.
15. Emre M, Aarsland D, Albanese A, *et al.* Rivastigmine for dementia associated with Parkinson's disease. *N Engl J Med* 2004;**351**:2509–18.
16. Ballard C, Lane R, Barone P, *et al.* Cardiac safety of rivastigmine in Lewy body and Parkinson's disease dementias. *Int J Clin Pract* 2006;**60**:639–45.
17. Poewe W, Wolters E, Emre M, *et al.* Long-term benefits of rivastigmine in dementia associated with Parkinson's disease: an active treatment extension study. *Mov Disord* 2005;**21**(4):456–61.
18. Oertel W, Poewe W, Wolters E, *et al.* Effects of rivastigmine on tremor and other motor symptoms in patients with Parkinson's disease dementia. A retrospective analysis of a double-blind trial and open-label extension. *Drug Saf* 2008;**31**:79–94.
19. Gurevich TY, Shabtai H, Korczyn A, *et al.* Effect of rivastigmine on tremor in patients with Parkinson's disease and dementia. *Mov Disord* 2006;**21**:1663–6.
20. Burn D, Emre M, McKeith I, *et al.* Effects of rivastigmine in patients with and without visual hallucinations in dementia associated with Parkinson's disease. *Mov Disord* 2006;**21**(11):1899–907.
21. Wesnes KA, McKeith I, Edgar C, *et al.* Benefits of rivastigmine on attention in dementia associated with Parkinson disease. *Neurology* 2005;**65**:1654–6.
22. Bronnick K, Ehrt U, Emre M, *et al.* Attentional deficits affect activities of daily living in dementia-associated with Parkinson's disease. *J Neurol Neurosurg Psychiatry* 2006;**77**:1136–42.
23. Aarsland D, Laake K, Larsen JP, Janvin C. Donepezil for cognitive impairment in Parkinson's disease: a randomised controlled study. *J Neurol Neurosurg Psychiatry* 2002;**72**:708–12.
24. Leroi I, Brandt J, Reich SG, *et al.* Randomized placebo-controlled trial of donepezil in cognitive impairment in Parkinson's disease. *Int J Geriatr Psychiatry* 2004;**19**(1):1–8.
25. Ravina B, Putt M, Siderowf A, *et al.* Donepezil for dementia in Parkinson's disease: a randomised, double blind, placebo controlled, crossover study. *J Neurol Neurosurg Psychiatry* 2005;**76**:934–9.
26. Dubois B, Tolosa E, Kulisevsky J, et al. Efficacy and safety of donepezil in the treatment o Parkinson's disease patients with dementia. Poster presented at AD–PD, Salzburg, 14–18 March 2007.
27. Rowan E, McKeith IG, Saxby BK, *et al.* Effects of donepezil on central processing speed and attentional measures in Parkinson's disease with dementia and dementia with Lewy bodies. *Dement Geriatr Cogn Disord* 2007;**23**:161–7.
28. Molloy SA, Rowan EN, O'Brien JT, *et al.* Effect of levodopa on cognitive function in Parkinson's disease with and without dementia and dementia with Lewy bodies. *J Neurol Neurosurg Psychiatry* 2006;**77**:1323–8.
29. Ridha BH, Josephs KA, Rossor MN. Delusions and hallucinations in dementia with Lewy bodies: worsening with memantine. *Neurology* 2005;**65**(3):481–2.
30. Sabbagh MN, Hake AM, Ahmed S, Farlow MR. The use of memantine in dementia with Lewy bodies. *J Alzheimers Dis* 2005;**7**(4):285–9.

31. Fox CG, Umoh G, Samuel M, *et al.* Memantine in Parkinson's disease dementia: clinical experience. *Mov Disorders* 2005;**20**(Suppl 10):P418.
32. Inzelberg R, Bonucelli U, Schechtman E, *et al.* Association between amantadine and the onset of dementia in Parkinson's disease. *Mov Disord* 2006;**21**:1375–9.
33. Sharma T, Anand R, Stocchi F, *et al.* Cognitive effects of safinamide in early Parkinson's disease (PD) patients. *Mov Disord* 2007;**22**(Suppl 16):S236.
34. Aarsland D, Bronnick K, Ehrt U, *et al.* Neuropsychiatric symptoms in patients with Parkinson's disease and dementia: frequency, profile and associated care giver stress. *J Neurol Neurosurg Psychiatry* 2007;**78**(1):36–42.
35. The Parkinson Study Group. Low-dose clozapine for the treatment of drug-induced psychosis in Parkinson's disease. *N Engl J Med* 1999;**340**:757–63.
36. The French Clozapine Parkinson Study Group. Clozapine in drug-induced psychosis in Parkinson's disease. *Lancet* 1999;**353**:2041–2.
37. Ondo WG, Levy JK, Vuong KD, *et al.* Olanzapine treatment for dopaminergic-induced hallucinations. *Mov Disord* 2002;**17**:1031–5.
38. Breier A, Sutton VK, Feldman PD, *et al.* Olanzapine in the treatment of dopamimetic-induced psychosis in patients with Parkinson's disease. *Biol Psychiatry* 2002;**52**:438–45.
39. Ellis T, Cudkowicz ME, Sexton PM, Growdon JH. Clozapine and risperidone treatment of psychosis in Parkinson's disease. *J. Neuropsychiatry Clin Neurosci* 2000;**12**:364–9.
40. Friedman JH, Fernandez HH. Atypical antipsychotics in Parkinson-sensitive populations. *J Geriatr Psychiatry Neurol* 2002;**15**:156–70.
41. Ondo WG, Tintner R, Voung KD, *et al.* Double-blind, placebo-controlled, unforced titration parallel tiral of quetiapine for dopaminergic-induced hallucinations in Parkinson's disease. *Mov Disord* 2005;**20**:958–63.
42. Rabey JM, Prokhorov T, Miniovitz A, *et al.* Effect of quetiapine in psychotic Parkinson's disease patients: a double-blind labeled study of 3 months duration. *Mov Disord* 2007;**22**:313–8.
43. Morgante L, Epifanio A, Spina E, *et al.* Quetiapine and clozapine in parkinsonian patients with dopaminergic psychosis. *Clin Nueropharmacol* 2004;**27**:153–6.
44. Merims D, Balas M, Peretz C, *et al.* Rater-blinded, prospective comparison: quetiapine versus clozapine for Parkinson's disease psychosis. *Clin Neuropharmacol* 2006;**29**(6): 331–7.
45. Fernandez HH, Trieschamann ME, Burke MA, *et al.* Long-term outcome of quetiapine use for psychosis among Parkinsonian patients. *Mov Disord* 2003;**18**:510–4.
46. Prohorov T, Klein C, Miniovitz A, *et al.* The effect of quetiapine in psychotic Parkinsonian patients with and without dementia. An open-labeled study utilizing a structured interview. *J Neurol* 2006;**253**:171–5.
47. Kurlan R, Cummings J, Raman R, Thal L; Alzheimer's Disease Cooperative Study Group. Quetiapine for agitation or psychosis in patients with dementia and parkinsonism. *Neurology* 2007;**68**:1356–63.
48. Goetz CG, Koller WC, Poewe W, *et al.* Drugs to treat dementia and psychosis. *Mov Disord* 2002;**17**(Suppl 4):120–7.
49. Weintraub D, Morales KH, Moberg PJ, *et al.* Antidepressant studies in Parkinsons's disease: a review and meta-analysis. *Mov Disord* 2005;**20**(9):1161–9.
50. Miyasaki JM, Shannon K, Voon V, *et al.* Practice Parameter: evaluation and treatment of depression, psychosis, and dementia in Parkinson disease (an evidence-based review): report of the Quality Standards Subcommittee of the American Academy of Neurology. *Neurology* 2006;**66**(7):996–1002.
51. Hogl B, Saletu M, Brandauer E, *et al.* Modafinil for the treatment of daytime sleepiness in Parkinson's disease: a double-blind, randomized, cross-over, placebo-controlled, polygraphic trial. *Sleep* 2002;**25**:905–9.
52. Adler CH, Caviness JN, Hentz JG, *et al.* Randomized trial of modafinil for treating subjective daytime sleepiness in patients with Parkinson's disease. *Mov Disord* 2003;**18**(3):287–93.
53. Nieves AV, Lang AE. Treatment of excessive daytime sleepiness in patients with Parkinson's disease with modafinil. *Clin Neuropharmacol* 2002;**25**(2):111–4.
54. Ondo WG, Fayle R, Atassi F, Jankovic J. Modafinil for daytime somnolence in Parkinson's disease: double blind, placebo controlled parallel trial. *J Neurol Neurosurg Psychiatry* 2005;**76**(12):1636–9.

Chapter 16
Psychosis in Parkinson's Disease

Joseph H. Friedman
Movement Disorders Program, Butler Hospital, and Department of Neurology, Warren Alpert Medical School of Brown University, Providence, RI, USA

Introduction

Psychotic symptoms occur in Parkinson's disease (PD) in three settings. Most commonly a patient with PD develops these problems while taking medications to improve motor function. Another common scenario is the PD patient who becomes demented, and as part of the dementia syndrome often compounded by PD medications, develops psychotic symptoms. Less common, but not often written about, is the patient with a primary psychotic disorder such as schizophrenia who develops PD [1].

Over the course of the twentieth century, the term "psychosis" has been variably defined. Psychotic symptoms refer to four general types of phenomena: hallucinations, delusions, thought disorder, and grossly disorganized or catatonic behavior [2]. In PD, psychosis primarily involves hallucinations and delusions [3–7]. The prevalence and features of thought disorder in PD have not been well studied and could easily be misdiagnosed in some patients. This is because patients with dementia and/or delirium, who are more likely to have psychotic symptoms, often have memory and attentional problems that manifest with vague tangential speech and illogicality due to inability to sustain a cogent thought [8]. This pattern of disturbance resembles a formal thought disorder. Abnormal motor behavior is intrinsic to PD and may or may not reflect a psychotic syndrome.

The term "psychotic," as applied to an individual, is not endorsed by psychiatrists. They prefer to employ the label "psychotic syndromes," which are those syndromes in which patients display psychotic symptoms. Until recently, the diagnosis of psychosis rested on the loss of reality testing, leading to impairment in social interactions accompanied by psychotic symptoms. Most non-psychiatrists are probably more comfortable with this outdated definition.

The DSM-IV-TR [2] definition of psychosis associated with a medical condition requires the presence of psychotic symptoms, hallucinations, or delusions in a patient who is not delirious. A group of experts, assembled to define the syndrome of psychosis in PD, characterized it by the presence of a psychotic symptom that was recurrent or continuous for at least 1 month without other evident explanations [9] (see Box 16.1). Hallucinations, in this definition, include "presence hallucinations" and illusions (see below). Three subtypes of psychosis were then defined: (a) with or without dementia; (b) with or without insight; (c) taking or not taking drug treatment for PD. Although the occurrence of psychosis in PD in patients not on anti-PD medications only rarely occurs [10,11], the recommended diagnostic criteria nevertheless include the taking of anti-PD medication as a modifying code.

Part of the problem with nomenclature at this time is the uncertain overlap between Parkinson's disease with dementia (PDD) and dementia with Lewy bodies (DLB). The diagnosis of DLB rests on the development of dementia before, or within 12 months of, the onset of parkinsonism, and is not necessarily a fundamentally different condition from PDD [12]. Although the cardinal features of DLB (episodes of unresponsiveness, marked fluctuations in level of cognitive dysfunction, parkinsonism) are often not present, especially early in the disease, the development of visual hallucinations prior to the institution of anti-PD medications is a major diagnostic clue that DLB is likely to be the correct diagnosis. Since the clinical and pathological overlap between DLB and PDD is most obvious in the settings of psychotic symptoms and dementia [13,14], the use of the modifying code, taking or not taking anti-PD medications, is important although arguable. There are very few data on the occurrence of hallucinations and delusions in PD patients not taking anti-PD medications [10,11] because it is usually difficult to stop medications in advanced PD patients where the problem is most common. During the 1980s, "drug holidays" [15,16] were used primarily to treat motor fluctuations but were occasionally used to treat psychotic symptoms. Psychotic features generally reverted during the drug

Parkinson's Disease: Non-Motor and Non-Dopaminergic Features, First Edition. Edited by C. Warren Olanow, Fabrizio Stocchi, and Anthony E. Lang.

Box 16.1 Proposed diagnostic criteria for PD associated psychosis

Characteristic symptoms
- Presence of at least one of the following symptoms:
  - Illusions
  - False sense of presence
  - Hallucinations
  - Delusions
- Primary diagnosis of PD meeting UK Brain Bank criteria
- Psychotic symptoms develop after onset of PD
- Duration of psychotic symptoms – 1 month as recurrent or continuous
- Exclusion of other causes such as DLB, primary psychiatric disorders, or a general medical condition, including delirium
- Associate features
  - With/without insight
  - With/without dementia
  - With/without treatment of PD (drug, surgical, other)

Modified from Ravina *et al.* [9]

holiday, but recurred when the drugs were reintroduced at similar doses. This treatment approach fell out of favor so that complete drug withdrawal is rarely performed now. Formal reports on the assessment of hallucinating patients who have been taken off their PD medications have not been published. In PD patients who develop hallucinations within the first year of starting PD medications, and are therefore most likely to be able to stop them without a major motor decline, most often have either primary psychiatric disease or an atypical parkinsonism [17].

Definitions

Hallucinations are sensory phenomena that occur in the absence of any reasonable source for the sensation. These may occur in each of the special senses, namely visual, auditory, olfactory, gustatory, or somatosensory, and may span more than one sense. A new term, "*minor hallucinations*," has been coined [9] to include transient visual hallucinations that are seen only in the peripheral field, and also "*presence hallucinations*," which are not in fact hallucinations, but rather a feeling that there is a person or animal nearby, usually behind the patient. When the patient turns to look at the hallucination or the person presumed to be behind him, there is nothing there.

Illusions refer to distorted sensory inputs, typically misperceiving one shape for another, seeing an animal in a shadow, mistaking a fire hydrant for a child, hearing voices when the sounds are something different. Illusions occur in normal people but not on a routine basis.

Table 16.1 Psychotic symptoms in two parallel drug treatment trials.

Symptom	USA	Europe	Total
Total enrollment	83	77	160
Hallucinations	82	75	98
Visual	81	74	97
Auditory	37	39	48
Tactile	20	16	23
Olfactory	18	7	16
Delusions	61	61	76
Stealing	32	21	33
Not my house	25	21	29
Infidelity	23	23	29
Abandonment	20	21	26
Spouse imposter	15	17	20

Data from Chou *et al.* [6].

Delusions are false or irrational beliefs. These are beliefs that cannot be argued away since they are not based on facts, and no matter how irrational the belief, they are considered indisputable by the affected.

Disordered thinking and *loose associations* are common problems in schizophrenia, referring to illogical thought processes which make a train of thought impossible to follow and empty of content. These do not occur in PD psychosis.

Clinical syndrome of Parkinson's disease psychosis (PDP)

Psychotic symptoms are fairly stereotypic in Parkinson's disease psychosis (PDP). Visual hallucinations are usually the first symptom and may remain the only symptom (see Table 16.1). Unlike the case of primary psychotic disorders such as schizophrenia, psychotic depression, or bipolar disease, hallucinations in PD are usually visual and devoid of emotional content. This latter fact is rarely mentioned in articles on psychotic symptoms in PD and is important. In schizophrenia, for example, the hallucinations are typically voices saying denigrating things about the patient. They are "ego syntonic," meaning that the content of the voices reflects the patient's emotional state. In PD, the hallucinations are typically benign and devoid of emotional connotation.

The visual hallucinations are generally complex and formed, usually in the form of people or animals [3,6,7,9, 18–22]. These are usually seen clearly (even when there are visual acuity problems) as if the person is actually present. Sometimes they are not clearly seen, even when nearby. They are usually silent, tend to appear when the environment is tranquil, and last from seconds to minutes. The hallucinated people generally do not interact with the patient, so that a PD patient may talk to the hallucination but the hallucination will usually ignore the patient as if the patient did not exist. The hallucinations typically disappear when the patient approaches. Interestingly, the hallucinations tend to be fixed for each patient. A patient sees three girls dressed in ballet costumes dancing on her driveway. This occurs two or three times each week, always the same girls dressed in the same outfits. Their behaviors may vary but there will always be some dancing of a similar type. Oftentimes the hallucinations occur outside the house so that there may be a question as to whether a vision is real or not. Scenes such as workmen digging up the garden, children playing in a tree, parades passing a house, are fairly typical of the kinds of hallucinations that PD patients experience. Visions of children are common. Seeing tiny creatures such as ants or bugs on a plain surface is not uncommon. Lilliputian figures are less common but not unusual, so that little people, otherwise normal in appearance, may be seen in a potted plant. In contrast, enlarged figures are rare. Usually the visions do not make sounds, even when they appear to be talking among themselves or slamming doors. Patients will occasionally see objects rather than living things, such as trucks, flowers, or statues.

Auditory hallucinations are less common, but can occur, particularly in people who also have visual hallucinations [23]. Sometimes there are conversations, which are usually appropriate to the hallucinated scene, in which the patient converses with the hallucination. In general, however, auditory hallucinations are completely different in nature to the visual. They are usually not as clearly perceived. Patients hear music or party sounds coming from another part of the house or the next house. They hear unclear voices in the corridor but the content is not intelligible.

Somatosensory hallucinations are very uncommon [6,7]. They usually consist of the feeling that bugs or small animals are crawling on the skin. Gustatory and olfactory hallucinations, are rare, but may also occur. Like the other hallucinations, they are intermittent, not sustained, and tend to be stereotypic for a single individual.

Delusions

Delusions in PD patients tend to be paranoid [6]. A particularly common delusion is of spousal infidelity, which is an extremely challenging problem both for the patient, who feels helpless and betrayed, and for the innocent accused, who reaps this accusation as the reward for years of solicitous care. Other common delusions common to other dementing illnesses include thinking that others are living in the house, that people are spying on them, that money is being stolen, and that objects are being moved around the house as an explanation for why things are so often misplaced (see Table 16.1). Rare delusional syndromes such as reduplication syndromes including Capgras's syndrome, in which people have been replaced by exact duplicates, or Cotard's syndrome, where the patients think that they are dead, have been described. Delusional misidentification syndromes generally appear in PD patients who are demented and also suffering from hallucinations [24]. One self-fulfilling delusion is that the family is trying to abandon the patient. Since psychosis is so stressful for caregivers, this may become reality [25–28]. Unlike schizophrenia, delusions of grandeur, thought broadcasting, religiosity, bizarre delusions (e.g., needing to wear aluminum hats to prevent radiowaves from controlling thoughts), thought control, and so on, do not occur.

"Secondary" delusion is a psychiatric term defining a fixed belief that is based on a fictitious observation that is perceived by the patient. These are not uncommon in PD with psychoses and frequently consist of the belief that hallucinations are real or intermittently real. In this setting, the patient insists that dinner be served to the hallucination, traps be set to catch the rodents that have started running around the kitchen, and salves be placed on the skin to deter the insects that are crawling on their body.

Differential diagnosis of psychosis (Box 16.2)

Delirium

The definition of delirium requires a change from baseline in attention coupled with increased confusion or disorientation, usually with fluctuations [8]. In the typical case of PDP, the sensorium is clear, the scores on cognitive tests such as the MMSE are unchanged from baseline. When a patient is "confused," disoriented, and hallucinating, the diagnosis is usually delirium, which has implications for treatment. The clinical problem is to distinguish the new level of confusion from the old, especially in a demented patient who fluctuates from day to day and from hour to hour. "Sundowning," a late afternoon, early evening syndrome of increased confusion in a demented person, is a delirious state. Behavioral

Box 16.2 Differential diagnosis of psychosis in PD

Dementia with Lewy bodies
REM intrusions
REM sleep behavior disorder
Vivid dreams
Primary psychiatric disorders
Bonnet's syndrome
Illusions?

symptoms in sundowning combine the problems of confusion, reduced attention and easy distractability, hallucinations, illusions, and sleep-related problems.

Dementia with Lewy bodies (DLB)

DLB is, of course, closely related to PDD, and is defined by the development of dementia prior to, or within 12 months of, the development of the classical motor features of PD. DLB can be associated with visual hallucinations even in an unmedicated state [12–14]. Based on the current definition, DLB can, on occasion, develop after the patient has begun anti-PD medications. Because PDD and DLB overlap to a great extent, it may be impossible to distinguish the two, although it remains uncertain that they are different disorders and do not simply represent extremes of a spectral disorder.

Sleep disorders

Probably the most important and difficult clinical distinction to make in a PD patient is between psychotic symptoms and sleep-related phenomena. Hallucinations and delusions tend to occur more frequently at night, which is when most patients become sleepy and are most prone to have vivid dreams and/or RBD features. Patients may be thought psychotic when they report peculiar happenings at night regardless of the cause. One consideration is simply vivid dreams [29–31]. These are common, and may occur sporadically or in relation to drug side effects. Patients may ask about a fire in the house next door, or comment on the commotion caused by the car accident down the street, which happened only in a dream. If the dream had a paranoid content such as a criminal invading the house it can be even more confusing, as the possibility of paranoid delusions must be excluded, and "secondary delusions" may develop whereby the patient believes that a problem related to a primary behavioral process is in fact real. REM sleep behavior disorder is a common problem in PD, particularly in men, and involves acting out of dreams that typically have a violent or physically active theme [32,33]. The patient might punch, kick, or scream during REM sleep, which could be readily misinterpreted by the spouse as a hallucination. The frequency of these spells in an individual person is highly variable and unpredictable, and it is not known what triggers such a spell. Dreams may also intrude into wakefulness in PD patients who are just about to fall asleep or are just waking up, causing them to experience hypnogogic and hypnopompic hallucinations [34]. The intrusion of dreams into a twilight state in a demented person makes it challenging to make a reliable clinical interpretation as to what they are actually experiencing.

Release hallucinations

Bonnet's syndrome is a benign form of "release hallucination" that typically occurs in elderly people with visual impairment [35,36]. These patients start seeing hallucinations with far greater clarity than they do real objects in their most affected visual field. This may develop abruptly after an acute loss or decrease in vision. The mental state is otherwise completely unchanged from the baseline. These hallucinations tend to be less stereotyped than those that are drug induced. They may also occur in deaf people, who develop auditory hallucinations.

Vignette: an 80-year-old man suffered mild visual hallucinations during the day and mild cognitive impairment. He awoke during the night convinced that burglars were in his house and coming into his room. He saw them, panicked and jumped out the window, breaking his arm.

Comment: this is a true example and it was never able to be determined if the patient awoke from a vivid dream or was hallucinating. The interpretation is important since the treatments are different.

Clinical course

Psychotic symptoms usually develop several years into the course of PD, 10 years or more in one study [7]. For many years it had been thought that there was a natural progression from vivid dreams to hallucinations to delusions, as reflected in the UPDRS question in Section 1 in which a score of 1 is given for vivid dreams and 2 for hallucinations, but this notion has been dispelled [29,30]. A connection between dream or sleep abnormalities has been hypothesized (REM intrusion hypothesis) [37], and supported by some data [38], but does not adequately explain the syndrome.

Although hallucinations may develop shortly after a drug is initiated or increased, they often develop on a background of stable medication doses that have been unchanged for years. When hallucinations occur within the first year of drug treatment, the patient generally has a primary psychiatric disorder, DLB, or another parkinsonian disorder [17]. Although hallucinations early on in their course generally cause little problem, they are generally harbingers of problems in the future of an evolving dementia. Thus, the concept of "benign hallucinations" that was popular until recently is no longer considered to represent an accurate depiction of the problem [39]. Most patients will continue to have hallucinations if medications are not changed, may go on to become demented, or may experience increasing psychotic symptoms. While all of these represent possible outcomes for hallucinating PD patients, the long-term outcome is highly variable. There are many examples of patients who suffer hallucinations which resolve with medication change and do not recur after 10 or more years without the need for anti-psychotic drugs.

Delusions typically occur in patients who already have hallucinations. The hallucinations and delusions may be consonant with each other, for example seeing people spying from outside the window. Alternatively, they may be unrelated such as seeing children playing in the yard, but thinking the spouse is having sexual liaisons in the house.

The implications of psychotic symptoms cannot be overemphasized. It is hard to fathom the distress caused to a relatively helpless patient by paranoid delusions. Caregiver stress [25–28] is markedly exacerbated by PD-related mental changes, particularly psychosis. The corollary of this observation is that behavioral abnormalities and psychosis are probably the single most important precipitant for nursing home placement [27,28]. Psychosis is also a predictor of increased mortality. In a small study of nursing home residents in Chicago before atypical anti-psychotics were available, there was 100% mortality within 2 years [40]. In the first multi-center study of low-dose clozapine [41], which enrolled subjects who were deemed to be so mentally ill that they would have been treated with a typical anti-psychotic if they did not have PD, six of 60 died within the course of the double-blind and open-label extension study which lasted only 4 months. None were attributed to the study drug. A long-term follow-up of the subjects who completed that trial revealed that 25% were dead, 68% were demented, and 69% were still psychotic 3 years later [42]. An Israeli group [43] performed a chart review on 32 PD patients who had been started on clozapine, and reported that 19 were still taking the medication at a 5 year follow-up. An American study which was prospective in nature found that of six subjects treated with quetiapine or clozapine only one was able to stop the anti-psychotic and three of the six had worse psychosis than when they started treatment [44]. In another study of 39 parkinsonian patients who were taking clozapine for psychosis, and which included some patients who did not have idiopathic PD (IPD), 15% had died by 5 years and 33% had been admitted to nursing homes [45], a poor outcome but better than in the first study of nursing home patients with 100% mortality at 2 years. Galvin, Pollack, and Morris reported that "visual hallucinations increase the risk of developing dementia 20-fold in comparison to PD patients who did not suffer hallucinations" [46], implying that visual hallucinations not only cause problems in and of themselves, but also carry the prognosis of an imminent dementia. These studies illustrate the poor outcomes that are frequently seen in PD patients who experience psychosis.

Measuring psychosis

There is no validated and universally accepted scale to measure psychosis in PD. A review of all of the 12 scales that have been used in published studies found them all to be suboptimal [47]. The most popularly used scales are subtests of the Neuropsychiatric Inventory (NPI) (a tool developed for and widely used in Alzheimer disease) [48], the Brief Psychiatric Rating Scale [49] (a tool used in schizophrenia trials), the Survey Assessment of Positive Symptoms [50] (another tool designed used in schizophrenia trials), the Parkinson's Psychosis Rating Scale [51], and the Clinical Global Impression Scale (CGI), which is a seven-point scale simply rating how ill the subject is [52]. While these rating instruments have held up rather well in the various studies, they have not been validated for assessing psychosis in PD and do not encompass the entire range of behaviors that should be considered. Most studies employ two or three of these scales to balance their lack of validation and their limitations.

Risk factors

Medications are the major risk factor for developing psychotic symptoms. Although psychotic symptoms were not specifically mentioned, the original placebo-controlled trial of L-dopa reported "psychic manifestations" in 10 of the 60 subjects [53]. Dopamine agonists have generally cause more hallucinations than L-dopa in trials comparing the two drugs for motor response [54]. Older age, dementia, duration of disease, REM sleep behavior disorder, and visual impairment [3,5,19,21,37,38] are also important risk factors. Polypharmacy may play a role, but this has not been formally studied.

Pathophysiology

There is clearly an increased risk of psychotic symptoms in PD patients with dementia [3]. This makes the overlap with DLB more complex. Lower scores on the MMSE in PD patients correlate with an increased risk of developing hallucinations when patients are placed on anti-parkinsonian medications [55]. Double-blind placebo-controlled trials also demonstrate an increase risk of hallucinations in patients treated with dopamine agonists compared with L-dopa [54]. Some reports have shown a correlation between impaired vision [19] and the development of visual hallucinations, suggesting an element of "release hallucinations" [35]. No such correlation has been reported between hearing impairment and auditory hallucinations, although this is more challenging to confirm as hearing loss is difficult to assess in dementia patients. However, decreased hearing has been associated with delusions in patients with dementia [56].

In a study of cognitively intact PD patients with visual hallucinations, deficits in tests of executive function have been demonstrated in comparison with non-hallucinators despite similar scores on the MMSE and short-term memory evaluations [57]. The executive problems involved "inhibitory" functions "thought to be particularly important for selective attention." This observation supports the hypothesis that deficits of attention combine with visual spatial dysfunction to cause hallucinations in these patients. It does not explain why the hallucinations tend to be stereotyped in each individual, or why they are so similar across all populations.

Pathological studies have demonstrated that visual hallucinations occur almost exclusively in patients with Lewy body diseases such as IPD and DLB. One report [58,59] noted Lewy bodies in the amygdala and parahippocampus of every hallucinator and their absence in non-hallucinators. In a study of 788 brains of people with parkinsonism, a history of hallucinations was associated with Lewy bodies in 93% of cases [60]. This is an important observation for at least two reasons. One is that the occurrence of hallucinations induced by anti-PD medications appears to be seen only in patients with IPD and DLB, not in the other parkinsonian conditions, similar to the striking difference in the occurrence of L-dopa dyskinesias. The second is that Lewy bodies, and more precisely their localization, hold a clue to the pathophysiology of hallucinations.

There have been limited numbers of studies examining what causes hallucinations in PD. Fenelon, Goetz, and Karenberg summarized the PD literature in the pre-L-dopa treatment and concluded that psychotic manifestations were probably exceedingly rare [10]. Thus, in PD, unlike DLB, psychotic symptoms appear to be primarily drug-induced. Perhaps most important is the demonstration [61] that hallucinations do not simply reflect elevated serum levels of a drug. PD patients who reported nightly visual hallucinations were hospitalized for a research study to determine the plasma levels of L-dopa which induced hallucinations. Subjects were given intravenous L-dopa that produced plasma levels higher than they would have experienced at home with oral medication, yet none developed hallucinations, indicating that the presence of L-dopa, even at a high levels in the serum, is not sufficient to cause hallucinations. The presence of hallucinations may be a state–trait phenomenon, requiring that a patient have a particular state of mind (usually quiet, alone, and unstimulated) and the drug. A single case report described a patient who reliably hallucinated minutes after he had L-dopa administered into a jejunal tube, suggesting that his hallucinations at least in this case did indeed parallel the blood level of the drug [62]. Another important observation concerning the pharmacology of hallucinations is that psychotic symptoms may long outlast the serum level of the drug which induced them, just as the beneficial motor effects of L-dopa may far outlast its serum levels [53].

Only a limited number of imaging studies have been performed on patients with hallucinations. A technetium brain SPECT scan was performed in a 72-year-old man with PD who had visual hallucinations and delusions. He had an MMSE of 23 and was taking amantadine, levodopa, bromocriptine, and trihexiphendyl [63]. The SPECT was obtained while the subject was delusional, and showed "increased regional cerebral blood flow (CBF) in the left superior, middle temporal, and inferior frontal gyri, and the apex of the right temporal lobe." When his hallucinations had resolved, the SPECT was repeated and showed decreased blood flow in both occipital lobes, as has been reported in demented PD patients who were not suffering hallucinations [64,65]. Another study of PD patients with visual hallucinations showed less CBF in the left temporal–occipital areas than in PD patient without visual hallucinations, but none of the scans were obtained while the patients were experiencing visual hallucinations [66]. PET scanning with fluorodeoxyglucose (FDG) showed an increased glucose metabolic rate in the left superior frontal gyrus in PD patients who had visual hallucinations, but again the scans were not obtained during the period when the patients were actually experiencing visual hallucinations [67].

Treatment

Psychotic symptoms in PD patients most often occur in relation to drug treatment. They may occur as part of a delirium, or can be triggered by infection or other toxic/metabolic derangements. The first step in developing a treatment regimen is to determine if there are precipitating factors and to treat them accordingly. The second step is to consider whether there might be alternative factors such as nightmares, REM intrusions (hypnogogic and hypnopompic hallucinations), or vivid dreams that might be mistaken for psychosis. Unfortunately, it is usually not clear if treatment will be effective for these types of problems. Bonnet's syndrome can also be considered, and is generally unresponsive to anti-psychotics and anti-convulsants. When there is no evident "medical" explanation for the psychosis in PD, it is almost always drug induced. The next treatment approach is therefore to consider a reduction in medication. There are no specific evidence-based data on how to taper medications in a PD patient with psychosis. A reduction in anti-parkinsonian medications can lead to an unacceptable worsening of motor function. For this reason, most authorities recommend first reducing or stopping any potential contributing drug that is not directly related to PD. These can include anti-cholinergic drugs that are used to treat bladder hyperactivity; whereas the newer such drugs are less prone to cause confusion or add to psychotic symptoms, the older drugs, particularly oxybutynin and tolteradine do so. Benzodiazepines and sedative hypnotics should be reduced or discontinued; a sedating anti-psychotic may be used to replace these. The tricyclic anti-depressants generally have anti-cholinergic properties and may aggravate psychosis, whereas selective serotonin reuptake inhibitors (SSRIs) and serotonin–norepinephrine reuptake inhibitors (SNRIs) are less likely to contribute to psychosis. At that stage, anti-parkinsonian drugs can be gradually reduced or stopped – usually beginning with anti-cholinergics and amantadine, and then moving on to dopamine agonists and levodopa as required. The approach to reducing PD medications is always individualized, based on the patient's needs. In general, my personal approach is borrowed from epileptologists – use as few drugs as possible in order to minimize toxicity. In terms of PD, this means using fewer drugs at higher doses in preference to more drugs at lower doses. If these approaches fail or are not well tolerated, then anti-psychotic agents can be considered. The American Academy of Neurology task force on treatment for Parkinson's disease recommended drug reduction followed by quetiapine as the first-line drug therapy, despite the lack of double-blind, placebo-controlled evidence to support this approach, followed by a trial of clozapine [68].

Although classical neuroleptics may be effective, they are generally not employed because of their potential to worsen parkinsonism and even induce a neuroleptic malignant syndrome. The first report on the use of an atypical anti-psychotic for treating psychosis in PD was published in 1985 by Scholz and Dichgans [69], who reported that four of five patients treated with clozapine showed a good response. Subsequently, a number of reports described outstanding results with clozapine in the treatment of psychosis in these patients [70,71]. There were few reports of worsening motor function and the drug was found to work exceedingly well in the PD population when used at extremely low doses in comparison with doses used in schizophrenia.

There have been two placebo-controlled, double-blind trials of clozapine in PD psychosis [41,72]. Although one was performed in the USA and the other in France, they had similar designs. Patients remained on their anti-PD medications, which were not changed during the trial, and were then treated with clozapine, starting at 6.25 mg per day or placebo, with weekly increases, as needed, to a ceiling dose of 50 mg q.h.s. This contrasts with patients who receive clozapine for schizophrenia, who often take the drug because they are refractory to other drugs, and generally take doses in the 600–900 mg per day range. In both the US and French clozapine trials, a number of measures of psychosis were used, since no universally accepted measure of psychosis in PD has been developed. Each measure, including global impression, showed clinically meaningful and statistically significant improvements. Equally importantly was the lack of worsened motor function. In fact, there was a non-statistically significant trend to improvement in motor function, due largely to clozapine having an anti-tremor effect in PD [73–75].

The effective doses of clozapine are very low in PD psychosis, making it unlikely that the benefit is related to dopamine blockade [76]. Rather, it has been speculated that a serotonin [5-hydroxytryptamine (5-HT)]2A receptor blockade is more important [77]. Phase II trials of pimavanserin, a 5HT2A inverse agonist, having been encouraging [78] and two Phase III trials are under way.

In early studies, clozapine was found to carry a 1–2% risk of agranulocytosis [79], which is not dose dependent. For this reason, patients who take clozapine require weekly complete blood counts for 6 months, then every other week for 6 months, and then once monthly. This makes the drug difficult to use because it may be inconvenient for patients to receive only enough medication to get them through to their next blood test. Sedation and orthostatic hypotension can be problems. Other side effects of clozapine, namely weight gain and a metabolic syndrome, appear not to occur at the low doses used in PD [80].

Following the release of clozapine, risperidone was introduced to the market as another atypical anti-psychotic drug. Unlike clozapine, however, risperidone was associated with dose-dependent motor side effects and prolactin increase [81,82], thus behaving more like a "typical" or first-generation anti-psychotic agent. The published reports on risperidone's effects on psychosis in patients with PD are all open-label observations, but are extremely interesting. Results span the spectrum of good anti-psychotic efficacy with no decline in motor function [83], to good psychotic efficacy with some motor worsening [84–87], to poor efficacy and dramatic declines in mobility [88,89]. Ford, Lynch, and Greene [88] and Rich, Friedman, and Ott [89] reported together that 11 of 12 parkinsonian patients were unable to tolerate the drug, even at low doses, due to motor decline. Because of the inconsistent benefits and the potential of the drug to induce motor worsening, the drug has not been widely used by PD experts.

The next atypical anti-psychotic to be marketed was olanzapine. Unlike the other atypicals, which improved psychosis but may not have been well-tolerated, olanzapine has not been shown to improve the psychosis. The first publication, on an open-label study, reported excellent benefit and tolerability [90]. For this reason, olanzapine has been the subject of at least four double-blind, placebo-controlled trials, and is the best studied of the anti-psychotic agents [91–93]. One was aborted by the safety monitoring committee due to worsened motor function [93]. The others found that psychosis was not improved and that motor function declined. There is, therefore, strong evidence that olanzapine is not a useful drug for PD psychosis and it is not regularly employed for this indication [91–93].

Quetiapine has attracted considerable attention because anti-psychotic benefits without motor deterioration were reported in a series of open-label studies, and there were no hematologic side effects [94–96]. The anti-psychotic benefit was thought to be good, but less robust than seen with clozapine [97]. Three double-blind trials have subsequently been published [98–100]. Two showed no efficacy for the psychosis and the other showed lack of inferiority to clozapine, suggesting, but not proving, efficacy [100]. No motor deterioration was observed. Despite this lack of confirmatory evidence, many physicians continue to use quetiapine, often as the first-line therapy. In a retrospective chart review of 87 patients, Fernandez *et al.* found the drug to be effective, with the mean dose being 65 mg per day [44]. A small chart review found no clear evidence of increased risk of diabetes in PD patients taking quetiapine [101], a concern associated with the use of other atypical anti-psychotics.

The release of aripiprazole generated expectations within the PD community of it being an ideal drug to treat PD psychosis. It has a purported effect as a partial dopamine agonist at the D2 receptor with a high 5-HT2/D2 ratio [102]. Based on this profile, it was hypothesized that the drug might have potent anti-psychotic effects but a better movement disorder side effect profile than other atypical anti-psychotics. To date, two open-label studies have been published concerning aripiprazole [103,104]. Unfortunately, even at doses as low as 1 mg per day, some patients experienced worsening of motor function. In the larger of the two reports [104], five of 14 subjects stopped the drug due to motor worsening at doses of 5 mg or less per day, and the study was aborted.

Ziprasidone is yet another anti-psychotic that has been examined for benefits in PD, but it has not been widely employed because of a possible QT interval increase, making it a potentially risky choice in a frail elderly population. In a review of its motor effects in primary psychotic disorders in patients without PD, the authors opined that its extrapyramidal side effect profile was somewhere between those of risperidone and quetiapine/clozapine [105]. All studies on this drug in PD patients have been open label. In one prospective study, no motor side effects were seen in 43 subjects [106], but in another five of 12 subjects had motor effects [107]. Further, one case report describes severe worsening in parkinsonism with the addition of the drug [108]. As with risperidone, open-label reports suggest that there is a wide biological variation in the potential of this drug to induce motor side effects.

Electroconvulsive therapy (ECT) is an accepted treatment for severe, refractory depression, whether psychotic symptoms are present or not. In a number of cases of depressed PD patients it has been noted to improve not only mood, but also motor function, although this benefit is not sustained. The motor benefit lasts from hours to weeks (personal observation). ECT has also rarely been reported to improve psychosis in PD patients who may or may not have had depressive psychoses [109,110]. It has also been reported to improve neuroleptic malignant-like symptoms following L-dopa withdrawal in a single patient [111]. My own limited experience with maintenance ECT is that the motor benefit is not renewed with the usual schedule of one ECT every few weeks, and it is not a recommended therapy for psychosis.

Drug holidays, a popular approach to treating a variety of PD medication-related problems in the late 1970s, particularly severe dyskinesias and "on–off," involved hospitalizing the patient, completely withdrawing the PD medications, and supporting the patient during a 7–14 day period without any PD medications. The theory was that striatal dopamine receptors that had been downregulated by chronic dopaminergic therapy would become normalized, allowing for a return to a good treatment response similar to that during the early years of treatment. The holidays did work, in that patients did well on much lower doses of drugs, and consequently had a reduced risk of psychosis. However, the benefit was short lived, so that within a few months the patient was back taking the same medications with the same motor and mental complications as before the drug holiday [15].

Cholinesterase inhibitors may have some value in treating hallucinations in PD patients [112], but have not been shown to be helpful for delusions, the most important aspect of the psychosis. In a large, placebo-controlled trial of rivastigmine in patients with PDD, the drug was mildly more effective in hallucinators than in those who did not have hallucinations, but did not significantly reduce the visual hallucinations themselves [113]. Other studies have revealed similar responses [114–122] with mild [112,118] or no [114] motor worsening. The difficulty with the cholinesterase inhibitors is that they appear to have only mild anti-hallucinatory properties and little effect on delusions, and they require many weeks to take effect. They are therefore of no benefit in urgent or emergency situations.

There are no data on the effect of memantine on psychosis in PD. Although memantine has been noted in dementia trials to improve certain behavioral complications of dementia such as agitation, irritability, appetite, and emotional lability, it has not been shown to improve psychotic symptoms specifically [123]. Memantine has, unfortunately, been suggested actually to worsen these symptoms in some patients with DLB [124] and Alzheimer's disease [125].

Deep brain stimulation (DBS) should probably not be used to treat PDP. As is the case with compulsive symptoms induced by dopamine agonists, DBS may allow for a reduction in anti-PD medications, which may therefore lead to relief from drug-induced behavior disorder, but DBS may cause psychiatric side effects, most commonly hypomania, which, superimposed on a patient already prone to have hallucinations and delusions, could produce major psychiatric decompensation. In many centers, psychotic symptoms are considered relative contraindications to DBS surgery [126] because of the potential for the procedure to induce behavioral complications, although this is only a mild problem in most cases.

Patients with primary psychosis and Parkinson's disease

There is no reason to believe that schizophrenia or other primary psychotic disorders, whether they represent a dopamine disorder or not [127], are protective against the development of IPD [1,128–130]. It is therefore possible that a patient could have PD superimposed on a primary psychiatric disorder, although these symptoms tend to be different to the psychotic features that occur in PD. There is virtually no literature on this subject.

The most common scenario for presentation of these patients to a neurologist is worsening or developing parkinsonism in a patient taking an anti-psychotic drug. Although the atypical anti-psychotics are associated with fewer extrapyramidal side effects than the first generation of anti-psychotic drugs, all but quetiapine and clozapine have the potential to cause or worsen parkinsonism [97]. The patient is then diagnosed with a Parkinson syndrome, thought to reflect either purely the extrapyramidal effects of the anti-psychotic or IPD exacerbated by the drug. Because it may take months for the parkinsonian side effects to resolve once the offending drug has been stopped, and it is sometimes not possible for the anti-psychotic to be changed, it is sometimes impossible ever to be certain whether the patient truly had PD or simply became increasingly sensitive to the parkinsonian drug side effects as occurs with age.

A single case report followed a schizophrenic patient from time of diagnosis of PD to autopsy, which confirmed the diagnosis of IPD [1]. The patient became psychotic with the introduction of bromocriptine, and was intolerant of very low doses of thioridazine. Clozapine was introduced and appeared to stabilize his schizophrenia. He tolerated adjustments of L-dopa and bromocriptine without psychiatric decompensation, and although he required several psychiatric admissions due to recurrences of paranoia with delusions that the FBI and CIA were spying on him, his psychiatric state was thought to have been better controlled on clozapine and anti-PD medications than it was on first-generation anti-psychotics prior to the diagnosis of IPD. There are other examples of PD in patients with schizophrenia where the diagnosis of PD has been confirmed by SPECT scanning [128–130]. I have personally followed five additional patients who had been diagnosed with either schizophrenia or schizoaffective disorder prior to the development of presumed IPD, none of whom appeared to have had psychotic fluctuations in temporal relationship to the adjustment of anti-PD medications (unpublished observations). Other reports confirm that both PD and schizophrenia can be adequately treated with the use of quetiapine or clozapine coupled with anti-parkinsonian medications.

Conclusions and treatment recommendations

Psychosis can be a disabling feature for PD patients, and its control has permitted increased levodopa doses to be employed and improved quality-of-life. A treatment algorithm might be as follows. First, rule out and treat other causes as appropriate. Second, stop or reduce as many psychoactive medications as possible. Third, reduce or stop anti-parkinsonian medications not thought to be necessary, particularly anti-cholinergics, amantadine, and dopamine agonists in that sequence. If symptoms persist, add quetiapine, starting at 12.5–25 mg q.h.s., increasing as needed, depending on tolerability and symptom response. The lowest dose that makes the problem either tolerable or disappear, with the fewest side effects, is the goal. If quetiapine is not effective at a tolerable dose, either stop it and start clozapine, beginning at 6.25–12.5 mg q.h.s., or, if the patient has been on quetiapine for a period of time, initiate clozapine as quetiapine is tapered. There is no value in obtaining clozapine levels. If quetiapine and clozapine are not tolerated at effective doses, then aripiprazole should be considered, and perhaps ECT. Once the patient's psychotic symptoms have been controlled, it is usually not possible to stop the anti-psychotic unless the anti-PD drugs have been significantly reduced [131]. In contrast, the addition of anti-psychotic medications may permit higher doses of anti-parkinsonian medications to be employed with better control of PD features.

References

1. Friedman JH, Fernandez HH. Autopsy follow up of a patient with schizophrenia and presumed idiopathic Parkinson's disease. *Clin Neuropharmacol* 2001;**24**:120–1.
2. American Psychiatric Association, *Diagnostic and Statistical Manual of Mental Disorders*, 4th edn, Text Revision, Washington, DC: American Psychiatric Association, 2000.
3. Fenelon G. Psychosis in Parkinson's disease: phenomenology, frequency, risk fators, and current understanding of pathophysiologic mechanisms. *CNS Spectr* 2008;**13**(3 Suppl 4): 18–25.

4. Kiziltan G, Ozekmekci S, Ertan S, *et al*. Relationship between age and subtypes of psychotic symptoms in Parkinson's disease. *J Neurol* 2007;**254**:448–52.
5. Aarsland D, Larsen JP, Cummings JL, Laake K. Prevalence and clinical correlates of psychotic symptoms in Parkinson disease: a community-based study. *Arch Neurol* 1999;**56**:595–601.
6. Chou KL, Messing S, Oakes D, *et al*. Drug induced psychosis in Parkinson's disease: phenomenology and correlations among psychosis rating instruments. *Clin Neuropharmacol* 2005;**28**:215–9.
7. Papapetropoulos S. Drug induced psychosis in Parkinson's disease: phenomenology and correlations among psychosis rating instruments. *Clin Neuropharmacol* 2006;**29**:59.
8. Brust JCM. Delirium. In: Jeste D, Friedman JH, eds. *Psychiatry for Neurologists*. Totowa, NJ: Humana Press, 2006: 307–13.
9. Ravina B, Marder K, Fernandez HH, *et al*. Diagnostic criteria for psychosis in Parkinson's disease. Report of an NINDS/NIMH work group. *Mov Disord* 2007;**22**:1061–8.
10. Fenelon G, Goetz CG, Karenberg A. Hallucinations in the prelevodopa era in Parkinson's disease. *Neurology* 2006;**66**:93–8.
11. Cummings JL. Neuropsychiatric complications of drug treatment in Parkinson's disease. In: Huber S, Cummings JL, eds. *Parkinson's Disease: Neurobehavioral Aspects*. New York: Oxford University Press, 1992: 313–27.
12. McKeith IG, Dickson DW, Lowe J, *et al*. Diagnosis and management of dementia with Lewy bodies: third report of the DLB Consortium. *Neurology* 2005;**65**:1863–72.
13. McKeith IG. Dementia with Lewy bodies. *Br J Psychiatry* 2002;**180**:144–7.
14. Weintraub D, Hurtig HI. Presentation and management of psychosis in Parkinson's disease and dementia with Lewy bodies. *Am J Psychiatry* 2007;**164**:1491–7.
15. Friedman JH. Drug holidays in the treatment of Parkinson's disease. A brief review. *Arch Intern Med* 1985:**145**:913–5.
16. Goetz CG, Tanner CM, Klawans HL. Drug holiday in the management of Parkinson disease. *Clin Neuropharmacol* 1982;**5**:351–64.
17. Goetz CG, Vogel C, Tanner C. Early dopaminergic drug-induced hallucinations in parkinsonian patients. *Neurology* 1998;**51**:811–4.
18. Fenelon G, Mahieux F, Huon R, Ziefler M. Hallucinations in Parkinson's disease. Prevalence, phenomenology and risk factors. *Brain* 2000;**123**:733–45.
19. Hoyroyd S, Currie L, Wooten GR. Prospective study of hallucinations and delusions in Parkinson's disease. *J Neurol Neurosurg Psychiatry* 2001;**70**:734–8.
20. Graham JM, Grunewald RA, Sagar HJ. Hallucinosis in idiopathic Parkinson's disease. *J Neurol Neurosurg Psychiatry* 1997;**63**:434–40.
21. Barnes J, David AS. Visual hallucinations in Parkinson's disease: a review and phenomenological survey. *J Neurol Neurosurg Psychiatry* 2001;**70**:727–33.
22. Sanchez-Ramos JR, Ortoll R, Paulson GW. Visual hallucninations associated with Parkinson's disease. *Arch Neurol* 1995;**53**:1265–8.
23. Inzelberg R, Kipervasser S, Korczyn AD. Auditory hallucinations in Parkinson's disease. *J Neurol Neurosurg Psychiatry* 1998;**64**:533–5.
24. Pagonabarraga J, Llebaria G, Garcia-Sanchez C, *et al*. A prospective study of delusional misidentification syndromes in Parkinson's disease with dementia. *Mov Disord* 2008;**23**:443–8.
25. Aarsland D, Larsen JP, Karlsen K, *et al*. Mental symptoms in Parkinson's disease are important contributors to caregiver distress. *Int J Geriat Psychiatry* 1999;**14**:866–74.
26. Goetz CG, Stebbins GT. Risk factors for nursing home placement in advanced Parkinson's disease. *Neurology* 1993;**43**:2227–9.
27. Aarsland D, Larsen JP, Tandbert E. Predictors of nursing home placement in PD: a population-based prospective study. *J Am Geriatr Soc* 2000;**48**:938–42.
28. Schrag A, Hovris A, Morley A, *et al*. Caregiver burden in parkinson's disease is closely associated with psychiatric symptoms, falls and disability. *Parkinsonism Relat Disord* 2006;**12**:35–41.
29. Pappert EJ, Boetz CG. Niederman FG, *et al*. Sleep fragmentation, and altered dream phenomena in PD. *Mov Disord* 1999;**14**:117–21.
30. Goetz CG, Wuu J, Curgian LM, Leurgans S. Hallucinations and sleep disorders in PD: six year prospective longitudinal study. *Neurology* 2005;**64**:81–6.
31. Sharf B, Moskowitz C, Lupton MD, Klawans HL. Dream phenomena induced by chronic levodopa therapy. *J Neural Transm* 1978;**43**:143–51.
32. Borek LL, Kohn R, Friedman JH. Mood and sleep in parkinson's disease. *J Clin Psychiatry* 2006;**67**:958–63.
33. De Cock VK, Vidailhet M, Leu S, *et al*. Restoration of normal motor control in Parkinson's disease during REM sleep. *Brain* 2007;**130**(Pt 2): 450–6.
34. Takata K, Inouye Y, Hazama H, Fukuma E Night-time hypnopompic visual hallucinations related to REM sleep behavior disorder. *Psychiatry Clin Neurosci* 1998;**52**: 207–9.
35. Cogan DG. Visual hallucinations as release phenomena. *Albrecht Von Graefes Arch Klin Exp Opthalmol* 1973;**188**: 139–50.
36. Teunisse RJ, Cruysberg JR, Hoefnagels WH, *et al*. Visual hallucinations in psychologically normal people: Charles Bonnet's syndrome. *Lancet* 1996;**347**:794–7.
37. Arnulf I, Bonnet AM, Damier P, *et al*. Hallucinations, REM sleep and Parkinson's disease: a medical hypothesis. *Neurology* 2000;**55**:281–8.
38. Nomura T, Inoue Y, Mitani H, *et al*. Visual hallucinations as REM sleep behavior disorder in patient with Parkinson's disease. *Mov Disord* 2003;**18**:812–7.
39. Goetz CG, Fan W, Leurgans S, *et al*. The malignant course of "benign hallucinations" in Parkinson disease. *Arch Neurol* 2006;**63**:713–6.
40. Goetz CG, Stebbins GT. Mortality and hallucinations in nursing home patients with advanced Parkinson's disease. *Neurology* 1995;**45**:45:669–71.
41. Parkinson Study Group. Low dose clozapine for the treatment of drug-induced psychosis in Parkinson's disease. *N Engl J Med* 1999;**340**:757–63.
42. Factor SA, Feustel PJ, Friedman JH, *et al*. Longitudinal outcome of Parkinson's disease patients with psychosis. *Neurology* 2003;**60**:1756–61.

43. Klein C, Gordon J, Pollak L, *et al.* Clozapine in Parkinson's disease psychosis: 5 year follow up review. *Clin Neuropharmacol* 2003;**26**:8–11.
44. Fernandez HH, Trieschmann ME, Burke MA, Friedman JH. Long-term outcome of quetiapine use for psychosis among parkinsonian patients. *Mov Disord* 2003;**18**:510–4.
45. Fernandez HH, Donnelly EM, Friedman JH. Long term outcome of clozapine use for psychosis in parkinsonian patients. *Mov Disord* 2004;**19**:831–3.
46. Galvin JE, Pollack J, Morris JC. Clinical phenotype of Parkinson's disease dementia. *Neurology* 2006;**67**:1605–11.
47. Fernandez HH, Aarsland A, Fenelon G, *et al.* Scale to assess psychosis in Parkinson's disease: critique and recommendations. *Mov Disord* 2008;**23**:484–500.
48. Cummings JL, Mega M, Gray K, *et al.* The Neuropsychiatric Inventory: comprehensive assessment of psychopathology in dementia. *Neurology* 1994;**44**:2308–14.
49. Overall JE, Gorham DR. The Brief Psychiatric Rating Scale (BPRS): recent developments in ascertainment and scaling. *Psychopharmacol Bull* 1988;**24**:97–9.
50. Andreasen N. *Scale for the Assessment of Positive Symptoms (SAPS).* Iowa City, IA: Department of Psychiatry,University of Iowa, 1984.
51. Friedberg G, Zoldan J, Melamed E. Parkinson Psychosis Rating Scale: a practical instrument for grading psychosis in parkinson's disease. *Clin Neuropharmacol* 1998;**21**:280–4.
52. Guy W, ed. *Clinical Global Impressions. ECDEU Assessment Manual for Psychopharmacology.* DHEW Publication No. (ADM)76-338. Rockville, MD: US Department of Health, Education and Welfare, 1976.
53. Yahr MD, Duvoisin RC, Schear MJ, *et al.* Treatment of parkinsonism with levodopa. *Arch Neurol* 1969;**21**:343–54.
54. Papapetropoulos S, Mash DC. Psychotic symptoms in parkinson's disease. From description to etiology. *J Neurol* 2005;**252**:753–64.
55. Biglan KM, Holloway RG, McDermott MP, *et al.* Risk factors for somnolence, edema and hallucinations in early Parkinson disease. *Neurology* 2007;**69**:187–95.
56. Ballard C, Bannister C, Graham C, *et al.* Association of psychotic symptoms in dementia sufferers. *Br J Psychiatry* 1995;**164**:537–40.
57. Barnes J, Boubert L. Executive functions are impaired in patients with Parkinson's disease with visual hallucinations. *J Neurol Neurosurg Psychiatry* 2008;**79**:190–2.
58. Harding AJ, Broe GA, Halliday GM. Visual hallucinations in Lewy body disease relate to Lewy bodies in the temporal lobe. *Brain* 2002;**125**:391–403.
59. Harding AJ, Stimson E, Henderson JM, Halliday GM. Clinical correlates of selective pathology in the amygdala of patients with Parkinson's disease. *Brain* 2002;**125**:2431–45.
60. Williams DR, Lees AJ. Visual hallucinations in the diagnosis of idiopathic Parkinson's disease: a retrospective autopsy study. *Lancet Neurol* 2005;**4**:605–10.
61. Goetz CG, Pappert EJ, Blasucci LM, *et al.* Intravenous levodopa in hallucinating Parkinson's disease patients: high-dose challenge does not precipitate hallucinations. *Neurology* 1998;**50**:515–7.
62. Friedman JH. Intravenous levodopa in hallucinating Parkinson's disease patients. *Neurology* 1999;**52**:219–20.
63. Kataoka H, Furiya Y, Morikawa M, *et al.* Increased temporal blood flow associated with visual hallucinations in Parkinson's disease with dementia. *Mov Disord* 2008;**23**:464–71.
64. Matsui H, Udaka F, Miyoshi T *et al.N*-Isopropyl-*p*-[^{123}I]iodoamphetamine single photon emission computed tomography study of Parkinson's disease with dementia. *Intern Med* 2005;**44**:1046–50.
65. Spampinato U, Habert MO, Mas JL, *et al.* [^{99m}Tc]-HM-PAO SPECT and cognitive impairment in Parkinson's disease: a comparison with dementia of the Alzheimer type. *J Neurol Neurosurg Psychiatry* 1991;**54**:787–92.
66. Okada K, Suyama N, Oguro H, *et al.* Medication-induced hallucination and cerebral blood flow in Parkinson's disease. *J Neurol* 1999;**246**:365–8.
67. Nagano-Saito A, Washimi Y, Arahata Y, *et al.* Visual hallucination in Parkinson's disease with FDG PET. *Mov Disord* 2004;**19**:801–6.
68. Miyasaki JM, Shannon K, Voon V, *et al.* Practice Parameter: evaluation and treatment of depression, psychosis, and dementia in Parkinson's disease (an evidence-based review): report of the Quality Standards Subcommittee of the American Academy of Neurology. *Neurology* 2006;**66**:996–1002.
69. Scholz E, Dichgans J. Treatment of drug induced exogenous psychosis in parkinsonism with clozapine and fluperlapine. *Eur Arch Psychiatry Neurol Sci* 1985;**235**:60–4.
70. Friedman JH, Max J, Swift R. Idiopathic Parkinson's disease in a chronic schizophrenic patient: long term treatment with clozapine and L-dopa. *Clin Neuropharmacol* 1987;**10**:470–5.
71. Friedman JH, Factor SA. Atypical antipsychotics in the treatment of drug-induced psychosis in Parkinson's disease. *Mov Disord* 2000;**15**:201–11.
72. Pollak P, Tison F, Rascol O, *et al.* Clozapine in drug induced psychosis in Parkinson's disease: a randomised placebo controlled study with open follow-up. *J Neurol Neurosurg Psychiatry* 2004;**75**:689–95.
73. Friedman JH, Lannon MC. Clozapine-responsive tremor in Parkinson's disese. *Mov Disord* 1990;**5**:225–9.
74. Friedman JH, Koller WC, Lannon MC, *et al.* Benztropine versus clozapine for the treatment of tremor in Parkinson's disease. *Neurology* 1997;**48**:1077–81.
75. Pakkenberg H, Pakkenberg B. Clozapine in the treatment of tremor. *Acta Neurol Scand* 1986;**73**:295–7.
76. Meltzer HY, Kennedy J, Dai J, *et al.* Plasma clozapine levels and the treatmentof L-DOPA-induced psychosis in Parkinson's disease: a high potency effect of clozapine. *Neuropsychopharmacology* 1995;**12**:39–45.
77. Meltzer HY, Li Z, Kaneda Y, Ichikawa J. Serotonin receptors: their key role in drugs to treat schizophrenia. *Prog Neuropsychopharmacol Biol Psychiatry* 2003;**27**:1159–72.
78. Revell S, Friedman JH, Mills RG, *et al.* A double blind, placebo controlled dose escalation trial of pimavanserin in Parkinson's disese and psychosis. *Neurology* 2008;**70**(Suppl 1): A284–5.
79. Alvir JM, Lieberman JA, Safferman AZ, *et al.* Clozapine-induced agranulocytosis. Incidence and risk factors in the United States. *N Engl J Med* 1993;**329**:162–7.
80. Fernandez H, Friedman J, Lansang M, *et al.* Diabetes mellitus among parkinsonian patients treated chronically with clozapine. *Parkinsonism Relat Disord* 2004;**10**:439–41.

81. Grant S, Fitton A. Risperidone: a review of its pharmacology and therapeutic potential in the treatment of schizophrenia. *Drugs* 1994;**43**:253–73.
82. Rustembegovic A, Sofic E, Wichart I. Serum prolactin, leptin, lipids and lipoprotein levels during antipsychotic treatment in Parkinson's disease and related psychosis. *Med Arh* 2006; **60**:211–2.
83. Workman RH Jr, Orengo CA, Bakey AA, *et al.* The use of risperidone for psychosis and agitation in in demented patients with Parkinson's disease. *J Neuropsychiatry Clin Neurosci* 1997;**9**:594–7.
84. Meco G, Alessandria A, Giustini P, Bonifati V. Risperidone in levodopa-induced psychosis in advanced Parkinson's disease:an open label, long-term study. *Mov Disord* 1997;**12**:610–2.
85. Mohr E, Mendis T, Heldebrand K, De Deyn PP. Risperidone in the treatment of dopamine-induced psychosis in Parkinson's disease: an open pilot trial. *Mov Disord* 2000;**15**:1230–7.
86. Leopold NA. Risperidone treatment of drug-related psychosis in patients with parkinsonism. *Mov Disord* 2000;**15**: 301–4.
87. Ellis T, Cudkowicz ME, Sexton PM, Growdon JH. Clozapine and risperidone treatment of psychosis in Parkinson's disease. *J Neuropsychiatry Clin Neurosci* 2000;**12**:364–9.
88. Ford B, Lynch T, Greene P. Risperidone in Parkinson's disease. *Lancet* 1994;**344**:681.
89. Rich SS, Friedman JH, Ott BR. Risperidone versus clozapine in the treatment of psychosis in 6 patients with Parkinson's disease and other akinetic rigid syndromes. *J Clin Psychiatry* 1995;**56**:556–9.
90. Wolters ECH, Jansen EN, Tuynman-Qua HG, Bergmans PL. Olanzapine in the treatment of dopaminomimetic psychosis in patients with Parkinson's disease. *Neurology* 1996;**47**:1085–7.
91. Breier A, Sutton VK, Feldman PD, *et al.* Olanzapine in the treatment of dopamimetic-induced psychosis in patients with Parkinson's disease. *Biol Psychiatry* 2002;**52**:438–45.
92. Ondo WG, Levy JK, Vuong KD, *et al.* Olanzapine treatment for dopaminergic-induced hallucinations. *Mov Disord* 2002;**17**:1031–5.
93. Goetz CG, Blasucci LM, Leurgans S, Pappert EJ. Olanzapine and clozapine: comparative effects on motor function in hallucinating PD patients. *Neurology* 2000;**55**:789–94.
94. Fernandez HH, Friedman JH, Jacques C, Rosenfeld M. Quetiapine for the treatment of drug-induced psychosis in Parkinson's disease. *Mov Disord* 1999;**14**:484–7.
95. Juncos JL, Roberts VJ, Evat ML, *et al.* Quetiapine improves psychotic symptoms and cognition in Parkinson disease. *Mov Disord* 2004;**19**:29–35.
96. Wijnen HH, van der Heijden, van Schendel FM, *et al.* Quetiapine in the elderly with parkinsonism and psychosis. *Eur Psychiatry* 2003;**18**:372–3.
97. Chou KL, Borek LL, Friedman JH. The management of psychosis in movement disorder patients. *Expert Opin Pharmacother* 2007;**8**:935–43.
98. Ondo WG, Tintner R, Voung KD, *et al.* Double-blind, placebo-controlled, unforced titration parallel trial of quetiapine for dopaminergic-induced hallucinations in Parkinson's disease. *Mov Disord* 2005;**20**:958–63.
99. Rabey JM, Prokhorov T, Miniovich A, Klein C. The effet of quetiapine in Parkinson's disease psychotic patients: a double-blind labeled study of three months duration. *Mov Disord* 2007;**22**:313–8.
100. Morgante L, Epifanio A, Spina E, *et al.* Quetiapine and clozaine in parkinsonian patients with dopaminergic psychosis. *Clin Neuropharmacol* 2004;**27**:153–6.
101. Fernandez HH, McCown MK, Romrell J, *et al.* New-onset diabetes mellitus among Parkinsonian patients treated with long-term quetiapine. *Drug Target Insights* 2008;**3**:27–9.
102. McGavin JH, Goa KL. Aripiprazole. *CNS Drugs* 2002;**16**: 779–86.
103. Fernandez HH, Trieschmann ME, Friedman JH. Aripiprazole for drug-induced psychosis in Parkinson disease: preliminary experience. *Clin Neuropharmacol* 2004;**27**:4–5.
104. Friedman JH, Berman RM, Goetz CG, *et al.* Open-label flexible-dose pilot study to evaluate the safety and tolerability of aripiprazole in patients with psychosis associated with Parkinson's disease. *Mov Disord* 2006;**21**:2078–81.
105. Wieden PJ, Uqbal N, Mendelowitz AJ, *et al.* Best clinical practice with ziprasidone: update after one year of experience. *J Psychiatr Pract* 2002;**8**:81–97.
106. Lopez del Val LJ, Santos S. Quetiapine and ziprasidone in the treatment of psychotic disorder in Parkinson's disease. *Rev Neurol* 2004;**39**:661–7.
107. Gomez-Esteban JC, Zaranz JJ, Velasco F, *et al.* Use of ziprasidone in parkinsonism patients with psychosis. *Clin Neuropharmacol* 2005;**28**:111–4.
108. Schinduette J, Trenkwalder C. Treatment of drug induced psychosis in Parkinson's disease with ziprasidone can induce severe dose-dependent off-periods and pathological laughing. *Clin Neurol Neurosurg* 2007;**109**:188–91.
109. Factor SA, Molho ES, Brown DL. Combined clozapine and electroconvulsive therapy for the treatment of drug induced psychosis in Parkinson's disease. *J Neuropsychiatry Clin Neurosci* 1995;**7**:304–7.
110. Shulman RB, Maintenance ECT in the treatment of Parkinson's disease. Therapy improves psychotic symptoms, physical function. *Geriatric* 2003;**58**:43–5.
111. Ozer F, Meral H, Aydin B, *et al.* Electroconvulsive therapy in drug induced psychiatric states and neuroleptic malignant syndrome. *J ECT* 2005;**21**:125–7.
112. Emre M, Aarsland D, Albanese A, *et al.* Rivastigmine for dementia associated with Parkinson's disease. *N Engl J Med* 2004;**351**:2509–18.
113. Burn D, Emre M, McKeith I, *et al.* Effects of rivastigmine in patients with and without hallucinations in dementia associated with Parkinson's disease. *Mov Disord* 2006;**21**:1899–907.
114. Hutchinson M, Fazzini E. Cholinesterase inhibition in Parkinson's disease. *J Neurol Neurosurg Psychiatry* 1996;**61**:324–5.
115. Fabbrini G, Barbanti P, Aurilia C, *et al.* Donepezil in the treatment of hallucinations and delusions in Parkinson's disease. *Neurol Sci* 2002;**23**:41–3.
116. Bergman J, Lerner V. Successful use of donepezil for the treatment of psychotic symptoms in patients with Parkinson's disease. *Clin Neuropharacol* 2002;**25**:107–10.
117. Kurita A, Ochiai Y, Kono Y, *et al.* The beneficial effect of donepezil on visual hallucinations in three patients with Parkinson's disease. *J Geriatr Psychiatry Neurol* 2003;**16**:184–8.

118. Aarsland D, Laake K, Larsen J, Janvin C. Donepezil for cognitive impairment in Parkinson's disease: a randomized controlled study. *J Neurol Neurosurg Psychiatry* 2002;**72**:708–12.
119. Ravina B, Putt M, Siderowf A, *et al*. Donepezil for dementia in Parkinson's disease: a randomised double blind, placebo controlled, crossover study. *J Neurol Neurosurg Psychiatry* 2005;**76**:934–9.
120. Aarsland D, Hutchinson M, Larsen JP. Cognitive, psychiatric and motor response to galantamine in Parkinson's disease with dementia. *Int J Geriatr Psychiatry* 2003;**18**:937–41.
121. Reading PJ, Luce AK, McKeith IG. Rivastigmine in the treatment of parkinsonian psychosis and cognitive impairment: preliminary findings from an open trial. *Mov Disord* 2001;**16**:1171–4.
122. Burn D, Emre M, McKeith IG, *et al*. Effects of rivastigmine in patients with and without visual hallucinations in dementia associated with Parkinson's disease. *Mov Disord* 2006;**21**:1899–907.
123. Zahodne LB, Fernandez HH. Course, prognosis, and management of psychosis in Parkinson's disease: are current treatments really effective? *CNS Spectr* 2008;**13**(Suppl 4):26–33.
124. Ridha BH, Josephs KA, Rossor MN. Delusions and hallucinations in dementia with Lewy bodies: worsening with memantine. *Neurology* 2005;**65**:481–2.
125. Monastero R, Camarda C, Pipia C, Camarda R. Visual hallucinations and agitation in Alzheimer's disease due to memantine: report of three cases. *J Neurol Neurosurg Psychiatry* 2007;**78**:546.
126. Voon V, Saint-Cyr J, Lozano AM, *et al*. Psychiatric symptoms in patients with Parkinson disease presenting for deep brain stimulation surgery. *J Neurosurg* 2005;**103**:246–51.
127. Seeman P, Schwarz J, Chen JF, *et al*. Psychosis pathways converge via D2 high dopamine receptors. *Synapse* 2006;**60**:319–46.
128. Winter C, Juckel G, Plotkin M *et al*. Paranoid schizophrenia and iodpathic Parkinson's disease do coexist: a challenge for clinicians. *Psychiatry Clin Neurosci* 2006;**60**:639.
129. Urban A, Libiger J, Hosak L, Kupka K. Comorbidity of parkinsonism and schizophrenia in a patient treated with clozapine. *Eur Psychiatry* 2003;**28**:258–9.
130. Schwarz J, Scherer J, Trenkealder C, *et al*. Reduced striatal dopaminergic innervation shown by IPT and SPECT in patients under neuroleptic treatment: need for levodopa therapy? *Psychiatry Res* 1998;**83**:23–8.
131. Fernandez HH, Trieschmann ME, Okun MS. Rebound psychosis: effect of discontinuation of antipsychotics in Parkinson's disease. *Mov Disord* 2004;**20**:104–5.

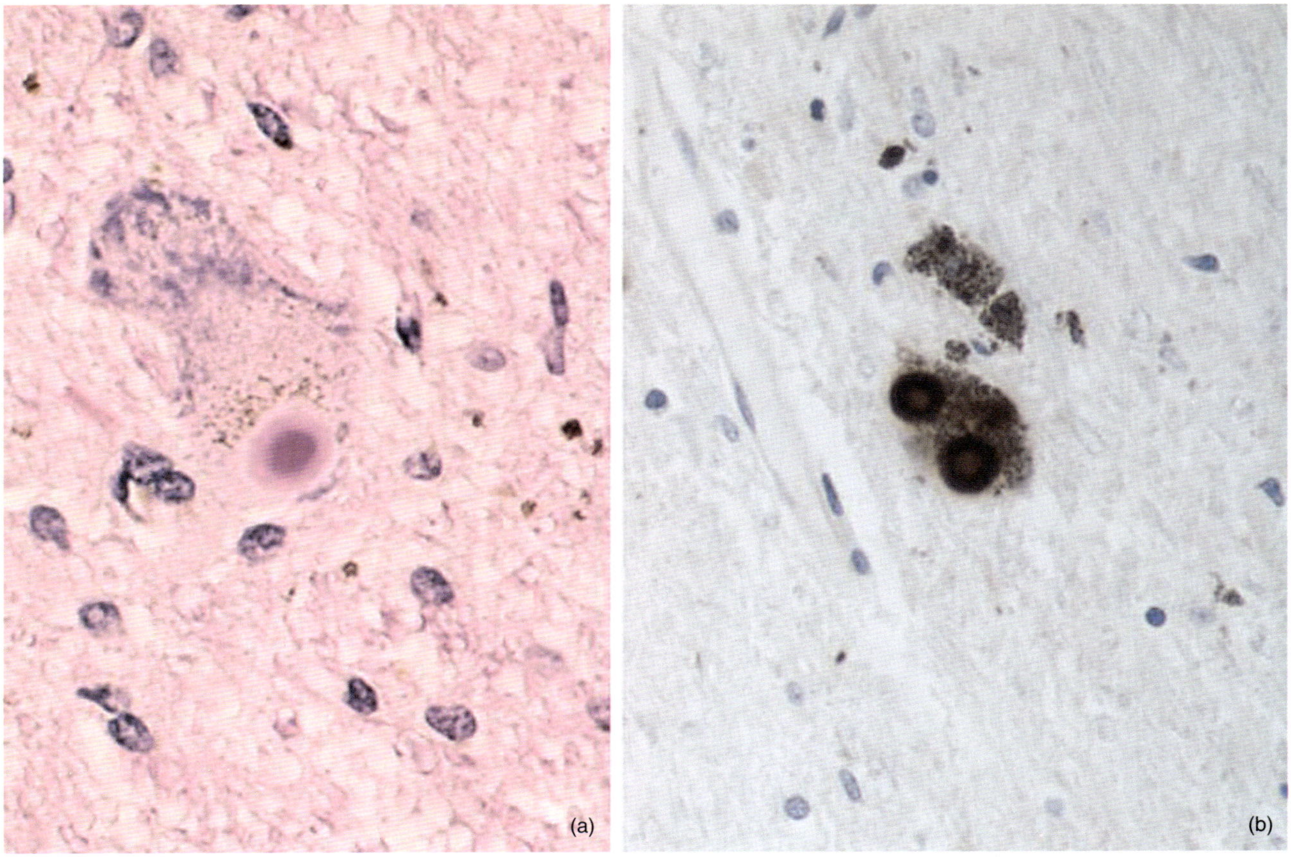

Plate 2.1 Substantia nigra pars compacta neurons with Lewy bodies; hematoxylin and eosin stain (a) and α-synuclein immunostain (b).

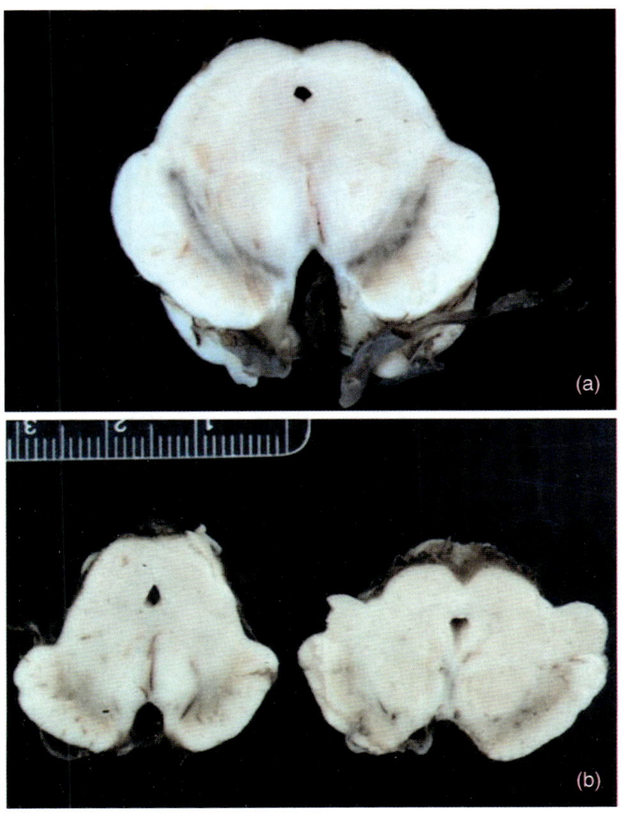

Plate 2.2 Gross appearance of the midbrain: transverse section of a normal control (a) and a case of Parkinson's disease (b).

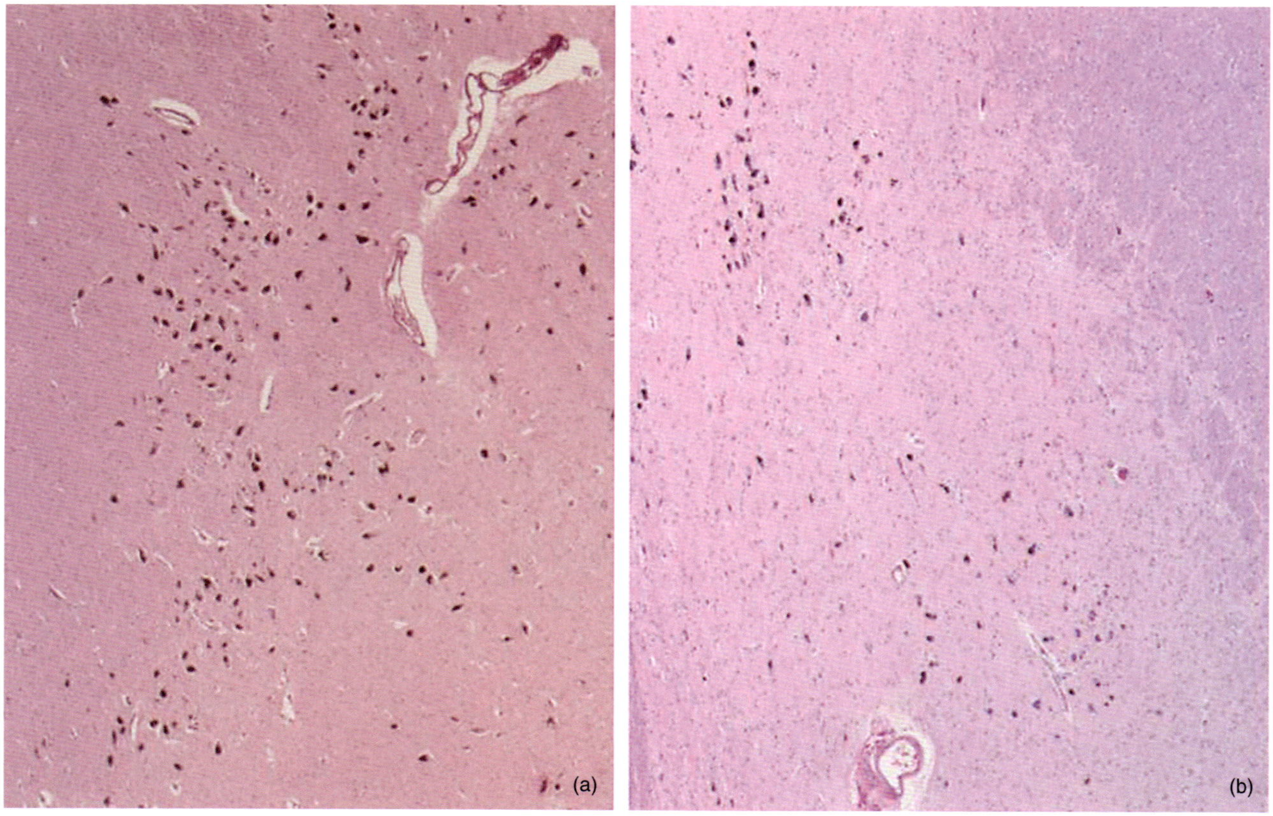

Plate 2.3 Substantia nigra pars compacta, hematoxylin and eosin stain, original magnification 20×: normal (a) and Parkinson's disease (b)

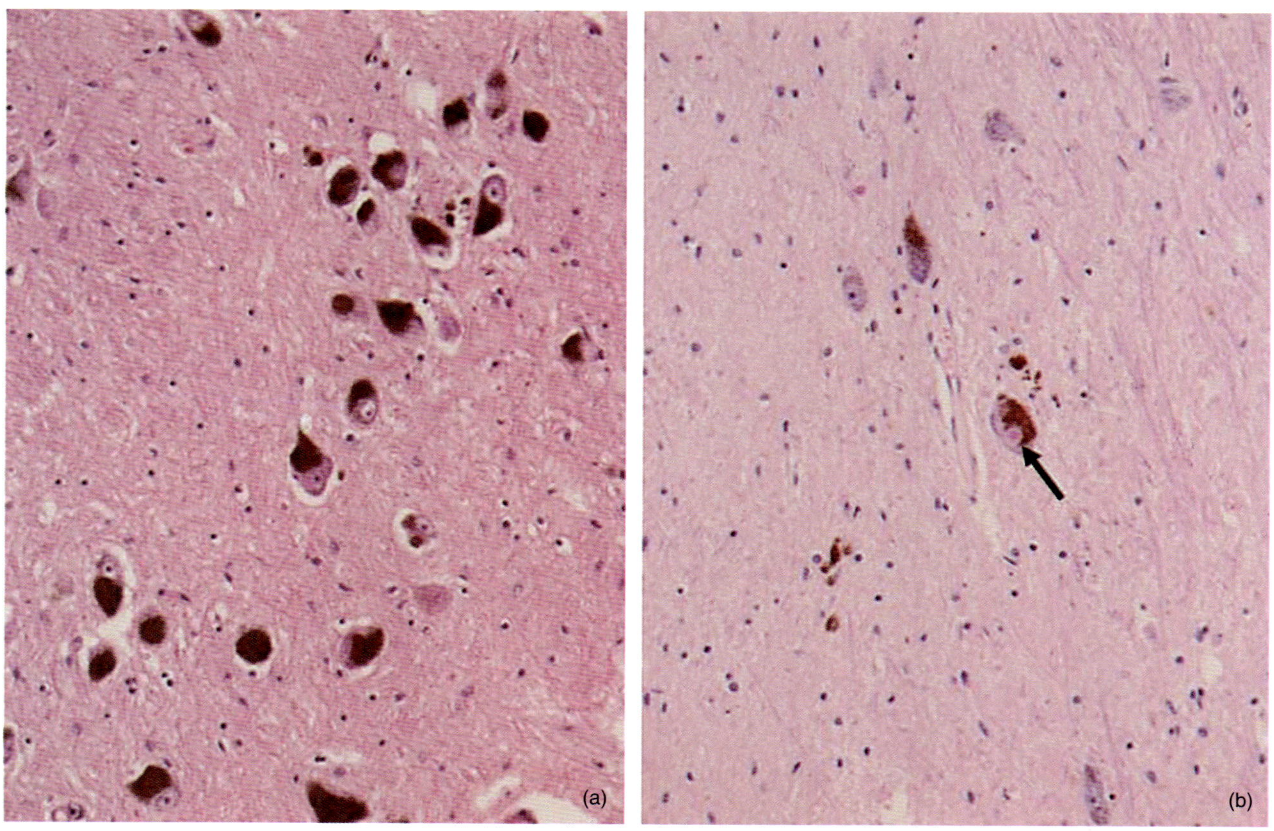

Plate 2.4 Substantia nigra pars compacta, hematoxylin and eosin stain, original magnification 180×: normal (a) and Parkinson's disease (b) showing loss of melanized neurons, incontinent pigment, and neuron with a Lewy body (arrow).

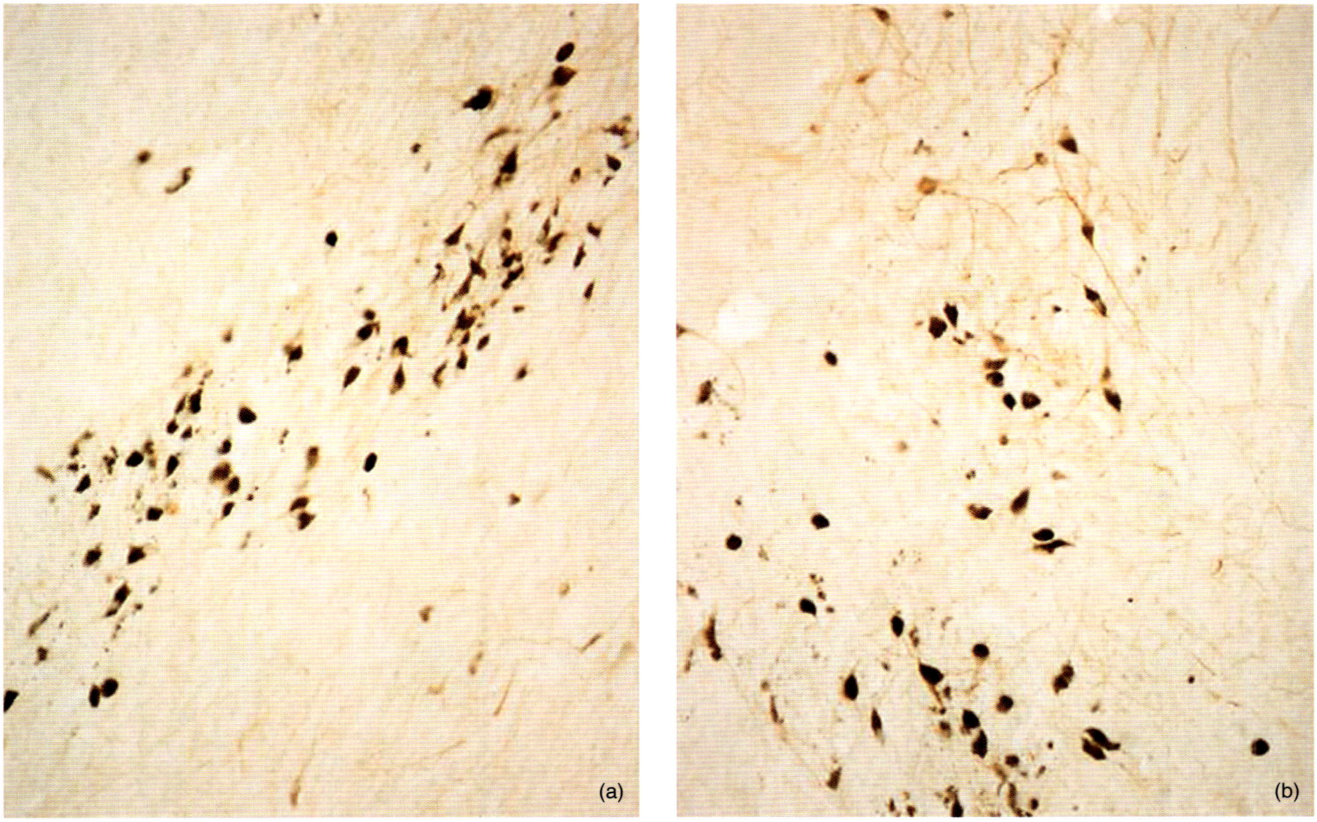

Plate 2.5 Normal substantia nigra pars compacta (a) and ventral tegmental area (b); tyrosine hydroxylase immunostain, 50 μm thick cryosection.

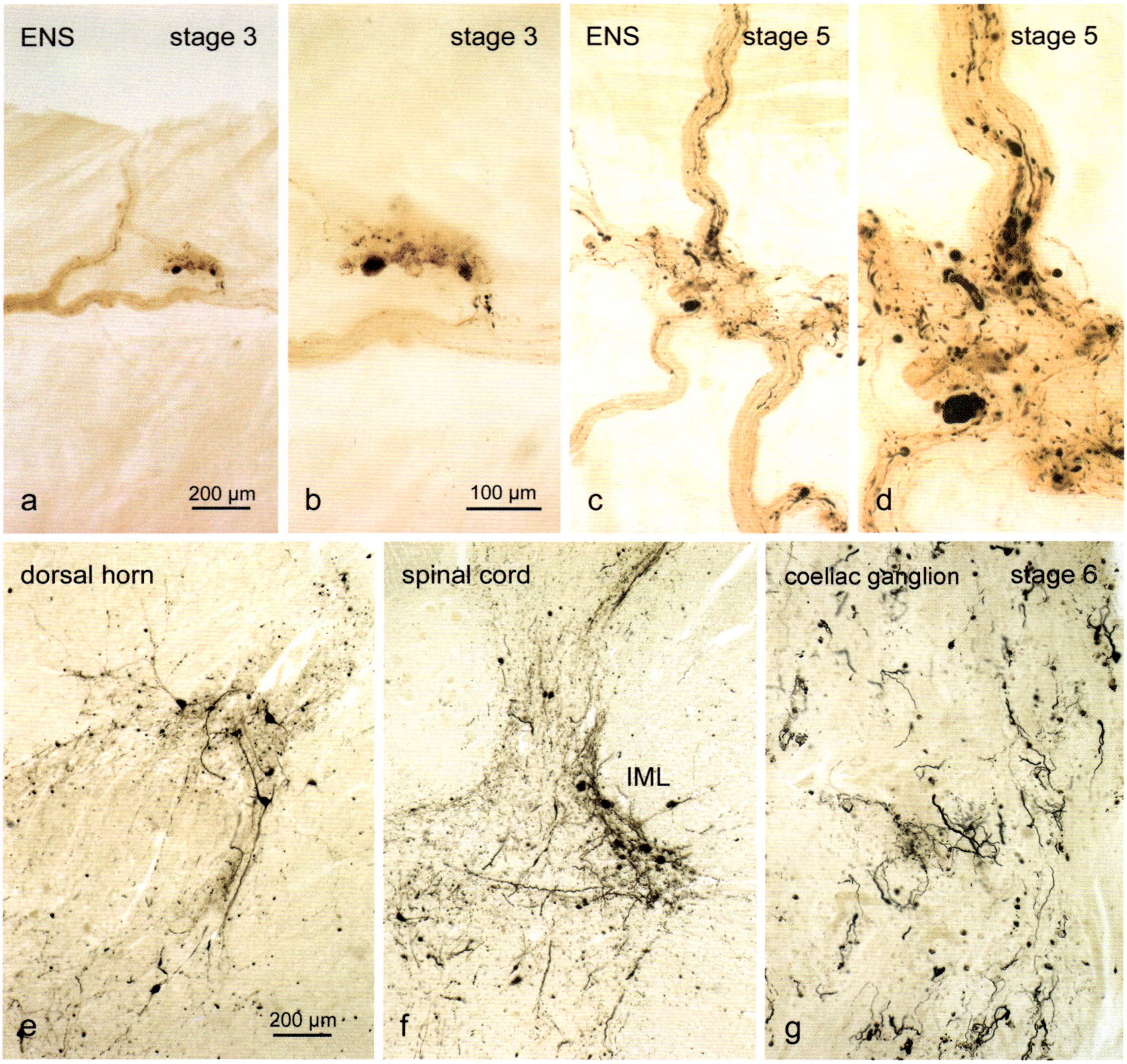

Plate 3.1 Lewy pathology in the enteric nervous system, spinal cord, and peripheral autonomic ganglia seen in immunoreactions against α-synuclein (100 μm sections, syn-1, Transduction and BD Bioscience Laboratories). (a–d) Gastric Auerbach plexus. (a, b) An intramural ganglion in a section cut tangentially to the surface of the gastric cardia from an asymptomatic individual with stage 3 brain pathology. Note that, at this early stage, α-synuclein aggregations almost completely fill individual axons within the fiber bundles interconnecting the ganglia. The micrograph in (b) shows a detail from (a). The scale bar in (a) is valid for (c), the bar in (b) is valid for (d). (c, d) In late-stage cases (here, stage 5), heavy involvement of the enteric nervous system is one of the reasons why so many patients experience gastrointestinal dysfunction. The micrograph in (d) shows a detail from (c) at higher magnification. (e) Lewy pathology in the dorsal horn at the level of the 10th thoracic segment at stage 5. The involvement of relatively large lamina I multipolar neurons predominates. The α-synuclein aggregates almost completely fill the somatodendritic domain of these cells. (f) Overview of the 12th thoracic segment of the spinal cord at stage 4 shows heavy involvement of the intermediolateral nucleus (IML). (g) Lewy neurites and Lewy bodies are distributed throughout the entire coeliac ganglion (stage 6). The scale bar in (e) is valid for (f) and (g).

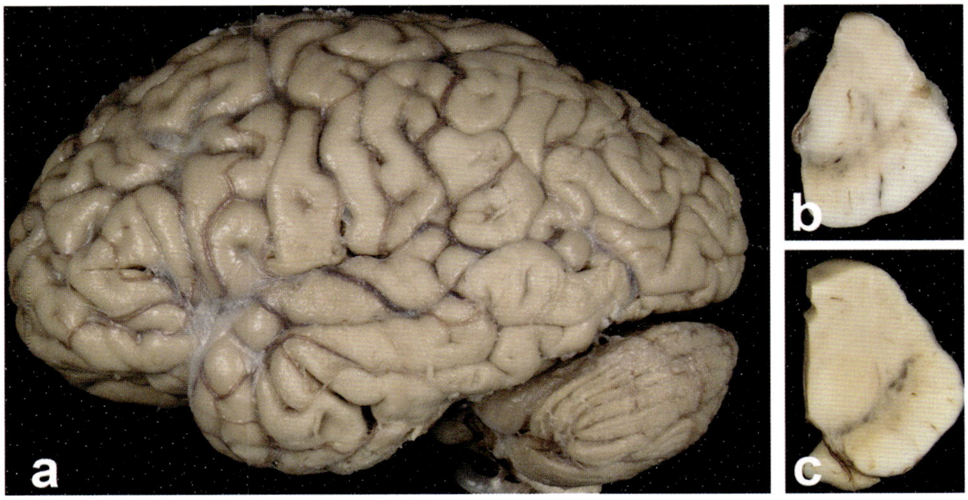

Plate 14.1 Macroscopic appearance of the brain in PDD shows no significant cortical atrophy over the convexity (a), but there is loss of neuromelanin pigmentation in the substantia nigra (b) compared with an age-matched neurologically normal control (c).

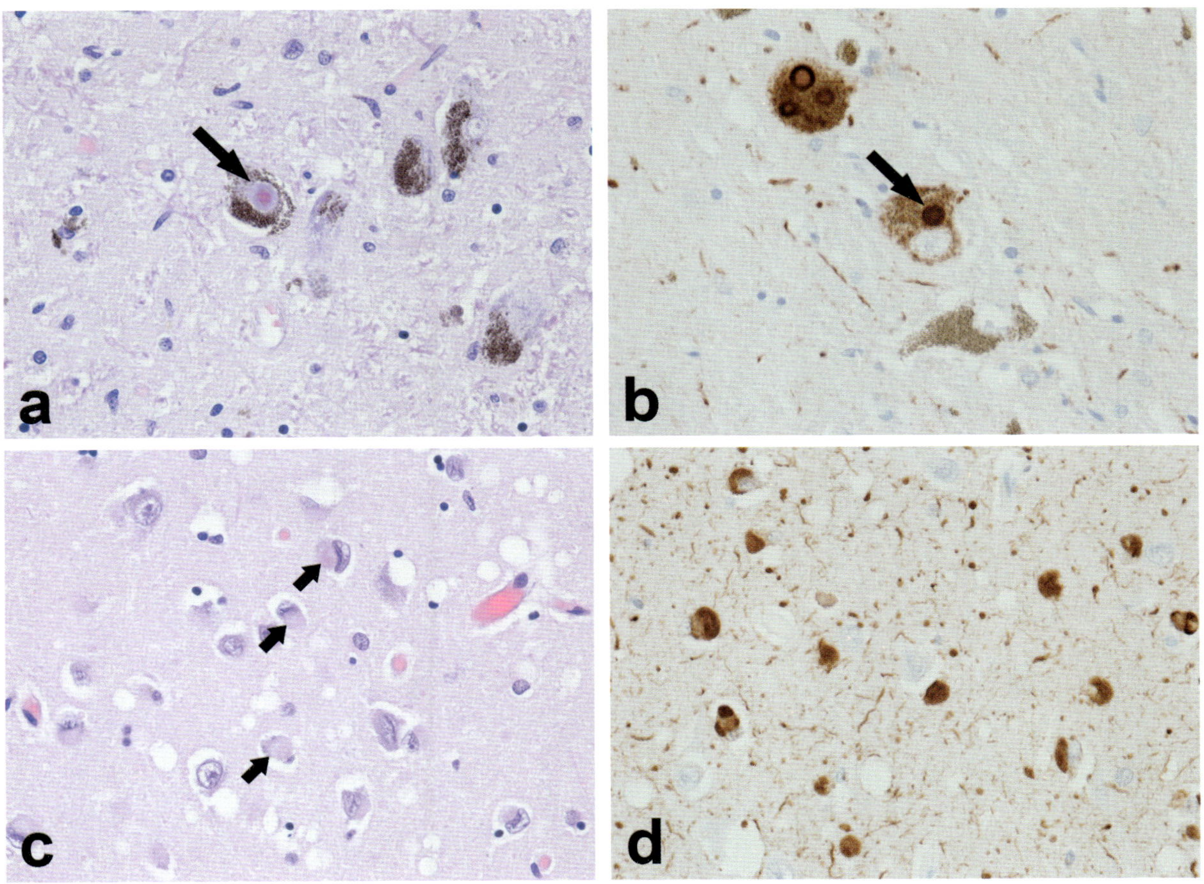

Plate 14.2 Lewy bodies in brainstem nuclei have a dense hyaline appearance [arrow in (a)] in pigmented neurons of the pars compacta of the substantia nigra. Immunohistochemistry for α-synuclein reveals Lewy bodies (arrow), and also more diffuse cytoplasmic immunoreactivity of affected neurons and scattered neuritic processes (b). Cortical type Lewy bodies (arrows) are difficult to detect with routine hematoxylin and eosin stains (c), but are clearly visible with α-synuclein immunohistochemistry (d). All images: original magnification $\times 400$.

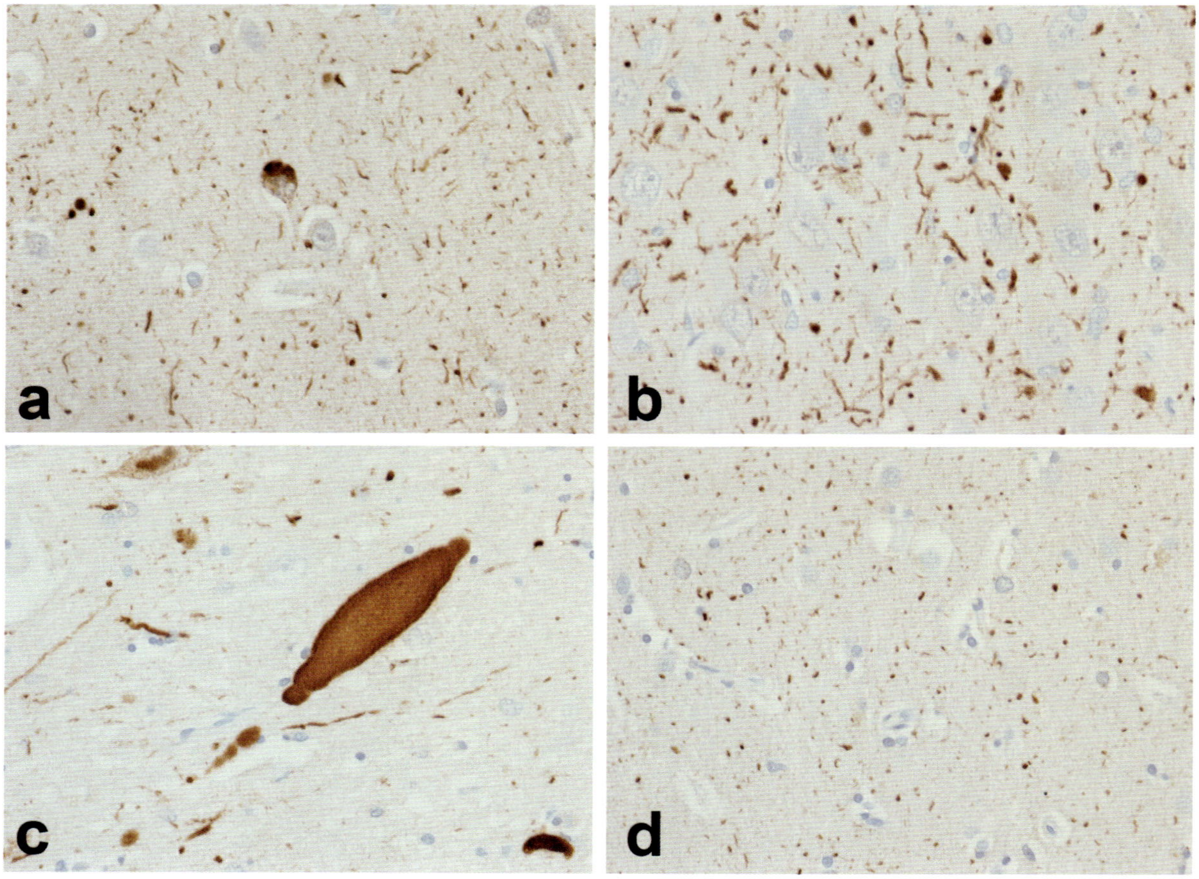

Plate 14.3 Neuritic pathology revealed by α-synuclein immunohistochemistry is widespread in PDD, including cerebral cortex (a), hippocampus (b), basal nucleus of Meynert (c), and striatum (d). All images: original magnification ×400.

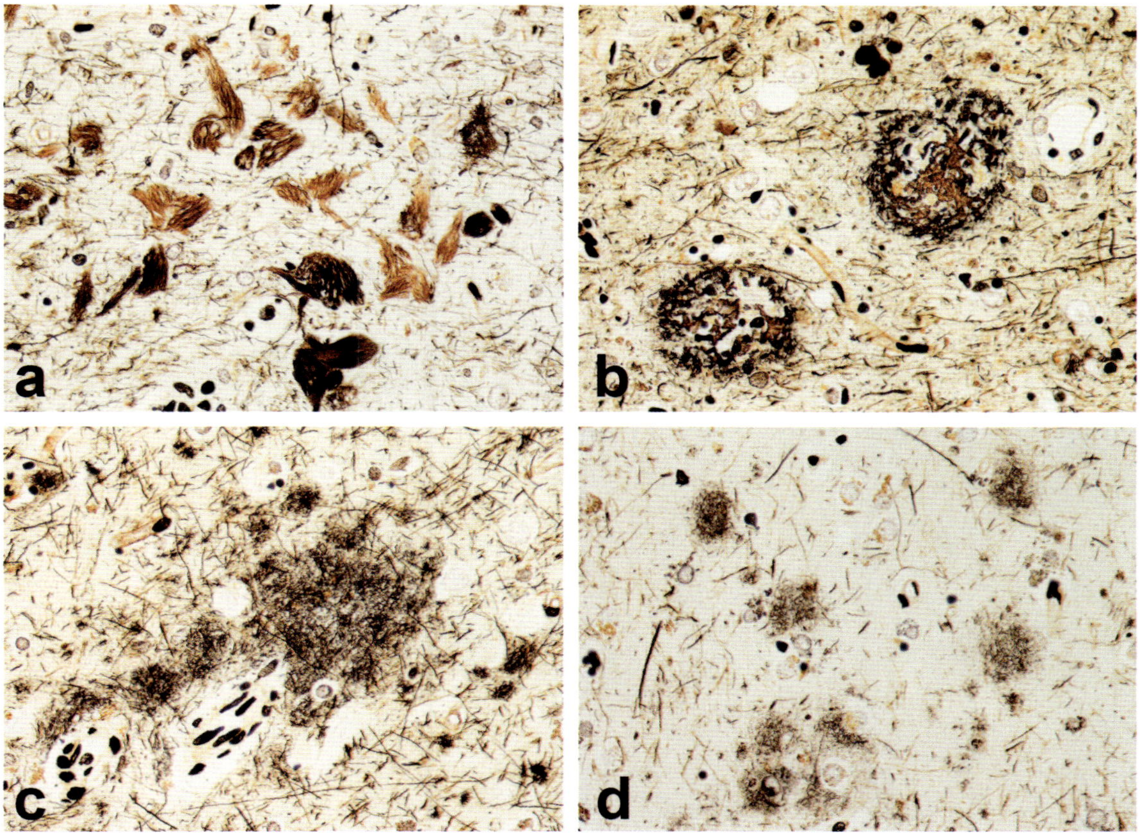

Plate 14.4 Alzheimer-type pathology in PDD is often characterized by medial temporal neurofibrillary tangles [entorrhinal cortex tangles (a)], neuritic plaques in amygdala (b), and diffuse type plaques in cortex (c) and striatum (d).

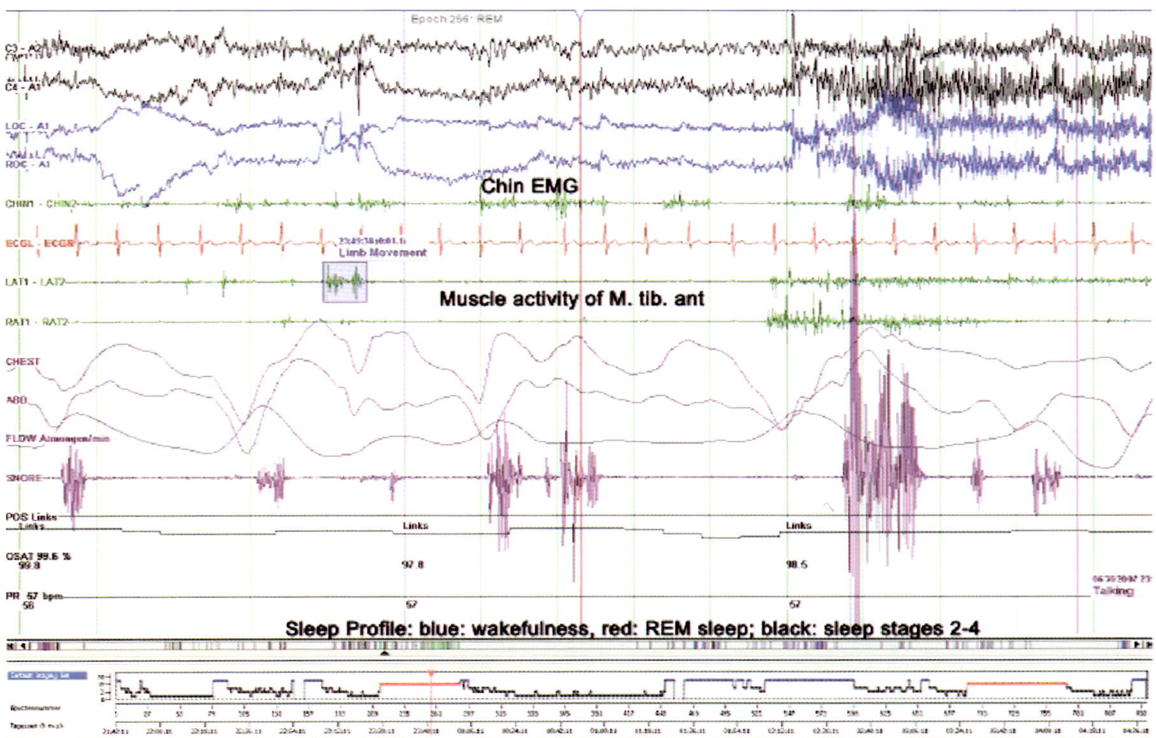

Plate 21.1 Polysomnographic recording of an RBD episode: lack of physiologic REM sleep atonia with muscle activity in the chin and tibialis anterior EMG during an REM sleep episode. The hypnogram shows disturbed sleep architecture and fragmentation of sleep with waking phases.

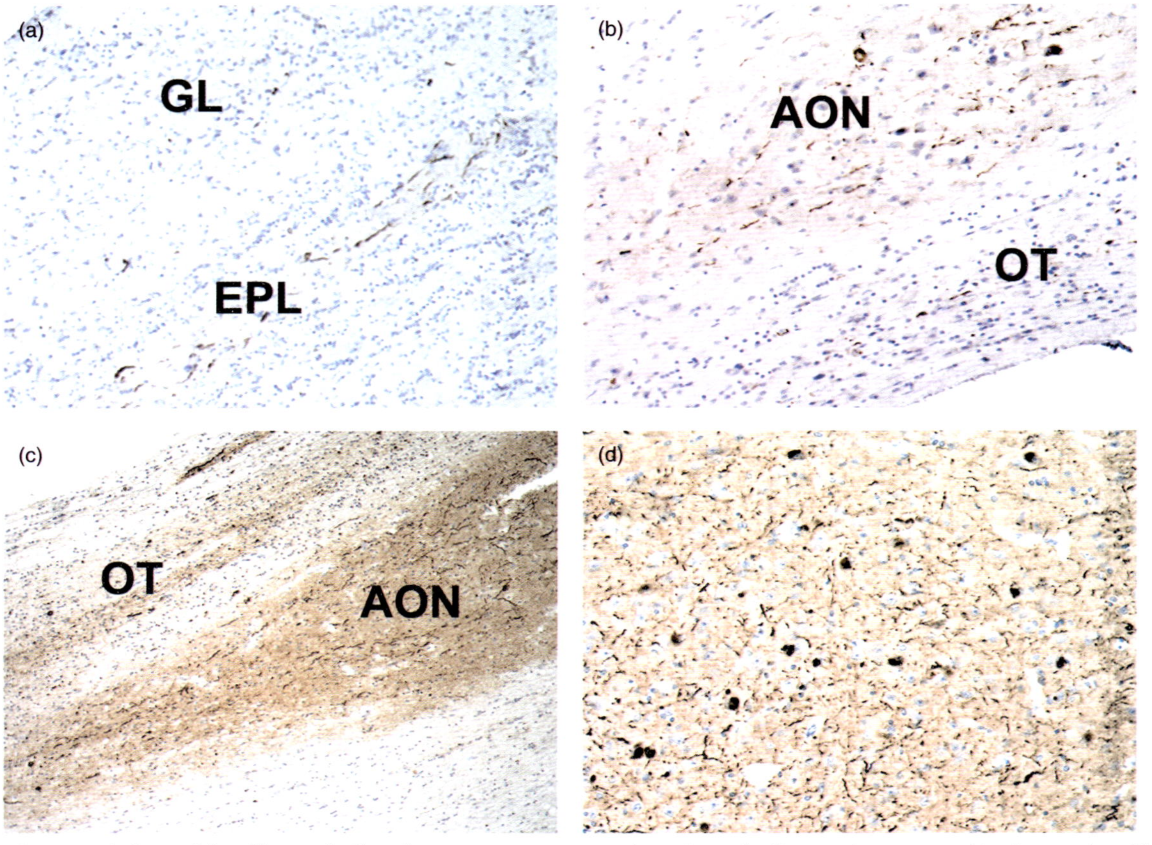

Plate 28.1 Lewy pathology of the olfactory bulb and tract. Immunostaining with antibodies to α-synuclein reveals Lewy pathology in the olfactory bulb and tract in patients with Parkinson's disease (PD) and incidental Lewy body disease (ILBD). (a) In a patient with ILBD, Lewy neurites are demonstrated in the external plexiform layer (EPL) and rarely in the glomerular layer (GL). (b) In the same patient, Lewy neurites and rare Lewy bodies are demonstrated in the anterior olfactory nucleus (AON) and Lewy neurites in the olfactory tract (OT). (c) In a patient with PD, higher burdens of Lewy pathology are demonstrated in the AON and OT. (d) Higher power magnification of the AON in another patient with PD reveals large numbers of Lewy bodies as well as Lewy neurites. Original magnification 200× (panels a, b, d) and 100× (panel c).

Chapter 17
Depression in Parkinson's Disease

Tiffini Voss & Irene Hegeman Richard
Department of Neurology, University of Rochester School of Medicine and Dentistry, Rochester, NY, USA

Introduction

Depression is a syndrome involving disturbances in emotional, cognitive, and physical functioning. Clinically important depressive symptoms affect an estimated 40–50% of Parkinson's disease (PD) patients during the course of their illness [1] and are associated with increased disability [2] and impaired quality-of-life [3]. The impact of depression in PD spreads beyond the individual, as depression and other non-motor symptoms are associated with increased caregiver distress [4]. From a societal perspective, the presence of depressive symptoms correlates with increasing annual health care costs [5] and is associated with increased inpatient admissions and outpatient visits [6]. Despite its frequency, the diagnosis and management of PD depression (dPD) can be challenging for several reasons. First, patients may under-report their symptoms due to lack of insight about their condition or the persistent stigma of mental health disorders. Second, many depressive symptoms can be readily mistaken for the motor manifestations of PD (for example, hypomimia and bradykinesia). Finally, both patients and physicians can operate under the misconception that depression is "normal" in the older population and in chronic illness and is therefore not amenable to further management.

This chapter addresses issues in the diagnosis of dPD, including its epidemiology and phenomenology. Recent insights into the pathophysiology of dPD are reviewed, and current avenues for therapy are presented. Although information is expanding in this area, further research is needed to improve our ability to manage this common and disabling feature of PD.

Diagnosis

Diagnostic criteria

Diagnostic criteria for a depressive episode are outlined in the *Diagnostic and Statistical Manual of Mental Disorders* (DSM-IV-TR) [7]. Core features for a depressive episode include (1) a pervasive negative disturbance in mood and (2) decreased ability to respond positively to normally pleasurable events (anhedonia), or diminished interest and motivation. Other features include worry, feeling hopeless or helpless, poor self-worth, guilt, and suicidal thoughts. Cognitive symptoms of indecisiveness and impaired concentration are common. Somatic features can be easily confused with PD symptoms and include sexual dysfunction, insomnia or hypersomnia, changes in appetite, diminished energy and motivation, and slowed movements or restlessness.

Depressive symptoms vary in severity and several types of depressive episodes exist, including major depression, minor depression, and dysthymia. Major depression involves the presence of many symptoms of depression, lasts more than 2 weeks, and is associated with functional impairment. In contrast, minor depression involves fewer symptoms overall. Dysthymia does not follow the episodic pattern of major and minor depression, but instead involves chronic depressive symptoms over a period of at least 2 years. Milder symptom constellations that do not fit any of these categories have been categorized as subsyndromal depression.

Although the DSM criteria have been essential in defining depression, they were not designed with PD individuals in mind and may not be valid for dPD. Several aspects of dPD raise the question of whether DSM criteria can be usefully applied to this population. One of the greatest challenges is to determine which symptoms are due to depression and which are features of PD. For example, slowed movement may represent bradykinesia, psychomotor slowing, or both. Impaired concentration and attention, fatigue, and sleep disturbances may be features of PD, even in the absence of depression. In addition, the life changes resulting from living with a chronic, progressive disorder can themselves trigger transient symptoms or adjustment reactions that may be difficult to separate from a more pervasive mood disorder.

To address the concerns regarding the application of DSM criteria to dPD, Marsh *et al.* published a report

Parkinson's Disease: Non-Motor and Non-Dopaminergic Features, First Edition. Edited by C. Warren Olanow, Fabrizio Stocchi, and Anthony E. Lang.

summarizing the efforts of a National Institute for Neurological Diseases (NINDS) and National Institute of Mental Health (NIMH) Working Group [8]. This group examined how the DSM criteria could be applied to dPD diagnosis and provided several recommendations for modifying the DSM criteria for dPD. Overall, an emphasis was placed on enhancing diagnostic reliability and sensitivity, with the acknowledgment that this carries the risk of inflating the prevalence of dPD. They made the following recommendations:

1 Include all symptoms that may be related to depression, regardless of potential etiology.

2 Eliminate "due to the effects of a general medical condition" as an exclusion criterion.

3 Require the presence of either depressed mood or anhedonia (but not simply diminished interest) as a core symptom for the diagnosis of minor depressive disorder. The current DSM criteria for minor depressive disorder can be met by exhibiting one core depressive symptom and one ancillary depressive symptom. The group's recommendation was made to avoid over-diagnosing minor depression since any PD patient with apathy (diminished interest) and bradykinesia (psychomotor retardation) but no other evidence of depression could meet criteria based solely on these two features.

4 Account for the motor state of the patient when performing a diagnostic assessment, preferably evaluating patients in their "on" state to reduce the impact of transient mood fluctuations.

5 Use informants to enhance data accuracy in cognitively impaired patients.

These modifications have the advantage of simplifying dPD diagnosis, since they do not require the clinician to judge the underlying etiology of a specific symptom before ascribing it to a mood disorder. Overall, the provisional criteria promise to enhance the reliability of dPD diagnosis and to clarify patient populations in research settings. However, they require validation and their use in clinical practice has not yet been studied.

Rating scales in dPD

Depression rating scales have been applied as a diagnostic tool in depression. Several rating scales have been created for the general population and have undergone validation and psychometric analysis. They are appealing because they are usually short and many can be completed by the patients themselves. However, all rating scales were designed to assess disease severity and response to treatment. No scale attempts to define the possible underlying etiology of the presenting symptoms or provides an assessment of whether the symptoms are related to the mood disorder or to another condition. Rating scales perform less well than the DSM criteria in diagnosing depression and currently cannot replace the structured interview.

The Quality Standards Subcommittee of the American Academy of Neurology (AAN) reviewed the validity of available depression rating scales in dPD as part of a more global practice parameter on the evaluation and treatment of several non-motor aspects of PD (depression, dementia, psychosis) [9]. Based on rigorous analytic criteria, only three studies were felt to be of sufficient strength to guide recommendations. The Beck Depression Inventory (BDI), a self-rated measure, and the Hamilton Depression Rating Scale (HDRS), an observer-rated measure, were both considered probably useful (Level B strength of evidence). The Montgomery–Asberg Depression Rating Scale (MADRS), an observer-rated measure, was considered possibly useful (Level C strength of evidence). No rating scale was established as definitely useful, and several other rating scales were not evaluated due to concerns about the methodologic quality of the respective studies.

Soon after the AAN parameter, the Movement Disorder Society Task Force on Rating Scales for Parkinson Disease published their analysis [10]. This group reviewed nine depression rating scales in common use in the PD population, identifying their use in PD, clinicometric properties, diagnostic accuracy, and suitability for use in research. Overall, the BDI and HDRS were considered to be the best, having been validated in PD populations. Both appeared to be useful both for screening purposes and for the assessment of symptom severity. No scale was established as a preferred rating scale for depression in cognitively impaired patients, although several scales were considered potentially useful, including the MADRS and the Geriatric Depression Rating Scale (GDS). Although the GDS was recognized as a valid depression screening instrument, there was insufficient evidence to judge its use as a measure of depression severity. Overall, depression rating scales can be useful in dPD, but many scales need further validation in this population. A summary of rating scales is presented in Table 17.1.

Differential diagnosis

Similarly to the assessment of depression in the general population, it remains important to consider other medical conditions (e.g., hypothyroidism) and medications (e.g., beta-blockers) that can occasionally induce depressive symptoms.

Anxiety, apathy, and dementia are all prevalent in PD and have considerable symptom overlap with dPD. Apathy is common in PD and can occur in the absence of depression [11]. Although both apathy and depression share features such as anhedonia, decreased motivation, and fatigue, it is important to recognize that the mood valence in apathy is neutral, whereas depression is defined by negative mood and associated with emotional suffering. Anxiety is common in patients with PD and may be particularly prominent among patients with

Table 17.1 Depression rating scales in PD.

Scale[a]	Rater	Suggested cut-off	Sensitivity	Specificity	PPV[b]	NPV[b]	Recommended use
HDRS (HAM-D)	Clinician	15/16	–	0.99	0.93	–	Diagnosis [75]
		13/14	0.88	0.89	0.74	0.96	Diagnosis [76]
		9/10	0.95	–	–	0.98	Screening [75]
MADRS	Clinician	14/15	–	–	–	–	Screening [77]
		17/18	–	–	–	–	Diagnosis [77]
BDI	Patient	8/9	0.92	0.52	–	–	Screening [78]
		16/17	0.42	0.98	–	–	Diagnosis [78]
HADS	Patient	10/11	–	–	–	–	Screening [10]
		23/24	–	–	–	–	Diagnosis [10]
GDS-30	Patient	9/10	0.81	0.84	–	–	Screening [79]
GDS-15	Patient	4/5	0.88	0.85	–	–	Screening [80]
SDS	Patient	Not specifically determined for dPD					
CSDD	Clinician	Not specifically determined for dPD					
CES-D	Patient	Not specifically determined for dPD					
UPDRS Part I	Clinician	2	–	–	–	–	Screening [10]

[a]HDRS, Hamilton Depression Rating Scale; MADRS, Montgomery–Asberg Depression Rating Scale; BDI, Beck Depression Inventory; HADS, Hospital Anxiety and Depression Scale; GDS, Geriatric Depression Scale; SDS, Zung Self-Rating Depression Scale; CSDD, Cornell Scale for Depression in Dementia; CES-D, Center for Epidemiologic Studies Depression Scale; UPDRS, Unified Parkinson Disease Rating Scale.
[b]PPV, positive predictive value; NPV, negative predictive value.

dPD, but the precise relationship between anxiety and depression in PD remains unclear [12,13] Depression is frequently associated with cognitive impairment, both in primary depression and in dPD [14]. It is important to separate depression and dementia in the older population, as the pseudo-dementia of depression is reversible with appropriate therapy.

Mood fluctuations are another disturbance of mood that is unique to PD and must be distinguished from dPD. Mood fluctuations, like motor fluctuations, develop in the setting of advancing disease and dopaminergic therapy. They are frequently accompanied by other non-motor fluctuations (e.g., anxiety, pain). They are defined as frequent shifts in mood that occur multiple times per day. These fluctuations can be dramatic, shifting from suicidality to euphoria within minutes. In between these shifts, individuals may have normal mood. In this way they differ from an individual with depression, in which there may be variations in symptom severity during the day, but mood is persistently low. Some patients experience both decreased and elevated mood, whereas others fluctuate only between normal and low mood. Isolated periods of abnormally elevated mood (without periods of low mood) appear to be uncommon [15]. Mood and anxiety fluctuations can occur independently, but are frequently seen together [16]. Mood and other non-motor fluctuations (e.g., anxiety) are increasingly recognized complications of advancing PD and can occur in up to 75% of patients with motor fluctuations. Although individuals with mood fluctuations are more likely than those without to have a history of depression or anxiety, fluctuations may also occur in those without a past or current psychiatric disorder [16].

Phenomenology

There are two lines of thought that motivate research into the phenomenology of dPD. In one, dPD is a fully distinct disorder from primary depression, with separate pathophysiology and risk factors. In the other, dPD shares the same pathophysiology as typical depression, but may display a different phenotype due to the modifying influence of Lewy body or other PD pathology. Overall, the available evidence suggests that dPD manifests with low energy and motivation, higher degrees of anxiety, and poor concentration, whereas the self-reproach, worry, and intense sadness of typical depression appear to be less common [17–19].

Epidemiology

The prevalence of dPD varies depending both on how depression is assessed and defined and on the source population studied. Although studies drawn from specialty clinics have reported a prevalence for major depression in PD of 25–40% [20,21], a community-based study reported a prevalence of only 7.7% [1]. Minor and mild depressive symptoms are much more common, occurring in up to 50% of PD individuals. A recent meta-analysis of 36 articles defined a weighted prevalence of 17% for major depression, 22% for minor depression, and 13% for dysthymia [22]. Depressive symptoms that were clinically significant, regardless of fulfillment of DSM criteria for a specific syndrome, were present in 35%. Early age of PD onset [23], cognitive impairment, and thought disorder are associated with an increased risk of dPD [24].

Depression has a negative impact on several aspects of PD. In a recent cohort study [25], depression was one of three factors (including cognitive function and functional independence) associated with declines in health-related quality-of-life (HRQOL) scores. PD depression results in increased disability [2], impairments in activities of daily living (ADL) [26], and impaired quality-of-life [3]. One case–control study demonstrated that depression was a significant predictor of 10-year mortality (HR 2.66, 95% CI 1.59–4.44) [27]. In a study examining 413 subjects with early untreated PD, depression was a significant predictor of impairment in ADLs and shortened time to needing symptomatic therapy for motor symptoms [28].

Etiology

The etiology of depression in PD remains unclear. However, the available evidence refutes the possibility that all depression in PD is merely a reaction to disability. One of the stronger lines of evidence comes from studies showing that depression can precede the onset of motor features and a diagnosis of PD by several years [29,30]. In addition, the presence and degree of depression are unrelated to disease severity, which would be expected if depression resulted only from increasing disability. In fact, the converse appears to be possible, in that having depression can worsen the perception of motor symptoms and increase disability at a given level of disease severity [28]. First-degree relatives of patients with PD also appear to be at increased risk of depressive and anxiety disorders in a population-based study, suggesting that PD and depression share susceptibility factors and arguing against depression being a reactive process [31].

Brain imaging and pathologic studies have attempted to delineate better the structures affected in dPD. Morphometric imaging has shown gray matter alterations in the bilateral orbitofrontal, bilateral rectal gyri, and right superior temporal lobes when comparing dPD with non-depressed PD [32]. Pathologically, depression is associated with more severe neuronal loss in the dorsal raphe nucleus compared with non-depressed PD patients [33]. Complementary work using transcranial sonography (TCS) and magnetic resonance imaging (MRI) demonstrated reduced echogenicity of the midline mesencephalon, particularly the raphe nuclei and nearby sagittal fiber tracts, in dPD compared with non-depressed PD [34]. The authors noted, however, that neither TCS nor MRI data support a correlation between signal intensity and severity of depression. In a single case report, stimulation of the left subthalamic nucleus was sufficient to induce acute and severe depressive symptoms in an individual with PD receiving deep brain stimulation (DBS) [35], but the networks and neurotransmitters involved in this dramatic response remain unclear. Taken together, the data suggest that dPD is associated with several changes in the brainstem structures with outputs to other cortical and subcortical limbic areas.

Neurotransmitter work has also implicated limbic systems in dPD. Dysfunction of the serotonergic system is widely recognized in typical depression, and several studies have examined the role of serotonin in dPD. Depressed individuals with PD have lower levels of serotonin metabolites in their CSF than non-depressed individuals [36]. Individuals with PD also have blunted responses to serotonergic challenge when compared with healthy controls, and this response is further reduced in PD subjects with depression ($p < 0.02$ in comparison with both healthy controls and to non-depressed PD subjects) [37]. Two studies of hospital-based subjects have shown a link between genetic polymorphisms affecting the serotonin transporter and depression [38] and anxiety in PD [39]. However, another study of a community-based cohort did not confirm this association [40]. In addition, a double-blind placebo-controlled cross-over study of transient serotonin depletion did not find any effect on mood symptoms in PD individuals, in contrast to changes seen in typical depression [41].

Because PD is classically considered as a disease of dopamine dysfunction, decreased dopamine activity has been examined as a potential cause of dPD. Functional imaging work involving the dopamine transporter (DAT) has suggested that both depression and anxiety are associated with decreased dopamine transport in the left putamen [42].

Functional neuroimaging of both dopamine and noradrenaline transporters suggests that depressed PD individuals have reduced binding in the locus coeruleus, mediodorsal and inferior thalamus, left ventral striatum, and right amygdala, when compared with non-depressed PD. Apathy scores correlated with the binding values in the ventral striatum, whereas anxiety scores correlated with multiple regions [43].

Acetylcholine is more typically associated with cognitive deficits in Alzheimer's disease. However, one study of acetylcholinesterase activity in dPD demonstrated that decreasing activity correlated with worsening depressive symptoms [44]. However, this group was not clinically diagnosed with depression, and whether the depressive symptoms in fact reflect pseudo-dementia is uncertain.

In summary, converging evidence suggests that disrupted connections between the basal ganglia, midbrain structures, and limbic and cortical areas are responsible for dPD, and that this disruption predominantly involves the monoamine neurotransmitter systems. The pathology underlying this process, however, is unknown.

Depression and deep brain stimulation

Conflicting data are available regarding the effect of DBS on mood. Although evidence for worsening of premorbid depression after DBS is limited, severe or uncontrolled depression is generally considered a contraindication to DBS surgery. Postoperative depression has been consistently reported in several study designs, but the prevalence varies widely from 1.5 to 25%, whereas suicide attempts range from 0.5 to 2.9% [45]. In a randomized trial of DBS in 156 PD patients, no significant differences were noted between groups on emotional wellbeing or depression rating scale scores [46]. Four subjects did, however, develop depression in the stimulation group, with one suicide, whereas none of the medical group developed depression.

Suicide after DBS is not limited to individuals with PD. A 2006 meta-analysis examined 546 studies of DBS at all anatomic locations for the following indications: PD (65.4% of studies), essential tremor (ET) (11.7%), dystonia (9.9%), other movement disorder (10.1%), and other, including chronic pain, epilepsy, and depression (3%) [47]. The overall prevalence of depression was 2.4%, with a prevalence of suicidal ideation or attempt of 0.3–0.7% and a completed suicide rate of 0.16–0.32%. Of the 32 subjects reporting suicidality, 26 had PD, four had dystonia, one had ET, and one had obsessive–compulsive disorder (OCD). The rate of completed suicides was highest in the group receiving thalamic stimulation (5.4%). Although the relative rate of suicidality may be higher in other populations, the increased incidence in PD is particularly concerning because suicide is uncommon despite the high prevalence of depression. Suicide after DBS may be related to a combination of altered mood and increased impulsivity, particularly in cases without a preoperative psychiatric history [48].

Another issue involving DBS and mood is whether anatomic location modifies the risk of developing depression or other mood disorders after DBS. In a recent analysis of adverse event (AE) reporting in DBS [49], mental status and behavioral AEs were more prevalent in subthalamic nucleus (STN) DBS than in globus pallidus interna (GPi) stimulation. However, most of the difference was due to confusion; depression rates appeared to be similar and uncommon for both anatomic sites (1.3% for STN versus 0.9% for GPi). In a systematic review of neuropsychiatric issues in DBS, neuropsychiatric side effects appeared to be more common with stimulation of STN than GPi [45]. However, this suggestion may simply reflect that STN is a more common target and more information is available regarding this placement location. Another possibility is that STN DBS permits a greater reduction in dopaminergic therapy for motor symptoms. In this setting, non-motor symptoms that may have been treated or masked by dopaminergic therapy may be uncovered as the medication is reduced.

DBS may affect other pathways involved in the control of emotions besides mood. An extended case series of STN stimulation noted significant worsening of apathy scores postoperatively, without changes in depression scores [50]. The subgroup of patients with apathy appeared to have electrodes located more ventrally and internally compared with the other group, suggesting a potential mechanistic influence of the STN on apathy symptoms. However, these findings require replication. Also, although DBS is effective at improving motor fluctuations, evidence for the effects of DBS on non-motor fluctuations is limited [51].

As noted above with regard to the effect of GPi versus STN DBS, mood effects seen after DBS implantation within the STN in particular may result not from stimulation, but from the withdrawal of dopaminergic medications (which are typically reduced by about 50%). One goal of DBS therapy is to reduce dyskinesias by reducing the amount of medication taken. However, it is becoming clear that DBS is not simply a replacement for L-dopa therapy. One study of acute mood effects noted that whereas medication and stimulation both improved motor and cognitive symptoms, only L-dopa had an effect on hedonia [52]. Other studies have demonstrated mood symptoms after medication withdrawal that improved when dopaminergic therapy was reintroduced [53]. Little information is available to distinguish between mood effects due to medication withdrawal versus stimulation. Taken together, these data suggest the need for more rigorous evaluation of mood disorders in the setting of DBS.

Management and prognosis

Antidepressant therapy

Evidence is limited regarding pharmacotherapy in dPD, and most available data come from small trials of varying quality. Consequently, in a 2006 practice parameter, the AAN could only recommend amitriptyline, a first-generation tricyclic anti-depressant (TCA). TCAs can be problematic in the elderly, however, given their side effect profile. In particular, their tendency to induce or worsen orthostatic hypotension and to cause anti-cholinergic effects (e.g., constipation, confusion) frequently result in poor tolerability among patients with PD. As a result, most patients with dPD are started on a selective serotonin reuptake inhibitor (SSRI). This tendency was confirmed in a large study of the US veteran population, in which individuals with PD depression were most commonly prescribed an SSRI (62.9%) or a newer non-SSRI such as venlafaxine and mirtazapine (20.6%), with low rates of TCA use (7.4%) [54]. Although case reports have described worsening of motor symptoms with the use of various SSRIs, motor deterioration is not found consistently in larger studies (Table 17.2) [55]. Although SSRIs appear effective in open-label studies, two randomized, placebo-controlled trials found that sertraline [56] and citalopram [57] were not effective. More recently, two pilot trials have re-examined TCAs and SSRIs for the treatment of dPD. One recently completed trial was a randomized, placebo-controlled study of paroxetine CR and nortriptyline involving 52 subjects [58]. At 8 weeks, nortriptyline was superior to placebo, but paroxetine CR was not. Another randomized, placebo-controlled trial involving 48 subjects with a 30-day follow-up period compared desipramine and citalopram, and found that desipramine was better than placebo at 2 weeks, but citalopram was not [59]. However, both anti-depressants were more effective than placebo at 4 weeks, and citalopram was better tolerated. These data suggest that TCAs may be equally or more effective than SSRIs in treating dPD and raise the concern that SSRIs may be ineffective in dPD.

Serotonin–norepinephrine reuptake inhibitors (SNRIs) may be a rational choice for dPD therapy given the impairments to the norepinephrine system seen in PD (see the section Etiology, above), and have the potential advantage of improved tolerability compared with TCAs. One case report described two patients with an incomplete response to SSRI treatment, both of whom achieved full remission after switching to milnacipran, an SNRI [60]. Reboxetine, another SNRI, was also effective in treating dPD resistant to amitriptyline and fluoxetine in a single case study [61]. To address better the question of optimal anti-depressant therapy in dPD, an NIH-funded, multicenter, randomized, placebo-controlled clinical trial comparing paroxetine (an SSRI) and venlafaxine (an SNRI) is currently under way [62].

Emerging evidence suggests that pramipexole may have anti-depressant effects, presumably due to its effect on D3 receptors. In an observational cohort of 657 PD patients, Lemke *et al.* noted a significant reduction in depression and anhedonia during treatment with pramipexole [63]. Rektorova *et al.* performed a prospective randomized single-blind study of pramipexole and pergolide and discovered an anti-depressant effect for pramipexole, but not pergolide [64]. A randomized open-label study of pramipexole and sertraline for depression found that both medications were effective in reducing depression scores [65]. However, all of these studies are limited by their open-label design, raising concerns about whether the results are influenced by the high placebo effect seen in clinical trials for depression. Pramipexole has also been shown to be effective in bipolar depression in a preliminary placebo-controlled trial [66], arguing that the response in PD is not simply due to improvement in motor functioning. A randomized, placebo-controlled trial of pramipexole for dPD is currently under way [67].

Other therapeutic modalities

There are few controlled trials involving other therapeutic modalities in the treatment of dPD. Still, preliminary studies have examined several potential options for therapy beyond anti-depressant medications. Cognitive behavioral treatment (CBT) aims to improve depression by educating the patient to identify maladaptive thoughts and encouraging positive cognitive techniques. Although data in PD are limited, in a pilot study CBT has been shown to reduce depression significantly, with roughly 10-point improvements in both the HAM-D and the BDI [68]. Electroconvulsive therapy can improve the motor symptoms of PD [69,70] and was effective for the specific treatment of medication-refractory PD depression in one case [71]. Bright light therapy has been shown to have a modest but statistically significant effect on both depression and tremor in a randomized sham-controlled study [72]. However, the study follow-up was only 2 weeks, and the long-term effects of this therapy in dPD are unknown.

In another small study of 15 patients, repetitive transcranial magnetic stimulation (rTMS) was examined as a potential treatment for dPD and found to result in significant improvements in both mood and motor functioning ("off" state only) that persisted at a 3-week follow-up visit [73]. A double-blind randomized trial with both placebo and sham controls evaluated the effects of rTMS versus fluoxetine on PD depression, and concluded that rTMS and fluoxetine had comparable efficacy [74]. These results are promising but need to be interpreted with caution in the light of more recent studies that have questioned the efficacy of SSRIs in the treatment of dPD.

Few data are available regarding the clinical course of dPD or predictors of severity, remission, or response to therapy. A recent secondary data analysis of 413 subjects with early untreated PD suggests that depressive symptoms may remain mild over time for most and that mild symptoms tend to remit (B. Ravina *et al.*, unpublished observations, July 2008). However, the presence of mild symptoms increases the risk of developing more severe symptoms. In addition, PD individuals with persistent depression appear to be undertreated, with only 11% receiving treatment at the highest recommend range and 33% receiving a second agent in one study [75].

Conclusion

Depression is a common neuropsychiatric co-morbidity in PD. Although most patients experience only mild symptoms, dPD is associated with significant declines in quality-of-life, worsened disability, and increased need

Table 17.2 Prospective trials of SSRIs, heterocyclics in dPD.

Study	Study design	*N*	Outcome measure used[a]	Results
Sertraline				
Antonini *et al.* (2006) [81]	Randomized, single-blind comparison of sertraline and amitriptyline on depression and quality-of-life	31	HDRS	Improvement in depression without changes in motor symptoms rating scale; only sertraline had positive effect on quality-of-life
Leentjens *et al.* (2003) [56]	Randomized, double-blind, placebo-controlled	12	MADRS	No effect
Hauser and Zesiewcz (1997) [82]	Open-label	15	BDI	Improvement in depression without changes in motor symptoms; 13% dropout due to adverse effects
Paroxetine				
Tesei *et al.* (2000) [83]	Open-label tolerability study	65	HDRS	Improvement in depression with 20% dropout due to adverse effects
Ceravolo *et al.* (2000) [84]	Open-label	33	HDRS	Improvement in depression; one subject had reversible worsening of tremor
Paroxetine CR				
Menza *et al.* (2008 [58]	Randomized, placebo-controlled study of paroxetine CR and nortriptyline	52	HDRS	Nortriptyline was superior to placebo, but paroxetine CR was not; no worsening of motor symptoms in either group
Citalopram				
Devos *et al.* (2008 [59]	Randomized, double-blind placebo-controlled comparison of desipramine and citalopram	48	MADRS	Both citalopram and desipramine improved symptoms; desipramine worked more quickly but had more mild adverse events. No significant worsening of motor symptoms
Menza *et al.* (2004) [57]	Open-label	10	HDRS	Improvement in depression and anxiety without motor impairment
Wermuth *et al.* (1998) [85]	Randomized, placebo-controlled trial	37	HDRS	No effect
Nefazodone, fluoxetine				
Avila *et al.* (2003) [86]	Randomized, unblinded comparison of nefazodone and fluoxetine on depression and motor symptoms	16	BDI	Both interventions improved depression, and nefazodone had beneficial effect on motor symptoms
Escitalopram				
Weintraub *et al.* (2006) [87]	Open-label, flexible dose	12	IDS	Improvement in depressive scores and global impression
Bupropion				
Goetz *et al.* (1984) [88]	Open-label, designed to examine motor symptoms	20	CGI-Change	5 out of 12 depressed patients improved on global impression scale; no impairment in motor symptoms
Mirtazapine	No controlled trials	–	–	–
Venlafaxine	No controlled trials	–	–	–
Duloxetine	No controlled trials	–	–	–
Reboxetine				
Pintor *et al.* (2006) [89]	Open-label, single-blind assessment	17	HDRS	Improvement in depression and anxiety, no impairment in motor symptoms

[a]IDS, Inventory of Depressive Symptomatology; CGI-Change, Clinical Global Impression – Change.

for therapy to address motor symptoms. Further research is needed to improve our understanding of the pathophysiology underlying dPD and provide additional prognostic information. The upcoming results of large and well-controlled clinical trials should help to guide therapy for depression in PD.

References

1. Tandberg E, Larsen JP, Aarsland D, Cummings JL. The occurrence of depression in Parkinson's disease: a community-based study. *Arch Neurol* 1996;**53**(2):175–9.
2. Weintraub D, Moberg PJ, Duda JE, *et al.* Effect of psychiatric and other nonmotor symptoms on disability in Parkinson's disease. *J Am Geriatr Soc* 2004;**52**(5):784–8.
3. Schrag A, Jahanshahi M, Quinn N. What contributes to quality-of-life in patients with Parkinson's disease? *J Neurol Neurosurg Psychiatry* 2000;**69**(3):308–12.
4. Aarsland D, Larsen JP, Karlsen K, *et al.* Mental symptoms in Parkinson's disease are important contributors to caregiver distress. *Int J Geriatr Psychiatry* 1999;**14**:866–74.
5. McCrone P, Allcock LM, Burn DJ. Predicting the cost of Parkinson's disease. *Mov Disord* 2007;**22**(6):804–12.
6. Chen P, Kales HC, Weintraub D, *et al.* Depression in veterans with Parkinson's disease: frequency, co-morbidity, and healthcare utilization. *Int J Geriatr Psychiatry* 2007;**22**(6):543–8.
7. American Psychiatric Association. *Diagnostic and Statistical Manual of Mental Disorders*, 4th edn. Washington, DC: American Psychiatric Association, 1994.
8. Marsh L, McDonald WM, Cummings J, Ravina B. NINDS/NIMH Work Group on Depression and Parkinson's Disease. Provisional diagnostic criteria for depression in Parkinson's disease: report of an NINDS/NIMH Work Group. *Mov Disord* 2006;**21**(2):148–58.
9. Miyasaki JM, Shannon K, Voon V, *et al.* Practice Parameter: evaluation and treatment of depression, psychosis, and dementia in Parkinson disease (an evidence-based review). Report of the Quality Standards Subcommittee of the American Academy of Neurology. *Neurology* 2006;**66**(7):996–1002.
10. Schrag A, Barone P, Brown RG, *et al.* Depression rating scales in Parkinson's disease: critique and recommendations. *Mov Disord* 2007;**22**(8):1077–92.
11. Kirsch-Darrow L, Fernandez HH, Marsiske M, *et al.* Dissociating apathy and depression in Parkinson disease. *Neurology* 2006;**67**(1):33–8.
12. Schiffer RB, Kurlan R, Rubin A. Evidence for atypical depression in Parkinson's disease. *Am J Psychiatry* 1988;**145**:1020–2.
13. Richard IH, Szegethy E, Lichter D, *et al.* Parkinson's disease: a preliminary study of yohimbine challenge in patients with anxiety. *Clin Neuropharmacol* 1999;**22**:172–5.
14. Costa A, Peppe A, Carlesimo GA, *et al.* Major and minor depression in Parkinson's disease: a neuropsychological investigation. *Eur J Neurol* 2006;**13**(9):972–80.
15. Black KJ, Hershey T, Hartlein JM, *et al.* Levodopa challenge neuroimaging of levodopa-related mood fluctuations in Parkinson's disease. *Neuropsychopharmacology* 2005;**30**(3):590–601.
16. Richard IH, Justus AW, Kurlan R. Relationship between mood and motor fluctuations in Parkinson's disease. *J Neuropsychiatry Clin Neurosci* 2001;**13**(1):35–41.
17. Richard IH. Apathy does not equal depression in Parkinson disease: why we should care. *Neurology* 2006;**67**(1):10–1.
18. Ehrt U, Brønnick K, Leentjens AFG, *et al.* Depressive symptom profile in Parkinson's disease: a comparison with depression in elderly patients without Parkinson's disease. *Int J Geriatr Psychiatry* 2006;**21**(3):252–8.
19. Weintraub D, Xie S, Karlawish J, Siderowf A. Differences in depression symptoms in patients with Alzheimer's and Parkinson's diseases: evidence from the 15-item Geriatric Depression Scale (GDS-15). *Int J Geriatr Psychiatry* 2007;**22**(10):1025–30.
20. Dooneief G, Mirabello E, Bell K, *et al.* An estimate of the incidence of depression in idiopathic Parkinson's disease. *Arch Neurol* 1992;**49**(3):305–7.
21. Cole SA, Woodard JL, Juncos JL, *et al.* Depression and disability in Parkinson's disease. *J Neuropsychiatry Clin Neurosci* 1996;**8**(1):20–5.
22. Reijnders JS, Ehrt U, Weber WE, *et al.* A systematic review of prevalence studies of depression in Parkinson's disease. *Mov Disord* 2008;**23**(2):183–9.
23. Giladi N, Treves TA, Paleacu D, *et al.* Risk factors for dementia, depression and psychosis in long-standing Parkinson's disease. *J Neural Transm* 2000;**107**(1):59–71.
24. Tandberg E, Larsen JP, Aarsland D, *et al.* Risk factors for depression in Parkinson disease. *Arch Neurol* 1997;**54**(5):625–30.
25. Marras C, McDermott MP, Rochon PA, *et al.* Predictors of deterioration in health-related quality-of-life in Parkinson's disease: results from the DATATOP trial. *Mov Disord* 2008;**23**(5):653–9.
26. Holroyd S, Currie LJ, Wooten GF. Depression is associated with impairment of ADL, not motor function in Parkinson disease. *Neurology* 2005;**64**(12):2134–5.
27. Hughes TA, Ross HF, Mindham RH, Spokes EG. Mortality in Parkinson's disease and its association with dementia and depression. *Acta Neurol Scand* 2004;**110**(2):118–23.
28. Ravina B, Camicioli R, Como PG, *et al.* The impact of depressive symptoms in early Parkinson disease. *Neurology* 2007;**69**(4):342–7.
29. Leentjens AFG, van den Akker M, Metsemakers JFM, *et al.* Higher incidence of depression preceding the onset of Parkinson's disease: a register study. *Mov Disord* 2003;**18**(4):414–8.
30. Schuurman AG, van den Akker M, *et al.* Increased risk of Parkinson's disease after depression: a retrospective cohort study. *Neurology* 2002;**58**(10):1501–4.
31. Arabia G, Grossardt BR, Geda YE, *et al.* Increased risk of depressive and anxiety disorders in relatives of patients with Parkinson disease. *Arch Gen Psychiatry* 2007;**64**(12):1385–92.
32. Feldmann A, Illes Z, Kosztolanyi P, *et al.* Morphometric changes of gray matter in Parkinson's disease with depression: a voxel-based morphometry study. *Mov Disord* 2008;**23**(1):42–6.
33. Paulus W, Jellinger K. The neuropathologic basis of different clinical subgroups in Parkinson's disease. *J Neuropath Exp Neurol* 1991;**50**:743–55.

34. Becker G, Berg D. Neuroimaging in basal ganglia disorders: perspectives for transcranial ultrasound. *Mov Disord* 2001;**16**(1):23–32.
35. Bejjani B, Damier P, Arnulf I, *et al*. Transient acute depression induced by high-frequency deep brain stimulation. *N Engl J Med* 1999;**340**(19):1476–80.
36. Mayeux R, Stern Y, Cote L, Williams JBW. Altered serotonin metabolism in depressed patients with Parkinson's disease. *Neurology* 1984;**34**:642–6.
37. Kostic VS, Lecic D, Doder M, *et al*. Prolactin and cortisol responses to fenfluramine in Parkinson's disease. *Biol Psychiatry* 1996;**40**:769–75.
38. Mossner R, Henneberg A, Schmitt A, *et al*. Allelic variation of serotonin transporter expression is associated with depression in Parkinson's disease. *Mol Psychiatry* 2001;**6**(3):350–2.
39. Menza MA, Palermo B, DiPaola R, *et al*. Depression and anxiety in Parkinson's disease: possible effect of genetic variation in the serotonin transporter. *J Geriatr Psychiatry Neurol* 1999;**12**:49–52.
40. Burn DJ, Tiangyou W, Allcock LM, *et al*. Allelic variation of a functional polymorphism in the serotonin transporter gene and depression in Parkinson's disease. *Parkinsonism Relat Disord* 2006;**12**(3):139–41.
41. Leentjens AF, Scholtissen B, Vreeling FW, Verhey FR. The serotonergic hypothesis for depression in Parkinson's disease: an experimental approach. *Neuropsychopharmacology* 2006;**31**(5):1009–15.
42. Weintraub D, Newberg AB, Cary MS, *et al*. Striatal dopamine transporter imaging correlates with anxiety and depression symptoms in Parkinson's disease. *J Nucl Med* 2005;**46**(2):227–32.
43. Remy P, Doder M, Lees A, *et al*. Depression in Parkinson's disease: loss of dopamine and noradrenaline innervation in the limbic system. *Brain* 2005;**128**:1314–22.
44. Bohnen NI, Kaufer DI, Hendrickson R, *et al*. Cortical cholinergic denervation is associated with depressive symptoms in Parkinson's disease and parkinsonian dementia. *J Neurol Neurosurg Psychiatry* 2007;**78**(6):641–3.
45. Voon V, Kubu C, Krack P, *et al*. Deep brain stimulation: neuropsychological and neuropsychiatric issues. *Mov Disord* 2006;**21**(Suppl 14):S305–27.
46. Deuschl G, Schade-Brittinger C, Krack P, *et al*. A randomized trial of deep brain stimulation for Parkinson's disease. *N Engl J Med* 2006;**355**(9):896–908.
47. Appleby BS, Duggan PS, Regenberg A, Rabins PV. Psychiatric and neuropsychiatric adverse events associated with deep brain stimulation: a meta-analysis of ten years' experience. *Mov Disord* 2007;**22**(12):1722–8.
48. Soulas T, Gurruchaga J, Palfi S, *et al*. Attempted and completed suicides after subthalamic nucleus stimulation for Parkinson's disease. *J Neurol Neurosurg Psychiatry* 2008;**79**(8):952–4.
49. Videnovic A, Metman LV. Deep brain stimulation for Parkinson's disease: prevalence of adverse events and need for standardized reporting. *Mov Disord* 2008;**23**(3):343–9.
50. Drapier D, Drapier S, Sauleau P, *et al*. Does subthalamic nucleus stimulation induce apathy in Parkinson's disease? *J Neurol* 2006;**253**(8):1083–91.
51. Witjas T, Kaphan E, Regis J, *et al*. Effects of chronic subthalamic stimulation on nonmotor fluctuations in Parkinson's disease. *Mov Disord* 2007;**22**(12):1729–34.
52. Witt K, Daniels C, Herzog J, *et al*. Differential effects of L-dopa and subthalamic stimulation on depressive symptoms and hedonic tone in Parkinson's disease. *J Neuropsychiatry Clin Neurosci* 2006;**18**(3):397–401.
53. Czernecki V, Schüpbach M, Yaici S, *et al*. Apathy following subthalamic stimulation in Parkinson disease: a dopamine responsive symptom. *Mov Disord* 2008;**23**(7):964–9.
54. Chen P, Kales HC, Weintraub D, *et al*. Antidepressant treatment of veterans with Parkinson's disease and depression: analysis of a national sample. *J Geriatr Psychiatry Neurol* 2007;**20**(3):161–5.
55. Gony M, Lapeyre-Mestre M, Montastruc JL; French Network of Regional Pharmacovigilance Centers. Risk of serious extrapyramidal symptoms in patients with Parkinson's disease receiving antidepressant drugs: a pharmacoepidemiologic study comparing serotonin reuptake inhibitors and other antidepressant drugs. *Clin Neuropharmacol* 2003;**26**(3):142–5.
56. Leentjens AF, Vreeling FW, Luijckx GJ, Verhey FR. SSRIs in the treatment of depression in Parkinson's disease. *Int J Geriatr Psychiatry* 2003;**18**(6):552–4.
57. Menza M, Marin H, Kaufman K, *et al*. Citalopram treatment of depression in Parkinson's disease: the impact on anxiety, disability, and cognition. *J Neuropsychiatry Clin Neurosci* 2004;**16**(3):315–9.
58. Menza M, Dobkin R, Marin H, *et al*. A controlled trial of antidepressants in patients with Parkinson's disease and depression. *Poster session presented at: 161st Annual Meeting of the American Psychiatric Association*, 3–8 May 2008, Washington, DC.
59. Devos D, Dujardin K, Poirot I, *et al*. Comparison of desipramine and citalopram treatments for depression in Parkinson's disease: a double-blind, randomized, placebo-controlled study. *Mov Disord* 2008;**23**(6):850–7.
60. Takahashi H, Kamata M, Yoshida K, *et al*. Remarkable effect of milnacipran, a serotonin–noradrenalin reuptake inhibitor (SNRI), on depressive symptoms in patients with Parkinson's disease who have insufficient response to selective serotonin reuptake inhibitors (SSRIs): two case reports. *Prog Neuropsychopharmacol Biol Psychiatry* 2005;**29**(2):351–3.
61. Lemke MR. Reboxetine treatment of depression in Parkinson's disease. *J Clin Psychiatry* 2000;**61**(11):872.
62. ClinicalTrials.gov. Study of antidepressants in Parkinson's disease (SAD-PD), http://clinicaltrials.gov/ct2/show/NCT00086190?term=sad+pd&rank=1 (updated 4 March 2008; accessed 28 July 2008).
63. Lemke MR, Brecht HM, Koester J, Reichmann H. Effects of the dopamine agonist pramipexole on depression, anhedonia and motor functioning in Parkinson's disease. *J Neurol Sci* 2006;**248**(1–2):266–70.
64. Rektorova I, Rektor I, Bares M, *et al*. Pramipexole and pergolide in the treatment of depression in Parkinson's disease: a national multicentre prospective randomized study. *Eur J Neurol*. 2003;**10**(4):399–406.
65. Barone P, Scarzella L, Marconi R, *et al*. Pramipexole versus sertraline in the treatment of depression in Parkinson's disease: a national multicenter parallel-group randomized study. J Neurol 2006;**253**(5):601–7.
66. Goldberg J, Burdick K, Endick C. Preliminary randomized, double-blind, placebo-controlled trial of pramipexole added to mood stabilizers for treatment-resistant bipolar depression. *Am J Psychiatry* 2004;**161**(3):564–6.

67. Barone P, Schapira AHV, Debieuvre CD, Massey D. Design of a randomized, placebo-controlled trial of pramipexole in patients with Parkinson's disease and depressive symptoms. *Mov Disord* 2008;**22**(S1):S199.
68. Dobkin RD, Allen LA, Menza M. Cognitive-behavioral therapy for depression in Parkinson's disease: a pilot study. *Mov Disord* 2007;**22**(7):946–52.
69. Pridmore S, Pollard C. Electroconvulsive therapy in Parkinson's disease: 30-month follow-up. *J Neurol Neurosurg Psychiatry* 1996;**61**:693–700.
70. Moellentine C, Rummans T, Ahlskog JE, *et al.* Effectiveness of ECT in patients with parkinsonism. *J Neuropsychiatry Clin Neurosci* 1998;**10**(2):187–93.
71. Chou KL, Hurtig HI, Jaggi JL, *et al.* Electroconvulsive therapy for depression in a Parkinson's disease patient with bilateral subthalamic nucleus deep brain stimulators. *Parkinsonism Relat Disord* 2005;**11**(6):403–6.
72. Paus S, Schmitz-Hubsch T, Wullner U, *et al.* Bright light therapy in Parkinson's disease: a pilot study. *Mov Disord* 2007; **22**(10):1495–8.
73. Epstein CM, Evatt ML, Funk A, *et al.* An open study of repetitive transcranial magnetic stimulation in treatment-resistant depression with Parkinson's disease. *Clin Neurophysiol* 2007;**118**(10):2189–94.
74. Fregni F, Santos CM, Myczkowski ML, *et al.* Repetitive transcranial magnetic stimulation is as effective as fluoxetine in the treatment of depression in patients with Parkinson's disease. *J Neurol Neurosurg Psychiatry* 2004;**75**(8):1171–4.
75. Weintraub D, Moberg PJ, Duda JE, *et al.* Recognition and treatment of depression in Parkinson's disease. *J Geriatr Psychiatry Neurol* 2003;**16**(3):178–83.
76. Naarding P, Leentjens AFG, van Kooten F, Verhey FRJ. Disease-specific properties of the Hamilton Rating Scale for depression in patients with stroke, Alzheimer's dementia, and Parkinson's disease. *J Neuropsychiatry Clin Neurosci* 2002;**14**(3): 329–34.
77. Leentjens AFG, Verhey FRJ, Lousberg R, *et al.* The validity of the Hamilton and Montgomery–Asberg depression rating scales as screening and diagnostic tools for depression in Parkinson's disease. *Int J Geriatr Psychiatry* 2000;**15**(7): 644–9.
78. Leentjens AF, Verhey FR, Luijckx GJ, Troost J. The validity of the Beck Depression Inventory as a screening and diagnostic instrument for depression in patients with Parkinson's disease. *Mov Disord* 2000;**15**(6):1221–4.
79. McDonald WM, Holtzheimer PE, Haber M, *et al.* Validity of the 30-item Geriatric Depression Scale in patients with Parkinson's disease. *Mov Disord* 2006;**21**(10):1618–22.
80. Weintraub D, Oehlberg KA, Katz IR, Stern MB. Test characteristics of the 15-item Geriatric Depression Scale and Hamilton Depression Rating Scale in Parkinson disease. *Am J Geriatr Psychiatry* 2006;**14**(2):169–75.
81. Antonini A, Tesei S, Zecchinelli A, *et al.* Randomized study of sertraline and low-dose amitriptyline in patients with Parkinson's disease and depression: effect on quality-of-life. *Mov Disord* 2006;**21**(8):1119–22.
82. Hauser RA, Zesiewicz TA. Sertraline for the treatment of depression in Parkinson's disease. *Mov Disord* 1997;**12**(5): 756–9.
83. Tesei S, Antonini A, Canesi M, *et al.* Tolerability of paroxetine in Parkinson's disease: a prospective study. *Mov Disord* 2000;**15**(5):986–9.
84. Ceravolo R, Nuti A, Piccinni A, *et al.* Paroxetine in Parkinson's disease: effects on motor and depressive symptoms. *Neurology* 2000;**55**:1216–8.
85. Wermuth L, Sorensen PS, Timm S, *et al.* Depression in idiopathic Parkinson's disease treated with citalopram: a placebo-controlled trial. *Nordic J Psychiatry* 1998;**52**(2):163–9.
86. Avila A, Cardona X, Martin-Baranera M, *et al.* Does nefazodone improve both depression and Parkinson disease? A pilot randomized trial. *J Clin Psychopharmacol* 2003;**23**(5): 509–13.
87. Weintraub D, Taraborelli D, Morales KH, *et al.* Escitalopram for major depression in Parkinson's disease: an open-label, flexible-dosage study. *J Neuropsychiatry Clin Neurosci* 2006; **18**(3):377–83.
88. Goetz C, Tanner C, Klawans H. Buproprion in Parkinson's disease. *Neurology* 1984;**34**:1092–4.
89. Pintor L, Baillès E, Valldeoriola F, *et al.* Response to 4-month treatment with reboxetine in Parkinson's disease patients with a major depressive episode. *Gen Hosp Psychiatry* 2006;**28**(1): 59–64.

Chapter 18
Anxiety Syndromes and Panic Attacks

Daniel Weintraub[1,2,3,4] *& Staci Hoops*[1]
[1]Department of Psychiatry, University of Pennsylvania, Philadelphia, PA, USA
[2]Department of Neurology, University of Pennsylvania, Philadelphia, PA, USA
[3]Parkinson's Disease Research, Education and Clinical Center (PADRECC), Veterans Affairs Medical Center, Philadelphia, PA, USA
[4]Mental Illness Research, Education and Clinical Center (MIRECC), Veterans Affairs Medical Center, Philadelphia, PA, USA

Introduction

A wide range of anxiety disorders have been reported to occur in Parkinson's disease (PD), including generalized anxiety disorder (GAD), panic attacks or disorders, social phobia, specific phobia, and, to a lesser degree, obsessive–compulsive disorder (OCD) [1,2].

Generalized anxiety disorder (GAD), as defined in the *Diagnostic and Statistical Manual of Mental Disorders* (DSM-IV-TR) [3], is characterized by excessive anxiety and worry about a number of activities and is associated with restlessness, fatigue, difficulty in concentrating, irritability, muscle tension, or sleep disturbance.

A *panic attack*, which by itself is not a psychiatric disorder, is characterized by a discrete period of intense fear or discomfort, in which a variety of symptoms develop abruptly and reach a peak within 10 min. The symptoms include palpitations, sweating, shaking, shortness of breath, dizziness, depersonalization, and fear of dying. *Panic disorder* is recurrent, unexpected panic attacks plus persistent concern about additional attacks, worry about the implications or consequences of attacks, or a significant change in behavior related to the attacks.

Social phobia is characterized by a marked and persistent fear of one or more social situations. The individual fears that he or she will act in a way (or show anxiety symptoms) that will be embarrassing, but also recognizes that the fear is excessive. DSM-IV-TR specifically states that individuals with social phobia may be vulnerable to a worsening of social anxiety and avoidance related to a general medical condition. However, if the social phobia symptoms are *limited* to concerns about the general medical condition, then by convention a diagnosis of social phobia is not made. Thus, if the patient only fears that his or her PD symptoms will cause embarrassment in public, then criteria for social phobia are not met.

Obsessive–compulsive disorder (OCD) is characterized by complaints of persistent or repetitive thoughts (obsessions) or behaviors (compulsions). The person feels compelled to continue the thoughts or behaviors, despite awareness that the thoughts or behaviors may be inappropriate, and feels distress if he or she stops them. OCD must be distinguished from both obsessive–compulsive personality disorder (OCPD) and impulse control disorders (ICDs). OCPD is a personality disorder characterized by orderliness, perfectionism, and mental and interpersonal control at the expense of flexibility, openness, and efficiency. ICDs are characterized by a failure to resist an impulse, drive, or temptation to perform a typically pleasurable activity that is ultimately harmful to the person or to others due to its excessive nature. ICDs that can occur in PD include compulsive gambling, buying, sexual behavior, and eating.

Specific phobia, formally known as *simple phobia*, is the most common of all anxiety disorders in the general population. It is characterized by an excessive or unreasonable fear that is cued by the presence or anticipation of a specific object or situation (e.g., flying, heights, animals, receiving an injection, seeing blood).

In addition to these formal psychiatric disorders, both general anxiety symptoms and discrete panic attacks have been reported to occur as part of "off" periods in PD patients with motor fluctuations [4]. These symptoms are typically classified as *non-motor fluctuations* (NMFs).

Epidemiology

General

It has been reported in cross-sectional studies that up to 25–50% of PD patients experience some type of anxiety symptoms or disorders [1,2,5], and these prevalence estimates far exceed those reported for anxiety disorders in the general population (5–15%) [1]. In addition, most comparison studies have found that anxiety disorders are

Parkinson's Disease: Non-Motor and Non-Dopaminergic Features, First Edition. Edited by C. Warren Olanow, Fabrizio Stocchi, and Anthony E. Lang.

more common in PD than in other neurological disorders (e.g., multiple sclerosis) [6] or medical illnesses (e.g., osteoarthritis) [5,7].

Specific anxiety disorders

Most studies have reported that the most common anxiety disorders in PD are panic disorder, phobic disorder, and GAD [5], and these disorders can be co-morbid [8]. However, there has been limited research into the prevalence of specific anxiety disorders in PD. One study of 90 PD patients reported that 30% of the patients met criteria for panic disorder, 11.1% for GAD, and 3.3% for OCD [9]. Only panic disorder was more common in PD patients than in an age- and sex-matched group, and co-morbid mood and anxiety disorders were more common in PD patients than in controls (19.3% versus 8.6%, respectively). In another study of 131 PD patients, 24% of the patients experienced recurrent panic attacks [10].

In a recent study that used a structured psychiatric interview to examine the frequency of social phobia and performance on the Liebowitz Social Anxiety Scale (LSAS) in PD [11], social phobia was diagnosed in 50% of a convenience sample of 90 PD patients at a movement disorder center. Approximately 80% of the patients who met criteria of social phobia had generalized social phobia (i.e., fearful of or avoiding four or more social situations).

One study that administered an OCD inventory to PD patients and normal controls found that PD patients with severe disease had more OCD symptoms (i.e., checking, doubting, and cleaning subscales) than controls, whereas no difference was detected for patients with milder disease [12]. Another study found that PD patients scored higher than controls on an OCD ordering subscale, but had less OCD symptoms overall than patients with Tourette's syndrome or non-PD patients diagnosed with OCD [13]. In contrast, another study found that neither OCD as a diagnosis nor OCD symptoms were more common in PD than in matched controls [14].

In a small study, the lifetime prevalence of specific phobia in PD patients was reported to be 35.7%, significantly higher than the lifetime prevalence in the general population (8.9%) based on the results of a large epidemiological study [15]. Interestingly, 80% of the PD patients reported to have a history of specific phobia had the onset of these symptoms prior to the onset of PD.

Non-motor fluctuations

Non-motor fluctuations (NMFs) have long been recognized as a feature of "off" periods in PD patients with motor fluctuations; commonly reported NMFs include depressive symptoms, anxiety symptoms, and slowness of thinking. In one of the few studies to study systematically a range of NMF in patients with motor fluctuations, fluctuating anxiety symptoms were reported in 66% of patients. Of this group, 88% reported experiencing increased anxiety during "off" periods, 3% in the "pre-off" period, and 9% reported that anxiety and motor fluctuations occurred independently [4].

Deep brain stimulation (DBS)

One recent review of neuropsychiatric complications of DBS treatment found that anxiety was rarely discussed in studies of surgical treatments of PD [16]. Another review of the neuropsychiatric complications of subthalamic nucleus (STN) DBS reported the occurrence of transient confusion, emotional reactivity, depression, psychosis, and apathy post-surgery, but there was no mention of anxiety symptoms or disorders [17]. The authors made a point of noting that interpreting the literature on the effects of DBS surgery on neuropsychiatric symptoms is complicated by several factors, including patient selection bias, assessment measurement bias, and lack of systematic consideration of confounding variables (e.g., changes in dopaminergic medications post-DBS surgery and psychosocial adjustment).

Impact of anxiety

A recent study that assessed the impact of neuropsychiatric symptoms on quality-of-life (QOL) using the Parkinson's Disease Questionnaire (PDQ-39) found that 77% of PD patients had symptoms consistent with one or more neuropsychiatric disorders [18]. Using the Hospital Anxiety and Depression Scale (HADS) with a predetermined cutoff point, 16.7% of patients reported clinically significant anxiety symptoms. When analyses were controlled for the severity of motor symptoms, increasing severity of anxiety (and also depression and hallucinations) was associated with poorer QOL.

In the aforementioned study of NMF, in which anxiety was the most commonly reported symptom, patients were asked to rate the level of disability and incapacity caused by each subgroup (i.e., motor, dysautonomic, mental, or sensory subgroup) [4]. The level of disability caused by psychic fluctuations correlated with the presence of fluctuating anxiety, and 28% of patients reported that NMFs were more disabling than motor fluctuations.

In a cholinesterase inhibitor treatment study of patients with PD with dementia (PDD), some patients were placed in a "mood" cluster based on elevated anxiety, depression, and apathy scores. The caregivers of these patients were found to have significantly higher caregiver distress scores [based on their Neuropsychiatric Inventory (NPI) scores] than the caregivers of patients without any neuropsychiatric co-morbidity [19].

Although there is little published research on the relative impact of anxiety symptoms on QOL, function, or caregiver distress in PD, clinical experience indicates that many patients with co-morbid anxiety and depression find the anxiety symptoms to be more distressing than depressive symptoms, perhaps due to their intensity, accompanying somatic complaints, and propensity to worsen parkinsonism (i.e., increased tremor).

Correlates and risk factors

Demographic

There has been limited reporting on the demographic correlates of anxiety disorders in PD. One study of 90 PD patients reported no association between the presence of anxiety disorders and either age or sex [9].

Psychiatric and cognitive

There is extensive overlap between anxiety and depressive symptoms or disorders in PD. Menza, Robertson-Hoffman, and Bonapace found that 92% of PD patients with an anxiety disorder also met criteria for a depressive disorder, and that 67% of those with a depressive disorder also had an anxiety disorder [5]. Another study of PD patients and age-matched spousal controls found that the combination of depression and anxiety best differentiated the two populations [20].

As depression has been more extensively researched and reported on in PD than in anxiety disorders, some experts have suggested that anxiety in PD is secondary to depression, and that the extensive overlap makes depression in PD distinct from idiopathic mood disorders [21]. However, this prioritizing of depression over anxiety (i.e., anxiety being a component of depression as opposed to being an independent disorder) is not based on any empirical evidence, and is also not consistent with the clinical observation that many PD patients find anxiety symptoms to be more distressing and disabling than depressive symptoms.

Definite conclusions about the relationship between anxiety and dementia in PD cannot be drawn due to limited research and mixed results. Most studies either have failed to comment on the cognitive status of their subjects, or demented patients were deliberately excluded. In one cholinesterase inhibitor treatment study of a large cohort of PDD patients, 49% of the patients were found to have anxiety based on caregiver-rated scores using the NPI [19]. Using cluster analysis, 11% of patients were part of a "mood" cluster, which included subjects with elevated depression, anxiety, and apathy scores. Patients in the mood cluster had higher MMSE scores than patients in the "agitation" cluster and a trend for higher scores than patients in the "psychosis" cluster. In addition, females were more likely to be in the mood cluster than in the unaffected group.

Excessive daytime sleepiness (EDS) has been shown to be independently associated with anxiety in PD [22,23]. In one study, anxiety was more strongly associated with EDS than cognitive impairment, levodopa equivalent daily dosage (LEDD), and even depression. The authors speculated that loss of striatal and limbic dopaminergic transmission in PD results in reduced inhibitory control over the amygdala, therefore leading to both anxiety and sleep disturbances, with the latter resulting in EDS [22].

PD characteristics

Although research has been limited, no clear correlation has been established between the presence of anxiety disorders and commonly examined clinical variables such as laterality of motor signs, tremor- versus akinetic-rigid-predominant symptoms, severity of disease, age of PD onset, or PD duration [8,9].

The strongest association between anxiety and PD features is the high frequency of anxiety symptoms reported as part of NMFs in patients with motor fluctuations. As previously mentioned, one study found that 66% of patients with motor fluctuations also reported anxiety as an NMF, with anxiety being the most common NMF [4]. In the study, there was an association between occurrence of NMFs and increasing severity of PD. In another study that assessed anxiety and parkinsonian disability [the latter using the self-rated Parkinson's symptom diary (PSD)], anxiety scores were significantly higher during "off" periods ($p < 0.03$), and the magnitude of anxiety correlated with changes in PSD scores ($p = 0.006$). Anxiety scores were also correlated with disease duration [24]. In a study of panic attacks in PD by Vázquez, Jiménez-Jiménez, and García-Urra [10], a significant relationship between panic attacks and both motor fluctuations and dyskinesias was reported. Additionally, patients with panic attacks had an earlier age of PD onset, more severe disease as measured by Hoehn and Yahr staging, and greater impairment in activities of daily living (ADLs).

In one of the few studies of OCD in PD, a significant correlation was found between both severity and duration of illness and the Maudsley obsessional–compulsive inventory (MOCI) total score. In this study, patients with mild PD did not report any obsessive–compulsive symptoms [12].

The relationship between DBS and anxiety, and also other psychiatric and cognitive symptoms, is complex. One study of 15 consecutive PD patients assessed 3 months before and both 3 and 6 months after DBS found an overall increase in apathy, but no significant change in anxiety symptoms [25]. The authors speculated that apathy and anxiety seemed to be incompatible, although this has not been formally evaluated in PD. Another study of 72 consecutive PD patients found that 15 months post-STN DBS 12% of patients reported an increase and 23% a decrease in severity of anxiety symptoms [26]. In another study that assessed a range of anxiety symptoms in the context of DBS, significant improvements overall were reported in depression, anxiety, and psychosocial functioning [27]. However, on closer examination, 23% reported improvement and 13% worsening on the

State Anxiety Inventory (STAI), 19% reported improvement and 19% worsening on an obsessive–compulsive measure [from the Symptom-Checklist 90-R (SCL-90-R)], and 6% noted improvement and 10% worsening of phobic anxiety (also from the SCL-90-R). The authors concluded that although STN stimulation can have a positive impact on psychiatric symptoms, some patients experience a worsening. It has also been noted that psychiatric symptoms, including anxiety, can worsen even in patients who experience a significant improvement in motor symptoms with DBS [28]. Another study tested stable STN DBS patients "on" and "off" stimulation and "on" and "off" PD medications (2 × 2 study design), and found no acute effect of either stimulation or medication on anxiety scores [29].

Proposed risk factors for worsening of psychiatric symptoms post-DBS include preoperative psychiatric disorders, direct surgical effects, stimulation effects, medication changes, and psychosocial adjustment [28,30]. In a study that assessed 40 consecutive PD patients presenting for DBS, 78% were found to have at least one lifetime or current psychiatric disorder, with a 40% prevalence rate of anxiety disorders (GAD, panic attacks, or social phobia) [30]. The authors concluded that a range of psychiatric symptoms are common in advanced PD patients who are experiencing a diminishing response to, or complications of, dopamine replacement therapy.

Autonomic dysfunction

In a study examining the association between autonomic symptoms, anxiety, and depression in PD and matched control subjects, numerous autonomic symptoms (postural dizziness, frequency of micturition, urinary hesitancy, constipation, dry mouth, impotence, and loss of libido) were more common in PD patients than in controls [31]. Interestingly, anxiety and depression were associated with self-reported autonomic symptoms, but not with objective measures of autonomic function. The authors suggested that anxiety and depression in some PD subjects are likely to be a "behavioral phenocopy" caused by autonomic failure (i.e., symptom overlap leading to misdiagnosis of anxiety and depressive disorders), and that this may help explain the limited response to antidepressant treatment in these patients [32].

Presentation

As mentioned previously, the four most commonly reported anxiety disorders in PD are GAD, panic disorder, social phobia, and OCD. No research suggests that the symptom profile for any of these disorders is different than that in the general population, as has been reported for depression [33].

When anxiety occurs as part of NMFs during "off" periods, patients may describe a sensation of feeling "trapped" as they become increasingly immobilized, with symptoms resolving with improvement in motor symptoms. However, motor and non-motor symptoms are not always correlated [34].

In a study assessing the concurrent validity of three anxiety inventories [the State–Trait Anxiety Inventory (STAI), the Hospital Anxiety Scale (HADS), and the Hamilton Anxiety Scale (Ham-A), the main characteristics of anxiety were "inability to relax," "restlessness or inability to feel calm," and "feeling tense" [35].

Etiology and pathophysiology

Premorbid personality traits and psychiatric disorders

Numerous studies comparing PD patients and matched controls have reported an increased prevalence of anxiety and depressive disorders in PD patients up to 20 years prior to PD onset [36,37]. In a recent systematic review of studies examining mental illness preceding PD onset, the authors reported on one case–control study and one cohort study examining pre-morbid anxiety and PD [38]. The case–control study found a significant positive association between a history of anxiety disorders and subsequent PD. The cohort study found a similar, although slightly less significant, association. The authors hypothesized that mid-life anxiety disorders involve neurobiological changes that increase susceptibility to the development of PD. This positive association between anxiety disorders in mid-life and subsequent development of PD suggests a neurobiological underpinning to anxiety in PD.

A recent retrospective study reviewed 433 cases of pathologically proven PD to ascertain presenting symptoms [39]. One-fifth of patients presented with exclusively non-motor symptoms (NMS), and 12.1% of those patients had depression or anxiety. Within 2 years of disease onset, 24.7% had developed depression or anxiety symptoms. Not surprisingly, patients presenting with NMS were more likely to have a delay in their PD diagnosis compared with patients presenting with motor symptoms (median interval = 1.6 years versus 1.0 years, respectively). These findings underscore the fact that a diagnosis of PD needs to be considered in the differential diagnosis of patients presenting with mid- or late-life anxiety symptoms.

There has also been widespread interest in the possibility of a "parkinsonian personality" that predates the onset of PD motor symptoms. In a recent review of this literature, the authors found only four studies that attempted to assess pre-morbid personality in PD patients [40]. Three of four studies with a control group reported personality differences between PD patients and controls, and found PD patients to be more cautious, apprehensive, self-reproaching, and less novelty seeking. In another study of over 7000 adults in the general population who completed the Minnesota Multiphasic Personality Inventory (MMPI) in the 1960s, subjects who scored in the top 25th percentile on "psychasthenia" (a measure of anxiety) were twice as likely (odds ratio = 1.95) to develop PD over the next 40 years as those in the bottom 75th percentile [41]. The "traits" studied overlapped with the symptoms of generalized anxiety disorder, so this research raises the possibility that patients who go on to develop PD are more likely to have an anxious temperament. Future research will need to determine if such traits are a risk factor for PD, an early manifestation of PD, or linked to PD via common risk factors or a common genetic predisposition.

Dopamine

There has been limited research on the association between anxiety symptoms and the use of anti-parkinsonian medications in PD. In a small study examining the correlates of anxiety disorders in PD patients, there were no differences between patients with and without an anxiety disorder in levodopa dosage or total levodopa exposure [8]. Another study of anxiety in PD found no correlation between levodopa dosage and severity of anxiety symptoms [5]. Yet another study reported that anxiety symptoms in PD patients were as common prior to levodopa initiation as after starting levodopa treatment [20]. Regarding other PD medications, a small study of levodopa-treated PD patients found no difference in anxiety symptoms based on the absence or presence of adjunctive PD medications, including dopamine agonists, MAO-B inhibitors, and anti-cholinergics [24]. Thus, other than in patients with motor fluctuations, it is not clear that any class of PD medications has a consistent effect on anxiety symptoms in PD.

In the general population, panic disorder is reported to be the least common of anxiety disorders in the elderly, and it is thought that most cases of panic disorder in the elderly have their onset earlier in adulthood [42]. In addition, late-onset panic disorder usually is associated with co-morbid psychiatric or medical disorders. These findings in the general population have been referenced to support the hypothesis that the development of panic attacks in a subset of PD patients is due to a shared neurobiological vulnerability between panic symptoms and PD [1]. The role of dopamine in the development of anxiety symptoms in PD is strongest for patients with "off" periods or NMFs. One study of panic attacks in PD found a correlation between panic attacks and earlier disease onset, earlier initiation of levodopa therapy, and higher levodopa dosages [10]. In this study, panic attacks occurred nearly always during "off" periods, and there was a positive correlation between the number of daily panic attacks, "fragmentation" of levodopa dosages, and number of fluctuations. This study is consistent with other reports of an association between anxiety symptoms and NMFs, particularly during the "off" state [1,4,43].

In general, anxiety symptoms occurring during "off" periods are reported to improve after levodopa intake. In an open-label levodopa infusion study, anxiety levels were high pre-infusion ("off" state), improved with infusion, and then worsened with levodopa wearing off. There was no correlation between improvement in motor function (tapping speed) and anxiety improvement, suggesting that the anti-anxiety effects of levodopa infusion were not a psychological response to improved motor function [44]. In a subsequent double-blind, placebo-controlled levodopa infusion study, levodopa (but not placebo) improved both anxiety symptoms and tapping speed, with improvements in anxiety often *preceding* improvement in motor symptoms [45]. Although there is not always a direct correlation between anxiety symptoms and "off" periods [34], overall the research suggests that NMFs in PD are probably due to the combination of dopamine depletion and the administration of short-lived dopaminergic drugs, which lead to pulsatile stimulation of striatal dopamine receptors, as has been proposed for the pathophysiology of motor fluctuations in PD [46].

Other neurotransmitters

The main neurotransmitters implicated in the pathogenesis of anxiety disorders in primary psychiatric populations are norepinephrine, serotonin, and γ-aminobutyric acid (GABA). Most selective serotonin reuptake inhibitors (SSRIs) and other anti-depressants with serotonergic reuptake inhibition properties also are approved for the treatment of a range of anxiety disorders, including generalized anxiety disorder, panic disorder, social phobia, and OCD. There is also evidence that cholecystokinin (CKK) may be involved in the pathogenesis of panic disorder [47], and that dopamine may have a role in the development of social phobia [48].

High levels of noradrenergic neuronal activity are related to the expression of anxiety and fear, and also to the somatic and cardiovascular symptoms that accompany panic anxiety states. Clinical investigations of yohimbine and clonidine, which increase and decrease, respectively, noradrenergic activity have found that panic disorder patients are more sensitive to their effects than healthy controls [49]. The suggestion that the noradrenergic system has a key role in the development of anxiety disorders is particularly interesting for PD patients, given the increasing awareness of noradrenergic dysfunction in PD [50], even early in the disease course [51]. Some experts suggest an interaction between the dopaminergic and noradrenergic systems in the etiology of panic attacks in PD, with falling levels of dopamine in the brain leading to a disinhibited firing of the norepinephrine-producing locus coeruleus, clinically manifested by a panic attack [10].

Alegret *et al.*'s study of OCD in PD found a correlation between duration and severity of disease and anxiety [12]. As only patients with severe PD demonstrated OCD symptoms, the authors hypothesized that OCD symptoms in PD are not directly related to the initial nigrostriatal dopaminergic deficiency which causes initial PD symptoms, but rather involves changes at the level of basal ganglia circuitry, including degeneration of corticostriatal circuitry in the advanced stages of the disease.

Brain regions

In a PET regional cerebral blood flow (rCBF) study of PD patients with motor fluctuations, some of whom also had NMFs (including anxiety symptoms), CBF was measured pre- and post-levodopa challenge [52]. Patients with mood fluctuations had decreased blood flow after levodopa challenge in several brain regions, including the posterior cingulate cortex and the medial frontal gyrus. The authors concluded that mood fluctuations, including anxiety, may arise in parkinsonian PD patients who have abnormal dopaminergic modulation of the caudate nucleus, anterior cingulate cortex, or orbitofrontal cortex, all of which innervate the posterior cingulate cortex, an area strongly linked to mood and anxiety and with known rCBF responsiveness to levodopa or D2-like dopamine receptor agonists.

In an [^{18}F]fluorodopa PET study examining the association between personality traits and dopaminergic function in PD, the harm-avoidance personality score (associated with anxiety and depression) was increased in PD patients compared with healthy controls. In addition, the PD patients' higher scores on this measure were associated with increased [^{18}F]fluorodopa uptake in the right caudate nucleus [53].

Genetics

Although there is no published research on the genetics of anxiety disorders in PD, indirect evidence for the genetic underpinnings of anxiety in PD comes from a recent case–control study which found that first-degree relatives of PD patients had an increased lifetime risk of both anxiety (hazards ratio = 1.55, 95% CI = 1.05–2.28) and depressive disorders [54]. These results were primarily driven by the relatives of patients with younger age at PD onset, and held true even after excluding those PD patients who had experienced depressive or anxiety disorders prior to the onset of their motor symptoms. These findings suggest that anxiety disorders and PD may share familial susceptibility factors (either genetic or nongenetic) and common pathogenetic mechanisms.

Assessment and diagnosis

Symptom overlap

As mentioned previously, there is evidence of symptom overlap between anxiety symptoms and common autonomic symptoms in PD [31]. Symptoms such as postural dizziness, frequency of micturition, urinary hesitancy, constipation, dry mouth, impotence, and loss of libido, all reported to occur commonly in PD, were associated with measures of anxiety. It is impossible to know if such symptoms in PD occur primarily in the context of an autonomic disorder or an anxiety disorder, but the overlap does highlight complexities in the diagnosis of anxiety disorders in PD. Symptom overlap has also been reported for depressive symptoms and core PD symptoms (e.g., psychomotor retardation, insomnia, weight loss, and fatigue), which led to a proposal for modified diagnostic criteria for depression in PD [33]. As part of these proposed criteria, a recommendation was made to use an inclusive approach (i.e., counting endorsed items towards a diagnosis of depression without trying to ascertain the etiology of the symptom) for rating depressive symptoms in PD, but no such similar recommendation exists for rating autonomic symptoms.

Rating scales

The Movement Disorder Society (MDS) recently commissioned a task force to critique and make recommendations regarding the use of anxiety rating scales in PD [55]. A systematic review was conducted to identify anxiety scales that have either been validated or used in patients with PD. Six anxiety rating scales were identified. These were the Beck Anxiety Inventory (BAI), the Hospital Anxiety and Depression Scale (HADS), the Zung Self-rating Anxiety Scale (SAS) and Anxiety Status Inventory (ASI), the Spielberger State Trait Anxiety Inventory (STAI), and the Hamilton Anxiety Rating Scale (HAM-A). In addition, item 5 of the NPI, which assesses anxiety, was included in the review.

The task force concluded that no scales met criteria to be "recommended," as essential clinimetric information is missing for all scales. All available anxiety scales tend to focus on symptoms of GAD and panic disorder and not on other anxiety disorders. However, since these are the most prevalent anxiety syndromes in PD, this is not a major limitation. Based on the item formulation, time frame, and clinimetric information, the BAI is more sensitive to episodic anxiety disorders, such as panic disorder, whereas the STAI is more focused towards sustained anxiety disorders, such as GAD. Since the time frame of the "state" subscale of the STAI is "right now," it may be assumed that it is not at all sensitive for panic disorder. Other scales have items that are less differentially focused towards either episodic or sustained anxiety disorders. A basic clinimetric question that is not limited to PD remains unanswered: can a single scale be reliable and valid for both episodic and sustained anxiety disorders?

Differential diagnosis

Terminologies for several distinct diagnostic categories are similar and can create confusion. GAD, panic disorder, social phobia, and OCD are all considered anxiety disorders in DSM-IV-TR. A range of impulsive–compulsive behaviors or disorders have been reported to occur in PD; impulse control disorders (ICDs), which include pathological gambling and related disorders reported to occur in PD (e.g., compulsive buying and sexual behavior), comprise a class of psychiatric disorders distinct from anxiety disorders. Obsessive–compulsive personality disorder is a pathological personality style characterized by a preoccupation with orderliness, perfectionism, and mental and interpersonal control, but does not include specific obsessions or compulsive behaviors that are necessary to meet criteria for OCD.

Diagnosis

There are DSM-IV-TR criteria for all of the anxiety disorders reported to occur in PD, including GAD, panic disorder, social phobia, and OCD, and the criteria can be applied informally in a clinical setting or as part of a structured diagnostic interview by a trained rater. Whereas *panic attacks* apply only to the occurrence of discrete episodes of intense fear or discomfort, a diagnosis of panic disorder requires both recurrent unexpected panic attacks and at least one of the following: persistent concern about additional attacks, worry about the implications or consequences of an attack, or a significant change in behavior related to the attacks. As panic attacks in PD occurring during "off" periods are often expected, it is not clear if this should preclude a diagnosis of panic disorder. DSM-IV-TR also specifically states that social phobia should not be diagnosed in a PD patient if the sole fear relates to PD symptoms (e.g., tremor) being observed in public. Also according to DSM-IV-TR, GAD should not be diagnosed if the anxiety symptoms occur exclusively during a mood disorder (e.g., major depressive episode), but it is not clear how to determine if the anxiety disorder or the mood disorder is primary.

Treatment

Published research

One recent double-blind crossover study examined the effects of immediate and controlled-release levodopa on mood and anxiety in PD patients with and without motor fluctuations. A dosage of levodopa was associated with improvement in anxiety scores in patients with motor fluctuations only, with no difference between immediate and controlled-release levodopa [56].

There are no published controlled treatment studies specifically for anxiety disorders in PD that tested either available anti-anxiety medications (e.g., benzodiazepines or selective serotonin reuptake inhibitors) or non-pharmacologic treatments. Most treatment evidence comes from secondary analyses of anxiety measures in depression treatment studies. For instance, in an open-label trial of citalopram for major depression in PD, on secondary analysis it was found that anxiety severity (as measured by the HAM-A) improved significantly over an 8-week course of treatment [57]. In an open-label study of escitalopram for major depression in PD, there was a suggestion for improvement in anxiety severity over the course of treatment, although the mean decrease in HAM-A score was only 22.2% [58]. Overall, there is a lack of research to guide clinical decision making, so most recommendations are made on the basis of clinical experience.

Regarding non-pharmacologic treatments, an open-label study of treatment-resistant depression in PD found that 2 weeks of left dorsolateral prefrontal repetitive transcranial magnetic stimulation (rTMS) was associated with a significant decrease in HAM-A scores [59]. In another rTMS study for major depression in PD, in which all subjects also met criteria for an anxiety disorder (panic disorder, GAD, or social phobia), rTMS was associated with trend improvement in both trait and state anxiety on the STAI [60]. In an uncontrolled study of 10–14 sessions of cognitive–behavioral therapy (CBT) for major depressive disorder in PD (including cases unresponsive to anti-depressant treatment), a significant decrease in STAI scores was reported both at the end of treatment and at a 1-month follow-up visit [61].

For PD patients with anxiety symptoms in the context of dementia, there is preliminary evidence from open-label studies that cholinesterase inhibitor treatment is associated with an improvement in neuropsychiatric symptoms, including anxiety [62].

Clinical experience

For patients who experience anxiety as an NMF during "off" states, PD medication adjustments (shortening the interval between levodopa dosages) or additions (e.g., COMT inhibitors, dopamine agonists, or MAO-B inhibitors) can decrease the duration and severity of motor fluctuations, although it is not known if these adjustments also improve psychiatric symptoms.

Newer anti-depressants [e.g., selective serotonin reuptake inhibitors (SSRIs) and serotonin–norepinephrine reuptake inhibitors (SNRIs)] are approved for the treatment of a range of anxiety disorders in the general population and, due to their favorable side effect profile and limited drug–drug interactions, they are commonly used as a first-line treatment for anxiety symptoms in PD. It may take several weeks for treatment effects to occur, and many patients do not experience significant improvement in anxiety symptoms with anti-depressant treatment. In addition, physicians must be cautious regarding the combined use of SSRIs or SNRIs with MAO-B inhibitors due to the potential induction of serotonin syndrome [1].

Despite the common treatment of anxiety symptoms with anti-depressants, anxiety in PD sometimes requires treatment with benzodiazepines, most commonly lorazepam, alprazolam, or clonazepam. Lorazepam does not undergo oxidative metabolism by the liver, so dosage adjustments are unnecessary in patients with liver impairment. Alprazolam is often perceived by patients as the most potent benzodiazepine, and is relatively non-sedating compared with other benzodiazepines. Finally, clonazepam has a long half-life that allows daily or twice-a-day dosaging; it is also used in PD patients with rapid eye movement behavior disorder (RBD). Benzodiazepines in PD must be started at a low dosage, titrated upwards slowly, and used at the lowest possible effective dosage, as possible side effects include sedation, cognitive impairment, and gait impairment.

References

1. Richard IH. Anxiety disorders in Parkinson's disease. *Adv Neurol* 2005;**96**:42–55.
2. Walsh K, Bennett G. Parkinson's disease and anxiety. *Postgrad Med J* 2001;**77**:89–93.
3. American Psychiatric Association. *Diagnostic and Statistical Manual of Mental Disorders*, 4th edn. Washington, DC: American Psychiatric Association, 2000.
4. Witjas T, Kaphan E, Azulay JP, *et al.* Nonmotor fluctuations in Parkinson's disease: frequent and disabling. *Neurology* 2002;**59**:408–13.
5. Menza MA, Robertson-Hoffman DE, Bonapace AS. Parkinson's disease and anxiety: comorbidity with depression. *Biol Psychiatry* 1993;**34**:465–70.
6. Schiffer RB, Kurlan R, Rubin A, *et al.* Evidence for atypical depression in Parkinson's disease. *Am J Psychiatry* 1988;**145**:1020–2.
7. Menza MA, Mark MH. Parkinson's disease and depression: the relationship to disability and personality. *J Neuropsychiatry Clin Neurosci* 1994;**6**:165–9.
8. Stein MB, Heuser IJ, Juncos JL, Uhde TW. Anxiety disorders in patients with Parkinson's disease. *Am J Psychiatry* 1990;**147**:217–20.
9. Nuti A, Ceravolo R, Piccinni A, *et al.* Psychiatric comorbidity in a population of Parkinson's disease patients. *Eur J Neurol* 2004;**11**:315–20.
10. Vazquez A, Jiménez-Jiménez FJ, García-Urra D. " Panic attacks" in Parkinson's disease. *Acta Neurol Scand* 1993;**87**: 14–8.
11. Kummer A, Cardoso F, Teixeira AL. Frequency of social phobia and psychometric properties of the Liebowitz social anxiety scale in Parkinson's disease. *Mov Disord* 2008;**23**:1739–43.
12. Alegret M, Junqué C, Valldeoriola F, *et al.* Obsessive–compulsive symptoms in Parkinson's disease. *J Neurol Neurosurg Psychiatry* 2001;**70**:394–6.
13. Müller N, Putz A, Kathmann N, *et al.* Characteristics of obsessive–compulsive symptoms in Tourette's syndrome, obsessive–compulsive disorder and Parkinson's disease. *Psychiatry Res* 1997;**70**:105–14.
14. Maia AF, Pinto AS, Barbosa ER, *et al.* Obsessive–compulsive symptoms, obsessive–compulsive disorder, and related disorders in Parkinson's disease. *J Neuropsychiatry Clin Neurosci* 2003;**15**:371–4.
15. Lauterbach EC, Freeman A, Vogel RL. Differential DSM-III psychiatric disorder prevalence profiles in dystonia and Parkinson's disease. *J Neuropsychiatry Clin Neurosci* 2004;**16**: 29–36.
16. Burn DJ, Tröster AI. Neuropsychiatric complications of medical and surgical therapies for Parkinson's disease. *J Geriatr Psychiatry Neurol* 2004;**17**:172–80.
17. Voon V, Kubu C, Krack P, *et al.* Deep brain stimulation: neuropsychological and neuropsychiatric issues. *Mov Disord* 2006;**21** (Suppl. 14): S305–26.
18. McKinlay A, Grace RC, Dalrymple-Alford JC, *et al.* A profile of neuropsychiatric problems and their relationship to quality of life for Parkinson's disease patients without dementia. *Parkinsonism Relat Disord* 2008;**14**:37–42.
19. Aarsland D, Brønnick K, Ehrt U, *et al.* Neuropsychiatric symptoms in patients with Parkinson's disease and dementia: frequency, profile and associated caregiver stress. *J Neurol Neurosurg Psychiatry* 2007;**78**:36–42.
20. Henderson R, Kurlan R, Kersun JM, Como P. Preliminary examination of the comorbidity of anxiety and depression in Parkinson's disease. *J Neuropsychiatry Clin Neurosci* 1992;**4**:257–64.
21. Cummings JL. Depression and Parkinson's disease: a review. *Am J Psychiatry* 1992;**149**:443–54.
22. Wegelin J, McNamara P, Durso R, *et al.* Correlates of excessive daytime sleepiness in Parkinson's disease. *Parkinsonism Relat Disord* 2005;**11**:441–8.
23. Borek LL, Kohn R, Friedman JH. Mood and sleep in Parkinson's disease. *J Clin Psychiatry* 2006;**67**:958–63.
24. Siemers ER, Shekhar A, Quaid K, Dickson H. Anxiety and motor performance in Parkinson's disease. *Mov Disord* 1993;**8**:501–6.
25. Drapier D, Drapier S, Sauleau P, *et al.* Does subthalamic nucleus stimulation induce apathy in Parkinson's disease? *J Neurol* 2006;**8**:1083–91.
26. Castelli L, Perozzo P, Ziegler M, *et al.* Chronic deep brain stimulation of the subthalamic nucleus for Parkinson's disease: effects on cognition, mood, anxiety and personality traits. *Eur Neurol* 2006;**55**:136–44.
27. Kalteis K, Standhardt H, Kryspin-Exner I, *et al.* Influence of bilateral Stn-stimulation on psychiatric symptoms and psychosocial functioning in patients with Parkinson's disease. *J Neural Transm* 2006;**9**:1191–206.
28. Houeto JL, Mesnage V, Mallet L, *et al.* Behavioral disorders, Parkinson's disease and subthalamic stimulation. *J Neurol Neurosurg Psychiatry* 2002;**72**:701–7.

29. Berney A, Panisset M, Sadikot AF, *et al.* Mood stability during acute stimulator challenge in Parkinson's disease patients under long-term treatment with subthalamic deep brain stimulation. *Mov Disord* 2007;**22**:1093–6.
30. Voon V, Saint-Cyr J, Lozano AM, *et al.* Psychiatric symptoms in patients with Parkinson disease presenting for deep brain stimulation surgery. *J Neurosurg* 2005;**103**:246–51.
31. Berrios GE, Campbell C, Politynska BE. Autonomic failure, depression and anxiety in Parkinson's disease. *Br J Psychiatry* 1995;**166**:789–92.
32. Weintraub D, Morales KH, Moberg PJ, *et al.* Antidepressant studies in Parkinson's disease: a review and meta-analysis. *Mov Disord* 2005;**20**:1161–9.
33. Marsh L, McDonald WM, Cummings JL, *et al.* Provisional diagnostic criteria for depression in Parkinson's disease: report of an NINDS/NIMH work group. *Mov Disord* 2006;**21**:148–58.
34. Richard IH, Justus AW, Kurlan R. Relationship between mood and motor fluctuations in Parkinson's disease. *J Neuropsychiatry Clin Neurosci* 2001;**13**:35–41.
35. Mondolo F, Jahanshahi M, Graná A, *et al.* Evaluation of anxiety in Parkinson's disease with some commonly used rating scales. *Neurol Sci* 2007;**28**:270–5.
36. Gonera EG, van't Hof M, Berger HJC, *et al.* Symptoms and duration of the prodromal phase in Parkinson's disease. *Mov Disord* 1997;**12**:871–6.
37. Shiba M, Bower JH, Maraganore DM, *et al.* Anxiety disorders and depressive disorders preceding Parkinson's disease: a case–control study. *Mov Disord* 2000;**15**:669–77.
38. Ishihara L, Brayne C. A systematic review of depression and mental illness preceding Parkinson's disease. *Acta Neurol Scand* 2006;**113**:211–20.
39. O'Sullivan SS, Williams DR, Gallagher DA, *et al.* Nonmotor symptoms as presenting complaints in Parkinson's disease: a clinicopathological study. *Mov Disord* 2008;**23**:101–6.
40. Ishihara L, Brayne C. What is the evidence for a premorbid parkinsonian personality: a systematic review. *Mov Disord* 2006;**21**:1066–72.
41. Bower JH, Grossardt BR, Maraganore DM, *et al.* The Mayo Clinic Cohort Study of Personality and Aging: results for Parkinson's disease. Neurology 2005;**64** (Suppl 1): A282–3 (Abstract).
42. Flint AJ. Epidemiology and comorbidity of anxiety disorders in the elderly. *Am J Psychiatry* 1994;**151**:640–9.
43. Riley D, Lang AE. The spectrum of levodopa-related fluctuations in Parkinson's disease. *Neurology* 1993;**43**:1459–64.
44. Maricle RA, Nutt JG, Carter JH. Mood and anxiety fluctuation in Parkinson's disease associated with levodopa infusion: preliminary findings. *Mov Disord* 1995;**10**:329–32.
45. Maricle RA, Nutt JG, Valentine RJ, *et al.* Dose–response relationship of levodopa with mood and anxiety in fluctuating Parkinson's disease: a double-blind, placebo-controlled study. *Neurology* 1995;**45**:1757–60.
46. Linazasoro G. Pathophysiology of motor complications in Parkinson disease: postsynaptic mechanisms are crucial. *Arch Neurol* 2007;**64**:137–40.
47. Hattori E, Ebihara M, Yamada K, *et al.* Identification of a compound short tandem repeat stretch in the 5′-upstream region of the cholecystokinin gene, and its association with panic disorder but not schizophrenia. *Mol Psychiatry* 2001;**6**: 465–70.
48. Tiihonen J, Kuikka J, Bergstromm K, *et al.* Dopamine reuptake site densities in patients with social phobia. *Am J Psychiatry* 1997;**154**:239–42.
49. Charney DS, Woods SW, Nagy LM, *et al.* Noradrenergic function in panic disorder. *J Clin Psychiatry* 1990;**51** (12, Suppl A): 5–11.
50. Rommelfanger KS, Weinshenker D. Norepinephrine: the redheaded stepchild of Parkinson's disease. *Biochem Pharmacol* 2007;**74**:177–90.
51. Braak H, Del Tredici K, Rüb U, *et al.* Staging of brain pathology related to sporadic Parkinson's disease. *Neurobiol Aging* 2003;**24**:197–210.
52. Black KJ, Hershey T, Hartlein JM, *et al.* Levodopa challenge neruoimaging of levodopa-related mood fluctuations in Parkinson's disease. *Neuropsychopharmacology* 2005;**30**:590–601.
53. Kaasinen V, Nurmi E, Bergman J, *et al.* Personality traits and brain dopaminergic function in Parkinson's disease. *Proc Natl Acad Sci USA* 2001;**98**:13272–7.
54. Arabia G, Grossardt BR, Geda YE, *et al.* Increased risk of depressive and anxiety disorders in relative of patients with Parkinson disease. *Arch Gen Psychiatry* 2007;**64**:1385–92.
55. Leentjens AFG, Dujardin K, Marsh L, *et al.* Anxiety rating scales in Parkinson's disease: critique and recommendations. *Mov Disord* 2008;**23**:2004–14.
56. Kulisevsky J, Pascual-Sedano B, Barbanoj M, *et al.* Acute effects of immediate and controlled-release levodopa on mood in Parkinson's disease: a double-blind study. *Mov Disord* 2007;**22**:62–7.
57. Menza MA, Marin H, Kaufman K, *et al.* Citalopram treatment of depression in Parkinson's disease: the impact on anxiety, disability, and cognition. *J Neuropsychiatry Clin Neurosci* 2004;**16**:315–9.
58. Weintraub D, Taraborelli D, Morales KH, *et al.* Escitalopram for major depression in Parkinson's disease: an open-label, flexible-dosage study. *J Neuropsychiatry Clin Neurosci.* 2006;**18**:377–83.
59. Epstein C, Evatt M, Funk A, *et al.* An open study of repetitive transcranial magnetic stimulation in treatment-resistant depression in Parkinson's disease. *Clin Neurophysiol* 2007;**118**:2189–94.
60. Kormos T. Efficacy of rTMS in the treatment of comorbid anxiety in depressed patients with Parkinson's disease. *Mov Disord* 2007;**22**:1836.
61. Dobkin RD, Allen LA, Menza M. Cognitive–behavioral therapy for depression in Parkinson's disease: a pilot study. *Mov Disord* 2007;**22**:946–52.
62. Thomas AJ, Burn DJ, Rowan EN, *et al.* A comparison of the efficacy of donepezil in Parkinson's disease with dementia and dementia with Lewy bodies. *Int J Geriatr Psychiatry* 2005;**20**:938–44.

Chapter 19
Dopamine Dysregulation Syndrome

Sean S. O'Sullivan & Andrew J. Lees
Reta Lila Weston Institute of Neurological Studies, Institute of Neurology, University College London, London, UK

Introduction

The dopamine dysregulation syndrome (DDS) is an uncommon behavioral complication of long-term dopaminergic therapy characterized by an inappropriate intake of dopamine replacement therapy (DRT) in excess of that required to control motor symptoms [1,2], and resulting in psychosocial handicaps similar to those seen in chronic psychostimulant substance users [3].

Phenomenology of DDS and associated behaviors

Cyclical mood disturbances in relation to L-dopa dosing were described over 36 years ago [4], and occasional case reports of L-dopa dependence have also appeared in the literature [5]. Dysphoria, anhedonia, fatigue, irritability, lassitude, sadness, anxiety, and panic [5–9] are the commonest psychologic sequelae seen during "off" periods whereas euphoria, hypomania, and aggression may be seen in the "on" state [2,5]. These psychologic fluctuations resemble the mood changes seen in bipolar depression but the swings occur from hour to hour rather than over months or years.

Dopamine dysregulation syndrome

Patients typically justify overuse of dopaminergic medication on the grounds of avoidance of distressing mood changes and a perceived ineffectiveness of their medication [10]. A minority of patients also acknowledge a subjective "kick." "rush," "buzz," or "high," particularly after short-acting drugs [11]. As drug treatment continues, socially harmful behaviors may appear and are often accompanied by severe interdose or biphasic dyskinesias [11–13]. A preoccupation with complex drug regimens is common and any attempt by the physician to reduce the medication dose is met with strong resistance. Hoarding of medicine and the purchase of additional dopaminergic treatment through the Internet or from private physicians is not uncommon. Some patients with DDS also exhibit impulse control disorders, although we do not consider these to be an integral part of the syndrome [2,14]. See Box 19.1 [11].

Impulse control disorders (ICDs)

ICDs are characterized by a failure to resist an impulse, drive, or temptation to perform, which may result in harm to the person or to others. Pathologic gambling (PG), kleptomania, intermittent explosive disorder, trichotillomania, and pyromania have all been reported [15]. Other ICDs without formal diagnostic criteria in the *Diagnostic and Statistical Manual of Mental Disorders*, 4th edition (DSM-IV-TR) [15] include excessive and inappropriate sexual behavior, compulsive binge eating with weight gain, and impulsive shopping [16–18]. These disorders may go unrecognized for a long time or be deliberately hidden from their families, potentially leading to tragic social consequences [19,20]. They are also underreported during consultations with physicians. ICDs in Parkinson's disease (PD) are reviewed in Chapter 20 and in a paper by Voon and Fox [21].

Phenomenology of punding behaviors and associated symptoms in Parkinson's disease

Punding was first described in amphetamine and cocaine addicts in 1972 [22], the term deriving from the Swedish slang for "block-head" used by addicts to describe their endless perseverations [23]. It is a complex, pointless, stereotyped motor activity carried out for many hours at the expense of all other behaviors. Common forms include the dismantling of technical equipment, cataloguing and sorting of collections, an intense fascination with mundane objects, tinkering with the car, long walks to nowhere special, and the conduction of extended monologues devoid of content [3]. Since the first description in 1994 of L-dopa-induced punding behaviors in a patient

Parkinson's Disease: Non-Motor and Non-Dopaminergic Features, First Edition. Edited by C. Warren Olanow, Fabrizio Stocchi, and Anthony E. Lang.

Box 19.1 Diagnostic criteria of DDS [11]

A Parkinson's disease with documented L-dopa responsiveness
B Need for increasing doses of dopamine replacement therapy (DRT) in excess of those normally required to relieve parkinsonian symptoms and signs
C Pattern of pathologic use: expressed need for increased DRT in the presence of excessive and significant dyskinesias despite being "on," drug hoarding or drug-seeking behavior, unwillingness to reduce DRT, absence of painful dystonias
D Impairment in social or occupational functioning: fights, violent behavior, loss of friends, absence from work, loss of job, legal difficulties, arguments or difficulties with family
E Development of hypomanic, manic, or cyclothymic affective syndrome in relation to DRT
F Development of a withdrawal state characterized by dysphoria, depression, irritability, and anxiety on reducing the level of DRT
G Duration of disturbance of at least 6 months

with PD, there has been increased interest in this phenomenon in PD patients on dopamine replacement therapies (DRT) [24].

These repetitive behaviors are diverse but share a number of common features. A failure of completion and the creation of a chaotic mess in the home were identified in all 17 patients in a study by Evans *et al.*, with 10/17 patients developing a fascination for collecting objects [3]. In their paper, the activities pursued by patients were often linked to previous occupations, for example, a seamstress repetitively sorted buttons, a joiner undertook repetitive and unnecessary home carpentry tasks, an IT consultant became increasingly fascinated by computer animation, and a musician composed hundreds of songs which he sang over and over again [3]. Unlike the reports of punding in amphetamine addicts [22], patients with PD do not describe their repetitive activities as being pleasurable [25]. If distracted from the intrusive behavior, patients soon became irritable and anxious if not allowed to resume their activity [3]. A few patients found punding calming and some spent a great deal of money on their "hobbies" [3]. Punding inevitably led to social avoidance, severe sleep deprivation, and disintegration of family relationships [3,26,27].

Punding is often associated with the dopamine dysregulation syndrome (DDS) and was seen in 10/17 cases of punding described by Evans *et al.* [3], a finding also seen in other case reports [28]. An association with impulse control disorders such as hypersexuality, PG, and compulsive eating has also been described in patients with punding behaviors [3,18,29].

Case Illustration

A 60-year-old man developed PD at the age of 53. There was a previous history of depression, with no history of alcohol or drug abuse. He responded well initially to L-dopa treatment, but within 4 years he was taking 700 mg of L-dopa, 1400 mg of entacapone, 9 mg of ropinirole, 300 mg of amantadine, and 20 mg of paroxetine per day. In the following 2–3 years, his family noted that he had developed a compulsion to copy pointlessly old videos on to blank DVDs. He would rise early and spend up to 10 h per day engrossed in this pastime, to the extent that he sometimes forgot to eat or take his medications. He would become irritable if interrupted. Prior to developing this fascination with DVDs he had spent time tinkering with his model train set, or using the Internet to investigate proposed purchases of second-hand cars. These activities were felt to be excessive by his family and led to disharmony. Around the same time he developed an increased libido and an increased craving for sweet foods. He had developed cyclic mood fluctuations. He described feeling depressed when "switching off," and then getting a "sudden burst of energy" after taking his tablets. He had begun to self-escalate his dopaminergic medications, despite increasing problems with dyskinesias and visual hallucinations. A gradual reduction of his dopaminergic medication over months led to gradual improvement.

Psychiatric disorders that may mimic punding

Punding needs to be clearly distinguished from obsessive–compulsive disorder (OCD) which has been reported in some studies to have a positive association with PD [30]. Certainly, the repetitive tidying and rearranging behaviors seen in some punders bear a phenomenologic similarity to the motor behavior of OCD and described in DSM-IV-TR when defining OCD [15]. However, intrusive distressing thoughts (obsessions) do not occur in punding [3]. Punding has more in common with habitual manipulations of the body, such as body rocking, trichotillomania, and head banging. Hypomania is a recognized complication of dopaminergic therapy [31], and the increased level of goal-focused activity, with a diminished need for sleep, seen in some punders engaged in their repetitive behaviors may be compatible with some of the DSM-IV-TR criteria for the diagnosis of a manic episode [15]. However, unlike mania, punders do not demonstrate features such as excessive talking or pressured speech, racing thoughts or flights of ideas, and grandiosity. Mania is also often associated with an indiscriminate enthusiasm for multiple tasks, whereas punders focus on a single motor behavior.

Epidemiology of the DDS and associated behaviors in PD

Epidemiology of DDS and ICDs in PD

The prevalence of DDS in the community is unknown, as the few published figures all refer to specialist referral centers. In a UK-based study, 15 (4.1%) out of 364 patients had DDS [11] and similar figures were obtained in an Italian movement disorders clinic with 3.4% of 202 patients showing evidence of dysregulation of their medication [14]. Both studies reported a higher proportion of young males, but this difference did not reach statistical difference. The lifetime prevalence of PG in PD has been estimated at 3.4%, which increases to 7.2% in patients taking dopamine agonists [32]. This figure contrasts with 0.42–2.5% in the general population [33,34]. The lifetime prevalence of pathologic hypersexuality in PD is said to be 2.4%, and compulsive shopping 0.7%, but these figures may be an underestimation [35]. There are no large studies to determine the prevalence of these disorders in a healthy non-PD population, although the prevalence of hypersexuality may be as high as 19% in fronto-temporal dementia and 15% in Alzheimer's disease [36]. Interpretation of the hypersexuality in PD is confounded by the recognized hyperlibidinous effects of dopaminergic medication.

Epidemiology of punding

Evans *et al.* performed a structured interview in patients on higher amounts of dopaminergic medications (>800 L-dopa equivalent units per day), from a total of 123 unselected patients with PD [3]. This study showed a prevalence of punding of 14%, of which almost 60% demonstrated patterns of compulsive medication use. Analyzing those patients taking increased dopaminergic medications revealed no differences in gender, age, or severity of PD compared with non-punders. In a prevalence study in a Canadian academic center, punding was identified in four of 291 patients with PD (1.4%) [37]. The authors suggest that this lower prevalence rate may be due to differences in medications between their unselected cohort and those of Evans *et al.*, which selected for patients using higher amounts of dopaminergic medications. In both studies, punding was observed in patients with PD exhibiting ICDs without DDS, emphasizing the degree of overlap between these behaviors [3,37]. It is highly likely that punding is under-diagnosed in the general neurologic clinic setting, because of a combination of low awareness and a reluctance of patients to divulge information about this behavior.

DDS as a substance dependence disorder or addiction

Difficulties exist in using current diagnostic criteria for substance dependence when this refers to the use of medication in a chronic progressive neurodegenerative condition. Physical dependence is defined as a state of adaptation that is manifested by a drug class specific withdrawal syndrome that can be produced by abrupt cessation, rapid dose reduction, decreasing blood level of the drug, and/or administration of an antagonist. Physical dependence and tolerance to prescribed drugs do not constitute sufficient evidence of addiction or substance dependence, as they are normal physiologic responses that often occur with the persistent use of certain medications [38]. The ICD-10 definition of dependence syndrome is "a cluster of behavioral, cognitive, and physiologic phenomena that develop after repeated substance use and that typically include a strong desire to take the drug, difficulties in controlling its use, persisting in its use despite harmful consequences, a higher priority given to drug use than to other activities and obligations, increased tolerance, and sometimes a physical withdrawal state" [39].

Patients with PD require dopaminergic medication to control motor handicap, which when taken correctly represents an "adaptive dependence" [10]. This is not always easily distinguished from maladaptive dependence or addiction, as defined by the ICD-10 or DSM-IV-TR criteria [15,39]. Similar difficulties are seen in defining addiction to opioids in chronic pain patients, with a recent review finding that the prevalence varied from 0 to 50% in chronic non-malignant pain patients and from 0 to 7.7% in cancer patients [38]. In PD, the development of physiologic tolerance to L-dopa is mediated by central pharmacokinetic and pharmacodynamic changes related to progressive dopaminergic denervation. Both tolerance and sensitization may be involved in the reduction in duration of motor response, the increase in baseline disability, the reduced time to onset of action, and the emergence of dyskinesias [40]. Severe continuous dyskinesias should alert the physician to the possibility of dopamine dysregulation, particularly when associated with complaints that the medication is not working adequately [1]. In patients with DDS, the dysphoric effects of wearing-off often precede any discernable physical changes [11].

In an attempt to distinguish between a "physiologic" adaptive dependence and a "pathologic" or maladaptive dependence in patients with PD, Bearn *et al.* performed structured psychiatric interviews [10]. DDS patients described avoidance of off-period non-motor symptoms as the most frequent reason for taking more medications, despite a significant number reporting that their medications had a negative impact on their quality-of-life. The study demonstrated maladaptive use of dopaminergic therapies in patients diagnosed with DDS, which fulfilled DSM-IV-TR criteria for substance dependence [15]. Because patients with DDS continued to use L-dopa despite clear evidence of harmful consequences, they were also felt to fulfill ICD-10 criteria for "addiction" [10,39].

Risk factors for dopamine dysregulation

Personality traits and age of drug exposure

Personality traits related to impulsivity and sensation seeking (ISS) have been consistently associated with drug dependence [41–43], drug craving [44], and vulnerability to relapse [45] in individuals with substance dependence. ISS traits which include novelty seeking [41] and sensation seeking [46] are thought to be mediated through mesocorticolimbic dopaminergic systems [47], Individuals scoring highly on ISS personality traits exhibit a wide range of responses to novel stimuli and cues predictive of reward, including positive affect (elation and expectation), increased energy, and enhanced psychomotor activity.

In contrast, the "parkinsonian personality" has been described as being industrious, anhedonic, obsessive, cautious, inflexible, and disinclined to take risks [48,49], traits which may precede the motor changes in PD by decades [50]. Individuals with PD frequently score highly on ratings of personality traits such as harm avoidance, and demonstrate low levels of novelty-seeking behaviors [49,51]. These personality characteristics in PD have been hypothesized as a reason why these individuals are less prone to start smoking and drink fewer caffeinated beverages [52,53]. The concept of a distinctive personality profile linked to PD is controversial and inevitably based on retrospective case–control studies, which are prone to recall bias [54].

Unlike the risk-averse personality traits seen in most cases of PD, the small subgroup of patients with DDS score higher on ISS ratings, have greater past experimental drug use, and have a history of higher pre-morbid alcohol intake than healthy controls and other patients with PD without DDS [55]. Similarly, patients with PD who develop PG score highly on ISS inventories and are more likely to have a personal or immediate family history of alcohol use disorders [56]. Higher impulsivity ratings are also associated with higher punding scores in patients without documented addictive tendencies [57].

ISS traits decline with age, and earlier age of exposure to potentially addictive drugs is known to influence subsequent development and severity of substance dependence [58]. Patients with DDS, ICDs, or punding tend to develop PD at a younger age than those who do not dysregulate [55,56,59]. Patients with PD who develop DDS are also more likely to have a history of depressive symptoms [55], which is not a consistent feature in PD patients with PG [56,59]. In contrast, patients who develop punding show a trend towards higher scores on the obsessive–compulsive inventory [3], although obsessive traits have not been specifically assessed in DDS. See Box 19.2 for clinical "green flags" for the development of DDS.

Box 19.2 Clinical "green flags" for the development of DDS in patients

Strong risk factors
Young-onset PD (age <45 years)
Previous history of alcohol or illicit drug abuse
Impulsive sensation seeking (ISS) personality traits, previous "risk-taking" activities

Probable contributors
History of depressive symptoms
Use of large amounts of rapidly-acting dopamine replacement therapies (rapid-release L-dopa formulations, bolus apomorphine injections)

Other features
Disabling dyskinesias often well tolerated by patient
Impulse control disorders
Punding
Hypomanic mood spells
Insomnia
Aggressive behavior

Genetic factors influencing personality and addictive behaviors

Various candidate genes have been linked with addiction and ISS traits. Candidate systems include the serotonergic system [60], the monoamine metabolism pathway (monoamine oxidase A and catechol *O*-methyltransferase), the noradrenergic system, and GABAergic and nitric oxide systems [61]. Research implicating genes in the dopaminergic system, involving members of the "D2-like" family of dopamine receptors, including DRD4 receptors, have been encompassed in a model known as the "reward deficiency syndrome" [62].

Variants of the dopamine D2 dopamine receptor (DRD2) gene, especially the TaqI A1 allele, may be involved in addiction, co-morbid anti-social personality disorder symptoms, and high novelty seeking [63]. This polymorphism may play a role in learning, particularly relating to the negative consequences of actions [64], and this reward-based decision making in TaqI A1-positive subjects may be influenced by DRT [65]. An association between DRD2 and DRD4 polymorphisms has been associated with increased impulsivity on a delay discounting task [66]. The TaqI A1 allele has been linked to alcoholism, cigarette smoking, and cocaine, opiate, and psychostimulant addiction [67–69]. DRD2 gene polymorphisms have also been linked to various behavioral addictions and ICDs, which may be of particular relevance to DDS. A study of pathologic gamblers found them to have a higher prevalence of the DRD2 A1 allele than controls, and this prevalence increased progressively among more severe gamblers [70]. A link between obesity, binge eating, and the DRD2 A1 allele has also been described [71,72]. However, it is also worth noting that a number of studies have failed to find an association between the D2-like family genes and personality traits [73–75]. D2-like family genes have been investigated in PD. A positive association between DRD2 polymorphisms and PD has been found in some [76–79] but not all studies [80–82]. Although one study has shown an association between D2 and D3 receptor polymorphisms and motor fluctuations [83], there are currently no published studies investigating an association between these polymorphisms and addictive behaviors in PD.

Brain-derived neurotrophic factor (BDNF) modulates synaptic transmission by regulating synaptogenesis and synaptic plasticity and efficacy [84], and is of potential relevance in addiction. Nucleus accumbens BDNF is an important modulator of cocaine's rewarding effects in the drug self-administration model, promoting the development and persistence of addictive behaviors [85]. BDNF polymorphisms have been investigated in addiction in humans, particularly involving a single nucleotide polymorphism (G196A) which results in either a valine or a methionine residue at codon 66. BDNF Val66Met has been associated with vulnerability to methamphetamine or heroin dependence, and may affect age of onset of substance abuse [86,87], in addition to affecting the response to amphetamines [88]. Studies have investigated this polymorphism in smokers and alcohol abusers [72,89–91], but not all studies on addiction have demonstrated positive association [92]. Previous studies have examined the possible role of BDNF polymorphisms in the pathogenesis of PD, given its established role as a trophic factor for dopaminergic neurons [93,94]. Although two studies in Oriental populations [95,96] have found such an association, this has not been reproduced for other ethnic groups [97,98]. There are currently no published studies investigating an association with BDNF polymorphisms and addictive behaviors in PD.

PD-related cognitive deficits

Cognitive processes that may be impaired in individuals with behavioral and substance addictions relate to psychologic systems that allow for responding based upon conditional associations between stimuli and reward, rapidly changing reinforcement contingencies, and future planning. These models are based upon a relative competition for behavioral control in the nucleus accumbens with inputs from the amygdala and prefrontal cortex that may gate competing response tendencies based upon associative learning and cognition [99]. The orbitofrontal cortex (OFC) is involved in sensory integration, in representing the affective value of reinforcers, and in decision making and expectation [100]. Jentsch and Taylor proposed that these regions of the frontal cortex are directly affected by prolonged exposure to potential drugs of abuse and that during drug self-administration, the synaptic release of dopamine increases in the amygdala, helping to establish associations with the rewarding qualities of the drug [101]. This frontal cognitive dysfunction reduces the ability to inhibit conditioned or unconditioned responses elicited by drugs and, when combined with the increased motivational properties of the drug resulting from limbic and amygdalar dysfunction, drug-seeking behavior occurs [102]. Frontal lesions are associated with other disinhibited behaviors, and a preference for immediate small rewards over delayed larger rewards [103]. Increased perseveration and other repetitive behaviors are seen following lesions in areas such as the dorsolateral prefrontal, lateral orbitofrontal, or ventromedial cortex [104].

Cognitive testing in addiction and in PG demonstrate impairments in decision-making, with dorsolateral prefrontal and orbitofrontal cortex dysfunctions particularly implicated [105]. Decreased activity of the OFC and the anterior cingulate gyrus has been found in imaging studies of addicts during drug withdrawal [106,107]. Areas such as the OFC ventral striatum and ventromedial prefrontal cortex are also activated by rewarding stimuli other than drugs of abuse. Pathologic gamblers appear to show less activation in the ventromedial prefrontal cortex in response to a guessing task [108], and in the orbitofrontal cortex, caudate/basal ganglia, and thalamus when looking at gambling-related imagery [109].

Impaired decision making in patients with PD is of relevance in the development of addictive behaviors. Examples of decision-making tests in which PD patients performed poorly include the Iowa Gambling Task (IGT), and executive function tests such as the Wisconsin Card-Sorting test and the Stroop test [110]. Patients with early (Hoehn and Yahr stage 1–2.5) PD also perform poorly in tests of prefrontal cortical dysfunction such as the IGT [111]. Functional magnetic resonance imaging (fMRI) has been used to investigate the neural mechanisms underlying reward prediction and reward outcome processing in unmedicated early PD (Hoehn and Yahr stage 1). Schott *et al.* found that healthy elderly participants and early PD patients had an absent mesolimbic reward prediction response, but increased mesolimbic activation to the reward feedback itself [112]. They suggested that healthy elderly and PD patients were less proficient in learning the predictive value of the reward cues despite preserved mesolimbic processing of reward prediction errors. These deficits may be related to disruption of the reciprocal loops between the striatum and structures in the prefrontal cortex following dopamine depletion.

Dopaminergic medications have been shown to influence cognitive function relevant to rewarding behaviors in PD. Frank, Seeberger, and O'Reilly demonstrated that medicated patients with PD displayed enhanced positive-feedback learning greater than that seen in normal controls [113]. Other frontal functions, such as probabilistic reversal learning, which involves the adaptation of behavior according to changes in stimulus–reward contingencies, are adversely affected by dopaminergic medications [114]. These findings support a "dopamine overdose hypothesis" where DRT causes over-stimulation of the ventral striatum, a brain region which is relatively spared in early-stage PD [115]. Non-medicated patients with PD show enhanced avoidance of negative stimuli, which may relate to the cautious, inflexible, and risk-aversive "parkinsonian personality" [113].

Chronic dopaminergic treatment subverts brain reward systems

In attempting to understand DDS, analogies have been drawn with compulsive psychostimulant use, where a drug's ability to induce pleasure or to help escape withdrawal from life stressors has been considered to be the root cause [2]. However, these models do not explain why most patients who develop DDS fail to recognize or acknowledge pleasurable effects from their medication. Lawrence, Evans, and Lees [2] have reviewed current models of addiction, including habit and hedonic theories, and suggest that Robinson and Berridge's incentive sensitization theory [116] best explains DDS.

A central mechanism in mesolimbic reward processing is phasic activity of dopamine-containing neurons in the ventral tegmental area and the medial substantia nigra. During unexpected rewards, the nucleus accumbens receives dopaminergic signals from these midbrain structures [117]. Stimuli that are repeatedly presented with reward, termed conditioned stimuli (CS+), are able to elicit phasic dopamine firing in the midbrain when presented alone, whereas stimuli that do not predict reward (CS–) do not elicit such a response [118]. Presentation of a CS+ leads to increased response speed compared with the presentation of a CS–, an effect that is modulated by ventral striatal dopamine [119]. Robinson and Berridge suggested that compulsive drug use stems from progressive neuroadaptations in the dopamine projections to the nucleus accumbens-related circuitry [120]. These include persistent changes in dopaminergic and GABAergic neurotransmission and the intracellular signaling pathways which they activate, with resultant changes in the morphologic appearance of the neurons [116,121]. Sensitization, causing a progressive increase in the rewarding effect of dopaminergic drugs with repeated use occurs, and the resulting neuroadaptations mediate a subcomponent of reward termed incentive salience, a component of normal appetite, which, when attributed to stimuli, causes them to become attractive and "wanted" [116,120]. Over time the pleasurable effects of drug taking disappear and instead the drugs become compulsively "wanted" or craved for [2,120].

Evidence of sensitization in DDS

Using molecular imaging with positron emission tomography (PET) and the dopamine D2/3 receptor ligand [^{11}C]raclopride, Evans *et al.* evaluated L-dopa-induced dopamine neurotransmission in the ventral striatum of patients with DDS compared with matched PD controls [122]. Patients with DDS exhibited enhanced L-dopa-induced ventral striatal dopamine release compared with L-dopa-treated patients with PD who were not compulsively taking dopaminergic drugs. The sensitized ventral striatal dopamine neurotransmission produced by L-dopa in these individuals correlated with self-reported compulsive drug "wanting" but not "liking" [122]. DDS patients in this study were also found to have a heightened responsivity to a small financial reward – further evidence that dopaminergic medications may cause a "motivational spillover" into other rewarding behaviors.

Further indirect evidence of sensitization comes from the frequent association with punding. These senseless repetitive behaviors resemble the stereotyped movements seen in animals treated with dopaminergic drugs including amphetamine and cocaine, and plastic changes in the striatum have been suggested to mediate these activities [123]. A link between punding and dyskinesias, independent of increased dopaminergic medication use, has also been reported [124]. This suggests that both phenomena may be due to drug-induced sensitization of neural systems mediating motor and behavioral function [125]. L-Dopa therapy stimulates both dopamine D1 and D2 receptor subtypes, both of which are involved in the development of stereotypies in animals [116,126].

Dopaminergic medication types and doses implicated in DDS and punding

L-Dopa is considered the most potent trigger for DDS in PD, but subcutaneous intermittent injections of apomorphine and oral dopamine agonists may also be responsible [13,14,127,128]. The potency and rapid action of L-dopa and apomorphine may be more likely to give the patient a subjective "high" and therefore increase the risk of excessive use [11]. Evans *et al.* showed that punders were taking higher daily amounts of dopaminergic medications than non-punders, and that all punders were using dopamine agonists [3]. This association between the use of dopamine agonists and punding has been reported by other authors, including "computer addictions"

[26,27], compulsive sorting, gardening, and musical instrument playing [18,29,57]. Withdrawal of agonist therapy has also been reported to lead to the rapid curtailment of punding in a few patients [129]. Punding behaviors have occasionally been described in patients taking L-dopa alone [3,130]. Interestingly, Miwa *et al.* described two cases of patients developing punding behaviors after commencement of the anti-psychotic quetiapine [131]. Although both patients were also on L-dopa, and one was on a dopamine agonist, the authors considered that the quetiapine was responsible for the punding.

ICDs in PD without addictive behaviors are much more associated with dopamine agonists (DAs) than L-dopa. PG is the impulse control disorder that has been most studied, and a recent review showed that over 98% of patients with PG were on DAs [59]. Some studies have implicated pramipexole as particularly likely to induce impulse control disorders, although this remains to be confirmed. This drug's increased affinity for D3 receptors, which are found predominantly in limbic regions and have been implicated in the addiction process, has been suggested as a possible explanation [132]. Reports linking PG particularly to agonists are potentially confounded by prescribing practices, as patients with younger ages of onset of PD might be more likely to be prescribed DAs and also more likely to develop ICD. A recent meta-analysis of the risk of PG on different DAs showed no significant differences, comparing pramipexole with ropinirole and non-ergot and ergot DAs [59].

Patients with DDS have much higher daily L-dopa doses than PD patients with similar motor deficits (frequently 2 g and exceptionally up to 4 g per day) [122,133]. In contrast, the total L-dopa equivalent dose (LED) including L-dopa and DAs used by patients with PG is not consistently elevated compared with disease-matched controls [32,134,135]. Animal studies suggest that intermittent (pulsatile) administration of various drugs affecting the dopaminergic system augment motor responses – interpreted as behavioral sensitization – whereas continuous steady-state round-the-clock administration produces tolerance [136,137]. However, locomotor sensitization has also been associated with continuous drug administration in some preclinical studies [138].

Box 19.3 Suggested screening questionnaire for punding

Do you have any hobbies or pastimes or activities you do repeatedly?
When did you become interested in your hobby (years)?
How many hours per day do you spend on your hobby?
Does your hobby interfere with sleep?
When engaged in your hobby, would you neglect to take food or your medications?
Do you have difficulties in finishing your hobby projects?
How do you feel if you are interrupted when you are engaged with your hobby (i.e., do you ever get angry or upset)?
Do you make a mess when you are pursuing your pastimes or hobbies?
Are you interested in your hobby only when "on"?
How many hours per day do you spend on the following?
- cleaning/tidying
- gardening or DIY
- collecting things
- repairing/dismantling, e.g., computers, television, radio (if yes, were you able to put them back together?)
- sorting, e.g., papers, through drawers/handbag
- on the computer
- crosswords/Sudoku puzzles, etc.

Management of DDS

Despite recent increasing awareness of dopamine dysregulation and punding, it is probable that these phenomena remain under-recognized or misinterpreted by physicians. Some patients find that they are able to extend their "on" periods by punding and may be reluctant to mention them during the consultation. Careful inquiry through the family in the absence of the patient may be required to bring important behavioral problems to light. In patients who continually complain that their medication is not working adequately, a careful assessment of their actual dosing regimen and level of adherence is advised. Young-onset patients should be warned of the small potential risk of developing ICDs, punding, and DDS before initiation of treatment. Some screening questions such as "How do you spend the day?" or "How many hours sleep do you get?" may reveal behavioral disturbances including punding. See Box 19.3.

An immediate gradual reduction of DRT is the first critical step in bringing DDS and punding under control and may meet with strong resistance from the patient who lacks insight into the disastrous consequences of his or her actions. The patient's family general practitioner and local pharmacist may all need to be involved in the institution of a stringent and carefully monitored rationing program [11]. "Booster" medications such as subcutaneous bolus doses of apomorphine and rapidly acting L-dopa formulations should be stopped completely [11]. Phased withdrawal of oral dopamine agonists is the first treatment adjustment in patients with ICDs, with a concomitant increase in L-dopa dosage if motor symptoms become severe and disabling [132,139]. Occasionally, hospital admission may be required for supervised drug reductions and the management of associated hypomanic, depressive, or paranoid psychotic episodes associated with DDS. Anti-psychotic medications such as quetiapine or aripiprazole should be considered, although trials on the efficacy of these specific treatments are lacking. If these are ineffective, clozapine with regular white cell monitoring should be considered. Dopaminergic drug reduction may occasionally precipitate a more severe depression or an anxiety state which requires intensive in-patient treatment with anti-depressants and behavioral therapy. There are currently no data available regarding the preferred anti-depressant types in treating DDS. Anti-depressants such as citalopram have been found useful in treating compulsive shopping in non-PD cases [140], but do not abolish compulsive DRT seeking and intake [141]. Caution may be required when using tricyclic anti-depressants, with reports on cocaine-addicted patients suggesting that these drugs may be associated with an increased risk of relapse [142]. Further, animal studies have implicated desipramine as a potential promoter of incentive sensitization [143]. Rarely, electroconvulsive therapy may be required [11].

Opiate antagonists and mood stabilizers such as lithium, valproate, and carbamazepine have been claimed to be useful in PG, but there is little experience with them in any of the impulse control disorders in PD [144,145]. Further research is required regarding these agents, particularly as valproate and lithium may be associated with an increased risk of parkinsonism [146,147]. A potential role for amantadine, a medication with dopaminergic effects, has also been suggested to be useful in cocaine users with high withdrawal severity [148]. Amantadine also has NMDA antagonistic properties, and is used as a treatment for L-dopa-induced dyskinesias [149]. Amantadine has recently been described as reversing punding in a patient with PD [150], and may warrant further investigation in clinical trials. No differences in the frequency of punding in amantidine and non-amantidine users was found by Evans *et al.* [3].

Currently, there are no published studies assessing psychologic interventions in DDS. Psychosocial treatments, including contingency management, relapse prevention, family-based approaches, and general cognitive behavior therapy (CBT), have been shown to be beneficial in treating substance use disorders [151–153]. CBT may be helpful for internet addictions [154] and ICDs such as PG [155,156]. In patients with severe DDS, shared care between neurologists and psychiatrists with expertise in drug dependency is important and pressure should be brought to bear by the family to persuade the patient to attend organizations such as Gamblers and Narcotics Anonymous [11].

Deep brain stimulation (DBS) surgery of the subthalamic nucleus (STN) or globus pallidus internus (GPi) may markedly improve "off"-medication motor symptoms, and STN DBS has the potential to allow significant dose reductions (on average by about 50%) [157]. A significant proportion of young-onset PD patients with severe refractory motor fluctuations suitable for DBS also have DDS or ICDs, and it is unclear at present what advice to give them with respect to the potential effects of surgery on their coexisting behavioral difficulties. There have been no prospective studies specifically looking at DBS and compulsive behaviors in PD, with current data available from case series only. In five patients, DDS failed to improve following DBS of the subthalamic nucleus [158,159], whereas in another 10 patients, DDS resolved or was dramatically improved [5,160]. Regarding ICDs and DBS, some authors have described improvements in well-screened PD patients with PG after bilateral STN DBS [19,161]. Others have reported ICDs developing or decompensating postoperatively [56,162–165], and preoperative DDS or ICDs may be a risk factor for postoperative suicide attempts [166]. Further research is required to identify factors which can predict those patients with DDS or ICDs who will derive benefit from DBS.

Conclusion

DDS is a relatively uncommon and still under-diagnosed iatrogenic neurobehavioral disorder often associated with devastating social sequelae. Further research is needed to identify at-risk groups, thereby facilitating more early effective intervention. DDS needs to be distinguished from the related ICD, which requires a somewhat different management approach and may have distinct if intertwined pathologic causes.

Acknowledgments

The preparation of this chapter was supported by the Reta Lila Weston Trust. The funding organization was not involved in the collection, management, analysis, and interpretation of the data, and preparation, review, or approval of the text.

References

1. Evans AH, Lees AJ. Dopamine dysregulation syndrome in Parkinson's disease. *Curr Opin Neurol* 2004;**17**(4):393–8.
2. Lawrence AD, Evans AH, Lees AJ. Compulsive use of dopamine replacement therapy in Parkinson's disease: reward systems gone awry? *Lancet Neurol* 2003;**2**(10):595–604.
3. Evans AH, Katzenschlager R, Paviour D, *et al.* Punding in Parkinson's disease: its relation to the dopamine dysregulation syndrome. *Mov Disord* 2004;**19**(4):397–405.

4. O'Brien CP, DiGiacomo JN, Fahn S, Schwarz GA. Mental effects of high-dosage levodopa. *Arch Gen Psychiatry* 1971;**24**(1):61–4.
5. Witjas T, Kaphan E, Azulay JP, *et al.* Nonmotor fluctuations in Parkinson's disease: frequent and disabling. *Neurology* 2002;**59**(3):408–13.
6. Hillen ME, Sage JI. Nonmotor fluctuations in patients with Parkinson's disease. *Neurology* 1996;**47**(5):1180–3.
7. Maricle RA, Valentine RJ, Carter J, Nutt JG. Mood response to levodopa infusion in early Parkinson's disease. *Neurology* 1998;**50**(6):1890–2.
8. Menza MA, Sage J, Marshall E, *et al.* Mood changes and "on–off" phenomena in Parkinson's disease. *Mov Disord* 1990;**5**(2):148–51.
9. Nissenbaum H, Quinn NP, Brown RG, *et al.* Mood swings associated with the "on–off" phenomenon in Parkinson's disease. *Psychol Med* 1987;**17**(4):899–904.
10. Bearn J, Evans A, Kelleher M, *et al.* Recognition of a dopamine replacement therapy dependence syndrome in Parkinson's disease: a pilot study. *Drug Alcohol Depend* 2004;**76**(3):305–10.
11. Giovannoni G, O'Sullivan JD, Turner K, *et al.* Hedonistic homeostatic dysregulation in patients with Parkinson's disease on dopamine replacement therapies. *J Neurol Neurosurg Psychiatry* 2000;**68**(4):423–8.
12. Merims D, Galili-Mosberg R, Melamed E. Is there addiction to levodopa in patients with Parkinson's disease? *Mov Disord* 2000;**15**(5):1014–6.
13. Spigset O, von Scheele C. Levodopa dependence and abuse in Parkinson's disease. *Pharmacotherapy* 1997;**17**(5):1027–30.
14. Pezzella FR, Colosimo C, Vanacore N, *et al.* Prevalence and clinical features of hedonistic homeostatic dysregulation in Parkinson's disease. *Mov Disord* 2005;**20**(1):77–81.
15. American Psychiatric Association. *Diagnostic and Statistical Manual of Mental Disorders*, 4th edn. Washington, DC: American Psychiatric Association, 2000.
16. Grant JE, Levine L, Kim D, Potenza MN. Impulse control disorders in adult psychiatric inpatients. *Am J Psychiatry* 2005;**162**(11):2184–8.
17. McElroy SL, Keck PE Jr, Pope HG Jr, *et al.* Compulsive buying: a report of 20 cases. *J Clin Psychiatry* 1994;**55**(6):242–8.
18. Nirenberg MJ, Waters C. Compulsive eating and weight gain related to dopamine agonist use. *Mov Disord* 2006;**21**(4): 524–9.
19. Molina JA, Sainz-Artiga MJ, Fraile A, *et al.* Pathologic gambling in Parkinson's disease: a behavioral manifestation of pharmacologic treatment? *Mov Disord* 2000;**15**(5):869–72.
20. Klos KJ, Bower JH, Josephs KA, *et al.* Pathological hypersexuality predominantly linked to adjuvant dopamine agonist therapy in Parkinson's disease and multiple system atrophy. *Parkinsonism Relat Disord* 2005;**11**(6):381–6.
21. Voon V, Fox SH. Medication-related impulse control and repetitive behaviors in Parkinson disease. *Arch Neurol* 2007;**64**(8):1089–96.
22. Rylander G. Psychoses and the punding and choreiform syndromes in addiction to central stimulant drugs. *Psychiatr Neurol Neurochir* 1972;**75**(3):203–12.
23. Schiorring E. Psychopathology induced by "speed drugs". *Pharmacol Biochem Behav* 1981;**14**(Suppl 1):109–22.
24. Friedman JH. Punding on levodopa. *Biol Psychiatry* 1994;**36**(5):350–1.
25. Fernandez HH, Friedman JH. Punding on L-dopa. *Mov Disord* 1999;**14**(5):836–8.
26. Fasano A, Elia AE, Soleti F, *et al.* Punding and computer addiction in Parkinson's disease. *Mov Disord* 2006;**21**(8): 1217–8.
27. Miyasaki JM, Al Hassan K, Lang AE, Voon V. Punding prevalence in Parkinson's disease. *Mov Disord* 2007;**22**(8) 1179–81.
28. Kummer A, Maia DP, Salgado JV, *et al.* Dopamine dysregulation syndrome in Parkinson's disease: case report. *Arq Neuropsiquiatr* 2006;**64**(4):1019–22.
29. Shapiro MA, Chang YL, Munson SK, *et al.* Hypersexuality and paraphilia induced by selegiline in Parkinson's disease: report of 2 cases. *Parkinsonism Relat Disord* 2006;**12**(6): 392–5.
30. Alegret M, Junque C, Valldeoriola F, *et al.* Obsessive–compulsive symptoms in Parkinson's disease. *J Neurol Neurosurg Psychiatry* 2001;**70**(3):394–6.
31. Factor SA, Molho ES, Podskalny GD, Brown D. Parkinson's disease: drug-induced psychiatric states. *Adv Neurol* 1995;**65**: 115–38.
32. Voon V, Hassan K, Zurowski M, *et al.* Prospective prevalence of pathologic gambling and medication association in Parkinson disease. *Neurology* 2006;**66**(11):1750–2.
33. Petry NM, Stinson FS, Grant BF. Comorbidity of DSM-IV pathological gambling and other psychiatric disorders: results from the National Epidemiologic Survey on Alcohol and Related Conditions. *J Clin Psychiatry* 2005;**66**(5):564–74.
34. Cunningham-Williams RM, Grucza RA, Cottler LB, *et al.* Prevalence and predictors of pathological gambling: results from the St. Louis personality, health and lifestyle (SLPHL) study. *J Psychiatr Res* 2005;**39**(4):377–90.
35. Voon V, Hassan K, Zurowski M, *et al.* Prevalence of repetitive and reward-seeking behaviors in Parkinson disease. *Neurology* 2006;**67**(7):1254–7.
36. Bathgate D, Snowden JS, Varma A, *et al.* Behaviour in frontotemporal dementia, Alzheimer's disease and vascular dementia. *Acta Neurol Scand* 2001;**103**(6):367–78.
37. Miyasaki JM, Al Hassan K, Lang AE, Voon V. Punding prevalence in Parkinson's disease. *Mov Disord* 2007;**22**(8):1179–81.
38. Hojsted J, Sjogren P. Addiction to opioids in chronic pain patients: a literature review. *Eur J Pain* 2007;**11**(5):490–518.
39. World Health Organization. *ICD-10 Version 2007*, http://www.who.int/classifications/apps/icd/icd10online/. Geneva: World Health Organization, 2007.
40. Colosimo C, Merello M, Hughes AJ, *et al.* Motor response to acute dopaminergic challenge with apomorphine and levodopa in Parkinson's disease: implications for the pathogenesis of the on-off phenomenon. *J Neurol Neurosurg Psychiatry* 1996;**60**(6):634–7.
41. Cloninger CR. A systematic method for clinical description and classification of personality variants. A proposal. *Arch Gen Psychiatry* 1987;**44**(6):573–88.
42. Hosak L, Preiss M, Halir M, *et al.* Temperament and character inventory (TCI) personality profile in methamphetamine abusers: a controlled study. *Eur Psychiatry* 2004;**19**(4):193–5.
43. Palmgreen P, Donohew L, Lorch EP, *et al.* Television campaigns and adolescent marijuana use: tests of sensation seeking targeting. *Am J Public Health* 2001;**91**(2):292–6.
44. Zilberman ML, Tavares H, el-Guebaly N. Relationship between craving and personality in treatment-seeking

women with substance-related disorders. *BMC Psychiatry* 2003;**3**:1.
45. Meszaros K, Lenzinger E, Hornik K, *et al.* The Tridimensional Personality Questionnaire as a predictor of relapse in detoxified alcohol dependents. The European Fluvoxamine in Alcoholism Study Group. *Alcohol Clin Exp Res* 1999;**23**(3): 483–6.
46. Zuckerman M. Sensation seeking and behavior disorders. *Arch Gen Psychiatry* 1988;**45**(5):502–4.
47. Leyton M, Boileau I, Benkelfat C, *et al.* Amphetamine-induced increases in extracellular dopamine, drug wanting, and novelty seeking: a PET/[^{11}C]raclopride study in healthy men. *Neuropsychopharmacology* 2002;**27**(6):1027–35.
48. Todes CJ, Lees AJ. The pre-morbid personality of patients with Parkinson's disease. *J Neurol Neurosurg Psychiatry* 1985;**48**(2):97–100.
49. Menza MA, Golbe LI, Cody RA, Forman NE. Dopamine-related personality traits in Parkinson's disease. *Neurology* 1993;**43**(3 Pt 1):505–8.
50. Poewe W, Karamat E, Kemmler GW, Gerstenbrand F. The premorbid personality of patients with Parkinson's disease: a comparative study with healthy controls and patients with essential tremor. *Adv Neurol* 1990;**53**: 339–42.
51. Fujii C, Harada S, Ohkoshi N, *et al.* Cross-cultural traits for personality of patients with Parkinson's disease in Japan. *Am J Med Genet* 2000;**96**(1):1–3.
52. Menza M. The personality associated with Parkinson's disease. *Curr Psychiatry Rep* 2000;**2**(5):421–6.
53. Evans AH, Lawrence AD, Potts J, *et al.* Relationship between impulsive sensation seeking traits, smoking, alcohol and caffeine intake, and Parkinson's disease. *J Neurol Neurosurg Psychiatry* 2006;**77**(3):317–21.
54. Ishihara L, Brayne C. What is the evidence for a premorbid parkinsonian personality: a systematic review. *Mov Disord* 2006;**21**(8):1066–72.
55. Evans AH, Lawrence AD, *et al.* Factors influencing susceptibility to compulsive dopaminergic drug use in Parkinson disease. *Neurology* 2005;**65**(10):1570–4.
56. Voon V, Thomsen T, Miyasaki JM, *et al.* Factors associated with dopaminergic drug-related pathological gambling in Parkinson disease. *Arch Neurol* 2007;**64**(2):212–6.
57. Lawrence AJ, Blackwell AD, Barker RA, *et al.* Predictors of punding in Parkinson's disease: results from a questionnaire survey. *Mov Disord* 2007;**22**(16):2339–45.
58. Chambers RA, Taylor JR, Potenza MN. Developmental neurocircuitry of motivation in adolescence: a critical period of addiction vulnerability. *Am J Psychiatry* 2003;**160**(6):1041–52.
59. Gallagher DA, O'Sullivan SS, Evans AH, *et al.* Pathological gambling in Parkinson's disease: risk factors and differences from dopamine dysregulation. An analysis of published case series. *Mov Disord* 2007;**22**(12):1757–63.
60. Kreek MJ, Nielsen DA, LaForge KS. Genes associated with addiction: alcoholism, opiate, and cocaine addiction. *Neuromol. Med* 2004;**5**(1):85–108.
61. Kreek MJ, Nielsen DA, Butelman ER, LaForge KS. Genetic influences on impulsivity, risk taking, stress responsivity and vulnerability to drug abuse and addiction. *Nat Neurosci* 2005;**8**(11):1450–7.
62. Blum K, Braverman ER, Holder JM, *et al.* Reward deficiency syndrome: a biogenetic model for the diagnosis and treatment of impulsive, addictive, and compulsive behaviors. *J Psychoactive Drugs* 2000;**32**(Suppl):i–iv, 1–112.
63. Blum K, Noble EP, Sheridan PJ, *et al.* Allelic association of human dopamine D2 receptor gene in alcoholism. *JAMA* 1990;**263**(15):2055–60.
64. Klein TA, Neumann J, Reuter M, *et al.* Genetically determined differences in learning from errors. *Science* 2007;**318**(5856):1642–5.
65. Cohen MX, Krohn-Grimberghe A, Elger CE, Weber B. Dopamine gene predicts the brain's response to dopaminergic drug. *Eur J Neurosci* 2007;**26**(12):3652–60.
66. Eisenberg DT, Mackillop J, Modi M, *et al.* Examining impulsivity as an endophenotype using a behavioral approach: a DRD2 TaqI A and DRD4 48-bp VNTR association study. *Behav Brain Funct* 2007;**3**: 2.
67. Blum K, Braverman ER, Wood RC, *et al.* Increased prevalence of the TaqI A1 allele of the dopamine receptor gene (DRD2) in obesity with comorbid substance use disorder: a preliminary report. *Pharmacogenetics* 1996;**6**(4):297–305.
68. Noble EP. D2 dopamine receptor gene in psychiatric and neurologic disorders and its phenotypes. *Am J Med Genet B Neuropsychiatr Genet* 2003;**116B**(1):103–25.
69. Comings DE, Ferry L, Bradshaw-Robinson S, *et al.* The dopamine D2 receptor (DRD2) gene: a genetic risk factor in smoking. *Pharmacogenetics* 1996;**6**(1):73–9.
70. Comings DE, Rosenthal RJ, Lesieur HR, *et al.* A study of the dopamine D2 receptor gene in pathological gambling. *Pharmacogenetics* 1996;**6**(3):223–34.
71. Fang YJ, Thomas GN, Xu ZL, *et al.* An affected pedigree member analysis of linkage between the dopamine D2 receptor gene TaqI polymorphism and obesity and hypertension. *Int J Cardiol* 2005;**102**(1):111–6.
72. Davis C, Levitan RD, Kaplan AS, *et al.* Reward sensitivity and the D2 dopamine receptor gene: a case–control study of binge eating disorder. Prog Neuropsychopharmacol *Biol Psychiatry* 2008;**32**(3):620–8.
73. Strobel A, Spinath FM, Angleitner A, *et al.* Lack of association between polymorphisms of the dopamine D4 receptor gene and personality. *Neuropsychobiology* 2003;**47**(1):52–6.
74. Gebhardt C, Leisch F, Schussler P, *et al.* Non-association of dopamine D4 and D2 receptor genes with personality in healthy individuals. *Psychiatr Genet* 2000;**10**(3):131–7.
75. Tsai SJ, Hong CJ, Yu YW, Chen TJ. Association study of catechol-*O*-methyltransferase gene and dopamine D4 receptor gene polymorphisms and personality traits in healthy young Chinese females. *Neuropsychobiology* 2004;**50**(2): 153–6.
76. Oliveri RL, Annesi G, Zappia M, *et al.* The dopamine D2 receptor gene is a susceptibility locus for Parkinson's disease. *Mov Disord* 2000;**15**(1):127–31.
77. Plante-Bordeneuve V, Taussig D, Thomas F, *et al.* Evaluation of four candidate genes encoding proteins of the dopamine pathway in familial and sporadic Parkinson's disease: evidence for association of a DRD2 allele. *Neurology* 1997;**48**(6):1589–93.
78. Grevle L, Guzey C, Hadidi H, *et al.* Allelic association between the DRD2 TaqI A polymorphism and Parkinson's disease. *Mov Disord* 2000;**15**(6):1070–4.
79. Juyal RC, Das M, Punia S, *et al.* Genetic susceptibility to Parkinson's disease among South and North Indians: I. Role

of polymorphisms in dopamine receptor and transporter genes and association of DRD4 120-bp duplication marker. *Neurogenetics* 2006;**7**(4):223–9.
80. Costa-Mallen P, Costa LG, Smith-Weller T, *et al.* Genetic polymorphism of dopamine D2 receptors in Parkinson's disease and interactions with cigarette smoking and MAO-B intron 13 polymorphism. *J Neurol Neurosurg Psychiatry* 2000;**69**(4):535–7.
81. Pastor P, Munoz E, Obach V, *et al.* Dopamine receptor D2 intronic polymorphism in patients with Parkinson's disease. *Neurosci Lett* 1999;**273**(3):151–4.
82. Tan EK, Tan Y, Chai A, *et al.* Dopamine D2 receptor TaqIA and TaqIB polymorphisms in Parkinson's disease. *Mov Disord* 2003;**18**(5):593–5.
83. Wang J, Liu ZL, Chen B. Association study of dopamine D2, D3 receptor gene polymorphisms with motor fluctuations in PD. *Neurology* 2001;**56**(12):1757–9.
84. Woo NH, Teng HK, Siao CJ, *et al.* Activation of p75NTR by proBDNF facilitates hippocampal long-term depression. *Nat Neurosci* 2005;**8**(8):1069–77.
85. Graham DL, Edwards S, Bachtell RK, *et al.* Dynamic BDNF activity in nucleus accumbens with cocaine use increases self-administration and relapse. *Nat Neurosci* 2007;**10**(8):1029–37.
86. Cheng CY, Hong CJ, Yu YW, *et al.* Brain-derived neurotrophic factor (Val66Met) genetic polymorphism is associated with substance abuse in males. *Brain Res Mol Brain Res* 2005; **140**(1–2):86–90.
87. Uhl GR, Liu QR, Walther D, *et al.* Polysubstance abuse-vulnerability genes: genome scans for association, using 1,004 subjects and 1,494 single-nucleotide polymorphisms. *Am J Hum Genet* 2001;**69**(6):1290–300.
88. Flanagin BA, Cook EH Jr, de Wit H. An association study of the brain-derived neurotrophic factor Val66Met polymorphism and amphetamine response. *Am J Med Genet B Neuropsychiatr Genet* 2006;**141B**(6):576–83.
89. Beuten J, Payne TJ, Ma JZ, Li MD. Significant association of catechol-*O*-methyltransferase (COMT) haplotypes with nicotine dependence in male and female smokers of two ethnic populations. *Neuropsychopharmacology* 2006;**31**(3):675–84.
90. Lang UE, Sander T, Lohoff FW, *et al.* Association of the met66 allele of brain-derived neurotrophic factor (BDNF) with smoking. *Psychopharmacology (Berl)* 2007;**190**(4):433–9.
91. Matsushita S, Kimura M, Miyakawa T, *et al.* Association study of brain-derived neurotrophic factor gene polymorphism and alcoholism. *Alcohol Clin Exp Res* 2004;**28**(11): 1609–12.
92. Itoh K, Hashimoto K, Shimizu E, *et al.* Association study between brain-derived neurotrophic factor gene polymorphisms and methamphetamine abusers in Japan. *Am J Med Genet B Neuropsychiatr Genet* 2005;**132B**(1):70–3.
93. Fumagalli F, Racagni G, Riva MA. Shedding light into the role of BDNF in the pharmacotherapy of Parkinson's disease. *Pharmacogenomics J* 2006;**6**(2):95–104.
94. Mogi M, Togari A, Kondo T, *et al.* Brain-derived growth factor and nerve growth factor concentrations are decreased in the substantia nigra in Parkinson's disease. *Neurosci Lett* 1999;**270**(1):45–8.
95. Masaki T, Matsushita S, Arai H, *et al.* Association between a polymorphism of brain-derived neurotrophic factor gene and sporadic Parkinson's disease. *Ann Neurol* 2003;**54**(2):276–7.
96. Momose Y, Murata M, Kobayashi K, *et al.* Association studies of multiple candidate genes for Parkinson's disease using single nucleotide polymorphisms. *Ann Neurol* 2002;**51**(1):133–6.
97. Hong CJ, Liu HC, Liu TY, *et al.* Brain-derived neurotrophic factor (BDNF) Val66Met polymorphisms in Parkinson's disease and age of onset. *Neurosci Lett* 2003;**353**(1):75–7.
98. Hakansson A, Melke J, Westberg L, *et al.* Lack of association between the BDNF Val66Met polymorphism and Parkinson's disease in a Swedish population. *Ann Neurol* 2003;**53**(6):823.
99. Jentsch JD, Roth RH, Taylor JR. Role for dopamine in the behavioral functions of the prefrontal corticostriatal system: implications for mental disorders and psychotropic drug action. *Prog Brain Res* 2000;**126**: 433–53.
100. Kringelbach ML. The human orbitofrontal cortex: linking reward to hedonic experience. *Nat Rev Neurosci* 2005;**6**(9): 691–702.
101. Jentsch JD, Taylor JR. Impulsivity resulting from frontostriatal dysfunction in drug abuse: implications for the control of behavior by reward-related stimuli. *Psychopharmacology (Berl)* 1999;**146**(4):373–90.
102. Koob GF, Le Moal M. Neurobiological theories of addiction. In: Koob GF, Le Moal M, eds. *Neurobiology of Addiction*. London: Elsevier, 2006: 381–4.
103. Roesch MR, Calu DJ, Burke KA, Schoenbaum G. Should I stay or should I go? Transformation of time-discounted rewards in orbitofrontal cortex and associated brain circuits. *Ann N Y Acad Sci* 2007;**1104**: 21–34.
104. Ridley RM, Clark BA, Durnford LJ, Baker HF. Stimulus-bound perseveration after frontal ablations in marmosets. *Neuroscience* 1993;**52**(3):595–604.
105. Brand M, Kalbe E, Labudda K, *et al.* Decision-making impairments in patients with pathological gambling. *Psychiatry Res* 2005;**133**(1):91–9.
106. Volkow ND, Fowler JS, Wolf AP, *et al.* Changes in brain glucose metabolism in cocaine dependence and withdrawal. *Am J Psychiatry* 1991;**148**(5):621–6.
107. Sekine Y, Minabe Y, Ouchi Y, *et al.* Association of dopamine transporter loss in the orbitofrontal and dorsolateral prefrontal cortices with methamphetamine-related psychiatric symptoms. *Am J Psychiatry* 2003;**160**(9):1699–701.
108. Reuter J, Raedler T, Rose M, *et al.* Pathological gambling is linked to reduced activation of the mesolimbic reward system. *Nat Neurosci* 2005;**8**(2):147–8.
109. Potenza MN, Steinberg MA, Skudlarski P, *et al.* Gambling urges in pathological gambling: a functional magnetic resonance imaging study. *Arch Gen Psychiatry* 2003;**60**(8):828–36.
110. Mimura M, Oeda R, Kawamura M. Impaired decision-making in Parkinson's disease. *Parkinsonism Relat Disord* 2006;**12**(3):169–75.
111. Perretta JG, Pari G, Beninger RJ. Effects of Parkinson disease on two putative nondeclarative learning tasks: probabilistic classification and gambling. *Cogn Behav Neurol* 2005;**18**(4):185–92.
112. Schott BH, Niehaus L, Wittmann BC, *et al.* Ageing and early-stage Parkinson's disease affect separable neural mechanisms of mesolimbic reward processing. *Brain* 2007;**130**(Pt 9): 2412–24.
113. Frank MJ, Seeberger LC, O'Reilly RC. By carrot or by stick: cognitive reinforcement learning in parkinsonism. *Science* 2004;**306**(5703):1940–3.

114. Swainson R, Rogers RD, Sahakian BJ, *et al.* Probabilistic learning and reversal deficits in patients with Parkinson's disease or frontal or temporal lobe lesions: possible adverse effects of dopaminergic medication. *Neuropsychologia* 2000;**38**(5):596–612.
115. Cools R, Barker RA, Sahakian BJ, Robbins TW. Enhanced or impaired cognitive function in Parkinson's disease as a function of dopaminergic medication and task demands. *Cereb Cortex* 2001;**11**(12):1136–43.
116. Robinson TE, Berridge KC. The psychology and neurobiology of addiction: an incentive-sensitization view. *Addiction* 2000;**95**(Suppl 2):S91–117.
117. Schultz W. Neural coding of basic reward terms of animal learning theory, game theory, microeconomics and behavioural ecology. *Curr Opin Neurobiol* 2004;**14**(2):139–47.
118. Schultz W, Dayan P, Montague PR. A neural substrate of prediction and reward. *Science* 1997;**275**(5306):1593–9.
119. Wyvell CL, Berridge KC. Intra-accumbens amphetamine increases the conditioned incentive salience of sucrose reward: enhancement of reward "wanting" without enhanced "liking" or response reinforcement. *J Neurosci* 2000;**20**(21):8122–30.
120. Robinson TE, Berridge KC. Addiction. *Annu Rev Psychol* 2003;**54**: 25–53.
121. Berke JD, Hyman SE. Addiction, dopamine, and the molecular mechanisms of memory. *Neuron* 2000;**25**(3):515–32.
122. Evans AH, Pavese N, Lawrence AD, *et al.* Compulsive drug use linked to sensitized ventral striatal dopamine transmission. *Ann Neurol* 2006;**59**(5):852–8.
123. Robbins T, Mittleman G, O'Brien C, Winn P. The neuropsychological significance of stereotypy induced by stimulant drugs. In: Cooper S, Dourish C, eds. *Neurobiology of Stereotyped Behaviour*. Oxford: Clarendon Press, 1990: 25–63.
124. Silveira-Moriyama L, Evans AH, Katzenschlager R, Lees AJ. Punding and dyskinesias. *Mov Disord* 2006;**21**(12):2214–7.
125. Graybiel AM, Canales JJ, Capper-Loup C. Levodopa-induced dyskinesias and dopamine-dependent stereotypies: a new hypothesis. *Trends Neurosci* 2000;**23**(10 Suppl):S71–7.
126. Chen JF, Moratalla R, Impagnatiello F, *et al.* The role of the D(2) dopamine receptor (D(2)R) in A(2A) adenosine receptor (A(2A)R)-mediated behavioral and cellular responses as revealed by A(2A) and D(2) receptor knockout mice. *Proc Natl Acad Sci USA* 2001;**98**(4):1970–5.
127. Tack E, De Cuypere G, Jannes C, Remouchamps A. Levodopa addiction. A case study. *Acta Psychiatr Scand* 1988;**78**(3):356–60.
128. Priebe S. Levodopa dependence: a case report. *Pharmacopsychiatry* 1984;**17**(4):109–10.
129. Kimber TE, Thompson PD, Kiley MA. Resolution of dopamine dysregulation syndrome following cessation of dopamine agonist therapy in Parkinson's disease. *J Clin Neurosci* 2008;**15**(2):205–8.
130. Kurlan R. Disabling repetitive behaviors in Parkinson's disease. *Mov Disord* 2004;**19**(4):433–7.
131. Miwa H, Morita S, Nakanishi I, Kondo T. Stereotyped behaviors or punding after quetiapine administration in Parkinson's disease. *Parkinsonism Relat Disord* 2004;**10**(3):177–80.
132. Dodd ML, Klos KJ, Bower JH, *et al.* Pathological gambling caused by drugs used to treat Parkinson disease. *Arch Neurol* 2005;**62**(9):1377–81.
133. O'Sullivan SS, Gallagher DA, Evans AH, *et al.* Dopamine dysregulation syndrome, impulse control disorders and subthalamic nucleus deep brain stimulation: a case series and literature review. *Mov Disord* 2007;**22**(S16, Suppl):S163.
134. Avanzi M, Baratti M, Cabrini S, *et al.* Prevalence of pathological gambling in patients with Parkinson's disease. *Mov Disord* 2006;**21**(12):2068–72.
135. Grosset KA, Macphee G, Pal G, *et al.* Problematic gambling on dopamine agonists: not such a rarity. *Mov Disord* 2006;**21**(12):2206–8.
136. Izenwasser S, French D. Tolerance and sensitization to the locomotor-activating effects of cocaine are mediated via independent mechanisms. *Pharmacol Biochem Behav* 2002;**73**(4): 877–82.
137. Blanchet PJ, Calon F, Martel JC, *et al.* Continuous administration decreases and pulsatile administration increases behavioral sensitivity to a novel dopamine D2 agonist (U-91356A) in MPTP-exposed monkeys. *J Pharmacol Exp Ther* 1995;**272**(2):854–9.
138. Trujillo KA, Kubota KS, Warmoth KP. Continuous administration of opioids produces locomotor sensitization. *Pharmacol Biochem Behav* 2004;**79**(4):661–9.
139. Mamikonyan E, Siderowf AD, Duda JE, *et al.* Long-term follow-up of impulse control disorders in Parkinson's disease. *Mov Disord* 2008;**23**(1):75–80.
140. Koran LM, Bullock KD, Hartston HJ, *et al.* Citalopram treatment of compulsive shopping: an open-label study. *J Clin Psychiatry* 2002;**63**(8):704–8.
141. Courty E, Durif F, Zenut M, Courty P, Lavarenne J. Psychiatric and sexual disorders induced by apomorphine in Parkinson's disease. *Clin Neuropharmacol* 1997;**20**(2):140–7.
142. Weiss RD. Relapse to cocaine abuse after initiating desipramine treatment. *JAMA* 1988;**260**(17):2545–6.
143. Nomikos GG, Damsma G, Wenkstern D, Fibiger HC. Chronic desipramine enhances amphetamine-induced increases in interstitial concentrations of dopamine in the nucleus accumbens. *Eur J Pharmacol* 1991;**195**(1):63–73.
144. Pallesen S, Molde H, Arnestad HM, *et al.* Outcome of pharmacological treatments of pathological gambling: a review and meta-analysis. *J Clin Psychopharmacol* 2007;**27**(4):357–64.
145. Iancu I, Lowengrub K, Dembinsky Y, *et al.* Pathological gambling: an update on neuropathophysiology and pharmacotherapy. *CNS Drugs* 2008;**22**(2):123–38.
146. Zadikoff C, Munhoz RP, Asante AN, *et al.* Movement disorders in patients taking anticonvulsants. *J Neurol Neurosurg Psychiatry* 2007;**78**(2):147–51.
147. Brandt-Christensen M, Kvist K, Nilsson FM, *et al.* Treatment with antidepressants and lithium is associated with increased risk of treatment with antiparkinson drugs: a pharmacoepidemiological study. *J Neurol Neurosurg Psychiatry* 2006;**77**(6):781–3.
148. Sofuoglu M, Kosten TR. Novel approaches to the treatment of cocaine addiction. *CNS Drugs* 2005;**19**(1):13–25.
149. Metman LV, Del Dotto P, LePoole K, *et al.* Amantadine for levodopa-induced dyskinesias: a 1-year follow-up study. *Arch Neurol* 1999;**56**(11):1383–6.
150. Kashihara K, Imamura T. Amantadine may reverse punding in Parkinson's disease – observation in a patient. *Mov Disord* 2008;**23**(1):129–30.

151. Dutra L, Stathopoulou G, Basden SL, *et al.* A meta-analytic review of psychosocial interventions for substance use disorders. *Am J Psychiatry* 2008;**165**(2):179–87.
152. Carroll KM, Onken LS. Behavioral therapies for drug abuse. *Am J Psychiatry* 2005;**162**(8):1452–60.
153. Stanton MD, Shadish WR. Outcome, attrition, and family–couples treatment for drug abuse: a meta-analysis and review of the controlled, comparative studies. *Psychol Bull* 1997;**122**(2):170–91.
154. Young KS. Cognitive behavior therapy with Internet addicts: treatment outcomes and implications. *Cyberpsychol Behav* 2007;**10**(5):671–9.
155. Oei TP, Gordon LM. Psychosocial factors related to gambling abstinence and relapse in members of gamblers anonymous. *J Gambl Stud* 2008;**24**(1):91–105.
156. Dowling N, Smith D, Thomas T. Treatment of female pathological gambling: the efficacy of a cognitive–behavioural approach. *J Gambl Stud* 2006;**22**(4):355–72.
157. Limousin P, Krack P, Pollak P, *et al.* Electrical stimulation of the subthalamic nucleus in advanced Parkinson's disease. *N Engl J Med* 1998;**339**(16):1105–11.
158. Houeto JL, Mesnage V, Mallet L, *et al.* Behavioural disorders, Parkinson's disease and subthalamic stimulation. *J Neurol Neurosurg Psychiatry* 2002;**72**(6):701–7.
159. Schupbach WM, Chastan N, Welter ML, *et al.* Stimulation of the subthalamic nucleus in Parkinson's disease: a 5 year follow up. *J Neurol Neurosurg Psychiatry* 2005;**76**(12):1640–4.
160. Bandini F, Primavera A, Pizzorno M, Cocito L. Using STN DBS and medication reduction as a strategy to treat pathological gambling in Parkinson's disease. *Parkinsonism Relat Disord* 2007;**13**(6):369–71.
161. Ardouin C, Voon V, Worbe Y, *et al.* Pathological gambling in Parkinson's disease improves on chronic subthalamic nucleus stimulation. *Mov Disord* 2006;**21**(11):1941–6.
162. Smeding HM, Speelman JD, Koning-Haanstra M, *et al.* Neuropsychological effects of bilateral STN stimulation in Parkinson disease: a controlled study. *Neurology* 2006;**66**(12):1830–6.
163. Smeding H, Goudriaan A, Foncke E, *et al.* Pathological gambling after bilateral STN stimulation in Parkinson disease. *J Neurol Neurosurg Psychiatry* 2007;**78**(5) 517–9.
164. Morgan JC, diDonato CJ, Iyer SS, *et al.* Self-stimulatory behavior associated with deep brain stimulation in Parkinson's disease. *Mov Disord* 2006;**21**(2):283–5.
165. Lu C, Bharmal A, Suchowersky O. Gambling and Parkinson disease. *Arch Neurol* 2006;**63**(2):298.
166. Voon V, Potenza MN, Thomsen T. Medication-related impulse control and repetitive behaviors in Parkinson's disease. *Curr Opin Neurol* 2007;**20**(4):484–92.

Chapter 20
Neurobiology of Impulse Control Disorders in Parkinson's Disease

Thomas D.L. Steeves[1], *Janis Miyasaki*[1], *Anthony E. Lang*[1,2], *& Antonio P. Strafella*[1,2,3]
[1]Toronto Western Hospital (Movement Disorders Centre) and [2]Toronto Western Research Institute, University Health Network (UHN), University of Toronto, Toronto, ON, Canada
[3]PET Imaging Centre, Centre for Addiction and Mental Health (CAMH), University of Toronto, Toronto, ON, Canada

Introduction

Impulse control disorders (ICDs) are a diverse group of behavioral pathologies characterized by a loss of voluntary control over impulses and drives that result in repetitive, self-destructive behavior. The range of disorders that comprise the ICDs is broad and, as currently defined by the *Diagnostic and Statistical Manual of Mental Disorders*, 4th edition, of the American Psychiatric Association (DSM-IV-TR) [1], includes such diverse conditions as compulsive eating, hypersexuality, trichotillomania, kleptomania, intermittent explosive disorder, and compulsive gambling; however, the extent to which ICDs reflect a common underlying pathophysiology still remains unclear.

A number of ICDs have been reported in the setting of Parkinson's disease (PD) treated with dopaminergic agents. These include hypersexuality [2–5], compulsive shopping [2–5], compulsive eating [6], and pathologic gambling [2,3,5,7]. The phenomenon appears to be primarily a class effect of the dopamine (DA) agonists with an unclear relationship to dosage [2,3,5,7]. Importantly for our understanding of these disorders, the emergence of ICDs with exposure to DA agonists is not restricted to patients with PD, but occurs in all conditions for which agonists are prescribed, including multiple system atrophy (MSA) [8,9] and restless legs syndrome [10–12]. Although these behaviors can have devastating psychosocial consequences, including divorce, imprisonment, and bankruptcy [13], many patients experience them as being internally consistent with their normal repertoire of thoughts and actions and therefore without subjective distress.

ICDs have been variously conceptualized as states of imbalance resulting from excessive drive, impairment of inhibition, or as disorders lying along spectrum extending from purely impulsive to compulsive behavior [14–16]. Other investigators have highlighted the similarities between ICDs and substance addiction, and have proposed that the ICDs should be included in a reward-based group that may best align with behavioral addiction [17–19]. Although the conceptualization of addiction itself continues to be debated, it can be viewed, on current evidence and in the most general terms, as a process that reflects dysfunction of a number of behavioral subsystems controlling the modulation of reward, appetitive urge, craving and salience, behavioral impulsivity, and the formation of habits [20,21]. This imperfect understanding of the neurobiology of addiction has also provided much of the conceptual framework that has guided investigations of ICDs in the general population. The emergence of ICDs in a relatively large number of PD patients exposed to DA agonists provides an opportunity to examine the phenomenology and neurobiology of these disorders and may in turn provide further insights into the pathophysiology of ICDs in the general population. This chapter attempts to summarize some of the current thinking and research relating to the ICDs that emerge in the setting of treatment with DA agonists.

Definitions and classifications

Addictions, obsessions, and compulsions are all characterized by loss of voluntary control over behavior that results in repetitious, self-destructive actions. The DSM-IV-TR likewise defines an ICD as a condition in which there is a failure to resist an impulse, drive, or temptation to perform an act that is harmful to oneself or to others [1]. The specific classification of ICDs, however, is an evolving one that does not necessarily reflect a coherent understanding of their pathophysiology. ICDs

Parkinson's Disease: Non-Motor and Non-Dopaminergic Features, First Edition. Edited by C. Warren Olanow, Fabrizio Stocchi, and Anthony E. Lang.

are currently classified in the DSM-IV-TR under disparate rubrics, such as substance abuse-related disorders, eating disorders, sexual and gender identity disorders, and anxiety disorders. Pathologic gambling and most of the ICDs associated with the dopaminergic agents used to treat PD are for the most part grouped under the heading "ICDs Not Elsewhere Classified (NEC)," which also includes a number of the disorders not typically seen in association with the dopaminergic agents, such as intermittent explosive disorder, kleptomania, pyromania, and trichotillomania. Conversely, the diagnostic criteria for pathologic gambling, one of the more common ICDs seen in association with dopaminergic agents, most closely resemble those for Substance Use Disorders, which is a distinct class in the DSM-IV-TR completely separate from the ICDs. Still other ICDs commonly seen in association with the DA agonists, including compulsive sexual behaviors, compulsive buying and shopping, and problematic Internet use, are classified as "ICDs Not Otherwise Specified," which is a separate subheading within ICDs NEC under consideration for inclusion as distinct disorders in the next iteration of the DSM [22,23].

A further distinction can be made between ICDs and two other pathologic behaviors seen in PD. These are punding, purposeless repetition of behavior first described in the setting of amphetamine abuse [24, 25], and the syndrome of compulsive medication use, also known as dopamine dysregulation syndrome (DDS) [26–28] or hedonistic homeostatic dysregulation syndrome [24,26,28,29]. Although the co-occurrence of ICDs in a small group of patients with DDS has been described and therefore suggests a mechanistic link between excess DA replacement therapy and ICDs, in most PD patients ICDs occur in the absence of DDS. The precise relationship between these two conditions therefore awaits an improved understanding of their neurobiology.

ICDs in PD

The increased reported incidence of ICDs in the PD population over the last decade has paralleled the popularization of the DA agonists for treatment of this condition [30,31]. However, the earliest publications describing what were probably ICDs in PD were rare instances of hypersexuality induced by levodopa monotherapy in PD patients [32]. Quinn *et al.* in 1983 were the first to report an ICD – again hypersexuality – developing in the setting of DA agonist therapy [33]. The association between ICDs and dopaminergic therapy, however, remained largely unrecognized until DA agonists became more widely available in the late 1990s. At this time, a number of case reports and limited case series describing pathologic gambling in association with agonists were published [34–36]; A number of other ICDs were subsequently described in association with agonists, including compulsive shopping [2–5,26], hypersexuality, also referred to as compulsive sexual behavior [4,5,8,30], compulsive computer use [37], and compulsive eating [6].

Epidemiology of ICDs in PD

Early studies evaluating the prevalence of ICDs in PD patients reported similar overall rates of pathologic gambling, hypersexuality, and compulsive shopping despite differing screening techniques and definitions of these disorders. Initial estimates of the prevalence of all ICDs in PD were reported to range from 5.9 to 6.6% of patients, [2,3,5,7,38]. However, the DOMINION study, the most recent and comprehensive evaluation of ICDs in PD, involving 3090 patients from 46 sites in North America, reported a 6 month prevalence of 13.6% [39]. The reported prevalence of ICDs on levodopa alone, 0.7%, versus on DA agonists, 13.7%, provides some measure of the relative contribution of DA agonists to the disorder [7].

The lifetime prevalence of pathologic gambling in PD reported in the early systematic studies from movement disorders clinics ranged from 3 to 8% [2,3,5,38]. The DOMINION study reported a 6 month prevalence of 6.4%. This is in contrast to the estimated 1.6% prevalence of PG in the North American population as a whole [40]. The incidence of compulsive shopping in PD has been reported to lie between 0.4 and 1.5% [3,4], considerably lower than the 5.8% prevalence estimated in the North American population [41]. However, most recently the DOMINION study reported a 6 month prevalence of 7.2%, making this the most common ICD observed in the PD population. The DOMINION study is also the only study to date to examine the prevalence of compulsive eating in treated PD, and reported a 6 month prevalence of 5.6% [39].

The reported prevalence of hypersexuality in PD has ranged from 2.4%, in a study based on a survey completed by patients, to 8.4%, based on a survey using a clinician-administered questionnaire [4]. Positive predictive values of the questionnaires were 48 and 92%, respectively, yet both studies were performed in the same clinic, demonstrating the degree to which incidence rates for sensitive topics may differ based on screening methods. The DOMINION study, which used the clinician-administered Minnesota Impulsive Disorder Interview (MIDI), documented a rate of hypersexuality of 4.4% [39].

Having one ICD appears to lower the threshold for developing another, and this suggests the potential for pathophysiologic similarities between disorders, with symptom expression depending on idiosyncratic, cultural, opportunistic, or individual susceptibilities among patients. However, just what form an ICD takes in treated

PD patients, as in the unmedicated general population, also seems to have much to do with a person's sex. Men are overwhelmingly over-represented among patients with hypersexuality, gambling, or substance abuse, outnumbering women by approximately 2:1; while women are far more prone to eating and shopping disorders.

Conceptualizing the ICDs

The extent to which ICDs constitute a homogeneous group of disorders representing common underlying pathophysiology remains unclear. The current debate over their conceptualization, however, has important implications for both their continued investigation and clinical management. ICDs have been variously conceptualized as states of imbalance resulting from excessive drive, and impairment of inhibition, alterations of reward processing, or a combination of these elements. Some authors have proposed that ICDs may exist within a spectrum of disordered behavior defined by extremes of purely impulsive to compulsive behavior [14–16].

A role for impulse dyscontrol

Impulsivity is a complex and multifaceted trait that features in many psychiatric disorders, including ICDs and addictions [42]. It can be defined in general terms as a predisposition towards rapid, unplanned reactions to internal or external stimuli with diminished regard to the negative consequences of those reactions, either to oneself or to others [43]. When impulsivity is present in moderation it is likely adaptive and leads to the pursuit of novel and beneficial opportunities; only when immediate stimuli are continuously pursued to the exclusion of long-term goals is the behavior deemed pathologic. Impulsivity likely makes multiple and varying contributions to individual ICDs [44]. For example, it may well contribute to ICDs from the very outset by facilitating behavioral experimentation. Once an ICD is established it may equally facilitate it. However, some authors have postulated that impulsivity is such a central feature of ICDs and addictions that it may well be their proximal cause rather than a more peripheral manifestation [14,15].

Most of the various constructs that attempt to describe impulsivity also parse it into a variety of sub-domains, for example, the ability to inhibit motor and pre-potent cognitive responses, to consider future consequences, and to avoid impulsive choice with a tendency to choose lower, immediate rewards over higher, delayed rewards. Studies of decision making and neurocognition in patients with ICDs have consistently identified similar deficits in decision making, with increased delayed discounting as the most characteristic feature [45–47]. Additional impairments of cognitive flexibility, higher order attention, and planning, have been reported in non-PD patients with pathologic gambling [44,48–50] and also in treated PD patients, where features of impulsivity are associated with increased probability of ICDs [51]. Both pathologic gambling and hypersexuality in PD patients are likewise associated with state-dependent impulsivity that is higher in the presence of dopaminergic medications [52].

A number of functional imaging studies have consistently identified neurophysiologic correlates to cognitive deficits observed in patients with ICDs. These commonly localize to portions of ventral medial prefrontal cortex that are felt to contribute to decision making and prediction of reward [53–60]. Decreased brain blood flow to these areas has likewise been reported in subjects with pathologic gambling relative to controls during the presentation of gambling cues [61] and also during simulated gambling [62].

Although features of impulsivity are common to both ICDs and addiction, the distinction between impulsivity and compulsivity can become blurred, and complex relationships seem to link the two [19,63]. Some investigators have proposed that although addictive behaviors may start as impulsive acts, they become progressively more compulsive and habitual over time. Several studies have suggested that the there may in fact be neural correlates to such a transition, as neural processing associated with addictive behaviors seems to migrate from ventral to dorsal striatal circuitry with progressive duration of disease [64–66].

However, key features differentiate impulse control disorders from compulsions as formally defined, and would argue against their classification as forms of obsessive–compulsive behavior. Although individuals with ICDs engage in repetitive behaviors, often provoked by strong urges that could be described as compulsions, the behaviors themselves are usually pleasurable or ego-syntonic; this is in contrast to the repetitive behaviors or rituals of OCD, which are often profoundly ego-dystonic and are generally performed in order to escape from displaced anxiety or from the specific fear of the negative consequence of not performing the acts [23,67,68].

ICDs as behavioral addictions

Multiple lines of evidence point to similarities between impulse control disorders and substance addiction, and a number of investigators have therefore proposed that ICDs should be included in a reward-based group that may best align with behavioral addictions [17–19,69]. Traditionally, scientists have confined the term addiction to describe responses to substances that foster physical dependence in the user, as evidenced by craving, increased tolerance, and withdrawal. The ICDs seen most commonly in association with treated PD – pathologic gambling, hypersexuality, and compulsive shopping, in addition to excessive use of dopaminergic agents themselves – share a number of clinical features with chemical addiction, including a strong urge or craving for the addictive stimulus, hedonic reward during attainment of the stimulus, and repetitive, compulsive, and poorly controlled behavior to obtain it despite adverse consequences and major impairments in life functioning as a result of doing so. Not uncommonly, patients with chemical and behavioral addictions will have made unsuccessful attempts to reduce the frequency with which they pursue the stimulus without success [70]. The development of tolerance and withdrawal, which are more commonly seen in substance abuse disorders, can also occasionally be seen in behavioral addictions [67]. Also, increasingly, both chemical and behavioral addictions are defined in behavioral terms – a trend reflected in the diagnostic criteria for ICDs, which overlap with those for substance dependence and include specific criteria relating to the development of tolerance and withdrawal, repeated unsuccessful attempts to cut back or quit the behaviors, and the negative impacts of the behavior on major areas of life.

The high rate of co-occurrence of ICDs and chemical addiction also suggests that these conditions may share genetic and neurobiologic underpinnings. For example, co-morbid substance abuse has been reported in 23–50% of patients with kleptomania [71,72] and in 30–46% of patients with compulsive shopping [72–74]. In patients with pathologic gambling, nicotine dependence approaches 70% [74], alcohol abuse or dependence 50–75% [75,76], and other drug abuse nears 40% [77].

Studies evaluating the genetics of ICDs in relation to addiction have been largely limited to evaluations of pathologic gambling and substance abuse, but likewise suggest some commonalities between the two disorders. Elevated rates of substance abuse disorders have been reported in first-degree relatives of patients with pathologic gambling. One twin study from the Vietnam Era Twin Registry demonstrated that 12% of genetic risk and 8% of non-shared environmental risk for pathologic gambling overlap with the genetic and environmental risks for alcohol dependence [78], suggesting that shared genetic vulnerability and familial factors may account for a portion of the combined risks for both pathologic gambling and substance abuse.

More specific genetic evaluations of candidate genes relating to ICDs and addictions have also been performed. The dopamine D_{2A1} allele of the D2 receptor has been implicated in an association study of both compulsive and addictive behaviors such as drug abuse, compulsive eating, smoking, and pathologic gambling [79,80]. Elevated rates of homozygosity of the dopamine *Dde I* allele of the D1 receptor has also been demonstrated in patients with pathologic gambling, tobacco smokers, and Tourette's syndrome [81]. An additional association has been reported between pathologic gambling and allelic variants of the *DRD4* gene [82,83].

Recent developments in the neuroscience of motivation and reward have suggested elements of a shared pathophysiology for ICDs and addiction and, importantly, have expanded the spectrum of stimuli that are known to activate common neural pathways regulating reward. In normal subjects, the activity and biochemistry of the brain do not appear to differ qualitatively when processing rewards derived directly from drugs of abuse or indirectly from behavioral stimuli. Monetary and sexual stimuli [84,85] and images of luxury consumer goods associated with wealth and social dominance [86] all illicit the same patterns of striatal activation as drugs of abuse, although the changes observed in response to direct stimulation from drugs are often significantly greater than for behavioral ones [87]. Accordingly, pathologic gamblers demonstrate the same patterns of activation in frontal limbic brain regions as do drug addicts when exposed to images of paraphernalia relating to their respective addictions, and several placebo-controlled studies have demonstrated that pathologic gamblers, like addicts, respond to drugs that block drug "highs" and inhibit craving, again suggesting that drugs of abuse and gambling stimulate the same biochemical pathways [88–90].

Models of behavioral addiction: theory and neurobiology

Much of the current thinking regarding the pathogenesis of ICDs has evolved from a more established body of theory and literature pertaining to the neurobiologic underpinnings of addiction [20,91,92]. The various models of addiction that have developed over the last 30 years have each emphasized different components of what is increasingly viewed as an addiction process. Accordingly, dysregulation of cognitive domains controlling the experience of pleasure and reward, incentive, habit formation, impulsivity, and executive function have each, at one time or another, been postulated as primary drives for addictive behavior.

Pleasure models of addiction

The earliest recorded theories of addiction date to classical antiquity. Aristotle was among the first to propose that the uncontrolled desire for pleasure was the basis for the destructive behaviors associated with addiction. The contemporary expression of this view is found in pleasure or hedonic theories of addiction, which have likewise assumed that the pursuit of pleasure is the primary drive for addictive behavior. Many patients with addictions do indeed report feelings of euphoria and joy when exposed to the stimuli to which they have become addicted, and this is equally true of many PD patients with ICDs.

One of the early variants of pleasure theory posits a "deficiency of reward" in addicted patients that renders them vulnerable to addiction by triggering a drive for rewarding substances or behaviors to stimulate reward circuits to a more normal level of activity [62,93]. In this context, it is interesting that some patients with PD show reduced brain activity in response to rewards [94] and a blunted euphoric response to methylphenidate compared with age-matched non-PD controls [95,96].

However, pleasure in addiction is not a universal finding, and for most conditions there is little evidence that individuals who ultimately develop addiction experience differences in behaviorally induced euphoria compared with individuals who do not [27]. This points to a general problem with pleasure theory: wanting the stimulus, which is the motivation to perform an addictive behavior, can be disassociated from liking the pleasurable effects that may or may not derive from it, and numerous studies have now demonstrated that neural correlates for the difference between wanting and liking also exist.

Hedonic homeostatic dysregulation

A further variation of hedonic models of addiction is based on the idea that addictive behaviors arise not only to generate pleasure, but also to avoid unpleasant withdrawal from pleasure when the stimulus is absent. A number of models fall into this general group. The first of these is the opponent process model [97]. According to this view, an addictive stimulus activates a primary response in brain reward circuits that is both pleasurable and dose dependent; this primary process then activates a secondary, unpleasant response whose purpose is to restore homeostasis. With repeated activation of these circuits, the secondary restorative process becomes strengthened and manifests as tolerance to the pleasurable sensations invoked by the primary process.

A variant of the opponent process model is the hedonic homeostatic dysregulation model proposed by Koob and Le Moal [97–99]. The key difference of this model is that after repeated stimulation the secondary or restorative process posited in the opponent model does not return to baseline between stimulus events, but resets the reward states of the individual to a lower level. This is expressed as dysphoria, irritability, and anxiety during abstinence. From a neurobiologic standpoint, this unpleasant state is felt to reflect reduced dopaminergic and possibly opioidergic function [100].

Incentive sensitization theory: the role of salience and craving

Yet other theories of addiction have placed less emphasis on the pleasurable aspects of addictive stimuli and greater emphasis on their incentive or motivational features. One of the major theories of addiction that has emerged within this framework is the incentive salience theory first proposed by Robinson and Berridge [101,102]. The theory proposes that repeated exposure to a rewarding stimulus produces progressive and persistent neuroadaptation that renders reward circuits hypersensitive to stimuli and thus increases the rewarding effect of a stimulus. This hypersensitivity upregulates a subcomponent of normal appetite called incentive salience, which can be loosely defined as the object's importance or desirability. The upregulation of salience occurs to the point of making it highly attractive and pathologically craved. This wanting of the stimulus is completely separate from the liking of it, which is closer to a sensory pleasure that may be mediated by a separate circuit and neurotransmitter system [103]. The distinction between wanting a stimulus and liking it is in agreement with our own clinical observations of PD patients with pathologic gambling, some of whom report giving in to their cravings to gamble with a sensation not of pleasure but of dread, fully aware of the negative consequences of their actions. Conversely, addictive behavior without conscious awareness of wanting the behavior has also been described [101,102].

Some attempts have been made to evaluate the neural substrates of salience and craving in subjects with ICDs in addition to chemical addiction. Hollander *et al.*, using [^{18}F]fluoro-2-deoxyglucose positron emission tomography (PET) to compare brain activation in patients with pathologic gambling during gambling tasks with and without monetary rewards, reported increased activation in sensory and limbic areas of the brain during rewarding tasks that they interpreted as reflecting the effects of greater salience associated with reward [104]. Crockford *et al.*, using fMRI to compare patients with pathologic gambling with control subjects viewing gambling-related materials, reported in pathologic gamblers heightened activation in dorsolateral prefrontal cortical areas that correlated with cravings induced by viewing the gambling-related material [105]. Likewise, a study evaluating both gambling urges in pathologic gamblers and cocaine cravings in cocaine-dependent subjects, each viewing images of stimuli related to their own addictions, demonstrated diminished activation of the ventral striatum in both patient groups compared with control subjects viewing the same imagery, again suggesting that the same neurobiologic substrate may generate cravings in both chemical dependence and behavioral addictions [17].

Habit theory

Habit theory is a more recent contribution to the theoretical framework of addictions. It emphasizes the role of learning in addiction, completely separate from the acquisition of salience. Habits are automatic actions that result from a learned, context-dependent association between a stimulus and a response. Emerging theories that incorporate the role of habit in addiction postulate a sequential process whereby the use of drugs or the performance of addictive behaviors initially starts as a response that is goal directed and based on the desire for pleasure. Neural processes of reinforcement then confer salience upon them, and reward-based learning then drives their subsequent conversion into overlearned habitual and compulsive behaviors over which the individual loses voluntary control [106,107].

It has been proposed that the anatomic correlate of habit formation may be a shift of neural processing from the ventral striatum, which is thought to regulate explicit learning of behavior [66], to the dorsolateral striatum and putamen, which may preferentially process automatic, stimulus–response behaviors [27]. Some evidence indicates that the development of addiction may localize to the same circuitry. For example, functional imaging studies of primates have demonstrated that repeated cocaine self-administration correlates initially with preferential activation of the ventral striatum that shifts over time to activation of the dorsal striatum with repeated self-administration of the drug [108].

However, a number of criticisms can be applied to habit theory as it pertains to behavioral addictions and ICDs, perhaps the most obvious of these being that there is a clear phenomenologic difference between the automatic, habitual actions which are the basis of study for most animal models of habit formation, and the strongly motivated and complex compulsions of human ICDs.

Functional anatomic substrates of addiction

Over the last two decades, a motivational circuitry associated with substance and behavioral addiction has been delineated in considerable detail [109]. Brain structures important in this process include the nucleus accumbens of the ventral striatum, which plays a central role in forming associations between stimuli and rewards, the amygdala, which assigns emotional significance to stimuli [20,110], and the orbitofrontal cortex which, along with the amygdala and anterior cingulate cortex, may encode expectations and learned associations of outcome [111,112]. Additional structures include the hippocampus, which provides a contextual memory of motivational stimuli, and the hypothalamic and septal nuclei, which provide appetitive drives, particularly for sexual and food stimuli [111,113].

Central to our current understanding of the neural basis of addictions is the dopaminergic mesolimbic pathway which projects from the ventral tegmental area of the midbrain to the nucleus accumbens of the ventral striatum [114]. The structure and connectivity of the nucleus accumbens may reflect a dual role for it in the acquisition and performance of behaviors. The shell of the nucleus accumbens makes reciprocal connections with the dopaminergic ventral tegmental area, which in turn projects to the amygdala, orbital frontal cortex, and the anterior cingulate cortex. Activation of the ventral tegmental area results in phasic release of DA into the nucleus accumbens shell, which appears to facilitate the formation of the initial associations between motivationally salient events and the environmental cues that predict them [115,116]. The core of the nucleus makes reciprocal connections with the orbitofrontal cortex and lateral amygdala and activates primarily during the performance of behaviors already learned in response to reinforcing or rewarding stimuli [20,91].

During the learning of an association between a stimulus and an outcome, the magnitude of phasic DA released in the nucleus accumbens shell varies monotonically with the magnitude of the unexpected reward. Subsequently, when a reward becomes learned or expected, phasic DA release decreases [117,118]. Importantly, however, in situations where the probability of an outcome is least known and there is thus high uncertainty of reward, DA release becomes tonic or continuous. The signal that alterations in DA release encodes, therefore, likely serves to update continuously the importance and value of any stimulus linked to and thus predicting a reward, and in this way the release of DA may be guiding the organism to select actions that maximize reward [119,120].

However, once the initial associations between a reward and the salient events that predict it have formed in the nucleus accumbens shell, a growing body of evidence suggests that the neural circuitry underlying this association then appears to migrate, first to the core of the nucleus accumbens, where conditioned reinforcement drives and imprints the association further [66,121], and then in the final stages of addiction as behavior solidifies into habit, to the dorsal striatum, where it is driven by inputs from the sensorimotor cortex and the septal hypothalamic nuclei [91,122]. The initiation and consolidation of addiction may therefore reflect a sequential shift from limbic, to associative, and finally sensorimotor and corticostriatal circuits. Within this postulated, dynamic anatomic framework, the specific events that generate addiction can be considered.

Potential roles for dopamine in ICDs and addiction

Abnormalities of the DA neurotransmitter system have been implicated in most of the disordered cognitive and behavioral domains that are a feature of both the addictions and the ICDs, including the regulation of reward, appetitive urge and craving, the concept of salience, behavioral impulsivity, and the formation of habits.

DA and reward

Most models of behavioral and chemical addiction that are based on reward theory incorporate the idea that a rewarding stimulus induces adaptive changes to neurotransmission in dopaminergic reward circuitry [123]. In contrast, the reward deficiency syndrome, which is a variant of reward theory, postulates an *a priori* hypodopaminergic state that renders individuals vulnerable to addiction by triggering a drive for rewarding substances or behaviors that normalizes DA release in reward circuits. Some experimental evidence has supported a role for possible hypofunction of the dopaminergic system in various forms of addiction. Low D2 receptor availability as demonstrated with [^{11}C]raclopride PET predicts subsequent increased cocaine self-administration in primates [124,125] and also liking for methylphenidate in non-addicted humans, again suggesting that this feature may mediate vulnerability to addiction [125]. Low striatal D2 receptor availability has likewise been demonstrated in subjects with morbid obesity and compulsive overeating [126].

However, a more extensive body of research has failed to show a direct role for DA in the mediation of the pleasure component of reward, as opposed to the motivation for it. In rodent models, for example, near total DA depletion induced by neurotoxins does not diminish characteristic facial expressions of pleasure to sweet taste even though it abolishes the motivation to eat; and in humans, dopaminergic blockade diminishes the self-reported craving for drugs but not the liking for them [103]. A number of authors have therefore proposed that the release of brain DA may code rather for the appetitive or motivating aspects of behavior, and that other neurotransmitters, such as opioids, may directly mediate the perception of pleasure associated with reward [127].

The role of dopamine in craving

The distinction between wanting a stimulus and liking the sensory pleasure derived from it is integral to the incentive salience sensitization theory of addiction [101,102]. The model proposes that repeated exposure to a rewarding stimulus produces progressive and persistent neuro-adaptation that specifically sensitizes or upregulates a subcomponent of normal appetite called "incentive salience" to the point of making it pathologically craved. Incentive salience can be loosely defined as the object's importance or desirability. This craving for a stimulus is completely separate from the liking of it, which is closer to a sensory pleasure that may be mediated by a separate circuit and neurotransmitter system [103]. Incentive sensitization can be further differentiated from theories that emphasize incentive learning in the formation of addiction [128,129]. The latter propose that the subject's unpleasant experience of and relief from the withdrawal state created by the absence of the stimulus increases its salience when it is subsequently re-encountered.

In the context of both of these forms of acquired incentive, Di Chiara and Bassareo have proposed that drugs that increase extracellular DA may "prime" DA release in reward circuits by bypassing the adaptive mechanisms that normally constrain its release in the nucleus accumbens shell [106]. This facilitates Pavlovian incentive learning, which in turn ingrains the abnormally high DA-releasing properties of the conditioned stimulus. The proposed behavioral correlate to this primed increase in incentive salience of a stimulus is the internal experience of craving for it. Sensitization in the context of addictions, however, does not appear to be an inevitable consequence of repeated exposure to a stimulus but is, rather, highly dependent on individual variability, learning, and contextual factors [101,102].

Dopamine in habit formation

A significant body of evidence has highlighted the role of striatal DA in the development and reinforcement of habits [107,130–132], which is also an area of interest in relation to the formation of behavioral addiction [106,107]. In primates, for example, the administration of cocaine, which induces release of DA and blocks its re-uptake, has been shown to impair the reversal of learned behaviors, and an analogous impairment has been documented in PD patients with the administration of levodopa [133].

However, the contribution of DA to the formation of habits is not in itself sufficient to explain why most patients with PD are free of ICDs. If exposure to dopaminergic agents were to induce ICDs through a universal mechanism of habit formation, "habitual" ICDs should be present in a much higher proportion of PD patients than is currently seen. To explain the variability in the expression of the disorder, one must therefore posit additional underlying pathology that renders individual PD patients susceptible to the habit-forming effects of agonists, for example, deficits from frontal cortical pathology that are seen relatively frequently in PD patients [134] and whose effects can be further exacerbated by the administration of dopaminergic agents [135,136].

Dopamine and impulsivity

Abnormalities of DA neurotransmission have also been implicated in the trait of impulsivity, which is a more general feature of behavioral and chemical addictions as well as ICDs. For example, PET studies of a rat model for impulsivity that also predicts high rates of cocaine self-administration demonstrates decreased D2/D3 receptor binding in the nucleus accumbens independently of DA release [65]. Similarly, PET studies in humans have demonstrated decreased striatal D2 receptor availability in abstinent drug addicts compared with non-drug-abusing control subjects – a finding associated with both reduced metabolism in the orbitofrontal cortex and deficits in impulse control [137].

Whether or not the changes observed in human studies are primary or secondary to chronic drug abuse remains open to question. Di Chiara and Bassareo postulated that chronic drug exposure may induce neuroadaptive changes in subcortical DA release that alters the function of prefrontal–striatal loops to impair impulse control and decision making [106]. Some evidence in support of this view comes form rodent models of addiction, where chronic high doses of methamphetamine have been shown to increase impulsive choice [138]. In this context, the finding that in treated PD patients pathologic gambling and hypersexuality are associated with state-dependent impulsivity that is higher in the presence of dopaminergic medications may be particularly relevant [52].

A role for non-dopaminergic neurotransmitter systems in ICDs

A number of clinical trials evaluating treatments for ICDs have implicated other, non-dopaminergic, neurotransmitter systems in the development of these disorders [139,140]. *N*-Acetylcysteine, an amino acid that is known to reduce synaptic release of glutamate and DA in the nucleus accumbens [141–143], has shown modest efficacy in treating both cocaine addiction [144] and pathologic gambling in non-PD patients [145]. Studies in animal models have likewise implicated both glutamate and its inhibitory metabolite GABA in the modulation of reward-seeking behaviors [146].

The opioid antagonists, naltrexone and nalmefene, have also demonstrated efficacy in treating impulse control disorders [89,147] and substance abuse disorders [148,149] in non-PD patients. The mu opioid system has been postulated to encode the neurochemical signal for reward, and one hypothesis to explain the contribution of the opioidergic system to these disorders is that individuals who are susceptible to ICDs may feel a more intense euphoria when performing rewarding behaviors, and this may in turn generate greater salience and craving for them. The possibility that such differences may have a genetic basis is suggested by the observation that individuals with a genetic predisposition to alcohol use have enhanced beta-endorphin release and euphoria after intake of alcohol [150].

Although a number of biochemical, pharmacologic, and genetic studies in both humans and animal models have suggested possible variation or dysfunction of the 5-HT neurotransmitter system in ICDs, in addition to addictions and impulsivity [151–154], overall, treatment studies with serotonergic agents have yielded only mixed results [147,155–157]. Most studies have demonstrated clinical improvements early in the course of treatment with both drug and placebo, suggesting treatment or placebo response rather than a specific drug effect.

Pathophysiology of ICDs in PD: potential roles for individual susceptibility, Parkinson's disease, and dopamine agonists

A number of studies have demonstrated that PD patients not uncommonly develop more than one ICD in response to treatment with DA agonists [6,9,158], which suggests the potential for a common underlying mechanism contributing to their development. Proposed pathogenic mechanisms for the emergence of ICDs in PD can be broadly separated into three potentially interacting processes: the first is the contribution of pre-morbid susceptibility to compulsive behaviors, completely separate from any effects of neurodegenerative disease or its treatment; the second is the contribution of PD itself to the behaviors, whether as a manifestation of a particular disease phenotype or genotype, or as a compensatory mechanism for the underlying disease process; the third is the potential contribution of dopaminergic agents to the behavior and their potential interaction with either of the above.

Individual susceptibility to disorders of impulse control

A potentially salient observation relating to the origin of impulse control disorders in the setting of dopaminergic medications is that they emerge only in a subset of patients, regardless of the underlying condition for which these drugs are used, whether it be for PD, MSA, or restless legs syndrome [8–10,12]. This suggests the existence at baseline of an underlying susceptibility within the population, completely separate from the co-occurrence of additional disease, although a potential interaction between a susceptibility to ICDs and underlying disease cannot be excluded. According to this view, the emergence of ICDs with exposure to dopaminergic agents could be viewed as a form of pharmacologic challenge, unmasking behavioral vulnerabilities latent in the general population.

Importantly for our understanding of the pathophysiology of ICDs in this group, a number of studies have now demonstrated that a history of the relevant behavior at a subsyndromal level is often associated with escalation of the same behavior to a level meeting diagnostic criteria for an ICD when patients are treated with DA agonists [5,6]. Likewise, a number of other cognitive, behavioral, and genetic features have been shown to differentiate patients with ICDs in the general population. For example, impulsivity and related temperamental constructs such as sensation and novelty seeking have been associated with ICDs in both PD [52,159] and non-PD populations [17,68,160]. Such traits are common in the population of pathologic gamblers with PD, but contrast strikingly with the low rate of novelty seeking seen in older [161–163] but not younger [161] patients with PD.

Genetic factors likely also play a considerable role in ICDs. A strong genetic predisposition has been noted for pathologic gambling [112,164] and additional genetic factors seem to be shared between pathologic gambling and alcohol dependence [165]. Likewise, pathologic gambling co-occurs with a broad range of psychiatric disorders which may also reflect genetic vulnerabilities held in common, including major depression, anxiety, adult antisocial behavior [166], and a number of personality disorders [75,77,167].

Additional associations with age and gender among the ICDs may point to underlying vulnerability for the expression of individual behaviors. For instance, in the general population, specific age groups have an increased likelihood of developing ICDs, with the highest rates typically seen in adolescents and young adults and lower frequencies seen thereafter [168,169]. Gender differences in the expression of ICDs also exist in both PD patients and in the general population. Men are more likely to have intermittent explosive disorder, pathologic gambling, and compulsive sexual behaviors, and women are more likely to exhibit compulsive buying and eating [4,6, 8,168,170]. The phenomenon of telescoping, a rapid progression from initial addiction to problematic pursuit of the stimulus, which is seen principally in women alcoholics, is also seen in women pathologic gamblers [171]. Additional cultural and societal factors seem to be linked to ICDs. For example, high rates of problem gambling have been reported in Asian immigrant populations where gambling is a popular pastime. The mechanism behind this finding may therefore reflect the effects of cultural exposure and opportunity.

Parkinson's disease-related factors

Another potential mechanism to explain the association of ICDs with treated PD is that PD pathology itself or the interaction between it and the dopaminergic medications used to treat its symptoms confers susceptibility to ICDs. The selective and unequal degeneration of DA projection fields typically seen in the disease has been proposed as a potential mechanism for this phenomenon [172–174]. In early PD, the most striking cell loss typically occurs in the ventral lateral tier of the substantia nigra pars compacta that projects to the dorsolateral putamen [175]. Variable and less pronounced loss of neurons occurs in other regions, such as the dorsal tier of the substantia nigra, which projects to the caudate, the retrorubral region, which projects to the hypothalamus, and in the ventral tegmental area, which projects to the nucleus accumbens, amygdala, hippocampus, motor, premotor, cingulate and pre-frontal cortices [172,175]. It is possible that patient-to-patient variability in these patterns of neurogeneration and the interaction between this an a medication effect could contribute to the variable expression of ICDs.

One example of how patient to patient variability could mediate susceptibility to ICDs can be seen in the interaction between young age of disease onset and the emergence of dyskinesias in treated PD patients [176,177]. This motor feature has been postulated to reflect either underlying neurobiologic differences in individual patients or predisposing genetic variants of the disease. Pathologic gambling, hypersexuality, and compulsive medication use are all likewise seen at a higher frequency in PD patients who have had a younger age of disease onset [5,52,159]. However, the higher novelty-seeking traits of younger patients combined with the relatively greater use of DA agonists at higher dosages in this population may equally provide an alternative explanation for the increased rate of ICDs observed in this group.

However, dopaminergic denervation does not appear to be a necessary condition for the emergence of ICDs upon exposure to DA agonists. The state of our current knowledge indicates that ICDs can occur in any individual treated with DA agonists for both non-neurodegenerative and non-parkinsonian disorders such as restless legs syndrome, and for other parkinsonian conditions such as MSA, for which the known neurodegenerative changes are very different from those of PD. These findings constitute relatively strong evidence against the ICDs emerging as a disease-specific effect.

Some investigators have proposed that the cognitive deficits typically seen in PD could likewise facilitate the development of ICDs. Indeed, a variety of studies have demonstrated distinct similarities between the deficits in planning and cognitive flexibility seen in unmedicated PD patients [178,179] and those of pathologic gambling subjects free of PD [44]. However, given the frequency with which deficits in executive function are observed in PD patients, one should expect to see a much higher frequency of ICDs within the population of PD patients as a whole, if impaired cognition did contribute significantly to the emergence of ICDs. Moreover, if disease-specific cognitive deficits did contribute to the emergence of ICDs, the personality profile of PD patients should if anything protect against ICDs. Pre-morbid patients with PD have lower rates of risk-taking behaviors such as smoking, caffeine, and alcohol use that are presumed to reflect the lower novelty-seeking traits of this population [180] that may itself be due to incipient ventral striatal pathology [181].

Potential roles of dopaminergic medications in the development of ICDs

A final proposed mechanism for the emergence of ICDs in treated PD is the potential contribution of dopaminergic agents themselves to the behavior. This includes the potential for their interaction with either pre-morbid susceptibility to impulse control disorders or the underlying disease process. The incidence of ICDs with DA agonists appears to be largely a class effect with an unclear relationship to dosage [2–5,7]. Onset or exacerbation of ICDs correlates with either initiation of treatment or dosage increases of DA agonists, and remission or reduction of the behavior correlate with reductions of agonist dosage 36,158,182,183]. Only a few studies have reported individual cases of ICDs emerging with levodopa monotherapy at high dose [34], treatment with monoamine oxidase (MAO) inhibitors [184], or deep brain stimulation (DBS) [185].

The mechanism whereby DA replacement therapy may induce ICDs is an active area of investigation. DA therapy is associated with a variety of psychomotor complications, including restlessness and insomnia, aggression, hypomania, hypersexuality, impulsivity, and vivid dreams [186,187]. These are complications similar to those seen after excessive use of psychomotor stimulants such as amphetamines and cocaine [188]. Dopaminergic medications could potentially stimulate compulsive behaviors at multiple levels, and several hypotheses have been advanced to explain the phenomenon, usually working within one or more theoretical frameworks for behavioral addiction. Proposed mechanisms have included differential DA receptor stimulation preferentially affecting limbic circuits regulating reward, the effects of continuous DA receptor stimulation conferring excessive salience to stimuli or impairing the withdrawal of salience, and a more specific priming effect of dopaminergic agents inducing excess release of DA in ventral striatal circuits to generate likewise increased salience and thus craving for the relevant stimulus.

Preferential stimulation of the DA D3 receptor subtype

One of the early hypotheses advanced to explain the development of ICDs in the setting of dopaminergic therapy proposed preferential stimulation of the DA D3 receptor subtype which is found predominantly in limbic regions of the brain. Much of the initial impetus for the hypothesis came from a few studies which suggested a specific association of ICDs with pramipexol, which has relatively higher specificity for D3 DA receptors than D2 receptors, which have a preferential striatal localization [62]. Additional evidence for the hypothesis was drawn from studies in animal models such as the 6-hydroxydopamine-lesioned rat, where repeated administration of levodopa triggers overexpression of DA D3 receptors in the nucleus accumbens [189], which is the same adaptation observed after repeated amphetamine administration in a non-lesioned rodent model of compulsive amphetamine use [189,190].

However, subsequent evaluations controlling for differences in the prescribing practices of agonists, which significantly favor pramipexol, and also the dosing of the drug in relation to other DA agonists, revealed only a broad association between ICDs and a variety of DA agonists, regardless of receptor affinities [2,3,5,7,52].

DA receptor stimulation altering the assignment of salience

Another mechanism whereby dopaminergic agents could induce ICDs is based on their potential to amplify the assignment of salience or interfere with its eventual withdrawal. DA release in the ventral striatum likely serves to update the value associated with any stimulus that predicts a reward in order to guide actions that maximize it [119,120]. During the learning of a task, the magnitude of DA release increases with the magnitude of an unexpected reward and suppresses when the expected reward is not received. In this context, excessive and continuous stimulation of DA receptors, in particular by long-acting DA agonists, could assign inappropriate salience in the setting of reward or counter an appropriate withdrawal of salience by preventing a natural suppression of dopaminergic stimulation after an unexpected absence of reward. Consistent with this view, a recent functional MRI study of healthy volunteers has demonstrated that administration of levodopa increases the expected value of stimuli, whereas D2 blockade with haloperidol decreases it [191].

Priming effects of dopaminergic agents associated with craving

An extensive literature describes the ability of DA and dopaminergic agents to prime and thus increase subsequent DA release in the nucleus accumbens in response to repeated stimuli. The phenomenon appears to be associated with increased salience and craving for the relevant stimuli [102,190]. Importantly, both drugs of abuse [20] and behaviors such as gambling [192] have been shown to prime DA release. Evans *et al.* have likewise demonstrated in an [^{11}C]raclopride PET evaluation that PD patients with DA dysregulation who crave medication in excess release elevated levels of DA in ventral striatal circuits compared with PD controls in response to a single dose of levodopa [159]. Importantly, for the incentive salience model, this hypersensitivity correlates with the self reported compulsive "wanting" of the drug but not the liking for it.

A related phenomenon is the ability of drugs with similar mechanisms of action to cross-prime for the release of DA induced by other drugs within the same class [193]. Importantly, the ability of drugs to cross-prime and upregulate the incentive salience of a variety of unrelated stimuli that are temporally correlated to them is also well documented. For example, studies in rodent models of addiction indicate that repeated exposure to psychostimulants such as amphetamine also increases the salience for other rewards such as food and sex that are presented at the same time [101,102,194,195]. Interestingly, the development of increased appetite for a given stimulus in a given animal seems highly dependent on environment and other individual factors, such as the animal's temperament. Animals that develop the strongest stimulant-induced sensitization for one reward therefore do not necessarily develop an appetite for other rewards in the same experimental paradigm and vice versa [195]. Zack and Poulos have likewise demonstrated that amphetamine increases the motivation for gambling in problem gamblers in a manner that is predicted by the severity of their gambling [196].

The parallels between this phenomenon and the development of behavioral addictions in patients treated with dopaminergic agents are self-evident. Rewarding stimuli such as money and images of luxury consumer goods associated with wealth and social dominance have been shown to activate accumbens circuitry and induce DA release [84]. A prominent feature of the ICDs that relate to these stimuli – compulsive gambling, shopping, and hypersexuality – is an intense craving for the behaviors consistent with increased incentive salience. In this context, one can postulate that the post-synaptic stimulation provided by DA agonists may mimic the sensitizing effects of amphetamine in ventral striatal circuits to prime DA release associated with these stimuli and so increase their incentive salience. For any individual, the specific stimuli that generate increased appetitive urge may depend very much on contextual cues and individual preferences for rewarding stimuli.

Implications for management

Reducing or discontinuing DA agonist therapy typically provides the most immediate and reliable relief from ICDs [6,8,197,198]. In most instances, resolution of ICDs can be achieved without compromise of motor function simply by supplementing with additional levodopa to maintain the total intake of levodopa daily equivalents [198]. Rarely in individual cases reducing the L-dopa dosage may be necessary to bring ICDs under control [33,170,197]. In some instances, despite supplementation with additional L-dopa during withdrawal of agonists, patients may experience a worsening of motor function. This may relate to the longer duration of action of the DA agonists, inadequate frequency of L-dopa dosing, or inadequate absorption of L-dopa, particularly if the drug is administered at mealtimes or in the sustained release formulation. In many patients, DA agonists also seem to provide an artificial but pleasurable feeling of wellbeing that is difficult to replicate with L-dopa alone. Switching from one DA agonist to another may occasionally improve symptoms of ICD, but this experience is relatively uncommon, and no agonist is known to carry a lower risk of inducing ICDs [6,197,199].

Non-pharmacologic measures targeted towards specific compulsive behaviors, such as restricting money and credit cards for patients with a compulsive shopping condition or, for those with a compulsive gambling problem, discontinuing Internet access and placing patients' names on regional lists of individuals banned from casinos. may be helpful, but such measures are rarely sufficient in isolation.

In patients for whom reduction of DA agonists has proved problematic, DBS surgery may be considered [200]. DBS surgery of the subthalamic nucleus (STN) in particular allows significant reductions in dopaminergic medications, on the order of 50% in most patients, whereas DBS surgery of the globus pallidus internus (GPI) typically has minimal effects on the need for medication [201–203]. However, specific regions within the STN regulating motivational, emotional, and cognitive circuits may also be affected by current spread, despite attempts to target motor symptoms [200], and STN DBS has rarely been reported to induce mania [204], impulse dyscontrol, and even impulsive suicide, despite excellent postoperative improvements in motor function [205, 206]. As for all surgical candidates, careful evaluation of the patient's cognitive status, psychiatric function, and social support is therefore mandatory prior to considering treatment.

Beyond reducing dopaminergic medications, little is known about optimal management of ICDs. Success with a number of alternative treatment strategies has been reported in PD patients with ICDs; however, these approaches have almost always been confounded by concomitant reductions in dopaminergic medications. An added complication is that in the non-PD population, high placebo response rates have been documented for treatment of conditions such as pathologic gambling [156] and compulsive shopping [207]. Several of the of the atypical neuroleptics, including quetiapine [8,208] and clozaril [209], which in modest doses typically do not worsen PD motor symptoms significantly, have been used successfully in open-label trials in PD patients to treat agonist-associated pathologic gambling and hypersexuality; however, in non-PD pathologic gamblers, controlled trials of DA receptor blockers have been shown to be ineffective [210,211]. Controlled trials of selective serotonin reuptake inhibitors (SSRIs) for pathologic gambling and compulsive buying in non-PD patients have likewise yielded mixed results [156,212]. Sodium valproate and lithium have been used successfully to treat ICDs in PD patients with and without associated mania [8]. Topiramate has been shown in a recent small, open-label study to be effective in PD patients with a variety of ICDs, including pathologic gambling, hypersexuality, compulsive buying, and compulsive eating [213].

The opioid antagonists naltrexone [90] and nalfedime [89] have been shown in controlled trials in non-PD patients to be effective for pathologic gambling and in open-label trials to be effective for the treatment of hypersexuality, compulsive shopping, and binge eating [214,215]. Somewhat surprisingly, the efficacy of these agents has not yet been reported in PD patients with ICDs on DA agonists.

Conclusion

The ICDs that emerge with exposure to dopaminergic treatment in PD are a fascinating group of behaviors that highlight the interactions between psychiatric and neurologic disorders and the somewhat arbitrary division between the two. Although the extent to which ICDs constitute a homogeneous group of disorders representing common underlying pathophysiology remains unclear, the continued debate over their conceptualization has important implications for both their continued investigation and clinical management.

Much of the current thinking regarding the pathogenesis of ICDs has evolved from a more established body of theory and literature pertaining to the neurobiologic underpinnings of addiction [20,91,92]. The various models of addiction that have developed over the last 30 years have each emphasized different components of what is increasingly viewed as an addiction process. Accordingly, dysregulation of cognitive domains controlling the experience of pleasure and reward, incentive, habit formation, impulsivity, and executive function have each, at one time or another, been postulated as primary drives for addictive behavior and have more recently been implicated as abnormalities central to the development of ICDs.

Abnormalities of the DA neurotransmitter system have been implicated in most of the behavioral features that are characteristic of addictions and ICDs as they are expressed in the general population, and the incidence of ICDs in PD patients appears to be largely a class effect of treatment with DA agonists. A potentially salient observation relating to the origin of impulse control disorders in the setting of dopaminergic treatment is that they emerge only in a subset of patients, regardless of the underlying condition for which these drugs are used, whether it be for PD, MSA, or restless legs syndrome. This suggests the existence at baseline of an underlying susceptibility within the population, completely separate from the co-occurrence of additional disease, although a potential interaction between a susceptibility to ICDs and underlying disease cannot be excluded. According to this view, the emergence of ICDs with exposure to dopaminergic agents could be viewed as a form of pharmacologic challenge, unmasking behavioral vulnerabilities latent in the general population. Dopaminergic medications could potentially stimulate compulsive behaviors at multiple levels, and several hypotheses have been advanced to explain the phenomenon, usually working within one or more theoretical frameworks for behavioral addiction. Proposed mechanisms include differential DA receptor stimulation preferentially affecting limbic circuits regulating reward, the effects of continuous DA receptor stimulation conferring excessive salience to stimuli or impairing its withdrawal, and a more specific priming effect of dopaminergic agents inducing excess release of DA in ventral–striatal circuits that likewise generates increased salience and thus craving for the relevant stimulus.

The study of the ICDs that are seen in PD patients on exposure to DA agonists provides a valuable clinical paradigm with which to evaluate the phenomenon of ICDs in general. It is hoped that ongoing studies in this area will provide useful insights into the neurobiologic basis of compulsions and addictions and suggest new avenues for the treatment of this challenging group of disorders.

References

1. American Psychiatric Association. *Diagnostic and Statistical Manual of Mental Disorders*, 4th edn. Washington, DC: American Psychiatric Association, 2000.
2. Grosset KA, Macphee G, Pal G, *et al*. Problematic gambling on dopamine agonists: not such a rarity. *Mov Disord* 2006;**21**(12): 2206–8.
3. Lu C, Bharmal A, Suchowersky O. Gambling and Parkinson disease. *Arch Neurol* 2006;**63**(2):298.
4. Voon V, Hassan K, Zurowski M, *et al*. Prevalence of repetitive and reward-seeking behaviors in Parkinson disease. *Neurology* 2006;**67**(7):1254–7.
5. Weintraub D, Siderowf AD, Potenza MN, *et al*. Association of dopamine agonist use with impulse control disorders in Parkinson disease. *Arch Neurol* 2006;**63**(7):969–73.
6. Nirenberg MJ, Waters C. Compulsive eating and weight gain related to dopamine agonist use. *Mov Disord* 2006;**21**(4): 524–9.

7. Voon V, Hassan K, Zurowski M, *et al.* Prospective prevalence of pathologic gambling and medication association in Parkinson disease. *Neurology* 2006;**66**(11):1750–2.
8. Klos KJ, Bower JH, Josephs KA, *et al.* Pathological hypersexuality predominantly linked to adjuvant dopamine agonist therapy in Parkinson's disease and multiple system atrophy. *Parkinsonism Relat Disord* 2005;**11**(6):381–6.
9. McKeon A, Josephs KA, Klos KJ, *et al.* Unusual compulsive behaviors primarily related to dopamine agonist therapy in Parkinson's disease and multiple system atrophy. *Parkinsonism Relat Disord* 2007;**13**(8):516–9.
10. Tippmann-Peikert M, Park JG, Boeve BF, *et al.* Pathologic gambling in patients with restless legs syndrome treated with dopaminergic agonists. *Neurology* 2007;**68**(4):301–3.
11. Quickfall J, Suchowersky O. Pathological gambling associated with dopamine agonist use in restless legs syndrome. *Parkinsonism Relat Disord* 2007;**13**(8):535–6.
12. Evans AH, Butzkueven H. Dopamine agonist-induced pathological gambling in restless legs syndrome due to multiple sclerosis. *Mov Disord* 2007;**22**(4):590–1.
13. Merims D, Giladi N. Dopamine dysregulation syndrome, addiction and behavioral changes in Parkinson's disease. *Parkinsonism Relat Disord* 2008;**14**(4):273–80.
14. Hollander E, Wong CM. Body dysmorphic disorder, pathological gambling, and sexual compulsions. *J Clin Psychiatry* 1995;**56**(Suppl 4):7–12; discussion 3.
15. Hollander E, Wong CM. Obsessive–compulsive spectrum disorders. *J Clin Psychiatry* 1995;**56**(Suppl 4):3–6; discussion 53–5.
16. McElroy SL, Hudson JI, Pope H Jr,et al. The DSM-III-R impulse control disorders not elsewhere classified: clinical characteristics and relationship to other psychiatric disorders. *Am J Psychiatry* 1992;**149**(3):318–27.
17. Potenza MN. Should addictive disorders include non-substance-related conditions? *Addiction* 2006;**101**(Suppl 1):142–51.
18. Holden C. " Behavioral" addictions: do they exist? *Science* 2001;**294**(5544):980–2.
19. Grant JE, Brewer JA, Potenza MN. The neurobiology of substance and behavioral addictions. *CNS Spectr* 2006;**11**(12):924–30.
20. Kalivas PW, Volkow ND. The neural basis of addiction: a pathology of motivation and choice. *Am J Psychiatry* 2005;**162**(8):1403–13.
21. Bergh C, Eklund T, Sodersten P, Nordin C. Altered dopamine function in pathological gambling. *Psychol Med* 1997;**27**(2):473–5.
22. Grant JE, Potenza MN. Impulse control disorders: clinical characteristics and pharmacological management. *Ann Clin Psychiatry* 2004;**16**(1):27–34.
23. Grant JE, Potenza MN. Compulsive aspects of impulse-control disorders. *Psychiatr Clin North Am* 2006;**29**(2):539–51, x.
24. Evans AH, Katzenschlager R, Paviour D, *et al.* Punding in Parkinson's disease: its relation to the dopamine dysregulation syndrome. *Mov Disord* 2004;**19**(4):397–405.
25. Miyasaki JM, Al Hassan K, Lang AE, Voon V. Punding prevalence in Parkinson's disease. *Mov Disord* 2007;**22**(8): 1179–81.
26. Giovannoni G, O'Sullivan JD, Turner K, *et al.* Hedonistic homeostatic dysregulation in patients with Parkinson's disease on dopamine replacement therapies. *J Neurol Neurosurg Psychiatry* 2000;**68**(4):423–8.
27. Lawrence AD, Evans AH, Lees AJ. Compulsive use of dopamine replacement therapy in Parkinson's disease: reward systems gone awry? *Lancet Neurol* 2003;**2**(10):595–604.
28. Pezzella FR, Colosimo C, Vanacore N, *et al.* Prevalence and clinical features of hedonistic homeostatic dysregulation in Parkinson's disease. *Mov Disord* 2005;**20**(1):77–81.
29. Borek LL, Friedman JH. Levodopa addiction in idiopathic Parkinson disease. *Neurology* 2005;**65**(9):1508.
30. Weintraub D, Potenza MN. Impulse control disorders in Parkinson's disease. *Curr Neurol Neurosci Rep* 2006;**6**(4):302–6.
31. Voon V, Fox SH. Medication-related impulse control and repetitive behaviors in Parkinson disease. *Arch Neurol* 2007;**64**(8):1089–96.
32. Barbeau A. L-Dopa therapy in Parkinson's disease: a critical review of nine years' experience. *Can Med Assoc J* 1969;**101**(13):59–68.
33. Quinn NP, Toone B, Lang AE, *et al.* Dopa dose-dependent sexual deviation. *Br J Psychiatry* 1983;**142**:296–8.
34. Molina JA, Sainz-Artiga MJ, Fraile A, *et al.* Pathologic gambling in Parkinson's disease: a behavioral manifestation of pharmacologic treatment? *Mov Disord* 2000;**15**(5):869–72.
35. Gschwandtner U, Aston J, Renaud S, Fuhr P. Pathologic gambling in patients with Parkinson's disease. *Clin Neuropharmacol* 2001;**24**(3):170–2.
36. Seedat S, Kesler S, Niehaus DJ, Stein DJ. Pathological gambling behaviour: emergence secondary to treatment of Parkinson's disease with dopaminergic agents. *Depress Anxiety* 2000;**11**(4):185–6.
37. Fasano A, Elia AE, Soleti F, *et al.* Punding and computer addiction in Parkinson's disease. *Mov Disord* 2006;**21**(8): 1217–8.
38. Avanzi M, Baratti M, Cabrini S, *et al.* Prevalence of pathological gambling in patients with Parkinson's disease. *Mov Disord* 2006;**21**(12):2068–72.
39. Weintraub D, Koester J, Potenza MN, *et al.* Dopaminergic therapy and impulse control disorders in Parkinson's disease: top line results of a cross-sectional study of over 3,000 patients. Presented at the 12th International Congress of Parkinson's Disease and Movement Disorders, Chicago, 22–26 June 2008.
40. Shaffer HJ, Hall MN, Vander Bilt J. Estimating the prevalence of disordered gambling behavior in the United States and Canada: a research synthesis. *Am J Public Health* 1999;**89**(9):1369–76.
41. Koran LM, Faber RJ, Aboujaoude E, *et al.* Estimated prevalence of compulsive buying behavior in the United States. *Am J Psychiatry* 2006;**163**(10):1806–12.
42. Evenden JL. Varieties of impulsivity. *Psychopharmacology (Berl)* 1999;**146**(4):348–61.
43. Moeller FG, Barratt ES, Dougherty DM, *et al.* Psychiatric aspects of impulsivity. *Am J Psychiatry* 2001;**158**(11): 1783–93.
44. Goudriaan AE, Oosterlaan J, de Beurs E, van den Brink W. Neurocognitive functions in pathological gambling: a comparison with alcohol dependence, Tourette syndrome and normal controls. *Addiction* 2006;**101**(4):534–47.
45. Bechara A, Damasio H. Decision-making and addiction (Part I): impaired activation of somatic states in substance

dependent individuals when pondering decisions with negative future consequences. *Neuropsychologia* 2002;**40**(10):1675–89.

46. Petry NM. Pathological gamblers, with and without substance use disorders, discount delayed rewards at high rates. *J Abnorm Psychol* 2001;**110**(3):482–7.
47. Cavedini P, Riboldi G, Keller R, *et al.* Frontal lobe dysfunction in pathological gambling patients. *Biol Psychiatry* 2002;**51**(4):334–41.
48. Kertzman S, Lowengrub K, Aizer A, *et al.* Stroop performance in pathological gamblers. *Psychiatry Res* 2006;**142**(1):1–10.
49. Rugle L, Melamed L. Neuropsychological assessment of attention problems in pathological gamblers. *J Nerv Ment Dis* 1993;**181**(2):107–12.
50. Specker SM, Carlson GA, Christenson GA, Marcotte M. Impulse control disorders and attention deficit disorder in pathological gamblers. *Ann Clin Psychiatry* 1995;**7**(4):175–9.
51. Isaias IU, Siri C, Cilia R, *et al.* The relationship between impulsivity and impulse control disorders in Parkinson's disease. *Mov Disord* 2008;**23**(3):411–5.
52. Voon V, Thomsen T, Miyasaki JM, *et al.* Factors associated with dopaminergic drug-related pathological gambling in Parkinson disease. *Arch Neurol* 2007;**64**(2):212–6.
53. Adinoff B, Devous MD Sr, Cooper DB, *et al.* Resting regional cerebral blood flow and gambling task performance in cocaine-dependent subjects and healthy comparison subjects. *Am J Psychiatry* 2003;**160**(10):1892–4.
54. Bechara A. Risky business: emotion, decision-making, and addiction. *J Gambl Stud* 2003;**19**(1):23–51.
55. Gottfried JA, O'Doherty J, Dolan RJ. Encoding predictive reward value in human amygdala and orbitofrontal cortex. *Science* 2003;**301**(5636):1104–7.
56. Grant S, Contoreggi C, London ED. Drug abusers show impaired performance in a laboratory test of decision making. *Neuropsychologia* 2000;**38**(8):1180–7.
57. London ED, Ernst M, Grant S, *et al.* Orbitofrontal cortex and human drug abuse: functional imaging. *Cereb Cortex* 2000;**10**(3):334–42.
58. Potenza MN, Leung HC, Blumberg HP, *et al.* An FMRI Stroop task study of ventromedial prefrontal cortical function in pathological gamblers. *Am J Psychiatry* 2003;**160**(11): 1990–4.
59. Tanaka SC, Doya K, Okada G, *et al.* Prediction of immediate and future rewards differentially recruits cortico-basal ganglia loops. *Nat Neurosci* 2004;**7**(8):887–93.
60. Tucker KA, Potenza MN, Beauvais JE, *et al.* Perfusion abnormalities and decision making in cocaine dependence. *Biol Psychiatry* 2004;**56**(7):527–30.
61. Potenza MN, Steinberg MA, Skudlarski P, *et al.* Gambling urges in pathological gambling: a functional magnetic resonance imaging study. *Arch Gen Psychiatry* 2003;**60**(8):828–36.
62. Reuter J, Raedler T, Rose M, *et al.* Pathological gambling is linked to reduced activation of the mesolimbic reward system. *Nat Neurosci* 2005;**8**(2):147–8.
63. Potenza MN. Impulsivity and compulsivity in pathological gambling and obsessive-compulsive disorder. *Rev Bras Psiquiatr* 2007;**29**(2):105–6.
64. Brewer JA, Potenza MN. The neurobiology and genetics of impulse control disorders: relationships to drug addictions. *Biochem Pharmacol* 2008;**75**(1):63–75.
65. Dalley JW, Fryer TD, Brichard L, *et al.* Nucleus accumbens D2/3 receptors predict trait impulsivity and cocaine reinforcement. *Science* 2007;**315**(5816):1267–70.
66. Yin HH, Knowlton BJ. The role of the basal ganglia in habit formation. *Nat Rev Neurosci* 2006;**7**(6):464–76.
67. Blanco C, Moreyra P, Nunes EV, *et al.* Pathological gambling: addiction or compulsion? *Semin Clin Neuropsychiatry* 2001;**6**(3):167–76.
68. Blaszczynski A, Steel Z, McConaghy N. Impulsivity in pathological gambling: the antisocial impulsivist. *Addiction* 1997;**92**(1):75–87.
69. Shaffer HJ. Strange bedfellows: a critical view of pathological gambling and addiction. *Addiction* 1999;**94**(10):1445–8.
70. Grant JE, Levine L, Kim D, Potenza MN. Impulse control disorders in adult psychiatric inpatients. *Am J Psychiatry* 2005;**162**(11):2184–8.
71. Grant JE, Kim SW. Clinical characteristics and associated psychopathology of 22 patients with kleptomania. *Compr Psychiatry* 2002;**43**(5):378–84.
72. McElroy SL, Pope HG Jr, Hudson JI, *et al.* Kleptomania: a report of 20 cases. *Am J Psychiatry* 1991;**148**(5):652–7.
73. Christenson GA, Faber RJ, de Zwaan M, *et al.* Compulsive buying: descriptive characteristics and psychiatric comorbidity. *J Clin Psychiatry* 1994;**55**(1):5–11.
74. Crockford DN, el-Guebaly N. Psychiatric comorbidity in pathological gambling: a critical review. *Can J Psychiatry* 1998;**43**(1):43–50.
75. Petry NM, Stinson FS, Grant BF. Comorbidity of DSM-IV pathological gambling and other psychiatric disorders: results from the National Epidemiologic Survey on Alcohol and Related Conditions. *J Clin Psychiatry* 2005;**66**(5):564–74.
76. McCormick RA, Russo AM, Ramirez LF, Taber JI. Affective disorders among pathological gamblers seeking treatment. *Am J Psychiatry* 1984;**141**(2):215–8.
77. Cunningham-Williams RM, Cottler LB, Compton WM III, Spitznagel EL. Taking chances: problem gamblers and mental health disorders – results from the St. Louis Epidemiologic Catchment Area Study. *Am J Public Health* 1998;**88**(7): 1093–6.
78. Shah KR, Eisen SA, Xian H, Potenza MN. Genetic studies of pathological gambling: a review of methodology and analyses of data from the Vietnam Era Twin Registry. *J Gambl Stud* 2005;**21**(2):179–203.
79. Blum K, Braverman ER, Wood RC, *et al.* Increased prevalence of the Taq I A1 allele of the dopamine receptor gene (DRD2) in obesity with comorbid substance use disorder: a preliminary report. *Pharmacogenetics* 1996;**6**(4):297–305.
80. Comings DE, Muhleman D, Ahn C, *et al.* The dopamine D2 receptor gene: a genetic risk factor in substance abuse. *Drug Alcohol Depend* 1994;**34**(3):175–80.
81. Comings DE, Gade R, Wu S, *et al.* Studies of the potential role of the dopamine D1 receptor gene in addictive behaviors. *Mol Psychiatry* 1997;**2**(1):44–56.
82. Comings DE, Gonzalez N, Wu S, *et al.* Studies of the 48 bp repeat polymorphism of the DRD4 gene in impulsive, compulsive, addictive behaviors: Tourette syndrome, ADHD, pathological gambling, and substance abuse. *Am J Med Genet* 1999;**88**(4):358–68.
83. Perez de Castro I, Ibanez A, Torres P, *et al.* Genetic association study between pathological gambling and a functional

DNA polymorphism at the D4 receptor gene. *Pharmacogenetics* 1997;**7**(5):345–8.

84. Koepp MJ, Gunn RN, Lawrence AD, *et al.* Evidence for striatal dopamine release during a video game. *Nature* 1998;**393**(6682):266–8.
85. Knutson B, Adams CM, Fong GW, Hommer D. Anticipation of increasing monetary reward selectively recruits nucleus accumbens. *J Neurosci* 2001;**21**(16):RC159.
86. Erk S, Spitzer M, Wunderlich AP, *et al.* Cultural objects modulate reward circuitry. *Neuroreport* 2002;**13**(18):2499–503.
87. Childress AR, Ehrman RN, Wang Z, *et al.* Prelude to passion: limbic activation by "unseen" drug and sexual cues. *PLoS ONE* 2008;**3**(1):e1506.
88. Grant JE, Kim SW, Hartman BK. A double-blind, placebo-controlled study of the opiate antagonist naltrexone in the treatment of pathological gambling urges. *J Clin Psychiatry* 2008;**1**:e1–7.
89. Grant JE, Potenza MN, Hollander E, *et al.* Multicenter investigation of the opioid antagonist nalmefene in the treatment of pathological gambling. *Am J Psychiatry* 2006;**163**(2): 303–12.
90. Kim SW, Grant JE, Adson DE, Shin YC. Double-blind naltrexone and placebo comparison study in the treatment of pathological gambling. *Biol Psychiatry* 2001;**49**(11):914–21.
91. Everitt BJ, Robbins TW. Neural systems of reinforcement for drug addiction: from actions to habits to compulsion. *Nat Neurosci* 2005;**8**(11):1481–9.
92. Volkow ND, Fowler JS, Wang GJ. The addicted human brain viewed in the light of imaging studies: brain circuits and treatment strategies. *Neuropharmacology* 2004;**47**(Suppl 1):3–13.
93. Blum K, Sheridan PJ, Wood RC, *et al.* The D2 dopamine receptor gene as a determinant of reward deficiency syndrome. *J R Soc Med* 1996;**89**(7):396–400.
94. Kunig G, Leenders KL, Martin-Solch C, *et al.* Reduced reward processing in the brains of parkinsonian patients. *Neuroreport* 2000;**11**(17):3681–7.
95. Cantello R, Aguggia M, Gilli M, *et al.* Major depression in Parkinson's disease and the mood response to intravenous methylphenidate: possible role of the "hedonic" dopamine synapse. *J Neurol Neurosurg Psychiatry* 1989;**52**(6):724–31.
96. Persico AM, Reich S, Henningfield JE, *et al.* Parkinsonian patients report blunted subjective effects of methylphenidate. *Exp Clin Psychopharmacol* 1998;**6**(1):54–63.
97. Solomon RL, Corbit JD. An opponent-process theory of motivation. II. Cigarette addiction. *J Abnorm Psychol* 1973;**81**(2):158–71.
98. Koob GF, Le Moal M. Drug abuse: hedonic homeostatic dysregulation. *Science* 1997;**278**(5335):52–8.
99. Koob GF, Le Moal M. Drug addiction, dysregulation of reward, and allostasis. *Neuropsychopharmacology* 2001;**24**(2):97–129.
100. Barr AM, Markou A, Phillips AG. A "crash" course on psychostimulant withdrawal as a model of depression. *Trends Pharmacol Sci* 2002;**23**(10):475–82.
101. Robinson TE, Berridge KC. Addiction. *Annu Rev Psychol* 2003;**54**:25–53.
102. Robinson TE, Berridge KC. The psychology and neurobiology of addiction: an incentive-sensitization view. *Addiction* 2000;**95**[Suppl 2(2)]:S91–117.
103. Berridge KC, Robinson TE. What is the role of dopamine in reward: hedonic impact, reward learning, or incentive salience? *Brain Res Brain Res Rev* 1998;**28**(3):309–69.
104. Hollander E, Pallanti S, Baldini Rossi N, *et al.* Imaging monetary reward in pathological gamblers. *World J Biol Psychiatry* 2005;**6**(2):113–20.
105. Crockford DN, Goodyear B, Edwards J, *et al.* Cue-induced brain activity in pathological gamblers. *Biol Psychiatry* 2005;**58**(10):787–95.
106. Di Chiara G, Bassareo V. Reward system and addiction: what dopamine does and doesn't do. *Curr Opin Pharmacol* 2007;**7**(1):69–76.
107. Everitt BJ, Dickinson A, Robbins TW. The neuropsychological basis of addictive behaviour. *Brain Res Brain Res Rev* 2001;**36**(2–3):129–38.
108. Porrino LJ, Lyons D, Smith HR, *et al.* Cocaine self-administration produces a progressive involvement of limbic, association, and sensorimotor striatal domains. *J Neurosci* 2004;**24**(14):3554–62.
109. Martin-Soelch C, Linthicum J, Ernst M. Appetitive conditioning: neural bases and implications for psychopathology. *Neurosci Biobehav Rev* 2007;**31**(3):426–40.
110. Everitt BJ, Cardinal RN, Parkinson JA, Robbins TW. Appetitive behavior: impact of amygdala-dependent mechanisms of emotional learning. *Ann N Y Acad Sci* 2003;**985**:233–50.
111. Parkinson JA, Cardinal RN, Everitt BJ. Limbic cortical–ventral striatal systems underlying appetitive conditioning. *Prog Brain Res* 2000;**126**:263–85.
112. Potenza MN, Xian H, Shah K, *et al.* Shared genetic contributions to pathological gambling and major depression in men. *Arch Gen Psychiatry* 2005;**62**(9):1015–21.
113. Swanson LW. Cerebral hemisphere regulation of motivated behavior. *Brain Res* 2000;**886**(1–2):113–64.
114. Nestler EJ, Aghajanian GK. Molecular and cellular basis of addiction. *Science* 1997;**278**(5335):58–63.
115. Mirenowicz J, Schultz W. Importance of unpredictability for reward responses in primate dopamine neurons. *J Neurophysiol* 1994;**72**(2):1024–7.
116. Schultz W. Behavioral theories and the neurophysiology of reward. *Annu Rev Psychol* 2006;**57**:87–115.
117. Christoph GR, Leonzio RJ, Wilcox KS. Stimulation of the lateral habenula inhibits dopamine-containing neurons in the substantia nigra and ventral tegmental area of the rat. *J Neurosci* 1986;**6**(3):613–9.
118. Ullsperger M, von Cramon DY. Error monitoring using external feedback: specific roles of the habenular complex, the reward system, and the cingulate motor area revealed by functional magnetic resonance imaging. *J Neurosci* 2003;**23**(10):4308–14.
119. Fiorillo CD, Tobler PN, Schultz W. Discrete coding of reward probability and uncertainty by dopamine neurons. *Science* 2003;**299**(5614):1898–902.
120. Hollerman JR, Schultz W. Dopamine neurons report an error in the temporal prediction of reward during learning. *Nat Neurosci* 1998;**1**(4):304–9.
121. Baler RD, Volkow ND. Drug addiction: the neurobiology of disrupted self-control. *Trends Mol Med* 2006;**12**(12):559–66.
122. Chambers RA, Taylor JR, Potenza MN. Developmental neurocircuitry of motivation in adolescence: a critical period of addiction vulnerability. *Am J Psychiatry* 2003;**160**(6):1041–52.

123. Wise RA. Dopamine, learning and motivation. *Nat Rev Neurosci* 2004;**5**(6):483–94.
124. Nader MA, Morgan D, Gage HD, *et al.* PET imaging of dopamine D2 receptors during chronic cocaine self-administration in monkeys. *Nat Neurosci* 2006;**9**(8):1050–6.
125. Volkow ND, Wang GJ, Fowler JS, *et al.* Brain DA D2 receptors predict reinforcing effects of stimulants in humans: replication study. *Synapse* 2002;**46**(2):79–82.
126. Volkow ND, Wang GJ, Telang F, *et al.* Low dopamine striatal D2 receptors are associated with prefrontal metabolism in obese subjects: possible contributing factors. *Neuroimage* 2008;**13**:13.
127. Barbano MF, Cador M. Opioids for hedonic experience and dopamine to get ready for it. *Psychopharmacology (Berl)* 2007;**191**(3):497–506.
128. Hutcheson DM, Everitt BJ, Robbins TW, Dickinson A. The role of withdrawal in heroin addiction: enhances reward or promotes avoidance? *Nat Neurosci* 2001;**4**(9):943–7.
129. Di Chiara G. Drug addiction as dopamine-dependent associative learning disorder. *Eur J Pharmacol* 1999;**375**(1–3):13–30.
130. Everitt BJ, Wolf ME. Psychomotor stimulant addiction: a neural systems perspective. *J Neurosci* 2002;**22**(9):3312–20.
131. Ito R, Dalley JW, Robbins TW, Everitt BJ. Dopamine release in the dorsal striatum during cocaine-seeking behavior under the control of a drug-associated cue. *J Neurosci* 2002;**22**(14):6247–53.
132. Jones GH, Mittleman G, Robbins TW. Attenuation of amphetamine-stereotypy by mesostriatal dopamine depletion enhances plasma corticosterone: implications for stereotypy as a coping response. *Behav Neural Biol* 1989;**51**(1):80–91.
133. Swainson R, Rogers RD, Sahakian BJ, *et al.* Probabilistic learning and reversal deficits in patients with Parkinson's disease or frontal or temporal lobe lesions: possible adverse effects of dopaminergic medication. *Neuropsychologia* 2000;**38**(5):596–612.
134. Jentsch JD, Taylor JR. Impulsivity resulting from frontostriatal dysfunction in drug abuse: implications for the control of behavior by reward-related stimuli. *Psychopharmacology (Berl)* 1999;**146**(4):373–90.
135. Cools R, Barker RA, Sahakian BJ, Robbins TW. Enhanced or impaired cognitive function in Parkinson's disease as a function of dopaminergic medication and task demands. *Cereb Cortex* 2001;**11**(12):1136–43.
136. Cools R, Barker RA, Sahakian BJ, Robbins TW. L-Dopa medication remediates cognitive inflexibility, but increases impulsivity in patients with Parkinson's disease. *Neuropsychologia* 2003;**41**(11):1431–41.
137. Volkow ND, Chang L, Wang GJ, *et al.* Low level of brain dopamine D2 receptors in methamphetamine abusers: association with metabolism in the orbitofrontal cortex. *Am J Psychiatry* 2001;**158**(12):2015–21.
138. Richards JB, Sabol KE, de Wit H. Effects of methamphetamine on the adjusting amount procedure, a model of impulsive behavior in rats. *Psychopharmacology (Berl)* 1999;**146**(4):432–9.
139. Cardinal RN, Winstanley CA, Robbins TW, Everitt BJ. Limbic corticostriatal systems and delayed reinforcement. *Ann N Y Acad Sci* 2004;**1021**:33–50.
140. Kreek MJ, Bart G, Lilly C, *et al.* Pharmacogenetics and human molecular genetics of opiate and cocaine addictions and their treatments. *Pharmacol Rev* 2005;**57**(1):1–26.
141. Baker DA, Xi ZX, Shen H, *et al.* The origin and neuronal function of *in vivo* nonsynaptic glutamate. *J Neurosci* 2002;**22**(20):9134–41.
142. Hu G, Duffy P, Swanson C, *et al.* The regulation of dopamine transmission by metabotropic glutamate receptors. *J Pharmacol Exp Ther* 1999;**289**(1):412–6.
143. McFarland K, Lapish CC, Kalivas PW. Prefrontal glutamate release into the core of the nucleus accumbens mediates cocaine-induced reinstatement of drug-seeking behavior. *J Neurosci* 2003;**23**(8):3531–7.
144. LaRowe SD, Mardikian P, Malcolm R, *et al.* Safety and tolerability of *N*-acetylcysteine in cocaine-dependent individuals. *Am J Addict* 2006;**15**(1):105–10.
145. Grant JE, Kim SW, Odlaug BL. *N*-Acetylcysteine, a glutamate-modulating agent, in the treatment of pathological gambling: a pilot study. *Biol Psychiatry* 2007;**62**(6):652–7.
146. Sofuoglu M, Kosten TR. Emerging pharmacological strategies in the fight against cocaine addiction. *Expert Opin Emerg Drugs* 2006;**11**(1):91–8.
147. Kim SW, Grant JE, Adson DE, *et al.* A double-blind placebo-controlled study of the efficacy and safety of paroxetine in the treatment of pathological gambling. *J Clin Psychiatry* 2002;**63**(6):501–7.
148. Mason BJ, Salvato FR, Williams LD, *et al.* A double-blind, placebo-controlled study of oral nalmefene for alcohol dependence. *Arch Gen Psychiatry* 1999;**56**(8):719–24.
149. Volpicelli JR, Alterman AI, Hayashida M, O'Brien CP. Naltrexone in the treatment of alcohol dependence. *Arch Gen Psychiatry* 1992;**49**(11):876–80.
150. Dackis C, O'Brien C. Neurobiology of addiction: treatment and public policy ramifications. *Nat Neurosci* 2005; **8**(11):1431–6.
151. Schlosser S, Black DW, Repertinger S, Freet D. Compulsive buying. Demography, phenomenology, and comorbidity in 46 subjects. *Gen Hosp Psychiatry* 1994;**16**(3):205–12.
152. Potenza MN. The neurobiology of pathological gambling. *Semin Clin Neuropsychiatry* 2001;**6**(3):217–26.
153. Mobini S, Chiang TJ, Ho MY, *et al.* Effects of central 5-hydroxytryptamine depletion on sensitivity to delayed and probabilistic reinforcement. *Psychopharmacology (Berl)* 2000;**152**(4):390–7.
154. Poulos CX, Parker JL, Le AD. Dexfenfluramine and 8-OH-DPAT modulate impulsivity in a delay-of-reward paradigm: implications for a correspondence with alcohol consumption. *Behav Pharmacol* 1996;**7**(4):395–9.
155. Blanco C, Petkova E, Ibanez A, Saiz-Ruiz J. A pilot placebo-controlled study of fluvoxamine for pathological gambling. *Ann Clin Psychiatry* 2002;**14**(1):9–15.
156. Grant JE, Kim SW, Potenza MN, *et al.* Paroxetine treatment of pathological gambling: a multi-centre randomized controlled trial. *Int Clin Psychopharmacol* 2003;**18**(4):243–9.
157. Hollander E, DeCaria CM, Finkell JN, *et al.* A randomized double-blind fluvoxamine/placebo crossover trial in pathologic gambling. *Biol Psychiatry* 2000;**47**(9):813–7.
158. Dodd ML, Klos KJ, Bower JH, *et al.* Pathological gambling caused by drugs used to treat Parkinson disease. *Arch Neurol* 2005;**62**(9):1377–81.
159. Evans AH, Lawrence AD, Potts J, *et al.* Factors influencing susceptibility to compulsive dopaminergic drug use in Parkinson disease. *Neurology* 2005;**65**(10):1570–4.

160. Petry NM. Substance abuse, pathological gambling, and impulsiveness. *Drug Alcohol Depend* 2001;**63**(1):29–38.
161. Jacobs H, Heberlein I, Vieregge A, Vieregge P. Personality traits in young patients with Parkinson's disease. *Acta Neurol Scand* 2001;**103**(2):82–7.
162. Kaasinen V, Nurmi E, Bergman J, *et al.* Personality traits and brain dopaminergic function in Parkinson's disease. *Proc Natl Acad Sci USA* 2001;**98**(23):13272–7.
163. Menza MA, Golbe LI, Cody RA, Forman NE. Dopamine-related personality traits in Parkinson's disease. *Neurology* 1993;**43**(3 Pt 1):505–8.
164. Eisen SA, Lin N, Lyons MJ, *et al.* Familial influences on gambling behavior: an analysis of 3359 twin pairs. *Addiction* 1998;**93**(9):1375–84.
165. Slutske WS, Eisen S, True WR, *et al.* Common genetic vulnerability for pathological gambling and alcohol dependence in men. *Arch Gen Psychiatry* 2000;**57**(7):666–73.
166. Slutske WS, Eisen S, Xian H, *et al.* A twin study of the association between pathological gambling and antisocial personality disorder. *J Abnorm Psychol* 2001;**110**(2):297–308.
167. Desai RA, Potenza MN. Gender differences in the associations between past-year gambling problems and psychiatric disorders. *Soc Psychiatry Psychiatr Epidemiol* 2008;**43**(3): 173–83.
168. McElroy SL, Keck PE Jr, Pope HG Jr, *et al.* Compulsive buying: a report of 20 cases. *J Clin Psychiatry* 1994;**55**(6):242–8.
169. Chambers RA, Potenza MN. Neurodevelopment, impulsivity, and adolescent gambling. *J Gambl Stud* 2003;**19**(1):53–84.
170. Uitti RJ, Tanner CM, Rajput AH, *et al.* Hypersexuality with antiparkinsonian therapy. *Clin Neuropharmacol* 1989;**12**(5):375–83.
171. Potenza MN, Kosten TR, Rounsaville BJ. Pathological gambling. *JAMA* 2001;**286**(2):141–4.
172. Forno LS. Neuropathology of Parkinson's disease. *J Neuropathol Exp Neurol* 1996;**55**(3):259–72.
173. Hornykiewicz O, Kish SJ. Biochemical pathophysiology of Parkinson's disease. *Adv Neurol* 1987;**45**:19–34.
174. Kish SJ, Shannak K, Hornykiewicz O. Uneven pattern of dopamine loss in the striatum of patients with idiopathic Parkinson's disease. Pathophysiologic and clinical implications. *N Engl J Med* 1988;**318**(14):876–80.
175. Damier P, Hirsch EC, Agid Y, Graybiel AM. The substantia nigra of the human brain. II. Patterns of loss of dopamine-containing neurons in Parkinson's disease. *Brain* 1999;**122**(Pt 8):1437–48.
176. Obeso JA, Olanow CW, Nutt JG. Levodopa motor complications in Parkinson's disease. *Trends Neurosci* 2000;**23**(10 Suppl):S2–7.
177. Fahn S. The spectrum of levodopa-induced dyskinesias. *Ann Neurol* 2000;**47**(4 Suppl 1):S2–9; discussion S11.
178. Cools R, Barker RA, Sahakian BJ, Robbins TW. Mechanisms of cognitive set flexibility in Parkinson's disease. *Brain* 2001;**124**(Pt 12):2503–12.
179. Cools R, Stefanova E, Barker RA, et al.. Dopaminergic modulation of high-level cognition in Parkinson's disease: the role of the prefrontal cortex revealed by PET. *Brain* 2002;**125**(Pt 3): 584–94.
180. Allam MF, Campbell MJ, Hofman A, *et al.* Smoking and Parkinson's disease: systematic review of prospective studies. *Mov Disord* 2004;**19**(6):614–21.
181. Evans AH, Lawrence AD, Potts J, *et al.* Relationship between impulsive sensation seeking traits, smoking, alcohol and caffeine intake, and Parkinson's disease. *J Neurol Neurosurg Psychiatry* 2006;**77**(3):317–21.
182. Witjas T, Baunez C, Henry JM, *et al.* Addiction in Parkinson's disease: impact of subthalamic nucleus deep brain stimulation. *Mov Disord* 2005;**20**(8):1052–5.
183. Pontone G, Williams JR, Bassett SS, Marsh L. Clinical features associated with impulse control disorders in Parkinson disease. *Neurology* 2006;**67**(7):1258–61.
184. Galvez-Jimenez N. Rasagiline and selegiline induced hypersexuality and other impulse control disorders (ICD) in Parkinson disease. Presented at the Impulse Control Disoders in Parkinson's Disease Workshop, 12–13 July 2007, Toronto.
185. Smeding HM, Goudriaan AE, Foncke EM, *et al.* Pathological gambling after bilateral subthalamic nucleus stimulation in Parkinson disease. *J Neurol Neurosurg Psychiatry* 2007;**78**(5):517–9.
186. Damasio AR, Lobo-Antunes J, Macedo C. Psychiatric aspects in Parkinsonism treated with L-dopa. *J Neurol Neurosurg Psychiatry* 1971;**34**(5):502–7.
187. Goodwin FK. Psychiatric side effects of levodopa in man. *JAMA* 1971;**218**(13):1915–20.
188. Wise RA, Bozarth MA. A psychomotor stimulant theory of addiction. *Psychol Rev* 1987;**94**(4):469–92.
189. Guillin O, Diaz J, Carroll P, *et al.* BDNF controls dopamine D3 receptor expression and triggers behavioural sensitization. *Nature* 2001;**411**(6833):86–9.
190. Berke JD, Hyman SE. Addiction, dopamine, and the molecular mechanisms of memory. *Neuron* 2000;**25**(3):515–32.
191. Pessiglione M, Seymour B, Flandin G, *et al.* Dopamine-dependent prediction errors underpin reward-seeking behaviour in humans. *Nature* 2006;**442**(7106):1042–5.
192. Loba P, Stewart SH, Klein RM, Blackburn JR. Manipulations of the features of standard video lottery terminal (VLT) games: effects in pathological and non-pathological gamblers. *J Gambl Stud* 2001;**17**(4):297–320.
193. Schenk S, Partridge B. Cocaine-seeking produced by experimenter-administered drug injections: dose–effect relationships in rats. *Psychopharmacology (Berl)* 1999;**147**(3): 285–90.
194. Engber TM, Susel Z, Juncos JL, Chase TN. Continuous and intermittent levodopa differentially affect rotation induced by D-1 and D-2 dopamine agonists. *Eur J Pharmacol* 1989;**168**(3):291–8.
195. Nocjar C, Panksepp J. Chronic intermittent amphetamine pretreatment enhances future appetitive behavior for drug- and natural-reward: interaction with environmental variables. *Behav Brain Res* 2002;**128**(2):189–203.
196. Zack M, Poulos CX. Amphetamine primes motivation to gamble and gambling-related semantic networks in problem gamblers. *Neuropsychopharmacology* 2004;**29**(1):195–207.
197. Gallagher DA, O'Sullivan SS, Evans AH, *et al.* Pathological gambling in Parkinson's disease: risk factors and differences from dopamine dysregulation. An analysis of published case series. *Mov Disord* 2007;**22**(12):1757–63.
198. Mamikonyan E, Siderowf AD, Duda JE, *et al.* Long-term follow-up of impulse control disorders in Parkinson's disease. *Mov Disord* 2008;**23**(1):75–80.

199. Driver-Dunckley E, Samanta J, Stacy M. Pathological gambling associated with dopamine agonist therapy in Parkinson's disease. *Neurology* 2003;**61**(3):422–3.
200. Okun MS, Foote KD. Subthalamic nucleus vs globus pallidus interna deep brain stimulation, the rematch: will pallidal deep brain stimulation make a triumphant return? *Arch Neurol* 2005;**62**(4):533–6.
201. Anderson VC, Burchiel KJ, Hogarth P, *et al.* Pallidal vs subthalamic nucleus deep brain stimulation in Parkinson disease. *Arch Neurol* 2005;**62**(4):554–60.
202. Rodriguez-Oroz MC, Obeso JA, Lang AE, *et al.* Bilateral deep brain stimulation in Parkinson's disease: a multicentre study with 4 years follow-up. *Brain* 2005;**128**(Pt 10):2240–9.
203. Volkmann J, Allert N, Voges J, *et al.* Long-term results of bilateral pallidal stimulation in Parkinson's disease. *Ann Neurol* 2004;**55**(6):871–5.
204. Frank MJ, Samanta J, Moustafa AA, Sherman SJ. Hold your horses: impulsivity, deep brain stimulation, and medication in parkinsonism. *Science* 2007;**318**(5854):1309–12.
205. Berney A, Vingerhoets F, Perrin A, *et al.* Effect on mood of subthalamic DBS for Parkinson's disease: a consecutive series of 24 patients. *Neurology* 2002;**59**(9):1427–9.
206. Burkhard PR, Vingerhoets FJ, Berney A, *et al.* Suicide after successful deep brain stimulation for movement disorders. *Neurology* 2004;**63**(11):2170–2.
207. Black DW. A review of compulsive buying disorder. *World Psychiatry* 2007;**6**(1):14–8.
208. Sevincok L, Akoglu A, Akyol A. Quetiapine in a case with Parkinson disease and pathological gambling. *J Clin Psychopharmacol* 2007;**27**(1):107–8.
209. Fernandez HH, Trieschmann ME, Burke MA, *et al.* Long-term outcome of quetiapine use for psychosis among parkinsonian patients. *Mov Disord* 2003;**18**(5):510–4.
210. Fong T, Kalechstein A, Bernhard B, *et al.* A double-blind, placebo-controlled trial of olanzapine for the treatment of video poker pathological gamblers. *Pharmacol Biochem Behav* 2008;**89**(3):298–303.
211. McElroy SL, Nelson EB, Welge JA, *et al.* Olanzapine in the treatment of pathological gambling: a negative randomized placebo-controlled trial. *J Clin Psychiatry* 2008;**69**(3):433–40.
212. Black DW. Compulsive buying disorder: a review of the evidence. *CNS Spectr* 2007;**12**(2):124–32.
213. Bermejo PE. Topiramate in managing impulse control disorders in Parkinson's disease. *Parkinsonism Relat Disord* 2008;**14**(5):448–9.
214. Bostwick JM, Bucci JA. Internet sex addiction treated with naltrexone. *Mayo Clin Proc* 2008;**83**(2):226–30.
215. Neumeister A, Winkler A, Wober-Bingol C. Addition of naltrexone to fluoxetine in the treatment of binge eating disorder. *Am J Psychiatry* 1999;**156**(5):797.

Chapter 21
Sleep Disorders in Parkinson's Disease

Friederike Sixel-Döring & Claudia Trenkwalder
Paracelsus-Elena-Klinik, Center for Parkinsonism and Movement Disorders, Kassel, Germany

Introduction

Patients suffering from Parkinson's disease (PD) frequently report a variety of nighttime problems including poor sleep quality [1]. In recent years, excessive daytime sleepiness and so-called paroxysmal sleep – an unexpected dozing-off – were associated with dopaminergic medication, and this resulted in transient restrictions in the use of non-ergot dopamine agonists for those patients who wanted to continue driving. However, James Parkinson in his first report on Parkinson's disease in 1817 already described an increase in disturbed sleep, daytime somnolence with mild confusion, and other signs of intense fatigue in advanced stages of the illness [2]. Today it is generally acknowledged that disordered sleep not only appears in advanced stages of the disease, but can also be an early symptom. Prior to the evolution of motor symptoms, patients may prodromally present with disruptions of dream sleep, thereby indicating that this feature could be highly significant for preclinical diagnosis. It has been recognized that the specific pathophysiology of PD *per se* will lead to disordered sleep and thus have an additional negative impact on daytime performance. A number of neurodegenerative, psychologic and pharmacologic factors may be involved in the somnopathy of parkinsonian patients, calling for special attention to be paid to diagnosis and treatment of their dyssomnia. The presence of sleep disorders can be established through an interview with the patient and his/her bed partner. Video-supported polysomnography (PSG) is recommended for clarifying sleep diagnosis, identifying the specific nocturnal problem, and choosing the right treatment.

Pathophysiologic aspects

Serotonergic neurons in the dorsal raphe nucleus, noradrenergic neurons in the locus coeruleus, and cholinergic neurons in the pedunculo-pontine region are regarded as crucial for sleep. Disturbances in these neural areas can lead to disruption of the sleep–wake rhythm. Likewise, alterations in the mesocorticolimbic system may produce sleep-wake abnormalities [3]. We also know that dopamine D1 receptor agonists are particularly likely to provoke electroencephalogram (EEG) desynchronizations and arousal reactions [4], whereas low doses of dopamine D1 and D2 receptor agonists work in a sleep-inducing fashion. This seems to be a function of the dopamine D2 autoreceptors, which play an important role in sleep mediation and indirectly take part in the regulation of sleep by influencing the firing rate of the ventral tegmental dopaminergic neurons [5]. The regulation of rapid eye movement (REM) sleep and, more importantly, its disruption, which manifests as REM sleep behavior disorder (RBD), has not yet been elucidated in humans (see Chapter 22). Recent experimental data from a rat model propose a putative on–off switch for the control of REM sleep [6]. According to this model, REM-off is activated by the ventrolateral part of the periaqueductal gray matter and the lateral pontine tegmentum. These regions are inhibited by GABAergic and galaninergic projections from the forebrain ventrolateral preoptic nucleus, thus inducing REM-on. The REM-off neurons in turn are activated by noradrenergic projections from locus coeruleus, serotonergic raphe nucleus, and hypocretinergic pathways from the lateral hypothalamus, thereby ending the period of REM sleep. REM-on and -off areas are mutually inhibitory with reciprocal interactions with each other. In the rat, projections from the sublaterodorsal nucleus to the medulla and the spinal cord with activation of inhibitory interneurons that hyperpolarize anterior horn motor neurons are held responsible for atonia during REM sleep. Braak *et al.* showed a characteristic ascension pattern of Lewy bodies and Lewy neurites as the specific pathologic–anatomic hallmarks of PD, affecting sleep-sensitive areas of the brainstem at the earliest "preclinical" stage [7], thereby explaining why sleep disorders such as RBD might precede the typical motor manifestation of the disease. It is therefore essential for sleep

Parkinson's Disease. Non-Motor and Non-Dopaminergic Features, First Edition. Edited by C. Warren Olanow, Fabrizio Stocchi, and Anthony E. Lang.

disorders to be recognized as an important non-motor feature of PD that can be present at all stages of the illness ranging from the preclinical to the advanced state.

Clinical symptoms

Parkinsonian patients often complain of difficulties in falling asleep and maintaining sleep, and also nocturnal immobility and RBD, as reported by bed partners. Sleep disorders undeniably worsen with the progression of PD. Up to 15% of PD patients show daytime sleepiness and paroxysmal sleep, which become more obvious during the course of the illness. Severe sleep disorders are primarily seen in elderly patients who already suffer from motor fluctuations and/or hallucinations [8]. See Table 21.1 and Figure 21.1 for aspects of PD that contribute to sleep–wake disturbances.

Disorders of initiating and maintaining sleep

Problems in falling asleep are likely related to an increased dosage of mainly dopamine agonists, and rarely to levodopa therapy. Fragmented sleep with loss of slow wave sleep and a subsequent increase in sleep stages 1 and 2, as well as an increase of arousals [9,10], are usually not predominant in early stages of the disease, but escalate with advancing neurodegeneration [11]. Patients will experience this as a problem of sleep maintenance, which can be further aggravated by dopaminergic overstimulation.

Nocturnal akinesia

Many patients complain about being unable to turn over at night, and have difficulties in getting up to go to the toilet. This nighttime immobility as a motor fluctuation is also a classic symptom of advanced PD. It is often associated with recurrent nocturnal tremor, periodic and non-periodic leg movements, and feelings of rigidity [1,12]. Nocturnal tremor typically occurs during sleep stage 1 or in waking phases at night; it can be very bothersome for the patient as it prevents him/her from going back to sleep. Simple or complex movements, such as blinking when falling asleep, blepharospasm, increased muscle contractility of the extremities during non-REM sleep, and so-called fragmented myoclonus of an extremity, are observed at varied intensity and frequency in parkinsonian patients while asleep.

Periodic leg movements in sleep (PLMS)

PLMS, like restless legs syndrome (RLS), is a frequent disorder that can, in severe cases, have a periodic limb movement index (PLMI) (the number of periodic limb

Table 21.1 Aspects of Parkinson's disease that contribute to sleep–wake disturbances (modified from Happe and Trenkwalder [12].

Reason	Predominant impairments
Neurochemical alterations of cholinergic, serotonergic, and noradrenergic systems and the neuropathologic changes of PD	Impaired sleep–wake control, reduced REM sleep Alterations of REM sleep control, "flip-flop" switch of REM sleep
Bradykinesia and rigidity	Reduction of normal body shifts during sleep with problem turning over in bed, leading to discomfort and awakenings; impaired ability to use the bathroom at night, and respiratory muscle dysfunction
Periodic and non-periodic movements	Increased motor activity – disturbs sleep continuity
PLMS, tremor, dystonia, drug-induced myoclonus	Arousals, pain with discomfort during lying down
Restless legs syndrome	Sleep onset problems, discrepancy between wish to move and immobility
REM sleep behavior disorder	Disrupted REM sleep, arousals, anxiety
Abnormal motor activity affecting respiratory and upper airway muscles	Breathing abnormalities during sleep such as sleep apnea syndrome, obstructive and/or central sleep apnea
Drug-related effects	Dopamine agonists: reduced total sleep time with increased time awake Anti-depressants: reduced REM sleep Various agents: reduced slow-wave sleep, nightmares, psychosis, hallucinosis
Depression and anxiety	Difficulty falling asleep, arousals, early morning awakening
Dementia and psychosis	Nocturnal episodes of confusion, "sundowning" with disturbed day-and-night rhythm
Nocturia	Increased time awake, problems of falling asleep again, nocturnal falls, discomfort

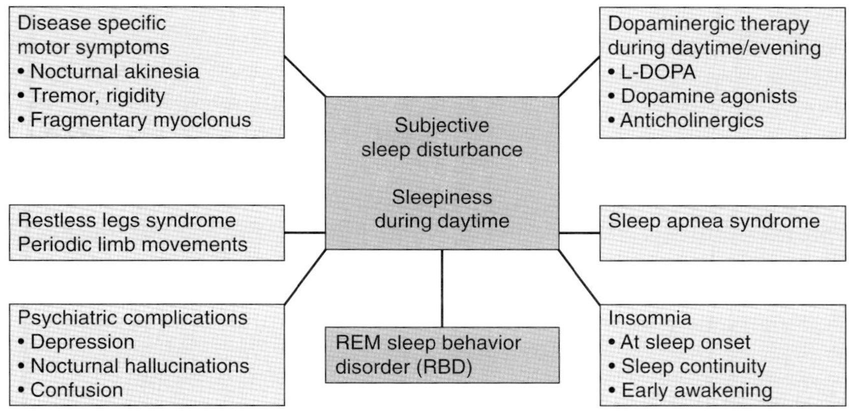

Figure 21.1 Sleep disturbance in parkinsonism.

movements per hour) of >100, thus considerably interfering with the course of sleep. PLMS can also cause arousals (PLMSA). PLMS in abundance, however, do not produce any EEG alterations. The debate is still open about the clinical relevance of PLMS in sleep disorders in PD patients. It is possible that PLMS-induced autonomic changes, such as heart rate alterations and blood pressure variations, are the only clinically significant parameters.

Sleep benefit

Although most PD patients with motor fluctuations wake in the "off" state, some patients experience sleep benefit and wake in the "on" state. Sleep benefit is characterized by a clear improvement in motor performance and in the general condition of the patient without a prior intake of dopaminergic agents. It lasts approximately 15–30 min and then gradually wears off. About one-third of PD patients experience this sleep-related symptom amelioration. The reasons for this improvement are not clear. A possible explanation could be a recovery of the dopaminergic system during the night [13].

REM sleep behavior disorder (RBD)

In the 1990s, Schenck and Mahowald described a so-called idiopathic RBD which was subsequently discovered to be predominantly associated with neurodegenerative diseases [14]. RBD is currently defined, in accordance with the International Classification of Sleep Disorders [15], as an increased tonicity of the chin muscles evidenced on PSG during REM sleep, along with clinical features such as movements (e.g., of the limbs) in REM sleep, and dream-related vocalizations (screaming, laughing, or singing while asleep) (Plate 21.1). These dream-enacting behaviors can result in patients harming themselves or others, and can cause them to fall out of bed without being able to recollect the incident afterwards [16,17]. The prevalence of RBD is higher than previously imagined: up to 90% of patients with multiple system atrophy [18] and up to 60% of patients with PD [19] are affected. Up to two-thirds of patients with idiopathic RBD may develop parkinsonism within 10 years of diagnosis [14]. As striatal dopamine transporters have been found to be reduced in idiopathic RBD, it has been suggested that RBD can in fact be a very early manifestation of a synucleinopathy that precedes the development of the more classic motor features of the particular disease [20]. Recent studies suggest that RBD in PD may be associated with cognitive impairment [21], and occurs predominantly in patients with the akinetic rigid form of the disease, suggesting the possibility of different underlying patterns of neurodegeneration in PD with and without RBD [22].

It is important to differentiate RBD from nocturnal psychosis or confused states since these disturbances are distinctly different in nature and pathogenesis, and require different therapeutic approaches [23]. It has so far been impossible to diagnose RBD reliably through the use of validated questionnaires. Therefore, it is important carefully to take the patient's sleep history through interviews with the patient and his/her bed partner, and to perform a video-supported PSG to establish the correct diagnosis. As RBD may be an early symptom of neurodegeneration, a timely diagnosis may allow the identification of preclinical PD patients prior to the development of motor disturbances [24,25]. This could permit the early introduction of neuroprotective therapies – should they become available – and perhaps prevent the emergence of motor symptoms.

Nocturnal respiratory disorders

As with all patients with disturbed sleep, PD patients can suffer from nocturnal breathing disorders that subsequently increase daytime sleepiness. Upper airway obstruction, possibly due to altered muscle tone in the oropharyngeal region, is thought to be most often responsible [26]. Nocturnal breathing disorders with central apneas, obstructive apneas, and hypoventilation episodes can be observed. PD patients appear to experience consequent autonomic disturbances more frequently than non-parkinsonian age-matched individuals. Furthermore, an akinetically fixed nocturnal posture with the patient lying on the back, as is often present in PD patients, will encourage upper airway obstruction. Stridor and laryngeal stenosis can also develop as a manifestation of a dystonic syndrome, particularly in patients with multiple system atrophy.

Excessive daytime sleepiness (EDS)

Excessive daytime sleepiness (EDS) is a well-known phenomenon in PD patients. After 20 years of disease duration, 70% of PD patients have EDS [27]. Although EDS may arise as a primary manifestation of PD reflecting the anatomic structures affected by the neurodegenerative process, nocturnal breathing disorders, nocturnal leg movements, fragmented sleep, and dopaminergic drugs can also each contribute to or exacerbate this problem [28]. Patients complain mainly of increasing tiredness, for example, and describe, that they nod off while eating or reading. Sudden onset "sleep attacks," that were formerly associated with the use of the non-ergot dopamine agonists pramipexole and ropinirole, have been proven to be a class effect attributable to all dopamine agonists currently employed in the management of PD [29]. A recent study using continuous sleep EEG monitoring showed that even patients without a history of sleep attacks also had microsleep episodes in the form of non-REM stage 1 and 2 intrusions into wakefulness during the day. Furthermore, the majority of these microsleep episodes were not perceived by the patients [30]. Recent studies show that daytime somnolence is further enhanced by sedative medications taken at night [31,32]. EDS can manifest as simply falling asleep while reading or watching TV but can also occur in more dangerous situations such as while the patient is driving. The issue of sleepiness should be addressed routinely in all PD patients, assisted by the use of appropriate scales such as the Epworth Sleepiness Scale (ESS) or the Parkinson's Disease Sleep Scale (PDSS) [33]. Individual counseling is recommended. Patients obviously need to be informed that they must refrain from driving if they suffer from daytime somnolence or episodes of paroxysmal sleep [34]. This may be a potential conflict with the patient for whom the ability to drive may be an important issue for maintaining quality-of-life and independence.

Diagnostic work-up

Experience shows that sleep problems rarely represent the main complaint of PD patients. However, up to 90% of patients will report sleep difficulties at some point during the course of their disease and it can be a troublesome problem. Since a variety of factors contribute to sleep disorders in PD patients, individual case histories with an assessment of sleep perception, assessment of sleep habits, and medication status should all be carefully reviewed. An interview with bed partners and/or family members and caregivers could yield important additional information. Specific questionnaires, such as the PDSS, can be used to provide a more accurate clinical picture [33].

Video-based polysomnography and multiple sleep latency (MSLT)

If the physician is unable to come to a clear diagnosis through clinical examination and by eliciting the patient's sleep history, the patient should be referred to a sleep laboratory for further examination. Synchronized video recording is specifically necessary to recognize and adequately assess RBD. MSLT can be useful in providing an objective measure of excess sleepiness in a patient where it is not clear from history by recording the length of time it takes for the person to fall asleep.

Treatment of sleep disorders

The aim of a thorough diagnostic work-up should be a specific treatment for the PD patient's sleep disturbance. It is necessary to establish whether disturbed sleep is mainly due to parkinsonian akinesia and motor symptoms, which generally require increased doses of dopaminergic medication, or alternatively whether the problems are due to increased fragmentation of sleep with insomnia and increased waking phases or nocturnal confusion with abnormal behaviors which are often caused by medications such as high-dose dopamine agonists, amantadine, anti-cholinergics, or selegiline and are best treated by a reduction in medication. RBD needs to be differentiated from nocturnal hallucinations, and treatable conditions such as RLS and sleep-disordered breathing (sleep apnea) should be identified.

Nocturnal akinesia

Increasing the dose of dopaminergic medication at night may ameliorate nocturnal akinesia and other parkinsonian features that interfere with sleep. Levodopa slow-release preparations in doses of 100–200 mg taken at bedtime are frequently recommended [35]. Long-acting dopamine receptor agonists [36] or continuous dopaminergic stimulation via transdermal application (ongoing trial with rotigotine patch) may also be useful, if slow-release formulations of levodopa are not sufficient. For patients in advanced stages of the disease who have severe motor fluctuations and dyskinesias, these measures may not be sufficient and may result in further sleep disruption with nocturnal exacerbation of PD symptoms and dyskinesia after the additional medication intake. For these patients, continuous dopaminergic stimulation via duodenal levodopa instillation or subcutaneous apomorphine infusion around the clock may prove beneficial [37], although here one must be concerned about the risk of developing tolerance with impaired motor responses. Deep brain stimulation of the subthalamic nucleus, which has been shown to reduce parkinsonian features effectively in advanced stages of PD, also can have a favorable impact on sleep quality and sleep architecture [38]. Some patients, however, complain about symptoms of nocturnal RLS after DBS and reduced dopaminergic medication. Those complaints can easily be managed, however, with one dosage of a nocturnal dopaminergic or even opioidergic medication (authors' personal observation).

RLS and PLMS

The treatment of choice for PLMS is increased dosing of dopaminergic agents. Interestingly, no case of augmentation has been observed in patients with PD and RLS. This may be because PD patients typically receive dopaminergic therapy during the daytime, which may prevent the emergence of augmentation in PD RLS patients compared with patients with idiopathic RLS. Another explanation, that is perhaps more likely, is that RLS in PD develops by way of a different pathophysiologic mechanism. In contrast to idiopathic RLS patients, PD patients have a proven dopamine deficiency that prevents them from developing dopaminergic overstimulation during the daytime, which could be one reason for augmentation in those with idiopathic RLS [39]. Clinical experience shows that PLMS, like RLS, can also be relieved by opiates such as tilidine slow release; however, published randomized controlled studies are lacking. The symptoms of RLS – associated with particularly unpleasant sensory symptoms in PD patients, not only when falling asleep but also during the night – can be managed with dopaminergic agents or with opiates, preferably in the slow-release form [36]. Aperiodic movements and fragmentary myoclonus are best treated with benzodiazepines, and will often benefit from a reduction in dopaminergic medication.

Insomnia

As mentioned above, insomnia in PD patients may be an adverse effect of PD medication. Administration late in the day of amantadine, anti-cholinergics, selegiline, and dopamine agonists can seriously impede the initiation of sleep and should then be avoided. Frightful hallucinations will add to this effect and also call for a reduction of nighttime dopaminergic medication. Concomitant depression is frequently found in PD patients and may induce or enhance insomnia [40]. In these cases, the administration of tricyclic anti-depressants or mirtazapine has been recommended [41,42]. It must be remembered, however, that the anti-cholinergic effects of tricyclic agents can contribute to nocturnal states of confusion in PD patients and their use should be restricted in patients with cognitive impairment.

Treatment of insomnia in PD patients includes the evaluation of psychosocial and behavioral issues as it would for non-PD patients. Special attention should be paid to sleep hygiene: patients should be advised to have regular bedtimes, and to avoid caffeine, alcohol, and physical effort in the evening. Intermittent administration of benzodiazepine receptor agonists such as zolpidem can be helpful for severe sleep initiation difficulty that cannot be addressed otherwise and that lead to additional impairment of daytime functioning (personal clinical experience). It is also essential to reduce the frequency of nocturia to avoid subsequent awakenings at night. Urologic agents can help to improve a patient's sleep at night. Longstanding insomnia may sometimes be linked to a prior abuse of benzodiazepines or benzodiazepine receptor agonists, prohibiting withdrawal of this medication.

Nocturnal abnormal behaviors

In the advanced stage of PD, nocturnal problems are predominantly governed by hallucinations and psychotic states at night. In the course of the illness up to 30% of patients will encounter vivid dreams and nightmares with hallucinations, especially if they are treated with dopamine agonists. These conditions can be extremely bothersome for patients and caregivers, as nighttime rest may be disturbed for every household member. Video-based PSG will allow for the differentiation of nocturnal psychotic states and RBD. For severe RBD the treatment of choice is clonazepam (0.5–2 mg). Clozapine as an anti-psychotic substance that does not induce adverse exrapyramidal side effects has been successfully studied in a controlled setting for treating hallucinations and psychotic states in PD [43]. Quetiapine has also been found to be efficient, although a double-blind, randomized study could not show a beneficial effect on drug-induced psychosis in PD, probably owing to a large drop-out rate in the trial [44]. It is generally used as the first-choice drug for the treatment of hallucinations and nocturnal psychosis (starting with a dose of 12.5 or 25 mg HS) as it avoids the risk of hematologic side effects seen with clozapine [45–47]. Both drugs can also enhance nighttime rest, as they induce sleepiness. Although no trials are available, low-dosage quetiapine is widely used to treat insomnia in PD patients. It may particularly be helpful in patients who do not tolerate benzodiazepines or anti-depressants, likely providing some anti-psychotic prophylaxis at the same time. In some cases, administration of low-dose clomethiazole before retiring may be a relevant therapeutic supplement. However, one must be aware that all drugs with a sedative effect may worsen sleep-disordered breathing.

Sleep-disordered breathing (SDB)

Concomitant SDB may distinctly worsen pre-existing daytime vigilance problems in PD patients. As a treatable cause it should be identified and addressed with nighttime ventilation therapy as in non-PD patients. As PD patients often have difficulties tolerating a mask for continuous positive airways pressure application, compliance may be a problem. Individual tailoring of therapy is necessary and much patience is required to adapt therapy to the individual patient. Adequate treatment of sleep-disordered breathing is a prerequisite for treating concurrent RBD with clonazepam or RLS with opiates, as the administration of these substances may worsen an obstructive or central sleep apnea syndrome. Successfully addressing a sleep apnea syndrome in PD patients may be of value in improving many tedious nocturnal problems such as nocturia, nocturnal confusion, and sleep disruption, with subsequent improvement in daytime performance.

Excessive daytime sleepiness (EDS)

The first steps in managing EDS in PD patients are to identify treatable causes and to improve sleep hygiene. If these measures, including nocturnal ventilation therapy and the reduction of sedative medication in the evening [48], do not sufficiently improve the condition, a psychostimulating therapy such as modafinil can be tried. However, not every patient benefits from this medication and differing results have been observed [49]. A recently published double-blind, placebo-controlled trial showed no significant positive effect of modafinil on EDS in PD patients [50]. It is important that physicians seek out EDS in PD patients. Patients should be advised about the risks, and refrain from driving until the problem has been satisfactorily managed.

Conclusion

Sleep fragmentation, PLMS, RLS, and RBD are common disease-related sleep disorders in PD and can be regarded as manifestations of Lewy body pathology in sleep-related areas of the brainstem. Nocturnal exacerbation of PD symptoms and SDB, insomnia due to depression, and side-effects of the many drugs taken by these patients may furthermore severely disturb the initiation and maintenance of sleep, enhancing EDS. Therefore, sleep disorders represent an important, multifactorial, non-motor symptom of the disease. A thorough diagnostic work-up including interviews with the patient and his/her bed partner and also video-supported PSG can establish the specific sleep diagnosis and facilitate therapy.

References

1. Lees AJ, Blackburn NA, Campbell VL. The nighttime problems of Parkinson's disease. *Clin Neuropharmacol* 1988;**11**:512–9.
2. Parkinson J. *An Essay on the Shaking Palsy*. London: Whittingham and Rowland: 1817.
3. Javoy-Agid F, Agid Y. Is the mesocortical dopaminergic system involved in Parkinson disease? *Neurology* 1980;**30**:1326–30.
4. Ongini E, Caporali MG, Massotti M. Stimulation of dopamine D-1 receptors by SKF 38393 induces EEG desynchronization and behavioral arousal. *Life Sci* 1985;**37**:2327–33.
5. Bagetta G, De Sarro G, Priolo E, Nistico G. Ventral tegmental area: site through which dopamine D2-receptor agonists evoke behavioural and electrocortical sleep in rats. *Br J Pharmacol* 1988;**95**:860–6.
6. Boeve BF, Silber MH, Saper CB, *et al*. Pathophysiology of REM sleep behaviour disorder and relevance to neurodegenerative disease. *Brain* 2007;**130**:2770–88.
7. Braak H, Del Tredici K, Rub U, de Vos RA, Jansen Steur EN, Braak E. Staging of brain pathology related to sporadic Parkinson's disease. *Neurobiol Aging* 2003;**24**:197–211.
8. Comella CL, Tanner CM, Ristanovic RK. Polysomnographic sleep measures in Parkinson's disease patients with treatment-induced hallucinations. *Ann Neurol* 1993;**34**:710–4.
9. Kales A, Ansel RD, Markham CH, *et al*. Sleep in patients with Parkinson's disease and normal subjects prior to and following levodopa administration. *Clin Pharmacol Ther* 1971;**12**:397–406.
10. Mouret J. Differences in sleep in patients with Parkinson's disease. *Electroencephalogr Clin Neurophysiol* 1975;**38**:653–7.
11. Wetter TC, Collado-Seidel V, Pollmacher T, *et al*. Sleep and periodic leg movement patterns in drug-free patients with Parkinson's disease and multiple system atrophy. *Sleep* 2000;**23**:361–7.
12. Happe S, Trenkwalder C. Sleep disorders and Parkinson's disease. In: Ebadi MS, Pfeiffer R, eds. *Parkinson's Disease*. Boca Raton, FL: CRC Press, 2005: 1050.
13. Hogl BE, Gomez-Arevalo G, Garcia S, *et al*. A clinical, pharmacologic, and polysomnographic study of sleep benefit in Parkinson's disease. *Neurology* 1998;**50**:1332–9.
14. Schenck CH, Mahowald MW. REM sleep behavior disorder: clinical, developmental, and neuroscience perspectives 16 years after its formal identification in sleep. *Sleep* 2002;**25**:120–38.
15. American Academy of Sleep Medicine. *The International Classification of Sleep Disorders : Diagnostic and Coding Manual*, 2nd edn. Westchester, IL: American Academy of Sleep Medicine, 2005.
16. Comella CL, Nardine TM, Diederich NJ, Stebbins GT. Sleep-related violence, injury, and REM sleep behavior disorder in Parkinson's disease. *Neurology* 1998;**51**:526–9.
17. Olson EJ, Boeve BF, Silber MH. Rapid eye movement sleep behaviour disorder: demographic, clinical and laboratory findings in 93 cases. *Brain* 2000;**123**(Pt 2):331–9.
18. Plazzi G, Cortelli P, Montagna P, *et al*. REM sleep behaviour disorder differentiates pure autonomic failure from multiple system atrophy with autonomic failure. *J Neurol Neurosurg Psychiatry* 1998;**64**:683–5.
19. Gagnon JF, Bedard MA, Fantini ML, *et al*. REM sleep behavior disorder and REM sleep without atonia in Parkinson's disease. *Neurology* 2002;**59**:585–9.

20. Eisensehr I, Linke R, Noachtar S, *et al.* Reduced striatal dopamine transporters in idiopathic rapid eye movement sleep behaviour disorder. Comparison with Parkinson's disease and controls. *Brain* 2000;**123**(Pt 6):1155–60.
21. Sinforiani E, Pacchetti C, Zangaglia R, *et al.* REM behavior disorder, hallucinations and cognitive impairment in Parkinson's disease: a two-year follow up. *Mov Disord* 2008;**23**:1441–5.
22. Postuma RB, Gagnon JF, Vendette M, *et al.* REM sleep behaviour disorder in Parkinson's disease is associated with specific motor features. *J Neurol Neurosurg Psychiatry* 2008;**79**: 1117–21.
23. Arnulf I, Bonnet AM, Damier P, *et al.* Hallucinations, REM sleep, and Parkinson's disease: a medical hypothesis. *Neurology* 2000;**55**:281–8.
24. Iranzo A, Molinuevo JL, Santamaria J, *et al.* Rapid-eye-movement sleep behaviour disorder as an early marker for a neurodegenerative disorder: a descriptive study. *Lancet Neurol* 2006;**5**:572–7.
25. Stiasny-Kolster K, Doerr Y, Moller JC, *et al.* Combination of "idiopathic" REM sleep behaviour disorder and olfactory dysfunction as possible indicator for alpha-synucleinopathy demonstrated by dopamine transporter FP-CIT-SPECT. *Brain* 2005;**128**:126–37.
26. Vincken WG, Gauthier SG, Dollfuss RE, *et al.* Involvement of upper-airway muscles in extrapyramidal disorders. A cause of airflow limitation. *N Engl J Med* 1984;**311**:438–42.
27. Hely MA, Reid WG, Adena MA, *et al.* The Sydney multicenter study of Parkinson's disease: the inevitability of dementia at 20 years. *Mov Disord* 2008;**23**:837–44.
28. Comella CL. Sleep disorders in Parkinson's disease: an overview. *Mov Disord* 2007;**22**(Suppl 17):S367–73.
29. Chaudhuri KR, Pal S, Brefel-Courbon C. "Sleep attacks" or "unintended sleep episodes" occur with dopamine agonists: is this a class effect? *Drug Saf* 2002;**25**:473–83.
30. Moller JC, Unger M, Stiasny-Kolster K, *et al.* Continuous sleep EEG monitoring in PD patients with and without sleep attacks. *Parkinsonism Relat Disord* 2009;**15**:238–41.
31. Happe S, Berger K. The association of dopamine agonists with daytime sleepiness, sleep problems and quality of life in patients with Parkinson's disease – a prospective study. *J Neurology* 2001;**248**:1062–7.
32. Moller JC, Rethfeldt M, Korner Y, *et al.* Daytime sleep latency in medication-matched parkinsonian patients with and without sudden onset of sleep. *Mov Disord* 2005;**20**:1620–2.
33. Chaudhuri KR, Pal S, DiMarco A, *et al.* The Parkinson's Disease Sleep Scale: a new instrument for assessing sleep and nocturnal disability in Parkinson's disease. *J Neurol Neurosurg Psychiatry* 2002;**73**:629–35.
34. Meindorfner C, Korner Y, Moller JC, *et al.* Driving in Parkinson's disease: mobility, accidents, and sudden onset of sleep at the wheel. *Mov Disord* 2005;**20**:832–42.
35. Koller WC, Hutton JT, Tolosa E, Capilldeo R. Immediate-release and controlled-release carbidopa/levodopa in PD: a 5-year randomized multicenter study. Carbidopa/Levodopa Study Group. *Neurology* 1999;**53**:1012–9.
36. Hogl B, Rothdach A, Wetter TC, Trenkwalder C. The effect of cabergoline on sleep, periodic leg movements in sleep, and early morning motor function in patients with Parkinson's disease. *Neuropsychopharmacology* 2003;**28**:1866–70.
37. Nyholm D. Pharmacokinetic optimisation in the treatment of Parkinson's disease : an update. *Clin Pharmacokinet* 2006;**45**: 109–36.
38. Mehta SH, Morgan JC, Sethi KD. Sleep disorders associated with Parkinson's disease: role of dopamine, epidemiology, and clinical scales of assessment. *CNS Spectr* 2008;**13**:6–11.
39. Paulus W, Trenkwalder C. Less is more: pathophysiology of dopaminergic-therapy-related augmentation in restless legs syndrome. *Lancet Neurol* 2006;**5**:878–86.
40. Chen JJ. Anxiety, depression, and psychosis in Parkinson's disease: unmet needs and treatment challenges. *Neurol Clin* 2004;**22**:S63–90.
41. Gordon PH, Pullman SL, Louis ED, *et al.* Mirtazapine in parkinsonian tremor. *Parkinsonism Relat Disord* 2002;**9**: 125–6.
42. Poewe W, Seppi K. Treatment options for depression and psychosis in Parkinson's disease. *J Neurol* 2001;**248**(Suppl 3):III 12–21.
43. The Parkinson Study Group. Low-dose clozapine for the treatment of drug-induced psychosis in Parkinson's disease. *N Engl J Med* 1999;**340**:757–63.
44. Rabey JM, Prokhorov T, Miniovitz A, *et al.* Effect of quetiapine in psychotic Parkinson's disease patients: a double-blind labeled study of 3 months' duration. *Mov Disord* 2007;**22**: 313–8.
45. Fernandez HH, Friedman JH, Jacques C, Rosenfeld M. Quetiapine for the treatment of drug-induced psychosis in Parkinson's disease. *Mov Disord* 1999;**14**:484–7.
46. Ondo WG, Tintner R, Voung KD, *et al.* Double-blind, placebo-controlled, unforced titration parallel trial of quetiapine for dopaminergic-induced hallucinations in Parkinson's disease. *Mov Disord* 2005;**20**:958–63.
47. Prohorov T, Klein C, Miniovitz A, *et al.* The effect of quetiapine in psychotic parkinsonian patients with and without dementia. An open-labeled study utilizing a structured interview. *J Neurol* 2006;**253**:171–5.
48. Braga-Neto P, da Silva-Junior FP, Sueli Monte F, *et al.* Snoring and excessive daytime sleepiness in Parkinson's disease. *J Neurol Sci* 2004;**217**:41–5.
49. Hogl B, Saletu M, Brandauer E, *et al.* Modafinil for the treatment of daytime sleepiness in Parkinson's disease: a double-blind, randomized, crossover, placebo-controlled polygraphic trial. *Sleep* 2002;**25**:905–9.
50. Ondo WG, Fayle R, Atassi F, Jankovic J. Modafinil for daytime somnolence in Parkinson's disease: double blind, placebo controlled parallel trial. *J Neurol Neurosurg Psychiatry* 2005;**76**:1636–9.

Chapter 22
Neuronal Mechanisms of REM Sleep and Their Role in REM Sleep Behavior Disorder

Jun Lu & Clifford B. Saper
Department of Neurology, Program in Neuroscience and Division of Sleep Medicine, Harvard Medical School and Beth Israel Deaconess Medical Center, Boston, MA, USA

Introduction

The regulation of REM (rapid eye movement) sleep was historically thought to be controlled by the interaction of brainstem monoaminergic and cholinergic neurons [1]. However, recent work has identified several additional components to the REM regulatory system, resulting in a new synthesis of REM sleep mechanisms [2,3]. These new observations have given rise to a greater understanding of the circuitry in the brainstem that is disordered during REM sleep behavior disorder (RBD) and other conditions of motor control related to REM sleep, such as cataplexy. In this chapter, we examine the underlying circuitry and then the ways in which it may be involved in different neurodegenerative disease states.

Overall control of wake–sleep switching

Early studies of the mechanism of maintaining a wakeful state used electrolytic lesions of the brainstem reticular formation to cause coma (for reviews, see [2,4]). This work gave rise to the "reticular activating system" theory by which the brainstem reticular formation was thought to activate the thalamus and hence the cerebral cortex. Subsequent studies refined this theory, to demonstrate that the waking signal actually emerges from well-characterized neurons with specific neurotransmitters in the upper brainstem, not the reticular formation, and that these neurons produce wakefulness by means of both projections to the thalamus as well as the hypothalamus, basal forebrain, and cerebral cortex (Figure 22.1). The largest source of inputs to the thalamus comes from cholinergic neurons in the pedunculopontine and laterodorsal tegmental nuclei, whereas the major source of the hypothalamic–basal forebrain–cortical pathway is monoaminergic neurons. These include the noradrenergic locus coeruleus, the serotoninergic dorsal and median raphe nuclei, dopaminergic neurons near the dorsal raphe nucleus, histaminergic neurons in the tuberomammillary nucleus in the posterior hypothalamus, and glutamatergic neurons in the parabrachial and precoeruleus areas. The last pathway is augmented by peptidergic (orexin or hypocretin) and glutamatergic neurons in the lateral hypothalamus and also by cholinergic and GABAergic basal forebrain neurons. The cholinergic input to the thalamus is most active during wakefulness and REM sleep, whereas firing in the monoaminergic system is most active during wakefulness, slows during slow wave or non-REM sleep, and stops during REM sleep. Thus, REM sleep is defined by a disparity of firing in the cholinergic system (active) and the monoaminergic system (halted).

Opposing the waking influence of the arousal system is a sleep-promoting system, including the ventrolateral preoptic nucleus (VLPO) in the hypothalamus [2]. These neurons contain the inhibitory neurotransmitters GABA and galanin, and they innervate all of the components of the ascending arousal systems so that they can turn them off in a coordinated fashion (Figure 22.2). Other sleep-promoting neurons in the median preoptic nucleus and basal forebrain probably also contribute to this response [5]. For example, neurons in the median preoptic nucleus may contribute to the accumulation of sleep pressure, with progressively greater firing during sleep deprivation to cause sleepiness. Neurons in the VLPO, by contrast, do not start firing until actual sleep onset, and so are thought to cause the actual inhibition of the arousal system that permits sleep to occur [6].

Interestingly, not only do the VLPO neurons inhibit the arousal systems, but they are also inhibited by many of the arousal systems (for a review, see [2]). The result is a mutually inhibitory interaction, which produces what electrical engineers call a "flip-flop switch" (Figure 22.3).

Parkinson's Disease: Non-Motor and Non-Dopaminergic Features, First Edition. Edited by C. Warren Olanow, Fabrizio Stocchi, and Anthony E. Lang.

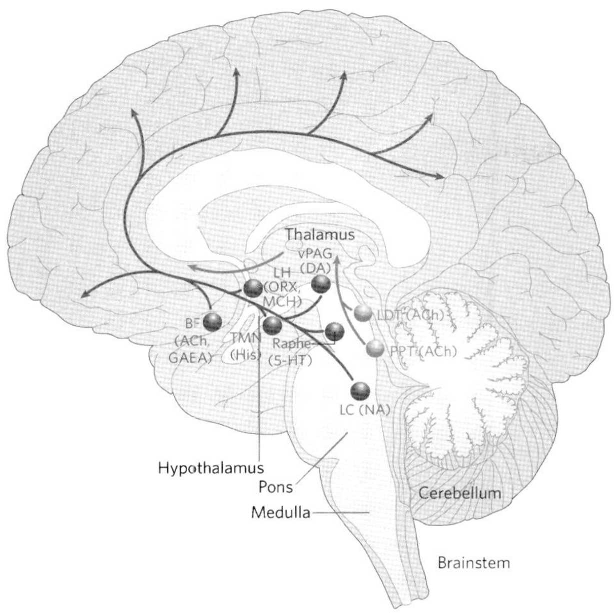

Figure 22.1 The ascending arousal system from the upper brainstem uses two main pathways. The major input to the thalamic relay and reticular nucleus originates from cholinergic neurons (Ach) in the pedunculopontine (PPT) and laterodorsal (LDT) tegmental nuclei. A second major pathway begins with monoaminergic neurons including noradrenergic (NE) neurons in the locus coeruleus (LC), serotoninergic (5-HT) neurons in the dorsal and median raphe nuclei, dopaminergic (DA) neurons in the ventral periaqueductal gray matter (vPAG), and histaminergic neurons (His) in the tuberomammillary nucleus (TMN). The axons from this pathway run through the lateral hypothalamus, where they are joined by additional inputs from the orexin (ORX) and melanin-concentrating hormone (MCH) neurons, and then run through the basal forebrain where cholinergic and GABA-containing neurons add to the pathway, which then terminates diffusely throughout the cerebral cortex. This second pathway is believed to activate cortical neurons, and both pathways are active during wakefulness. During non-REM sleep, firing in both pathways decreases. However, in REM sleep, the cholinergic neurons again fire briskly, but the monoaminergic neurons stop firing completely. The activation of thalamic transmission to a cerebral cortex that is not fully aroused is believed to be the basis for dreaming in REM sleep. Reproduced from Fuller, Gooley, and Saper [26] with permission from Nature Publishing Group.

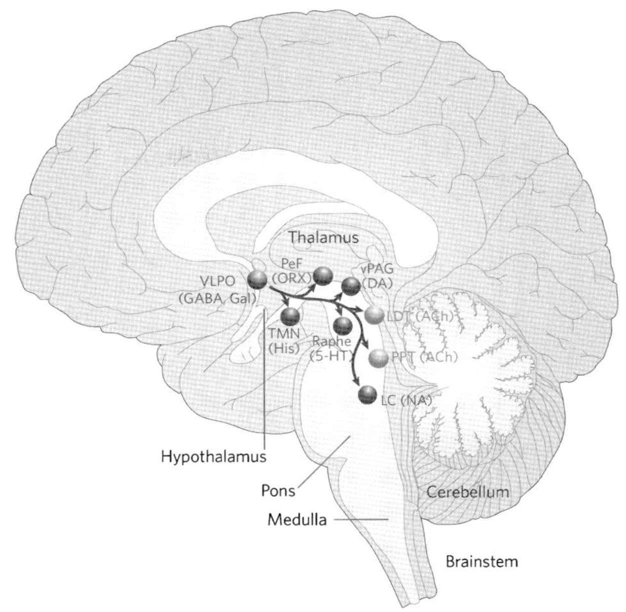

Figure 22.2 The ventrolateral preoptic nucleus (VLPO) sends descending projections containing both galanin (Gal) and GABA to the components of the ascending arousal system. Both galanin and GABA are believed to have inhibitory effects on their targets, allowing the VLPO to turn down activity broadly in the ascending arousal system like a master switch. Other abbreviations as in Figure 22.1. Reproduced from Fuller, Gooley, and Saper [26] with permission from Nature Publishing Group.

This configuration is used for circuits when the designer wants to insure rapid and complete state transitions. As one side of the switch gains ascendancy over the other, it rapidly turns the other side off, and resistance collapses. This configuration is useful for wake–sleep state transitions, where homeostatic or circadian forces would otherwise cause slow oscillation between wake and sleep states, resulting in individuals spending most of their lives in a half-asleep state, which would not be adaptive, for example, in finding food or avoiding predators. As a result, mammalian brains have evolved flip-flop switches to insure that minimal time is spent in state switching, and the individual is almost always either awake or asleep.

One problem with flip-flop switches is that they can occasionally be activated at the wrong time, which could also have negative consequences (e.g., falling asleep if one became slightly bored while driving). As a result, the mammalian brain contains a secondary system, using the orexin (also called hypocretin) family of neuropeptides, that activate neurons on the waking side of the switch [2]. The result, which is predictable from mathematical models of flip-flop switches, is that the switch is stabilized in both states (i.e., there is enhancement of consolidated wakefulness, resulting in the accumulation of sufficient homeostatic sleep drive to cause consolidated sleep as well). We now understand that the disorder of narcolepsy is due to loss of most of the orexin neurons. The result is that the switch becomes destabilized in both states (i.e., narcoleptics not only fall asleep too easily when awake, but they wake up too often during sleep). This instability in both states is a mathematically predictable outcome from weakening one side of a flip-flop switch.

REM sleep state switching

The identification of the cholinergic and monoaminergic brainstem neuronal systems, and the effects of cholinergic

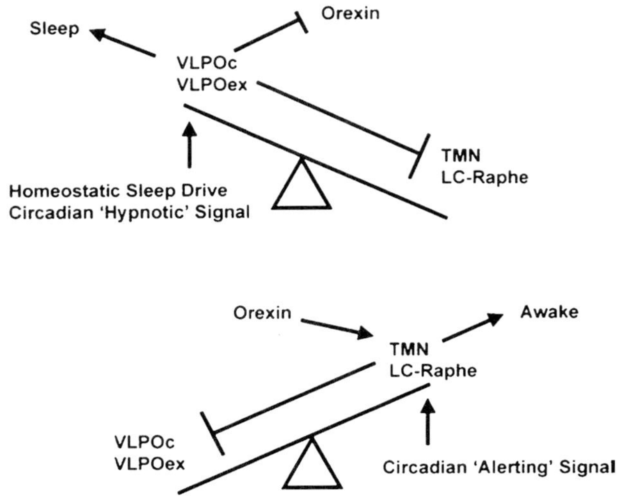

Figure 22.3 A summary drawing of the wake–sleep flip-flop switch. During wakefulness, the monoaminergic neurons in the ascending arousal system (TMN, LC, raphe) inhibit the VLPO neurons, whereas during sleep the VLPO inhibits the arousal system neurons. This mutual inhibition sets up the conditions for a flip-flop switch, which makes more rapid and complete transitions than would be the case as the homeostatic and circadian drives change much more slowly and gradually. However, such a switch can sometimes make unwanted transitions (such as falling asleep too easily while driving). The orexin neurons provide an additional component to the system that reinforces the waking state. Mathematical models demonstrate that by adding additional weight to the wake side of the switch, the switch is stabilized in both positions. Removal of the orexin neurons in narcolepsy destabilizes the switch, so that patients not only fall asleep too often when they are awake, but wake up too often when they are asleep. Abbreviations as in Figures 22.1 and 22.2. Reproduced from Fuller, Gooley, and Saper [26] with permission from Nature Publishing Group.

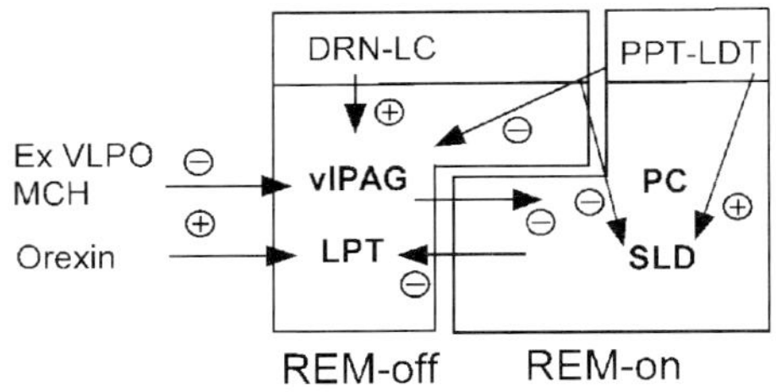

Figure 22.4 A model for a REM sleep state switch. The ventrolateral periaqueductal gray matter (vlPAG) and lateral pontine tegmentum (LPT) contain GABAergic REM-off neurons that inhibit REM sleep. They project to the nearby REM-on area, consisting of neurons in the sublaterodorsal nucleus (SLD) and precoeruleus area (PC) that drive REM sleep. GABAergic neurons in the SLD project back to inhibit the REM-off neurons during REM sleep. As a result, this mutually inhibitory relationship forms a flip-flop switch, ensuring rapid transitions from non-REM to REM sleep and back. Other inputs that regulate REM sleep may do so by modulating the switching neurons. For example, the GABAergic neurons in the extended VLPO and the melanin-concentrating hormone (MCH) neurons in the lateral hypothalamus may activate REM sleep by inhibiting the REM-off population, while the orexin neurons may prevent REM sleep by activating the same target. The serotoninergic neurons in the dorsal raphe nucleus (DRN) and noradrenergic neurons in the locus coeruleus (LC) appear to project to both sides of the switch, but are likely to excite the REM-off neurons and inhibit the REM-on neurons, as they prevent REM sleep. Cholinergic neurons in the pedunculopontine (PPT) and laterodorsal (LDT) tegmental nuclei also project to both sides of the REM switch, but are likely to have the opposite effects as monoamines, as injections of muscarinic agonist drugs increase REM sleep. Modified from Lu *et al.* [8].

and monoaminergic drugs, led early theorists to hypothesize that there was an inhibitory interaction between cholinergic and monoaminergic systems [1,7]. This model was driven by the observation that drugs such as anti-depressants, which decrease the reuptake of norepinephrine, serotonin, or both, reduce the amount of time spent in REM sleep, whereas injection of cholinergic agonists into the pontine tegmentum causes a REM-like state. However, there are problems with this model, not the least of which is that lesions of neither the monoaminergic nor the cholinergic cell groups have much effect on the amount of REM sleep achieved [2]. In other words, the presence of either type of neurotransmitter can influence or modulate REM sleep, but neither is necessary to drive it.

Recently, Lu *et al.* proposed a somewhat different model [8], based upon their own work and that of the groups of Luppi [9] and Sakai [10], which hypothesizes that REM state switching involves mutually inhibitory GABAergic interactions (Figure 22.4). By following the output from the inhibitory neurons in the VLPO that promote REM sleep, they identified a target area at the junction of the midbrain and pons that is adjacent to the dorsal raphe nucleus and just rostral to the laterodorsal and pedunculopontine tegmental nuclei [2]. This area contains presumably inhibitory REM-off neurons that inhibit the firing of REM-on neurons. When these neurons, located in the ventrolateral periaqueductal gray matter (vlPAG) and lateral pontine tegmentum (LPT), are inhibited with muscimol, animals enter a REM-like state. The GABAergic neurons in the vlPAG and LPT send their axons to a nearby region, which in rats and mice is ventral to the laterodorsal tegmental nucleus [and hence is called the sublaterodorsal nucleus (SLD)] and in cats and humans is ventral to the locus coeruleus (LC, hence the subcoeruleus area, SLC, or LC pars alpha). SLD neurons are predominantly active during REM sleep, and activating these neurons with glutamate agonists or disinhibiting them with bicuculline [10,11] produces REM-like states. The SLD in turn was found to contain GABAergic neurons that sent their axons back to the vlPAG-LPT. This mutual GABAergic, inhibitory interaction sets up the conditions for a REM flip-flop switch (Figure 22.4).

We believe that this flip-flop switch may be the main REM switching mechanism. The influence of the cholinergic and monoaminergic systems may, therefore, be predominantly on this GABA–GABA mutually inhibitory switch. We initially posited that cholinergic neurons may inhibit the vlPAG-LPT, as injections of carbachol at this level of the brainstem result in continuous REM sleep in cats. Monoaminergic neurons may also act on these neurons, to reinforce their firing and thus prevent REM states. However, it is also possible that these neurotransmitters may have the opposite effects on the REM-on neurons, and it is likely that these powerful modulators do both (see Figure 22.4).

REM atonia systems

Embedded within both the REM-on and REM-off GABAergic populations are glutamatergic neurons, which may be the effector neurons, as both populations of neurons project directly to the spinal cord [8]. The REM-off glutamatergic neurons in the LPT appear to target motor neurons directly (J. Lu and C.B. Saper, unpublished observations; see Figure 22.5). This input may support motor tone in addition to locomotion, as injections of excitatory drugs into the LPT cause animals to walk. These neurons may represent the long-sought midbrain locomotor region, a site first identified in decerebrate cats where electrical stimulation would cause locomotion on a treadmill.

In contrast, the REM-on glutamatergic neurons in the SLD also project to the brainstem and spinal cord, but they terminate on inhibitory interneurons, which are thought to project to motor neurons [8]. This pathway is thought to provide the motor inhibition during REM sleep. However, the withdrawal of glutamatergic motor tone from silencing of the LPT may also play a major role in REM atonia [12].

A dominant theory in the past was that the excitatory neurons in the subcoeruleus area would target mainly inhibitory interneurons in the medial medullary reticular formation to cause atonia [13]. However, cell-specific lesions in the medial medullary reticular formation in both rats and cats fails to block REM atonia [8,14]. Although the GABA and glycinergic motor inhibitory neurons in the medial medulla may, in fact, contribute to REM atonia, they are not necessary for it to occur. In addition, glutamatergic neurons in the medial medullary reticular formation may target spinal interneurons (J. Lu, unpublished observations), providing a fourth pathway for reinforcing REM atonia (see Figure 22.5).

Pathologic conditions of the REM atonia system

The destabilization of the REM atonia system in patients with narcolepsy who lose the orexin neurons has been

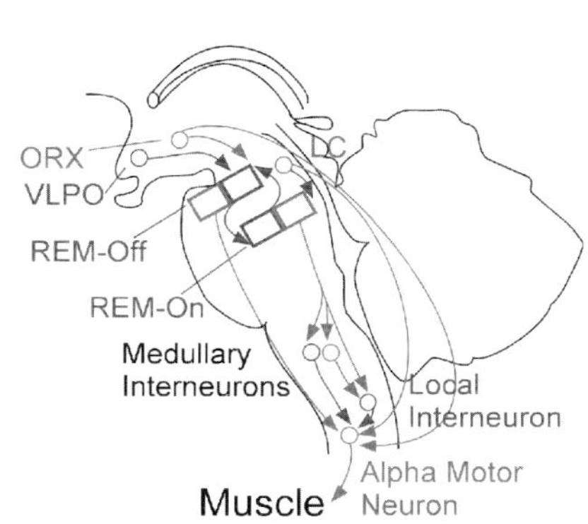

Figure 22.5 A summary diagram illustrating the proposed REM switch and its relationship to pathways that regulate motor tone. The heart of the REM switch is represented by two populations of mutually inhibitory GABAergic neurons (represented in black) in the upper pons, one of which is REM-off and the other REM-on. The REM-off neurons are inhibited by the ventrolateral preoptic nucleus (VLPO, also black because they are inhibitory) to induce REM sleep and excited by the orexin neurons (in gray) to prevent onset of REM onset directly from wakefulness. Orexin neurons also project directly to alpha motor neurons, and provide excitatory tone during waking states. Each side of the REM switch also contains excitatory glutamatergic neurons (represented in gray). The REM-off glutamatergic neurons project directly to motor neurons in the spinal cord and increase motor tone. These neurons are also important for motor tone during waking states. The loss of this excitatory input during REM sleep contributes to atonia. At the same time, the glutamatergic neurons in the REM-on area send descending projections to the medulla and spinal cord that ultimately activate inhibitory interneurons (black) projecting to alpha motor neurons. Thus, when the REM-on pathway is firing, there is active hyperpolarization of motor neurons. In addition, the locus coeruleus (LC) noradrenergic neurons are REM-off cells that inhibit the glutamatergic REM-on cells during non-REM states, and also provide excitatory drive to motor neurons. Withdrawal of this input during REM sleep may also contribute to the maintenance of atonia.

hinted at above. Not only is the main wake–sleep flip-flop switch destabilized, but also the REM switch (for a review, see [2]). Because the REM atonia neurons are a separate population from those that produce other features of REM sleep (dreaming, eye movements), they may be activated separately in patients with narcolepsy. The occurrence of REM atonia during waking is called cataplexy, and is one of the most disturbing features of the disease.

The problem in REM behavior disorder is essentially the opposite: damage to the REM atonia system allows the emergence of motor behaviors during REM sleep [8]. A similar condition has been produced in animals by lesions of the SLD in rodents [8] or SLC in cats [15,16]. This state is sometimes called "REM without atonia," but this term is really an oversimplification. Like patients with RBD, the animals actually do go into atonia most of the time during REM sleep. However, they intermittently show large motor jerks, similar to myoclonic jerks, and occasionally will express more complete behaviors, which are usually lunges or fighting behaviors in rodents. More complex behaviors such as the mouse-hunting behavior that has been recorded in cats [15,16] are not seen in rats or mice. Recordings of humans with RBD in the sleep laboratory show that the individuals do go into an atonic state during REM sleep but break out of it intermittently for predominantly brief episodes of motor activity, with lunges, striking out, and sometimes more complete violent or fighting behaviors also. However, complex behavioral sequences, such as are seen in cats with subcoeruleus lesions, are rarely seen in the sleep laboratory setting. Reports of such behaviors in other settings are complicated by the possibility that they may represent other parasomnias, such as sleepwalking, which occur mainly during non-REM states. The patient with REM behavior disorder, when awakened following an episode of motor activity, generally reports a very vivid and often violent dream, and the content of the dream often matches the physical activity that was observed. The reason why these behaviors are most commonly fragmentary, and why they are typically so violent, is not yet understood.

However, the similarity of "REM without atonia" in animals and RBD in humans has suggested that this disorder in humans is due to the loss of SLC neurons that are involved in producing the atonic response. Several case reports in humans show RBD associated with lesions in the SLC area [17]. However, this hypothesis remains a conjecture, as no pathologic examination of the brain has confirmed the location of the lesion with respect to the REM atonia cell groups in humans, nor has a good marker for glutamatergic neurons in humans been available. {Staining of neurons with antisera against the vesicular glutamate transporter 2 (VGLUT2) has been reported in human brainstem [18], but in our hands this staining does not match the distribution of VGLUT2 mRNA patterns in other species, and no VGLUT2 antiserum that we have tested will reliably stain neuronal cell bodies in other species.}

RBD is also distinguished by a high proportion of the patients eventually developing Parkinson's disease (PD) [19]. Studies by several different groups indicate that about 50% of idiopathic RBD patients will develop PD by 10–15 years after diagnosis of RBD [20,21]. Interestingly, this proportion keeps increasing with time, and has reached 80% in the University of Minnesota series by 20–25 years (C.H. Schenk and M.W. Mahowald, personal communication). These observations suggest that idiopathic RBD in most cases is a pre-morbid marker for PD, but that the motor disorder may be delayed by decades. These exciting observations may give movement disorder doctors the opportunity to study the early development of PD, and perhaps to prevent the later motor manifestations.

The early onset of RBD compared with motor signs in PD is consistent with the observations by Braak *et al.* that PD may begin in the brainstem and gradually ascend with time, in most cases not reaching the level of motor symptoms until about midway through the disease [22]. The SLC is lower in the brainstem than the substantia nigra, and is said by Braak *et al.* to contain α-synuclein deposits along with the locus coeruleus in stage II–III. It is not yet clear whether the α-synuclein deposition reported in the SLC is in glutamatergic neurons that cause REM atonia, but this would be an important hypothesis to investigate.

Is the hypertonia and gait disorder of Parkinson's disease caused by disinhibiting the LPT?

The extrapyramidal motor system is generally thought to contain a descending branch from the internal segment of the globus pallidus and substantia nigra pars reticularis that innervates the pedunculopontine tegmental nucleus. This branch is thought to have a relationship with postural tone and gait. The basis for this claim comes from early work by Nauta and Mehler [23], who thought that the descending pallidal projection in monkeys terminated near the pedunculopontine nucleus. More detailed tracer studies by Rye *et al.* in rats [24] and by Shink, Sidibe, and Smith in monkeys [25], however, show that the descending extrapyramidal projection does *not* innervate the pedunculopontine cholinergic neurons, but instead terminates in a region just ventromedial to the cholinergic neurons, which Rye *et al.* called the midbrain extrapyramidal area (MEA). The MEA is a hypocellular region, occupied by relatively small interneurons, whose connections are not known. Just medial and ventral to the MEA is the LPT, however, which contains a dense population of spinally projecting glutamatergic neurons.

Studies by Lu and colleagues suggest that it is these LPT glutamatergic neurons, which are not only REM-off, but tone-on neurons, that may play a key role as a link in the extrapyramidal system (J. Lu, D. Sherman, P.M. Fuller, and C.B. Saper, unpublished observations). This site is immediately adjacent to the pedunculopontine tegmental nucleus and the MEA, and hence electrodes placed in the "pedunculopontine tegmental nucleus" for deep brain stimulation in PD patients, almost certainly can access all three areas. It will be very important to identify clearly the actual sites of stimulation in these patients, so the relative contributions of these cell groups to motor tone, and its improvement with deep brain stimulation, can be sorted out.

Note added in proof: For a more extensive review of sleep switch circuitry and mathematical modeling, see: Saper CB, Fuller PM, Pedersen NP, Lu J, Scammell TE. Sleep state switching. *Neuron* 2010;**68**:1023–42.

References

1. McCarley RW. Neurobiology of REM and NREM sleep. *Sleep Med* 2007;**8**:302–330.

2. Saper CB, Scammell TE, Lu J. Hypothalamic regulation of sleep and circadian rhythms. *Nature* 2005;**437**:1257–63.
3. Sapin E, Lapray D, Berod A, *et al.* Localization of the brainstem GABAergic neurons controlling paradoxical (REM) sleep. *PLoS ONE* 2009;**4**:e4272.
4. Posner JB, Saper CB, Schiff ND, Plum F. *Plum and Posner's Diagnosis of Stupor and Coma*, 4th edn. New York: Oxford University Press, 2008.
5. Gvilia I, Xu F, McGinty D, Szymusiak R. Homeostatic regulation of sleep: a role for preoptic area neurons. *J Neurosci* 2006;**26**:9426–33.
6. Szymusiak R, Alam N, Steininger TL, McGinty D. Sleep–waking discharge patterns of ventrolateral preoptic/anterior hypothalamic neurons in rats. *Brain Res* 1998;**803**:178–88.
7. Pace-Schott EF, Hobson JA. The neurobiology of sleep: genetics, cellular physiology and subcortical networks. *Nat Rev Neurosci* 2002;**3**:591–605.
8. Lu J, Sherman D, Devor M, Saper CB. A putative flip-flop switch for control of REM sleep. *Nature* 2006;**441**:589–94.
9. Boissard R, Fort P, Gervasoni D, *et al.* Localization of the GABAergic and non-GABAergic neurons projecting to the sublaterodorsal nucleus and potentially gating paradoxical sleep onset. *Eur J Neurosci* 2003;**18**:1627–39.
10. Crochet S, Onoe H, Sakai K. A potent non-monoaminergic paradoxical sleep inhibitory system: a reverse microdialysis and single-unit recording study. *Eur J Neurosci* 2006;**24**: 1404–12.
11. Boissard R, Gervasoni D, Schmidt MH, *et al.* The rat ponto-medullary network responsible for paradoxical sleep onset and maintenance: a combined microinjection and functional neuroanatomical study. *Eur J Neurosci* 2002;**16**:1959–73.
12. Burgess C, Lai D, Siegel J, Peever J. An endogenous glutamatergic drive onto somatic motoneurons contributes to the stereotypical pattern of muscle tone across the sleep–wake cycle. *J Neurosci* 2008;**28**:4649–60.
13. Morales FR, Sampogna S, Yamuy J, Chase MH. c-fos expression in brainstem premotor interneurons during cholinergically induced active sleep in the cat. *J Neurosci* 1999;**19**:9508–18.
14. Sastre JP, Sakai K, Jouvet M. Are the gigantocellular tegmental field neurons responsible for paradoxical sleep? *Brain Res* 1981;**229**:147–61.
15. Morrison AR. Paradoxical sleep without atonia. *Arch Ital Biol* 1988;**126**:275–90.
16. Sastre JP, Jouvet M. Oneiric behavior in cats. *Physiol Behav* 1979;**22**:979–89 (in French).
17. Boeve BF, Silber MH, Saper CB, *et al.* Pathophysiology of REM sleep behaviour disorder and relevance to neurodegenerative disease. *Brain* 2007;**130**:2770–88.
18. Benarroch EE, Schmeichel AM, *et al.* Depletion of putative chemosensitive respiratory neurons in the ventral medullary surface in multiple system atrophy. *Brain* 2007;**130**:469–75.
19. Mahowald MW. Does "idiopathic" REM sleep behavior disorder exist? *Sleep* 2006;**29**:874–5.
20. Schenck CH, Bundlie SR, Mahowald MW. Delayed emergence of a parkinsonian disorder in 38% of 29 older men initially diagnosed with idiopathic rapid eye movement sleep behaviour disorder. *Neurology* 1996;**46**:388–93.
21. Postuma RB, Gagnon JF, Vendette M, *et al.* Quantifying the risk of neurodegenerative disease in idiopathic REM sleep behavior disorder. *Neurology* 2009;**72**(25):1296–300.
22. Braak H, Del Tredici K, Rub U, *et al.* Staging of brain pathology related to sporadic Parkinson's disease. *Neurobiol Aging* 2003;**24**:197–211.
23. Nauta WJ, Mehler WR. Projections of the lentiform nucleus in the monkey. *Brain Res* 1966;**1**:3–42.
24. Rye DB, Saper CB, Lee HJ, Wainer BH. Pedunculopontine tegmental nucleus of the rat: cytoarchitecture, cytochemistry, and some extrapyramidal connections of the mesopontine tegmentum. *J Comp Neurol* 1987;**259**:483–528.
25. Shink E, Sidibe M, Smith Y. Efferent connections of the internal globus pallidus in the squirrel monkey: II. Topography and synaptic organization of pallidal efferents to the pedunculopontine nucleus. *J Comp Neurol* 1997;**382**:348–63.
26. Fuller PM, Gooley JJ, Saper CB. Neurobiology of the sleep–wake cycle: sleep architecture, circadian regulation, and regulatory feedback. *J Biol Rhythms* 2006;**21**:482–93.

Chapter 23
REM Sleep Behavior Disorder and Neurodegenerative Disorders

Mark W. Mahowald, Carlos H. Schenck, & Michel A. Cramer Bornemann
Minnesota Regional Sleep Disorders Center and Hennepin County Medical Center, University of Minnesota Medical School, Minneapolis, MN, USA

Introduction

Rapid eye movement (REM) sleep behavior disorder (RBD) is one of the most common parasomnias, which are undesirable experiential or motor phenomena arising from the sleep period. Parasomnias can conveniently be divided into two major categories: those representing abnormalities of sleep states *per se*, and those due to abnormalities of various organ systems taking advantage of the sleep state to declare themselves. The primary sleep parasomnias can be divided into three categories: those arising from non-rapid eye movement (NREM) sleep such as disorders of arousal (confusional arousals, sleepwalking, or sleep terrors), those arising from REM sleep [REM sleep behavior disorder (RBD)], and those not respecting sleep states such as head-banging, bruxism, and enuresis. The secondary sleep parasomnias may be classified by the organ system involved such as central nervous system (nocturnal seizures) [1]. RBD is the most common primary REM sleep parasomnia and typically presents with violent and potentially injurious complex motor behaviors arising from the sleep period.

RBD was predicted by animal experiments in 1965: cats with bilateral perilocus coeruleus lesions demonstrated prominent motor activity during REM sleep [2]. The cat animal model has been extended to the rat [3]. The persistence of muscle tone during REM sleep is termed REM sleep without atonia (RWA).

Demographics

The prevalence of RBD is greater than initially suspected. A recent telephone survey of over 4900 individuals between the ages of 15 and 100 years indicated an overall prevalence of violent behaviors in general during sleep of 2%, one-quarter of which were likely due to RBD, giving an overall prevalence of RBD of 0.5% [4]. Another survey estimated the prevalence of REM sleep behavior to be 0.38% in elderly individuals [5].

Clinical features

The typical complaint of a patient with RBD is violent dream-enacting behaviors which are potentially injurious to the individual or bed partner [6,7]. There are acute and chronic forms of RBD. Acute RBD is almost always induced by medications [most commonly tricyclic antidepressants, monoamine oxidase inhibitors (MAOIs), and serotonin-specific reuptake inhibitors (SSRIs)] or associated with withdrawal (alcohol, barbiturates, and meprobamate) [6,8]. The chronic form of RBD has two striking demographic characteristics: it is overwhelmingly a disorder affecting older individuals (above age 50) and men (80–90%), although females and virtually all age groups may be affected [9,10]. One-quarter of patients have a prodrome, often lengthy, involving subclinical behavioral release during sleep. Few patients with RBD have histories of childhood sleepwalking or sleep terrors.

RBD most frequently presents with the complaint of dramatic, violent, potentially injurious motor activity during sleep. These behaviors include talking, yelling, swearing, grabbing, punching, kicking, jumping, and running out of the bed. Injuries to the individual or bed partner are not uncommon and include ecchymoses, lacerations, and fractures. The violence of the sleep-related behavior is often discordant with the waking personality. The increased aggressive dream content experienced by patients with RBD is not associated with increased daytime aggressiveness [11]. The reported motor activity usually correlates with remembered dream mentation, leading to the complaint of "acting out my dreams." Less

Parkinson's Disease: Non-Motor and Non-Dopaminergic Features, First Edition. Edited by C. Warren Olanow, Fabrizio Stocchi, and Anthony E. Lang.

frequently, the primary complaint is one of sleep interruption. The duration of behaviors is generally brief, and upon awakening from an episode there is usually a rapid return of alertness and orientation. Some patients adopt extraordinary measures to prevent injury during sleep: they may tether themselves to the bed with a rope or belt, sleep in sleeping bags, or sleep on a mattress on the floor in a room without furniture. RBD behaviors occur *within* REM sleep, often without associated tachycardia, and not during arousals from REM sleep. Complex RBD behaviors are generally aggressive or exploratory, and never appetitive (feeding, sexual). Despite the impressive behavioral and EMG motor activity, few patients with RBD complain of excessive sleep disruption and daytime fatigue.

Due to its association with REM sleep, the timing of the behaviors during the sleep period ranges from 90 min after sleep onset to the final awakening in the morning. RBD rarely occurs during daytime naps in that REM sleep during naps is exceptional. There may be a prodromal period lasting years or decades of progressively more prominent sleep talking, yelling, or limb jerking during sleep. Many patients with RBD report that dreams have become more vivid and "action packed" coincident with the onset of the dream-enacting behavior. The frequency of the episodes ranges from once every few weeks to multiple nightly episodes [12]. Complications include fractures, lacerations, ecchymoses, and subdural hematomas [9,13]. Sleep-related violence may have forensic science implications [14].

Case example: RBD and parkinsonism

A 58-year-old happily married man without psychiatric history presented with his wife with a 7-year history of throwing himself out of bed during sleep and hurting himself and his wife while acting-out "crazy dreams." His dreams had become more vivid, intense, and "nasty" with dreamed passers-by on the street suddenly confronting him, making derogatory comments, grabbing him, throwing punches, kicking him, and pulling out weapons while threatening to kill him. His wife noticed that most nights he was moving his arms, legs, and body during sleep. During his dream enactments, he would shout, pound the mattress, punch his wife, leap out of bed, and run around the room. These episodes became more frequent (3–5 nights weekly) over time, and always began at least 2 h after falling asleep. He usually awakened rapidly from these episodes, and immediately would be fully oriented and report a dream. His wife was aware that he was acting completely out-of-character from his typical, pleasant, daytime personality. Several months before presenting to the sleep center, the patient noticed that he was starting to have problems buttoning his shirt, his balance and gait were becoming unsteady, and he had a shuffling gait. When he turned around, it was becoming more of a "military" maneuver ("en bloc" movements), with rigidity and loss of his usual fluid movements. He smiled less, hardly blinked his eyes any more, and seemed to have a much less expressive face. A resting tremor was not observed, however. A neurologist diagnosed Parkinson's disease (PD), and initiated therapy with levodopa, which rapidly ameliorated some of his PD symptoms, but without any suppression of his dream-enacting behaviors at night. There was no history of alcohol or substance abuse, and he had never been treated with anti-depressants or other psychotropic medications. His Epworth Sleepiness Scale score of 9 was normal. His Mini Mental State Examination score was 30/30.

The patient was studied at a hospital-based sleep laboratory while not taking any medication. The polysomnographic (PSG) recording was accompanied by continuous, time-synchronized audio-visual monitoring, with a sleep technologist in continuous attendance. Abnormal findings occurred only in REM sleep, with prominent loss of submental electromyographic (EMG) atonia during all four REM sleep periods, accompanied by frequent bursts of high-voltage, phasic EMG twitching, with gross limb movements and complex behaviors. Whenever the sleep technologist entered his room during these behaviors, he rapidly became alert and oriented, and reported dreaming just before awakening. The dreams "were my typical dreams that I have at home, people becoming instant terrorists, attacking me or chasing me on a street, and I have to fight back or run for my life." Clinical sleep-disordered breathing was not detected during the PSG study (AHI <4 per hour), and no clinical or EEG seizure-like activity was detected.

The patient was treated with clonazepam, 0.5 mg at bedtime, and at 1 month follow-up the patient and his wife reported full control of complex and violent dream-enacting behaviors, with only minimal limb jerking persisting that was of no clinical importance.

Pathophysiology

Wakefulness, REM sleep, and NREM sleep are each associated with a number of physiologic variables that usually occur in concert to produce a fully declared state. REM sleep contains two types of variables: tonic (occurring throughout the REM period) and phasic (occurring intermittently during an REM period). Tonic elements include a desynchronized EEG and somatic muscle atonia (sparing the diaphragm). Phasic REM elements include rapid eye movements, middle ear muscle activity, and extremity twitches.

Somatic muscle atonia is one of the defining characteristics of REM sleep. The supraspinal mechanisms responsible for REM atonia originate in the perilocus coeruleus-alpha nucleus in the pons that excite neurons of the nucleus reticularis magnocellularis in the medulla, which then transmit descending inhibitory projections – more powerful than the competing descending excitatory projections – to the spinal alpha motoneurons, resulting in hyperpolarization and thence muscle atonia. This atonia is felt to be mediated by glycine [15] and may be influenced by medullary enkephalinergic neurons [16]. (The prevailing hypothesis that REM atonia is due to glycinergic inhibition has recently been questioned [17].) Therefore, "REM atonia" represents an active paralysis involving specific neuronal circuitry, and not passive relaxation of somatic muscles (sparing the diaphragm, permitting respiration during REM sleep). During normal REM sleep, the motor system is paralyzed at the level of the spinal motoneurons, but highly activated at higher levels of the neuraxis [15]. Loss of muscle tone during REM sleep is very complex, and has been shown to be due to a combination of activation of brainstem motor inhibitory systems and inactivation of brainstem facilitatory systems [18,19]. Multiple areas of the brainstem may influence muscle tone during REM sleep [18]. Sleep–wake states may oscillate rapidly or their component physiologic variables may become dissociated. In rare patients, the dissociation may be so severe that, polygraphically, sleep–wake states cannot be differentiated at all [20–22].

In RBD, the REM sleep state is incomplete: all elements are present except the atonia, permitting motor activity to occur that parallels dream mentation generated by the activated REM sleep state. The observed motor activity may result from either impairment of tonic REM muscle atonia or from increased phasic locomotor drive during REM sleep. Although the original animal model was produced with lesions of the locus coeruleus region, it is clear from later animal studies that the atonia of REM sleep is determined or influenced by a number of brainstem regions [23,24]. In animal studies, the degree of aggression associated with RWA may be influenced by additional lesions of the nervous system [25].

However, loss of REM atonia is alone insufficient to permit complex behaviors during REM sleep. Presumably, there must also be disinhibition of motor pattern generators in the mesencephalic locomotor region to result in over-excitation of phasic motor activity with behavioral release during REM [26]. Studies in dogs by Lai and Siegel revealed a co-localization of the atonia and locomotor systems of REM sleep in the pons, providing an anatomic basis for the simultaneous dysregulation of these two systems in RBD [27]. Animal models suggest that abnormalities at multiple levels of the central nervous system may produce RWA and RBD (i.e., mice lacking the histamine H3 receptor [28] and cats with neurotoxic lesions of the ventral mesopontine junction [29]).

Neuroimaging studies indicate dopaminergic abnormalities in RBD. SPECT studies have found reduced striatal dopamine transporters [30,31], and decreased striatal dopaminergic innervation has been reported [32]. Decreased blood flow in the upper portion of the frontal lobe and pons has been reported [33], as has functional impairment of brainstem neurons [34]. PET and SPECT studies have revealed decreased nigrostriatal dopaminergic projections in patients with multiple system atrophy and RBD [35]. Decreased blood flow in the upper portion of the frontal lobe and pons has been found in one MRI and SPECT study [33]. Impaired cortical activation as determined by electroencephalographic spectral analysis in patients with idiopathic RBD supports the relationship between RBD and neurodegenerative disorders [36].

[^{123}I]MIBG cardiac scintigraphy assesses the function of adrenergic neurons and may serve to differentiate among various neurodegenerative conditions. Cardiac [^{123}I}MIBG findings are similar among idiopathic RBD and the syndromes of PD and dementia with Lewy bodies, and are different from those with progressive supranuclear palsy and multiple system atrophy [37].

One intriguing explanation for the dissociation of behavior from consciousness has been proposed by Tassinari *et al.*, who suggested that the behaviors are generated by locomotor centers (LMCs) released during REM sleep [38]. This dissociation of the LMCs from the parent state of REM or NREM sleep would explain the presence of complex motor behavior seen in both RBD and disorders of arousal.

Epidemiology and associated conditions

The chronic form of RBD is idiopathic in 25–60% of occurrences. The remainder are associated with various degenerative neurologic disorders, most notably with the synucleinopathies [PD (including juvenile PD)], dementia with Lewy body disease, multiple system atrophy (Shy–Drager syndrome, striatonigral degeneration, olivopontocerebellar degeneration), and pure autonomic failure [39–42].

Systematic study of patients with neurologic syndromes indicates that RBD and RWA may be far more prevalent than previously suspected. Initially, the chronic form of RBD was felt to be predominantly idiopathic; however, systematic longitudinal monitoring of patients with RBD suggests that up to two-thirds will eventually manifest symptoms of neurodegenerative disorders, most notably the synucleinopathies. RBD often precedes the appearance of other symptoms of these disorders by more than a decade [43–53].

Combined animal and human studies have identified physiologic and anatomic links between RBD and neurodegenerative disorders, leading to the proposal that neurodegeneration can begin in either the rostroventral midbrain or the ventral mesopontine junction and progressively extend to the rostral or caudal part of the brainstem. When the lesion starts in the ventral mesopontine region, RBD will develop first, but when the lesion initially involves the rostroventral midbrain, PD will be the initial manifestation [54]. A recent study in which lesions of the ventral mesopontine junction, which is proximate to the substantia nigra, resulted in RWA in the cat suggests a link between RBD and PD [55]. The fact that severity of loss of cholinergic pedunculopontine tegmental/laterodorsal tegmental nuclei neurons in dementia with Lewy bodies and multiple system atrophy do not correlate with the presence or absence of RBD suggests that other mechanisms are involved [56].

Although the prevalence of RBD in PD is unknown, subjective reports indicate that 25% of patients with PD have behaviors suggestive of RBD or sleep-related injurious behaviors, and PSG studies found RBD in up to 47% of patients with PD with sleep complaints [57–60]. In one large series of patients with multiple system atrophy (MSA), 90% were found to have RWA and 69% had clinical RBD [61]. In another, nearly half had RBD [62]. The presence of RBD may differentiate pure autonomic failure from MSA with autonomic failure [63]. The finding of incidental Lewy body disease in one patient asymptomatic for PD suggests that this condition may explain idiopathic RBD in some older patients [64]. The presentation of RBD and dementia is suggestive enough of dementia with Lewy body disease that RBD has been proposed as one of the core diagnostic features of dementia with Lewy body disease [65]. Selegiline or mirtazapine prescribed for patients with PD and cholinergic agents for Alzheimer's disease may trigger RBD in these populations [66–69].

The link between PD and RBD is supported by the fact that impaired olfactory and color discrimination is common to both [70,71]. Also, the possible presence of cognitive deficits and slowing in the waking electroencephalogram in idiopathic RBD share common features with dementia with Lewy body disease [72–74]. RBD is also seen in non-synucleinopathy-related PD, in Guadeloupian parkinsonism, and progressive supranuclear palsy (tauopathies) [75–77]. The clinical features of RBD are identical in the idiopathic cases and in those with PD or multiple system atrophy [78]. Interestingly, there is a striking (77%) male predominance in patients with PD who display RBD [79]. To date, no reliable tests have been shown to identify which subgroup of patients with idiopathic RBD is prone to develop PD [80]. In longitudinal studies, the frequency of RBD in patients with PD varied over time and was associated with male sex, less parkinsonism, and higher levodopa equivalent dose [81]. RBD has been found to be more common in non-tremor-predominant PD and to precede the appearance of PD when the PD began after the age of 50 years [82].

The waking motor impairments of PD may improve or even normalize during REM sleep-related movements in PD RBD patients. In a study of 53 patients with PD RBD who slept with bed partners, 100% reported improvement of at least one of the following during RBD episodes: faster, stronger, or smoother movements; more intelligible, louder, or better articulated speech; or normalization of facial expression. Furthermore, 38% of bed partners reported that movements were "much better" even in the most disabled PD patients. The responsible mechanisms for these fascinating observations remain obscure [83].

Other reported associations include mitochondrial encephalomyopathy, normal pressure hydrocephalus, Tourette's syndrome, Machado–Joseph disease (spinocerebellar ataxia type 3), cerebellopontine angle tumors, group A xeroderma, multiple sclerosis, ischemic or hemorrhagic cerebrovascular disease, focal brain lesions, autism, Mobius syndrome, voltage-gated potassium channel autoimmunity, and Guillain–Barré syndrome [84–99]. RBD is present in over half of cases of narcolepsy, may be an early feature in childhood cases, and may even be the presenting feature [100–104]. Furthermore, tricyclic anti-depressants, MAOIs, and SSRIs, prescribed to treat cataplexy, can trigger or exacerbate RBD in this population. The demographics (age and sex) of RBD in narcolepsy conform to those of narcolepsy, indicating that RBD in these patients is yet another manifestation of state boundary dyscontrol seen in narcolepsy [105]. The recent description of low levels of ventricular CSF orexin/hypocretin levels and orexin/hypocretin cell loss in PD may provide an interesting link between the increased prevalence of RBD in both narcolepsy and PD and may help explain the hypersomnia [106–108]. Cases of narcolepsy with RBD due to inflammatory lesions of the brain add further support to the relationship between these two disorders [109,110]. An interesting aside is that the olfactory discrimination abnormality seen early in patients with RBD who are likely to develop a synucleinopathy is also present in patients with narcolepsy-associated RBD [111,112]. The demographics of RBD in narcolepsy are strikingly different from those in "idiopathic" ("cryptogenic") RBD, namely, much younger individuals with equal sex representation [102]. Furthermore, narcolepsy is not generally considered to be a neurodegenerative disorder. Ongoing monitoring of these patients may be very interesting.

The overwhelming male predominance of RBD (not seen in the associated neurodegenerative disorders) raises the intriguing question of hormonal influences, as suggested in male aggression studies in both animals and humans [113–115]. Another possible explanation for the male predominance is sex differences in brain development and aging [116–118]. There is evidence for a sex difference on the effects of sex steroids on the development of the locus coeruleus in rats [119]. However, serum sex hormone levels are normal in idiopathic RBD or RBD associated with PD [120,121].

Diagnosis (clinical and laboratory evaluation)

A detailed review of the sleep–wake complaints should be followed by a medical, neurologic, and psychiatric history and examination. Information from a bed partner is most valuable. As it is often impossible to differentiate RBD from other parasomnias by history alone, formal PSG study is mandatory. Such PSG studies must be more extensive than those performed for many other sleep disorders, with an expanded EEG montage, monitors for movements of all four extremities, continuous technologist observation, and audiovisual recording. Periodic leg movements are more frequent in RBD [122]. A PSG scoring system for RBD in neurodegenerative disorders has been developed and automated programs for assessment are under development [123–126].

Diagnostic criteria are (1) history of problematic sleep behavior (or videotaped documentation of such behavior), (2) polygraphic evidence of excessive augmentation of chin electromyogram tone or of excessive chin or limb electromyogram twitching, and (3) absence of seizure activity on the EEG. Other common findings include a high percentage of slow-wave sleep and frequent periodic and aperiodic extremity movements during NREM sleep [12]. A single night of recording is generally sufficient to establish the diagnosis, because REM sleep PSG abnormalities are usually present even when a behavioral episode does not occur [127,128]. Typical PSG findings are shown in Figure 23.1.

Additional neurologic or psychiatric evaluations such as CT or MRI brain scans, waking EEG, evoked potential studies, and neuropsychologic tests are warranted only if there is evidence by history or examination suggesting a psychiatric disorder or a structural abnormality of the central nervous system.

Regardless of sex, age, or presence/absence of an underlying neurologic disorder, the PSG and behavioral features of RBD are indistinguishable. This suggests the presence of a final common pathway in RBD that can be accessed by a wide variety of pathologic states. It is important to remember that RBD is a clinical syndrome associated with a characteristic PSG finding – RWA. Finding RWA on a PSG recording does not necessarily mean that the patient has clinical RBD. RWA without the clinical symptoms of dream-enacting behaviors may be seen in many other conditions, including narcolepsy and neurodegenerative disorders such as PD and MSA, or may be a medication effect (particularly with SSRIs and tricyclic anti-depressants) [105,129,130].

Differential diagnosis

Differential diagnosis includes sleepwalking, sleep terrors, nocturnal seizures, psychogenic dissociative states, post-traumatic stress disorder, nocturnal panic disorder, delirium, and malingering. Confusional arousals with behaviors that may mimic RBD can occur with nocturnal seizures, obstructive sleep apnea, sleep-related gastroesophageal reflux, or periodic limb movement disorder [131–134]. Previously undiagnosed RBD occurring in a patient in the intensive care unit may be particularly difficult to diagnose [135].

Treatment

The acute form of RBD is self-limited following discontinuation of the offending medication or completion of withdrawal. About 90% of patients with chronic RBD respond well to clonazepam administered 30 min prior to sleep time. The dose ranges from 0.5 to 2.0 mg, and there has been little, if any, tendency to develop tolerance, dependence, abuse, or adverse sleep effects despite years of continuous administration and efficacy [136,137]. Interestingly, despite a dramatic clinical response to clonazepam, polygraphically there is little change in the muscle tone during REM sleep following effective treatment [138]. Clearly, clonazepam does not restore REM atonia. Melatonin at doses up to 12 mg at bedtime or pramipexole may also be effective [139–142]. Although tricyclic anti-depressants may sometimes induce or potentiate RBD, imipramine has been reported to be effective in three clonazepam-resistant cases [143]. Likewise, there are reports of response to an SSRI (paroxetine) [144,145]. Carbamazepine has been effective in one case report [146]. Levodopa may be effective, particularly in cases where RBD is the harbinger of PD [147]. There have been anecdotal reports of response to gabapentin, MAOIs, donepezil, and clonidine [148,149]. In RBD associated with narcolepsy, the tricyclic anti-depressants or MAOIs administered for cataplexy may be continued, and clonazepam added [105]. The treatment of medication-induced or PD-associated RBD is the same as for idiopathic RBD [44]. Pallidotomy has been effective in one case of RBD associated with PD, whereas chronic bilateral subthalamic stimulation was not [150–152]. Interestingly, an isolated episode of RBD has been reported immediately following left subthalamic electrode implantation for the treatment of PD [153]. Underlying obstructive sleep apnea should be ruled out before prescribing clonazepam [154]. The treatment of PD-associated RBD

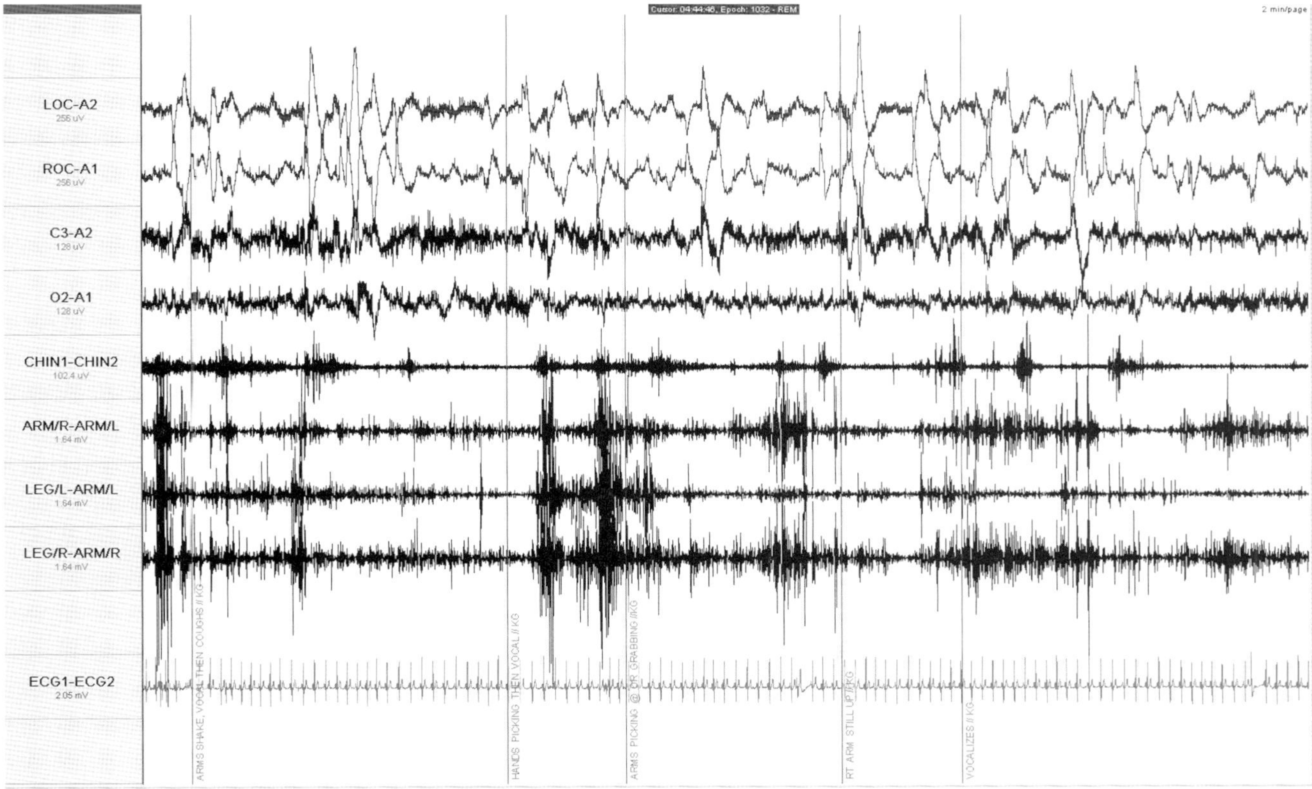

Figure 23.1 Two minute epoch of REM sleep in a patient with RBD and Parkinson's disease. Note the prominent increased tonic and phasic EMG activity of the submental, arm, and leg muscles associated with motor activity and vocalizations. LOC, left outer canthus; ROC, right outer canthus; C3, left central EEG; O2, right occipital EEG; A1, left mastoid; A2, right mastoid; chin, submental EMG; arm, extensor digitorum EMG; leg, anterior tibialis EMG; ECG, electrocardiogram.

is the same as for idiopathic RBD [155]. Interestingly, there may be spontaneous improvement in RBD symptoms with progression of the underlying neurodegenerative condition [156].

RBD variations

A likely related condition is "agrypnia excitata," a recently described syndrome characterized by generalized overactivity associated with loss of slow-wave sleep, mental oneiricism (inability to initiate and maintain sleep with wakeful dreaming), and marked motor and autonomic sympathetic activation seen in such diverse conditions as delirium tremens, Morvan's fibrillary chorea, and fatal familial insomnia [157–160]. Oneiric dementia is likely a related condition [161]. Agrypnia excitata is similar to "status dissociatus," which may be the most extreme form of RBD, appearing to represent the complete breakdown of state-determining boundaries. The abnormal motor and verbal nocturnal behaviors of status dissociatus may respond to treatment with clonazepam [20,21].

Perspectives

Systematic sequential follow-up of patients with RBD revealed that for many, if not most, the initial symptom of dream-enacting behaviors was a harbinger of a neurodegenerative disorder, particularly the synucleinopathies – especially PD – often preceding and predicting other symptoms by many years. With continued follow-up, the percentage of RBD patients developing neurodegenerative conditions continues to grow, leading to the suggestion that the term "idiopathic RBD" be abandoned for "cryptogenic RBD" – the implication being that if RBD patients are followed long enough, the underlying culprit will eventually declare itself [162].

Our concept of neurodegenerative disorders is changing, aided by new diagnostic techniques. There is mounting evidence that in some neurodegenerative conditions, changes in neurologic function are actually identifiable years if not decades before the more classical clinical manifestation. PD is an excellent example. Subtle changes in a number of areas (sleepiness, visual discrimination, olfactory discrimination, EEG slowing, neurocognitive decline, cerebral blood flow, autonomic function, depression, and RBD) may be present years before the appearance of tremor, bradykinesia, rigidity, and postural instability [39,71,163–169]. This would stand to reason, as the idea that PD is due to a pure dopamine deficiency is patently overly simplistic. The true PD pathology involves diverse parts of the nervous system, likely beginning in the medullary and olfactory bulb regions, with abnormalities of numerous neurotransmitters and neuropeptide systems [170,171]. Lai and Siegel offered speculation as to why some patients may present with one symptom and others with different symptoms [54]. The complexity and vagaries of PD are such that it has recently been suggested that it be thought of as a "centrosympathomyenteric neuronopathy" [172]. One haunting unanswered question is: why are individuals with neurodegenerative disorders who exhibit RBD overwhelmingly male, when the underlying disorders affect both sexes equally? RBD, often induced by commonly prescribed medications (particularly SSRIs), is now commonplace [173]. This raises the interesting if not worrisome question: is medication-induced RBD a harbinger of things to come?

Conclusion

In summary, RBD is an REM sleep-related parasomnia, presenting with potentially violent or injurious behaviors. "Idiopathic" RBD is becoming progressively scarce (and may cease to exist) as more patients with RBD are being thoroughly evaluated and followed. Drug-induced RBD is becoming increasingly common, and non-drug-induced RBD is clearly very often a harbinger of a developing neurodegenerative condition – particularly a synucleinopathy. Oneiric symptoms reminiscent of RBD should lead to closer scrutiny of sleep in other neurologic conditions [158,174]. Rigorous study of these relationships affords an exciting opportunity for basic scientists and sleep medicine clinicians to expand our understanding of both sleep and neurologic function.

References

1. Mahowald MW, Ettinger MG. Things that go bump in the night – the parasomnias revisited. *J Clin Neurophysiol* 1990;**7**:119–43.
2. Jouvet M, Delorme F. Locus coeruleus et sommeil paradoxal. *C R Seances Soc Biol Filiales* 1965;**159**:895–9.
3. Sanford LD, Cheng CS, *et al.* Sleep and behavior in rats with pontine lesions producing REM without atonia. *Sleep Res Online* 2001;**4**:1–5.
4. Ohayon MM, Caulet M, *et al.* Violent behavior during sleep. *J Clin Psychiatry* 1997;**58**:369–76.
5. Chiu HFK, Wing YK, *et al.* Sleep-related injury in the elderly – an epidemiological study in Hong Kong. *Sleep* 2000;**23**:513–7.
6. Schenck CH, Mahowald MW. REM sleep behavior disorder: clinical, developmental, and neuroscience perspectives 16 years after its formal identification in sleep. *Sleep* 2002;**25**:120–30.
7. Olson EJ, Boeve BF, *et al.* Rapid eye movement sleep behaviour disorder: demographic, clinical and laboratory findings in 93 cases. *Brain* 2000;**123**:331–9.
8. Parish JM. (2007) Violent dreaming and anti-depressant drugs: or how paroxetine made me dream that I was fighting Saddam Hussein. *J Clin Sleep Med* **3**, 529–31.
9. Schenck CH, Hurwitz TD, *et al.* REM sleep behavior disorder: a report on a series of 96 consecutive cases and a review of the literature. *J Sleep Res* 1993;**2**:224–31.
10. Sheldon SH, Garey A, *et al.* REM-sleep motor disorder in children. *Sleep Res* 1994;**23**:173.
11. Fantini ML, Corona A, *et al.* Increased aggressive dream content without increased daytime aggressiveness in REM sleep behavior disorder. *Neurology* 2005;**65**:1010–5.
12. Mahowald MW, Schenck CH. REM sleep behavior disorder. In: Kryger MH, Dement W, Roth T, eds. *Principles and Practice of Sleep Med*, 2nd edn. Philadelphia: Saunders, 1994: 574–88.
13. Dyken ME, Lin-Dyken DC, *et al.* Violent sleep-related behavior leading to subdural hemorrhage. *Arch Neurol* 1995;**52**:318–21.
14. Cramer Bornemann MA, Mahowald MW, *et al.* Parasomnias. Clinical features and forensic implications. *Chest* 2006;**130**:605–10.
15. Lopez-Rodriguez F, Kohlmeier K, *et al.* State dependency of the effects of microinjection of cholinergic drugs into the nucleus pontalis oralis. *Brain Res* 1994;**649**:271–81.
16. Fort P, Rampon C, *et al.* Anatomical demonstration of a medullary enkephalinergic pathway potentially implicated in the oro-facial muscle atonia of paradoxical sleep in the cat. *Sleep Res Online* 1998;**1**:102–8.
17. Brooks PL, Peever JH. Glycinergic and $GABA_A$-mediated inhibition of somatic motoneurons does not mediate rapid eye movement sleep motor atonia. *J Neurosci* 2008;**28**: 3535–45.
18. Mileykovskiy BY, Kiyashchenko LI, *et al.* Activation of pontine medullary motor inhibitory regions reduces discharge in neurons located in the locus coeruleus and the anatomical equivalent of the midbrain locomotor region. *J Neurosci* 2000;**20**:8551–8.
19. Mileykovskiy BY, Kiyashchenko LI, *et al.* Cessation of activity in red nucleus neurons during stimulation of medial medulla in decerebrate rats. *J Physiol* 2002;**543**:997–1006.
20. Mahowald MW, Schenck CH. Status dissociatus - a perspective on states of being. *Sleep* 1991;**14**:69–79.
21. Mahowald MW, Schenck CH. Dissociated states of wakefulness and sleep. *Neurology* 1992;**42**:44–52.
22. Mahowald MW, Schenck CH. Evolving concepts of human state dissociation. *Arch Ital Biol* 2001;**139**:269–300.
23. Lai YY, Siegel JM. Muscle tone suppression and stepping produced by stimulation of midbrain and rostral pontine reticular formation. *J Neurosci* 1990;**10**:2727–34.
24. Schenkel E, Siegel JM. REM sleep without atonia after lesions of the medial medulla. *Neurosci Lett* 1989;**98**:159–65.
25. Zagrodzka J, Hedberg CE, *et al.* Contrasting expressions of aggressive behavior released by lesions of the central nucleus of the amygdala during wakefulness and rapid

eye movement sleep without atonia in cats. *Behav Neurosci* 1998;**112**:589–602.

26. Morrison AR. Paradoxical sleep without atonia. *Arch Ital Biol* 1988;**126**:275–289.
27. Lai YY, Siegel JM. Medullary regions mediating atonia. *J Neurosci* 1988;**8**:4790–4796.
28. Dugovic C, Koehl M, *et al.* Sleep in mice lacking the histamine H3 receptor. A putative genetic animal model for REM sleep behavior disorder. *Sleep* 2002;**25**(Abstr Suppl):A114.
29. Lai Y, Shalita T, *et al.* Neurotoxic lesions of the ventral mesopontine junction induces hypersomnia and muscle hyperactivity during sleep – an animal model of PLMD and RBD. *Sleep* 2002; **25**(Abstr Suppl):A62.
30. Eisensehr I, Linke R, *et al.* Reduced striatal dopamine transporters in idiopathic rapid eye movement sleep behavior disorder. Comparison with Parkinson's disease and controls. *Brain* 2000;**123**:1155–60.
31. Eisensehr I, Linke R, *et al.* Increased muscle activity during rapid eye movement sleep correlates with decrease of striatal presynaptic dopamine transporters. IPT and IBZM SPECT imaging in subclinical and clinically manifest idiopathic REM sleep behavior disorder, Parkinson's disease, and controls. *Sleep* 2003;**26**:507–12.
32. Albin RL, Koeppe RA, *et al.* Decreased striatal dopaminergic innervation in REM sleep behavior disorder. *Neurology* 2000;**55**:1410–2.
33. Shirakawa S-I, Takeuchi N, *et al.* Study of image findings in rapid eye movement sleep behavioral disorder. *Psychiatry Clin Neurosci* 2002;**56**:291–2.
34. Miyamoto M, Miyamoto T, *et al.* Brainstem function in rapid eye movement sleep behavior disorder: the evaluation of brainstem function by proton MR spectroscopy (^{1}H-MRS). *Psychiatry Clin Neurosci* 2000;**54**:350–1.
35. Gilman S, Koeppe RA, *et al.* REM sleep behavior disorder is related to striatal monoaminergic deficit in MSA. *Neurology* 2003;**61**:29–34.
36. Fantini ML, Gagnon JF, *et al.* Slowing of electroencephalogram in rapid eye movement sleep behavior disorder. *Ann Neurol* 2003;**53**:774–80.
37. Miyamoto T, Miyamoto M, *et al.* Reduced cardiac ^{123}I-MIBG scintigraphy in idiopathic REM sleep behavior disorder. *Neurology* 2006;**67**:2236–8.
38. Tassinari CA, Rubboli G, *et al.* Central pattern generators for a common semiology in fronto-limbic seizures and in parasomnias. A neuroethologic approach. *Neurol Sci* 2005;**26**:s225-s232.
39. Gagnon J-F, Postuma RB, *et al.* Rapid-eye-movement sleep behaviour disorder and neurodegenerative diseases. *Lancet Neurol* 2006;**5**:424–32.
40. Iranzo A, Molinuevo JL, *et al.* Rapid-eye-movement sleep behavior disorder as an early marker for neurodegenerative disorder: a descriptive study. *Lancet Neurol* 2006;**5**: 572–7.
41. Weyer A, Minnerop M, *et al.* REM sleep behavioral disorder in pure autonomic failure (PAF). *Neurology* 2006;**66**:608–9.
42. Kashihara K, Ohno M, *et al.* Frequent nocturnal vocalization in pure autonomic failure. *J Int Med Res* 2008;**36**:489–95.
43. Boeve BF, Silber MH, *et al.* Association of REM sleep behavior disorder and neurodegenerative disease may reflect an underlying synucleinopathy. *Mov Disord* 2001;**16**:622–30.
44. Schenck CH, Bundlie SR, *et al.* Delayed emergence of a parkinsonian disorder in 38% of 29 older men initially diagnosed with idiopathic rapid eye movement sleep behavior disorder. *Neurology* 1996;**46**:388–93.
45. Kimura K, Tachibana N, *et al.* Subclinical REM sleep behavior disorder in a patient with corticobasal degeneration. *Sleep* 1997;**20**:891–4.
46. Tachibana N, Kimura K, *et al.* REM sleep without atonia at early stage of sporadic olivopontocerebellar atrophy. *J Neurol Sci* 1995;**132**:28–34.
47. Tachibana N, Kimura K, *et al.* REM sleep motor dysfunction in multiple system atrophy. *Sleep Res* 1995;**24A**:415.
48. Tison F, Wenning GK, *et al.* REM sleep behavior disorder as the presenting symptom of multiple system atrophy. *J Neurol Neurosurg Psychiatry* 1995;**58**:379–80.
49. Turner RS, Chervin RD, *et al.* Probable diffuse Lewy body disease presenting as REM sleep behavior disorder. *Neurology* 1997;**49**:523–7.
50. Pareja JA, Caminero AB, *et al.* A first case of progressive supranuclear palsy and pre-clinical REM sleep behavior disorder presenting as inhibition of speech during wakefulness and somniloquy with phasic muscle twitching during REM sleep. *Neurologia* 1996;**11**:304–6.
51. Montplaisir J, Petit D, *et al.* Sleep and quantitative EEG in patients with progressive supranuclear palsy. *Neurology* 1997;**49**:999–1003.
52. Boeve BF, Silber MH, *et al.* Synucleinopathy pathology often underlies REM sleep behavior disorder and dementia or parkinsonism. *Neurology* 2003;**61**:40–5.
53. Boeve BF, Silber MH, *et al.* Pathophysiology of REM sleep behavior disorder and relevance to neurodegenerative disease. *Brain* 2007;**130**:2770–88.
54. Lai Y-Y, Siegel JM. Physiological and anatomical link between Parkinson-like disease and REM sleep behavior disorder. *Mol Neurobiol* 2003;**27**:137–51.
55. Lai Y-Y, Hsieh K-C, *et al.* Neurotoxic lesions at the ventral mesopontine junction change sleep time and muscle activity durng sleep: an animal model of motor disorders in sleep. *Neuroscience* 2008;**154**:431–43.
56. Schmeichel AM, Buchhalter LC, *et al.* Mesopontine cholinergic neuron involvement in Lewy body dementia and multiple system atrophy. *Neurology* 2008;**70**:368–73.
57. Comella CL, Nardine TM, *et al.* Sleep-related violence, injury, and REM sleep behavior disorder in Parkinson's disease. *Neurology* 1998;**51**:526–9.
58. Eisensehr I, von Lindeiner H, *et al.* REM sleep behavior disorder in sleep-disordered patients with versus without Parkinson's disease: is there a need for polysomnography? *J Neurol Sci* 2001;**186**:7–11.
59. Gagnon J-F, Bedard M-A, *et al.* REM sleep behavior disorder and REM sleep without atonia in Parkinson's disease. *Neurology* 2002;**59**:585–9.
60. Scaglione C, Vignatelli L, *et al.* REM sleep behaviour disorder in Parkinson's disease: a questionnaire-based study. *Neurol Sci* 2005;**25**:316–21.
61. Plazzi G, Corsini R, *et al.* REM sleep behavior disorders in multiple system atrophy. *Neurology* 1997;**48**:1094–7.
62. Ghorayeb I, Yekhlef F, *et al.* Sleep disorders and their determinants in multiple system atrophy. *J Neurol Neurosurg Psychiatry* 2002;**72**:798–800.

63. Plazzi G, Cortelli P, *et al.* REM sleep behavior disorder differentiates pure autonomic failure from multiple system atrophy with autonomic failure. *J Neurol Neurosurg Psychiatry* 1998;**64**:683–5.
64. Uchiyama M, Isse K, *et al.* Incidental Lewy body disease in a patient with REM sleep behavior disorder. *Neurology* 1995;**45**:709–12.
65. Ferman TJ, Boeve BF, *et al.* Dementia with Lewy bodies may present as dementia and REM sleep behavior disorder without parkinsonism or hallucinations. *J Int Neuropsychol Soc* 2002;**8**:904–14.
66. Louden MB, Morehead MA, *et al.* Activation by selegiline (Eldepryle) of REM sleep behavior disorder in parkinsonism. *W Virginia Med J* 1995;**91**:101.
67. Carlander B, Touchon J, *et al.* REM sleep behavior disorder induced by cholinergic treatment in Alzheimer's disease. *J Sleep Res* 1996;**5**(Suppl 1):28.
68. Ross JS, Shua-Haim JR. Aricept-induced nightmares in Alzheimer's disease: 2 case reports. *J Am Geriatr Soc* 1998; **46**:119–20.
69. Onofrj M, Luciano AL, *et al.* Mirtazapine induces REM sleep behavior disorder (RBD) in parkinsonism. *Neurology* 2003;**60**:113–5.
70. Staisny-Kolster K, Doerr Y, *et al.* Combination of "idiopathic" REM sleep behaviour disorder and olfactory dysfunction as possible indicator for alpha-synucleinopathy demonstrated by dopamine transporter FP-CIT-SPECT. *Brain* 2005;**128**: 126–37.
71. Postuma RB, Lang AE, *et al.* Potential early markers of Parkinson disease in idiopathic REM sleep behavior disorder. *Neurology* 2006;**66**:845–51.
72. Terzaghi M, Sinforiani E, *et al.* Cognitive performance in REM sleep behaviour disorder: a possible early marker of neurodegenerative disease? *Sleep Med* 2008;**9**:343–51.
73. Postuma RB, Gagno J-F, *et al.* Cognition in REM sleep behavior disorder – a window into preclinical dementia? *Sleep Med* 2008;**9**:341–2 (Editorial).
74. Massicotte-Marquez J, Decary A, *et al.* Executive dysfunction and memory impairment in idiopathic REM sleep behavior disorder. *Neurology* 2008;**70**:1250–7.
75. Kumru H, Santamaria J, *et al.* Rapid eye movement sleep behavior disorder in Parkinsonism with *PARKIN* mutations. *Ann Neurol* 2004;**56**:599–603.
76. Arnulf I, Merino-Andreu M, *et al.* REM sleep behavior disorder and REM without atonia in patients with progressive supranuclear palsy. *Sleep* 2005;**28**:349–54.
77. Cochen De Cock V, Lannuzel A, *et al.* REM sleep behavior disorder in patients with Guadeloupean parkinsonism, a tauopathy. *Sleep* 2007;**30**:1026–32.
78. Iranzo A, Santamaria J, *et al.* Characteristics of idiopathic REM sleep behavior disorder and that associated with MSA and PD. *Neurology* 2005;**65**:247–52.
79. Ozekmekci S, Apaydin H, *et al.* Clinical features of 35 patients with Parkinson's disease displaying REM sleep behavior disorder. *Clin Neurol Neurosurg* 2005;**107**:306–9.
80. Unger MM, Moller JC, *et al.* Assessment of idiopathic rapid-eye-movement sleep disorder by transcranial sonography, olfactory function test, and FP-CIT-SPECT. *Mov Disord* 2008;**23**:596–9.
81. Gjerstad MD, Boeve B, *et al.* Occurrence and clinical correlates of REM sleep behaviour disorder in patients with Parkinson's disease over time. *J Neurol Neurosurg Psychiatry* 2008;**79**:387–91.
82. Kumru H, Santamaria J, *et al.* Relation between subtype of Parkinson's disease and REM sleep behavior disorder. *Sleep Med* 2008;**8**:779–83.
83. De Cock VC, Vidailhet M, *et al.* Restoration of normal motor control in Parkinson's disease during REM sleep. *Brain* 2007;**130**:450–6.
84. Bianchin MM, Ferreira NP, *et al.* Dissociated sleep components in a patient with a pontomesencephalic astrocytoma. *Ann Neurol* 1997;**42**:470 (Abstract).
85. Plazzi G, Montagna P. Remitting REM sleep behavior disorder as the initial sign of multiple sclerosis. *Sleep Med* 2002;**3**:437–9.
86. Nozawa T, Sato Y, *et al.* Polygraphic findings in mitochondrial encephalo-myopathy. *Sleep Res* 1995;**24A**:403.
87. Uchiyama M, Tanaka K, *et al.* REM sleep behavior disorder in a case with normal pressure hydrocephalus. *Jpn J Psychiatry Neurol* 1991;**45**:935–6.
88. Trajanovic NN, Shapiro CM, *et al.* REM sleep behavior disorder in patients with Tourette's syndrome. *Sleep Res* 1997;**26**:524.
89. Kohyama J, Shimohira M, *et al.* Motor disturbance during REM sleep in group A xeroderma pigmentosum. *Acta Neurol Scand* 1995;**92**:91–5.
90. Fukutake T, Shinotoh H, *et al.* Homozygous Machado–Joseph disease presenting as REM sleep behaviour disorder and prominent psychiatric symptoms. *Eur J Neurol* 2002;**9**:97–100.
91. Zambelis T, Paparrigopoulos T, *et al.* REM sleep behavior disorder associated with a neurinoma of the left pontocerebellar angle. *J Neurol Neurosurg Psychiatry* 2002;**72**:821–2.
92. Kimura K, Tachibana N, *et al.* A discrete pontine ischemic lesion could cause REM sleep behavior disorder. *Neurology* 2000;**55**:894–5.
93. Thirumalai SS, Shubin RA, *et al.* Rapid eye movement sleep behavior disorder in children with autism. *J Child Neurol* 2002;**17**:173–8.
94. Friedman JH. Presumed rapid eye movement behavior disorder in Machado–Joseph disease (spinocerebellar ataxia type 3). *Mov Disord* 2002;**17**:1350–3.
95. Syed BH, Rye DB, *et al.* REM sleep behavior disorder and SCA-3 (Machado–Joseph disease). *Neurology* 2003;**60**: 148.
96. Anderson K, Shneerson J, *et al.* Mobius syndrome in association with the REM sleep behaviour disorder. *J Neurol Neurosurg Psychiatry* 2007;**78**:659–60.
97. Iranzo A, Aparicio J. A lesson from anatomy: focal brain lesions causing REM sleep behavior disorder. *Sleep Med* 2009;**10**:9–12.
98. Xi Z, Luning W. REM sleep behavior disorder in a patient with pontine stroke. *Sleep Med* 2009;**10**:143–6.
99. Iranzo A, Graus F, *et al.* Rapid eye movement sleep behavior disorder and potassium channel antibody-associated limbic encephalitis. *Ann Neurol* 2005;**59**:178–82.
100. Bonakis A, Howard RS, *et al.* Narcolepsy presenting as REM sleep behaviour disorder. *Clinical Neurol Neurosurg* 2008;**110**:518–20.

101. Mattarozzi K, Bellucci C, *et al.* Clinical, behavioural and polysomnographic correlates of cataplexy in patients with narcolepsy/cataplexy. *Sleep Med* 2008;**9**:425–33.
102. Nightingale S, Orgill JC, *et al.* The association between narcolepsy and REM behavior disorder (RBD). *Sleep Med* 2005;**6**:253–8.
103. Dauvilliers Y, Rompre S, *et al.* REM sleep characteristics in narcolepsy and REM sleep behavior disorder. *Sleep* 2007;**30**:844–9.
104. Nevsimalova S, Prihodova I, *et al.* REM sleep behavior disorder (RBD) can be one of the first symptoms of childhood narcolepsy. *Sleep Med* 2007;**8**:784–6.
105. Schenck CH, Mahowald MW. Motor dyscontrol in narcolepsy: rapid-eye-movement (REM) sleep without atonia and REM sleep behavior disorder. *Ann Neurol* 1992;**32**:3–10.
106. Thannickal TC, Lai Y-Y, *et al.* Hypocretin (orexin) cell loss in Parkinson's disease. *Brain* 2007;**130**:1586–95.
107. Fronczek R, Overeem S, *et al.* Hypocretin (orexin) loss in Parkinson's disease. *Brain* 2007;**130**:1577–85.
108. Drouot X, Moutereau S, *et al.* Low levels of ventricular CSF orexin/hypocretin in advanced PD. *Neurology* 2003;**61**:540–3.
109. Compta Y, Iranzo A, *et al.* REM sleep behavior disorder and narcoleptic features in anti-Ma2-associated encephalitis. *Sleep* 2007;**30**:767–9.
110. Mathis J, Hess CJ, *et al.* Isolated mediotemporal lesion causing narcolepsy and rapid eye movement sleep behaviour disorder; a case evidencing a common pathway in narcolepsy and rapid eye movement sleep behaviour disorder. *J Neurol Neurosurg Psychiatry* 2007;**78**:427–9.
111. Stiasny-Kolster K, Doerr Y, *et al.* Combination of "idiopathic" REM sleep behavior disorder and olfactory dysfunction as possible indicator for alpha-synucleinopathy demonstrated by dopamine transporter FP-CIT-SPECT. *Brain* 2005;**128**:126–37.
112. Stiasny-Kolster K, Clever S-C, *et al.* Olfactory dysfunction in patients with narcolepsy with and without REM sleep behavior disorder. *Brain* 2007;**130**:442–9.
113. Goldstein M. Brain research and violent behavior. *Arch Neurol* 1974;**30**:1–34.
114. Moyer KE. Kinds of aggression and their physiological basis. *Commun Behav Biol* 1968;**2** (Pt A), 65–87.
115. Ramirez JM. Hormones and aggression in childhood and adolescence. *Aggression Violent Behav* 2003;**8**:621–44.
116. Coffey CE, Licke JF, *et al.* Sex differences in brain aging. A quantitative magnetic resonance imaging study. *Arch Neurol* 1998;**55**:169–79.
117. Patwardhan AJ, Eliez S, *et al.* Brian morphology in Klinefelter syndrome. *Neurology* 2000;**54**:2218–23.
118. Cosgrove KP, Mazure CM, *et al.* Evolving knowledge of sex differences in brain structure, function, and chemistry. *Biol Psychiatry* 2007;**62**:847–55.
119. Guillamon A, de Blas MR, *et al.* Effects of sex steroids on the development of the locus coeruleus in rats. *Dev Brain Res* 1988;**40**:306–10.
120. Iranzo A, Santamaria J, *et al.* Absence of alterations in serum sex hormone levels in idiopathic REM sleep behavior disorder. *Sleep* 2007;**30**:803–6.
121. Chou KL, Moro-de-Casillas ML, *et al.* Testosterone not associated with violent dreams or REM sleep behavior disorder in men with Parkinson's. *Mov Disord* 2007;**22**:411–4.
122. Manconi M, Ferri R, *et al.* Time structure analysis of leg movements during sleep in REM sleep behavior disorder. *Sleep* 2007;**30**:1779–85.
123. Consens FB, Chervin RD, *et al.* Validation of a polysomnographic score for REM sleep behavior disorder. *Sleep* 2005;**28**:993–7.
124. Burns JW, Consens FB, *et al.* EMG variance during polysomnography as an assessment for REM sleep behavior disorder. *Sleep* 2007;**30**:1771–8.
125. Mayer G, Kesper K, *et al.* Quantification of tonic and phasic muscle activity in REM sleep behavior disorder. *J Clin Neurophysiol* 2008;**25**:48–55.
126. Ferri R, Manconi M, *et al.* A quantitative statistical analysis of the submentalis muscle EMG amplitude during sleep in normal controls and pateints with REM sleep behavior disorder. *J Sleep Res* 2008;**17**:89–100.
127. Zhang J, Lam SP, *et al.* Diagnosis of REM sleep behavior disorder by video-polysomnographic study: is one night enough? *Sleep* 2008;**31**:1179–85.
128. Bliwise DL, Rye DB. Elevated PEM (phasic electromyographic metric) rates identify rapid eye movement behavior disorder patients on nights without behavioral abnormalities. *Sleep* 2008;**31**:853–7.
129. Schenck CH, Mahowald MW, *et al.* Prominent eye movements during NREM sleep and REM sleep behavior disorder associated with fluoxetine treatment of depression and obsessive–compulsive disorder. *Sleep* 1992;**15**:226–35.
130. Schutte S, Doghramji K. REM behavior disorder seen with venlafaxine (Effexor). *Sleep Res* 1996;**25**:364.
131. D'Cruz OF, Vaughn BV. Nocturnal seizures mimic REM behavior disorder. *Am J Electroneurodiagn Technol* 1997;**37**:258–64.
132. Mahowald MW, Schenck CH. Parasomnia purgatory – the epileptic/non-epileptic interface. In: Rowan AJ, Gates JR, eds. *Non-Epileptic Seizures*, 2nd edn. Boston: Butterworth-Heinemann, 2000: 71–94.
133. Nalamalapu U, Goldberg R, *et al.* Behaviors simulating REM behavior disorder in patients with severe obstructive sleep apnea. *Sleep Res* 1996;**25**:311.
134. Iranzo A, Santamaria J. Severe obstructive sleep apnea/hypopnea mimicking REM sleep behavior disorder. *Sleep* 2005;**28**:203–6.
135. Schenck CH, Mahowald MW. Injurious sleep behavior disorders (parasomnias) affecting patients on intensive care units. *Intens Care Med* 1991;**17**:219–24.
136. Schenck CH, Mahowald MW. Polysomnographic, neurologic, psychiatric, and clinical outcome report on 70 consecutive cases with REM sleep behavior disorder (RBD): sustained clonazepam efficacy in 89.5% of 57 treated patients. *Cleve Clin J Med* 1990;**57**(Suppl):S9–23.
137. Schenck CH, Mahowald MW. Long-term, nightly benzodiazepine treatment of injurious parasomnias and other disorders of disrupted nocturnal sleep in 170 adults. *Am J Med* 1996;**100**:333–7.
138. Watanabe T, Sugita Y. REM sleep behavior disorder (RBD) and dissociated REM sleep. *Nippon Rinsho (Jpn J Clin Med)* 1998;**56**:433–8.
139. Anderson KN, Jamieson S, *et al.* REM sleep behaviour disorder treated wtih metalonin in a patient with Alzheimer's disease. *Clin Neurol Neurosurg* 2008;**110**:492–5.

140. Boeve BF, Silber MH, *et al.* Melatonin for treatment of REM sleep behavior disorder in neurologic disorders: results in 14 patients. *Sleep Med* 2003;**4**:281–4.
141. Fantini ML, Gagno J-F, *et al.* The effects of pramipexole in REM sleep behavior disorder. *Neurology* 2003;**61**:1418–20.
142. Schmidt MH, Koshal VB, *et al.* Use of pramipexole in REM sleep behavior disorder. *Sleep Med* 2006;**7**:418–23.
143. Matsumoto M, Mutoh F, *et al.* The effects of imipramine on REM sleep behavior disorder in 3 cases. *Sleep Res* 1991;**20A**:351.
144. Takahashi T, Mitsuya H, *et al.* Opposite effect of SSRIs and tandospirone in the treatment of REM sleep behavior disorder. *Sleep Med* 2008;**9**:317–9.
145. Yamamoto K, Uchimura N, *et al.* Evaluation of the effects of paroxetine in the treatment of REM sleep behavior disorder. *Sleep Biol Rhythms* 2006;**4**:190–2.
146. Bamford C. Carbamazepine in REM sleep behavior disorder. *Sleep* 1993;**16**:33.
147. Tan A, Salgado M, *et al.* Rapid eye movement sleep behavior disorder preceding Parkinson's disease with therapeutic response to levodopa. *Mov Disord* 1996;**11**:214–6.
148. Mike ME, Kranz AJ. MAOI suppression of R.B.D. refractory to clonazepam and other agents. *Sleep Res* 1996;**25**:63.
149. Ringman JM, Simmons JH. Treatment of REM sleep behavior disorder with donepezil: a report of three cases. *Neurology* 2000;**55**:870–1.
150. Rye DB, Dempsay J, *et al.* REM-sleep dyscontrol in Parkinson's disease: case report of effects of elective pallidotomy. *Sleep Res* 1997;**26**:591.
151. Iranzo A, Valldeoriola F, *et al.* Sleep symptoms and polysomnographic architecture in advanced Parkinson's disease after chronic bilateral subthalamic stimulation. *J Neurol Neurosurg Psychiatry* 2002;**72**:661–4.
152. Arnulf I, Bejjani BP, *et al.* Improvement of sleep architecture in PD with subthalamic stimulation. *Neurology* 2000;**55**:1732–4.
153. Piette T, Mescola P, *et al.* A unique episode of REM sleep behavior disorder triggered during surgery for Parkinson's disease. *J Neurol Sci* 2007;**253**:73–6.
154. Schuld A, Kraus T, *et al.* Obstructive sleep apnea syndrome induced by clonazepam in a narcoleptic patient with REM-sleep-behavior disorder. *J Sleep Res* 1999;**8**:321–2.
155. Schenck CH, Bundlie SR, et al. Delayed emergence of a parkinsonian disorder in 38% of 29 older men initially diagnosed with idiopathic rapid eye movement sleep behaviour disorder [erratum appears in *Neurology* 1996;**46**(6):1787]. *Neurology* 1996;**46**:388–93.
156. Tachibana N, Oka Y. Longitudinal change in REM sleep components in a patient with multiple system atrophy associated with REM sleep behavior disorder: paradoxical improvement of nocturnal behaviors in a progressive neurodegenerative disease. *Sleep Med* 2004;**5**:155–8.
157. Lugaresi E, Provini F. Agrypnia excitata: clinical features and pathophysiological implications. *Sleep Med Rev* 2001;**5**: 313–22.
158. Montagna P, Lugaresi E. Agrypnia excitata: a generalized overactivity syndrome and a useful concept in the neurophysiology of sleep. *Clin Neurophysiol* 2002;**113**:552–60.
159. Plazzi G, Montagna P, *et al.* Polysomnographic study of sleeplessness and onericisms in the alcohol withdrawal syndrome. *Sleep Med* 2002;**3**:279–82.
160. Provini F, Cortelli P, *et al.* Fatal insomnia and agrypnia excitata: sleep and the limbic system. *Rev Neurol (Paris)* 2008;**164**: 692–700.
161. Cibula JE, Eisenschenk S, *et al.* Progressive dementia and hypersomnolence with dream-enacting behavior. Oneiric dementia. *Arch Neurol* 2002;**59**:630–4.
162. Fantini ML, Ferini-Strambi L, *et al.* Idiopathic REM sleep behavior disorder. Toward a better nosologic definition. *Neurology* 2005;**64**:780–6.
163. Abbott RD, Ross GW, *et al.* Excessive daytime sleepiness and the subsequent development of Parkinson disease. *Neurology* 2006;**65**:1442–6.
164. Arnulf I. Excessive daytime sleepiness in parkinsonism. *Sleep Med Rev* 2005;**9**:185–200.
165. Boeve BF, Saper CB. REM sleep behavior disorder. A possible early marker for synucleinopathies. *Neurology* 2006;**66**:796–7 (Editorial).
166. Wolters EC. Variability in the clinical expression of Parkinson's disease. *J Neurol Sci* 2008;**266**:197–203.
167. Lieberman A. Depression in Parkinson's disease – a review. *Acta Neurol Scand* 2006;**113**:1–8.
168. Ross GW, Petrovitch H, *et al.* Association of olfactory dysfunction with rish for future Parkinson's disease. *Ann Neurol* 2008;**63**:167–73.
169. Tolosa E, Compta Y, *et al.* The premotor phase of Parkinson's disease. *Parkinsonism Relat Disord* 2007;**13**:S2–7.
170. Jellinger KA. Recent developments in the pathology of Parkinson's disease. *J Neural Transm Suppl* 2002;**62**:347–76.
171. Braak H, Tredici D, *et al.* Staging of the intracerebral inclusion body pathology associated with idiopathic Parkinson's disease (preclinical and clinical stages). *J Neurol* 2002;**249**(Suppl 3):III/1–5.
172. Langston JW. The Parkinson's complex: parkinsonism is just the tip of the iceberg. *Ann Neurol* 2006;**59**:591–6.
173. Schenck CH, Mahowald MW. REM sleep parasomnias. *Neurol Clin* 2005;**23**:1107–26.
174. Josephs KA, Silber MH, *et al.* Neurophysiologic studies in Morvan syndrome. *J Clin Neurophysiol* 2004;**21**:440–5.

Chapter 24
Gastrointestinal and Swallowing Disturbances in Parkinson's Disease

Ronald F. Pfeiffer
Department of Neurology, University of Tennessee Health Science Center, Memphis, TN, USA

Introduction

That individuals with Parkinson's disease (PD) may develop gastrointestinal (GI) dysfunction has been known since the first description of the disease by James Parkinson in 1817 [1]. He clearly described drooling, dysphagia, and bowel dysfunction in some individuals who were the subjects of his report. Perceptively, he attributed drooling to difficulty in swallowing and even described both facets of bowel dysfunction – decreased bowel movement frequency and difficulty with the act of defecation – that are now known to be characteristic of PD.

However, during the one and a half centuries following Parkinson's treatise, very little was written about GI dysfunction in PD, as attention focused almost exclusively on the motor aspects of the disorder. Interest in the GI system began to resurface in the 1960s [2] and since 1990; has undergone a veritable explosion. The ensuing flood of information has led to increased recognition and understanding of the clinical manifestations, but also to new and exciting discoveries about the origin of PD itself.

Basic mechanisms of swallowing and GI function

Control of GI function is mediated by interaction between components of the central, autonomic, and enteric nervous systems (see review by Cersósimo and Benarroch [3]). Dating back to the classic experiments of Penfield and Jasper [4] and more recent work by others [5,6], cortical localization for some aspects of GI function has been identified, including centers for hunger, vomiting, swallowing, salivation, and defecation. These centers communicate with specific brainstem nuclei, which in turn provide information to and receive information from the enteric nervous system (ENS), primarily via the parasympathetic and sympathetic components of the autonomic nervous system.

While the primary cortical center for control of volitional swallowing is in the lateral motor cortex within the inferior precentral gyrus, activation of additional areas has been noted during swallowing utilizing positron emission tomography [6–8]. The supplementary motor area may play a role in preparation for volitional swallowing, the anterior cingulate cortex in monitoring autonomic and vegetative functions, and the anterior insula in allowing gustatory and other intraoral sensations to modulate swallowing. Cerebellar activation also occurs during swallowing, presumably playing a role in coordination, timing, and sequencing of swallowing.

A central pattern generator, which contains the programs that direct the precise sequential movements of the various muscles involved with swallowing, exists in the brainstem and directly regulates swallowing [9]. The central pattern generator has two major neuronal subdivisions; a dorsomedial group of neurons located in the medial reticular formation of the rostral medulla and the reticulum adjacent to the nucleus tractus solitarius [10,11]. It is involved with the initiation and organization of the swallowing sequence [8]. A ventrolateral group of cells lies near the nucleus ambiguus and serves as a connecting pathway to motor nuclei such as the nucleus ambiguus and the dorsal motor nucleus of the vagus (DMV), which innervate the striated muscles of the pharynx and upper esophagus. A role for the pedunculopontine tegmental nucleus in swallowing has also been proposed [12].

Parasympathetic innervation of the stomach, small intestine, and proximal colon originates in the dorsal motor nucleus of the vagus and is carried to the gut via the vagus nerve [13], while the parasympathetic supply of the middle and distal colon derives from the sacral parasympathetic nucleus of the spinal cord and travels to the gut via sacral nerves [14]. Sympathetic supply to the entire GI tract arises from neurons of the

Parkinson's Disease: Non-Motor and Non-Dopaminergic Features, First Edition. Edited by C. Warren Olanow, Fabrizio Stocchi, and Anthony E. Lang.

intermediolateral column of the spinal cord from the T5 to L3 levels.

The parasympathetic and sympathetic nerves deliver their information to neurons that comprise the ENS, which is organized into two major ganglionated plexuses that consist of numerous ganglia extensively interconnected by nerve bundles, producing "the appearance of a flat meshwork with nodes (ganglia) at junctions in the mesh" [15]. The deeper myenteric (Auerbach's) plexus, which lies between the longitudinal and circular smooth muscle layers of the gut, controls the activity of smooth muscle within the GI tract, whereas the more superficial and delicate submucosal (Meissner's) plexus, which is located in the submucous coat of the intestine, is more involved with the regulation of mucosal secretion and blood flow.

The ENS contains approximately 100 million neurons, which is roughly comparable to the number of neurons within the spinal cord [16]. A variety of neuronal types is represented in the ENS, including afferent neurons, interneurons, and efferent neurons. Acetylcholine is the predominant excitatory neurotransmitter, whereas inhibitory neurons utilize a variety of neurotransmitters such as nitric oxide, vasoactive intestinal polypeptide (VIP), and others [17,18]. Dopaminergic neurons also are present within the ENS [19,20] and are inhibitory in character. Glial cells actually outnumber neurons within the ENS by a ratio of approximately 4:1 and may be involved not only in mechanical support but also in a variety of other gut activities, including neurotransmission, immunologic function, homeostasis, and possibly even motility [21–23]. Of particular note are the interstitial cells of Cajal, which are neither neurons nor smooth muscle cells, but probably derived from fibroblasts [15,24]. They are responsible for slow wave activity that serves a pacemaker function in generating propulsive muscle contractions within the gut. Thus, gut motility is largely governed from within the ENS itself, with modulation but not direct control from the central nervous system (CNS). Just as the striated pharyngeal muscles involved with swallowing are under direct control of a central pattern generator within the brainstem, so the striated muscles involved with rectoanal function (external anal sphincter and puborectalis) are also controlled from centers external to the ENS.

Pathology of GI dysfunction in PD

Although motor dysfunction in PD may be due to the extensive damage to nigrostriatal dopaminergic neurons, it has become increasingly clear that damage is not confined to the substantia nigra and even extends beyond the CNS. In fact, the initial pathologic manifestations of PD may originate completely outside the CNS, within the ENS. The work of Braak and colleagues has revolutionized this concept. In a series of reports, they have provided evidence that in PD the first changes within the CNS occur in two locations – the olfactory bulb/anterior olfactory nucleus and the DMV – and that the pathologic process gradually spreads from the DMV in a cephalad fashion up the brainstem, eventually reaching the substantia nigra when the motor features of PD first become evident [25–28]. The same group has taken things one step further and provided evidence that the very earliest changes in PD, in the form of α-synuclein immunoreactive aggregations, may actually develop within the gastric myenteric and submucosal plexuses and that the pathologic process subsequently ascends the vagus nerve by retrograde transmission, ultimately arriving at the DMV where the pathologic process within the CNS is initiated [29]. Braak and colleagues made the point that axons from the submucosal plexus extend and terminate within the mucosal lamina propria, where they are only micrometers away from the gut lumen, separated by only a single layer of epithelial cells, and thus potentially susceptible to attack by potential pathologic agents within the GI tract [28,29]. Even before the investigations by Braak and colleagues, other investigators had identified the presence of pathology within the ENS in individuals with PD. Qualman *et al.* described the presence of Lewy bodies in the esophagus of individuals with PD in 1984 [30]; others subsequently demonstrated the presence of Lewy bodies in other parts of the ENS [31–36]. While Lewy bodies were found most frequently in VIP neurons, Singaram *et al.* also demonstrated dopaminergic neuronal loss within the colonic myenteric plexus in PD [19]. Dopaminergic neurons have subsequently been reported to constitute 14–20% of neurons within the ENS [37].

More recent work with animal models of parkinsonism has also demonstrated involvement of the ENS. Loss of ENS dopaminergic neurons has been documented after intraperitoneal [18,38,39] and intravenous [40] administration of MPTP. In contrast, nigral administration of 6-hydroxydopamine increased the number of ENS dopaminergic neurons [38]. Mice overexpressing human wild-type α-synuclein demonstrate altered colonic motility with decreased fecal output [41]. In addition, intragastric administration of a selective proteasome inhibitor in rats resulted in the appearance of α-synuclein-immunopositive intracytoplasmic inclusions and activated microglia within the DMV [42].

Building on the theory that PD may have its genesis within the gut and based on reports of an association between PD and a history of gastric or duodenal ulcer disease [43–45], it has been proposed that *Helicobacter pylori* may be the etiologic agent in PD [46], perhaps generating its effect via immunologic mechanisms [47–51]. Firm proof and general acceptance of this hypothesis, however, are still lacking. Epidemiologic studies also suggest that

Box 24.1 Gastrointestinal dysfunction in Parkinson's disease

Dental deterioration
Salivary excess
Dysphagia
Gastroparesis
Intestinal dysmotility
Anorectal dysfunction

GI involvement may be a very early feature of PD. The Honolulu–Asia Aging Study, a community-based study of Japanese-American men, noted that those with a bowel movement frequency of less than one per day had a 2.7-fold greater risk of developing PD than men with daily bowel movements and were four times more likely to develop PD than men with two or more daily bowel movements [52]. Weight loss has also been reported in PD patients prior to the onset of motor dysfunction by some [53,54], but not all, investigators [55].

Clinical features

GI dysfunction in PD covers a broad array of features, which extend the entire length of the GI tract (Box 24.1). In a seminal survey in which 98 persons with PD were compared with 50 comparably aged spousal controls [56], and in a subsequent reports [57–69], Edwards and colleagues described five features of GI dysfunction that characterize PD. These are reviewed below.

Dental deterioration

Individuals with PD experience a number of problems that might lead to an increased frequency of dental, periodontal, and oral health problems. Rigidity and bradykinesia can impair the ability to perform the repetitive motions necessary for brushing the teeth, and levodopa-induced dyskinesia involving the oral musculature and jaw may interfere with dentures and compromise oral hygiene. Both saliva accumulation and dry mouth can occur in the setting of PD and can damage teeth. Some individuals also experience a craving for and consumption of sweets. In a survey of 104 individuals with PD compared with 191 controls, Nakayama, Washio, and Mori found that individuals with PD experienced more problems with oral health [70]. Loss of teeth was more prevalent, as were chewing difficulties and denture discomfort. Increased periodontal pathology, presumably due to inadequate oral hygiene, has also been noted [71]. In another study, 98% of PD patients wore dentures and all had extensive dental problems [72]. Not all reports paint such a gloomy dental picture. Kennedy *et al.* reported that individuals with PD who crave sweets did not demonstrate an increase in anaerobic microflora compared with PD patients who did not experience such craving and with normal controls, although the levels of *Streptococcus mutans* were higher in PD patients overall and mucositis was more common [73]. Surprisingly, Swedish and Japanese investigators have documented fewer decayed, missing, or filled teeth, and more remaining teeth, compared with a control group in the Swedish report and with both national statistics and a control group in two Japanese studies [74–76].

Other oral problems have also been described in persons with PD. Bruxism may develop, both as a feature of PD itself and as a complication of levodopa therapy [77,78]. Temporomandibular joint dysfunction and even mandibular dislocation have occurred [79,80]. The presence of a burning sensation within the mouth was present in 24% of responders in a survey of PD patients [81]. The etiology of the burning sensation is uncertain.

Box 24.2 Treatment of salivary excess

Sublingual ipratropium
Sublingual atropine ophthalmic solution
Botulinum toxin injections

Saliva

Excess saliva is a common and often frustrating problem for individuals with PD [82–84]. Although generally not dangerous, the drooling that sometimes occurs because of the excess saliva can be embarrassing and make affected individuals reluctant to participate in social activities. Surveys have documented excess saliva in 70–78% of persons with PD, compared with 6% of controls [2,56], with men affected more frequently than women [85]. Although the term sialorrhea, which means excessive salivation, is often used to describe this problem, it is a misnomer because saliva production actually is decreased in PD [86–89] and saliva accumulation results from infrequent and inefficient swallowing [90].

A variety of treatment approaches have been employed to reduce saliva accumulation and drooling in individuals with PD (Box 24.2). Anti-cholinergic drugs, such as trihexyphenidyl and benztropine, have been used, but in addition to making saliva more tenacious, these drugs are associated with cognitive impairment, urinary retention, and constipation, making their use somewhat problematic. Local application of anti-cholinergic drugs such as sublingual ipratropium spray [91] or atropine ophthalmic drops [92], has been successfully employed in an effort to reduce systemic anti-cholinergic toxicity. Investigations of other similar strategies are also in progress.

Another promising treatment approach is the use of botulinum toxin injections into salivary glands to reduce saliva production. Bushara first suggested this a as a possible treatment approach for individuals with amyotrophic lateral sclerosis and drooling [93] and it was first employed in PD patients by Bhatia, Münchau and Brown in 1999; [94]. Numerous subsequent positive reports on PD have been published, including several double-blind, placebo-controlled protocols [95–97]. Although parotid gland injection has most often been utilized, injection of submandibular glands, which are responsible for approximately 70% of unstimulated daily saliva production, has also been successfully employed [98]. Both botulinum toxin type A and type B have been utilized successfully, although most investigators have used type A, and reported that duration of benefit ranges from 7 weeks to 7 months [99]. A wide dose range has been employed in treating salivary excess with type A botulinum toxin, ranging from five units per side for the parotid [100] to 225 units per side for combined parotid and submandibular gland injection [95]. Ultrasound guidance is employed by some investigators. Few serious adverse effects have been reported, but dry mouth, dysphagia due to weakened pharyngeal muscles, infection of the injected gland, local pain, recurrent jaw dislocation, and facial nerve and artery damage have occurred [99,101]. Surgical approaches, such as tympanic neurectomy, have been advocated for excessive drooling refractory to other treatments, but are accompanied by significant drawbacks such as loss of taste on the anterior two-thirds of the tongue, and may not provide permanent reduction in saliva production [102].

Dysphagia

A number of studies have assessed the frequency with which patients with PD perceive difficulty in swallowing, with reports ranging from 30% to over 80% [2,56,103,104]. Objective studies, typically using the modified barium swallow (MBS), are even more striking, with abnormalities noted in 75–97% of PD patients [105–107]. Subclinical dysphagia may be present in individuals with early PD [105,108,109] and the development of dysphagia appears to be independent of both disease duration and severity [110]. Dysphagia has been described as the initial clinical manifestation of PD [111]. However, in a study of 83 individuals with pathologically confirmed parkinsonism, the median time to the appearance of dysphagia was 130 months in the 17 individuals with PD – far longer than in other forms of parkinsonism – and the development of dysphagia or dysarthria within 1 year of symptom onset virtually excluded a diagnosis of PD [112]. Dysphagia in PD most often is due to oropharyngeal dysfunction, but impaired esophageal dysfunction may also be responsible (Box 24.3).

Box 24.3 Dysphagia

Oral
- Impaired tongue control and mobility
- Delayed initiation of swallowing

Pharyngeal
- Misdirected swallows
- Pharyngeal and vallecular stasis
- Reflux of material from vallecular and pyriform sinuses
- Cricopharyngeal dysfunction
- Zenker's diverticulum formation

Esophageal
- Slowed transit
- Segmental and diffuse spasm
- Repetitive spontaneous contractions
- Ineffective or tertiary contractions
- Aperistalsis
- Esophageal dilatation
- Reduced lower esophageal sphincter pressure
- Achalasia

Oropharyngeal dysphagia

A variety of abnormalities of oropharyngeal function have been identified in individuals with PD [109,113–119]. In general, oropharyngeal transit time is prolonged. Within the oral phase, alterations in lingual control and oral mobility, due to rigidity and bradykinesia of the oral musculature, may result in impaired bolus formation. Initiation of swallowing may also be delayed and it may take repeated tongue pumping and several attempts to clear the food bolus. Even then, residual food may be left in the mouth. Further difficulties may then await the food bolus in the pharynx. Pharyngeal dysmotility may result in misdirected swallows, pharyngeal and vallecular stasis, vallecular residue, and even reflux of material from the vallecular and pyriform sinuses into the mouth.

Dysfunction of the cricopharyngeal muscle, which serves as the upper esophageal sphincter, is yet another potential source of dysphagia in PD. The cricopharyngeus normally maintains tonic contraction, relaxing during swallowing in response to the piston-like propulsive force of the tongue as it drives the food bolus into the pharynx. In some individuals with PD, however, the propulsive force generated by the tongue may simply be insufficient to trigger cricopharyngeus relaxation, with consequent impairment of swallowing [110]. Alternatively, the cricopharyngeal muscle itself may demonstrate impaired ability to relax [120], which may result in cricopharyngeal bar formation and consequent difficulty in swallowing [121]. Cricopharyngeal dysfunction may develop more frequently in PD than is generally recognized. In the experience of one group of investigators, 22% of individuals with PD referred for evaluation of dysphagia were found to have cricopharyngeal bars or Zenker's diverticulae; the latter considered a consequence of incomplete cricopharyngeal relaxation [122].

The abnormalities of pharyngeal function that result in dysphagia can also lead to the potentially more serious problem of aspiration. Impaired effectiveness of voluntary cough to clear material that has entered the airway has been documented in PD and may further increase the risk of aspiration [123]. The frequency of aspiration in individuals with PD ranges from 15 to 56% [105,110,113,115,116]. Aspiration may be accompanied by symptoms such as coughing or choking when eating or drinking, but may also occur without eliciting any obvious symptoms. Such asymptomatic, or silent, aspiration occurs in 15–33% of PD patients [105,109,115]. In light of this, it is surprising that the risk of pneumonia is less than expected in persons with PD [124,125].

Esophageal dysphagia

The presence of Lewy bodies within the esophageal myenteric plexus [30,32] would seem to predict esophageal dysfunction in PD. Esophageal dysfunction is a less frequent, but still an important cause of dysphagia in PD, with varying reports on frequency. Videofluoroscopic abnormalities have been reported in as few as 5% and as many as 86% of PD patients [59,106,116,126, 127], while esophageal manometry, another method of measuring esophageal function, demonstrates abnormalities in 61–73% of individuals [128,129]. An extensive array of abnormalities has been delineated, including slowed esophageal transit, both segmental and diffuse esophageal spasm, repetitive spontaneous contractions of the proximal esophagus, ineffective or tertiary contractions with air trapping, aperistalsis, esophageal dilatation, and reduced lower esophageal sphincter pressure [106,122,126–131]. The last finding may result in the development of gastroesophageal reflux symptoms in addition to dysphagia.

Achalasia is characterized by the absence of esophageal peristalsis and failure of the lower esophageal sphincter to relax. The concurrent appearance of both achalasia and PD in some individuals has prompted suggestions of a possible etiologic relationship [132–134]. Lewy bodies have been identified in the myenteric plexus and even in the substantia nigra of individuals with achalasia, and involvement of the DMV is also present in both disorders [30,131].

Evaluation of dysphagia

The MBS test has become the standard test for evaluation of oropharyngeal dysphagia in PD. Other diagnostic modalities, such as electromyography [12] and pharyngeal manometry [135], are also utilized, but primarily on a research basis. It is important to remember, however, that MBS does not evaluate esophageal function. Therefore, if the MBS does not reveal an explanation for dysphagia in an individual with PD, further evaluation of esophageal function via videofluoroscopy and perhaps esophageal manometry is appropriate. Some have advocated the radionuclide esophageal transit test as a useful measure for evaluating esophageal function in PD [136]. Additional diagnostic modalities such as high-resolution manometry, esophageal electrical impedance, and intraluminal ultrasound imaging [137] have been used to evaluate esophageal function, but no specific reports on PD have been published.

Treatment of dysphagia

There is no universally effective treatment for dysphagia in PD. Appropriate treatment depends in part on the location of the dysfunction. Responsiveness of oropharyngeal dysphagia to dopaminergic medication has been documented [138–141], but others have noted objective improvement in only 33–50% of patients following levodopa or apomorphine administration [105,107,142], and one study suggested that levodopa may actually reduce swallowing efficiency [143]. Investigations with anti-cholinergic drugs have similarly produced conflicting results [130,144].

A wide variety of non-pharmacologic therapies for dysphagia in PD has been utilized, but very few have been adequately evaluated [145,146]. Two large studies compared chin-down swallowing with drinking thickened (with either nectar or honey) liquids in a head-neutral position in persons with PD or dementia with aspiration. Honey-thickened liquids were more effective in an initial assessment, but no superiority of one method over the other in preventing pneumonia was demonstrated over a longer time span [124,147]. Expiratory muscle strength training was reported to be effective in decreasing aspiration in a small pilot study [123].

Targeted treatment of cricopharyngeal dysfunction can be very effective. Impaired cricopharyngeal relaxation with consequent cricopharyngeal bar formation can be relieved surgically by cricopharyngeal myotomy [121]. Non-surgical treatment via botulinum toxin injection into the cricopharyngeus has also been successfully employed [99,148]. In both instances, it is important to evaluate esophageal motility and lower esophageal sphincter function prior to treatment, since abnormalities of either would leave the patient at increased risk for aspiration [121].

Dysphagia due to esophageal dysfunction is especially difficult to treat. Improvement in esophageal function has been reported following apomorphine injection [149,150], but formal studies have not been undertaken. Similarly, botulinum toxin injections have been employed in treating achalasia, but not specifically in PD [99,151]. Sildenafil has also been proposed as a potentially beneficial treatment for spastic esophageal disorders, but has not been studied in persons with PD [152,153].

In individuals with severe, intractable dysphagia or aspiration in whom adequate nutrition or medication administration has become impossible, percutaneous endoscopic gastrostomy (PEG) placement may rarely become necessary [60]. It is also important to remember that PEG does not completely eliminate the risk of aspiration, since saliva is still being produced and swallowed and malfunctioning lower and upper esophageal sphincters may still allow gastric contents to ascend the esophagus and be aspirated, especially if intragastric pressure is elevated. The advisability of performing PEG placement if the individual has advanced dementia has been questioned [154].

Gastroparesis

In their study, Edwards *et al.* reported that 24% of 98 PD subjects experienced nausea [56]. Their inclination was to attribute the nausea to anti-PD medication, but nausea occurred in 16% of patients not receiving treatment. Furthermore, 43% of untreated subjects had a sense of bloating. This led them to suggest that at least in untreated individuals these symptoms might be secondary to impaired gastric emptying. Impaired gastric emptying was first documented in elderly individuals, including persons with PD, compared with younger healthy volunteers [155,156]. Impaired gastric motility in PD, with significant delay in gastric emptying time, has subsequently been confirmed by multiple investigators [157–164] and is present in the majority of individuals with PD, approaching 100% [162]. Prominent variability in gastric emptying rate among PD patients has been noted [159,165]. Impairment of gastric emptying correlates with disease severity as measured by motor dysfunction, but not with age or gender [162,164]. Some investigators report more pronounced impairment of gastric emptying in individuals who display motor response fluctuations [158], whereas others report that gastric emptying is slower in individuals with a smooth response to levodopa, and actually accelerates, or pseudonormalizes, in individuals with motor response fluctuations [159]. The clinical consequences of gastroparesis in PD have not been extensively evaluated. A sense of bloating, nausea, vomiting, early satiety, weight loss, and even malnutrition may occur in the setting of PD, although they have not been directly connected to the presence of gastroparesis. Certainly, in individuals with PD who are experiencing these symptoms and in whom no other explanation for the symptoms has been forthcoming, gastroparesis should be considered.

Alterations in gastric emptying in individuals with PD have also been shown to impact levodopa absorption and plasma levodopa levels. Since levodopa absorption occurs primarily in the proximal small intestine rather than in the stomach [166–169], any delay in gastric emptying will also delay levodopa absorption. This, in turn, may lead to a delayed clinical response to an administered dose of levodopa. To complicate matters further, dopa decarboxylase is present within the gastric mucosa and can convert levodopa trapped in the stomach into dopamine, which in turn can delay gastric emptying even further [170–172]. This is because there are dopamine receptors within the stomach and dopamine can serve as an inhibitory modulator of gastroduodenal motility [173,174]. Impaired gastric emptying has, therefore, been suggested to be one cause of motor response fluctuations in PD patients, especially when onset of action of a dose of levodopa is delayed or when complete dose failure occurs [175–179].

Evaluation of gastroparesis

Scintigraphic methods are most frequently used to measure gastric emptying [180,181], but other modalities have also been employed. Some investigators favor the sodium [^{13}C]octanoate breath test because of its simplicity [162,182]. Although not directly measuring gastric emptying, electrogastrography has also been utilized in evaluating gastric function in PD and has demonstrated a variety of rhythmic disturbances [160,161,183–185].

Treatment of gastroparesis

In conditions such as diabetes mellitus, where gastroparesis often occurs, metoclopramide is utilized because it accelerates gastric emptying, presumably through its ability to block dopamine receptors within the stomach. However, metoclopramide is contraindicated in PD because it crosses the blood–brain barrier and also blocks dopamine receptors within the brain. Domperidone is a peripheral D2 dopamine receptor antagonist but does not cross the blood–brain barrier to any significant extent [186–188]. It can, therefore, be safely used in persons with PD and has been demonstrated to improve gastroparesis and levodopa absorption in this setting [189–191], although care should be exercised since rare instances of domperidone producing extrapyramidal dysfunction have been reported [187]. Unfortunately, domperidone is not available in the United States. Cisapride, tegaserod, and mosapride are serotonin 5-HT4 receptor agonists that stimulate the release of acetylcholine within the ENS and possess prokinetic qualities [192–194]. All three have demonstrated effectiveness in improving gastroparesis, cisapride and mosapride specifically in individuals with PD [165,195]. However, concerns regarding potential cardiotoxicity have limited or precluded the availability of cisapride and tegaserod in many countries.

Other pharmacologic approaches to the treatment of gastroparesis are also under investigation, though not specifically for PD (Box 24.4). The macrolide antibiotic erythromycin is also a motilin agonist that has been

Box 24.4 Treatment of gastroparesis

Dopamine receptor antagonists
- Domperidone*

Serotonin 5-HT4 receptor agonists
- Cisapride[a]
- Tegaserod[a]
- Mosapride[a]

Motilin agonists
- Erythromycin
- Mitemcinal[b]
- Mirtazapine

Botulinum toxin injection of pyloric sphincter
Ghrelin agonists[b]
PEG tube placement
Gastric electrical stimulation

[a]Limited or restricted availability.
[b]Experimental agents.

shown to accelerate gastric emptying [196–198]. Concerns regarding prolonged administration of an antibiotic, however, have led to the development of other motilin agonists, such as mitemcinal, for which prokinetic activity has also been demonstrated [199,200]. Mirtazapine was reported to improve gastric emptying in a single individual in whom conventional treatments had failed [201], but formal investigation of this agent for the treatment of gastroparesis has not been undertaken. Botulinum toxin injection into the pyloric sphincter is another treatment approach that has been employed in an effort to ameliorate gastroparesis, but large, controlled trials are still needed to confirm its efficacy [202,203]. The demonstration that the hormone ghrelin can accelerate gastric emptying points to the potential of ghrelin agonists as a treatment for gastroparesis [204–206].

Drug delivery methods that bypass the stomach altogether may be employed in individuals with severe gastroparesis in whom less invasive methods have not provided relief. Treatment approaches such as duodenal delivery of a levodopa gel via PEG, subcutaneous infusion of a dopamine agonist such as apomorphine or lisuride, and transdermal administration of the dopamine agonist rotigotine have been or might be utilized in this regard [65,179,207,208]. However, formal studies specifically in PD patients with documented gastroparesis are lacking. Gastric electrical stimulation is yet another approach that is undergoing investigation as a potential treatment for gastroparesis but has not been employed in patients with PD [209,210].

Intestinal dysmotility

Small intestine

The small intestine in PD is largely terra incognita. Very few laboratory studies have investigated small intestinal function in the setting of experimental parkinsonism. The administration of MPTP to rats has been reported to produce disruption of the migrating myoelectric complex, which would be expected to alter peristaltic activity within the small intestine [211]. Salsolinol, a tetrahydroisoquinoline derivative, did not affect intestinal myoelectric activity in the fasting state, but did alter the response to gastric distension, suggesting a direct effect on gastroduodenal reflexes [212,213].

Clinical studies of small intestinal function in PD are equally sparse. Perhaps the earliest recognition of involvement in PD was the report of Lewitan, Nathanson, and Slade in 1951 of dilatation of the small intestine, along with megacolon, in a patient with PD [214]. More recently, pronounced prolongation of orocecal transit time, unrelated to disease duration or severity, was documented in 15 PD patients compared with 15 age- and sex-matched controls [215]. Although the orocecal transit time is a measure of combined gastric and small intestinal transit, the results are very suggestive of small intestinal involvement in PD. Additional studies by the same investigators demonstrated reduced absorption of mannitol, but not lactulose, in PD subjects, suggesting an alteration in the enterocyte brush border membrane [215]. The clinical ramifications of these studies are unclear. The presence of altered absorptive capability within the small intestine might account for progressive weight loss that can occur in PD [216,217]. It is also tempting to speculate that the sense of bloating of which some PD patients bitterly complain, especially during "off" periods, might be related to small intestinal dysmotility, although this has never been evaluated.

Colon

Decreased bowel movement frequency is the most familiar aspect of GI dysfunction in PD. Reports documenting the frequency with which constipation occurs in PD show broad variability. Some of the variability can be explained by the changing definition of what actually constitutes constipation. In older studies, performed in an era when the definition of constipation was less than one bowel movement per day, constipation was reported to be present in 50–67% of PD patients [2,218]. More recent studies, which use a definition of constipation of fewer than three bowel movements weekly, indicate a frequency in the range 20–29% [56,219], although others continue to document frequencies of 59–77% [220,221].

Impairment of colonic motility is the primary physiologic basis for decreased bowel movement frequency in PD. Slowed colonic transit of fecal material has been documented by multiple investigators. Reported colon transit times in PD patients range from 44 to 130 h or longer [59,222–224]. A colon transit time of 82.4 min in one study was presumably a typographical error and should be 82.4 h [225]. In all studies, however, the reported average colon transit time for PD patients is significantly longer than in normal controls, typically over twice as long [59,225]. Jost and Schimrigk indicated that prolonged transit time is present in as many as 80% of individuals with PD [222], whereas Edwards *et al.* noted two subgroups within their PD subjects – one with normal colon transit times comprising 42% of subjects and the other 58% with markedly prolonged transit times [59]. Constipation gradually becomes more severe as PD progresses [56,226], but prolongation of colon transit time may be present in individuals with early, untreated PD [224]. Ashraf *et al.* noted that constipation may precede the development of the motor features of PD in some individuals [227], a finding consistent with reports from the Honolulu–Asia Aging Study [52,228].

Evaluation of constipation

The solid marker colon transit test is the standard method of analysis [229]. It is non-invasive and no preparation is necessary, although patients should not use laxatives or enemas or take other medications known to affect GI motility during the study. There are several variations in how the study can be carried out [229], but all employ ingestion of radiopaque markers followed after some interval by an abdominal X-ray with counting of the number of markers remaining in the colon used to calculate the colon transit time. Segmental colon transit times can also be calculated, but are of limited value. It is worth noting, however, that this method of measuring colon transit time actually includes orocecal and colon transit [229].

Treatment of constipation

Relatively few studies have addressed treatment of constipation in PD. Hence most treatment is based on experience gained from treating constipation in other conditions and is largely empirical [230,231] (Box 24.5). Edwards *et al.* administered a dietary questionnaire to participants in their study and noted that daily fiber intake in PD patients was noticeably less than the recommended amount, although they did not quantify fiber intake separately for constipated versus non-constipated patients [56]. In a controlled trial, psyllium was found to be effective in increasing stool weight and bowel movement frequency, but did not alter colon transit time [227]. Other investigators have noted increased plasma levodopa levels and improved motor function in PD patients placed on a diet rich in insoluble fiber [232]. Although achieving adequate fiber consumption by dietary measures alone might be preferable, supplementation with substances such as psyllium or methylcellulose can be employed and has been shown to reduce laxative consumption [233]. Regardless of its source, combining fiber with adequate fluid intake is important. A recent recommendation by the American Dietetic Association is that the daily consumption of fiber should be 25 g for adult women and 38 g for adult men [234].

Box 24.5 Treatment of slow transit constipation

Increased fiber and fluid
Stool softeners
Osmotic laxatives
- Poly(ethylene glycol)
- Lactulose
- Sorbitol

Prokinetic agents
- Cisapride[a]
- Tegaserod[a]
- Mosapride[a]
- Prucalopride[a]
- Lubiprostone

Other agents
- Pyridostigmine
- Colchicine
- Misoprostol
- NT-3[b]

[a] Limited or restricted availability.
[b] Not available.

If adequate fiber and fluid do not relieve constipation, addition of a stool softener such as docusate may be useful. If constipation persists, an osmotic laxative such as sorbitol, lactulose, and polyethylene glycol (macrogol) may be added to the treatment regimen. The last preparation has been specifically studied and its effectiveness documented in patients with PD [235,236]. Osmotic laxatives can be taken on either an as-needed or a daily basis. Although irritant laxatives, such as senna, are readily available to patients without prescription, daily use of such agents should probably be avoided because chronic daily use might cause myenteric plexus damage, although such damage has not been definitively proven. The intermittent use of enemas is acceptable when other measures fail.

In recent years, a variety of prokinetic agents that accelerate colon transit, particularly 5-HT4 agonists, have been introduced into treatment. Both cisapride [237,238] and tegaserod [239,240] improved constipation in PD patients, but concerns regarding potential cardiotoxicity resulted in the removal of both from many markets. Mosapride and prucalopride, which are more selective serotonin 5-HT4 agonists and believed to have less risk of producing cardiac arrhythmia, have both been shown to improve slow transit constipation [241–244], but only mosapride has been specifically evaluated in PD patients [245] and neither is as yet approved. Lubiprostone is a prokinetic agent that works by activating chloride channels on GI epithelial cells and inducing fluid secretion into the intestinal lumen [246]. It has been found to be effective in the treatment of constipation [247], but it has not been specifically evaluated in individuals with PD.

Anecdotal reports have described the effectiveness of oral pyridostigmine [248] and intravenous neostigmine [249] in relieving constipation in individuals with PD. A small single-blind study of pyridostigmine in patients with autonomic neuropathy reported possible improvement of symptoms and colon transit in a subset of subjects [250], but no formal studies with either of these two agents in PD have been undertaken. Colchicine was reported to alleviate constipation in three individuals with PD [251], but no formal studies were subsequently undertaken. The efficacy of neurotrophin-3 in a small double-blind study of PD patients with constipation was reported in abstract form, but the agent was abandoned [252]. Misoprostol, a prostaglandin analog that is known to stimulate colonic motility, particularly in the left colon, has been reported to be effective in ameliorating chronic constipation but has not been evaluated in PD subjects [253]. In cases where megacolon or volvulus has developed, surgical treatment in the form of colectomy may become necessary, but this is very rare in the setting of PD [254,255].

Anorectal dysfunction

In their 1991; survey study, Edwards *et al.* distinguished two components of bowel dysfunction in the setting of PD – decreased frequency and difficulty with the act of defecation itself – and noted that the latter component was the more prevalent [56]. Defecatory dysfunction was experienced by 67% of PD patients compared with 29% who were troubled by decreased bowel movement frequency. Others have confirmed these findings and documented that defecatory dysfunction may be present both in patients with early and in those with advanced PD [224,256]. Difficulty with the act of defecation is due to dysfunction of the anorectal musculature and is characterized by excessive straining while attempting to defecate, pain upon defecation, and a sense of incomplete emptying. As with swallowing, successful defecation depends on the coordinated action of a surprising number of muscles. Reflex relaxation of the internal anal sphincter and both voluntary and reflexive relaxation of the external anal sphincter and pelvic floor musculature, especially the puborectalis muscle, must all occur, while production of adequate rectosigmoid tone to allow funneling of the fecal contents through the anal canal and contraction of the abdominal muscles, diaphragm, and even the glottic muscles to increase intra-abdominal pressure must also take place to facilitate evacuation [257,258].

Mathers and colleagues were the first to document failure to relax of the external anal sphincter and puborectalis muscles during attempted defecation in PD patients experiencing defecatory dysfunction [259,260], a finding subsequently confirmed by others, and noted to be present in 31% of individuals tested [59]. The puborectalis muscle forms the anorectal angle and its relaxation during defecation allows opening or widening of the anorectal angle to facilitate evacuation [258]. Mathers and colleagues suggested that failure of these muscles to relax was actually a dystonic phenomenon [259,260]. It is worth noting, however, that failure of the puborectalis muscle to relax during defecation may occur in normal individuals and some investigators have suggested that it may simply be a laboratory artifact due to the rather artificial nature of laboratory testing [261,262].

PD patients may also demonstrate lower basal sphincter pressure and difficulty in sustaining sphincter pressure during testing with anorectal manometry [59,221, 263–265]. A variety of other abnormalities of sphincter function, such as lower sphincter pressure on voluntary squeezing, lower sustained squeeze pressure, and short squeeze duration, have also been noted during anorectal manometric testing of PD patients but not in individuals with chronic idiopathic constipation or in normal controls [263]. Distinctive abnormalities, such as unusual phasic contractions of the sphincter muscles during voluntary contraction and a hypercontractile response of the external anal sphincter and puborectalis muscles on rectosphincteric (rectoanal inhibitory) reflex testing, with contraction of the muscles instead of the expected relaxation, have also been documented in PD patients [59,221, 264,265].

Evaluation of defecatory dysfunction

Anorectal manometry and fluoroscopic defecography are, perhaps, the most widely employed methods for evaluating anal sphincter function. Anal sphincter electromyography, MRI, anal endosonography, and other ultrasonographic procedures may also be utilized. However, all of these methods require sophisticated equipment or training and are not always readily available for routine patient evaluation.

Treatment of defecatory dysfunction

Relatively few studies specifically addressing the treatment of defecatory dysfunction in persons with PD have been published (Box 24.6). A broader supply of information from studies of persons with other causes of

Box 24.6 Potential treatments for anorectal dysfunction

Botulinum toxin injections
Apomorphine
Biofeedback training
Sacral nerve stimulation

defecatory dysfunction is available, but its applicability to individuals with PD is untested. Biofeedback training is advocated by some investigators for individuals with dysynergic defecation [266,267], although others report that biofeedback retraining is of dubious benefit [268]. Sacral nerve stimulation has been successfully employed in treating both slow transit and rectal outlet constipation in preliminary studies, but has not been extensively evaluated [269]. Neither of these treatment approaches, however, has been evaluated specifically in PD patients. Surgical treatments are also used in some types of defecatory dysfunction, but are probably not appropriate for individuals with PD. Botulinum toxin injections into the puborectalis muscle under transrectal ultrasonographic guidance have been pioneered by Albanese and colleagues in patients with PD [270–272]. In the most recent of these open label trials, Cadeddu *et al.* reported symptomatic improvement in defecation in 56% of study subjects at 2 months following injection, with widening of the anorectal angle during straining evident on defecography [272]. Waning of improvement was evident in the majority of individuals within 4 months. No significant adverse effects were reported, but fecal incontinence and a variety of other complications have been reported in other disorders [273], and perianal thrombosis has occurred following botulinum toxin injection into the external anal sphincter for treatment of anal fissure [274].

The fact that improvement in measures of anorectal function may be evident in some individuals with PD and motor fluctuations when they are "on" compared with when they are "off" [264], suggests that dopaminergic medications might be of value in the treatment of defecatory dysfunction. Indeed, some persons with PD are aware that it is easier for them to have a bowel movement when they are "on" than when they are "off." Experimental experience with subcutaneous apomorphine injections supports this idea. Improvement in measures of anorectal function, including anorectal manometry, anal sphincter electromyography, and defecography, has been noted [260,275], although actual clinical trials to confirm efficacy have not been undertaken.

Conclusion

GI dysfunction in PD occurs frequently and may involve virtually all levels of the GI tract. Symptoms of GI dysfunction may appear early in the course of the disease, and may even precede the development of the classic motor features of PD. Recent investigations have raised the possibility that GI involvement may even play an integral role in the genesis of the disorder. The growing importance of GI dysfunction in PD makes it imperative that neurologists become familiar with the nature and character of GI symptoms that may arise in their PD patients, so that these GI problems can be promptly recognized and appropriate treatment or referral initiated expeditiously.

References

1. Parkinson J. *An Essay on the Shaking Palsy*. London: Whittingham and Rowland, 1817.
2. Eadie MJ, Tyrer JH. Alimentary disorder in parkinsonism. *Australas Ann Med* 1965;**14**: 13–22.
3. Cersósimo MG, Benarroch EE. Neural control of the gastrointestinal tract: implications for Parkinson's disease. *Mov Disord* 2008;**23**:1065–75.
4. Penfield WG, Jasper H. *Epilepsy and the Functional Anatomy of the Human Brain*. Boston: Little, Brown, 1954.
5. Hunter PC, Crameri J, Austin S, *et al.* Response of parkinsonian swallowing dysfunction to dopaminergic stimulation. *J Neurol Neurosurg Psychiatry* 1997;**63**:579–83.
6. Hamdy S, Rothwell JC, Brooks DJ, *et al.* Identification of the cerebral loci processing human swallowing with $H_2{}^{15}O$ PET activation. *J Neurophysiol* 1999;**81**:1917–26.
7. Zald DH, Pardo JV. The functional neuroanatomy of voluntary swallowing. *Ann Neurol* 1999;**46**:281–6.
8. Schaller BJ, Graf R, Jacobs AH. Pathophysiological changes of the gastrointestinal tract in ischemic stroke. *Am J Gastroenterol* 2006;**101**:1655–65.
9. Jean A. Brain stem control of swallowing: neuronal network and cellular mechanisms. *Physiol Rev* 2001;**81**:929–69.
10. Miller AJ. Swallowing: neurophysiologic control of the esophageal phase. *Dysphagia* 1986;**2**:72–82.
11. Hunter PC, Crameri J, Austin S, *et al.* Response of parkinsonian swallowing dysfunction to dopaminergic stimulation. *J Neurol Neurosurg Psychiatry* 1997;**63**:579–83.
12. Alfonsi E, Versino M, Merlo IM, *et al.* Electrophysiologic patterns of oral-pharyngeal swallowing in parkinsonian syndromes. *Neurology* 2007;**68**:583–9.
13. Travagli RA, Hermann GE, Browning KN, *et al.* Brainstem circuits regulating gastric function. *Annu Rev Physiol* 2006;**68**:279–305.
14. Brading AF, Ramalingam T. Mechanisms controlling normal defecation and the potential effects of spinal cord injury. *Prog Brain Res* 2006;**152**:345–58.
15. Quigley EMM, Conklin JL. The "big" brain and the "little" brain: interactions between the enteric and central nervous systems in the regulation of gut function. In: Quigley EMM, Pfeiffer RF, eds. *Neuro-Gastroenterology*. Philadelphia: Butterworth Heinemann, 2004:3–14.
16. Camilleri M, Bharucha AE. An overview of gastrointestinal dysfunction in diseases of central and peripheral nervous systems. In: Quigley EMM, Pfeiffer RF, eds. *Neuro-Gastroenterology*. Philadelphia: Butterworth Heinemann, 2004:35–57.
17. Johnson LR. Gastrointestinal Physiology. St. Louis, MO: Mosby, 2001.
18. Anderson G, Noorian AR, Taylor G, *et al.* Loss of enteric dopaminergic neurons and associated changes in colon motility in an MPTP mouse model of Parkinson's disease. *Exp Neurol* 2007;**207**:4–12.

19. Singaram C, Ashraf W, Gaumnitz EA, *et al.* Dopaminergic defect of enteric nervous system in Parkinson's disease patients with chronic constipation. *Lancet* 1995;**346**: 861–4.
20. Li ZS, Pham TD, Tamir H, *et al* Enteric dopaminergic neurons: definition, developmental lineage, and effects of extrinsic denervation. *J Neurosci* 2004;**24**:1330–9.
21. Rühl A, Nasser Y, Sharkey KA. Enteric glia. *Neurogastroenterol Motil* 2004;**16**(Suppl 1):44–9.
22. Rühl A. Glial cells in the gut. *Neurogastroenterol Motil* 2005;**17**:777–90.
23. Bassotti G, Villannaci V, Antonelli E, *et al.* Enteric glial cells: new players in gastrointestinal motility? *Lab Invest* 2007;**87**:628–32.
24. Wu JJ, Rothman TP, Gershon MD. Development of the interstitial cell of Cajal: origin, kit dependence and neuronal and nonneuronal sources of kit ligand. *J Neurosci Res* 2000;**59**:384–401.
25. Del Tredici K, Rüb U, de Vos RAI, *et al.* Where does Parkinson disease pathology begin in the brain? *J Neuropathol Exp Neurol* 2002;**61**:413–26.
26. Braak H, Del Tredici K, Rüb U, *et al.* Staging of brain pathology related to sporadic Parkinson's disease. *Neurobiol Aging* 2003;**24**:197–211.
27. Braak H, Ghebremedhin E, Rüb U, *et al.* Stages in the development of Parkinson's disease-related pathology. *Cell Tissue Res* 2004;**318**:121–34.
28. Hawkes CH, Del Tredici K, Braak H. Review: Parkinson's disease: a dual-hit hypothesis. *Neuropathol Applied Neurobiol* 2007;**33**:599–614.
29. Braak H, de Vos RAI, Bohl J, *et al.* Gastric α-synuclein immunoreactive inclusions in Meissner's and Auerbach's plexuses in cases staged for Parkinson's disease-related brain pathology. *Neurosci Lett* 2006;**396**:67–72.
30. Qualman SJ, Haupt HM, Yang P, *et al.* Esophageal Lewy bodies associated with ganglion cell loss in achalasia. Similarity to Parkinson's disease. *Gastroenterology* 1984;**87**:848–56.
31. Kupsky WJ, Grimes MM, Sweeting J, *et al.* Parkinson's disease and megacolon: concentric hyaline inclusions (Lewy bodies) in enteric ganglion cells. *Neurology* 1987;**37**:1253–5.
32. Wakabayashi K, Takahashi H, Takeda s, *et al.* Parkinson's disease: the presence of Lewy bodies in Auerbach's and Meissner's plexuses. *Acta Neuropathol* 1988;**76**:217–21.
33. Wakabayashi K, Takahashi H, Takeda S, *et al.* Lewy bodies in the enteric nervous system in Parkinson's disease. *Arch Histol Cytol* 1989;**52**(Suppl):191–4.
34. Wakabayashi K, Takahashi H, Ohama E, *et al.* Parkinson's disease: an immunohistochemical study of Lewy body-containing neurons in the enteric nervous system. *Acta Neuropathol* 1990:**79**:581–3.
35. Wakabayashi K, Takahashi H, Ohama E, *et al.* Lewy bodies in the visceral autonomic nervous system in Parkinson's disease. *Adv Neurol* 1993;**60**:609–12.
36. Takeda S, Yamazaki K, Miyakawa T, *et al.* Parkinson's disease with involvement of the parasympathetic ganglia. *Acta Neuropathol* 1993;**86**:397–8.
37. Anlauf M, Schäfer MK, Eiden L, *et al.* Chemical coding of the human gastrointestinal nervous system: cholinergic, VIPergic, and catecholaminergic phenotypes. *J Comp Neurol* 2003;**459**:90–111.
38. Tian Y-M, Chen X, Luo D-Z, *et al.* Alteration of dopaminergic markers in gastrointestinal tract of different rodent models of Parkinson's disease. *Neuroscience* 2008;**153**:634–44.
39. Natale G, Kastsiuchenka O, Pasquali L, *et al.* MPTP- but not methamphetamine-induced parkinsonism extends to catecholamine neurons in the gut. *Ann N Y Acad Sci* **1** 2008;**139**:345–9.
40. Chaumette T, Lebouvier T, Aubert P, *et al.* Neurochemical plasticity in the enteric nervous system of a primate animal model of experimental Parkinsonism. *Neurogastroenterol Motil* 2009;**21**:215–22.
41. Wang L, Fleming SM, Chesselet MF, *et al.* Abnormal colonic motility in mice overexpressing human wild-type alpha-synuclein. *Neuroreport* 2008;**19**:873–6.
42. Miwa H, Kubo T, Suzuki A, *et al.* Intragastric proteasome inhibition induces alpha-synuclein-immunopositive aggregations in neurons in the dorsal motor nucleus of the vagus in rats. *Neurosci Lett* 2006;**401**:146–9.
43. Strang RR. The association of gastro-duodenal ulceration and Parkinson's disease. *Med J Aust* 1965;**1**:842–3.
44. Szabo S. Dopamine disorder in duodenal ulceration. *Lancet* 1979;**ii**:880–2.
45. Ma L, Zhang L, Gao XH, *et al.* Dietary factors and smoking as risk factors for PD in a rural population in China: a nested case–control study. *Acta Neurol Scand* 2006;**113**:278–81.
46. Altschuler E. Gastric *Helicobacter pylori* infection as a cause of idiopathic Parkinson disease and non-arteric anterior optic ischemic neuropathy. *Med Hypotheses* 1996;**47**:413–4.
47. Dobbs SM, Dobbs RJ, Weller C, *et al.* Link between *Helicobacter pylori* infection and idiopathic parkinsonism. *Med Hypotheses* 2000;**55**:93–8.
48. Dobbs RJ, Dobbs SM, Weller C, *et al.* Role of chronic infection and inflammation in the gastrointestinal tract in the etiology and pathogenesis of idiopathic parkinsonism. Part 1: eradication of *Helicobacter* in the cachexia of idiopathic parkinsonism. *Helicobacter* 2005;**10**:267–75.
49. Bjarnason IT, Charlett A, Dobbs RJ, *et al.* Role of chronic infection and inflammation in the gastrointestinal tract in the etiology and pathogenesis of idiopathic parkinsonism. Part 2: response of facets of clinical idiopathic parkinsonism to *Helicobacter pylori* eradication. A randomized, double-blind, placebo-controlled efficacy study. *Helicobacter* 2005;**10**:276–87.
50. Weller C, Charlett A, Oxlade NL, *et al.* Role of chronic infection and inflammation in the gastrointestinal tract in the etiology and pathogenesis of idiopathic parkinsonism. Part 3: predicted probability and gradients of severity of idiopathic parkinsonism based on *H. pylori* antibody profile. *Helicobacter* 2005;**10**:288–97.
51. Weller C, Oxlade N, Dobbs SM, *et al.* Role of inflammation in gastrointestinal tract in aetiology and pathogenesis of idiopathic parkinsonism. *FEMS Immunol Med Microbiol* 2005;**44**:129–35.
52. Abbott RD, Petrovitch H, White LR, *et al.* Frequency of bowel movements and the future risk of Parkinson's disease. *Neurology* 2001;**57**:456–62.
53. Chen H, Zhang SM, Hernán MA, *et al.* Weight loss in Parkinson's disease. *Ann Neurol* 2003;**53**:676–9.
54. Logroscino G, Sesso HD, Paffenbarger RS Jr, *et al.* Body mass index and risk of Parkinson's disease: a prospective cohort study. *Am J Epidemiol* 2007;**166**:1186–90.

55. Ragonese P, D'Amelio M, Callari G, *et al.* Body mass index does not change before Parkinson's disease onset. *Eur J Neurol* 2008;**15**:965–8.
56. Edwards LL, Pfeiffer RF, Quigley EMM, *et al.* Gastrointestinal symptoms in Parkinson's disease. *Mov Disord* 1991;**6**:151–6.
57. Edwards LL, Quigley EMM, Hofman R, *et al.* Gastrointestinal dysfunction in Parkinson's disease: frequency and pathophysiology. *Neurology* 1992;**42**:726–32.
58. Edwards LL, Quigley EMM, Hofman R, *et al.* Gastrointestinal symptoms in Parkinson's disease: 18 month follow-up study. *Mov Disord* 1993;**8**:83–6.
59. Edwards LL, Quigley EMM, Harned RK, *et al.* Characterization of swallowing and defecation in Parkinson's disease. *Am J Gastroenterol* 1994;**89**:15–25.
60. Quigley EMM. Gastrointestinal dysfunction in Parkinson's disease. *Semin Neurol* 1996;**16**:245–50.
61. Quigley EMM. Epidemiology and pathophysiology of gastrointestinal manifestations in Parkinson's disease. In: Corazziari E, ed. *NeUroGastroenterology*. Berlin: Walter deGruyter, 1996:167–78.
62. Pfeiffer RF. Gastrointestinal dysfunction in Parkinson's disease. *Clin Neurosci* 1998;**5**:136–46.
63. Pfeiffer RF, Quigley EMM. Gastrointestinal motility problems in patients with Parkinson's disease: epidemiology, pathophysiology and guidelines for management. *CNS Drugs* 1999;**11**:435–48.
64. Quigley EMM. Gastrointestinal features. In: Factor SA, Weiner WJ, eds. *Parkinson's Disease: Diagnosis and Clinical Management*. New York: Demos, 2002:87–93.
65. Pfeiffer RF. Gastrointestinal dysfunction in Parkinson's disease. *Lancet Neurol* 2003;**2**:107–15.
66. Pfeiffer RF, Quigley EMM. Gastrointestinal dysfunction in diseases of the cerebral hemispheres and movement disorders. In: Quigley EMM, Pfeiffer RF, eds. *Neuro-Gastroenterology*. Philadelphia: Butterworth Heinemann, 2004:59–81.
67. Pfeiffer RF. Gastrointestinal dysfunction in Parkinson's disease. In: Ebadi M, Pfeiffer RF, eds. *Parkinson's Disease*. Boca Raton, FL: CRC Press, 2005:259–73.
68. Pfeiffer RF. Intestinal dysfunction. In: Pfeiffer RF, Bodis-Wollner I, eds. *Parkinson's Disease and Nonmotor Dysfunction*. Totowa, NJ: Humana Press, 2005:115–25.
69. Quigley EMM. Gastrointestinal features. In: Factor SA, Weiner WJ, eds. *Parkinson's Disease: Diagnosis and Clinical Management*. New York: Demos, 2008:99–105.
70. Nakayama Y, Washio M, Mori M. Oral health conditions in patients with Parkinson's disease. *J Epidemiol* 2004;**14**:143–50.
71. Schwarz J, Heimhilger E, Storch A. Increased periodontal pathology in Parkinson's disease. *J Neurol* 22006;**53**: 608–11.
72. Anastassiadou V, Katsarou Z, Naka O, *et al.* Evaluating dental status and prosthetic need in relation to medical findings in Greek patients suffering from idiopathic Parkinson's disease. *Eur J Prosthodont Restor Dent* 2002;**10**:63–8.
73. Kennedy MA, Rosen S, Paulson GW, *et al.* Relationship of oral microflora with oral health status in Parkinson's disease. *Spec Care Dentist* 1994;**14**:164–8.
74. Persson M, Osterberg T, Granérus AK, *et al.* Influence of Parkinson's disease on oral health. *Acta Odontol Scand* 1992;**50**:37–42.
75. Fukayo S. Dental status in outpatients with Parkinson's disease. *Nippon Eiseigaku Zasshi* 2002;**57**:585–90 (in Japanese).
76. Fukayo S, Nonaka K, Shimizu T, *et al.* Oral health of patients with Parkinson's disease: factors related to their better dental status. *Tohoku J Exp Med* 2003;**201**:171–9.
77. Srivastava T, Ahuja M, Srivastava M, *et al.* Bruxism as a presenting feature of Parkinson's disease. *J Assoc Physicians India* 2002;**50**:457.
78. Magee KR. Bruxisma related to levodopa therapy. *JAMA* 1970;**214**:147.
79. Minagi S, Matsunaga T, Shibata T, *et al.* An appliance for management of TMJ pain as a complication of Parkinson's disease. *Cranio* 1998;**16**:57–9.
80. Sayama S, Fujimoto K, Shizuma N, *et al.* Habitual mandibular dislocation in two patients with Parkinson's disease. *Rinsho Shinkeigaku* 1999;**39**:849–51 (in Japanese).
81. Clifford TJ, Warsi MJ, Burnett CA, *et al.* Burning mouth in Parkinson's disease sufferers. *Gerodontology* 1998;**15**:73–8.
82. Merello M. Sialorrhoea and drooling in patients with Parkinson's disease: epidemiology and management. *Drugs Aging* 2008;**25**:1007–19.
83. Kalf JG, Smit AM, Bloem BR, *et al.* Impact of drooling in Parkinson's disease. *J Neurol* 2007;**254**:1227–32.
84. Chou KL, Evatt M, Hinson V, *et al.* Sialorrhea in Parkinson's disease: a review. *Mov Disord* 2007;**22**:2306–13.
85. Scott B, Borgman A, Engler H, *et al.* Gender differences in Parkinson's disease symptom profile. *Acta Neurol Scand* 2000;**102**:37–43.
86. Proulx M, de Courval FP, Wiseman MA, *et al.* Salivary production in Parkinson's disease. *Mov Disord* 2005;**20**:204–7.
87. Tumilasci OR, Cersósimo MG, Belforte JE, *et al.* Quantitative study of salivary secretion in Parkinson's disease. *Mov Disord* 2006;**21**:660–7.
88. Bagheri H, Damase-Michel C, Lapeyre-Mestre M, *et al.* A study of salivary secretion in Parkinson's disease. *Clin Neuropharmacol* 1999;**22**:213–5.
89. Bateson MC, Gibberd FB, Wilson RS. Salivary symptoms in Parkinson disease. *Arch Neurol* 1973;**29**:274–5.
90. Nóbrega AC, Rodrigues B, Torres AC, *et al.* Is drooling secondary to a swallowing disorder in patients with Parkinson's disease? *Parkinsonism Relat Disord* 2008;**14**:243–5.
91. Thomsen TR, Galpern WR, Asante A, *et al.* Ipratropium bromide spray as treatment for sialorrhea in Parkinson's disease. *Mov Disord* 2007;**22**:2268–73.
92. Hyson HC, Johnson AM, Jog MS. Sublingual atropine for sialorrhea secondary to parkinsonism: a pilot study. *Mov Disord* 2002;**17**:1318–20.
93. Bushara KO. Sialorrhea in amyotrophic lateral sclerosis: a hypothesis of a new treatment – botulinum toxin A injections of the parotid glands. *Med Hypotheses* 1997;**48**:337–9.
94. Bhatia KP, Münchau A, Brown P. Botulinum toxin is a useful treatment in excessive drooling of saliva. *J Neurol Neurosurg Psychiatry* 1999;**67**:697.
95. Mancini F, Zangaglia R, Cristina S, *et al.* Double-blind, placebo-controlled study to evaluate the efficacy and safety of botulinum toxin type A in the treatment of drooling in parkinsonism. *Mov Disord* 2003;**18**:685–8.
96. Ondo WG, Hunter C, Moore W. A double-blind placebo-controlled trial of botulinum toxin B for sialorrhea in Parkinson's disease. *Neurology* 2004;**62**:37–40.

97. Lagalla G, Millevolte M, Capecci M, *et al.* Botulinum toxin type A for drooling in Parkinson's disease: a double-blind, randomized, placebo-controlled study. *Mov Disord* 2006;**21**:704–7.
98. Kalf JG, Smit AM, Bloem BR, *et al.* Botulinum toxin A for drooling in Parkinson's disease: a pilot study to compare submandibular to parotid gland injections. *Parkinsonism Relat Disord* 2007;**13**:532–4.
99. Truong DD, Jost WH. Botulinum toxin: clinical use. *Parkinsonism Relat Disord* 2006;**12**:331–55.
100. Friedman A, Potulska A. Quantitative assessment of parkinsonian sialorrhea and results of treatment with botulinum toxin. *Parkinsonism Relat Disord* 2001;**7**:329–32.
101. O'Sullivan JD, Bhatia KP, Lees AJ. Botulinum toxin A as treatment for drooling saliva in PD. *Neurology* 2000;**55**:606–7.
102. Mullins WM, Gross CW, Moore JM. Long-term follow-up of tympanic neurectomy for sialorrhea. *Laryngoscope* 1979;**89**:1219–23.
103. Clarke CE, Gullaksen E, Macdonald S, *et al.* Referral criteria for speech and language therapy assessment of dysphagia caused by idiopathic Parkinson's disease. *Acta Neurol Scand* 1998;**97**:27–35.
104. Leopold NA, Kagel MC. Prepharyngeal dysphagia in Parkinson's disease. *Dysphagia* 1996 **11**:14–22.
105. Bushmann M, Dobmeyer SM, Leeker L, *et al.* Swallowing abnormalities and their response to treatment in Parkinson's disease. *Neurology* 1989;**39**:1309–14.
106. Leopold NA, Kagel MC. Pharyngo-esophageal dysphagia in Parkinson's disease. *Dysphagia* 1997;**12**:11–8.
107. Fuh JL, Lee RC, Wang SJ, *et al.* Swallowing difficulty in Parkinson's disease. *Clin Neurol Neurosurg* 1997;**99**:106–12.
108. Potulska A, Friedman A, Królicki L, *et al.* Swallowing disorders in Parkinson's disease. *Parkinsonism Relat Disord* 2003;**9**:349–53.
109. Bird MR, Woodward MC, Gibson EM, *et al.* Asymptomatic swallowing disorders in elderly patients with Parkinson's disease: a description of findings on clinical examination and videofluoroscopy in sixteen patients. *Age Aging* 1994;**23**:251–4.
110. Ali GN, Wallace KL, Schwartz R, *et al.* Mechanisms of oral–pharyngeal dysphagia in patients with Parkinson's disease. *Gastroenterology* 1996;**110**:383–92.
111. Thomas M, Haigh RA. Dysphagia, a reversible cause not to be forgotten. *Postgrad Med J* 1995;**71**:94–5.
112. Müller J, Wenning GK, Verny M, *et al.* Progression of dysarthria and dysphagia in postmortem-confirmed parkinsonian disorders. *Arch Neurol* 2001;**58**:259–64.
113. Nagaya M, Kachi T, Yamada T, *et al.* Videofluorographic study of swallowing in Parkinson's disease. *Dysphagia* 1998;**13**:95–100.
114. Silbiger ML, Pikielney R, Donner MW. Neuromuscular disorders affecting the pharynx. Cineradiographic analysis. *Invest Radiol* 1967;**2**:442–8.
115. Robbins JA, Logemann JA, Kirshner HS. swallowing and speech production in Parkinson's disease. *Ann Neurol* 1986;**19**:283–7.
116. Stroudley J, Walsh M. Radiological assessment of dysphagia in Parkinson's disease. *Br J Radiol* 1991;**64**:890–3.
117. Logemann J, Blonsky ER, Boshes B. Lingual control in Parkinson's disease. *Trans Am Neurol Assoc* 1973;**98**, 276–8.
118. Monte FS, da Silva- Júnior FP, Braga-Neto P, *et al.* Swallowing abnormalities and dyskinesia in Parkinson's disease. *Mov Disord* 2005;**20**:457–62.
119. Ertekin C, Tarlaci S, Aydogdu I, *et al.* Electrophysiological evaluation of pharyngeal phase of swallowing in patients with Parkinson's disease. *Mov Disord* 2002;**17**: 942–9.
120. Williams RBH, Wallace KL, Ali GN, *et al.* Biomechanics of failed deglutitive upper esophageal sphincter relaxation in neurogenic dysphagia. *Am J Physiol Gastrointest Liver Physiol* 2002;**283**:G16–26.
121. Born LJ, Harned RH, Rikkers LF, *et al.* Cricopharyngeal dysfunction in Parkinson's disease: role in dysphagia and response to myotomy. *Mov Disord* 1996;**11**:53–8.
122. Byrne KG, Pfeiffer R, Quigley EM. Gastrointestinal dysfunction in Parkinson's disease. A report of clinical experience at a single center. *J Clin Gastroenterol* 1994;**19**:11–6.
123. Pitts T, Bolser D, Rosenbek J, *et al.* Voluntary cough production and swallow dysfunction in Parkinson's disease. *Dysphagia* 2008;**23**:297–301.
124. Robbins JA, Gensler G, Hind J, *et al.* Comparison of 2 interventions for liquid aspiration on pneumonia incidence: a randomized trial. *Ann Intern Med* 2008;**148**:509–18.
125. Wintzen AR, Badrising UA, Roos RA, *et al.* Dysphagia in ambulant patients with Parkinson's disease: common, not dangerous. *Can J Neurol Sci* 1994;**21**:53–6.
126. Eadie MJ, Tyrer JH. Radiological abnormalities of the upper part of the alimentary tract in parkinsonism. *Australas Ann Med* 1965;**14**:23–7.
127. Gibberd FB, Gleeson JA, Gossage AAR, *et al.* Oesophageal dilatation in Parkinson's disease. *J Neurol Neurosurg Psychiatry* 1974;**37**:938–40.
128. Bassotti G, Germani U, Pagliaricci S, *et al.* Esophageal manometric abnormalities in Parkinson's disease. *Dysphagia* 1998;**13**:28–31.
129. Castell JA, Johnston BT, Colcher A, *et al.* Manometric abnormalities of the oesophagus in patients with Parkinson's disease. *Neurogastroenterol Motil* 2001;**13**:361–4.
130. Penner A, Druckerman LJ. Segmental spasms of the esophagus and their relation to parkinsonism. *Am J Dig Dis* 1942;**9**:282–6.
131. Johnston BT, Colcher A, Li Q, *et al.* Repetitive proximal esophageal contractions: a new manometric finding and a possible further link between Parkinson's disease and achalasia. *Dysphagia* 2001;**16**:186–9.
132. Sonnenberg A, Massey BT, McCarty DJ, *et al.* Epidemiology of hospitalization for achalasia in the United States. *Dig Dis Sci* 1993;**38**:233–44.
133. Mitani M, Kawamoto K, Funakawa I, *et al.* A case of esophageal achalasia followed by Parkinson's disease. *Rinsho Shinkeigaku* 2005;**45**:607–9 (in Japanese).
134. Trugman JM, Quinn CC, Shaffer HA. Esophageal disorders and surgery. In: Biller J, ed. *The Interface of Neurology and Internal Medicine*. Philadelphia: Lippincott Williams & Wilkins, 2008:217–21.
135. Hila A, Castell JA, Castell DO. Pharyngeal and upper esophageal sphincter manometry in the evaluation of dysphagia. *J Clin Gastroenterol* 2001;**33**:355–61.
136. Lin WY, Kao CH, Wang SJ, *et al.* Radionuclide esophageal transit test in the detection of esophageal dysmotility

in Parkinson's disease. *Gaoxiong Yi Xue Ke Xue Za Zhi* 1994;**10**:438–43.

137. Dogan I, Mittal RK. Esophageal motor disorders: recent advances. *Curr Opin Gastroenterol* 2006;**22**:417–22.
138. Cotzias GC, Papavasiliou PS, Gellene R. Modification of parkinsonism – chronic treatment with L-dopa. *N Engl J Med* 1969;**280**:337–45.
139. Paulson GD, Tafrate RH. Some "minor" aspects of parkinsonism, especially pulmonary function. *Neurology* 1970;**20**(12 Part 2):14–7.
140. Nowack WJ, Hatelid JM, Sohn RS. Dysphagia in parkinsonism. *Arch Neurol* 1977;**34**:320.
141. Lieberman AN, Horowitz L, Redmond P, *et al.* Dysphagia in Parkinson's disease. *Am J Gastroenterol* 1980;**74**:157–60.
142. Tison F, Wiart L, Guatterie M, *et al.* Effects of central dopaminergic stimulation by apomorphine on swallowing disorders in Parkinson's disease. *Mov Disord* 1996;**11**:729–32.
143. Lim A, Leow L, Huckabee ML, *et al.* A pilot study of respiration and swallowing integration in Parkinson's disease: "on" and "off" levodopa. *Dysphagia* 2008;**23**:76–81.
144. Bramble MG, Cunliffe J, Dellipiani AW. Evidence for a change in neurotransmitter affecting oesophageal motility in Parkinson's disease. *J Neurol Neurosurg Psychiatry* 1978;**41**: 709–12.
145. Deane KH, Whurr R, Clarke CE, *et al.* Non-pharmacological therapies for dysphagia in Parkinson's disease. *Cochrane Database Syst Rev* 2001;**1**:CD002816.
146. Baijens LWJ, Speyer R. Effects of therapy for dysphagia in Parkinson's disease: systematic review. *Dysphagia* 2009;**24**:91–102.
147. Logemann JA, Gensler G, Robbins J, *et al.* A randomized study of three interventions for aspiration of thin liquids in patients with dementia or Parkinson's disease. *J Speech Lang Hear Res* 2008;**51**:173–83.
148. Restivo DA, Palmeri A, Marchese-Ragona R. Botulinum toxin for cricopharyngeal dysfunction in Parkinson's disease. *N Engl J Med* 2002;**346**:1174–5.
149. Wang SJ, Chia LG, Hsu CY, *et al.* Dysphagia in Parkinson's disease. Assessment by solid phase radionuclide scintigraphy. *Clin Nucl Med* 1994;**19**:405–7.
150. Kempster PA, Lees AJ, Crichton P, *et al.* Off-period belching due to a reversible disturbance of oesophageal motility in Parkinson's disease and its treatment with apomorphine. *Mov Disord* 1989;**4**:47–52.
151. Jankovic J. Disease-oriented approach to botulinum toxin use. *Toxicon* 2009;**54**:614–23.
152. Bortolotti M, Mari C, Lopilato C, *et al.* Effects of sildenafil on esophageal motility of patients with idiopathic achalasia. *Gastroenterology* 2000;**118**:253–7.
153. Fox M, Sweis R, Wong T, *et al.* Sildenafil relieves symptoms and normalizes motility in patients with oesophageal spasm: a report of two cases. *Neurogastroenterol Motil* 2007;**19**:798–803.
154. Cervo FA, Bryan L, Farber S. To PEG or not to PEG: a review of evidence for placing feeding tubes in advanced dementia and the decision-making process. *Geriatrics* 2006;**61**:30–5.
155. Evans MA, Broe GA, Triggs EJ, *et al.* Gastric emptying rate and the systemic availability of levodopa in the elderly parkinsonian patient. *Neurology* 1981;**31**:1288–94.
156. Evans MA, Triggs EJ, Cheung M, *et al.* Gastric emptying rate in the elderly: implications for drug therapy. *J Am Geriatr Soc* 1981;**29**:201–5.
157. Sula M, Hardoff R, Giladi N, *et al.* Gastric emptying time and gastric motility in patients with untreated Parkinson's disease. *Mov Disord* 1996;**11**(Suppl 1):167 (Abstract).
158. Djaldetti R, Baron J, Ziv I, *et al.* Gastric emptying in Parkinson's disease: patients with and without response fluctuations. *Neurology* 1996;**46**:1051–4.
159. Hardoff R, Sula M, Tamir A, *et al.* Gastric emptying time and gastric motility in patients with Parkinson's disease. *Mov Disord* 12001;**6**:1041–7.
160. Krygowska-Wajs A, Lorens K, Thor P, *et al.* Gastric electromechanical dysfunction in Parkinson's disease. *Funct Neurol* 2000;**15**:41–6.
161. Soykan I, Lin Z, Bennett JP, *et al.* Gastric myoelectrical activity in patients with Parkinson's disease: evidence of a primary gastric abnormality. *Dig Dis Sci* 1999;**44**:927–31.
162. Goetze O, Wieczorek J, Mueller T, *et al.* Impaired gastric emptying of a solid test meal in patients with Parkinson's disease using ^{13}C-sodium octanoate breath test. *Neurosci Lett* 2005;**375**:170–3.
163. Thomaides T, Karapanayiotides T, Zoukos Y, *et al.* Gastric emptying after semi-solid food in multiple system atrophy and Parkinson disease. *J Neurol* 2005;**252**:1055–9.
164. Goetze O, Nikodem AB, Wiezcorek J, *et al.* Predictors of gastric emptying in Parkinson's disease. *Neurogastroenterol Motil* 2006;**18**:369–75.
165. Djaldetti R, Koren M, Ziv I, *et al.* Effect of cisapride on response fluctuations in Parkinson's disease. *Mov Disord* 1995;**10**:81–4.
166. Rivera-Calimlim L, Dujovne CA, Morgan JP, *et al.* Absorption and metabolism of L-dopa by the human stomach. *Eur J Clin Invest* 1971;**1**:313–20.
167. Wade DN, Mearrick PT, Morris JL. Active transport of L-dopa in the intestine. *Nature* 1973;**242**:463–5.
168. Sasahara K, Nitanai T, Habara T, *et al.* Dosage form design for improvement of bioavailability of levodopa V: absorption and metabolism of levodopa in intestinal segments of dogs. *J Pharm Sci* 1981;**70**:1157–60.
169. Nutt JG, Fellman JH. Pharmacokinetics of levodopa. *Clin Neuropharmacol* 1984;**7**:35–49.
170. Levein NG, Thörn SE, Wattwil M. Dopamine delays gastric emptying and prolongs orocaecal transit time in volunteers. *Eur J Anaesthesiol* 1999;**16**:246–50.
171. Valenzuela JE. Dopamine as a possible neurotransmitter in gastric relaxation. *Gastroenterology* 1976;**71**:1019–22.
172. Berkowitz DM, McCallum RW. Interaction of levodopa and metoclopramide on gastric emptying. *Clin Pharmacol Ther* 1980;**27**:414–20.
173. Schuurkes JA, Van Nueten JM. Is dopamine an inhibitory modulator of gastrointestinal motility? *Scand J Gastroenterol Suppl* 1981;**67**:33–6.
174. Van Nueten JM, Schuurkes JA. Studies on the role of dopamine and dopamine blockers in gastroduodenal motility. *Scand J Gastroenterol Suppl* 1984;**96**:89–99.
175. Djaldetti R, Ziv I, Melamed E. Impaired absorption of oral levodopa: a major cause for response fluctuations in Parkinson's disease. *Isr J Med Sci* 1996;**32**:1224–7.

176. Kurlan R, Rothfield KP, Woodward WR, *et al.* Erratic gastric emptying of levodopa may cause "random" fluctuations of parkinsonian mobility. *Neurology* 1988;**38**:419–21.
177. Melamed E, Zoldan J, Galili-Mosberg R, *et al.* Current management of motor fluctuations in patients with advanced Parkinson's disease treated chronically with levodopa. *J Neural Transm Suppl* 1999;**56**:173–83.
178. Deleu D, Ebinger G, Michotte Y. Clinical and pharmacokinetic comparison of oral and duodenal delivery of levodopa/carbidopa in patients with Parkinson's disease with a fluctuating response to levodopa. *Eur J Clin Pharmacol* 1991;**41**:453–8.
179. Nyholm D, Lennernäs H. Irregular gastrointestinal drug absorption in Parkinson's disease. *Expert Opin Drug Metab Toxicol* 2008;**4**:193–203.
180. Waseem S, Moshiree B, Draganov PV. Gastroparesis: current diagnostic challenges and management considerations. *World J Gastroenterol* 2009;**15**:25–37.
181. Abell TL, Camilleri M, Donohoe K, *et al.* Consensus recommendations for gastric emptying scintigraphy: a joint report of the American Neurogastroenterology and Motility Society and the Society of Nuclear Medicine. *Am J Gastroenterol* 2008;**103**:753–63.
182. Müller T, Erdmann C, Bremen D, *et al.* Impact of gastric emptying on levodopa pharmacokinetics in Parkinson disease patients. *Clin Neuropharmacol* 2006;**29**:61–7.
183. Lu CL, Shan DE, Chen CY, *et al.* Impaired gastric myoelectrical activity in patients with Parkinson's disease and effect of levodopa treatment. *Dig Dis Sci* 2004;**49**:744–9.
184. Naftali T, Gadoth N, Huberman M, *et al.* Electrogastrography in patients with Parkinson's disease. *Can J Neurol Sci* 2005;**32**:82–6.
185. Chen CL, Lin HH, Chen SY, *et al.* Utility of electrogastrography in differentiating Parkinson's disease with or without gastrointestinal symptoms: a prospective controlled study. *Digestion* 2005;**71**:187–91.
186. Laduron PM, Leysen JE. Domperidone, a specific *in vitro* dopamine antagonist, devoid of *in vivo* central dopaminergic activity. *Biochem Pharmacol* 1979;**28**:2161–5.
187. Barone JA. Domperidone: a peripherally acting dopamine 2-receptor antagonist. *Ann Pharmacother* 1999;**33**:429–40.
188. Reddymasu SC, Soykan I, McCallum RW. Domperidone: review of pharmacology and clinical applications in gastroenterology. *Am J Gastroenterol* 2007;**102**:2036–45.
189. Shindler JS, Finnerty GT, Towlson K, *et al.* Domperidone and levodopa in Parkinson's disease. *Br J Clin Pharmacol* 1984;**18**:959–62.
190. Soykan I, Sarosiek I, Shifflett J, *et al.* Effect of chronic oral domperidone therapy on gastrointestinal symptoms and gastric emptying in patients with Parkinson's disease. *Mov Disord* 1997;**12**:952–7.
191. Jost WH. Gastrointestinal motility problems in patients with Parkinson's disease. Effects of antiparkinsonian treatment and guidelines for management. *Drugs Aging* 1997;**10**:249–58.
192. Wiseman LR, Faulds D. Cisapride. An updated review of its pharmacology and therapeutic efficacy as a prokinetic agent in gastrointestinal motility disorders. *Drugs* 1994;**47**:116–52.
193. Degen L, Matzinger D, Merz, M, *et al.* Tegaserod, a 5HT4 receptor partial agonist, accelerates gastric emptying and gastrointestinal transit in healthy male subjects. *Aliment Pharmacol Ther* 2001;**15**:1745–51.
194. Mine Y, Yoshikawa T, Oku S, *et al.* Comparison of effect of mosapride citrate and existing 5-HT4 receptor agonists on gastrointestinal motility *in vivo* and *in vitro*. *J Pharmacol Exp Ther* 1997;**283**:1000–8.
195. Asai H, Udaka F, Hirano M, *et al.* Increased gastric motility during 5-HT4 agonist therapy reduces response fluctuations in Parkinson's disease. *Parkinsonism Relat Disord* 2005;**11**:499–502.
196. Weber FH Jr, Richards RD, McCallum RW. Erythromycin: a motilin agonist and gastrointestinal prokinetic agent. *Am J Gastroenterol* 1993;**88**:485–90.
197. Maganti K, Onyemere K, Jones MP. Oral erythromycin and symptomatic relief of gastroparesis: a systematic review. *Am J Gastroenterol* 2003;**98**:259–63.
198. Dhir R, Richter JE. Erythromycin in the short- and long-term control of dyspepsia symptoms in patients with gastroparesis. *J Clin Gastroenterol* 2004;**38**:237–42.
199. Yogo K, Onoma M, Ozaki K, *et al.* Effects of oral mitemcinal (GM-611), erythromycin, EM-574, and cisapride on gastric emptying in conscious rhesus monkeys. *Dig Dis Sci* 2008;**53**:912–8.
200. Onoma M, Ozaki K, Yogo K, et al. Mitemcinal (GM-611), an orally active motilin receptor agonist, improves delayed gastric emptying in a canine model of diabetic gastroparesis. *Clin Exp Pharmacol Physiol* 2008;**35**:788–96.
201. Kim SW, Shin IS, Kim JM, *et al.* Mirtazapine for severe gastroparesis unresponsive to conventional prokinetic treatment. *Psychosomatics* 2006;**47**:440–2.
202. Coleski R, Anderson MA, Hasler WL. Factors associated with symptom response to pyloric injection of botulinum toxin in a large series of gastroparesis patients. *Dig Dis Sci* 2009;**54**:2634–42.
203. DeSantis ER, Huang S. Botulinum toxin type A for treatment of refractory gastroparesis. *Am J Health Syst Pharm* 2007;**64**:2237–40.
204. Peeters TL. Central and peripheral mechanisms by which ghrelin regulates gut motility. *J Physiol Pharmacol* 2003; **54**(Suppl 4):95–103.
205. Peeters TL. Potential of ghrelin as a therapeutic approach for gastrointestinal motility disorders. *Curr Opin Pharmacol* 2006;**6**:553–8.
206. Venkova K, Greenwood-Van Meerveld B. Application of ghrelin to gastrointestinal diseases. *Curr Opin Investig Drugs* 2008;**9**:1103–7.
207. Nyholm D, Lewander T, Johansson A, *et al.* Enteral levodopa/carbidopa infusion in advanced Parkinson disease: long-term exposure. *Clin Neuropharmacol* 2008;**31**:63–73.
208. Samanta J, Hauser RA. Duodenal levodopa infusion for the treatment of Parkinson's disease. *Expert Opin Pharmacother* 2007;**8**:657–64.
209. Brody F, Vaziri K, Saddler A, *et al.* Gastric electrical stimulation for gastroparesis. *J Am Coll Surg* 2008;**207**:533–8.
210. Gumaste V, Baum J. Treatment of gastroparesis: an update. *Digestion* 2008;**78**:173–9.
211. Eaker EY, Bixler GB, Dunn AJ, *et al.* Chronic alterations in jejunal myoelectric activity in rats due to MPTP. *Am J Physiol* 1987;**253**:G809–15.

212. Banach T, Zurowski D, Kania D, *et al.* Myoelectrical activity of small intestine in rats with experimental Parkinson's disease. *Folia Med Cracov* 2005;**46**:119–24.
213. Banach T, Zurowski D, Gil K, *et al.* Peripheral mechanisms of intestinal dysmotility in rats with salsolinol induced experimental Parkinson's disease. *J Physiol Pharmacol* 2006;**57**:291–300.
214. Lewitan A, Nathanson L, Slade WR Jr. Megacolon and dilatation of the small bowel in parkinsonism. *Gastroenterology* 1951;**17**:367–74.
215. Davies KN, King D, Billington D, *et al.* Intestinal permeability and orocaecal transit time in elderly patients with Parkinson's disease. *Postgrad Med J* 1996;**72**:164–7.
216. Abbott RA, Cox M, Markus H, *et al.* Diet, body size and micronutrient status in Parkinson's disease. *Eur J Clin Nutr* 1992;**46**:879–84.
217. Chen H, Zhang SM, Hernán MA, *et al.* Weight loss in Parkinson's disease. *Ann Neurol* 2003;**53**:676–9.
218. Schwab RS, England AC. Parkinson's disease. *J Chronic Dis* 1958;**8**:488–509.
219. Siddiqui MF, Rast S, Lynn, MJ, *et al.* Autonomic dysfunction in Parkinson's disease: a comprehensive symptom survey. *Parkinsonism Relat Disord* 2002;**8**:277–84.
220. Kaye J, Gage H, Kimber A, *et al.* Excess burden of constipation in Parkinson's disease: a pilot study. *Mov Disord* 2006;**21**:1270–3.
221. Stocchi F, Badiali D, Vacca L, *et al.* Anorectal function in multiple system atrophy and Parkinson's disease. *Mov Disord* 2000;**15**:71–6.
222. Jost WH, Schimrigk K. Constipation in Parkinson's disease. *Klin Wochenschr* 1991;**69**:906–9.
223. Jost WH, Schimrigk K. The effect of cisapride on delayed colon transit time in patients with idiopathic Parkinson's disease. *Wien Klin Wochenschr* 1994;**106**:673–6.
224. Jost WH, Schrank B. Defecatory disorders in de novo Parkinsonians – colon transit and electromyogram of the external anal sphincter. *Wien Klin Wochenschr* 1998;**110**:535–7.
225. Sakakibara R, Odaka T, Uchiyama T, *et al.* Colonic transit time and rectoanal videomanometry in Parkinson's disease. *J Neurol Neurosurg Psychiatry* 2003;**74**:268–72.
226. Sakakibara R, Shinotoh H, Uchiyama T, *et al.* Questionnaire-based assessment of pelvic organ dysfunction in Parkinson's disease. *Auton Neurosci* 2001;**92**:76–85.
227. Ashraf W, Pfeiffer RF, Park F, *et al.* Constipation in Parkinson's disease: objective assessment and response to psyllium. *Mov Disord* 1997;**12**:946–51.
228. Abbott RD, Ross GW, Petrovitch H, *et al.* Bowel movement frequency in late life and incidental Lewy bodies. *Mov Disord* 2007;**22**:1581–6.
229. Lin HC, Prather C, Fisher RS, *et al.* Measurement of gastrointestinal transit. *Dig Dis Sci* 2005;**50**:989–1004.
230. Wiesel PH, Norton C, Brazzelli M. Management of faecal incontinence and constipation in adults with central neurological diseases. *Cochrane Database Syst Rev* 2001;**4**:CD002115.
231. Coggrave M, Wiesel PH, Norton C. Management of faecal incontinence and constipation in adults with central neurological diseases. *Cochrane Database Syst Rev* 2006;**2**:CD002115.
232. Astarloa R, Mena MA, Sánchez V, *et al.* Clinical and pharmacokinetic effects of a diet rich in insoluble fiber on Parkinson disease. *Clin Neuropharmacol* **1** 1992;**5**:375–80.
233. Sturtzel B, Mikulits C, Gisinger C, *et al.* Use of fiber instead of laxative treatment in a geriatric hospital to improve the well-being of seniors. *J Nutr Health Aging* 2009;**13**:136–9.
234. Slavin JL. Position of the American Dietetic Association: health implications of dietary fiber. *J Am Diet Assoc* 2008;**108**:1716–31.
235. Zangaglia R, Martignoni E, Glorioso M, *et al.* Macrogol for the treatment of constipation in Parkinson's disease. A randomized placebo-controlled study. *Mov Disord* 2007;**22**:1239–44.
236. Eichhorn TE, Oertel WH. Macrogol 3350/electrolyte improves constipation in Parkinson's disease and multiple system atrophy. *Mov Disord* 2001;**16**:1176–7.
237. Jost WH, Schimrigk K. Cisapride treatment of constipation in Parkinson's disease. *Mov Disord* 1993;**8**:339–43.
238. Jost WH, Schimrigk K. Long-term results with cisapride in Parkinson's disease. *Mov Disord* 1997;**12**:423–5.
239. Sullivan KL, Staffetti JF, Hauser RA, *et al.* Tegaserod (Zelnorm) for the treatment of constipation in Parkinson's disease. *Mov Disord* 2006;**21**:115–6.
240. Morgan JC, Sethi KD. Tegaserod in constipation associated with Parkinson's disease. *Clin Neuropharmacol* 2007;**30**:52–4.
241. Quigley EM, Vandeplassche L, Kerstens R, *et al.* Clinical trial: the efficacy, impact on quality of life, and safety and tolerability of prucalopride in severe chronic constipation – a 12-week, randomized, double-blind, placebo-controlled study. *Aliment Pharmacol Ther* 2009;**29**:315–28.
242. Camilleri M, Kerstens R, Rykx A, *et al.* A placebo-controlled trial of prucalopride for severe chronic constipation. *N Engl J Med* 2008;**358**:2344–54.
243. Tack J, van Outryve M, Beyens G, *et al.* Prucalopride (Resolor) in the treatment of severe chronic constipation in patients dissatisfied with laxatives. *Gut* 2009;**58**:357–65.
244. Curran MP, Robinson DM. Mosapride in gastrointestinal disorders. *Drugs* 2008;**68**:981–91.
245. Liu Z, Sakakibara R, Odaka T, *et al.* Mosapride citrate, a novel 5-HT4 agonist and partial 5-HT3 antagonist, ameliorates constipation in parkinsonian patients. *Mov Disord* 2005;**20**:680–6.
246. Rivkin A, Chagan L. Lubiprostone: chloride channel activator for chronic constipation. *Clin Ther* 2006;**28**:2008–21.
247. Johanson JF, Morton D, Geenen J, *et al.* Multicenter, 4-week, double-blind, randomized, placebo-controlled trial of lubiprostone, a locally-acting, type-2 chloride channel activator, in patients with chronic constipation. *Am J Gastroenterol* 2008;**103**:170–7.
248. Sadjadpour K. Pyridostigmine bromide and constipation in Parkinson's disease. *JAMA* 1983;**249**:1148.
249. Koornstra JJ, Klaver NS, ter Maaten JC, *et al.* Neostigmine treatment of acute pseudo-obstruction of colon (Ogilvie syndrome). *Ned Tijdschr Geneeskd* 2001;**145**:586–9 (in Dutch).
250. Bharucha AE, Camilleri M, Burton D, *et al.* Pilot study of pyridostigmine in constipated patients with autonomic neuropathy. *Clin Auton Res* 2008;**18**:194–202.
251. Sandyk R, Gillman MA. Colchicine ameliorates constipation in Parkinson's disease. *J R Soc Med* 1984;**77**:1066.
252. Pfeiffer RF. Effect of NT-3 on bowel function in Parkinson's disease. *Mov Disord* 2002;**17**:S223 (Abstract).
253. Roarty TP, Weber F, Soykan I, *et al.* Misoprostol in the treatment of chronic refractory constipation: results of a long-term open label trial. *Aliment Pharmacol Ther* 1997;**11**:1059–66.

254. Caplan LH, Jacobson HG, Rubenstein BM, *et al.* Megacolon and volvulus in Parkinson's disease. *Radiology* 1965;**85**:73–9.
255. Rosenthal MJ, Marshall CE. Sigmoid volvulus in association with parkinsonism. Report of four cases. *J Am Geriatr Soc* 1987;**35**:683–4.
256. Bassotti G, Maggio D, Battaglia E, *et al.* Manometric investigation of anorectal function in early and late stage Parkinson's disease. *J Neurol Neurosurg Psychiatry* 2000;**68**:768–70.
257. Crowell MD. Pathogenesis of slow transit and pelvic floor dysfunction: from bench to bedside. *Rev Gastroenterol Disord* 2004;**4**(Suppl 2):S17–27.
258. Wald A. Anorectal and pelvic floor dysfunction. In: Quigley EMM, Pfeiffer RF, eds. *Neuro-Gastroenterology*. Philadelphia: Butterworth Heinemann, 2004:255–71.
259. Mathers SE, Kempster PA, Swash M, *et al.* Constipation and paradoxical puborectalis contraction in anismus and Parkinson's disease: a dystonic phenomenon? *J Neurol Neurosurg Psychiatry* 1988;**51**:1503–7.
260. Mathers SE, Kempster PA, Law PJ, *et al.* Anal sphincter dysfunction in Parkinson's disease. *Arch Neurol* 1989;**46**:1061–4.
261. Voderholzer WA, Neuhaus DA, Klauser AG, *et al.* Paradoxical sphincter contraction is rarely indicative of anismus. *Gut* 1997;**41**:258–62.
262. Schouten WR, Briel JW, Auwerda JJ, *et al.* Anismus: fact or fiction? *Dis Colon Rectum* 1997;**40**:1033–41.
263. Ashraf W, Pfeiffer RF, Quigley EM. Anorectal manometry in the assessment of anorectal function in Parkinson's disease: a comparison with chronic idiopathic constipation. *Mov Disord* 1994;**9**:655–63.
264. Ashraf W, Wszolek ZK, Pfeiffer RF, *et al.* Anorectal function in fluctuating (on–off) Parkinson's disease: evaluation by combined anorectal manometry and electromyography. *Mov Disord* 1995;**10**:650–57.
265. Normand MM, Ashraf W, Quigley EM, *et al.* Simultaneous electromyography and manometry of the anal sphincters in parkinsonian patients: technical considerations. *Muscle Nerve* 1996;**19**:110–1.
266. Rao SS. Dyssynergic defecation and biofeedback therapy. *Gastroenterol Clin North Am* 2008;**37**:569–86.
267. Kairaluoma M, Raivio P, Kupila J, *et al.* The role of biofeedback therapy in functional proctologic disorders. *Scand J Surg* 2004;**93**:184–90.
268. Farid M, El Monem HA, Omar W, *et al.* Comparative study between biofeedback retraining and botulinum neurotoxin in the treatment of anismus patients. *Int J Colorectal Dis* 2009;**24**:115–20.
269. Holzer B, Rosen HR, Novi G, *et al.* Sacral nerve stimulation in patients with severe constipation. *Dis Colon Rectum.* 2008;**51**:524–9.
270. Albanese A, Maria G, Bentivoglio AR, *et al.* Severe constipation in Parkinson's disease relieved by botulinum toxin. *Mov Disord* 1997;**12**:764–6.
271. Albanese A, Brisinda G, Bentivoglio AR, *et al.* Treatment of outlet obstruction constipation in Parkinson's disease with botulinum neurotoxin A. *Am J Gastroenterol* 2003;**98**:1439–40.
272. Cadeddu F, Bentivoglio AR, Brandara F, *et al.* Outlet type constipation in Parkinson's disease: results of botulinum toxin treatment. *Aliment Pharmacol Ther* 2005;**22**:997–1003.
273. Madaliński MH, Slawek J, Duzyński W, *et al.* Side effects of botulinum toxin injection for benign anal disorders. *Eur J Gastroenterol Hepatol* 2002;**14**:853–6.
274. Jost WH, Schanne S, Mlitz H, *et al.* Perianal thrombosis following injection therapy into the external anal sphincter using botulinum toxin. *Dis Colon Rectum* 1995;**38**:781.
275. Edwards LL, Quigley EM, Harned RK, *et al.* Defecatory function in Parkinson's disease: response to apomorphine. *Ann Neurol* 1993;**33**:490–3.

Chapter 25
Bladder Dysfunction in Parkinson's Disease and Other Parkinsonism

Fabrizio Stocchi[1], *Margherita Torti*[1], *Giovanni Palleschi*[2], & *Antonio Carbone*[2]
[1]Institute of Neurology, IRCCS San Raffaele Pisana, Rome, Italy
[2]Institute of Urology, University "La Sapienza," Rome, Italy

Introduction

Bladder dysfunction is very common in patients with Parkinson's disease (PD) and parkinsonism. A recent international survey using the Non Motor Questionnaire (NMSQuest) to assess non-motor symptoms of PD found that 56% of 545 patients answered positively to the question, "have you experienced a sense of urgency to pass urine which makes you rush to the toilet?," and nocturia was reported by 62%. It emerged from the study that "urinary" complaints had the highest percentage of positive responses of all nine symptom domains examined [1,2]. Another study showed that urinary symptoms are significantly more common in PD patients than in age-matched control group [3]. Better and earlier characterization of bladder dysfunctions can also help to differentiate between idiopathic PD and other parkinsonisms such as multiple system atrophy (MSA) [4]. This chapter reviews the symptoms, pathophysiology, prevalence, diagnosis, and treatment of bladder dysfunction in PD and atypical parkinsonism.

Symptoms and pathophysiology

Symptoms

It is widely accepted that the complaint of urinary urgency reflects underlying detrusor overactivity. Detrusor overactivity is the commonest urodynamic abnormality in PD patients suffering from symptoms of overactive bladder such as urinary frequency, urinary urgency, nocturia, and incontinence [4]. However, symptoms of voiding difficulty such as hesitancy, abnormal stream, difficulty voiding, and a sensation of incomplete emptying may also occur [3]. The explanation for difficulty with voiding may be related to an impaired relaxation or bradykinesia of the urethral sphincter and a delayed relaxation of the pelvic floor with a consequent bladder outflow obstruction. This problem is more common in patients with advanced disease and can be reversed by apomorphine or levodopa (Figure 25.1) [4,5]. Nocturia appears to be a particular problem for patients with PD. In the NMSQuest study, nocturia was the commonest non-motor symptom, being reported by 62% of patients [1]. The reason for the frequency of this complaint has not been properly elucidated, and possibly relates to increased output at night, reduced bladder capacity, or impairment of sleep. Moreover, during the night patients are commonly undertreated, and it is appreciated that urinary urgency is more common during the "off" state. PD patients also suffer from impairment of sleep and restlessness during the night, which can aggravate the problem. See Table 25.1

Pathophysiology

The nature and cause of bladder symptoms in PD patients are becoming clearer, as the role of cortical, basal ganglia, and brainstem structure in the control of bladder function has become better understood. It is also now appreciated that dopamine receptors play an important role in bladder control. Physiological bladder control is dependent on the correct functioning of various structures, including suprapontine and pontine centers, spinal connections between the pons, the lumbo-sacral cord/plexus, and peripheral nerves. Any damage in these circuits that control the lower urinary tract can disrupt the physiological relation between these centers, leading to impairment in the normal vesico-urethral function.

The lower urinary tract consists of two major components, the bladder and the urethra, which play critical roles in the opposite functions of storage and voiding of urine. During bladder filling, any tendency for contraction of the detrusor smooth muscle in the bladder

Parkinson's Disease: Non-Motor and Non-Dopaminergic Features, First Edition. Edited by C. Warren Olanow, Fabrizio Stocchi, and Anthony E. Lang.

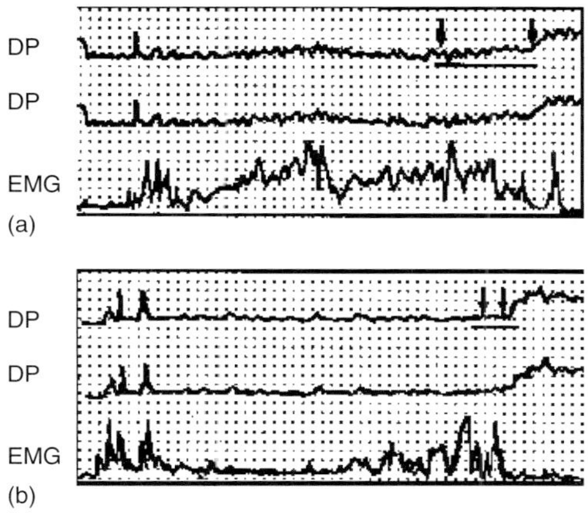

Figure 25.1 Delayed pelvic floor relaxation and the effect of apomorphine: urodynamic evaluation in a patients with advanced PD. (a) The patient is in the "off" state. The first arrow indicates the moment when the patient was asked to void and the second arrow the moment when he was able to start micturation. The bar indicates the delay. (b) A bolus of apomorphine has been given now the patient is "on". It is evident the latency reduction between the first and the second arrow. DP, detrusorial pressure (cmH_2O); EMG, EMG trace (mV).

wall is inhibited, while urethral smooth and striated muscle sphincters are contracted to prevent leakage. The high bladder wall compliance of the bladder helps to keep intravesical pressure low. When the first sensation or urge to void is reached (approximately 300 ml of bladder volume), reflex control of detrusor contractions invokes various mechanisms to suppress unwanted bladder contractions whilst maintaining a closed urethra. During voiding, the opposite occurs: complete relaxation of the sphincters and a sustained detrusor contraction to ensure that urine is expelled efficiently from the bladder (Figure 25.2a). The bladder is innervated by cholinergic (parasympathetic) nerves which promote contraction and noradrenergic (sympathetic) fibers which promote relaxation. The urethra is also innervated by noradrenergic (sympathetic – hypogastric nerve) and cholinergic (somatic – pudendal nerve) fibers. Reflexes mediated by the hypogastric nerves begin to operate at low bladder pressure, whereas pudendal–pelvic interaction is more important for detrusor inhibition at higher pressures during the storage of urine [6–10].

Table 25.1 Detrusor overactivity

Detrusor overactivity	Impaired relaxation or bradykinesia of the urethral sphincter
Urinary frequency	Difficulty voiding
Urinary urgency	Hesitancy and abnormal stream
Nocturia	Sensation of incomplete emptying
Incontinence	Intermittency and straining

The bladder control center resides in the dorsolateral area of the pons. The medial portion is known as the pontine micturition center (PMC) and projects to parasympathetic nuclei in the sacral intermediate cell column and innervates the detrusor muscle. The lateral part is called the pontine continence center (PCC) and projects to Onuf's nucleus in the sacral cord. Detrusor contraction is initiated by the excitatory pathway from the PMC to sacral bladder motoneurons and is mediated by the glutamate transmitter. The relaxation of the urethral sphincter at the beginning of micturition is caused by the inhibition of motoneurons in Onuf's nucleus and is mediated by GABA and glycine. Voiding functions seem to be facilitated by higher brain structures in the hypothalamus and prefrontal cortex (Figure 25.3). The hypothalamic preoptic area projects to the PMC and is probably responsible for the initiation of micturition. The prefrontal cortex and the anterior cingulate gyrus are involved in mechanisms such as attention and response selection. It has been suggested that forebrain lesions can cause incontinence due to an attention deficit that interferes with patients' ability to recognize that they have a full bladder [11–17].

The basal ganglia normally have an inhibitory effect on the micturition reflex. In PD, where the basal ganglia are affected, the bladder becomes hyperactive. The micturition reflex is under the influence of dopamine (D1 inhibitory and D2 facilitatory) and γ-aminobutyric acid (GABA inhibitory). The loss of dopaminergic neurons in the substantia nigra (SN) and the associated reduction of striatal dopamine levels causes a reduction of the D1 inhibitory output leading to detrusorial overactivity [18] (Figure 25.2b). Moreover, in the late stages of disease, the degeneration of the inhibitory dopaminergic neurons in the lateral SN is more prominent than in the ventral tegmental area (VTA), which has a facilitatory action on the micturition reflex. The disequilibrium between these two pathways causes detrusor hyperactivity leading to urinary urgency and frequency [19,20]. Dopaminergic drugs and deep brain stimulation can improve bladder function, emphasizing the role of the basal ganglia in bladder control [21–23].

The prevalence of urinary dysfunctions in PD patients is reported to range from 38 to 71%, although a large number of these studies included elderly patients and were published before the diagnosis of MSA was recognized [23–27]. Understanding the extent to which PD can contribute to urinary tract dysfunction is made difficult by the fact that older men may have an obstructive component to their symptoms due to benign prostatic hypertrophy and older women may be affected by stress urinary incontinence. Furthermore, a form of idiopathic detrusor over-activity may affect men and women over 65 years of age due to brain ischemia [28–31].

Recent reviews report that the prevalence of bladder disorders in PD patients diagnosed with modern criteria

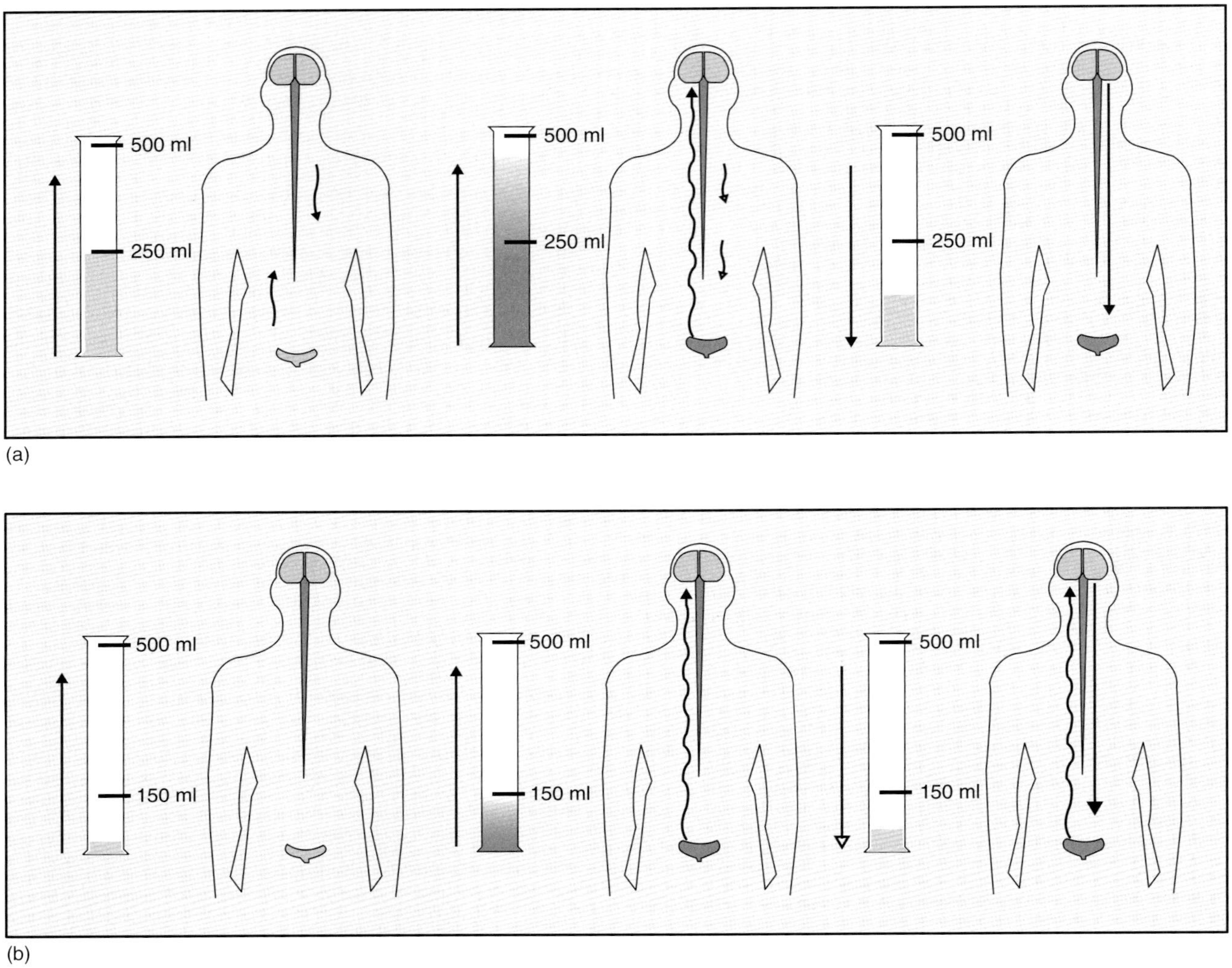

Figure 25.2 (a) Normal bladder filling and voiding; (b) overactive bladder.

ranges from 27 to 63.9% using validated questionnaires, or 53% in men and 63% in women using a non-validated questionnaire that included a urinary incontinence category [32,33]. All of these values are significantly higher than in healthy controls. There is also a different prevalence in older and younger PD patients [34–36]. A recent international survey using the NMSQuest to assess non-motor symptoms of PD found that 56% of the 545 patients with a mean Hoehn and Yahr stage of 2.5 answered positively to the question, "have you experienced a sense of urgency to pass urine which makes you rush to the toilet?" [1]. Similarly, 62% of patients answered positively to the question, "have you experienced getting up regularly at night to pass urine?" [1].

Lower urinary tract symptoms can be distinguished as being irritative or obstructive. The irritative symptoms are caused by an overactive bladder leading to urgency (33–54%), frequency (16–39%), and urge incontinence. The last symptom is usually associated with and aggravated by poor mobility [32,33]. Nocturia is the most frequent of the irritative symptoms and involves more than 60% of the PD population. A real assessment of the incidence of nocturia is made difficult by the fact that a large group of PD patients have sleep disorders and it can be difficult to distinguish between nocturnal polyuria, nocturnal storage problems, and voiding after wakening [37,38]. The obstructive symptoms arise from obstructed voiding and are characterized by hesitancy, poor flow, and dripping. About 70% of female PD patients complain of urgency and urge incontinence but can also complain of obstructive symptoms. Male PD patients seem to be more affected by bladder dysfunction; they complain mainly of obstructive symptoms. Urinary urgency is also frequent since obstructed voiding can lead to infection and an overactive bladder. Many of these patients suffer also from benign prostatic hypertrophy, making it difficult to delineate the true frequency of these symptoms [32,33].

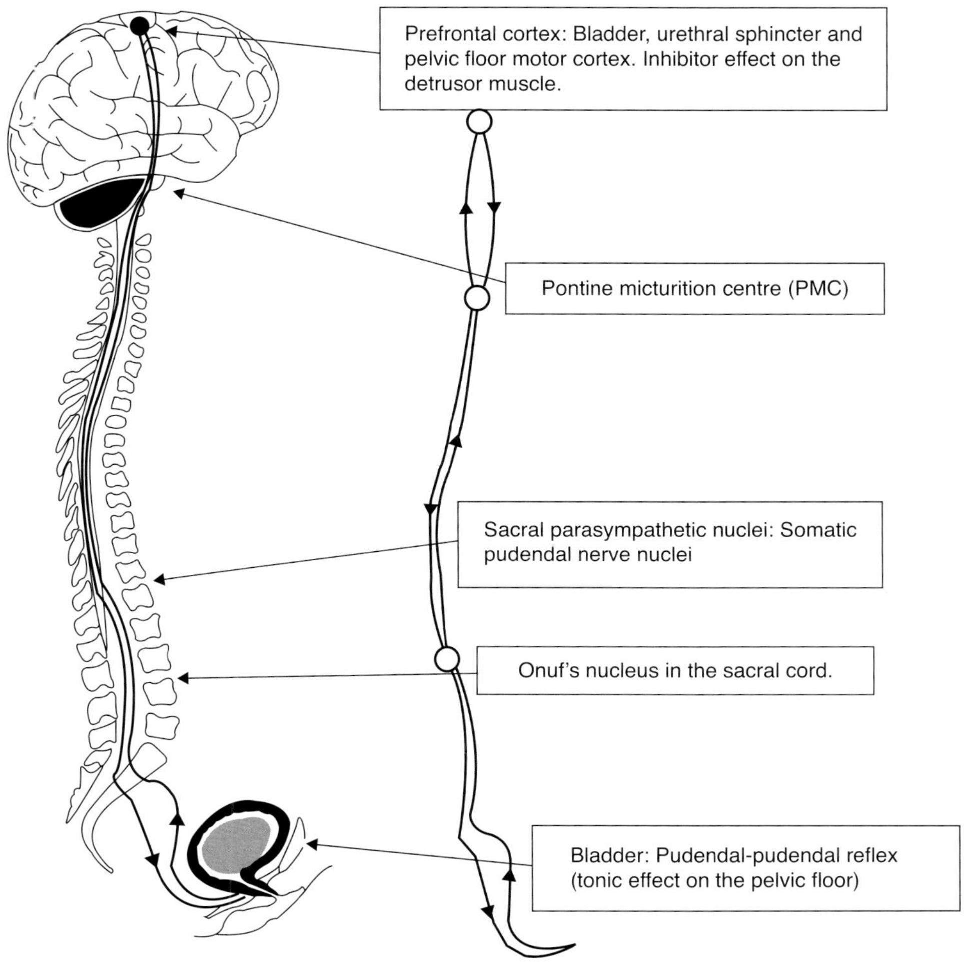

Figure 25.3 The bladder control center resides in the dorsolateral area of the pons. The medial part is called the pontine micturition center (PMC) and projects to the sacral parasympathetic nuclei in the sacral intermediate cell column and innervates the detrusor muscle. The lateral part is called the pontine continence center (PCC) and projects to Onuf's nucleus in the sacral cord. Detrusor contraction is initiated by the excitatory pathway from the PMC to sacral bladder motoneurones and is mediated by glutamate. The relaxation of the urethral sphincter at the beginning of micturition is caused by the inhibition of motoneurones in Onuf's nucleus and is mediated by GABA and glycine. The voiding functions seem to be facilitated by higher brain structures: the hypothalamus and prefrontal cortex.

Lower urinary tract symptoms usually appear some years after the onset of motor symptoms and after treatment for PD has started. Several studies show a correlation between increasing disease severity and increasing bladder problems [1,3]. Araki and colleagues found that voiding dysfunction progressively developed at advanced stages (with Hoehn and Yahr stage of the disability $\geq$3) and were correlated with the severity of the disease rather than with disease duration or age [39,40]. A study using single photon emission computed tomography (SPECT) imaging of dopamine transporter also showed a correlation between urinary dysfunction and nigrostriatal degeneration [41]. Another study showed that the severity of bladder symptoms correlated with the relative degree of degeneration of the caudate nucleus compared with the putamen [42]. However, Campos-Sousa *et al.* found that only the age of the patients correlated with urinary dysfunction [43].

Anti-parkinsonian medication can also affect bladder function. It would seem that the effect of medication does not correlate with the age of the patient or the stage of the disease, but only with the degree of nigrostriatal dopaminergic degeneration. In *de novo* PD patients, the administration of subcutaneous apomorphine and levodopa increases bladder capacity and improves voiding, reducing bladder outflow obstruction. Whereas hyperreflexic patients seem to improve with apomorphine, and to a lesser extent with levodopa, these drugs have no effect on hyporeflexic patients. These findings support the notion that bladder hyperreflexia in PD is related to dopaminergic lesions whereas non-dopaminergic lesions are responsible for bladder hyporeflexia [5,44].

In fluctuating patients, the effect of dopaminergic drugs can be unpredictable. Various studies have shown that in fluctuating patients, detrusor overactivity can worsen with levodopa in some patients but lessen in others. Uchiyama *et al.* demonstrated that in advanced PD, levodopa exacerbates detrusor activity during the filling phase but seems to improve bladder emptying through increased detrusor activity [45]. With regard to the overactive bladder, some reports demonstrate a storage facilitating effect of dopaminergic drugs with prevalent D1 receptor stimulation [46]. Kuno *et al.* demonstrated a reduction in nocturia after administration of pergolide [47] and an improvement of obstructive features with pergolide has been described. Several factors can explain this conflicting behavior in advanced PD patients. When levodopa is administered, it may first stimulate D2 autoreceptors, which can facilitate the micturition reflex. In PD patients on longstanding treatment with levodopa, dopamine receptors are downregulated and potential hypersensitivity may occur. Bladder overactivity may also involve an activation of D2 receptors in the spinal cord [45,46].

Genetic and atypical parkinsonisms

Bladder dysfunction can also be found in a genetic type of parkinsonism. Spira *et al.* reported an Australian family of Greek origin with a parkinsonian syndrome and an Ala53Thr α-synuclein gene mutation [48]. Five out of nine siblings were affected; the average age of onset was 45 years and the initial symptoms were variable, including resting tremor, bradykinesia, and gait disturbance. Affected family members responded well to levodopa, developed progressive cognitive impairment, and had disease duration of 5–16 years. However, there were several additional features not previously reported in families with this gene mutation. These features included severe central hypoventilation, orthostatic hypotension, prominent myoclonus, and urinary incontinence. These additional clinical features suggest that the Ala53Thr α-synuclein mutation can produce more widespread pathology and clinical dysfunction than typical idiopathic Parkinson's disease.

In contrast to patients with α-synuclein mutations, no urinary tract disorders were seen in a large Japanese family with autosomal recessive juvenile parkinsonism (AR-JP) associated with mutations of the *Parkin* gene (*PARK2*). Pathology in these cases is characterized by relatively restricted neuronal loss largely confined to the SN and the absence of Lewy bodies (LBs) [49]. Similarly, urinary problems were not seen in patients with the *PARK6* form of early-onset parkinsonism [50]. The lack of urological problems in these genetic forms of parkinsonism may reflect a more restrictive pathology than found in patients with idiopathic PD.

The onset of urinary symptoms in relation to the timing of other neurological symptoms is fundamentally different in MSA from what occurs in PD. Retrospective studies indicate that approximately 60% of patient with MSA develop urinary symptoms, either preceding or at the time of the presentation of parkinsonism [4,51–53]. The severity of incontinence in patients with MSA is more marked than that in patients with PD and many of these patients seek urological advice early in the course of their disease. It is not unusual to see patients with MSA undergo urological surgery (transurethral resection of prostate in men or anti-incontinence procedures in women), with subsequent worsening of urinary control before the diagnosis of MSA has been made. In some cases, urological clinical and instrumental evaluation may distinguish between patients affected by idiopathic PD and MSA [54].

Bladder dysfunctions have a higher prevalence in MSA patients than in PD patients, ranging from 45 to 95%. The characteristic symptoms are urgency 63–67%, frequency 33–45%, and incontinence, and these can eventually affect the whole population of MSA patients [52,53]. Incomplete bladder emptying is a major factor contributing to incontinence in MSA, and a raised post-micturition residual volume is much more likely in MSA than PD [4]. It is thought that detrusor hyperreflexia is due to cell loss in the midbrain, whereas incomplete bladder emptying and poor flow are due to loss of parasympathetic drive on the detrusor, following atrophy of preganglionic cells in the intermediolateral cell columns in the spinal cord. The balance of these pathophysiologic changes may flip during the course of the disease; whereas early on symptoms due to detrusor hyperreflexia predominate, as the disease progresses symptoms may change to those of incomplete bladder emptying. Postmortem studies of patients with MSA demonstrated a selective loss of anterior horn cells in Onuf's nucleus, which results in denervation of the urethral sphincter [55,56]. This, together with the detrusor hyperreflexia, can explain the high rate of incontinence and urgency incontinence that are found in these patients. Postural hypotension with compensatory supine hypertension at night leading to increased glomerular filtration and alteration in the production of atrial natriuretic peptide may also contribute to increased nocturnal frequency [57].

Two small studies have analyzed the characteristic of bladder dysfunctions in progressive supranuclear palsy (PSP) and have found that urgency, urgency incontinence, and high volume of residual urine are common features in this disease [58,59]. The frequency of urinary incontinence in PSP was 85.7% compared with 38.7% in PD. Vesicourethral function studies showed hyposensitivity and detrusor hyperreflexia with residual urine due to impaired detrusor contraction in the micturition phase. The combination of impaired contraction and hyposensitivity makes it more difficult to prevent urinary incontinence in PSP than in PD. Dementia and impaired ADLs that are frequently present in PSP worsen the ability of a patient to control incontinence.

In corticobasal ganglionic degeneration (CBD), nocturia and incontinence also occur more frequently than in healthy controls. Urinary symptoms appear 1–3 years after the onset of the disease and are more common in patients with longer disease duration (>5 years) and in patients with a forced grasp reflex. Nocturnal frequency is common and tends to be the initial urinary symptom, followed by urinary incontinence, urinary urgency, diurnal frequency, and difficulty in voiding. CBD patients show various other abnormalities, including decreased bladder capacity, detrusor overactivity (DO), detrusor hypocontractility on voiding, and low compliance detrusor [60]. Since decreased bladder capacity and DO are common in symptomatic patients, lesions in the supranuclear parasympathetic system are thought to be mainly responsible. In patients with DLB, episodes of urgency and urge incontinence are more prominent than in patients with PD. These symptoms correlate with DO and Hoehn and Yahr scores [61]. Duration of parkinsonian motor symptoms was significantly longer in PD than in DLB, suggesting faster progression of motor impairment in patients with DLB than in PD [62].

Diagnosis: urological assessment

Many PD patients need urologic assessment during the course of their disease due to the development of urinary symptoms. Urologists must determine if urinary disorders are the consequence of the neurological condition or are due to other primary urologic pathologies (such as benign prostatic hyperplasia in men or genital prolapse in women). A careful neurological and urological history and physical examination are essential in order to achieve this goal. In the physical examination, rectal exploration in men and genital examination in women must be included. The clinical assessment can be improved using standardized voiding questionnaires, which help to define better the type and severity of symptoms. Various voiding questionnaires have been evaluated in PD and the reliability of some of these has been demonstrated (such as the International Prostate Symptom Score) [33]. In particular, Palleschi *et al.* have shown that the OAB-q (Overactive Bladder Questionnaire), a specific questionnaire developed to diagnose overactive bladder, is also reliable in PD patients and its outcome has a significant correlation with instrumental findings even during drug therapy [63]. Bladder, prostate, and renal ultrasound examination can be of value in excluding or diagnosing various organic pathologic conditions of the urinary apparatus which may be the cause of the patient's symptoms (e.g., benign prostatic hyperplasia, urinary stones, prostatic cancer). They can also be used to evaluate residual urine after micturation. Urine examination and culture are required to rule out the presence of urinary tract infection and/or hematuria.

PD or MSA patients with urinary disorders often present with irritative symptoms suggestive of overactive bladder (a symptom syndrome characterized by urinary frequency and urinary urgency with or without urinary incontinence); however, in some cases, these symptoms are combined with obstructive disorders secondary to detrusor hypo-contractility, which may develop in advanced stages of the disease (characterized by weak stream, incomplete bladder emptying, and chronic urinary retention). The complexity of this clinical and pathological condition needs to be assessed by urodynamic investigation combined with external urethral sphincter electromyography. This instrumental tool categorizes the type of bladder dysfunction and is essential in order to determine the correct therapy. Several studies clearly describe the urodynamic and sphincter EMG findings in PD and MSA subjects [64], and both can be useful in differential diagnosis. PD patients can present with a normal urodynamic pattern (if there is less severe disease of relatively short duration) or they may have detrussor hyperactivity of neurogenic origin with a normal sphincter function. Two urodynamic patterns have been identified in PD: hyperreflexia with vesico-sphincteric synergy and hyperreflexia with vesico-sphincteric synergy and incomplete pelvic floor relaxation [4]. Urodynamic evaluation is usually abnormal in MSA patients even in the very early stage of the disease. PD and MSA subjects may also be evaluated by video-urodynamic examination. In this test, contrastography is performed during the urodynamic study to diagnose/exclude vesico-urethral reflux and to show the presence of an open bladder neck during the bladder filling phase suggestive of internal sphincter denervation. Using video-urodynamic studies, Sakakibara *et al.* found abnormalities in 72% of patients with PD and in 100% of those with MSA [65]. An open bladder neck at the start of filling, suggestive of internal sphincter denervation, was present in 53% of MSA patients, but not in PD patients. EMG and sphincter motor unit potential analysis showed neurogenic motor unit potentials in 5% of patients with PD and in 93% of those with MSA, again suggesting the predominance of external sphincter denervation in MSA patients. Detrusor–external sphincter dyssynergia was observed in 47% of MSA patients. Post-micturition residual greater than 100 ml was present in 47% of patients with MSA. The authors concluded that patients with PD had less severe urinary dysfunction compared with MSA patients. Internal or external sphincter denervation was very common in MSA patients but very rare in PD patients. The findings of post-micturition residual greater than 100 ml, detrusor–external sphincter dyssynergia, open bladder neck at the start of bladder filling, and neurogenic sphincter motor unit potentials are all highly suggestive of MSA.

Treatment

Urinary symptoms and bladder dysfunction severely affect the quality-of-life of PD patients. The aim of neurologists and urologists in treating PD patients with urinary disorders is to improve quality-of-life and preserve the upper urinary tract from damage (chronic renal failure). PD subjects with bladder disorders mostly present irritative symptoms suggestive of overactive bladder secondary to neurogenic detrusor overactivity, whose treatment is based on specific items described by ICI (International Consultation on Incontinence) addressing the treatment of overactive detrusor and incontinence [32]. Based on these guidelines, patients with mild symptoms may be treated by conservative approaches consisting of behavioral treatment, pelvic floor exercises, and electric stimulation; however, there are no specific data available today on the results of these approaches in patients with PD or MSA. Antimuscarinics are the most frequently prescribed drugs for overactive bladder. There are several drugs available: oxibutinin, tolterodine, trospium, solifenacin, and other molecules which are currently under study in randomized clinical trials. Antimuscarinics are competitive antagonists of muscarinic receptors at the detrusor level in the bladder and consequently they reduce urgency and micturition frequency. However it is important to balance the therapeutic benefits with side effects. A dry mouth due to the blocking of M3 receptors in the salivary glands and constipation due to the blocking of both M2 and M3 receptors in bowel are common. Adverse cognitive events from anti-muscarinics are a concern, particularly in the elderly. An investigation performed by Loran *et al.* evaluated the efficacy of antimuscarinics (oxibutinin, tolterodine, and trospium) in 64 PD subjects with detrusor overactivity. This clinical and urodynamic study demonstrated symptomatic improvement in all subjects who had undergone anti-muscarinic therapy [66].

There is some information regarding the relationship between L-dopa administration and bladder symptoms. Brusa *et al.* compared the acute versus the chronic effect of L-dopa on bladder function in patients with mild and drug naive PD with urinary urgency [67]. They concluded that acute L-dopa administration worsened bladder symptoms, whereas chronic administration was associated with an improvement of symptoms and in cystometric capacity. An effect of dopaminergic treatment on bladder function in PD patients has also been observed by others. Winge *et al.* evaluated the nature of voiding complaints, findings, and effects of L-dopa medication on bladder control in 32 individuals. They found that most patients experienced significant improvement of their voiding disorder, but the effects of dopaminergic treatment on bladder control and urodynamic parameters were unpredictable in an individual patient [46].

Herzog *et al.* performed a urodynamic study in 11 PD patients who had previously undergone bilateral subthalamic nucleus stimulation. They demonstrated a significant improvement in urinary symptoms and bladder function (increased cystometric capacity) [23]. Finazzi Agrò *et al.* similarly demonstrated a decrease in detrusor hyperreflexia after 9 months of continuous subthalamic stimulation [22]. A small study performed on 29 PD patients showed that tibial neurostimulation repeated for 30 min every 12 weeks also induced an improvement in detrusor overactivity [68].

Botulinum toxin treatment may be considered in cases of severe detrusor overactivity. This approach appears to be promising for individuals with neurogenic detrusor overactivity, but controlled trials are needed [69]. Alpha-adrenergic blockers (tamsulosin, alfuzosin, doxazosin) may also be used to try to improve urinary flow and reduce post-micturition residual. Desmopressin spray can be effective in reducing nocturia, but should not be used in subjects over 60 years old because of the risk of hyponatremia with consequent confusion.

PD subjects with obstructive symptoms and benign prostatic hyperplasia who do not respond to pharmacologic treatment can be considered for surgery [70]. In these patients, a specific urodynamic test with sphincter EMG assessment must be performed preoperatively to try to identify those subjects with a high risk of post-surgical incontinence. Staskin, Vardi, and Siroky showed, in a retrospective analysis, that there was a clear association between preoperative normal voluntary sphincter control and postoperative urinary continence in PD individuals submitted to transurethral prostatectomy [71]. In this study, five out of six patients who were continent preoperatively (83%) but had abnormal sphincter control became incontinent after transurethral prostatectomy, compared with one out of 24 (4.2%) who had normal preoperative sphincter control. However, a more recent study which looked at the effect of radical prostatectomy for prostate cancer included 20 men with PD and demonstrated that the rate of incontinence was the same in that group as in the general population, concluding that those with PD were not at particular risk [72]. Particular caution should be used with MSA subjects because of the high risk of postoperative incontinence secondary to urethral sphincter dysfunction.

Possible treatments to be explored in the future include serotoninergic drugs [73], tramadol, because of its positive effects in experimental animals [74], and sacral neuromodulation.

Conclusion

Urinary symptoms with poor bladder control can be one of the most common and troublesome non-motor symptoms of PD and other parkinsonisms. Neurogenic bladder symptoms usually occur late in the course of PD but can present in the very early stages of MSA. Anti-muscarinic medication is currently the mainstay of treatment, but it should be used with caution because of possible peripheral and central side effects. In case of drug failure, newer approaches, such as botulin toxin or sacral stimulation, may be considered. A PD patient with mild disease may be considered for prostatic surgery if cystometry confirms outflow obstruction.

References

1. Martinez-Martin P, Schapira AH, Stocchi F. Prevalence of nonmotor symptoms in Parkinson's disease in an international setting; study using nonmotor symptoms questionnaire in 545 patients. *Mov Disord* 2007;**22**:1623–9.
2. Chaudhuri KR, Martinez-Martin P, Schapira AH. International multicenter pilot study of the first comprehensive self-completed nonmotor symptoms questionnaire for Parkinson's disease: the NMSQuest study. *Mov Disord* 2006;**21**:916–23.
3. Sakakibara R, Shinotoh H, UchiyamaT, *et al.* Questionnaire-based assessment of pelvic organ dysfunction in Parkinson's disease. *Auton Neurosci* 2001;**92**:76–85.
4. Stocchi F, Carbone A, Inghilleri M, *et al.* Urodynamic and neurophysiological evaluation in Parkinson's disease and multiple system atrophy. *J Neurol Neurosurg Psychiatry* 1997;**62**: 507–11.
5. Christmas TJ, Kempster PA, Chapple CR, *et al.* Role of subcutaneous apomorphine in parkinsonian voiding dysfunction. *Lancet* 1988;**ii**:1451–53.
6. De Groat WC. Neural control of the urinary bladder and sexual organs. In Mathias CJ, Bannister R, eds. *Autonomic Failure*. New York: Oxford University Press, 1999: 151–65.
7. Blok BF, Holstege G. The central control of micturition and continence: implication for urology. *Br J Urol Int* 1999;**83**(Suppl 2):1–6.
8. International Federation of Association of Anatomists. *Terminologia Anatomica: International Anatomical Terminology*. Stuttgart: Georg Thieme, 1998.
9. Athwal BS, Berkley KJ, Hussain I, *et al.* Brain responses to changes in bladder volume and urge to void in healthy men. *Brain* 2001;**124**:369–77.
10. Blok BF. Central pathways controlling micturition and urinary continence. *Urology* 2002;**59**:13–7.
11. Blok BF, Holstege G. Ultrastructural evidence for a direct pathway from the pontine micturition centre to the parasympathetic preganglionc motoneurons of the bladder of the cat. *Neurosci Lett* 1997;**222**:195–8.
12. Matsumoto G, Hisamitsu T, De Groat WC. Role of glutamate and NMDA receptors in the descending limb of the spinobulbospinal micturition reflex pathway of the rat. *Neurosci Lett* 1995;**183**:58–61.
13. Blok BF, van Maarseveen JT, Holstege G. Electrical stimulation of the sacral dorsal gray commissure evokes relaxation of the external urethral sphincter in the cat. *Neurosci Lett* 1998;**249**:68–70.
14. Blok BF, de Weerd H, Holstege G. The pontine micturition centre projects to sacral cord GABA immunoreactive neurons in the cat. *Neurosci Lett* 1997;**233**:109–12.
15. Sie JA, Blok BF, de Weerd H, Holstege G. Ultrastructural evidence for the direct projection from the pontine micturition center to glycine-immunoreactive neurons in the sacral dorsal gray commissure in the cat. *J Comp Neurol* 2001;**429**:631–7.
16. Blok BF, Holstege G. The central nervous system control of micturition in cat and humans. *Behav Brain Res* 1998;**92**: 119–25.
17. Blok BF, de Weerd H, Holstege G. Ultrastructural evidence for a paucity of projections from the lumbosacral cord to the pontine micturition center or M-region in the cat: a new concept for the organization of micturition reflex with the periacqueductal gray as central relay. *J Comp Neurol* 1995;**359**: 300–9.
18. Seki S, Igawa Y, Kaidoh K, *et al.* Role of dopamine D1 and D2 receptors in the micturition reflex in conscious rats. *Neurourol Urodyn* 2001;**20**:105–13.
19. Holstege G. Descending motor pathways and the spinal motor system: limbic and non-limbic components. *Prog Brain Res* 1991;**87**:307–421.
20. Ancrew J, Mathan PW. Lesion of the anterior frontal lobes and disturbances of micturition and defaecation. *Brain* 1964;**87**:233–62.
21. Winge K, Werdelin LM, Nielsen KK, Stimple H. Effectcs of dopaminergic treatment on bladder function in Parkinson's disease. *Neurourol Urodyn* 2004;**23**:689–96.
22. Finazzi Agrò E, Peppe A, D'Amico A, *et al.* Effect of subthalamic nucleus stimulation on urodynamic findings in patients with Parkinson's disease. *J Urol* 2003;**169**:1388–91.
23. Herzog J, Weiss PH, Assmus A, *et al.* Subthalamic stimulation modulates cortical control of urinary bladder in Parkinson's disease. *Brain* 2006;**129**:3366–75.
24. Andersen JT, Disturbances of bladder and urethral function in Parkinson's disease. *Int Urol Nephrol* 1985;**17**:35–41.
25. Berger Y, Blaivas JG, DeLaRocha ER, Salinas JM. Urodynamic findings in Parkinson's disease. *J Urol* 1987;**138**:836–8.
26. Hattori T, Yasuda K, Kita K, Hirayama K. Voiding dysfunctions in Parkinson's disease. *JPN J Psychiatry Neurol* 1992;**46**:181–6.
27. Pavlakis AJ, Siroki MB, Goldstein I, Krane RJ. Neuro-urologic findings in Parkinson's disease. *J Urol* 1983;**129**:80–3.
28. Grey R, Stern G, Malone-Lee J. Lower urinary tract dysfunction in Parkinson's disease: changes related to age and not disease. *Age Ageing* 1995;**24**:499–504.
29. Aranda B, Perrigot M, Mazieres L, Pierrot-Deseilligny E. Bladder sphincters disorders in Parkinson's disease. *Rev Neurol* 1983;**139**:283–8.
30. Dmochowski RR. Female voiding dysfunction and movement disorders. *Int Urogynecol J Pelvic Floor Dysfunct* 1999;**10**:144–51.
31. Galloway NT. Urethral sphincter abnormalities in parkinsonisms. *Br J Urol* 1983;**55**:691–3.
32. Winge K, Fowler JC. Bladder dysfunction in Parkinsonism: mechanism, prevalence, symptoms and management. *Mov Disord* 2006;**21**:737–45.

33. Sakakibara R, Uchiyama T, Yamanishi T, *et al.* Bladder and bowel dysfunction in Parkinson's disease. *J Neural Transm* 2008;**115**:443–60.
34. Sakakibara R, Shinotoh H, UchiyamaT, *et al.* Questionnaire-based assessment of pelvic organ dysfunction in Parkinson's disease. *Auton Neurosci* 2001;**92**:76–85.
35. Lemack GE, Dewey RB, Roehrborn CG, *et al.* Questionnaire-based assessment of bladder dysfunction in patients with mild to moderate Parkinson's disease. *Urology* 2000;**56**:250–4.
36. Campos-Sousa RN, Quagliato E, da Silva BB, *et al.* Urinary symptoms in Parkinson's disease: prevalence and associated factors. *Arq Neuropsychiatry* 2003;**61**:359–63.
37. Kumar S, Bhatia M, Behari M. Sleep disorders in Parkinson's disease. *Mov Disord* 2002;**17**:775–81.
38. Van Kerrenbroeck P, Abrams P, Chaikin D, *et al.* The standardisation of terminology in nocturia: report of Standardization Sub-committee of the International Continence Society. *Neurourol Urodyn* 2002;**21**:179–83.
39. Araki I, Kuno S. Assessment of voiding dysfunctions in Parkinson's disease by the international prostate symptom score. *J Neurol Neurosurg Psychiatry* 2000;**68**:429–33.
40. Araki I, Kitahara M, Oida T, Kuno S. Voiding dysfunctions in Parkinson's disease: urodynamic abnormalities and urinary symptoms. *J Urol* 2000;**164**:1640–3.
41. Sakakibara R, Shinotoh H, UchiyamaT, *et al.* SPECT imaging of the dopamine transporter with [^{123}I]-beta-CIT reveals marked decline of nigrostriatal dopaminergic function in Parkinson's disease with urinary dysfunction. *J Neurol Sci* 2001;**187**: 55–9.
42. Winge K, Friberg L, Werderlin L, *et al.* Relationship between nigrostriatal dopaminergic degeneration, urinary symptoms and bladder control in Parkinson's disease. *Eur J Neurol* 2005;**12**:842–50.
43. Campos-Sousa RN, Quagliato E, da Silva BB, *et al.* Urinary symptoms in Parkinson's disease: prevalence and associated factors. *Arq Neuropsychiatry* 2003;**61**:359–63.
44. Aranda B, Cramer P. Effects of apomorphine and L-dopa on the parkinsonian bladder. *Neurourol Urodyn* 1993;**12**:203–9.
45. Uchiyama T, Sakakaibare R, Hattori T, Yamanishi T. Short term effect of a single levodopa dose on micturition disturbance in Parkinson's disease patients with the wearing off phenomenon. *Mov Disord* 2003;**18**:573–8.
46. Winge K, Werderlin LM, Nielsen KK, Stimpel H. Effects of dopaminergic treatment on bladder function in Parkinson's disease. *Neurourol Urodyn* 2004;**23**:689–96.
47. Kuno S, Mizuta E, Yamasaki S, Araki I. Effects of pergolide on nocturia in Parkinson's disease: three female cases selected from over 400 patients. *Parkinsonism Relat Disord* 2004;**10**:181–7.
48. Spira PJ, Sharpe DM, Halliday G, *et al.* Clinical and pathological features of a Parkinsonian syndrome in a family with an Ala53Thr alpha-synuclein mutation. *Ann Neurol* 2001;**49**: 313–9.
49. Ishikawa A, Tsuji S. Clinical analysis of 17 patients in 12 Japanese families with autosomal-recessive type juvenile parkinsonism. *Neurology* 1996;**47**:160–6.
50. Bentivoglio AR, Cortelli P, Valente EM, *et al.* Phenotypic characterization of autosomal recessive PARK6-linked parkinsonism in three unrelated Italian families. *Mov Disord* 2001;**16**:999–1006.
51. Beck RO, Betts CD, Fowler CJ. Genitourinary dysfunction in multiple system atrophy: clinical features and treatment in 62 cases. *J Urol* 1994;**151**:1336–41.
52. Kirby R, Fowler C, Gosling J, Bannister R. Urethro-vesical dysfunction in progressive autonomic failure with multiple system atrophy. *J Neurol Neurosurg Psychiatry* 1986;**49**:554–62.
53. Sakakibara R, Hattori T, Tojo M, *et al.* Micturitional disturbances in multiple system atrophy. *J Psychiatry Neurol* 1993;**47**:591–8.
54. Chandiramani VA, Palace J, Fowler CJ. How to recognize patients with parkinsonism who should not have urological surgery. *Br J Urol* 1997;**80**:100–14.
55. Burn DJ, Jaros E. Multiple system atrophy: cellular and molecular pathology. *Mol Pathol* 2001;**54**:419–26.
56. Wenning GK, Geser F, Stampfer-Kountchev M, Tison F. Multiple system atrophy: an update. *Mov Disord* 2003;**18**(Suppl 6): S34–42.
57. Endo K, Shirai K, Sakakibara R. Multiple system atrophy and the syndrome of inappropriate secretion of antidiuretic hormone. *Mov Disord* 2008;**23**:1325–6.
58. Sakakibara R, Hattori T, Tojo M, *et al.* Micturitional disturbance in progressive supranuclear palsy. *J Auton Nerv Syst* 1993;**45**:101–6.
59. Wakatsuki A, Tsujihata M, Miyake O, *et al.* Comparison of the vesicourethral function between progressive supranuclear palsy and Parkinson's disease. *Hinyokika Kiyo* 1993;**39**:523–8.
60. Sakakibara R, Uchiyama T, Yamanishi T, Hattori T. Urinary function in patients with corticobasal degeneration: comparison with normal subjects. *Neurourol Urodyn* 2004;**23**:154–8.
61. Sakakibara R, Ito T, Uchiyama T. Lower urinary tract function in dementia of Lewy body type. *J Neurol Neurosurg Psychiatry* 2005;**76**:729–32.
62. Ransmayr GN, Holliger S, Schletterer K, *et al.* Lower urinary tract symptoms in dementia with Lewy bodies, Parkinson's disease and Alzheimer disease. *Neurology* 2008;**70**: 299–303.
63. Palleschi G, Pastore AL, Stocchi F, *et al.* Correlation between the Overactive Bladder questionnaire (OAB-q) and urodynamic data of Parkinson disease patients affected by neurogenic detrusor overactivity during antimuscarinic treatment. *Clin Neuropharmacol* 2006;**29**:220–9.
64. Stocchi F, Barbato L, Carbone A, *et al.* Urodynamic study in the differential diagnosis between multiple system atrophy and Parkinson's disease. *Adv Neurol* 1993;**60**:434–7.
65. Sakakibara R, Hattori T, Uchiyama T, Yamanishi T. Videourodynamic and sphincter motor unit potential analyses in Parkinson's disease and multiple system atrophy. *J Neurol Neurosurg Psychiatry* 2001;**7**:600–6.
66. Loran OB, Fedorova NV, Mazurenko DA, Khitarishvili EV. Comparative assessment of combined therapy of neurogenic hyperactivity of detrusor in patients with Parkinson's disease. *Urologiia* 2006;(2):37–9,41.
67. Brusa L, Petta F, Pisani A, *et al.* Central acute D2 stimualtion worsens bladder function in patients with mild Parkinson's disease. *Neurology* 2007;**68**:1455–9.
68. Krivoborodov GG, Gekht AB, Korshunova ES. Tibial neuromodulation in the treatment of neurogenic detrusor hyperactivity in patients with Parkinson's disease. *Urologiia* 2006;(4):3–6.

69. Giannantoni A, Mearini E, Del Zingaro M, *et al.* Botulinum A toxin in the treatment of neurogenic detrusor overactivity: a consolidated field of application. *BJU Int* 2008;**102**(Suppl 1): 2–6.
70. Merimsky E, Canetti R. Prostate adenomectomy in patients with Parkinson's disease. *J Urol (Paris)* 1982;**88**:253–4.
71. Staskin DS, Vardi Y, Siroky MB. Post-prostatectomy continence in the parkinsonian patient: the significance of poor voluntary sphincter control. *J Urol* 1988;**140**:117–8.
72. Routh JC, Crimmins CR, Leibovich BC, Elliot DS. Impact of Parkinson's disease on continence after radical prostatectomy. *Urology* 2006;**68**:575–7.
73. Sakakibara R, Ito T, Uchiyama T, *et al.* Effects of milnacipran and paroxetine on overactive bladder due to neurologic diseases: a urodynamic assessment. *Urol Int* 2008;**81**:335–9.
74. Pehrson R, Andersson KE. Tramadol inhibits rat detrusor overactivity caused by dopamine receptor stimulation. *J Urol* 2003;**170**:272–5.

Chapter 26
Orthostatic Hypotension in Parkinson's Disease

Uday Muthane[1] *& Christopher J. Mathias*[2]

[1]Parkinson and Aging Research Foundation, Bangalore, India
[2]Autonomic and Neurovascular Medicine Unit, Imperial College London at St Mary's Hospital, and Autonomic Unit, National Hospital for Neurology and Neurosurgery, Queen Square, and Institute of Neurology, University College London, London, UK

Introduction

It is now increasingly recognized that autonomic dysfunction is a common feature in patients with Parkinson's disease (PD). This may affect various organs innervated by the autonomic nervous system, and result in abnormalities of cardiovascular, bowel, bladder, sexual, and sudomotor function. Orthostatic (postural) hypotension (OH) is of particular clinical relevance as it can lead to disability and morbidity, and can even contribute to mortality; importantly, it can be readily measured. OH may occur in the initial phases of parkinsonian syndromes such as multiple system atrophy (MSA) and is increasingly recognized in patients with idiopathic PD. This chapter focuses on the pathophysiologic basis of OH in PD, definition, clinical manifestations, investigation, and management of OH, with a particular emphasis on PD.

Pathophysiologic basis of OH in PD

Autopsies in "normal" elderly individuals, who do not have clinical features of PD during life, show that α-synuclein deposits occur in the dorsal motor nucleus of the vagus, the Locus coeruleus, and in the peripheral autonomic nervous system in the absence of change in the substantia nigra pars compacta. In Braak *et al.*'s neuropathologic staging of PD, α-synuclein deposits were found in autonomic nuclei before they were detected in nigral neurons [1]. These findings suggest that not only does autonomic dysfunction occur in PD, but also it may be one of the earliest manifestations, preceding the onset of the classic motor features of the disease.

The autonomic nervous system controls blood pressure (BP) and heart rate (HR) on a beat-by-beat basis by way of the baroreceptor reflex, with afferent, central, and efferent pathways transmitted via vagal innervation of the heart and sympathetic innervation to the heart and blood vessels. Close control exerted by the autonomic nervous system is needed in various situations in daily life, especially when standing upright due to the effect of gravitational forces. When OH results from autonomic failure (as there may be neurogenic and non-neurogenic components), the site of lesion may be on the afferent side (unlikely in PD), central [which is more likely in conditions such as MSA and PD), or due to impairment of efferent pathways (which is more common in PD and diffuse Lewy body disease (DLBD) than in MSA] [2]. The precise reasons for the probable central and efferent abnormalities in PD are not known; based on the findings of Braak and colleagues of Lewy bodies and Lewy neurites in central neurons and pathways, autonomic ganglia, and post-ganglionic sympathetic pathways, it may be that protein misfolding and accumulation are a contributing factor.

In both PD and MSA, the response to postural challenge while standing can result in a fall in BP, with variable changes in HR and a diminished or absent compensatory rise in levels of plasma noradrenaline (NA), reflecting impaired sympathetic activity. In PD, basal levels of NA may be below normal, suggesting a post-ganglionic sympathetic lesion. This contrasts with MSA, where basal NA levels are usually normal, because of a pre-ganglionic sympathetic lesion. However, in both PD and MSA there is an abnormal response to postural challenge because of sympathetic failure, albeit of differing causes, with a diminished rise in plasma NA when upright.

Cardiac sympathetic efferent nerve activity can be assessed non-invasively using imaging techniques, such as *m*-[^{123}I]iodobenzylguanidine (MIBG) with scintiscanning or 6-[^{18}F]fluorodopamine using positron tomography. These techniques suggest that in PD there is loss of myocardial sympathetic nerve terminals that are primarily post-synaptic, unlike in MSA, where

Parkinson's Disease: Non-Motor and Non-Dopaminergic Features, First Edition. Edited by C. Warren Olanow, Fabrizio Stocchi, and Anthony E. Lang.

post-ganglionic sympathetic terminals are preserved [3–6]. 6-[^{18}F]Fluorodopamine scanning in an LRRK2 mutation patient showed no detectable myocardial radioactivity despite near-normal perfusion on *N*-ammonia scanning, thus favoring loss of sympathetic nerves throughout the left ventricular myocardium [7]. These studies suggest that cardiac scanning may be useful in differentiating PD from MSA, and may also be useful in detecting cardiac sympathetic involvement in the pre-motor stages of PD.

Cardiac sympathetic nerve involvement in PD is supported by tyrosine hydroxylase immunohistochemistry studies showing reduced innervation compared with normal controls and patients with incidental Lewy body (iLB) disease. TH-immunoreactive fiber numbers correlate with the severity of PD, Hoehn and Yahr clinical stage, and disease duration [8,9]. α-Synuclein-positive neurites can be found in the epicardium in PD and iLB but not in normal controls, suggesting that cardiac sympathetic degeneration and α-synuclein pathology develop in the pre-motor phase of PD and increase with disease duration and severity [8]. The finding of aggregates of α-synuclein in peripheral autonomic neurons in individuals with iLB suggests that peripheral autonomic changes may precede the onset of the more classical pathologic changes of PD [10]. This is supported by the observation that 80% of patients with PD have decreased MIBG uptake on myocardial scintigraphy, suggesting that sympathetic cardiac denervation commonly occurs [11,12]. In addition, PD-related neuropathology is also found in the insular cortex, a central site of autonomic control, and correlates with the occurrence of OH [13].

Definition of OH and clinical manifestations of OH

Orthostatic hypotension is defined as a fall in systolic BP of 20 mmHg or more, or a fall in diastolic BP of 10 mmHg or more, on either standing or with head-up tilt to at least 60° (Figure 26.1). There are many causes of OH [14]. Neurogenic OH results from disease affecting the autonomic

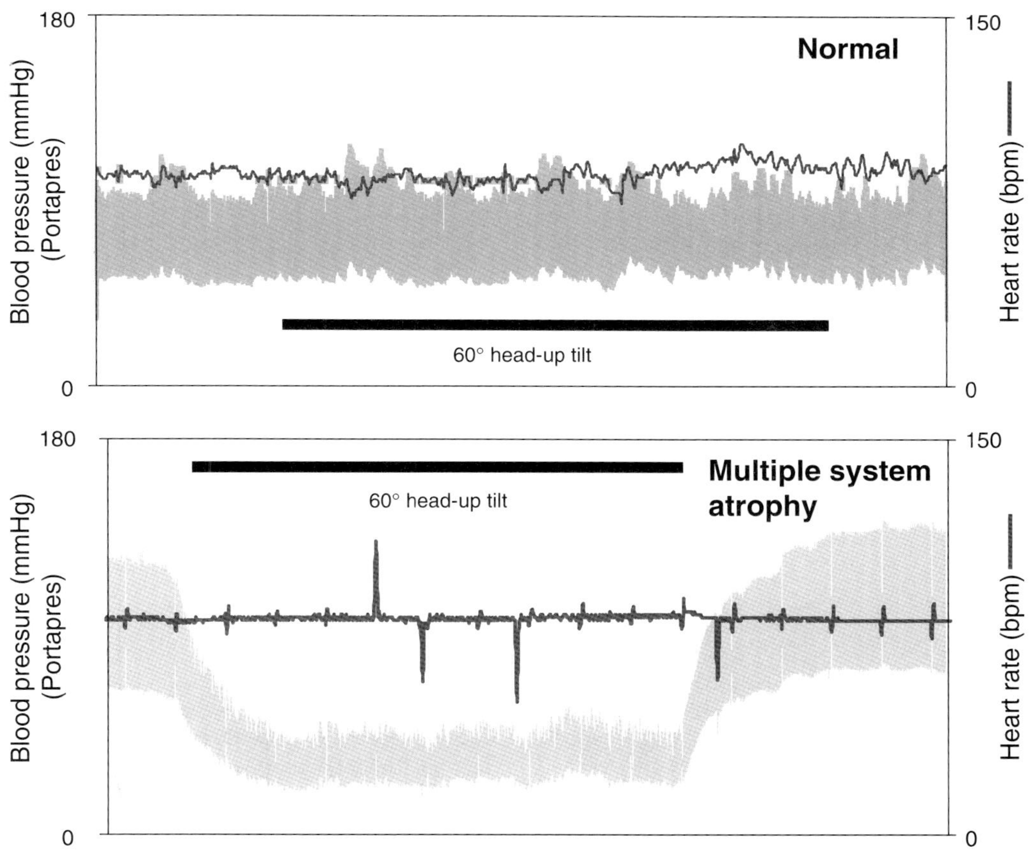

Figure 26.1 Blood pressure and heart rate measured continuously before, during, and after 60° head-up tilt in a normal subject and in a subject with OH due to autonomic failure caused by MSA. In the normal subject there is no fall in blood pressure during head-up tilt, unlike in a subject with autonomic failure in whom blood pressure falls promptly and remains low with a blood pressure overshoot on return to the horizontal. In this subject there is only a minimal change in heart rate despite the marked blood pressure fall. Data from Mathias and Galizia [41].

nervous system within the brain, spinal cord, periphery, or at multiple sites, which often is irreversible. In primary disorders, there is no clear etiology or association, as in pure autonomic failure (PAF) and MSA. Secondary causes include genetic disorders (familial dysautonomia), enzyme deficiencies (dopamine β-hydroxylase deficiency), or association with another clearly defined disease state such as diabetes mellitus. A variety of drugs can also cause OH by direct pharmacologic effects on the autonomic nervous system, or by causing an autonomic neuropathy. Non-neurogenic OH includes disorders that reduce intravascular fluid volume, impair function of the heart, or dilate blood vessels.

The prevalence and incidence of OH in PD have been debated. Recent studies indicate that a number of factors, including age, duration of disease, drug therapy, and co-morbidity, influence the presence and severity of OH. Whereas it was previously thought that the incidence and frequency of OH in PD was relatively low, it is now recognized that as many as 60% of PD patients have OH, with many symptomatic. A recent study in PD indicates that the accepted temporal period of 3 min in measuring OH may not apply in PD, as the BP in some can fall progressively after 3 min of standing or head-up tilt (Figure 26.2). Thus, limiting measurements to a 3 min time period may underestimate the true prevalence and clinical significance of OH in PD patients [15].

A variety of clinical symptoms may occur when the BP falls on standing, as outlined in Box 26.1. In some patients this may result in syncope, drop attacks, and falls, sometimes with little warning, suggesting a precipitous fall in BP. In these cases, it may be that additional factors unmask or exaggerate OH, especially in the presence of an abnormal autonomic baroreflex. These could include food, alcohol, drugs, and other causes, as outlined in Box 26.2. Some patients may have documented OH, but do not report symptoms, probably because they have a gradual fall in BP when upright and that the problem has been present for a period of time, thus allowing for compensatory mechanisms to develop. Despite lack of symptoms, BP measurements should routinely be obtained in the clinic while lying flat and standing upright; when possible, head-up tilt testing should be performed in an autonomic laboratory. The importance of routine and regular

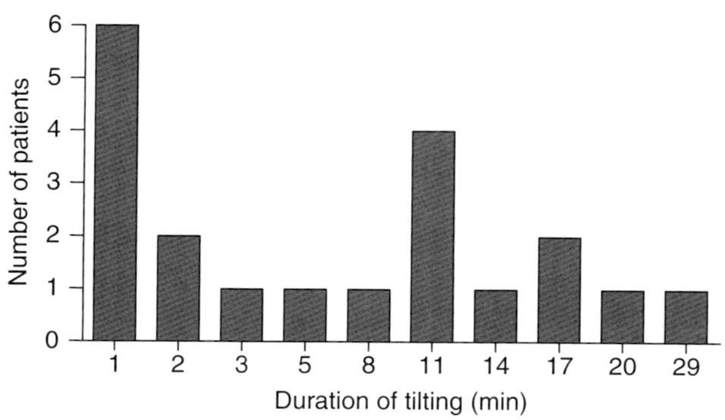

Figure 26.2 Frequency of orthostatic hypotension (OH) after head-up tilting in Parkinson's disease. OH frequently occurs after 3 min (the recommended duration for recording OH). Reproduced from Jamnadas-Khoda *et al.* [15] with permission from John Wiley & Sons, Inc.

Box 26.1 Symptoms resulting from orthostatic hypotension and impaired perfusion of various organs

Cerebral hypoperfusion
- **Dizziness**
- **Visual disturbances**
  - *Blurred vision – tunnel vision*
  - *Scotoma*
  - *Graying out – blacking out*
  - *Color defects*
- **Loss of consciousness**
- **Cognitive deficits**

Muscle hypoperfusion
- **Paracervical and suboccipital ("coathanger") ache**
- **Lower back/buttock ache**

Renal hypoperfusion
- **Oliguria**

Non-specific
- **Weakness, lethargy, fatigue**
- **Falls**

Adapted from Mathias *et al.* [14].

Box 26.2 Factors that influence orthostatic hypotension

Speed of positional change
Time of day (worse in the morning)
Prolonged recumbency
Warm environment (hot weather, hot bath)
Raised intrathoracic pressure – micturition, defecation, or coughing
Water ingestion[a]
Food and alcohol ingestion
Physical exertion
Physical maneuvers and positions (bending forward, abdominal compression, leg crossing, squatting, activating calf muscle pump)[b]
Drugs with vasoactive properties

[a] This raises blood pressure in autonomic failure.
[b] These maneuvers usually reduce the postural fall in blood pressure in neurogenic causes of orthostatic hypotension, unlike the others.
Adapted from Mathias *et al.* [14].

Box 26.3 Possible causes of orthostatic hypotension in a patient with parkinsonism

Side effects of anti-parkinsonian drugs
L-Dopa, bromocriptine, pergolide
L-Dopa and COMT inhibitors (tolcapone)
MAO-B inhibitor – selegeline
Coincidental disease causing autonomic dysfunction
Diabetes mellitus
Coincidental drug treatment for co-morbid conditions

Hypertension:	Antihypertensives
Prostatic hypertrophy:	α-Adrenoceptor blockers
Ischemic heart disease:	Vasodilators
Cardiac failure:	Diuretics
Erectile failure:	Sildenafil

Autonomic failure
Multiple system atrophy
Parkinson's disease with autonomic failure
Diffuse Lewy body disease

Adapted from Mathias *et al.* [14].

testing for OH and other types of autonomic dysfunction is illustrated by several studies indicating detection of OH and other features of autonomic dysfunction even in asymptomatic PD patients [15,16].

In PD, OH is more likely in older subjects and may be due to, or aggravated by, drugs to treat the underlying parkinsonian syndrome, or used in the management of associated diseases such as hypertension, cardiac problems, and benign prostatic hypertrophy (Box 26.3). There may be considerable variability in the basal supine level of BP and in the extent of postural fall that occurs when the autonomic nervous system is malfunctioning, with greater changes in the morning, after a meal, following physical exertion, and in hot weather. In such patients, non-neurogenic causes must also be considered, especially as they can worsen neurogenic OH. Also, OH is more common (50.3%) in parkinsonian patients who demonstrate the posture and gait instability (PIGD) phenotype [16,17]. The early occurrence of clinically significant OH in a parkinsonian patient, particularly if associated with bladder and erectile dysfunction, should alert one to the possibility of MSA.

Investigation of OH

In PD, it is important to establish if OH is present at diagnosis, and then at intervals. If OH is recorded, autonomic testing is needed to determine whether it is neurogenic or non-neurogenic. Appropriate investigations depends on the suspected cause, the underlying deficits, and any other associated disorders. Neurogenic causes of OH require a multi-pronged approach for evaluation, best conducted in an autonomic laboratory experienced in dealing with a variety of autonomic disorders. Box 26.4 outlines the screening tests that are used to evaluate cardiovascular autonomic function; additional tests may be needed.

Box 26.4 Investigation of neurogenic orthostatic hypotension

Head-up tilt (60°)[a]; **Standing**[a]; **Valsalva maneuver**[a]
Pressor stimuli* (isometric exercise, cold pressor, mental arithmetic)
Heart rate responses – to deep breathing[a], hyperventilation[a], standing[a], head-up tilt[a]
Liquid meal challenge
Modified exercise testing
Carotid sinus massage

[a]Indicates screening autonomic tests routinely used in our London units. Gravitational stress (head-up tilt and standing) may be combined with measurement of plasma noradrenaline and adrenaline, as a marker of sympathetic neural and humoral activation.
Adapted from Mathias and Bannister [43].

Laboratory investigation of autonomic function should be performed in PD for at least three purposes:

1 To determine if autonomic function is normal or abnormal, to record the degree of OH if present, and to help establish the correct diagnosis.
2 To evaluate the degree of autonomic dysfunction if detected, with emphasis on determining the site of the lesion and the related functional deficits.
3 To ascertain the precise cause of the autonomic dysfunction in relation to the individual's clinical features, so as to determine the need for further investigations, prognosis, and appropriate management strategies.

In the clinic, OH should be measured ideally with the patient lying down and standing, or sitting if standing is not possible. Sufficient time needs to be set aside for such BP readings to be achieved. Precautionary safety measures should be in place if BP falls precipitously when the subject is upright. It may be difficult to accomplish this in a clinical setting, particularly in patients who are frail and immobile; if OH is suspected it may be ideal to investigate the patient in a dedicated autonomic laboratory. In the laboratory, head-up tilt to 60° is used as the postural stimulus, and particularly if the neurologic deficit is severe or hypotension makes it difficult for the patient to stand. Protective bands secure the patient and electrically operated beds enable a rapid return to the horizontal position. In this setting, BP and HR can be accurately measured using non-invasive techniques, many of which are automated and provide a printout at preset intervals.

Autonomic function screening tests (which also include head-up tilt and standing) should be used to determine the site and extent of the cardiovascular autonomic abnormality. The response to a Valsalva maneuver, during which intrathoracic pressure is raised to a maximum of 40 mmHg, depends on the integrity of the entire baroreflex pathway. Changes in heart rate alone may provide a useful guide. Stimuli that raise BP, such as isometric exercise (sustained hand grip for 3 min), the cold pressor test (immersing the hand in ice for 90 s), and mental arithmetic (using serial –7 or –17 subtraction), activate different afferent or central pathways which stimulate the sympathetic outflow. The heart rate responses to postural change, deep breathing (sinus arrhythmia), and hyperventilation assess cardiac parasympathetic innervation and function of the cardiac vagus nerve.

Additional investigations may be needed to determine factors causing or contributing to OH and syncope. These include responses to ingestion of food, exercise, and in some (such as the elderly where the cause of collapse or loss of consciousness after initial testing is unclear), the cardiovascular autonomic responses to carotid sinus massage, after ensuring that there is no carotid disease. To assess postprandial hypotension, the supine and upright cardiovascular responses to a balanced liquid meal containing carbohydrate, protein, and fat are measured before and 45 min after the meal [18]. To evaluate exercise-induced hypotension, responses are obtained during graded incremental supine exercise using a bicycle ergometer while supine to avoid gravitational effects, with measurement of postural responses before and after exercise.

Intermittent ambulatory BP and heart rate recordings over a 24 h period using a small, computerized, lightweight device are of particular value in determining the effects of various stimuli of daily life, especially in the home setting. It is essential that appropriate protocols are followed with a diary of events linked to recordings to determine the effects of postural change, food, and activity. It is important to record symptoms of OH, especially postural dizziness and falls [19]. Ambulatory recordings are especially useful in detecting BP changes at different times of the day, and in response to various tasks and stimuli in daily life; thus a meal could cause substantial hypotension, especially when the patient is standing, whereas the reverse, hypertension, may occur while lying supine, as in bed at night. The lability of BP, especially if OH is severe, occasionally may result in hypoxic–ischemic injury in watershed areas of the brain in those with a compromised cerebral circulation. OH may contribute to cognitive disturbances, often transient if related to the fall in BP, and also to motor disturbances in PD [20]. Supine hypertension occurs more commonly in PD with OH (94.7%) than PD without OH (31.6%) [20]. Supine hypertension is also more likely to occur in PD with OH treated with pressor agents that have a long duration, such as fludrocortisone; 24 h ambulatory recordings are particularly helpful in monitoring the effects of therapy (Figure 26.3).

Plasma NA provides a measure of sympathetic neural activity and plasma adrenaline of adrenal medullary activity. In pure autonomic failure (PAF), the supine basal levels of plasma NA are low and suggest a distal lesion. This contrasts with MSA, where supine levels are often within the normal range as the lesions are central in origin. In both PAF and MSA, there is an attenuation or lack of the compensatory rise in plasma NA during head-up tilt, indicating impairment of sympathetic neural activity [21]. Some patients with PD have low baseline NA levels, similar to PAF.

Pharmacologic challenge combined with hormonal measurements provides diagnostic information. The central actions of clonidine, through the hypothalamus and anterior pituitary, stimulate the release of growth hormone in normal subjects and also patients with PAF and idiopathic PD who have distal autonomic lesions. In contrast, there is no response in MSA, where the lesions are central [22]. Advances in technology have also permitted non-invasive measurement of autonomic cardiac innervation and function (as previously described with MIBG and fluorodopamine scanning), and blood flow to various regions. Various spectral techniques assess cardiovascular autonomic function but are mainly used in research laboratories [8]. Invasive techniques that measure total body and regional NA spill-over in the heart, splanchnic, renal, and cerebral circulations are used experimentally, but not in routine clinical practice.

Associated factors to consider in OH associated with PD

There are a number of additional factors described further below because they aid the understanding, investigation, and management of OH in PD.

Postprandial hypotension

In normal subjects, BP does not change after a meal despite the release of vasodilatory gastrointestinal and pancreatic hormones. There is an increase in splanchnic blood flow with compensatory cardiac and regional hemodynamic responses mediated by the autonomic nervous system which maintains BP. In PD, however, food can cause a fall in BP and worsen parkinsonian symptoms [18] (Figure 26.4). Carbohydrates are more likely to lower BP than fat or protein in autonomic failure, but it is not clear whether this applies to PD. In elderly PD patients, postprandial hypotension is more frequent (82% compared with 41% in controls) than OH (13% versus

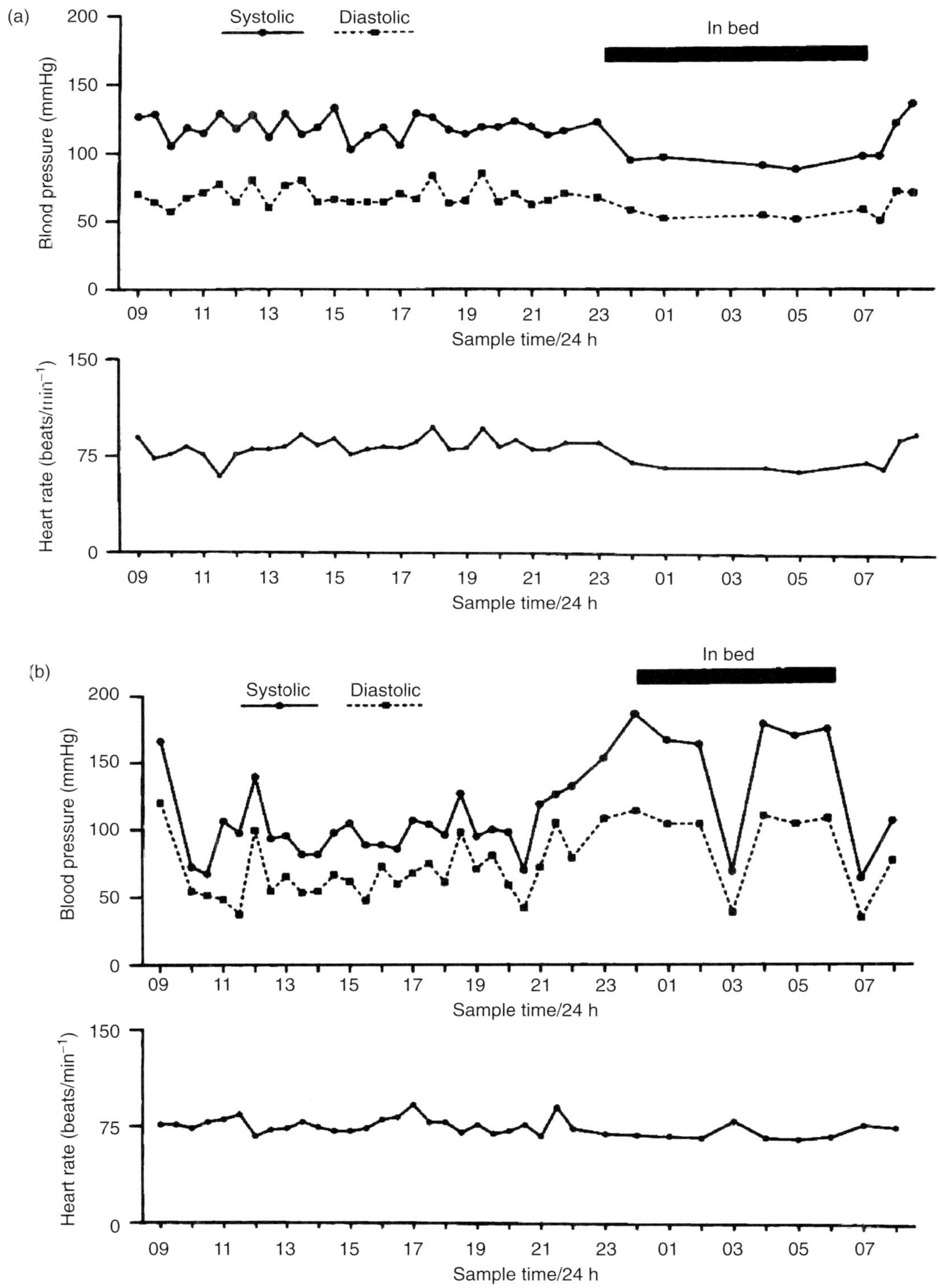

Figure 26.3 Twenty-four hour non-invasive ambulatory blood pressure profile, showing systolic and diastolic blood pressure and heart rate at intervals through the day and night. (a) The changes in a normal subject with no postural fall in blood pressure; there was a fall in blood pressure at night while asleep, with a rise in blood pressure on waking. (b) The marked fluctuations in blood pressure in a patient with autonomic failure; The marked falls in blood pressure are usually the result of postural changes, either sitting or standing. Supine blood pressure, particularly at night, is elevated. Getting up to micturate causes a marked fall in blood pressure (at 0300 h). There is a reversal of the diurnal changes in blood pressure. There are relatively small changes in heart rate, considering the marked changes in blood pressure. Reproduced from Mathias and Bannister [43] with permission from Oxford University Press.

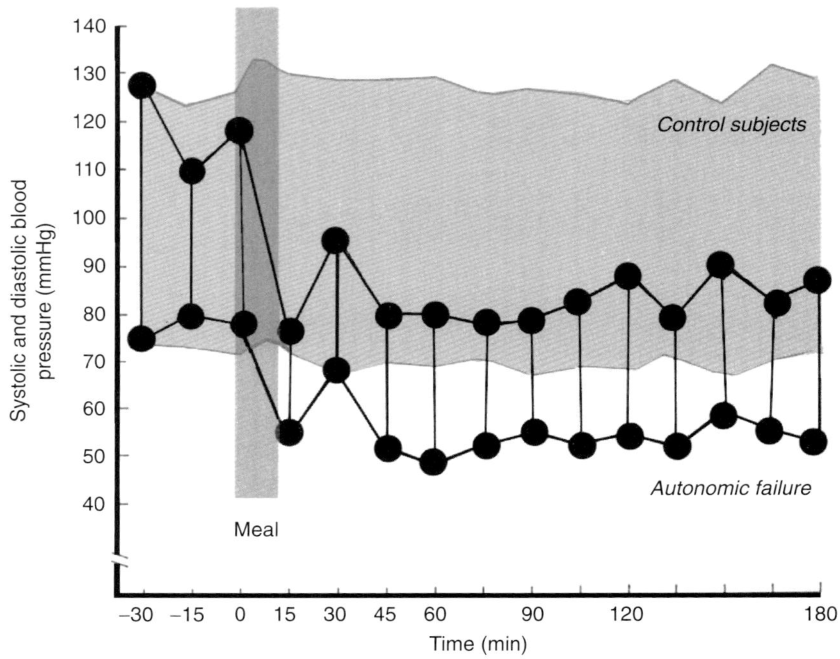

Figure 26.4 Supine systolic and diastolic blood pressure before and after a standard meal in a group of normal subjects (stippled area) and in a patient with autonomic failure. Blood pressure does not change in the normal subjects after a meal taken while lying flat. In the patient there is a rapid fall in blood pressure to levels around 80/50 mmHg, which remains low while in the supine position over the 3 h observational period. Reproduced from Mathias and Bannister [42] with permission from Oxford University Press.

6% in controls), while L-dopa does not appear to worsen either [18].

Exercise-induced hypotension

Modest exertion in normal subjects causes vasodilatation in exercising skeletal muscles and a compensatory increase in sympathetic activity to the vasculature of non-exercising muscles and other organs, thereby maintaining BP. In PD, exercise usually causes only a small fall in BP and does not unmask OH. However, in autonomic failure, exercise even in the supine position without the additional effect of gravity lowers BP even during exercise, as is commonly observed in MSA [23] (Figure 26.5). Some patients develop a marked fall in BP while exercising in the upright posture, whereas in others BP is maintained while walking but falls, with corresponding symptoms of OH, when they stand still after they stop walking. This is because the calf muscles act as a secondary cardiac pump that helps maintain BP while exercising. This lack of compensation is a factor contributing to OH. Although

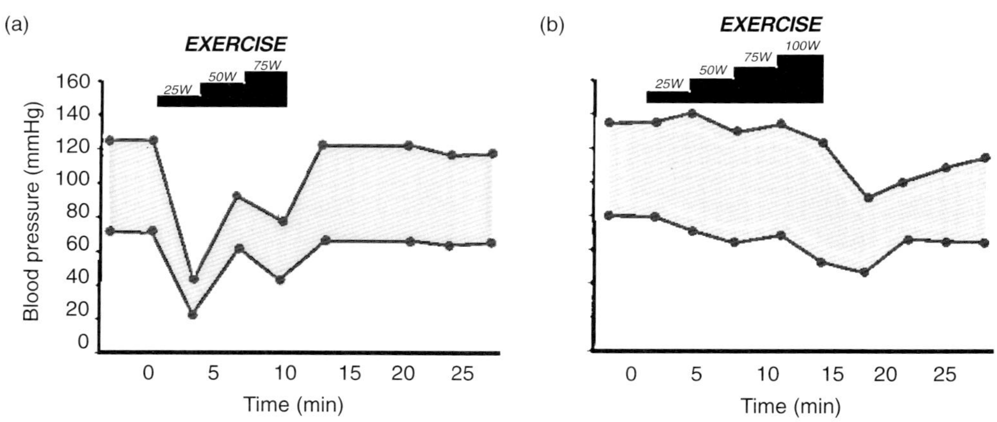

Figure 26.5 Systolic and diastolic blood pressure in two patients with autonomic failure before, during and after bicycle exercise performed with the patient in the supine position at different workloads, ranging from 25 to 100 W. In the patient in (a) there is a marked fall in blood pressure on initiating exercise; she had to crawl upstairs because of severe exercise-induced hypotension. In the patient in (b), there are minor changes in blood pressure during exercise, but a marked decrease soon after stopping exercise. This patient was usually asymptomatic while walking, but developed postural symptoms when he stopped walking and stood still. It is likely that the decrease in blood pressure post-exercise was a result of vasodilatation in exercising skeletal muscle that was not opposed by the calf muscle pump. Data from Mathias and Williams [44].

treadmill aerobic exercise for 3 months improves gait impairment in PD, patients will need to be monitored, as falls may be due to a reduction in BP [24]. Water ingestion prior to exercise may improve post-exercise orthostatic tolerance [25].

OH and dementia in PD

Recent studies in PD suggest that OH increases the risk of dementia [16,26]. There is also a higher incidence of cardiovascular symptoms in PD with dementia than in those without dementia [23,27]. There may be a number of reasons for this apparent association. There is no evidence that treating OH improves cognitive dysfunction in PD.

Hypotension induced by anti-parkinsonian drugs

In PD, L-dopa, dopamine agonists, and other dopaminergic agents, including selegiline, can cause vasodilatation and either cause OH or worsen pre-existing OH. In 148 PD patients with no other medical co-morbidity, BP and HR have been measured after acute L-dopa challenge which in some caused supine hypotension and OH [28]; patients who developed supine hypotension or OH after an acute L-dopa challenge were at greater risk of OH while on chronic dopaminergic therapy (Figure 26.6).

Effect of STN-DBS and OH

The motor improvement that occurs following deep brain stimulation of the subthalamic nucleus (STN-DBS) often results in a reduction in anti-parkinsonian medication, but this does not appear to protect against the development of cardiovascular autonomic failure in PD [29,30]. Conversely, the presence of preoperative cardiovascular autonomic dysfunction does not preclude a beneficial motor effect of STN-DBS in PD [30–32].

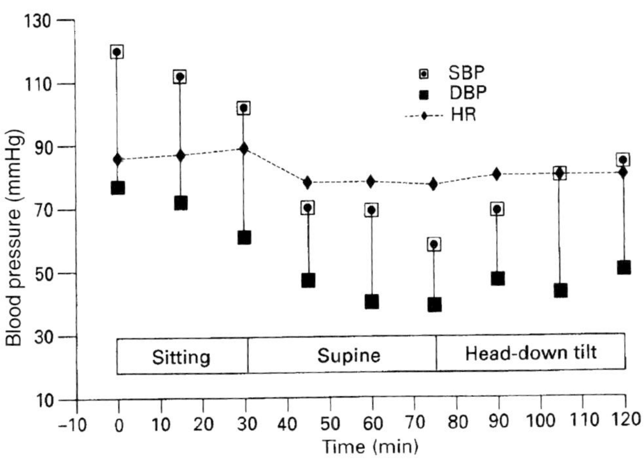

Figure 26.6 Systolic and diastolic blood pressure in a patient with parkinsonian features before and after a standard levodopa challenge (250 mg of levodopa along with 25 mg of carbidopa). The patient was initially seated but his blood pressure fell, and was so low that he needed to be laid horizontal and then head down. On further investigation the patient had autonomic failure and the final diagnosis was the parkinsonian form of multiple system atrophy. Data from Mathias [45].

Management of OH in PD

The appropriate management of OH in PD reduces troublesome symptoms, aids mobilization, prevents falls, and also reduces morbidity and sometimes even death consequent to a fall. In addition, treatment of OH allows more effective utilization of anti-parkinsonian drugs to achieve better control of PD motor symptoms when the limiting factor is symptomatic OH. Thus treatment and prevention of OH can markedly influence the quality-of-life in PD patients. Management is dependent not only on the recognition and measurement of OH, but on controlling the various factors which may contribute to OH. It is important that patients, families, and caregivers, including supporting therapists and physicians, are aware of these aspects, as this aids effective holistic management.

Management can be divided into non-pharmacologic and pharmacologic measures (Box 26.5) [33]. Treatment of both neurogenic and non-neurogenic factors may be

Box 26.5 Approaches to the management of orthostatic hypotension in PD

NON-PHARMACOLOGICAL MEASURES

To be avoided

- Sudden head-up postural change (especially on waking)
- Prolonged recumbency
- Straining during micturition and defecation
- High environmental temperature (including hot baths)
- Severe exertion
- Large meals (especially with refined carbohydrate)
- Alcohol
- Drugs with vasodepressor properties

To be introduced

- Head-up tilt during sleep
- Small, frequent meals
- High salt intake
- Judicious exercise (including swimming)
- Body positions and maneuvers

To be considered

- Elastic stockings
- Abdominal binders
- Water ingestion

PHARMACOLOGICAL MEASURES

Starter drug	Fludrocortisone
Sympathomimetics	Ephedrine, midodrine, L-DOPS
Specific targeting	Octreotide, desmopressin

Adapted from Mathias *et al.* [14].

required, depending on the underlying pathophysiologic processes responsible for OH in an individual patient. It should be emphasized that the management of non-neurogenic factors (such as dehydration and blood loss), is essential, as they can exacerbate neurogenic OH. It is also important to emphasize to all involved in PD care that the use of non-pharmacologic measures is an essential component of treatment, even when pharmacologic therapies are employed. As no single drug can completely mimic the full complement of actions of the sympathetic nervous system in different situations, a multi-pronged therapeutic approach is usually required.

Non-pharmacologic measures can be divided into factors to avoid, to institute, and to consider. They include simple measures such as avoiding rapid postural change. This is especially important in the morning when getting out of bed because the supine blood pressure tends to be at its lowest at this time, probably because nocturnal polyuria reduces intravascular fluid volume. Prolonged bed rest and recumbency, especially post-operatively, should be avoided. Head-up tilt at night is beneficial and probably reduces salt and water loss by stimulating the renin–angiotensin–aldosterone system or by activating other hormonal, neural, or local renal hemodynamic mechanisms, which reduce recumbency-induced diuresis. When head-up tilt is impractical or the degree of tilt achieved inadequate, nocturnal polyuria and nocturia can be reduced with the anti-diuretic agent desmopressin given at night only. Straining during micturition and bowel movement should be avoided. In hot weather, elevation of body temperature caused by impaired thermoregulatory mechanisms such as sweating may cause vasodilatation. Ingestion of alcohol or large meals, especially those with a high carbohydrate content, may cause postprandial hypotension and aggravate postural hypotension. Physical maneuvers such as leg crossing, squatting, sitting in the knee–chest position, and abdominal compression may be of value in reducing OH. Devices that prevent venous pooling during standing may help, and include lower limb elastic stockings and abdominal binders. Ingestion of 500 ml of water raises BP substantially in primary autonomic failure; this may be of value, although the later diuresis may be troublesome, especially in patients who have associated bladder disturbances [34].

The non-pharmacologic measures described above may need to be supplemented by drugs to sustain BP when upright. The major mechanisms by which they act are outlined in Box 26.6. It is important to consider that in autonomic failure there may be enhanced responses to pressor and depressor agents; the former may result in severe hypertension, especially when supine, whereas vasodepressor substances may cause marked hypotension.

A valuable starter drug is fludrocortisone, usually administered in a low dose (0.1 or 0.2 mg) at night; it probably acts by retaining salt and water, and by increasing the pressor sensitivity of blood vessels. Fludrocortisone occasionally, in higher doses, can cause ankle edema and hypokalemia, but these are not likely to occur at the low doses recommended. If nocturnal polyuria is not reduced by head-up tilt, fludrocortisone can be combined with desmopressin, a vasopressin-2 receptor agonist with potent antidiuretic but minimal direct pressor activity. Doses of 5–40 mg intranasally or 100–400 mg orally administered at night reduce the diuresis. Plasma sodium must be monitored to exclude hyponatremia and water intoxication [35].

Drugs that mimic the activity of NA, either directly or indirectly, include ephedrine and midodrine. Ephedrine acts both directly and indirectly, and is of value when symptoms are due to central or incomplete autonomic lesions, as in MSA. In peripheral sympathetic lesions (as in PAF or some PD), it may have minimal or no effect. A

Box 26.6 Outline of the major mechanisms by which a variety of drugs may reduce orthostatic hypotension

Reducing salt loss/plasma volume expansion
- Mineralocorticoids (fludrocortisone)

Reducing nocturnal polyuria
- V_2-receptor agonists (desmopressin)

Vasoconstriction- sympathetic
- Act on resistance vessels (ephedrine, midodrine, phenylephrine, norepinephrine, clonidine, tyramine with monoamine oxidase inhibitors, yohimbine, L-dihydroxyphenylserine)
- Act on capacitance vessels (dihydroergotamine)

Vasoconstriction – non-sympathomimetic
- V_1 receptor agents (terlipressin)

Ganglionic nicotinic-receptor stimulation
- Anticholinesterase inhibitors

Preventing vasodilatation
- Prostaglandin synthetase inhibitors (indomethacin, flurbiprofen)
- Dopamine receptor blockade (metoclopramide, domperidone)
- β_2-Adrenoceptor blockade (propranolol)

Preventing postprandial hypotension
- Adrenosine receptor blockade (caffeine)
- Peptide release inhibitors (somatostatin analog: octreotide)

Increasing cardiac output
- Beta-blockers with intrinsic sympathomimetic activity (pindolol, xamoterol)
- Dopamine agonists (ibopamine)

Increasing red cell mass
- Erythropoietin

Adapted from Mathias *et al.* [14].

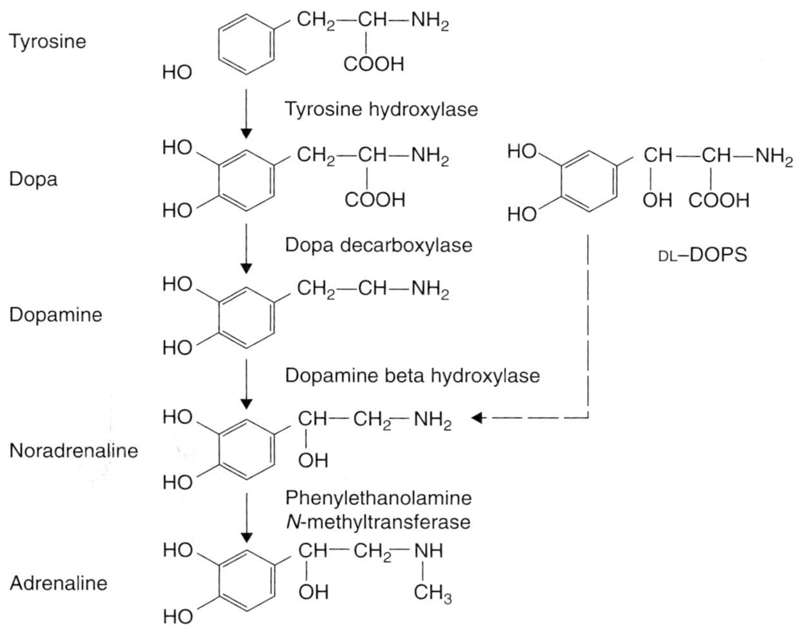

Figure 26.7 Biosynthetic pathway in the formation of adrenaline and noradrenaline. The structure of DL-DOPS (droxidopa) is shown on the right. It is converted directly to noradrenaline by dopa decarboxylase, thus bypassing dopamine β-hydroxylase. Reproduced from Mathias *et al.* [46] with permission from Oxford University Press.

dose of 15 mg three times daily initially can be increased to 30 or 45 mg three times daily, although central side effects may limit the use of the higher doses. Midodrine, which is converted to the active metabolite desglymidodrine, acts directly on α-adrenoceptors on blood vessels to increase vascular resistance and thus raise BP, and is more likely to be effective when OH is due to peripheral lesions.

Supine hypertension may occur in chronic autonomic failure and be made worse by treatment of OH; very occasionally only it may cause cerebral hemorrhage, myocardial ischemia, or cardiac failure. This may be a greater problem with certain drug combinations, such as tyramine and monoamine oxidase inhibitors (such as tranylcypromine and moclobemide), which block tyramine metabolism and prolong its actions. Supine hypertension may increase symptoms of cerebral ischemia during subsequent postural change, probably through an unfavorable resetting of cerebral autoregulatory mechanisms. To prevent these problems, head-up tilt, omission of the evening dose of vasopressor agents, a pre-bedtime snack to induce postprandial hypotension, and even nocturnal use of a short-acting hypotensive agent may be considered. Treatment approaches need to be tailored to the needs and response of the individual patient.

Various therapeutic approaches have been used to reduce postprandial hypotension. Caffeine may act by blocking vasodilatory adenosine receptors; a dose of 250 mg, the equivalent of two cups of coffee, may be of benefit. The somatostatin analog octreotide, which inhibits the release of a variety of gastrointestinal tract peptides, including those with vasodilatory properties, has been successfully used. It also may partly reduce postural- and exercise-induced hypotension, but does not appear to enhance nocturnal (supine) hypertension [36,37]. The need for subcutaneous administration with this drug is a drawback. Ingestion of carbohydrates influences the fall of BP, and drugs that reduce glucose absorption may attenuate postprandial hypotension.

Newer approaches to the management of OH in PD

The NA replacement drug DL-DOPS (DL-*threo*-3,4-dihydroxyphenylserine, droxidopa) has been used successfully in PD with OH. It can be given orally, unlike NA, which is denatured in the gastrointestinal tract. Droxidopa has a structure similar to that of NA but with an additional carboxyl group; it is converted to NA by the enzyme dopa decarboxylase (Figure 26.7). It is likely to have both neuronal and extraneuronal effects, with a direct effect on target organs similar to the natural transmitter NA [33]. Droxidopa has been shown to be of value in the treatment of neurogenic OH in MSA, PAF, and PD [38–40]. Concurrent use of dopa decarboxylase inhibitors (usually administered with L-dopa) does not appear, at the doses used, to reduce the conversion of droxidopa to NA and thus reduce its pressor effects in PD with OH.

STN-DBS has been reported to be associated with improvement in OH, but further studies are required to determine whether this is due to a reduction in potentially hypotensive dopaminergic medications.

Conclusion

In PD, it is important to identify and manage hypotension as appropriate treatment is associated with clinical benefits and reduced morbidity and mortality. This involves defining the anatomic and functional causes of OH so as to tailor the management to individual needs. Educating patients, their family, caregivers, and associated healthcare professionals is of importance.

Acknowledgment

Some of the original work reported in this chapter was supported by a collaborative grant from the Wellcome Trust, London, UK.

References

1. Braak H, Del Tredici K, Rub U, *et al.* Staging of brain pathology related to sporadic Parkinson's disease. *Neurobiol Aging* 2003;**24**(2):197–211.
2. Mathias CJ. Autonomic diseases: clinical features and laboratory evaluation. *J Neurol Neurosurg Psychiatry* 2003;**74**(Suppl 3):iii31–41.
3. Orimo S, Ozawa E, Nakade S, *et al.* ^{123}I-metaiodobenzylguanidine myocardial scintigraphy in Parkinson's disease. *J Neurol Neurosurg Psychiatry* 1999;**67**: 189–94.
4. Tipre DN, Goldstein DS. Cardiac and extracardiac sympathetic denervation in Parkinson's disease with orthostatic hypotension and in pure autonomic failure. *J Nucl Med* 2005;**46**(11):1775–81.
5. Courbon F, Brefel-Courbon C, Thalamas C, *et al.* Cardiac MIBG scintigraphy is a sensitive tool for detecting cardiac sympathetic denervation in Parkinson's disease. *Mov Disord* 2003;**18**:890–7.
6. Goldstein DS, Li ST, Kopin IJ. Sympathetic neurocirculatory failure in Parkinson disease: evidence for an etiologic role of alpha-synuclein. *Ann Intern Med* 2001;**135**(11):1010–1.
7. Goldstein DS, Imrich R, Peckham E, *et al.* Neurocirculatory and nigrostriatal abnormalities in Parkinson disease from LRRK2 mutation. *Neurology* 2007;**69**(16):1580–4.
8. Fujishiro H, Frigerio R, Burnett M, *et al.* Cardiac sympathetic denervation correlates with clinical and pathologic stages of Parkinson's disease. *Mov Disord* 2008;**23**(8):1085–92.
9. DelleDonne A, Klos KJ, Fujishiro H, *et al.* Incidental Lewy body disease and preclinical Parkinson disease. *Arch Neurol* 2008;**65**(8):1074–80.
10. Minguez-Castellanos A, Chamorro CE, Escamilla-Sevilla F, *et al.* Do alpha-synuclein aggregates in autonomic plexuses predate Lewy body disorders?: a cohort study. *Neurology* 2007;**68**(23):2012–8.
11. Orimo S, Takahashi A, Uchihara T, *et al.* Degeneration of cardiac sympathetic nerve begins in the early disease process of Parkinson's disease. *Brain Pathol* 2007;**17**(1):24–30.
12. Orimo S, Uchihara T, Nakamura A, *et al.* Axonal alpha-synuclein aggregates herald centripetal degeneration of cardiac sympathetic nerve in Parkinson's disease. *Brain* 2008;**131**(Pt 3):642–50.
13. Papapetropoulos S, Mash DC. Insular pathology in Parkinson's disease patients with orthostatic hypotension. *Parkinsonism Relat Disord* 2007;**13**(5):308–11.
14. Mathias CJ. Autonomic dysfunction. In: Clarke C, Howard R, Rossor M, Shorvon S, eds. *Neurology. A Queen Square Textbook.* Oxford: Wiley-Blackwell, 2009: 871–92.
15. Jamnadas-Khoda J, Koshy S, Mathias CJ, *et al.* Are current recommendations to diagnose orthostatic hypotension in Parkinson's disease satisfactory? *Mov Disord* 2009;**24**(12): 1747–51.
16. Wullner U, Schmitz-Hubsch T, Antony G, *et al.* Autonomic dysfunction in 3414 Parkinson's disease patients enrolled in the German Network on Parkinson's disease (KNP e.V.): the effect of ageing. *Eur J Neurol* 2007;**14**(12):1405–8.
17. Allcock LM, Kenny RA, Burn DJ. Clinical phenotype of subjects with Parkinson's disease and orthostatic hypotension: autonomic symptom and demographic comparison. *Mov Disord* 2006;**21**(11):1851–5.
18. Thomaides T, Bleasdale-Barr K, Ray Chaudhuri K, *et al.* Cardiovascular and hormonal responses to liquid food challenge in idiopathic Parkinson's disease, multiple system atrophy, and pure autonomic failure. *Neurology* 1993;**43** 900–4.
19. Senard JM. Prevalence of orthostatic hypotension in Parkinson's disease. *J Neurol Neurosurg Psychiatry* 1997;**63**:584–9.
20. Senard JM, Rai S, Lapeyre-Mestre M, *et al.* Prevalence of orthostatic hypotension in Parkinson's disease. *J Neurol Neurosurg Psychiatry* 1997;**63**(5):584–9.
21. Mathias CJ, Bannister R. *Investigation of Autonomic Disorders. Autonomic Failure. A Textbook of Clinical Disorders of the Autonomic Nervous System.* Oxford: Oxford University Press, 1999: 169–95.
22. Mathias CJ, Kimber J, Watson L, Muthane U. Is clonidine-growth hormone stimulation a good test to differentiate multiple system atrophy from idiopathic Parkinson's disease? *J Neurol* 2002;**249**(4):488–9.
23. Idiaquez J, Benarroch EE, Rosales H, *et al.* Autonomic and cognitive dysfunction in Parkinson's disease. *Clin Auton Res* 2007;**17**(2):93–8.
24. Skidmore FM, Patterson SL, Shulman LM, *et al.* Pilot safety and feasibility study of treadmill aerobic exercise in Parkinson disease with gait impairment. *J Rehabil Res Dev* 2008;**45**(1): 117–24.
25. Humm AM, Mason LM, Mathias CJ. Effects of water drinking on cardiovascular responses to supine exercise and on orthostatic hypotension after exercise in pure autonomic failure. *J Neurol Neurosurg Psychiatry* 2008;**79**(10):1160–4.
26. Allan LM, Ballard CG, Rowan EN, Kenny RA. Incidence and prediction of falls in dementia: a prospective study in older people. *PLoS One* 2009;**4**(5):e5521.
27. Peralta C, Stampfer-Kountchev M, Karner E, *et al.* Orthostatic hypotension and attention in Parkinson's disease with and without dementia. *J Neural Transm* 2007;**114**(5):585–8.
28. Sarangmath N, Dodaballapur SK, Mathias CJ, Muthane UB. Levodopa-induced hypotension in multiple system atrophy and Parkinson's disease: characteristics and factors that predict its occurrence. *Mov Disord* 2004;**19**(Suppl 9):S334.

29. Witjas T, Kaphan E, Regis J, *et al.* Effects of chronic subthalamic stimulation on nonmotor fluctuations in Parkinson's disease. *Mov Disord* 2007;**22**(12):1729–34.
30. Ludwig J, Remien P, Guballa C, *et al.* Effects of subthalamic nucleus stimulation and levodopa on the autonomic nervous system in Parkinson's disease. *J Neurol Neurosurg Psychiatry* 2007;**78**(7):742–5.
31. Stemper B, Beric A, Welsch G, *et al.* Deep brain stimulation improves orthostatic regulation of patients with Parkinson disease. *Neurology* 2006;**67**(10):1781–5.
32. Holmberg B, Corneliusson O, Elam M. Bilateral stimulation of nucleus subthalamicus in advanced Parkinson's disease: no effects on, and of, autonomic dysfunction. *Mov Disord* 2005;**20**(8):976–81.
33. Mathias CJ. Autonomic diseases: management. *J Neurol Neurosurg Psychiatry* 2003;**74**(Suppl 3):iii42–7.
34. Mathias CJ, Young TM. Water drinking in the management of orthostatic intolerance due to orthostatic hypotension, vasovagal syncope and the postural tachycardia syndrome. *Eur J Neurol* 2004;**11**(9):613–9.
35. Mathias CJ, Young TM. Plugging the leak – benefits of the vasopressin-2 agonist, desmopressin, in autonomic failure. *Clin Auton Res* 2003;**13**:85–7.
36. Smith GDP, Alam M, Watson LP, Mathias CJ. Effects of the somatostatin analogue, octreotide, on exercise induced hypotension in human subjects with chronic sympathetic failure. *Clin Sci* 1995;**89**:367–373.
37. Alam M, Smith GDP, Bleasdale-Barr K, *et al.* Effects of the peptide release inhibitor, octreotide, on daytime hypotension and on nocturnal hypertension in primary autonomic failure. *J Hypertens* 1995;**13**:1664–9.
38. Maruyama W, Naoi M, Narabayashi H. Study on the metabolism of droxidopa in humans. *Rinsho Shinkeigaku* 1994;**34**(10):991–5 (in Japanese).
39. Mathias CJ, Senard JM, Braune S, *et al.* L-*threo*-Dihydroxyphenylserine (L-*threo*-DOPS; droxidopa) in the management of neurogenic orthostatic hypotension: a multi-national, multi-center, dose-ranging study in multiple system atrophy and pure autonomic failure. *Clin Auton Res* 2001;**11**(4):235–42.
40. Mathias CJ. L-Dihydroxyphenylserine (droxidopa) in the treatment of orthostatic hypotension: the European experience. *Clin Auton Res* 2008;**18**(Suppl 1):25–9.
41. Mathias CJ, Galizia GJ. Orthostatic hypotension and orthostatic intolerance. In: Jameson JL, De Groot LJ, eds. *Endocrinology Adult and Pediatric*, Vol. II. Philadelphia: Saunders Elsevier, 2010: 2063–82.
42. Mathias CJ, Bannister R. Postprandial hypotension in autonomic disorders. In: Mathias CJ, Bannister R, eds. *Autonomic Failure. A Textbook of Clinical Disorders of the Autonomic Nervous System*, 4th edn. Oxford: Oxford University Press, 2002: 283–95.
43. Mathias CJ, Bannister R. Investigation of autonomic disorders. In: Mathias CJ, Bannister R, eds. *Autonomic Failure. A Textbook of Clinical Disorders of the Autonomic Nervous System*, 4th edn. Oxford: Oxford University Press, 2002: 169–95.
44. Mathias CJ, Williams AC. The Shy Drager syndrome (and multiple system atrophy). In: Calne DB, ed. *Neurodegenerative Diseases*, 1st edn. Philadelphia: Saunders, 1994: 743–68.
45. Mathias CJ. Autonomic dysfunction. In: Evans JG, ed. Oxford Textbook of Geriatric Medicine. Oxford: Oxford University Press, 2000: 833–52.
46. Mathias CJ, Bannister R, Cortelli P, *et al.* Clinical autonomic and therapeutic observations in two siblings with postural hypotension and sympathetic failure due to an inability to synthesize noradrenaline from dopamine because of a deficiency of dopamine beta-hydroxylase. *Q J Med (New Ser)* 1990;**278**:617–33.

Chapter 27
Sexual Dysfunction

Kimberly Pargeon, Karen Anderson, & William J Weiner
Department of Neurology, University of Maryland Medical Center, Baltimore, MD, USA

Introduction

Virtually all patients with Parkinson's disease (PD) experience some degree of autonomic instability. This can affect a number of organ systems, the most common being bladder, bowel, cardiovascular, and sexual functions [1]. The neuroanatomic basis for these problems includes alterations in the basal ganglia, hypothalamus, brainstem, sympathetic ganglia, and spinal cord [2]. Sexual dysfunction has received less attention than many other of the non-motor symptoms, although it has been the focus of some studies. These studies have primarily focused on hyposexual behavior in men with PD, such as erectile dysfunction, although sexual problems can also occur in women. Recent studies have also drawn attention to impulse control disorders that can be seen in association with current PD therapies and which include hypersexual behaviors. This chapter reviews hyposexual and hypersexual dysfunction, commonly seen in both men and women with PD.

Sexual dysfunction and PD

Autonomic dysfunction affects a variety of organ systems in PD and can be seen in as many as 80% of patients with PD [3]. While most attention has focused on the cardiovascular (orthostasis and dysrhythmias), gastrointestinal (constipation and sialorrhea), and urologic (urinary urgency, incomplete bladder emptying) systems, sexual dysfunction is also a common, but often neglected, problem [3,4]. In a comparison of 48 men with PD with 32 healthy, non-parkinsonian control subjects, the most common autonomic symptoms in PD patients were erectile dysfunction, incomplete bladder emptying, constipation, dysphagia, and orthostatic dizziness; 89% of PD patients reported at least one symptom of autonomic dysfunction compared with 43% of controls ($p < 0.05$). More specifically, 60.4% of PD patients reported erectile dysfunction compared with 37.5% in the control group [4].

Another study examined pelvic organ dysfunction using a questionnaire to evaluate urogenital functions in PD patients, including bladder, bowel, and sexual function. They found that the completion rate was higher for questions of bladder and bowel function than for sexual function, especially for men, suggesting that patients were less willing to discuss issues related to sexual dysfunction. Of reported problems, PD patients noted high rates of decreased libido and sexual intercourse, and for men, decreased erection and ejaculation [5]. Interestingly, ratings of dissatisfaction were significantly higher for those with bladder and bowel dysfunction than for those with sexual dysfunction, despite their higher prevalence. A significant association has been found between sexual dysfunction and patient age in patients with PD [5,6].

The etiology of sexual dysfunction in PD is multifactorial. One possible contributing factor could be the impairment in the motor functions that occur in PD, including tremor, rigidity, bradykinesia, and postural instability. However, it remains unclear as to whether the motor symptoms of PD pose a unique impediment to continued sexual function. Lipe *et al.* [7] compared 41 married male patients with PD with 27 age-matched, married men with arthritis. Ratings of disease severity were made with disease- and field-appropriate measures and both groups completed the same self-administered scales of sexual function. For both groups, sexual function declined with increased severity of disease ($p \leq 0.05$) and with worsening depression ($p < 0.01$). Although PD patients reported increased difficulties with arousal, there were no significant differences in the scores between the two groups on sexual functioning or in individual categories of desire, orgasm, frequency of sexual encounters per month, or satisfaction. Unfortunately, this particular study evaluated global functioning in both groups, and did not seek to discern the effects of the specific motor symptoms in PD on sexual dysfunction.

It also remains uncertain as to whether the sexual dysfunction that occurs in PD is particular to this disorder, or if it is a symptom that occurs generally in

Parkinson's Disease: Non-Motor and Non-Dopaminergic Features, First Edition. Edited by C. Warren Olanow, Fabrizio Stocchi, and Anthony E. Lang.

neurodegenerative conditions. Non-motor fluctuations that may occur in autonomic, cognitive, and psychiatric features may be a possible clue. For instance, Witjas *et al.* [8] assessed frequency and disability related to non-motor fluctuations (NMF) in PD compared to motor fluctuations (MF). Fifty PD patients with motor fluctuations answered a structured questionnaire grading their degree of disability due to NMF focusing on 54 non-motor symptoms divided into three subgroups (dysautonomic, cognitive, and psychiatric). All patients had at least one type of NMF, and these were most often associated with the "off" state. The total number of NMFs was correlated with the degree of MF; the most frequent NMFs were anxiety, drenching sweats, slowing of thinking, fatigue, and akathisia. Approximately a quarter of patients reported that NMFs resulted in greater disability than MFs. Importantly, sexual disorders were endorsed in 10% of patients during the "on" state but 50% during the "off" state, suggesting some specific role for PD features in the development of sexual dysfunction in these patients.

Non-motor symptoms, particularly psychologic factors, may adversely affect sexual function in PD patients, but may not be the primary clinical focus of most office visits. Jacobs, Vieregge, and Vieregge [9] evaluated sexual function and attitudes regarding sexuality among younger PD patients. A total of 121 patients with a mean age of 45 years were compared with 126 age- and sex-matched control subjects using a multiple choice questionnaire evaluating sexual attitudes, emotions regarding sexual practices, personal sexual function, and general health perception. They found that patients with PD had significantly higher rates of depression and unemployment than control subjects. They also found that PD patients were more often dissatisfied with their sexual lives, especially if they were male. Patients reporting sexual dissatisfaction also had higher ratings for depression than those who rated themselves as sexually satisfied.

There is high co-morbidity between PD and psychiatric disorders [10–12], which may contribute to sexual dysfunction, as in the general population. Prevalence rates for depression in PD patients vary widely from approximately 10 to 40% and can vary depending on the severity of depression [10]. Depression can adversely affect libido and sexual performance for both the patient and his or her partner [5,13]. Motor fluctuations inherent in the disease process may also alter the timing of sexual intercourse, as patients may have more "on" time in the morning as opposed to the evening. Further, there may be direct or indirect effects of anti-Parkinson's medications that may either decrease [14] or increase [15–18] sexual behaviors. In addition, patients can have profound cognitive impairment, even psychosis, which can be stressful to caregivers and impact on all aspects of the sexual and personal relationships [13].

Given this potential for significant strain on the relationship between the patient and their spouse or partner, it is surprising that few studies have specifically addressed this aspect of sexual function. Brown *et al.* [19] evaluated factors affecting sexual dysfunction in both PD patients and their partners, using self-reporting measures. They specifically looked at gender differences between male and female patients and their spouses. They found that the ratings of marital and sexual satisfaction for both patients and spouses were significantly lower when the patient was male. In fact, overall, 68% of male patients and 64% of female spouses, as compared with 36% of female patients and 27% of male spouses, reported moderate to severe sexual problems. There were no significant differences found in reported autonomic dysfunction or depression between the male and female patients.

Hyposexual behaviors

Men

Erectile dysfunction

The most widely investigated area of sexual dysfunction in men with PD is erectile dysfunction. This also appears to be one of the most prevalent problems, with estimates of approximately 60% compared with 37.5% in the general population [20]. It also appears to affect younger patients and may be an early symptom, occurring within the first few years of diagnosis. However, at least one study reported that patients with erectile dysfunction were 3.8 times more likely to develop PD than those with good erectile function ($p < 0.0001$), based upon analysis of 32 616 patients from a database covering a period 1986–2002 [21]. The authors suggested that erectile dysfunction was associated with a higher risk of developing PD.

Pathogenesis

Erectile function is centrally mediated by dopaminergic stimulation and involves both the mesocortical and mesolimbic pathways, which can be affected in PD. These pathways converge in the paraventricular nucleus (PVN) in the hypothalamus, which can also be diffusely affected. These inputs are relayed to the spinal cord and the peripheral autonomic nerves, which innervate the penis [3]. Studies have suggested that dopaminergic fibers exist in virtually all laminae in the spinal cord [3]. Since the motor symptoms of PD are not usually appreciated until there is approximately 70% loss of dopaminergic neurons in the substantia nigra, it might be reasonable to explain erectile dysfunction prior to the onset of PD motor symptoms on the basis of extranigral dopamine loss. However, it does not establish that erectile dysfunction is a risk factor for PD.

Further support for dopamine having central control of erectile function is found in studies with apomorphine. This is primarily a D2 dopamine-non-selective receptor agonist that can activate neurons in the PVN and medial preoptic area of the hypothalamus [3,22]. These seem to affect oxytocinergic cell bodies located in the PVN, which in turn project to areas outside the hypothalamus, including the hippocampus, medulla, and spinal cord. These appear to activate central pro-erectile pathways via nitric oxide signaling, resulting in erection [22]. Activation of these areas with a sublingual form of apomorphine has been shown to improve erectile dysfunction, and was the first centrally acting agent approved for the treatment of erectile dysfunction for this reason. Intermittent subcutaneous injections of apomorphine have primarily been used for treatment of motor fluctuations of PD [3], and interestingly have been reported to induce erections.

Diagnostic approach

A way to facilitate initial discussion of erectile dysfunction in patients who are reluctant to volunteer that they have sexual symptoms can be the use of screening questionnaires, such as the International Index of Erectile Dysfunction (IIEF) or the Erectile Dysfunction Inventory of Treatment Satisfaction (erectile dysfunctionITS) [23]. This will not, of course, substitute for a more thorough evaluation, but may bring the problem to the attention of the treating physician. A complete medical history, reflecting all other chronic medical diseases, such as diabetes, hypertension, and endocrine diseases, that can be associated with erectile dysfunction is vital. Attention should also be paid to any prior spinal cord injuries or prior surgeries that might have affected the prostate or the sacral region. A complete psychosocial assessment should also be obtained, including basic screening for depression and anxiety, in addition to accurate tobacco, alcohol, and illicit drug use. It is extremely important to obtain a complete list of all of the patient's medications, as a number of commonly used medications can contribute to erectile dysfunction. These can include anti-depressants and anti-hypertensives, particularly beta-blockers [24]. Of course, a complete physical examination should be performed, including a genitourinary evaluation.

Screening laboratories should include serum chemistry, lipid panel, TSH, testosterone, LH, FSH, and prolactin [24]. Nocturnal penile tumescence studies can be performed in the context of a sleep laboratory; however, there are some devices that have been modified for use at home [23,24]. Consultation with a urologist is an important component of evaluation and treatment. Intracorporal injection of prostaglandin E can induce erections and therefore can be used to evaluate hemodynamic characteristics with color Doppler ultrasonography. This technique can be used to look at the patency of the vascular system and may be helpful in ruling out ischemic etiologies that are also common in this age group [23].

Treatment

Subcutaneous administration of apomorphine, a centrally acting non-selective D2 agonist, is approved in most countries as a rescue agent for the treatment of motor fluctuations in PD [3]. It was also recently developed in a sublingual formulation in both 2 and 4 mg dosing for the treatment of erectile dysfunction. Another centrally acting agent that can be used in the treatment of erectile dysfunction is pergolide mesylate, a centrally acting ergolinic dopamine agonist with high affinity to the hD (2S) subtype of D2 dopamine receptors, but lower affinity for hD (2L) receptors [3]. It has been shown to be effective for treating the motor symptoms of PD both as monotherapy in early disease and in combination with levodopa for patients with more advanced disease. It also appears to be effective in the treatment of erectile dysfunction as it had unique action on those dopamine receptors located in the PVN of the hypothalamus. However, it was withdrawn from the market in 2007 because of its associations with cardiac valvulopathies [25,26]. Ropinirole is a selective D2 receptor agonist which also acts centrally. One case report has suggested that it may also have some benefit for erectile dysfunction in patients with PD [3]. It should be remembered, however, that many of the centrally acting dopamine agonists have also been implicated in pathologic hypersexual behaviors [15–18].

Therapeutic interventions for erectile dysfunction in PD can also be directed at intracavernosal pathways. One of the more widely used treatment modalities for men suffering from erectile dysfunction, not limited to PD, are the oral therapies currently on the market. The first of these approved by the US Food and Drug Administration for the treatment of erectile dysfunction was sildenafil citrate (Viagra). This medication acts peripherally by inhibiting phosphodiesterase-5 in corpus cavernosum smooth muscle [23]. Raffaele *et al.* [27] evaluated the efficacy of sildenafil in patients with both PD and depression and found that 84.8% of patients showed improved ability to achieve and maintain erections. In addition, 75% of patients reported improvement in depression. Another therapeutic modality is direct intracavernosal injections. One agent is prostaglandin E1, which can directly dilate the smooth muscle of the corpus cavernosum in the penis [23]. This should be used for patients who do not respond to oral therapies. The dosage should be increased gradually to avoid prolonged erections [3]. One difficulty with this medication is that is requires manual dexterity for injection into the corpus cavernosum prior to intercourse. Patients with advanced disease often require their partners to administer the injections.

Other treatment modalities include vacuum assist devices, surgical approaches, or psychotherapy. Vacuum assist devices are relatively non-invasive and consist of a cylinder, pump, and constriction ring. These should be employed for intercourse for only about 15 min duration as there can be complications associated with ischemia [23]. These devices also require manual dexterity, which can be problematic for patients with PD. Surgical procedures involving revascularization can be considered in cases with associated ischemia. However, these are often not curative and also carry the risks associated with microsurgery [24]. Finally, in psychogenic erectile dysfunction, psychotherapy can be considered as a primary therapy or can be performed in conjunction with any of the aforementioned therapies. Overall goals include decreasing performance anxiety by increasing the patient's repertoire of sexual activities that do not require erection for penetration. In order for this type of therapy to be successful, it may require cooperation from the patient's sexual partner [24]. In the discussion below of hyposexual dysfunction in women, there will be a more specific discussion of a type of psychotherapy that can be employed for patients with sexual dysfunction.

Premature ejaculation

Although erectile dysfunction is more common in patients with PD, one study suggested that premature ejaculation (PE) can also pose a significant problem, with 40.6% of respondents reporting this as a concern [28]. Premature ejaculation is thought to be related to disruptions of serotonergic transmission. There is also some suggestion that PE is related to dysfunction of both peripheral and central oxytocinergic neurons, the latter of which are located in the supraoptic and the paraventricular nuclei of the hypothalamus [28]. This anatomic region was implicated when discussing erectile dysfunction and has connections with other dopaminergic-containing neurons. Current definitions of PE are somewhat limited as they focus on the patient's complaint, as opposed to actual clear latency times that delineate the definition. New definitions proposed for upcoming editions of both the DSM and ICD codes will likely focus on the duration of symptoms, and also the latency time for intravaginal ejaculation [27].

Selective serotonin reuptake inhibitors (SSRIs) have been found to be to be efficacious for the treatment of premature ejaculation. On-demand or daily tricyclic anti-depressants, such as clomipramine, have also been shown to be effective; however, the side effect profile for tricyclic anti-depressants may not be advantageous for patients with PD [29]. Other alternatives include on-demand oral phosphodiesterase-5 inhibitors, such as sildenafil citrate. Another agent is tramadol, which acts centrally as an analgesic, combining activation of μ-opioid receptors and reuptake inhibition of both serotonin and norepinephrine [30]. This can be taken as needed (50 mg), but approximately one-quarter of patients experienced side effects in one study [31].

Women

Sexual dysfunction in women with PD has received significantly less research attention than for men. One study questioned 75 patients with PD regarding sexual dysfunction, 32 of whom were women. Although 21.9% of women reported pre-morbid sexual dysfunction, which may have been a contributory factor, the women surveyed reported significant impairment with arousal (87.5%), difficulty reaching orgasm (75.0%), low sexual desire (46.9%), and sexual dissatisfaction (37.5%) [28]. Welsh, Hung, and Waters [32] compared 27 women with PD with community age-matched controls with similar marital status. Women with PD were more depressed than control subjects ($p = 0.009$). Overall, the authors also found that in comparison to controls, PD patients were less satisfied with their sexual relationship ($p = 0.005$), including their sexual partners ($p = 0.005$). Women with PD reported increased anxiety and/or inhibition during sexual activities ($p = 0.04$), more difficulties with vaginal tightness ($p = 0.03$), and increased problems with involuntary urination ($p = 0.03$) [32]. Brown *et al.* [19] compared married male and female Parkinson's patients and their spouses with self-report measures of sexual dysfunction. Ratings of dysfunction were found to be significantly higher for both patient and spouse when the patient was male. Despite higher rates of vaginismus and anorgasmia for female spouses, rates for these in female PD patients were still 27 and 36%, respectively, although the sample size was small ($n = 11$).

Diagnostic approach

Female sexual dysfunction can be classified into one of four categories: hypoactive or sexual desire disorders, sexual arousal disorders, orgasmic disorders, and sexual pain disorders [33,34]. Appropriate classification of the disorder requires an open communication between the physician and patient regarding issues pertaining to sexual dysfunction, and may require involvement of the patient's partner in the discussion if appropriate. A complete history should be performed, including prior surgical history, with particular reference to pelvic surgeries. Discussion of other chronic medical illnesses, including endocrine diseases, atherosclerotic risk factors, and psychiatric disorders, should be explored. Brief psychosocial history should be performed, including any illicit drug use and alcohol intake, and also past history of sexual abuse or trauma. A complete physical examination should be performed, including genitourinary examination. Laboratory testing should be performed, including complete blood count, serum chemistry, lipid panel, TSH, FSH, and LH, and also hormone levels including estrogen, testosterone, and DHEA [35]. Screening measures should be performed for psychiatric disorders, including depression and anxiety [33]. The patient may be referred back to her primary care physician or an obstetrician/gynecologist for a more thorough examination of specific areas.

Treatment

Treatment will depend on the type of sexual dysfunction identified. If the etiology involves an organic cause, treatment should involve focus on the underlying disease, as there can be co-morbid medical problems in patients with PD. For hypoactive sexual disorders, consideration should be given to hormone replacement, which could include estrogen, testosterone, and DHEA. This can also be helpful for sexual arousal disorders, as can lubrication and vibrators, among other devices [33]. For orgasmic disorders, vibrators can also be used, as can Kegel exercises. Sexual pain disorders require thorough evaluation to rule out an underlying organic cause. Once this has been excluded, it should be determined at which point pain occurs during intercourse and treatment should then be directed accordingly. For instance, pain with friction could be treated with lubricants, whereas pain with deep penetration could be treated with relaxation techniques or changes in positioning [33].

Often, it is not practical for these issues to be addressed within the context of a neurologic visit for PD. Once the topic has been broached, patients can be given appropriate literature and referrals to physicians with expertise in this field. Some even suggest referral to a trained therapist with specialization in sexual dysfunction, particularly if there are related psychologic issues [34]. One model of sexual therapy and counseling was suggested by Annon in 1976 and is abbreviated the PLISSIT model [34]. The first aspect is the "permission (*P*)" phase, where the therapist creates a comfortable climate for the patient to voice and discuss his or her concerns. The second phase is called "limited information (*LI*)," where specific sexual concerns are addressed and any misconceptions are corrected. In the "specific suggestions (*SS*)" phase, a sexual history is obtained and the patient is given specific instructions on how to address these problems. In the final phase, "intensive therapy (*IT*)," more specialized therapy is provided for any issues that may be complicating the patient's recovery, such as a co-morbid psychiatric diagnosis [34].

Hypersexual behaviors

Hypersexual behaviors have been well documented as an apparent side effect of dopaminergic therapy. Pathologic hypersexuality was defined by Kaplan, Saddock, and Grebb in 1994 as follows: "The need for sexual behavior consumes so much money, time, concentration, and energy that the patient describes himself as out of control; intrusive unwanted paraphiliac thoughts prevent concentration on other life demands and are the source of anxiety; and orgasm does not produce satiety in the way it typically does for age mates." [36] This type of sexual behavior is considered an impulse control disorder (ICD), and in the same family as pathologic gambling, compulsive shopping, and excessive eating. The true prevalence of such behaviors is unclear, but it is likely that these behaviors are under-reported given the associated social stigma. Hence it is important that physicians be aware of possible warning signs and query these behaviors when warranted. Unfortunately, they may not come to a physician's attention until there is functional impairment or even criminal involvement.

Repetitive and reward-seeking behaviors

The prevalence of ICDs is unclear and there is variability in the reported rates in the literature, ranging from 6.6 to 13.7% [16,37]. However, the numbers of patients included in most studies are small and, in general, all types of impulse control disorders are included in these reports. In one study [16] of 297 PD patients, the lifetime prevalence of pathologic hypersexuality was 2.4%. Based upon this finding and those of a previous study, the authors estimated that the overall prevalence for ICDs was 13.7% for patients on dopamine agonists [16]. A few studies have also attempted to look at the patient characteristics that may be predictive for developing ICDs. For instance, Voon *et al.* [38] evaluated 21 patients with idiopathic PD with pathologic gambling receiving dopamine agonists and compared them with 42 patients with idiopathic PD without compulsive behaviors. They found that the patients with both PD and pathologic gambling had younger age at onset of PD, higher incidence of medication-induced hypomania or mania, personal or family history of alcohol use disorder, and higher novelty-seeking behaviors. These behaviors appear to occur more commonly in males [39] and there has been a suggestion that smoking may be a risk factor specifically for hypersexuality [39]. Pontone *et al.* [40] found a prevalence of ICDs of 9%, which was significantly associated with taking dopamine agonists ($p < 0.0001$). They also found that symptoms of depressed mood, irritability, and appetite changes, and also disinhibition, were more common in patients with ICDs.

Effects of Parkinson's medications

Although dopamine agonists have been implicated as possible causative agents in hypersexual behaviors and other ICDs, many studies suggest that these behaviors are seen when dopamine agonists are used as adjunctive therapy to levodopa [15,40]. These behaviors have also been witnessed with levodopa and dopamine agonist monotherapy [15–17]. There are also some studies that suggest that there may be a dose effect; however, this has not been consistently demonstrated [15]. The most commonly implicated dopamine agonists are pramipexole, ropinirole, and pergolide, although this may be a function of prescribing practices [15,18]. Prior studies also implicated bromocriptine and apomorphine [15]. Time of symptom onset after the initiation of therapy is also not clearly addressed in the literature. One study found an average time of symptom onset of 8 months after the addition of dopamine agonists in 14 patients [15], although the range was from 1 month to 1 year.

The types of hypersexual behaviors cited in the literature have varied widely and most of the descriptions are in the form of case reports [18,35,40]. One of the more common behaviors reported is increased and excessive demand for sexual intercourse with one's partner, even at inappropriate times. This may extend to excessive masturbation or viewing of pornography, or perhaps hypersexual interest in seemingly nonsexual situations. Patients may proposition others sexually in inappropriate situations or circumstances (e.g., a family member or friend who is not his or her spouse). Patients may also have delusional thoughts, such as belief that one's spouse is being unfaithful. There can also be instances of illegal behaviors, including exhibitionism, pedophilia, solicitation of prostitutes, and even rape. Various paraphilias have also been cited, including an example of a 51-year-old patient who exhibited frotteurism (a form of unsolicited groping) 3 years after starting treatment with pergolide [18].

Hypersexual behaviors and ICDs in general certainly do not occur in all patients with PD, which raises the question of why they occur in particular patients. Dopamine, in addition to dopamine agonists, appears to play a role in reward-seeking behaviors. For instance, positron emission tomography (PET) studies have shown strong activation in dopamine-rich areas of the mesodiencephalic junction and ventral tegmental area in healthy volunteers during orgasm and ejaculation [41]. The most commonly implicated dopamine agonists, pramipexole, ropinirole, and pergolide, appear to have a higher affinity for D3 receptors, which also are in higher concentration in the limbic regions of the brain [15,17].

One difficulty with many of the studies is that they involve small sample sizes and are largely retrospective. In addition, most patients tend to be male. Treatments cited in the literature have had variable responses and are reflective of the trial-and-error methodology inherent in clinical practice, as opposed to randomized controlled trials. Some cases improved with reduction or cessation of dopamine agonists [15,18,42]. Other patients have required the addition of anti-psychotic medications, particularly atypical anti-psychotics, including clozapine, olanzapine, and quetiapine [15,18,42]. The treatment recommendations from these studies are limited by their retrospective nature and the relatively small numbers of patients. In addition, there is wide variability in terms of the type of dopamine agonist administered. There is also great variability in the concurrent level of levodopa therapy and the underlying risk factors. The DOMINION study, a prospective examination of ICDs including hypersexuality, is currently ongoing and will provide useful prevalence data for these behaviors [43].

Effects of surgical procedures on sexual function

The prefrontal–subcortical or medial orbitofrontal–basal ganglia circuit regulates many motivated behaviors, including sexual function, and is associated with the striatum, ventral pallidum, and mediodorsal thalamus [44,45]. Lesions in this circuit can produce behavioral disinhibition, impulsivity, poor judgment, and emotional lability, in addition to sexually inappropriate behaviors [44]. There have been specific reports in the literature of patients experiencing hypersexual behavior after pallidal surgery or placement of deep brain stimulators (DBS) for treatment of PD [44,46].

Roane *et al.* [44] reported a 57-year-old man with a longer than 20-year history of PD and no prior psychiatric history. This patient underwent stereotactically guided right-sided pallidotomy, improving his left-sided motor symptoms. Later, he underwent placement of DBS in the left GPi to control right-sided dyskinesias and other motor symptoms. Although he showed improvement of his motor symptoms including dyskinesias, he developed hypersexual behavior approximately 5 months after placement of the DBS. This included excessive masturbation, demands for sexual intercourse with his wife in the middle of the night, threats to find a prostitute, and inappropriate remarks to others, including younger female relatives. He also had evidence of marked anxiety and mania. Ultimately, he was hospitalized and treated with clozapine, which controlled his hypersexual behavior.

Romito *et al.* [46] reported two additional patients who underwent bilateral DBS placement in the subthalamic nuclei (STN) for treatment of advanced PD. Both patients showed improvement of their motor symptoms even before the electrodes were activated and were ultimately weaned off of their anti-parkinsonian medications. However, the first patient developed mania and hypersexual behaviors 2 days after implantation (1 day prior to initiation of stimulation); the other patient developed similar symptoms 3 days after implantation and a few hours after stimulation was implemented. In both cases, the hypersexual behavior did not improve when stimulation was briefly turned off, although motor symptoms significantly worsened. Ultimately, manic symptoms resolved without treatment within 3 months in the first patient and after 8 months in the second patient. Both patients required continuation of the STN stimulation to treat the motor symptoms of PD.

Another study [47] examined changes in sexual wellbeing in men and women with PD who underwent bilateral implantation of STN DBS. Instead of finding evidence of hypersexual behavior, male patients showed significant improvements in pre-morbid sexual dissatisfaction, whereas female patients did not demonstrate any significant changes. Anatomic differences in electrode placement may explain the variability in response of sexual function to DBS surgery. Previous studies have noted that discrete lesions in this prefrontal–subcortical circuit, which include the STN, thalamus (paramedian), and pallidum, can result in hypersexual behavior [45]. It is likely that there is some disruption to this circuit which may contribute to these behaviors; it is unclear why these behaviors may spontaneously remit with continued improvement in motor symptoms.

Conclusion

Sexual dysfunction is common in PD, and can be highly disruptive and emotionally distressing to both the patient his or her partner. Symptoms of sexual dysfunction are often inadequately addressed by physicians. Approximately 80% of patients with PD have complaints of autonomic dysfunction [3], which can manifest primarily as hyposexual behaviors. In men, this often presents as erectile dysfunction, which can actually precede the diagnosis of PD [21]. For women, symptoms are recognized less often and the mechanisms responsible for their occurrence in PD are not as well understood, although there seems to be an association with co-morbid depression [32]. Treatment for hyposexual disorders is similar to that for those without PD. Hypersexual behaviors are most commonly related to dopaminergic therapy, and may relate to effects of these medications on limbic regions of the brain [15]. Treatment includes reduction or cessation of medication, or addition of an atypical anti-psychotic medication [15,18,42]. The most important thing for all patients with PD suffering from sexual dysfunction is for physicians to offer an open and nonjudgmental environment for discussing such issues. Recognition of warning signs or associated symptoms, such as depression, may be the keys to offering effective therapeutic options.

References

1. Paulson HL, Stern MB. Clinical manifestations of Parkinson's disease. In: Watts RL, Koller WC, eds. *Movement Disorders: Neurologic Principles and Practice*, 2nd edn. New York: McGraw-Hill Medical Publishing, 2004: 233–45.
2. Singer C, Weiner WJ. Sexual dysfunction in Parkinson's disease. In: Singer C, Weiner WJ, eds. *Sexual Dysfunction*. New York: Futura Publishing, 1994: 119–34.
3. Papatsoris AG, Deliveliotis C, Singer C, Papepetropoulos S. Erectile dysfunction in Parkinson's disease. *Urology* 2006; **67**:447–51.
4. Singer C, Weiner WJ, Sanchez-Ramos JR. Autonomic dysfunction in men with Parkinson's disease. *Eur Neurol* 1992;**32**(3): 134–40.
5. Sakakibara R, Shinotoh H, Uchiyama T, *et al.* Questionnaire-based assessment of pelvic organ dysfunction in Parkinson's disease. *Autonom Neurosci* 2001;**92**(1–2):76–85.
6. Wullner U, Schmitz-Hubsch T, Antony G, *et al.* Autonomic dysfunction in 3414 Parkinson's disease patients enrolled in the German Network on Parkinson's disease (KNP e.V.): the effect on ageing. *Eur J Neurol* 2007;**14**(12):1405–8.
7. Lipe H, Longstreth WT, Bird TD, Lind M. Sexuality in Parkinson's disease. *Neurology* 1989;**39**(Suppl 1):320.
8. Witjas T, Kaphan E, Azulay JP, *et al.* Nonmotor fluctuations in Parkinson's disease. *Neurology* 2002;**59**:408–20.
9. Jacobs H, Vieregge A, Vieregge P. Sexuality in youg patients with Parkinson's disease: a population based comparison with healthy controls. *J Neurol Neurosurg Psychiatry* 2000;**69**:550–2.
10. Thanvi BR, Munshi SK, Vijaykumar N, Lo TCN. Neuropsychiatric non-motor aspects of Parkinson's disease. *Postgrad Med J* 2003;**79**:561–5.
11. Scott B, Borgman A, Engler H, *et al.* Gender differences in Parkinson's disease symptom profile. *Acta Neurol Scand* 2000;**102**:37–43.
12. Leentjens AFG, Van denAkker M, Metsemakers JFM, *et al.* Higher incidence of depression preceding the onset of Parkinson's disease: a register study. *Mov Disord* 2003;**18**(4):414–8.
13. Lauterbach EC. The neuropsychiatry of Parkinson's disease and related disorders. *Psychiatric Clin North Am* 2004;**27**:801–25.
14. Cleeves L, Findley LJ. Bromocriptine induced impotence in Parkinson's disease. *Br Med J* 1987;**29**(6594):367–8.
15. Klos KJ, Bower JH, Josephs KA, *et al.* Pathological hypersexuality predominantly linked to adjuvant dopamine agonist therapy in Parkinson's disease and multiple system atrophy. *Parkinsonism Relat Disord* 2005;**11**:381–6.
16. Voon V, Hassan K, Zurowski M, *et al.* Prevalence of repetitive and reward-seeking behaviors in Parkinson disease. *Neurology* 2006;**67**:1254–7.
17. Black KJ, Friedman JH. Repetitive and impulsive behaviors in treated Parkinson disease. *Neurology* 2006;**67**:1118–9.
18. Cannas A, Solla P, Floris GL, *et al.* Aberrant sexual behaviours in Parkinson's disease during dopaminergic treatment. *J Neurol* 2007;**254**:110–2.
19. Brown RG, Jahanshahi M, Quinn N, Marsden CD. Sexual function in patients with Parkinson's disease and their partners. *J Neurol Neurosurg Psychiatry* 1990;**53**:480–6.
20. Singer C, Weiner WJ, Sanchez-Ramos J, Ackerman M. Sexual function in patients with Parkinson's disease. *J Neurol Neurosurg Psychiatry* 1991;**54**(10):942.
21. Gao X, Chen H, Schwarzchild MA, *et al.* Erectile function and risk of Parkinson's disease. *Am J Epidemiol* 2007;**166**(12):1446–50.
22. Montorsi F, Perani D, Anchisi D, *et al.* Apomorphine-induced brain modulation during sexual stimulation: a new look at

central phenomena related to erectile dysfunction. *Int J Impotence Res* 2003;**15**:203–9.
23. Nehra A, Moreland RB. Neurologic erectile dysfunction. *Urologic Clin North Am* 2001;**28**(2):289–308.
24. Kirby RS. Impotence: diagnosis and management of male erectile dysfunction. *Br Med J* 1994;**308**:957–61.
25. Van Camp G, Flamez A, Cosyns B, *et al.* Treatment of Parkinson's disease with pergolide and relation to restrictive valvular heart disease. *Lancet* 2004;**363**(9416):1179–83.
26. Zanettini R, Antonini A, Gatto G, et al.Valvular heart disease and the use of dopamine agonists for Parkinson's disease. *N Engl J Med* 2007;**356**(1):39–46.
27. Raffaele R, Vecchio I, Giammusso B, *et al.* Efficacy and safety of fixed-dose oral sildenafil in the treatment of sexual dysfunction in depressed patients with idiopathic Parkinson's disease. *Eur Urol* 2002;**41**:382–6.
28. Bronner G, Royter V, Korczyn AD, Giladi N. Sexual dysfunction in Parkinson's disease. *J Sex Marital Ther* 2004;**30**(2):95–105.
29. Frisina PG, Tenenbaum HR, Borod JC, Foldi NS. The effects of antidepressants in Parkinson's disease: a meta-analysis. *Int J Neurosci* 2008;**118**(5):667–82.
30. Waldinger MD. Premature ejaculation: definition and drug treatment. *Drugs* 2007;**67**(4):547–68.
31. Safarinejad MR, Hosseini SY. Safety and efficacy of tramadol in the treatment of premature ejaculation: a double-blind, placebo-controlled, fixed-dose, randomized study. *J Clin Psychopharmacol* 2006;**26**:27–31.
32. Welsh M, Hung L, Waters CH. Sexuality in women with Parkinson's disease. *Mov Disord* 1997;**12**(6):923–7.
33. Brassil DF, Keller M. Female sexual dysfunction: definitions, causes, and treatment. *Urol Nurs* 2002;**22**(4):237–44,284.
34. Ohl LE. Essentials of female sexual dysfunction from a sex therapy perspective. *Urol Nurs* 2007;**27**(1):57–64.
35. Salonia A, Munarriz RM, Naspro R, *et al.* Women's sexual dysfunction: a pathophysiological review. *BJU Int* 2004;**93**:1156–64.
36. Kaplan HI, Saddock BJ, Grebb JA. *Synopsis of Psychiatry*, 7th edn. Baltimore, MD: Williams & Wilkins, 1994.
37. Weintraub D, Siderowf AD, Potenza MN, *et al.* Association of dopamine agonist use with impulse control disorders in Parkinson Disease. *Arch Neurol* 2006;**63**:969–73.
38. Voon V, Thomsen T, Miyasaki JM, *et al.* Factors associated with dopaminergic drug-related pathological gambling in Parkinson disease. *Arch Neurol* 2007;**64**:212–6.
39. Merims D, Giladi N. Dopamine dysregulation syndrome, addiction and behavioral changes in Parkinson's disease. *Parkinsonism Relat Disord* 2008;**14**:273–80.
40. Pontone G, Williams JR, Bassett SP, Marsh L. Clinical features associate with impulse control disorders in Parkinson disease. *Neurology* 2006;**67**:1258–61.
41. Rees PM, Fowler CJ, Maas CP. Sexual dysfunction in men and women with neurological disorders. *Lancet* 2007;**369**:512–25.
42. Cannas A, Solla P, Floris G, *et al.* Hypersexual behavior, frotteurism and delusional jealousy in a young parkinsonian patient during dopaminergic therapy with pergolide: a rare case of iatrogenic paraphilia. *Progr Neuro-Psychopharmacol Biol Psychiatry* 2006;**30**(8):1539–41.
43. Boehringer Ingelheim Pharmaceuticals. Preliminary DOMINION study report dated 14 March 2008, Abstract for Poster at the Movement Disorders Society 12th International Congress of Parkinson's Disease and Movement Disorders (Chicago, IL, June 2008).
44. Roane DM, Yu M, Feinberg TE, Rogers JD. Hypersexuality after pallidal surgery in Parkinson disease. *Neuropsychiatr, Neuropsychol Behav Neurol* 2002;**15**(4):247–51.
45. Spinella M. Hypersexuality and dysexecutive syndrome after a thalamic infarct. *Int J Neurosci* 2004;**114**:1581–90.
46. Romito LM, Raja M, Daniele A, *et al.* Transient mania with hypersexuality after surgery for high-frequency stimulation of the subthalamic nucleus in Parkinson's disease. *Mov Disord* 2002;**17**(6):1371–4.
47. Castelli L, Perozzo P, Genesia ML, *et al.* Sexual well being in parkinsonian patients after deep brain stimulation of the subthalamic nucleus. *J Neurol Neurosurg Psychiatry* 2004;**75**: 1260–4.

Chapter 28
Olfactory Dysfunction

John E. Duda & Matthew B. Stern
Parkinson's Disease Research, Education and Clinical Center (PADRECC), Philadelphia Veterans Affairs Medical Center, and Department of Neurology, University of Pennsylvania School of Medicine, Philadelphia, PA, USA

Introduction

In his description of the eponymous disorder that now bears his name, James Parkinson, in his remarkable monograph of 1817, stated that there was "the absence of injury to the senses" [1]. At least for olfaction, this was thought to be the case until 1975, when Ansari and Johnson first reported that olfactory dysfunction was a common symptom in Parkinson's disease (PD) [2]. Since that time, recognition of the importance of this feature in the clinical phenotype of PD has left the realm of fascinomas, has become a focus of attention of ongoing research, and has become a clinically relevant finding. Research is now focused on the potential of olfactory dysfunction to be a biomarker for PD, a key component of a possible pre-motor diagnostic screening paradigm, and, finally, as a potential therapy-independent marker of disease progression. With a prevalence approaching 100%, olfactory dysfunction is more common among PD patients than at least one of the cardinal motor features, resting tremor [3–5]. Smell loss in PD is robust enough to be easily measured by standard quantitative tools, with deficits in all areas of olfaction – odor discrimination, odor identification, and odor detection threshold [6] – and has the sensitivity and specificity to justify its use in the diagnostic evaluation of parkinsonism [7]. In addition, although olfactory dysfunction was thought for years to be a static process, not correlating with disease duration or stage, recent studies have shown that careful sample selection with close follow-up intervals may reveal progression of olfactory dysfunction over time, at least in the early stages of the illness. Demonstrating the time course of olfactory loss in PD is important to our understanding of the pre-motor phase of PD, and for identifying a population of at-risk patients during a stage of the illness when intervention with disease-modifying properties might be more likely to be efficacious. Finally, in one of the seminal observations in the past 10 years of PD research, Braak and colleagues proposed a previously unrecognized progression of Lewy pathology through sequentially vulnerable brain regions and suggested that the olfactory system is a possible induction site of that cascade [8]. This observation has engendered pathophysiologic hypotheses for PD that include a central role for the olfactory system and the possibility that exogenous agents gain access to the central nervous system via olfactory pathways.

Assessing smell loss in PD

Olfactory dysfunction is an attractive biomarker for PD because of its high prevalence among PD patients and also its relative ease of testing compared with other putative biomarkers such as neuroimaging of the dopamine system. Several different modalities have been developed for the assessment of olfactory impairment in PD, most with commercially available instruments, enabling a shift from primarily the research setting to the movement disorder clinic (see Table 28.1). Olfactory identification has been the most widely used assessment of olfaction and by far the most commonly used instrument is The University of Pennsylvania Smell Identification Test (UPSIT), developed by Doty *et al.* in 1984 [9]. The UPSIT has been validated as a reliable method of quantifying olfactory identification in numerous different conditions and maladies, has been translated into several languages, and has been administered to hundreds of thousands of persons [10]. In this 40-item test, the patient is asked to scratch the surface of the testing card and identify the microencapsulated odor released from four possible written choices, so that it is a forced choice test. The UPSIT was formally modified to include only 12 items as the Cross-Cultural Smell Identification Test (CC-SIT, also known as the Brief Smell Identification Test), addressing some concerns that certain of the 40 odors were unlikely to be recognized by non-Western populations [11]. In addition, in order to assure that cognitive dysfunction is not interfering with the performance of the UPSIT, Doty, Deems, and Stellar

Parkinson's Disease: Non-Motor and Non-Dopaminergic Features, First Edition. Edited by C. Warren Olanow, Fabrizio Stocchi, and Anthony E. Lang.

Table 28.1 Commonly available psychophysical assessments of olfaction for subjects with Parkinson's disease.

Olfactory modality	Description	Commonly available assessment instruments[a]
Odor identification	Assesses the ability to identify specifically a presented odor, usually from a list of several choices	UPSIT (40 items; commercially termed the SIT); Sniffin' Sticks (16 items); Brief SIT (also known as CC-SIT; 12 items); Brief SIT Version B (developed specifically for Parkinson's disease; 12 items); Q-SIT (3 items); Pocket Smell Test (3 items)
Odor detection threshold	Assesses the minimal concentration at which a given odor can be reliably detected	Sniffin' Sticks; Odor Threshold Test; Toyota & Takagi Olfactometer Test
Odor discrimination	Assesses the ability to discriminate whether two presented odors are identical or not	Sniffin' Sticks; Odor Memory Test
Odor memory	Assesses the ability to remember previously presented odors after a delay interval	Odor Memory Test
Sniff magnitude	Assesses olfaction by measuring the reflex-like reduction in sniffing that occurs when a malodor is encountered	Sniff Magnitude Test

[a]UPSIT, University of Pennsylvania Smell Identification Test; SIT, Smell Identification Test; B-SIT, Brief Smell Identification Test; CC-SIT, Cross-Cultural Smell Identification Test; Q-SIT, Quick Smell Identification Test. Sniffin' Sticks available from Heinrich Burghart, Hamburg, Germany; Toyota & Takagi Olfactometer Test available from Daiichi-Yakuhin, Tokyo, Japan; all other tests available from Sensonics, Haddon Heights, NJ (www.sensonics.com).

developed the Picture Identification Test (PIT), which is in the same format as the UPSIT but utilizes pictures of objects rather than microencapsulated odors [3].

Although not originally developed for the assessment of olfaction specifically in PD, the UPSIT has been the most commonly used method in studies of olfaction in PD (see Table 28.2). Over the years, even though Doty, Bromley, and Stern have demonstrated a close relationship between the number of UPSIT items and its reliability [12], several groups have attempted to identify a subset of UPSIT items that would be more economical to administer and possibly have better predictive value in diagnosing PD. In 1997, Hawkes, Shephard, and Daniel examined 70 PD subjects and 70 age- and sex-matched control subjects and compared the sensitivity and specificity of all 40 UPSIT items [5]. They determined that the best discriminator between PD subjects and control subjects was a combination of results from two odor identifications, specifically those assessing identification of pizza, which primarily represents the odor of oregano, and wintergreen. This combination achieved a sensitivity of 90% and a specificity of 86% and was not improved by inclusion of a third UPSIT odor. In 2003, Double *et al.* utilized the CC-SIT to avoid cultural odor identification problems in Australian participants and assessed performance in 49 non-demented PD subjects and 52 age- and sex-matched controls. Utilizing discriminant function analysis, they determined that five specific odors (gasoline, banana, pineapple, smoke, and cinnamon) discriminated PD subjects from controls better than the entire CC-SIT [4]. Finally, a recent study by Bohnen *et al.* administered UPSITs and dopamine transporter–PET examinations to 27 PD patients and 27 age- and sex-matched control subjects. Analysis of individual UPSIT odors identified three (banana, licorice, and dill pickle) that correlated better with dorsal striatal and nigral dopamine transporter (DAT) activity than the full 40-item test results [13]. Given the low level of concordance between these studies for the odors identified as discriminatory and the absence of confirmatory studies for all of these determinations in large independent cohorts, the search for a better "PD UPSIT" continues. To assist in this process, Sensonics (Haddon Heights, NJ, USA), the manufacturer of the UPSIT, has generated a newer version of the Brief Smell Identification Test, Version B, which includes most of the 12 best discriminating odors in the analysis by Hawkes, Shephard, and Daniel [5].

Although modalities other than odor identification, including odor discrimination, odor detection threshold, and odor recognition memory, have been used in PD research for some time, readily available methods to assess these modalities have only become available more recently. The olfactory testing method developed by Hummel *et al.*, called Sniffin' Sticks (Heinrich Burghart, Hamburg, Germany), uses pen-like devices to test odor detection threshold, odor discrimination, and odor identification [14]. The patient sniffs the pen, which delivers successive concentrations of *n*-butanol for detection threshold testing, 16 pairs of odorants for odor discrimination, and 16 single odorants for identification from four stated choices. This has become the second most common olfactory assessment in PD and there are advantages and disadvantages to using either the UPSIT, similar products, or the Sniffin' Sticks (see Box 28.1). One significant drawback to the Sniffin' Sticks, the necessity of having trained personnel administer the test, has been partially alleviated by the development of a protocol for self-administration of the smell identification portion of the

Table 28.2 Summary of olfactory clinical studies in Parkinson's disease[a].

Study	*N*	Type of test	*p*-Value
Ansari and Johnson, 1975	22	Threshold	0.05
Korten and Meulstee, 1980	80	Questionnaire	0.001
Ward *et al.*, 1983	72	Odor detection; threshold D; odor discrimination	0.01; 0.03; Nst
Corwin and Serby, 1985	5	UPSIT – modified	Nst
Serby *et al.*, 1985	5	UPSIT – modified	0.05
Quinn *et al.*, 1987	78	threshold D	0.001
Doty *et al.*, 1988	81	UPSIT; threshold D	0.001; 0.001
Kesslak *et al.*, 1988	18	UPSIT; odor matching	0.05; Nst
Doty *et al.*, 1989	47	UPSIT	0.001
Bostantjopoulou *et al.*, 1991	44	Threshold D; odor naming	0.001; 0.01
Murofushi *et al.*, 1991	18	Threshold D; threshold R	0.01, 0.05
Doty *et al.*, 1992a	13	UPSIT; threshold R	0.005; 0.001
Doty *et al.*, 1992b	40	UPSIT	0.001
Hawkes and Shephard, 1993	96	UPSIT	0.0001
Stern *et al.*, 1994	118	UPSIT	0.001
Doty *et al.*, 1995	180	UPSIT	0.001
Lehrner *et al.*, 1995	13	Threshold D; odor ID; odor memory	Nr; Nr; Nr
Barz *et al.*, 1997	31	Odor discrimination; odor ID; OERP	Nr; 0.001; 0.05
Hawkes, *et al.*, 1997	96	UPSIT; OERP	0.0001; 0.001
Ahlskog *et al.*, 1998	9	UPSIT – modified	0.01
Hawkes and Shephard, 1998	155; 36	UPSIT; OERP	0.0001; Nst
Daum *et al.*, 2000	40	Sniffin' Sticks; threshold D	0.001; 0.001
Montgomery *et al.*, 2000a	18	UPSIT	0.001
Montgomery *et al.*, 2000b	58	UPSIT	0.001
Berendse *et al.*, 2001	16	B-SIT, disc., threshold D	0.001
Sobel *et al.*, 2001	20	UPSIT; threshold D (vanillin); threshold D (propionic acid)	0.0001; 0.007; 0.003
Tissingh *et al.*, 2001	41	B-SIT; odor discrimination; threshold D	0.001; 0.001; 0.001
Zucco *et al.*, 2002	6	Odor matching; identification	0.001; –
Muller *et al.*, 2002	50	Sniffin' Sticks	0.0001
Double *et al.*, 2003	49	B-SIT	0.001
Henderson *et al.*, 2003	52	Questionnaire	0.001
Hudry *et al.*, 2003	24	ID and ratings	0.001
Evidente *et al.*, 2004	20	UPSIT	0.001
Katzenschlager *et al.*, 2004	13	UPSIT	0.0001
Khan *et al.*, 2004	18	UPSIT	0.0001
Ondo and Lai, 2004	60	UPSIT	0.0007
Ponsen *et al.*, 2004	361	B-SIT, discrimination, threshold D	0.001
Hummel *et al.*, 2005	11	Sniffin' Sticks	Nst
Maaras *et al.*, 2005	26	UPSIT	0.001
Lee *et al.*, 2006	26	B-SIT	0.001
Bohnen *et al.*, 2007	27	UPSIT	0.0001
Ferreira *et al.*, 2007	138	UPSIT	0.001
Kim *et al.*, 2007	64	B-SIT	0.001
Lee *et al.*, 2007	24	B-SIT	0.001
Lotsch *et al.*, 2007	102	Sniffin' Sticks	0.001
Louis *et al.*, 2007	1078	UPSIT	0.001
Masaoka *et al.*, 2007	10	T&T threshold R	0.001
Quaqliato *et al.*, 2007	50	B-SIT	0.0001
Bohnen *et al.*, 2008	45	UPSIT	0.0001
Djaldelli *et al.*, 2008	18	threshold D	0.0001
Goldstein *et al.*, 2008	77	UPSIT	0.0001
Hawkes, 2008	266	UPSIT	0.0001
Herting *et al.*, 2008	27	Sniffin' Sticks	Nst
Ross *et al.*, 2008	2267	UPSIT	0.0001
Shah *et al.*, 2008	149	UPSIT	0.0001

[a]The growth of olfactory function as a research tool is apparent from the number of studies conducted in the past several years compared with the previous three decades. The *p*-values indicate poorer performance in the PD patients.

[b]*N*, number of subjects; UPSIT, University of Pennsylvania Smell Identification Test; Nr, not reported; Nst, no statistical test. The Sniffin' Sticks battery usually consists of a composite score of tests of odor identification, odor detection threshold, and odor discrimination.

Modified from Doty RL, *Handbook of Olfaction and Gustation* [87], in which the references to the studies cited can be found.

Box 28.1 Comparison between the UPSIT and Sniffin' Sticks

UPSIT

Advantages

- Most widely used research tool with validity in many patient populations
- Largest pool of normative data
- Can be administered without supervision
- Can be mailed
- Low cost per subject for small numbers of subjects
- Available in multiple languages
- Available in culturally sensitive subtest and also a version specifically designed for use in PD
- Availability of picture identification test to assess cognitive abilities
- Convenient web-based ordering

Disadvantages

- Only assesses olfactory identification
- Some batch-to-batch variance in strength of odorants
- High cost for large numbers of subjects

Sniffin' Sticks

Advantages

- Can assess odor identification, odor discrimination, and odor threshold detection
- Odor identification assessment has 16 items, so can be done faster in isolation than UPSIT
- Same odorants used repeatedly on different subjects so costs lower for large numbers of subjects

Disadvantages

- High up-front cost and high cost per subject for low numbers of subjects
- Full assessment must be administered by trained technician
- Not readily available online

examination [15]. In addition, it has been demonstrated that the olfactory threshold portion of the Sniffin' Sticks assessment may be administered repeatedly over a short time span reliably [16].

In addition to the UPSIT and Sniffin' Sticks, there are several other commercially available instruments for the assessment of olfaction that have recently been discussed in detail elsewhere [17]. For the assessment of odor detection threshold, the Smell Threshold Test (Sensonics) utilizes variable concentrations of phenylethyl alcohol in a seven-reversal, single-staircase threshold procedure to provide reliable detection of odor threshold with normative data for each decade of age [18]. The only commercially available assessment of odor memory is the Odor Memory Test (Sensonics), which is a 12-item test incorporating microencapsulated odors similarly to the UPSIT in a non-verbal screen of odor discrimination and memory that provides scores for variable delays from 10, 30, and 60 s [19]. The test has high test–retest reliability but has not been validated in PD subjects to date. Finally, in what has been described as an assessment of olfactory dysfunction which minimizes dependence on language and cognitive abilities, the Sniff Magnitude Test (Sensonics) measures the reflex-like reduction in sniffing that occurs when a malodor is encountered [20]. The Sniff Magnitude Test has been shown to have general agreement with the UPSIT [21,22] and may represent a valid modality for the assessment of olfaction in PD patients with cognitive impairment.

Another method of assessing olfactory function, olfactory event-related potentials (OERPs), can be obtained in response to olfactory stimulants, offering a method of quantifying olfaction that is independent of sniff volume or odor memory. The OERP has several peaks, including the P1 and P3 responses, which are thought to correlate with activity at the olfactory bulb and the olfactory cortex, respectively. The time to these responses has been shown to be clearly slowed in subjects with PD without a reduction in amplitude [5,23,24]. Limiting the use of OERPs is EEG contamination by slow wave activity, patient compliance required by long (30–40 s) inter-stimulus intervals, and the difficulty in interpreting a negative OERP in the setting of functional anosmia [25].

Although many olfactory assessment modalities, including odor identification, odor discrimination, odor detection threshold, and sniff magnitude, have been demonstrated to be impaired in PD, a previous meta-analysis suggested no significant difference between testing modalities in PD subjects [26]. However, there is a growing consensus that the use of more than one modality at a time may be indicated. Indeed, several recent studies have shown that different domains may be affected disproportionately [6,27]. Potagas *et al.* used unique tests of odor discrimination and identification to demonstrate a preferential decline in odor identification rather than odor detection, invoking an impairment in odor memory, but the novel methods of determining these deficits make this study difficult to validate against others [27]. However, other authors have reiterated the concept that designing tests of multiple olfactory domains is more effective for screening assessments [28,29]. Indeed, a recent study compared assessment strategies of olfaction, using the identification, discrimination, and threshold subsets of the Sniffin' Sticks protocol, in over 100 PD patients and over 2000 control subjects [30]. In a principal components analysis, they found two components in both the control and PD patients; one was loaded from all subtests, whereas the second was primarily loaded from odor threshold assessment, suggesting that combined assessment with multiple components, especially threshold testing, may be the most appropriate strategy.

Interestingly, it has been noted that decreased sniffing amplitude in PD may confound our ability to test olfaction. Sobel *et al.* assessed PD patients with the UPSIT before and after they were given instructions to take deep inspirations and reported that patients may miss 2–3 points out of 40 on the UPSIT by impaired sniffing alone [31].

The development of olfactory dysfunction as a biomarker of early PD

Often, in the clinic setting, it is very difficult to differentiate early idiopathic PD from other secondary or atypical causes of parkinsonism, particularly before assessment of response to dopaminergic therapies, when many subjects are recruited into *de novo* trials of neuroprotection. Therefore, in assessing the clinical utility of any marker of early PD, it is important to consider how well a test discriminates idiopathic PD from other causes of parkinsonism. To that end, olfactory dysfunction has been shown to help in the differentiation of PD from other causes of parkinsonism, so that patients presenting with parkinsonian signs but preserved olfaction should suggest consideration of either secondary or atypical parkinsonian syndromes. Specifically regarding atypical parkinsonian disorders, olfaction is felt to be less impaired in multiple system atrophy (MSA) compared with idiopathic PD [28], and patients with progressive supranuclear palsy (PSP) and corticobasal degeneration (CBD) appear to have preserved olfaction [28,32]. Based on these observations, a recent evidence-based practice parameter from the American Academy of Neurology stated that olfactory testing should be considered to differentiate PD from PSP and CBD, but not PD from MSA [7]. However, the methodology used to make this determination has been called into question [33]. In an analysis by McKinnon *et al.*, the authors critically examined the evidence available to answer the question, "What is the diagnostic accuracy of olfactory testing for differentiation of IPD from other diseases presenting with parkinsonism? [33]" Their conclusion was that because most of the evidence to date has been derived from small studies, some with questionable validity, "the diagnostic accuracy of olfactory testing for differentiating PD from other disorders is insufficient to justify its routine clinical use." Therefore, further studies in large community-based populations of patients with parkinsonian disorders, preferably with longitudinal olfactory assessments and autopsy confirmation of diagnosis, are needed to resolve these concerns.

One of the major concerns with the assessment of olfactory dysfunction as a biomarker of PD is the relative nonspecificity of impairment in elderly patients who are subject to other neurodegenerative disorders that may also affect olfaction. However, while olfactory dysfunction has also been demonstrated in AD, patients with dementia with Lewy bodies (DLB) have even greater impairments in olfaction, lending significance to the role of Lewy pathology in olfactory dysfunction [5,34,35]. Based on this assumption, it would be expected that non-degenerative causes of parkinsonism have intact olfaction, as is the case in vascular parkinsonism [36] and MPTP-induced parkinsonism [37]. In addition, Khan *et al.* found that a cohort of parkin-positive PD patients had better olfaction than idiopathic PD patients, supporting the concept of parkin-associated PD as a separate entity without Lewy bodies (LBs) [38]. Similarly, there have been two studies of olfactory dysfunction in drug-induced parkinsonism. Hensiek, Bhatia, and Hawkes noted that low UPSIT scores identified those patients who did not recover after cessation of the offending drug and suggested that the neuroleptic medications were causing an "unmasking" of an underlying idiopathic PD [39]. In a recent study by Kruger *et al.*, Sniffin' Sticks were used to demonstrate that depressed patients who were exposed to D2-blocking neuroleptic medications and developed extrapyramidal symptoms had significantly lower olfactory scores than either depressed patients who were exposed to D2-blocking neuroleptic medications and did not develop extrapyramidal symptoms or depressed patients who were not exposed to D2-blocking neuroleptic medications [40]. The authors suggested that olfactory dysfunction may be drug induced in patients with depression with sensitivity toward developing extrapyramidal symptoms, possibly due to latent basal ganglia dysfunction such as PD. They also raised the intriguing possibility that in the future, patients might have their olfaction assessed prior to exposure to D2-blocking neuroleptic medications to determine which patients are likely to develop extrapyramidal symptoms.

One of the best paradigms for assessing the utility of olfactory testing in the identification of a cohort at risk for developing PD is in studies of relatives of PD patients. Multiple studies by Berendse and Ponsen's group of their cohort of asymptomatic first-degree relatives of PD patients have shown that hyposmia was frequently the only clinical finding in relatives who would go on to develop PD [41,42]. They showed that in their cohort of asymptomatic relatives of PD patients, 10% of those with idiopathic hyposmia and SPECT abnormalities at baseline went on to develop clinical PD at a 2-year follow-up whereas none of the normosmic relatives did so [42]. Another powerful conclusion of these studies was that normosmic relatives of PD patients demonstrated a risk of developing PD lower than that of the general population. In a study of unaffected twins of idiopathic PD patients, olfactory testing was not sensitive enough to detect those that would develop PD at a 7-year follow-up evaluation [43]. In addition, in studies that showed olfactory dysfunction to be predictive of development of PD, the follow-up time was 1, 2, or 4 years, suggesting that olfactory dysfunction may only occur a short time prior to the onset of other PD symptoms [41,42,44,45]. In another study of 173 first-degree relatives of PD patients, Siderowf *et al.* were able to demonstrate a direct relationship between olfactory performance and lifetime caffeine intake, with subjects who drank more than two cups of caffeinated beverages per day having significantly better UPSIT scores than those who drank less than one cup per day [46]. As lower caffeine intake is known to be associated with an increased risk of developing PD [47], this represents an association between two known risk factors for PD in first-degree relatives of PD patients. Further research will determine whether assessing a combination of these risk factors will increase our ability to predict future development of PD.

In one of the few large, prospectively assessed, community-based cohorts of the elderly who have had olfactory assessments, Ross *et al.* demonstrated that impaired olfaction can predate clinical PD by at least 4 years [48]. The study, entitled the Honolulu–Asian Aging Study, assessed olfactory identification in 2267 elderly men of Japanese ancestry who were free of clinical PD and dementia at the time of testing, and then followed them for up to 8 years for incident PD. Their results revealed that men in the lowest quartile of olfactory performance had an odds ratio of 5.2 for development of PD within the next 4 years compared with men in the top two quartiles [48]. Interestingly, in a subset of 164 men from the same study who expired and were submitted to autopsy, Ross *et al.* were able to demonstrate that olfactory dysfunction also correlated with incidental Lewy body disease (ILBD), which they defined as subjects who had no history of PD or DLB and yet had LBs in the substantia nigra or locus coeruleus [49]. In this study, age-adjusted relative odds of having ILBD for men in the lowest tertile of olfactory identification performance was 11 times higher than those in the highest tertile.

The possible rapid degeneration of the olfactory system early in the course of PD may provide one explanation for why olfactory dysfunction has traditionally been observed to be a static phenomenon in PD. Although initially described as unrelated to the progression of motor dysfunction in PD [3], olfactory dysfunction was found to correlate with PD subtype by Stern *et al.* when they observed that olfaction was more impaired in those patients with "malignant" PD [Hoehn and Yahr (H&Y) Stage III or greater] than in patients with "benign" PD (H&Y Stage II or less for 4 or more years) [50]. Recent studies have suggested that an even closer link may be found between PD progression and olfactory dysfunction. Tissingh *et al.* found that odor discrimination loss was related to disease severity [29], whereas Hummel showed that OERPs correlated with Webster scores of disability due to PD [51]. In a cross-sectional analysis of 194 patients with early PD defined as H&Y Stage III or less, we found that after controlling for age, inverse correlations existed between UPSIT score and both disease duration and UPDRS motor scores [52]. In addition, 61% of PD patients scored in the anosmic range, with near total loss of sense of smell. We suggest that these correlations were possible, and contrary to previous studies, because of the exclusion of patients in the later stages of disease that might limit the ability to demonstrate a relationship due to a "basement effect" of poor olfactory function. However, these cross-sectional studies provide only a suggestion of a relationship between disease duration and olfactory dysfunction and the few longitudinal assessments of olfactory dysfunction in PD patients yield contradictory results. In a study with five *de novo* PD patients reported by Muller *et al.*, olfaction was tested three times in the first year after diagnosis [28]. Each of the three patients who demonstrated hyposmia on initial testing also showed a decline in olfactory function with these repeated tests. However, a recently published report of longitudinal assessment of olfactory dysfunction in 27 patients with PD with a mean follow-up time of over 4 years found that sequential assessment with Sniffin' Sticks revealed that there was significant variability in progression with some patients developing functional anosmia over time and others demonstrating improvements over time [53]. This study included patients with disease duration up to 19 years and was not autopsy confirmed, although the findings suggest a complex relationship in some patients with PD between disease duration and olfactory function. These findings necessitate further evaluation with larger sample sizes and autopsy corroboration of diagnosis to examine the possibility that progression of olfactory dysfunction may be demonstrable, at least in early PD, and potentially may serve as a medication-independent marker of disease progression for future trials of disease-modifying therapies.

The ability to detect early PD invariably increases when multiple psychometric tests are used together or in combination with imaging studies. Montgomery, Lyons, and Koller found that specificity for early PD could be increased to 92%, with 68% sensitivity, when combining tests of motor function, mood, and olfaction [54]. More recently, Siderowf *et al.* demonstrated a correlation between striatal dopaminergic loss seen with TRODAT-SPECT imaging and odor identification impairment in early PD [55]. Although advanced neuroimaging studies such as PET and SPECT are able to demonstrate dopaminergic loss in the brain, such investigations are currently too expensive to be widely implemented in screening paradigms. Recently, cardiac MIBG-SPECT has been utilized in differentiating between idiopathic PD and other parkinsonian syndromes, and has been shown to correlate closely with olfactory dysfunction in PD, independent of motor symptoms [56–58]. However, this assessment is not widely available outside Japan and, like cerebral functional imaging, is too expensive to serve as a screening instrument for PD. Transcranial sonography however, is potentially widely available and less invasive than PET or SPECT, and can identify hyperechogenicity in the substantia nigra of PD that is felt to be a marker of PD vulnerability [59]. Imaging in combination with olfactory testing has been used in several studies with success at identifying patients who would later develop other signs or symptoms of PD [42,44,45]. Sommer *et al.* used nigral hyperechogenicity on transcranial sonography to identify which patients of those presenting with idiopathic olfactory loss should receive SPECT scans, with 50% of these patients demonstrating dopaminergic loss on SPECT imaging [45].

Many studies have sought to find changes in cognitive, sensory or motor processing that, although subtle, may be predictors of development of future PD. Possible indicators have included neurocognitive tests, behavioral or mood changes, sensory complaints, REM sleep behavior disorder, and non-specific musculoskeletal pain [60–62]. Siderowf and Stern have described olfaction and other early non-motor signs as part of the "Parkinson's Disease at Risk Syndrome (PARS)" [63]. These data indicate that olfactory dysfunction will likely be a component of any panel of non-motor symptoms used as a screening tool to identify individuals at risk for developing PD who warrant further investigation.

The neuropathology of olfactory dysfunction in PD

Olfactory impairment in PD has been postulated to be caused by multiple different pathologic alterations observed throughout the olfactory system. Perhaps the most widely accepted hypothesis is that olfactory dysfunction is secondary to degeneration of neurons in the olfactory bulb with the accumulation of Lewy bodies and Lewy neurites [64,65] (see Plate 28.1). Lewy bodies and Lewy neurites are protein aggregates formed from insoluble α-synuclein and other proteins that occur in the cell soma and cell processes, respectively. These aggregates of insoluble proteins, collectively referred to as Lewy pathology, displace other intracellular structures and may lead to an interruption of axonal transport, axonal degeneration, and eventual demise of the affected neuron [66]. The significance of Lewy pathology was highlighted in a landmark body of work by Del Tredici, Braak, and colleagues, which was the first large scale attempt to develop a staging system of Lewy neurodegeneration in the human brain [8,67,68]. Largely, the traditional limitations of human neuropathologic assessment were circumvented by the use of large numbers of brains representing the breadth of human Lewy neurodegeneration, especially many cases of ILBD in which there had been no obvious evidence of clinical parkinsonism during life. In brains from ILBD subjects there was at least mild Lewy neurodegeneration. In these cases, it became clear that the earliest predilection sites of those examined were in the dorsal motor nucleus of the vagal/glossopharangeal nuclei, the intermediate reticular nucleus and the olfactory bulb and anterior olfactory nucleus. In a comprehensive assay of Lewy pathology in the brains of 110 patients, including 41 with clinical PD and 69 with ILBD, Braak and colleagues developed a staging system of the progression of Lewy pathology (see Chapter 3). This staging system was determined by comparing the regional distribution of pathology throughout the brain and brainstem and assuming that if the pathology progresses in a stepwise fashion, brains with less pathology in more restricted distributions would represent earlier pathologic stages. In this system, six stages were delineated, with stages 1 and 2 representing "preclinical" stages, stages 3 and 4 representing early "clinical" stages when typical motor features of PD are expected to arise, and stages 5 and 6 representing later stages with widespread pathology, frequently characterized by the development of dementia and other late non-motor symptoms.

It is possible to speculate that the initial Braak LB staging system delineated LB induction sites within the brainstem and olfactory system because of a lack of investigation of more peripheral nervous system tissues, including spinal cord and peripheral autonomic nervous system tissues. Indeed, Braak *et al.* suggested that this pathology may be the real induction sites for LB pathology in a separate report [69] in which they detailed the evidence for involvement of enteric nervous system tissues in idiopathic PD, and proposed a scheme by which each succeeding stage of Lewy pathology predilection sites is connected synaptically to nuclear areas involved in the previous stage. Interestingly, however, a similar scenario cannot be proposed for Lewy pathology in the olfactory system as no evidence of Lewy pathology specific to PD was seen in the first neurons in the olfactory pathway, the olfactory receptor neurons of the olfactory epithelium [70]. In this report, Lewy neurites were observed in the olfactory epithelium of patients with PD but were also observed in control subjects and no LBs were observed. It is possible that the lack of LB deposition in the olfactory receptor neurons may be due to the relatively short lifespan of these cells, which are continuously regenerated by basal cells throughout life.

Beyond the anterior olfactory nucleus and olfactory bulb, Lewy pathology has been demonstrated in the olfactory-related cortices in PD and ILBD. Silveira-Moriyama *et al.* examined the primary olfactory cortices including the olfactory tubercle, the frontal piriform cortex, and the temporal piriform cortex in seven cases of ILBD, 10 cases of PD and four healthy controls; they observed Lewy pathology in each area in all cases of ILBD and PD, but none of the controls [71]. Similarly, Braak *et al.* recognized that while Lewy pathology aggregated within periamygdaloid, piriform, and entorhinal cortices, they did not immediately spread to adjacent cortex unrelated to olfactory processing [67].

It would seem that the neuropathologic spread of Lewy pathology to the olfactory cortex may underlie the spectrum of olfactory deficits present, in the same way that cortical Lewy pathology correlates with dementia in PD [72]. True anosmia is somewhat rare in PD; even those patients most impaired in odor identification are still able to detect some strong odors, indicating that impairment in identification may involve cognitive processes beyond that of detection threshold. Indeed, major deficits in cognitive judgment regarding different odors has been observed in patients with PD [73].

The mechanism by which Lewy pathology in the olfactory bulb and anterior olfactory nucleus leads to impaired olfaction has yet to be elucidated. In fact, the olfactory bulb and tract are ideally suited for neuropathologic investigation into the pathophysiology of Lewy neurodegeneration because it is one of the few easily dissectible preparations that include the dendritic arborization, cell soma, axon, and axon terminal of neurons selectively vulnerable to Lewy pathology. Given the emphasis on dopaminergic denervation for the motor symptoms of PD, early studies examined the dopaminergic innervation of olfactory structures and found that the olfactory tubercle is severely depleted of dopamine in PD [74]. However, olfactory dysfunction does not respond to dopaminergic medication, so that dysfunction of dopaminergic projections to the olfactory system is either not causative or olfactory system neurons may be damaged early enough that no response is possible by the time anti-parkinsonian medications are typically prescribed [75]. In addition, as mentioned previously, there are several conditions with similar degrees of dopaminergic denervation of nigrostriatal and mesolimbic pathways, including atypical parkinsonian disorders such as progressive supranuclear palsy and MPTP intoxication, that do not have significant olfactory dysfunction [32,76]. Interestingly, most dopaminergic neurons in the olfactory bulb, the periglomerular dopaminergic neurons, are not know to be susceptible to the deposition of LBs, but rather it is the anterior olfactory neurons and possibly mitral and tufted neurons that are selectively vulnerable [64,77]. Regarding the dopaminergic neurons of the olfactory bulb, two studies have investigated the number of dopaminergic neurons in the olfactory bulb of PD patients and controls using stereologic assessment [78,79]. Huisman, Uylings, and Hoogland showed an unexpected doubling of tyrosine hydroxylase-positive periglomerular neurons in PD cases compared with healthy controls [78]. As dopamine is known to inhibit transmission between axons of olfactory receptor neurons and dendrites of mitral cells in the olfactory bulb in animal models, the authors hypothesized that a tonic inhibition of olfactory neurotransmission occurs, related to a compensatory increase in dopamine receptors in extranigral sites [80,81]. However, the same group more recently reported in a follow-up study with twice as many subjects that there was no difference in the number of dopaminergic neurons between male and female PD patients and male control subjects [79]. Female control subjects did have significantly fewer dopaminergic neurons than male controls for unclear reasons, but there was significant variability, even within controls, with as few as zero and as many as 60 000 dopaminergic neurons. Therefore, PD does not clearly alter the number of dopaminergic neurons in the olfactory bulb, at least in men, and intrabulbar dopamine concentrations are clearly not the sole reason for olfactory dysfunction in PD.

In addition to Lewy pathology, several other pathologic alterations have been demonstrated in the olfactory pathway of patients with PD and have been suggested to result in olfactory impairment. In the anterior olfactory nucleus, for example, Pearce, Hawkes, and Daniel demonstrated significant loss of neurons in the anterior olfactory nucleus that correlated with disease duration [64]. Similarly, in the olfactory bulb, Hoogland, van den Berg, and Huisman have demonstrated morphologic alterations that may contribute to olfactory dysfunction in PD [82]. These include misrouted olfactory projection fibers from the olfactory receptor neurons that normally terminate in the glomerular layer, occasionally terminating in the external plexiform layer of PD patients and elderly controls as well as ectopic glomeruli in the external plexiform layer that are specific to PD olfactory bulbs. The significance of these alterations and the relationship to Lewy pathology deposition remain to be determined.

The role of olfactory system pathology in PD pathophysiology

As the prevalence of olfactory dysfunction in PD has become better accepted, several hypotheses have arisen regarding the possibility that the olfactory system itself is central to the pathophysiology of PD. The olfactory system, with its unique neuronal privilege of entering the brain from the outside world without intervening synapses, seems remarkably poised for the delivery of external pathogens to the central nervous system [69]. The resulting olfactory vector hypothesis of PD pathophysiology suggests that an external agent enters the brain through the olfactory epithelium and sets in place a cascade of pathology that is spread via trans-synaptic transmission into primary olfactory cortices and finally into brainstem nuclei responsible for causing the motor symptoms of PD [83,84]. In a recent review, Doty makes it clear that many agents, including viruses, bacteria, prions, and a variety of exogenous toxins, may enter the brain via the olfactory epithelium and, in some cases, spread to brain areas classically associated with PD pathology [83]. Hawkes, Del Tredici, and Braak have proposed a modification of the classic olfactory vector hypothesis to include the possibility that a pathogen may gain access to the brain via two related routes, first via the olfactory epithelium, and second via the vagus nerve after invasion of axons of Meissner's plexus neurons in the digestive tract after swallowing infected nasal secretions [85]. This would, in theory, rectify aspects of the olfactory vector hypothesis with the progression of Lewy pathology suggested by Braak and colleagues, which includes early involvement of the peripheral autonomic nervous system and dorsal motor nucleus of the vagus. However, in an attempt to alleviate the need for an enteric pathogen transmitting an agent to the neurons of the dorsal motor nucleus, Lerner and Bagic reviewed anatomic connections between the olfactory system and brainstem nuclei and suggested that a preponderance of pathways leading to the dorsal motor nucleus may engender selective vulnerability to these neurons in a top-down fashion also [86]. Intriguing as these hypotheses are, they remain speculative until further research identifies the putative exogenous agents and demonstrates a capacity for exposure to induce Lewy neurodegeneration in susceptible neurons.

Conclusion

Due to its high prevalence early in the course of PD, olfactory dysfunction serves as a biomarker of the premotor state, and may eventually be viewed as a marker of very early disease progression. Currently, olfactory testing offers an inexpensive, reliable method for screening those patients already known to be at risk (such as family members of PD patients), and discriminating between PD and other parkinsonian syndromes. Insights obtained from a greater understanding of the pathophysiology of olfactory dysfunction in PD may also lead to greater understanding of the mechanism of Lewy neurodegeneration. Most importantly, understanding the evolution of olfactory impairment in early PD will shed light on the earliest pathologic changes in PD, which will provide the clues needed for much earlier detection when therapeutic interventions are more likely to be effective at slowing the inexorable progression to eventual neurologic disability.

References

1. Parkinson J. *An Essay on the Shaking Palsy*. London: Whittingham and Rowland, 1817.
2. Ansari KA, Johnson A. Olfactory function in patients with Parkinson's disease. *J Chron Dis* 1975;**28**:493–7.
3. Doty RL, Deems DA, Stellar S. Olfactory dysfunction in parkinsonism: a general deficit unrelated to neurologic signs, disease stage, or disease duration. *Neurology* 1988;**38**:1237–44.
4. Double KL, Rowe DB, Hayes M, *et al.* Identifying the pattern of olfactory deficits in Parkinson disease using the brief smell identification test. *Arch Neurol* 2003;**60**:545–9.
5. Hawkes CH, Shephard BC, Daniel SE. Olfactory dysfunction in Parkinson's disease. *J Neurol Neurosurg Psychiatry* 1997;**62**:436–46.
6. Mesholam RI, Moberg PJ, Mahr RN, Doty RL. Olfaction in neurodegenerative disease: a meta-analysis of olfactory functioning in Alzheimer's and Parkinson's diseases. *Arch Neurol* 1998;**55**:84–90.
7. Suchowersky O, Reich S, Perlmutter J, *et al.* Practice Parameter: diagnosis and prognosis of new onset Parkinson disease (an evidence-based review): report of the Quality Standards Subcommittee of the American Academy of Neurology. *Neurology* 2006;**66**:968–75.
8. Del Tredici K, Rub U, de Vos RA, *et al.* Where does parkinson disease pathology begin in the brain? *J Neuropathol Exp Neurol* 2002;**61**:413–26.
9. Doty RL, Shaman P, Kimmelman CP, Dann MS. University of Pennsylvania Smell Identification Test: a rapid quantitative olfactory function test for the clinic. *Laryngoscope* 1984;**94**:176–8.
10. Doty RL. Clinical studies of olfaction. *Chem Senses* 2005; **30**(Suppl 1):i207–9.
11. Doty RL, Avron M, Lee W. Development of the 12-item cross-cultural smell identification test (CC-SIT). *Laryngoscope* 1996;**106**:353–6.
12. Doty RL, Bromley SM, Stern MB. Olfactory testing as an aid in the diagnosis of Parkinson's disease: development of optimal discrimination criteria. *Neurodegeneration* 1995;**4**:93–7.
13. Bohnen NI, Gedela S, Kuwabara H, *et al.* Selective hyposmia and nigrostriatal dopaminergic denervation in Parkinson's disease. *J Neurol* 2007;**254**:84–90.
14. Hummel T, Sekinger B, Wolf SR, *et al.* 'Sniffin' sticks': olfactory performance assessed by the combined testing of odor identification, odor discrimination and olfactory threshold. *Chem Senses* 1997;**22**:39–52.

15. Mueller CA, Grassinger E, Naka A, *et al.* A self-administered odor identification test procedure using the "Sniffin' Sticks." *Chem Senses* 2006;**31**:595–8.
16. Albrecht J, Anzinger A, Kopietz R, *et al.* Test-retest reliability of the olfactory detection threshold test of the Sniffin' sticks. *Chem Senses* 2008;**33**:461–7.
17. Doty RL. Office procedures for quantitative assessment of olfactory function. *Am J Rhinol* 2007;**1**:460–73.
18. Wudarski TJ, Doty RL. Comparison of detection threshold values determined using glass sniff bottles and plastic squeeze bottles. *Percept Mot Skills* 2004;**98**:192–6.
19. Choudhury ES, Moberg P, Doty RL. Influences of age and sex on a microencapsulated odor memory test. *Chem Senses* 2003;**28**:799–805.
20. Frank RA, Dulay MF, Gesteland RC. Assessment of the Sniff Magnitude Test as a clinical test of olfactory function. *Physiol Behav* 2003;**78**:195–204.
21. Frank RA, Dulay MF, Niergarth KA, Gesteland RC. A comparison of the sniff magnitude test and the University of Pennsylvania Smell Identification Test in children and nonnative English speakers. *Physiol Behav* 2004;**81**:475–80.
22. Tourbier IA, Doty RL. Sniff magnitude test: relationship to odor identification, detection, and memory tests in a clinic population. *Chem Senses* 2007;**32**:515–23.
23. Barz S, Hummel T, Pauli E, *et al.* Chemosensory event-related potentials in response to trigeminal and olfactory stimulation in idiopathic Parkinson's disease. *Neurology* 1997;**49**:1424–31.
24. Thesen T, Murphy C. Reliability analysis of event-related brain potentials to olfactory stimuli. *Psychophysiology* 2002;**39**: 733–8.
25. Lotsch J, Hummel T. The clinical significance of electrophysiological measures of olfactory function. *Behav Brain Res* 2006;**170**:78–83.
26. Mesholam RI, Moberg PJ, Mahr RN, Doty RL. Olfaction in neurodegenerative disease: a meta-analysis of olfactory functioning in Alzheimer's and Parkinson's diseases. *Arch Neurol* 1998;**55**:84–90.
27. Potagas C, Dellatolas G, Ziegler M, *et al.* Clinical assessment of olfactory dysfunction in Parkinson's disease. *Mov Disord* 1998;**13**:394–9.
28. Muller A, Reichmann H, Livermore A, Hummel T. Olfactory function in idiopathic Parkinson's disease (IPD): results from cross-sectional studies in IPD patients and long-term follow-up of *de-novo* IPD patients. *J Neural Transm* 2002;**109**:805–11.
29. Tissingh G, Berendse HW, Bergmans P, *et al.* Loss of olfaction in *de novo* and treated Parkinson's disease: possible implications for early diagnosis. *Mov Disord* 2001;**16**:41–6.
30. Lotsch J, Reichmann H, Hummel T. Different odor tests contribute differently to the evaluation of olfactory loss. *Chem Senses* 2008;**33**:17–21.
31. Sobel N, Thomason ME, Stappen I, *et al.* An impairment in sniffing contributes to the olfactory impairment in Parkinson's disease. *Proc Natl Acad Sci USA* 2001;**98**:4154–9.
32. Wenning GK, Shephard B, Hawkes C, *et al.* Olfactory function in atypical parkinsonian syndromes. *Acta Neurol Scand* 1995;**91**:247–50.
33. McKinnon JH, Demaerschalk BM, Caviness JN, *et al.* Sniffing out Parkinson disease: can olfactory testing differentiate Parkinsonian disorders? *Neurologist* 2007;**13**:382–5.
34. McShane RH, Nagy Z, Esiri MM, *et al.* Anosmia in dementia is associated with Lewy bodies rather than Alzheimer's pathology. *J Neurol Neurosurg Psychiatry* 2001;**70**:739–43.
35. Olichney JM, Murphy C, Hofstetter CR, *et al.* Anosmia is very common in the Lewy body variant of Alzheimer's disease. *J Neurol Neurosurg Psychiatry* 2005;**76**:1342–7.
36. Katzenschlager R, Zijlmans J, Evans A, *et al.* Olfactory function distinguishes vascular parkinsonism from Parkinson's disease. *J Neurol Neurosurg Psychiatry* 2004;**75**:1749–52.
37. Doty RL, Singh A, Tetrud J, Langston JW. Lack of major olfactory dysfunction in MPTP-induced parkinsonism. *Ann Neurol* 1992;**32**:97–100.
38. Khan NL, Katzenschlager R, Watt H, *et al.* Olfaction differentiates parkin disease from early-onset parkinsonism and Parkinson disease. *Neurology* 2004;**62**:1224–6.
39. Hensiek AE, Bhatia K, Hawkes CH. Olfactory dysfunction in drug induced parkinsonism. *J Neurol* 2000;**247**:303.
40. Krüger S, Haehner A, Theim C, Hummel T. Neuroleptic-induced parkinsonism is associated with olfactory dysfunction. *J Neurol* 2008;**255**:1574–9.
41. Berendse HW, Booij J, Francot CM, *et al.* Subclinical dopaminergic dysfunction in asymptomatic Parkinson's disease patients' relatives with a decreased sense of smell. *Ann Neurol* 2001; **50**:34–41.
42. Ponsen MM, Stoffers D, Booij J, *et al.* Idiopathic hyposmia as a preclinical sign of Parkinson's disease. *Ann Neurol* 2004;**56**:173–81.
43. Marras C, Goldman S, Smith A, *et al.* Smell identification ability in twin pairs discordant for Parkinson's disease. *Mov Disord* 2005;**20**:687–93.
44. Haehner A, Hummel T, Hummel C, *et al.* Olfactory loss may be a first sign of idiopathic Parkinson's disease. *Mov Disord* 2007;**22**:839–42.
45. Sommer U, Hummel T, Cormann K, *et al.* Detection of presymptomatic Parkinson's disease: combining smell tests, transcranial sonography, and SPECT. *Mov Disord* 2004;**19**:1196–202.
46. Siderowf A, Jennings D, Connolly J, *et al.* Risk factors for Parkinson's disease and impaired olfaction in relatives of patients with Parkinson's disease. *Mov Disord* 2007;**22**:2249–55.
47. Ross GW, Abbott RD, Petrovitch H, *et al.* Association of coffee and caffeine intake with risk of Parkinson's disease. *JAMA* 2000;**283**:2674–9.
48. Ross GW, Petrovitch H, Abbott RD, *et al.* Association of olfactory dysfunction with risk for future Parkinson's disease. *Ann Neurol* 2008;**63**:167–73.
49. Ross GW, Petrovitch H, Abbott RD, *et al.* Association of olfactory dysfunction with risk for future Parkinson's disease. *Ann Neurol* 2008;**63**:167–73.
50. Stern MB, Doty RL, Dotti M, *et al.* Olfactory function in Parkinson's disease subtypes. *Neurology* 1994;**44**:266–8.
51. Hummel T. Olfactory evoked potentials as a tool to measure progression of Parkinson's Disease. In: Chase T, Bedard B, eds. *Focus on Medicine: New Developments in the Drug Therapy of Parkinson's disease*. Blackwell Science, Oxford, 1999:47–53.
52. Hower RE, Rick JH, Balderston CC, *et al.* Olfactory dysfunction and Parkinson's disease progression. *Neurology* 2008; **70**(Suppl 1):A397.

53. Herting B, Schulze S, Reichmann H, *et al.* A longitudinal study of olfactory function in patients with idiopathic Parkinson's disease. *J Neurol* 2008;**255**:367–70.
54. Montgomery EB Jr, Lyons K, Koller WC. Early detection of probable idiopathic Parkinson's disease: II. A prospective application of a diagnostic test battery. *Mov Disord* 2000;**15**:474–8.
55. Siderowf A, Newberg A, Chou KL, *et al.* [^{99m}Tc]TRODAT-1 SPECT imaging correlates with odor identification in early Parkinson disease. *Neurology* 2005;**64**:1716–20.
56. Braune S, Reinhardt M, Bathmann J, *et al.* Impaired cardiac uptake of *meta*-[^{123}I]iodobenzylguanidine in Parkinson's disease with autonomic failure. *Acta Neurol Scand* 1998;**97**:307–14.
57. Lee PH, Yeo SH, Kim HJ, Youm HY. Correlation between cardiac ^{123}I-MIBG and odor identification in patients with Parkinson's disease and multiple system atrophy. *Mov Disord* 2006;**21**:1975–7.
58. Yoshita M. Differentiation of idiopathic Parkinson's disease from striatonigral degeneration and progressive supranuclear palsy using iodine-123 *meta*-iodobenzylguanidine myocardial scintigraphy. *J Neurol Sci* 1998;**155**:60–7.
59. Behnke S, Berg D, Becker G. Does ultrasound disclose a vulnerability factor for Parkinson's disease? *J Neurol* 2003;**250**(Suppl 1):I24–7.
60. Horstink MW, Morrish PK. Preclinical diagnosis of Parkinson's disease. *Adv Neurol* 1999;**80**:327–33.
61. Koller WC, Langston JW, Hubble JP, *et al.* Does a long preclinical period occur in Parkinson's disease? *Geriatrics* 1991;**46**(Suppl 1):8–15.
62. Wolters EC, Francot C, Bergmans P, *et al.* Preclinical (premotor) Parkinson's disease. *J Neurol* 2000;**247**(Suppl 2):II103–9.
63. Siderowf A, Stern MB. Preclinical diagnosis of Parkinson's disease: are we there yet? *Curr Neurol Neurosci Rep* 2006;**6**:295–301.
64. Pearce RK, Hawkes CH, Daniel SE. The anterior olfactory nucleus in Parkinson's disease. *Mov Disord* 1995;**10**:283–7.
65. Kranick SM, Duda JE. Olfactory dysfunction in Parkinson's disease. *Neurosignals* 2008;**16**:35–40.
66. Duda JE. Pathology and neurotransmitter abnormalities of dementia with Lewy bodies. *Dement Geriatr Cogn Disord* 2004;**17**(Suppl 1):3–14.
67. Braak H, Del Tredici K, Rub U, *et al.* Staging of brain pathology related to sporadic Parkinson's disease. *Neurobiol Aging* 2003;**24**:197–211.
68. Braak H, Bohl JR, Muller CM. Stanley Fahn Lecture 2005. The staging procedure for the inclusion body pathology associated with sporadic Parkinson's disease reconsidered. *Mov Disord* 2006;**21**:2042–51.
69. Braak H, Rub U, Gai WP, Del Tredici K. Idiopathic Parkinson's disease: possible routes by which vulnerable neuronal types may be subject to neuroinvasion by an unknown pathogen. *J Neural Transm* 2003;**110**:517–36.
70. Duda JE, Shah U, Arnold SE, *et al.* The expression of alpha-, beta-, and gamma-synucleins in olfactory mucosa from patients with and without neurodegenerative diseases. *Exp Neurol* 1999;**160**:515–22.
71. Silveira-Moriyama L, Holton J, Kingsbury A, *et al.* Regional differences in the severity of Lewy body pathology across the olfactory cortex. *Neurosci Lett* 2009;**453**:77–80.
72. Hurtig HI, Trojanowski JQ, Galvin J, *et al.* Alpha-synuclein cortical Lewy bodies correlate with dementia in Parkinson's disease. *Neurology* 2000;**54**:1916–21.
73. Hudry J, Thobois S, Broussolle E, *et al.* Evidence for deficiencies in perceptual and semantic olfactory processes in Parkinson's disease. *Chem Senses* 2003;**28**:537–43.
74. Bogerts B, Hantsch J, Herzer M. A morphometric study of the dopamine-containing cell groups in the mesencephalon of normals, Parkinson's patients and schizophrenics. *Biol Psychiatry* 1983;**18**:951–69.
75. Doty RL, Stern MB, Pfeiffer C, *et al.* Bilateral olfactory dysfunction in early stage treated and untreated idiopathic Parkinson's disease. *J Neurol Neurosurg Psychiatry* 1992;**55**:138–42.
76. Doty RL, Singh A, Tetrud J, Langston JW. Lack of major olfactory dysfunction in MPTP-induced parkinsonism. *Ann Neurol* 1992;**32**:97–100.
77. Daniel SE, Hawkes CH. Preliminary diagnosis of Parkinson's disease by olfactory bulb pathology. *Lancet* 1992;**340**:186.
78. Huisman E, Uylings HB, Hoogland PV. A 100% increase of dopaminergic cells in the olfactory bulb may explain hyposmia in Parkinson's disease. *Mov Disord* 2004;**19**:687–92.
79. Huisman E, Uylings HB, Hoogland PV. Gender-related changes in increase of dopaminergic neurons in the olfactory bulb of Parkinson's disease patients. *Mov Disord* 2008;**23**:1407–13.
80. Duchamp-Viret P, Coronas V, Delaleu JC, *et al.* Dopaminergic modulation of mitral cell activity in the frog olfactory bulb: a combined radioligand binding–electrophysiological study. *Neuroscience* 1997;**79**:203–16.
81. Hsia AY, Vincent JD, Lledo PM. Dopamine depresses synaptic inputs into the olfactory bulb. *J Neurophysiol* 1999;**82**:1082–5.
82. Hoogland PV, van den Berg R, Huisman E. Misrouted olfactory fibres and ectopic olfactory glomeruli in normal humans and in Parkinson and Alzheimer patients. *Neuropathol Appl Neurobiol* 2003;**29**:303–11.
83. Doty RL. The olfactory vector hypothesis of neurodegenerative disease: is it viable? *Ann Neurol* 2008;**63**:7–15.
84. Hawkes CH, Shephard BC, Daniel SE. Is Parkinson's disease a primary olfactory disorder? *QJM* 1999;**92**:473–80.
85. Hawkes CH, Del Tredici K, Braak H. Parkinson's disease: a dual-hit hypothesis. *Neuropathol Appl Neurobiol* 2007;**33**:599–614.
86. Lerner A, Bagic A. Olfactory pathogenesis of idiopathic Parkinson disease revisited. *Mov Disord* 2008;**23**:1076–84.
87. Doty RL. Odor perception in neurodegenerative diseases. In: Doty RL, ed. *Handbook of Olfaction and Gustation*, 2nd edn. New York: Marcel Dekker, 2003; 479–503.

Chapter 29
Pain and Paresthesia in Parkinson's Disease

Shen-Yang Lim[1] *& Andrew H. Evans*[2]
[1]Faculty of Medicine, University of Malaysia, Kuala Lumpur, Malaysia
[2]Department of Neurology, Royal Melbourne Hospital, Parkville, Victoria and Department of Medicine, University of Melbourne, Australia

Introduction

Charcot noted in 1877 that "paralysis agitans is not only an extraordinarily sad disease in that it robs patients of the use of their limbs ... it is also a cruel disease since it causes distressing sensations." Pain is defined as an unpleasant or distressing sensory experience, whereas paresthesias are abnormal (usually non-painful and superficial) sensations. Pain is a frequent complaint in Parkinson's disease (PD) patients. It adversely affects health-related quality-of-life [1,2], and in a minority of patients may even overshadow the motor symptoms of PD [3–5]. It interferes with the ability of patients to participate in their activities of daily living [6], for example, by further impairing mobility [7,8]. Pain can contribute significantly to sleep disturbance due to frequent awakenings [9]. Major depression is much more common in patients with pain compared to those without [9]; some patients have even considered suicide because of their pain [10]. In many patients, pain is also associated with anxiety and even panic [11]. Conversely, it has been reported that paresthesias, which are often intermittent, are generally easily tolerated by patients and may not add to parkinsonian disability [12]. In this chapter, we describe the epidemiology, clinical features, and mechanisms of sensory (mainly pain) syndromes in PD, and provide a framework for evaluating and treating these symptoms.

Epidemiology of sensory symptoms in PD

The prevalence of sensory complaints in PD

Sensory or painful syndromes affect approximately *two-thirds* of PD patients (Table 29.1). In studies where an attempt was made to determine the etiology of painful symptoms, between 29 and 63% of PD patients were thought to have pain directly related to PD. Incidentally, pain is also reported by about half of patients with multiple system atrophy (MSA) [13], and is more common in MSA-P (predominantly parkinsonian subtype) than in MSA-C (predominantly cerebellar subtype) [14].

Studies comparing pain in PD patients to age-matched controls

Older age is associated with an increased propensity for painful conditions (e.g., rheumatologic/orthopedic) [15,16]. Studies of elderly people have found that about 70% experience pain [15,17]. However, in PD pain does not relate to older age [1,6,16,18–20] and is more prevalent – and more severe [1,2,16] – compared with age-matched controls. Karlsen *et al.* found that 67% of PD patients reported pain problems compared with 39% of healthy elderly controls matched for age and sex [21]. Riley *et al.* surveyed 150 consecutive PD patients and 60 age- and sex-matched controls and found a higher incidence of frozen shoulder in the PD group (13% versus 2%) [22]. Etchepare *et al.* reported a 60% point prevalence of thoracic/lumbar back pain in a group of 104 PD patients compared with 23% in a matched control group of chronically ill patients [16]. Radicular symptoms including pain are also more common in PD patients than non-PD neurologic controls (36% versus 11%) [23].

Gender differences

With a few exceptions [24,25], no gender difference in the frequency of pain complaints has been found in PD patients [6,8,18,26,27]. Burning mouth syndrome was reported to be 1.7 times more common in women patients [28]. and genital pain may also be more common in women [29].

Pain in early- and later-stage PD

With a few exceptions [2,30], no correlation has been found between the presence or severity of pain and

Parkinson's Disease: Non-Motor and Non-Dopaminergic Features, First Edition. Edited by C. Warren Olanow, Fabrizio Stocchi, and Anthony E. Lang.

Table 29.1 Frequency of sensory complaints in PD: unless noted otherwise (see footnotes), these were studies of patients attending movement disorders clinics.

		Frequency of sensory symptoms (%)			
Study	Sample size	Overall	Unrelated to PD	PD-related	Definition used
Snider *et al.* [24]	105	–	4	43[h]	Primary sensory symptoms (i.e., without an apparent somatic cause; patients with arthritis or diabetes excluded; painful muscle spasm or cramps secondary to sustained muscle contraction also excluded)
Koller [12]	50	–	–	38[i]	Primary sensory symptoms (patients with musculoskeletal disease or diabetes excluded)
Goetz *et al.* [6]	95	–	–	46	Pain that patients believed was directly related to their PD
Karlsen *et al.* [30][a]	233	67	–	–	Pain dimension of the Nottingham Health Profile
Honey *et al.* [112][b]	50	–	–	42	Pain attributable to PD
Shulman *et al.* [149]	99	–	–	63	Commonly experienced pain, numbness, tingling, or burning in association with PD
Vela *et al.* [27]	50	64	–	–	Pain
Quittenbaum and Grahn [1][c]	55	68	–	–	Aching/pain during the last month
Mott *et al.* [25][d]	444	64	–	–	Pain
Giuffrida *et al.* [18]	388	67	–	–	Sensory or painful syndromes
Lee *et al.* [19]	123	85	64	63	Pain
Tinazzi *et al.* [20]	117	40	–	–	Pain (duration $\geq$2 months)
Martinez-Martin *et al.* [224]	545	–	–	29	Unexplained pains (not due to known conditions such as arthritis) (NMSQuest)
da Silva *et al.* [8]	50	56	–	–	Pain
Negre-Pages *et al.* [2][e]	450	62	25[f]	37	Chronic pain (3 months duration)
Lim *et al.* [84]	50	–	–	48[g]	Commonly experienced pain which the patient attributed to PD

[a]Unselected community-based group of PD patients.
[b]Patients with medically refractory motor features presenting for pallidotomy.
[c]County hospital neurology clinic.
[d]PD support group members.
[e]General neurological practice.
[f]Mainly osteoarthritis.
[g]2/12 (17%) of the stable responders, 9/15 (60%) of the fluctuators (without dyskinesia), and 13/23 (57%) of the dyskinetic patients.
[h]Pain 29%; tingling 22%; numbness 21%; burning 11%.
[i]Numbness 24%; tingling 16%; pain and achiness 12%; coldness 12%; burning 2%.

disease duration or disease stage (as measured by the severity of motor features) [6,8,16,18–20,31]. The frequency of pain complaints in PD is thought to have a bimodal distribution [8,18]. There seems to be an initial peak of painful symptoms prior to or at the onset of PD [18]. For example, Riley *et al.* found that the peak incidence of frozen shoulder was during the 2 years prior to the onset of other clinical symptoms (11/19 cases) [22]. In many patients, pain resolves with initiation of antiparkinsonian treatment [3,8,22].

A second peak occurs later in the disease course, in conjunction with the development of motor fluctuations and dyskinesia [11,20], and possibly also as a consequence of accumulating PD pathology. For example, one study using multivariate analysis found that PD patients with pain had an odds ratio of 5.7 of having motor response complications (MRCs) compared with those without pain [20]. Other investigators have reported similar findings [2,25,27]. Further indirect support for a link between MRC and pain phenomena is that PD patients with chronic pain have younger age [6] and younger disease onset [2]. MRCs are also strongly linked to younger age of PD onset [32,33]. Furthermore, pain is also more commonly experienced by MSA patients with MRC (relative risk 1.63) [13].

Table 29.2 Relative proportions of sensory symptoms in PD.

Pain type	Goetz *et al.* [6]	Honey *et al.* [112]	Giuffrida *et al.* [18]	Tinazzi *et al.* [20]
No. of patients with sensory symptoms	43	21	269	47
Rheumatic				
Musculoskeletal	74%	76%	94% ("muscular")	47%
Joint	–	–	51% ("osteoarticular")	–
Somatic pain exacerbated by rigidity or involuntary movements of PD	14%	29%	–	–
Dystonic pain	28%	19%	–	66%
Radicular/neuritic pain (localized to the territory of a nerve root or nerve)	14%	0%	8% (localized or less-defined "neurogenic" pain)	9%
Primary parkinsonian (central) pain	0%	10% ("dysesthetic" pain – poorly localized, burning)		4%
Akathitic discomfort	2%	–	10% (akathisia or RLS)	–
RLS	–	–		–

The following case example, taken from a series by Riley and Lang (patient 1) [34], illustrates a pattern that is not infrequently encountered in clinical practice. A 62-year-old woman had a 3 year history of pain and stiffness in her neck and upper back, which had been diagnosed as "fibrositis." When signs of parkinsonism were found 3 years later, and L-dopa commenced, she experienced a marked improvement of her motor function and soon became pain free for the first time in years. However, she developed dyskinesia and motor response fluctuations. She had pain, where the skin over her legs felt extremely sensitive "like a fresh sunburn," together with pronounced parkinsonism and episodic severe depression each time her medication wore off. The "off" period pain resolved whenever her L-dopa took effect.

Phenomenology of PD-related pain

The spectrum of sensory symptoms experienced by PD patients is wide. Features to consider include the time course, location, quality and severity of pain, and impact of anti-parkinsonian medication, including relationship to motor fluctuations (e.g., "off" period or biphasic dystonia or "on" period chorea).

Topography

Every localization of pain has been described in PD [4], and in some patients the pain may be poorly localized [24,35–37]. The most commonly painful sites are the back, legs, and shoulders [2,19,20,25]. In the majority of cases, the pain occurs on the side more affected by parkinsonism [12,20,22,24,37,38]. Pain may adopt unusual distributions, such as a "pseudoradiculopathy" (radiating from the hip or shoulder down the affected limb) [3,39], oral (tongue, palate, lip or gum), or genital pain syndromes [28,29], chest pain [3,11], and upper or lower abdominal discomfort [3,11]. Apart from occasional cases of painful dystonic spasms involving the neck and jaw, headaches and facial pain syndromes are relatively rarely encountered in PD patients [3,18].

Clinical features

Quality/categorization of sensory symptoms

Discomforting sensations encompass a range of symptoms and include aching, cramping, stiffness, numbness, tingling, burning, coldness, and itching, and may be accompanied by motor restlessness [12,18,24]. A classification of sensory symptoms is given in Table 29.2. Published series are in general agreement on the prevalence of sensory symptoms in PD, but there is less consistency on the *proportion* of patients in each of the various categories. In contrast to the study by Goetz *et al.* (where pain was almost completely accounted for by somatic pain, due to musculoskeletal disease or dystonia) [6], other investigators have found high rates of "*primary*" sensory symptoms (see Table 29.1 – Snider *et al.* and Koller *et al.*). This discrepancy is no doubt at least partly accounted for by differing *definitions* of "central" or "primary parkinsonian" sensations. Ford described this type of painful sensation as follows: "Burning, tingling, formication; relentless, bizarre quality; location not confined to root or nerve territory; not explained by rigidity or dystonia; may fluctuate with medication effect" [4]. However, given that PD patients typically demonstrate hyperalgesia, it could be argued that a "central" component may be involved in most if not all types of pain experienced by PD patients. One may see patients whose pain has a clear nociceptive basis (e.g., secondary to lumbar disc herniation), but is aggravated during "off" medication periods [40].

Pain severity

Using a pain severity scale of 0–100, patients in the study by Goetz *et al.* reported a mean pain score of 56 [6]. In a study by Lee *et al.* using similar methodology, mean pain score was 39 (median 37) [19]. Significantly, 50% of patients in this series said their pain was moderate or dominating their day.

Fluctuations in relation to the L-dopa cycle

Pain fluctuates with parkinsonian disability in one- to two-thirds of PD patients [6,18], and usually (in almost 90% of cases) occurs in the motor-"off" phase (with or without dystonia) [5,6]. Less commonly, patients identify pain in the "off"-to-"on" (beginning-of-dose) switch, during L-dopa's peak effect, or at the time of the "on"-to-"off" (end-of-dose) switch [3,5]. Some patients report that the most incapacitating type of fluctuations (motor or non-motor) is the sensory ones [5].

Dystonic pain

Painful dystonic spasms tend to occur in the limbs most affected by parkinsonism [41] and are often accompanied by visible dystonia [6]. The toes and feet are mostly involved (e.g., inversion of the foot, toe curling, extension or flexion of the big toe), but dystonic pain can also involve the neck or jaw [39,41]. Dystonic pain is more common in the "off" phase [41]. but in patients with biphasic dyskinesia it can be most distressing at the beginning or end of dose [3,42]. The prevalence of dystonia correlates with the duration of dopaminergic treatment, but younger patients may occasionally experience it as their first motor symptom [41,43,44].

Neurobiology of pain

Pain may be categorized etiologically as nociceptive/inflammatory or neuropathic (also called neurogenic). Nociceptive pain is triggered by tissue injury; examples include arthritis and visceral pain. On the other hand, neuropathic pain is caused by damage to or dysfunction of the (central or peripheral) nervous system [45]. Causes of central neuropathic pain include stroke, multiple sclerosis, and PD [46]. Patients with neuropathic pain may report combinations of spontaneous (i.e., stimulus-independent) pain and abnormal evoked pain (termed "allodynia" when triggered by normally innocuous stimuli, and "hyperalgesia" when it is an exaggerated response to a stimulus that would normally cause pain) [47]. The basic categorization into nociceptive versus neuropathic pain – although not always straightforward [48,49] – may have clinical significance; for example, neuropathic pain may not respond as well as nociceptive pain to nonsteroidal anti-inflammatory agents or opioids, but can be more effectively treated by drugs that modulate nervous system function [47,50,51].

Ascending pathways

Nociceptive information is carried from peripheral pain receptors by small-diameter Aδ and C fibers. Upon entering the gray matter of the spinal cord, these axons synapse mainly in layers I (marginal zone) and V of the dorsal horn. Second-order sensory neurons then cross over in the spinal cord anterior commissure to ascend in the spinothalamic tract (Figure 29.1). The main relay for the

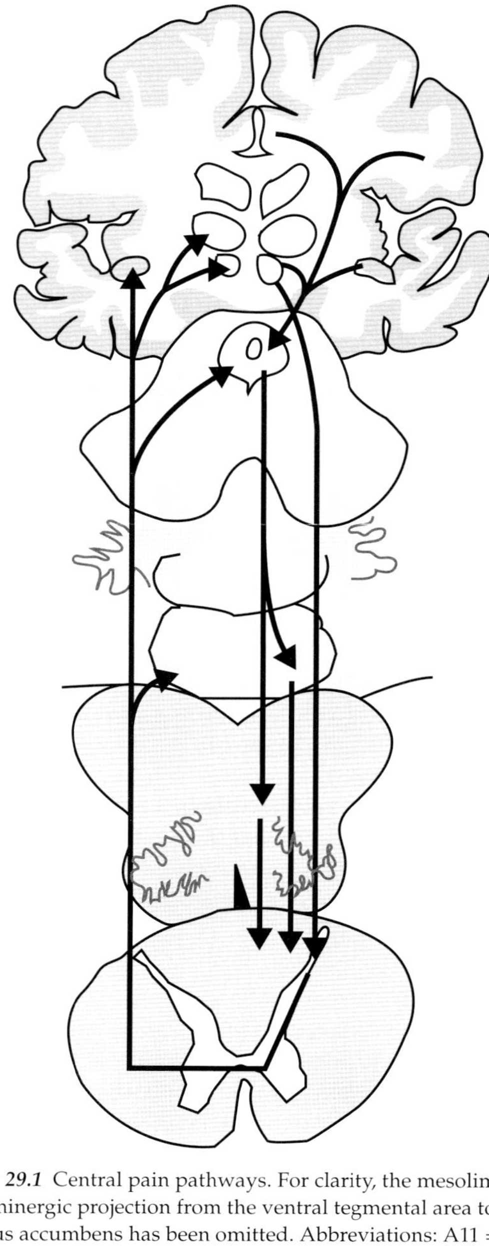

Figure 29.1 Central pain pathways. For clarity, the mesolimbic dopaminergic projection from the ventral tegmental area to the nucleus accumbens has been omitted. Abbreviations: A11 = A11 cell group in the dorsal hypothalamus/caudal thalamus; ACC = anterior cingulate cortex; DH = dorsal horn of spinal cord; LC = locus coeruleus; PAG = midbrain periaqueductal gray; PbN = parabrachial nucleus; RVM = rostral ventral medulla; SM = spinomesencephalic; SR = spinoreticular; ST = spinothalamic.

spinothalamic tract is the ventral posterior lateral nucleus (VPL) of the thalamus, which in turn relays somatosensory inputs to the cerebral cortex. In addition, the spinothalamic tract projects to intralaminar thalamic and medial thalamic nuclei; these projections, together with the spinoreticular tract (projecting to the parabrachial nucleus and locus coeruleus) are probably responsible for mediating the emotional and arousal aspects of pain [52–54]. The spinomesencephalic tract projects to the midbrain periaqueductal gray (PAG). Together, these ascending (spinothalamic, spinoreticular, and spinomesencephalic) pathways make up the anterolateral system.

Central modulation of pain

Brainstem-descending pain-inhibitory pathways include the PAG, which inhibits pain transmission in the dorsal horn via a relay called the rostral ventral medulla (RVM) or nucleus raphe magnus (part of the raphe nuclei of serotonergic neurons), and the A5 and locus coeruleus cell groups in the pontine tegmentum (which send noradrenergic projections to the dorsal horn) [50,55]. Higher order cerebral structures receive and integrate nociceptive information to regulate behavior and are also potential sources of (direct and indirect) influence on nociceptive processing in the dorsal horn [52,55]. There may be inputs, for example, to the PAG from pain-related cortical areas such as the somatosensory areas, the insular cortex, and anterior cingulate cortex (ACC) [52,55]. Other subcortical sites that may play a role in pain modulation include the nucleus accumbens (NAcc) (and other nuclei of the basal ganglia) [26,56,57–59], thalamus [56], hypothalamus (e.g., diencephalospinal dopaminergic pathway, projecting – uncrossed – from the dopaminergic A11 cell group in the dorsal hypothalamus/caudal thalamus to the dorsal horn at all spinal levels) [42,60–63], amygdala [55–57,64], and cerebellum [65]. For example, mesolimbic dopaminergic neurons projecting from the ventral tegmental area (VTA) to the NAcc form part of a potent pain-suppression system; enhanced dopamine release from terminals in the NAcc triggered by stress or noxious stimuli has been shown in animal studies to result in suppression of tonic pain of similar magnitude to high-dose morphine [66,67].

Dimensions of pain experience

Pain experience results from a complex integration of sensory-discriminative (e.g., perception of location and intensity of pain), affective–motivational (e.g., feelings of unpleasantness, with motivational properties of escape), cognitive–evaluative (e.g., learning to avoid similar stimuli in the future), and autonomic–neuroendocrine (e.g., induction of flight or fight responses) processes [53,68]. These different dimensions of the pain experience are mediated by different areas of the brain [52,69,70]. For example, activation of the lateral thalamus and S1/S2 somatosensory cortex seems to be preferentially associated with the sensory-discriminative aspect of pain. The intralaminar thalamic and medial thalamic nuclei, ACC, and anterior insular cortex (components of the limbic system) are more involved in the affective–emotional aspect of pain [52,69,70]. Systems mediating affective aspects of painful experiences overlap with limbic systems functionally mapped to a range of affective disturbances. Human brain imaging investigations of anxiety, fear, dysphoria, depression, and pain, and studies involving exposure to pleasant or unpleasant images, music, touch, or taste, have all implicated the subcallosal anterior cingulate region (BA 25) [71–78]. Medial temporal and prefrontal areas may be related to more cognitive aspects of pain, and structures such as the insular cortex, amygdala, hypothalamus, and brainstem nuclei are involved in the autonomic response to painful stimulation [52,53,55, 79–81]. There is a growing literature on the extensive interactions between the nociceptive and autonomic nervous systems at all levels of neuraxis, which has been reviewed elsewhere [81–83].

Mechanisms of PD-related pain

The etiologic basis of PD-related pain is multifactorial, with varying degrees of contribution from peripheral (motor/mechanical) and central sources (Figure 29.2). Central mechanisms include derangement of intrinsic pain-modulating (i.e., anti-nociceptive) monoaminergic systems [50], in addition to plastic central nervous system (CNS) changes induced by chronic anti-parkinsonian medication treatment [20,84].

CNS pathology of PD

Although the pathology of PD is defined by neuronal loss in the substantia nigra, there has been increasing

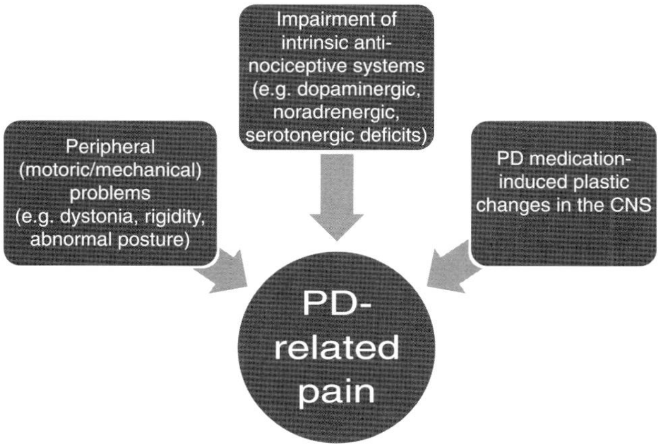

Figure 29.2 The etiological basis of PD-related pain is multifactorial, with varying degrees of contribution from peripheral and central mechanisms.

Table 29.3 Pain-processing structures involved in PD. PAG = midbrain periaqueductal gray.

Structures	Braak stage
Spinal cord lamina I	3, possibly earlier [83]
Lower brainstem (e.g., locus coeruleus, raphe nuclei)	2 [88]
Upper brainstem (e.g., PAG, parabrachial nucleus, pedunculopontine nucleus)	3–4 [88,225–228]
Hypothalamus	3 [88]
Thalamus (especially medial thalamic and intralaminar nuclei)	4 [86–88]
Limbic structures (e.g., amygdala, insula, anterior cingulate gyrus)	3–4 [88]

recognition of the pathologic changes that also occur in a range of extra-nigral sites in both the central and peripheral nervous systems [85], including many of the structures discussed above that are important in pain processing (Table 29.3). Lesions or dysfunction of systems that under normal conditions transmit noxious information from the dorsal horn of the spinal cord to the cerebral cortex can lead to central pain [46]. It has been suggested that the incidence of central pain is highest with lesions in the dorsal horn, followed by lower brainstem and thalamic lesions, regions that are *consistently* involved in PD [83,86–88]. However, clinico-anatomic studies are lacking and the precise anatomico-pathologic substrates for central parkinsonian pain remain speculative. Conduction along peripheral and central pain pathways, as tested by laser stimuli (selectively activating pain receptors in the skin, and recording laser-evoked potentials over the scalp), is normal in PD patients with primary central pain [37]. A peripheral neuropathic component is unlikely, given the absence of pathologic findings in peripheral somatosensory nerves [24]. Although there are case reports of peripheral neuropathy in juvenile PD (e.g., due to *Parkin* disease), this entity is clinically distinct from sporadic/idiopathic PD [89,90].

Pain due to central dopaminergic deficiency

Treatment of PD patients with dopaminergic agents may be dramatically effective in alleviating pain. Furthermore, experiments using evoked pain have found reduced pain threshold and tolerance (i.e., allodynia and hyperalgesia) in PD patients compared with non-PD subjects [84,91,92]. One study also found a lack of habituation of sympathetic sudomotor responses to repeated pain stimuli in PD patients with primary central pain (suggesting an autonomic hyper-reactivity to pain inputs) [37]. These abnormalities are more prominent in patients reporting spontaneous pain [37,91,93], and on the side with worse parkinsonism [37,84,91]. The importance of dopaminergic deficit as a causal factor in PD-related pain is implied by the normalization of these abnormalities after L-dopa administration seen in most [37,84,92,94,95], although not all [91,96], studies. Moreover, a PET study demonstrated that overactivation of cortical areas involved in processing sensory-discriminative and affective–motivational dimensions of pain in the untreated state is reduced after L-dopa administration [92]. A role for dopamine in pain modulation is further supported by observations that far more patients with parkinsonism induced by neuroleptics (dopamine receptor blockers) report pain compared with patients receiving other psychotropic medications [97], and dopaminergic therapy has been used to treat a variety of painful conditions in non-PD patients, including chronic thalamic pain [98], burning mouth syndrome [99], restless legs syndrome [100], diabetic neuropathy [101], fibromyalgia [102], and metastatic cancer [103]. Some authors have found that the analgesic effect of L-dopa may be dose dependent [94,104]. The site of action of exogenously administered dopamine has been hypothesized to involve the mesolimbic system [84]. Other possible sites of dopamine-mediated inhibition of nociceptive activity include the thalamus [105–107] and diencephalospinal pathway [42,60–63].

Non-dopaminergic mechanisms

Nevertheless, there remains a *majority* of patients with PD in whom initiation or modification of dopaminergic therapy does not abolish pain. This includes *de novo* patients in whom dopaminergic therapy ameliorates parkinsonism (i.e., the motor disorder) [35], and even patients in whom motor and sensory symptoms *fluctuate* in response to L-dopa (i.e., these patients do not obtain pain relief with additional administration of L-dopa) [50]. In an experimental setting (after overnight withdrawal of PD medications), we found reduced pain intensity and unpleasantness in 42% of 50 patients following the administration of a dose of L-dopa [in 17% of the stable responders, 53% of the fluctuators (without dyskinesia), and 48% of the dyskinetic patients; differences between groups did not reach statistical significance] [84]. In a series by Djaldetti *et al.*, spontaneous pain responded to L-dopa challenge in only 20% (3/15) of fluctuating patients [91]. In other studies, only 28% of (surveyed) patients reported that PD medication relieved their pain [8,27] (wearing-off and dyskinesia present in 53% and 25% of patients in the latter study). Lee *et al.* [19] reported that only 10% of pain complaints were improved by PD medication, and at the end of the spectrum, a study by Giuffrida *et al.* [18] found that pain present at the beginning of the disease resolved in only 3% of patients during the course of the disease. The observed lack of response to dopaminergic agents in many patients is perhaps not unexpected, considering the widespread involvement of *non*-dopaminergic structures in PD (Table 29.2).

Abnormalities of noradrenergic and serotonergic pathways descending to the spinal cord are assumed to have relevance for pain perception in PD [3,50], given that serotonin and noradrenaline are the major neurotransmitters in the inhibitory modulation of pain through descending pathways. Widespread loss of brain serotonergic innervation is a feature of PD [108], and reduced serotonin metabolite [5-hydroxyindoleacetic acid (5-HIAA)] in cerebrospinal fluid (CSF) (thought to indicate impaired central serotonin metabolism) has been demonstrated in non-depressed PD patients with pain, compared with those without pain and healthy volunteers [50,93] (CSF 5-HIAA is also reduced in depressed PD patients) [109]. In a placebo-controlled, double-blinded study, Cantello *et al.* reported on the potent analgesic effect of i.v. methylphenidate (which enhances adrenergic and serotonergic transmission) in PD patients with a fluctuating motor (in addition to pain) response to L-dopa, noting, however, that this effect was abolished by pretreating patients with a β-blocker or serotonin antagonist [50]. Dopaminergic and non-dopaminergic systems also interact; for example, it has been suggested that morphine and codeine may be synthesized in the body from L-dopa or dopamine [110], and lesioning the nigrostriatal dopaminergic system in rats prevents (the normal) tail pinch-induced increases in forebrain serotonin output [111].

Pain *directly* attributable to the motor features of PD (dystonia, rigidity, chorea, tremor, and postural abnormalities)

Dystonic pain is likely to be musculogenic in origin [112]. In support of this, Pacchetti *et al.* reported on the complete disappearance of painful foot dystonia in 70% of patients treated with botulinum toxin injections into the affected muscles (the mechanism of analgesia presumably relates to reduction of tonic muscle contraction) [113,114]. In other patients, pain appears to be secondary to *parkinsonian rigidity* in axial or limb muscles [6]. However, this explanation does not seem adequate in many patients with painful complaints, in whom rigidity is often relatively minor [24,50]. Three decades ago, Snider *et al.* found very similar rigidity scores for patients with and without sensory symptoms (1.37 ± 0.15 versus 1.31 ± 0.14, respectively, scored on a scale of 0 to 4 for increasing rigidity), and suggested that the motor deficit of PD accounts for only a small proportion of sensory symptoms [24]. The observation that pain usually occurs ipsilateral to the limb first and more affected by parkinsonism [12,20,22,24,38] does not necessarily, in our view, argue for a muscular origin. There are some data to suggest that *lateralization* of PD pathology may not be unique to the motor (nigrostriatal) system [115,116]. and it is theoretically possible that pain systems (e.g., mesolimbic pathway or serotonergic/noradrenergic pathways) [50] in PD may be more affected ipsilateral to the side with greater nigral pathology. Supporting this contention are cases in which pain precedes ipsilateral development of PD motor symptoms [12,24,38]. Conversely, there are patients with severe rigidity who do not have pain [112].

Somatic pain may be *exacerbated by repetitive movements* (dyskinesia or parkinsonian tremor), e.g., neck chorea triggering painful arthritis or cervical radiculopathy [3,6,112], or symptoms of median neuropathy secondary to severe tremor [6]. About 50% of patients with radicular/neuritic pain in the series by Goetz *et al.* related this type of pain to being "on," although it is not clear if this was due to dyskinetic movements. In this series, 85% of patients reported no consistent relationship between joint pain and motor fluctuations.

Postural abnormalities of PD (e.g., stooped posture) may sometimes contribute to pain [6]. In one study, 77% of patients with camptocormia (i.e., extreme spinal flexion deformity) reported mild-to-moderate low back pain [117]. This could result from paraspinal muscle hypertonia [117], or the postural abnormality may cause mechanical stress on soft tissues (and contribute to lumbar disc herniation) and bone structures [23]. The simple stooped posture of PD (i.e., not extreme camptocormia) may be enough to exaggerate low back pain in many patients.

Pain due to anti-parkinsonian medication-induced plastic changes

Patients initially treated with dopaminergic medications experience a stable response throughout the day. They do not perceive a change in their parkinsonian symptoms from one dose of medication to the next. However, the repeated pulsatile stimulation of striatal dopamine receptors inherent in the oral treatment of PD induces plastic changes in basal ganglia circuits that can lead to the development of pharmacologic sensitization and tolerance [118,119]. Augmentation of motor (and also some non-motor) responses and the emergence of dyskinesia are generally considered to be sensitization phenomena [119–122]; in contrast, shortening of the duration of medication effect with repeated dopaminergic drug dosing is considered to result from the development of drug tolerance [119]. Because the human striatum also has a central role in processing nociceptive information [26], we tested the hypothesis that plastic changes may also occur in pain responses in patients with dyskinesia and found that after a standard L-dopa challenge, dyskinetic patients experienced large increases in cold pain threshold (48%) and tolerance (66%) that were absent in stable responders (Figure 29.3) [84]. Consistent with this notion, parkinsonian monkeys with dyskinesia display pathologic metabolic activity in limbic and associative-related structures, and not simply in motor parts of the basal ganglia [123]. In addition to its role in pain modulation, the mesolimbic dopamine system mediates various aspects of reward and motivation [124]. Neuroplastic

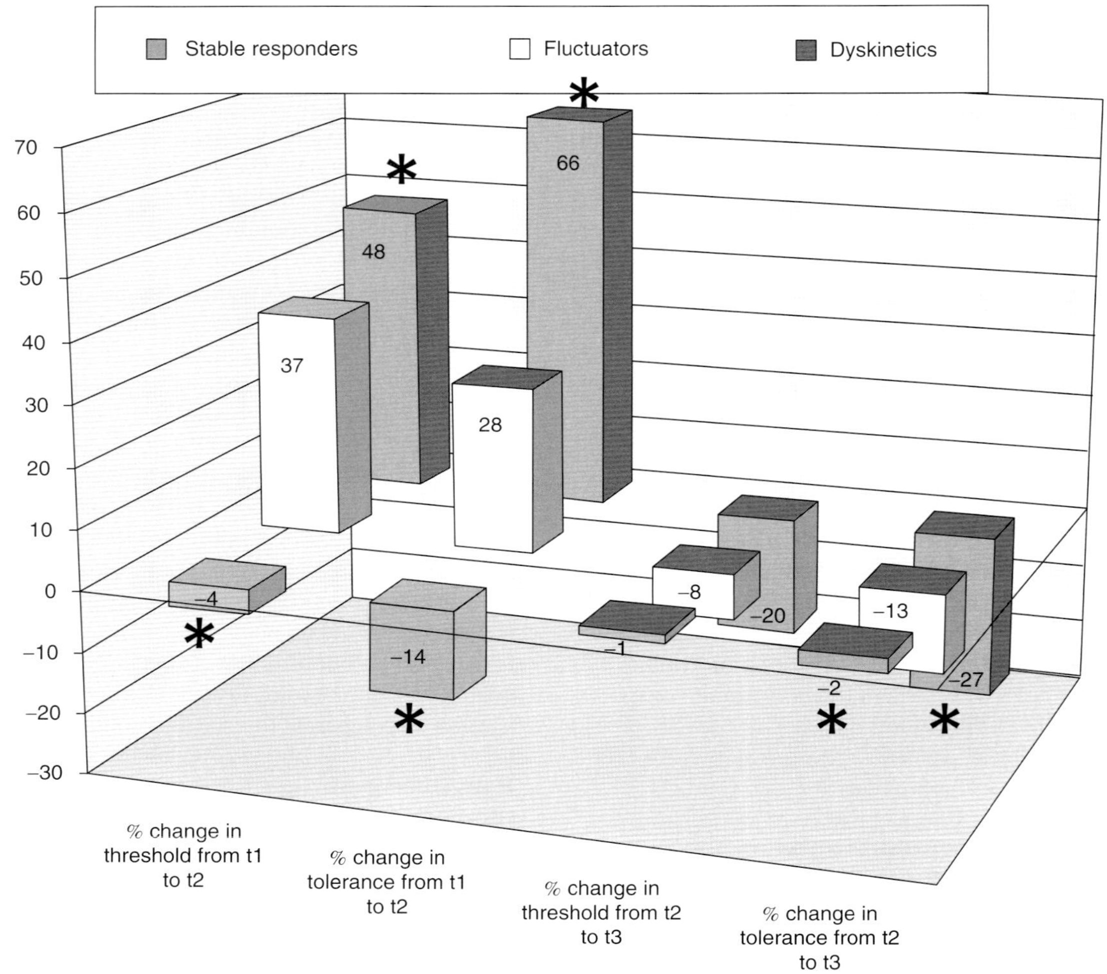

Figure 29.3 Mean percentage change in threshold and tolerance from t1 to t2, and from t2 to t3 in the stable responder, fluctuator, and dyskinetic groups. For clarity, error bars have been omitted, but are given as follows (mean ± standard error, from left to right, starting from the front row: −4 ± 11, −14 ± 5, −1 ± 10, −2 ± 5, 37 ± 19, 28 ± 18, −8 ± 11, −13 ± 8, 48 ± 12, 66 ± 20, −20 ± 7, −27 ± 6). Asterisks (*) indicate significant differences between the dyskinetic and stable responder groups according to repeated-measures ANOVA and *post hoc t*-tests. t1, 12 h off dopaminergic medication; t2, full "on" state at least 60 min after L-dopa; t3, 6 h post-L-dopa.

changes within this system were recently demonstrated in a group of PD patients compulsively overusing dopaminergic drugs and exhibiting disabling dyskinesia [125]. Taken together, we postulated that the increased pain threshold and tolerance observed in dyskinetic patients when "on" may reflect a process of sensitization to the analgesic and motivational effects of L-dopa [84].

It is intriguing to consider the possibility that *intermittent* administration of dopaminergic drugs that have analgesic effects may lead to a hyperalgesic state and predispose PD patients with dyskinesia to chronic pain in the same way that administration of opioids can sometimes paradoxically aggravate pain (the phenomenon of opioid-induced hyperalgesia) [126–128]. The motivational effects of drug withdrawal are central to negative reinforcement models of addiction in which the motivation to compulsively use drugs of addiction is driven by a desire to avoid the aversive affective state associated with withdrawal [129–131]. According to this theory, the acutely rewarding properties of psychostimulant drugs inevitably generate a withdrawal syndrome as the body seeks to restore its "hedonic equilibrium." Activation of corticotropin releasing factor (CRF)-containing neurons in the amygdala may mediate the negative emotional symptoms and also many of the somatic symptoms that occur upon drug withdrawal [132]. Given that the dopaminergic drugs used to treat PD share some of the psychomotor-activating properties of stimulant drugs such as amphetamines and cocaine [133,134], it is possible to speculate that recruitment of brain anti-reward systems, as an opponent process to excessive reward system activation by dopaminergic drugs, may be responsible for many of the symptoms seen in PD patients as dopaminergic medication effect wears off. Resolution of intractable "off" period pain during dopaminergic "drug holidays" (see below) is consistent with this theory [3,41,42,135,136]. Further, distressing chronic pain alone has been reported to powerfully motivate the compulsive self-administration of dopaminergic drugs in a PD patient [137].

Genetic factors

Recent animal and human studies suggest that genetic factors are linked to individual differences in pain experience. For example, polymorphisms in the gene for catechol-*O*-methyltransferase (COMT), an enzyme that delays the breakdown of dopamine, influence sensitivity to experimental pain, the risk of developing temporomandibular joint disorder (a common chronic pain condition), and also the clinical efficacy of opioid treatment [56,138,139]. In another study, a "pain-protective" haplotype of the gene for GTP cyclohydrolase (*GCH1*), the rate-limiting enzyme for tetrahydrobiopterin (BH4) synthesis (an essential cofactor for catecholamine, serotonin, and nitric oxide production), was associated with less pain following discectomy for persistent radicular low back pain, and reduced experimental pain sensitivity [140]. Genetic factors have not been studied in relation to PD-related pain.

Diagnosis and management

Proper recognition

Some reports have highlighted the problem of delayed diagnosis of PD (and sometimes inappropriate or invasive investigations and treatments) when patients present first with pain. Greater awareness of this possibility among physicians (general practitioners, geriatricians, neurologists, orthopedists, and rheumatologists) should facilitate earlier diagnosis and appropriate management [7,141,142]. In particular, patients presenting with frozen shoulder with no obvious precipitating factors should be assessed for signs of early parkinsonism, such as bradykinesia [22].

In evaluating pain complaints where PD has already been diagnosed, one of the physician's first tasks is to determine whether the pain syndrome represents a condition requiring further investigations or specific treatment (e.g., myelopathy, focal neuropathy). In some cases, it may be appropriate to seek specialty consultation (rheumatologic, orthopedic, vascular, etc.) [4]. One of the difficulties in diagnosing PD-related pain is the lack of specific clinical features or diagnostic tests; the diagnosis often is inferred by excluding other causes. No universally accepted clinical diagnostic criteria for neuropathic pain exist [48,49] and, unlike most causes of neuropathic pain which typically exhibit both *negative* [46] and positive sensory phenomena in the same area innervated by damaged nervous system pathways [143], the bedside sensory examination in patients with central parkinsonian pain typically does *not* reveal sensory deficits [2,3,12,24,35,50,61,91]. In one series, most cases of pain considered to be "directly related" to PD were reported as "vague painful sensations" that did not correspond to well-defined syndromes [2]. Just as in patients exhibiting a complicated motor response to L-dopa, an L-dopa challenge test can sometimes help to clarify the relationship of the sensory complaint to the patient's medication cycle (e.g., documenting that pain occurs mainly as an end-of-dose or "off" phenomenon).

Even with proper recognition, management of PD-related pain is often challenging. This is similar to the situation with chronic neuropathic pain in general, where the response to treatments is often inadequate [144] – this may reflect the existence of different neuronal pain mechanisms in an individual patient [145]. Nevertheless, the management goal should be to provide relief and comfort so that patients experience the best possible quality-of-life in spite of the disease. The treatment of pain is important not only for relief of discomfort, but also because pain may further exacerbate the reduced mobility of PD patients [7,8] and other co-morbidities such as depression and anxiety. Studies indicate that pain is undertreated in PD patients [2,19,23,146], and this may be particularly true for PD-related pain [2]. One author found that one-fifth of PD patients reporting moderate to severe constant pain or pain dominating their day were on no analgesics. Many patients with PD are elderly and many are cognitively impaired; in non-PD populations, these factors are associated with insufficient treatment of pain [36,147], possibly due to perceived risks of pharmacotherapy [17]. Nevertheless, one study of non-demented subjects showed lower analgesic consumption among patients with PD-related pain compared with non-PD subjects, despite greater pain intensity and impact on quality-of-life [2].

Patient education and support

Physicians should bear in mind that psychosocial factors are a major component of the experience of chronic pain [143]. Patient education and support are critical components of successful management, including careful explanation of the cause of pain and the treatment plan. Studies in patients with PD or pain have shown that expectation of treatment outcome is important to the production of optimum therapeutic effects (attributable, at least in part, to a "placebo" effect); this in turn is strongly influenced by the doctor–patient interaction [148]. Notably, one large study found that many PD patients experiencing pain perceived that their general practitioners did not understand what it is like to live with the disease [25].

Treatment of co-morbidities

Particular attention should be paid to identifying coexisting co-morbidities such as depression, anxiety, and sleep disturbances, which may act synergistically to increase disability [2,143,149]. One study showed that depression accounted for *most* of the variance in pain severity [31]. Anti-depressant medication may be indicated and selective serotonin reuptake inhibitors (SSRIs), which have a favorable side effect profile, are typically first choice in PD patients [150] and may also alleviate anxiety [151]. Tricyclic anti-depressants may be useful for treating depression in patients with chronic pain [6] and may also improve disturbed sleep [143]. Low-dose quetiapine can be helpful for insomnia [152].

Patients exhibiting prominent dysphoric "off" symptoms (including pain, depression, anxiety, panic attacks, chest pressure, palpitations, tachypnea, and profuse sweating), apparently disproportionate to the degree of "off" state motor dysfunction, should be carefully screened for the dopamine dysregulation syndrome (DDS). The treatment of DDS has been reviewed elsewhere [133,153]. In general, rescue L-dopa or injections of apomorphine should be avoided in patients thought to be susceptible to addiction.

Non-pharmacologic approaches to treat pain

Many patients manage pain by physical means, for example, massage, stretching, exercise, heat, or cold packs [19]. In cases where pain appears to be related to postural or other biomechanical abnormalities, rehabilitation may have a role [154]; for example, physical therapy may ameliorate back pain and increase autonomy in these patients. In one study of PD patients with camptocormia, wearing a corset was effective in reducing back pain and was well tolerated [117]. The use of complementary medicine therapies is common in patients with PD [155], but their role in symptom management remains unproven. Acupuncture may have a role in the treatment of some pain syndromes [156], but the evidence for this in PD is limited at present [157,158].

Pharmacologic approaches to treating pain – effective management of PD

Pain may be dramatically improved by effective treatment of parkinsonian motor symptoms [3]. Many patients report an improvement in pain when anti-parkinsonian therapy is initiated [3,8,22], a classic example being frozen shoulder [22]. Pain that fluctuates in parallel with motor fluctuations can be managed by modifying anti-parkinsonian therapy [3,20]. In cases where pain is associated with the "off" medication state, maximizing "on" time may help [20,159]. Strategies include an increase in the dose or frequency of L-dopa or addition of controlled-release L-dopa, a COMT inhibitor, or a longer-acting agent such as a dopamine agonist or MAO-B inhibitor. Apomorphine rescue injections may be dramatically effective in aborting severe "off" period pain within a few minutes [136,160]. Although, to our knowledge, the effect on pain of continuous subcutaneous apomorphine infusion or enteral (intraduodenal) infusion of L-dopa has not been specifically studied, these treatments typically result in substantial improvements in motor response fluctuations and dyskinesia [161,162]. Camptocormia is usually not greatly modified by PD medications [117], although some authors have reported on axial dystonia (occurring as an end-of-dose or "off" phenomenon) responding to increased L-dopa dose [163,164]. Pain aggravated by choreiform dyskinesia (which typically occurs as a peak-dose phenomenon) may be ameliorated by using anti-dyskinesia treatments (reduction of L-dopa, or use of amantadine, infusional therapies, or functional neurosurgery) [3]. Nevertheless, there remains a *majority* of patients in whom initiation or modification of dopaminergic therapy does not alleviate pain.

Transient L-dopa withdrawal ("drug holiday") has been reported to result in resolution of severe fluctuating dystonic [41,42,135] and non-dystonic [3,136] pain. For example, Quinn *et al.* described a patient who had severe "off" period abdominal and bilateral non-dystonic leg pain who was much happier remaining off L-dopa permanently (and being severely immobile as a result), but pain free [3]. However, this practice has been mostly relegated to the past because of the potential for precipitating serious events such as a neuroleptic-like malignant syndrome [165], and also limited efficacy – pain (like severe motor fluctuations) may reappear within a few days of treatment reinitiation [3].

Analgesic agents

There are very few clinical trial data concerning analgesic medication choice for PD-related pain that does not respond to optimization of anti-parkinsonian treatment. Guidance is available mainly from studies of *other* causes of neuropathic pain, although it is possible that different types of neuropathic pain respond differently to treatments [144]. Individual variation in response to medications used to treat neuropathic pain is substantial and unpredictable [144], and combination treatment is often required because of the limited efficacy of single agents [51]. Readers are referred to papers by Dworkin and colleagues for further details about management of neuropathic pain in general [143,144]. The treatment of somatic or nociceptive pain should proceed along the usual lines and has also been reviewed elsewhere [166]. The highly favorable risk/benefit ratio of acetaminophen (paracetamol) justifies a role for this agent as a near-routine background analgesic, notwithstanding the type of pain involved [166].

First-line agents for neuropathic pain

To our knowledge, there have been only two published clinical trials of treatment for PD-related pain (using duloxetine and clozapine) [167,168]. In an open-label study of duloxetine [a serotonin–norepinephrine reuptake inhibitor (SNRI)], *non*-depressed PD patients with pain of suspected central origin that did not respond to optimization of anti-parkinsonian treatment responded to this agent at doses of 30–60 mg daily [167]. However, the well-known strong placebo effect in PD patients means that controlled studies are required [169]. Venlafaxine is also efficacious for neuropathic pain in non-PD patient populations [166]. In addition to SNRIs, other recommended first-line treatments for neuropathic pain include tricyclic anti-depressants (TCAs) [29] and calcium channel $\alpha 2$-δ ligands (gabapentin or pregabalin). Gabapentin and pregabalin have good tolerability and may improve sleep [144] and restless legs symptoms [170–172]. Moreover, gabapentin has been reported to improve parkinsonism [173–175], although there is a case report of this agent inducing dyskinesia in PD [176].

Second-line agents (144)

Opioids also have demonstrated efficacy in neuropathic pain [143], and there are case reports of efficacy in PD-related pain [10]. However, meperidine (pethidine) can induce parkinsonism in neurologically normal subjects [177,178]. Morphine is probably less likely than meperidine to worsen parkinsonism in PD patients [40]. There is a potential for precipitating confusion or hallucinations [11], and constipation, a very common symptom in PD [179], usually requires concurrent management. Tramadol, an SNRI with a major metabolite that is a μ-opioid agonist [143]. was reported in one PD patient to improve dramatically chronic diffuse burning pain and major depression that fluctuated in relation to L-dopa dosing [137]. The risk of addiction to these agents is thought to be low in neuropathic pain patients without a history of substance abuse, and we are not aware of any reports of opioid addiction in PD patients. However, "poly-substance" abuse in the context of dopamine agonist treatment and behavioral addictions has been reported rarely [180]. Besides treatment with direct-acting dopamine agonists, red flags that may aid in identifying patients at higher risk for addictions include male gender, a personal or family history of substance dependence or impulse control disorders, younger age at PD onset, and early emergence of dyskinesia [181,182].

Third-line medications

These include other anti-epileptic agents. Again, the side effect profile should be considered in treatment selection, such as the potential for valproate to induce parkinsonism and cognitive impairment [183,184]. There is some evidence to support the use of cannabinoids for neuropathic pain secondary to multiple sclerosis [185]. One concern is the potential for these agents to precipitate psychosis [186], a common problem in the more advanced stages of PD. In a small, open-label study, clozapine improved severe "cramp-like" parkinsonian pain unresponsive to manipulations of anti-parkinsonian therapy by $\geq$60% [168]. Clozapine has also been reported to alleviate oral and genital pain in PD [29]. A major disadvantage of using this agent is the requirement for long-term blood monitoring.

Pain clinic management

For patients who have not responded adequately to pharmacologic management or those who have pain that is associated with a high level of disability or distress, consultation with a pain specialist or referral to a multidisciplinary pain management center may be helpful.

Treatments for dystonia

Agents that have been used successfully to treat parkinsonian dystonia include amantadine [187], clonazepam [188], baclofen [43,189], anti-cholinergics [135], lithium [3], clozapine [168,190], and gabapentin [174]. Pacchetti *et al.* described complete the disappearance of painful foot dystonia in 70% of patients treated with botulinum toxin injections into the affected muscles [113]. In another series, seven of 10 PD patients with dystonic clenched fist experienced pain relief with this treatment [191]. Camptocormia caused by rectus abdominis contraction can also sometimes be ameliorated by botulinum toxin injections [117,192]. More invasive approaches to treat pain may be considered when simpler methods fail.

Electroconvulsive therapy (ECT)

Snider *et al.* reported on a PD patient with severe medication-resistant truncal burning and depression who improved dramatically with ECT; otherwise, reports are lacking in PD [24]. ECT is an accepted treatment for treatment-resistant PD depression and may also improve psychosis and parkinsonism [193–195]. There are case reports of successful treatment of a variety of chronic pain syndromes in non-PD patients using ECT [196–199]. Some authors found that ECT has analgesic properties independent of its effect on improving depression [197,198].

Rheumatologic/orthopedic procedures

In patients with true rheumatologic disorders, procedures such as steroid injections and joint surgery (e.g., knee or hip replacement for severe osteoarthritis) can relieve pain and/or improve function [200–202]. For example, one study reported that 93% (62/67) of patients had no or only slight pain after hip joint replacement after a follow-up of at least 2 years [201]. However, there may be higher rates of complications including immobilization-related lower limb dystonia/contracture [202,203] and infections (urinary tract infections, pneumonia) [201], and some studies have reported longer hospitalizations [204] and possibly higher mortality in operated PD patients [201]. Anti-parkinsonian medications should be resumed without delay postoperatively, and this will also facilitate physical therapy.

Functional neurosurgery

Deep brain stimulation (DBS) surgery has become an established treatment for advanced PD [205], with multiple studies providing compelling evidence for a long-term effect on motor symptoms [206–208]. The majority of studies suggest that subthalamic nucleus (STN) DBS is superior to globus pallidus internus (GPi) DBS in improving the cardinal motor features of PD [209], and bilateral STN DBS has become the procedure of choice at most centers. Severe fluctuations in motor response to L-dopa remain the primary indication for treating PD patients with DBS, but important changes in non-motor symptoms (including pain) are also seen postoperatively. In one study selecting PD patients with severe dystonia, STN DBS reduced "off" period dystonia and related pain by 90 and 66%, respectively, at 6 months post-surgery [210]. Loher *et al.* reported comparable improvements in "off" period dystonia and pain with GPi DBS [211]. The benefit of DBS on these symptoms appeared very early (immediately, or within several days). Loher *et al.* concluded that disabling "off" period dystonia alone may be considered a good indication for functional neurosurgery.

Witjas *et al.* reported striking improvements in a range of non-motor fluctuations at 1 year post-STN DBS. The greatest reductions were in pain and sensory fluctuations (improvement reported by 84% of patients) (note that the analysis excluded "off" period dystonic pain) [212]. Whether the improvement in non-motor fluctuations relates to a direct effect of stable (i.e., non-fluctuating) STN inhibition or to a process of striatal desensitization due to reduced L-dopa intake [121,213,214], or both, is currently not known. Nevertheless, complete elimination of medication post-STN DBS clearly is not necessary for marked alleviation of dyskinesia or motor and non-motor fluctuations [212–214].

Although in most surgical centers lesional surgery has largely been surpassed by DBS surgery (one major reason for this is the relatively high risk of adverse outcomes with bilateral lesions), in many parts of the world scarce medical resources will dictate the practice of lesional surgery as a viable alternative [215]. Unilateral pallidotomy can provide lasting motor benefit [216]. In a prospective study, Honey *et al.* found a significant reduction in pain scores 6 weeks after unilateral pallidotomy, with a beneficial (and bilateral) effect still seen at 1 year [112]. Improvement was seen in somatic pain (e.g., arthritis or tendonitis triggered by tremor or dyskinesia) and musculoskeletal pain. However, the beneficial effect on dystonic pain was sustained in only half of the patients at 1 year and dysesthesias did not improve (only two patients had this to begin with). In another study, de Bie *et al.* found that patients with pain resulting from parkinsonism often reported relief of pain contralateral to the pallidotomy, but the improvement of sensory complaints did not achieve statistical significance; in this study, postoperative assessment was performed a median of 5 months after surgery [217]. Baron *et al.* reported improvement in pain and discomfort in 10 of 12 patients at 6 months but not at 1 year post-surgery [218].

Chronic epidural motor cortex stimulation (MCS)

MCS was first introduced to relieve refractory pain; experience with a few hundred patients in open-label studies indicates that 50–60% of patients with medically refractory neuropathic pain may benefit from the procedure [219]. MCS has also been suggested as a possible new treatment method for movement disorders, including PD [220]; this approach would be simpler and safer than DBS of the basal ganglia. Some authors have reported impressive reduction of painful dystonia after MCS [221];) however, data regarding its efficacy in ameliorating parkinsonian motor symptoms are conflicting, with recent studies reporting no motor benefit [222,223].

Acknowledgments

Dr Shen-Yang Lim wishes to acknowledge the mentoring provided by senior colleagues in the pain field: Dr Michael J. Farrell, Associate Professor Stephen J. Gibson, and Professor Robert D. Helme.

References

1. Quittenbaum BH, Grahn B. Quality of life and pain in Parkinson's disease: a controlled cross-sectional study. *Parkinsonism Relat Disord* 2004;**10**:129–36.
2. Negre-Pages L, Regragui W, Bouhassira D, *et al.*; DoPaMiP Study Group. Chronic pain in Parkinson's disease: the cross-sectional French DoPaMiP survey. *Mov Disord* 2008;**23**:1361–9.
3. Quinn NP, Koller WC, Lang AE, Marsden CD. Painful Parkinson's disease. *Lancet* 1986;**i**:1366–9.
4. Ford B. Pain in Parkinson's disease. *Clin Neurosci* 1998;**5**:63–72.
5. Witjas T, Kaphan E, Azulay JP, *et al.* Nonmotor fluctuations in Parkinson's disease: frequent and disabling. *Neurology* 2002;**59**(3):408–13.
6. Goetz CG, Tanner CM, Levy M, *et al.* Pain in Parkinson's disease. *Mov Disord* 1986;**1**:45–9.
7. Sekeff-Sallem FA, Barbosa ER. Diagnostic pitfalls in Parkinson's disease: case report. *Arq Neuropsiquiatr* 2007;**65**:348–51.

8. da Silva EG, Viana MA, Quagliato EMAB. Pain in Parkinson's disease: analysis of 50 cases in a clinic of movement disorders. *Arq Neuropsiquiatr* 2008;**66**:26–9.
9. Goetz CG, Wilson RS, Tanner CM, Garron DC. Relationships among pain, depression, and sleep alterations in Parkinson's disease. *Adv Neurol* 1987;**45**:345–7.
10. Shang AB, King SA. Parkinson's disease, depression, and chronic pain. *Hosp Commun Psychiatry* 1991;**42**:1162–3.
11. Factor SA, Molho ES. Emergency department presentations of patients with Parkinson's disease. *Am J Emerg Med* 2000;**18**:209–15.
12. Koller WC. Sensory symptoms in Parkinson's disease. *Neurology* 1984;**34**:957–9.
13. Tison F, Wenning GK, Volonte MA, *et al.* Pain in multiple system atrophy. *J Neurol* 1996;**243**:153–6.
14. Schrag A, Geser F, Stampfer-Kountchev M, *et al.* Health-related quality of life in multiple system atrophy. *Mov Disord* 2006;**21**:809–15.
15. Elliott AM, Smith BH, Penny KI, *et al.* The epidemiology of chronic pain in the community. *Lancet* 1999;**354**:1248–52.
16. Etchepare F, Rozenberg S, Mirault T, *et al.* Back problems in Parkinson's disease: an underestimated problem. *Joint Bone Spine* 2006;**73**:298–302.
17. Gagliese L, Melzack R. Chronic pain in elderly people. *Pain* 1997;**70**:3–14.
18. Giuffrida R, Vingerhoets FJ, Bogousslavsky J, Ghika J. Syndromes douloureux de la maladie de Parkinson (Pain in Parkinson's disease). *Rev Neurol* 2005;**161**:407–18.
19. Lee MA, Walker RW, Hildreth TJ, Prentice WM. A survey of pain in idiopathic Parkinson's disease. *J Pain Symptom Manage* 2006;**32**:462–9.
20. Tinazzi M, Del Vesco C, Fincati E, *et al.* Pain and motor complications in Parkinson's disease. *J Neurol Neurosurg Psychiatry* 2006;**77**:822–5.
21. Karlsen KH, Larsen JP, Tandberg E, Maland JG. Quality of life measurements in patients with Parkinson's disease: a community-based study. *Eur J Neurol* 1998;**5**:443–50.
22. Riley D, Lang AE, Blair RDG, *et al.* Frozen shoulder and other shoulder disturbances in Parkinson's disease. *J Neurol Neurosurg Psychiatry* 1989;**52**:63–6.
23. Broetz D, Eichner M, Gasser T, *et al.* Radicular and nonradicular back pain in Parkinson's disease: a controlled study. *Mov Disord* 2007;**22**:853–6.
24. Snider SR, Fahn S, Isgreen WP, Cote LJ. Primary sensory symptoms in parkinsonism. *Neurology* 1976;**26**:423–9.
25. Mott S, Kenrick M, Dixon M, Bird G. Pain as a sequela of Parkinson disease. *Aust Fam Physician* 2004;**33**:663–4.
26. Chudler EH, Dong WK. The role of the basal ganglia in nociception and pain. *Pain* 1995;**60**:3–38.
27. Vela L, Facca A, Lyons K, Lieberman AN. Pain and Parkinson's disease. *Mov Disord* 2002;**17**(Suppl 5):154–5.
28. Clifford TJ, Warsi MJ, Burnett CA, Lamey PJ. Burning mouth in Parkinson's disease sufferers. *Gerodontology* 1998;**15**:73–8.
29. Ford B, Louis ED, Greene P, Fahn S. Oral and genital pain syndromes in Parkinson's disease. *Mov Disord* 1996;**11**:421–6.
30. Karlsen KH, Larsen JP, Tandberg E, Maland JG. Influence of clinical and demographic variables on quality of life in patients with Parkinson's disease. *J Neurol Neurosurg Psychiatry* 1999;**66**; 431–5.
31. Starkstein SE, Preziosi TJ, Robinson RG. Sleep disorders, pain, and depression in Parkinson's disease. *Eur Neurol* 1991;**31**:352–5.
32. Quinn N, Critchley P, Marsden CD. Young onset Parkinson's disease. *Mov Disord* 1987;**2**:73–91.
33. Kumar N, Van Gerpen JA, Bower JH, Ahlskog JE. Levodopa-dyskinesia incidence by age of Parkinson's disease onset. *Mov Disord* 2005;**20**:342–66.
34. Riley DE, Lang AE. The spectrum of levodopa-related fluctuations in Parkinson's disease. *Neurology* 1993;**43**:1459–64.
35. Schott GD. Pain in Parkinson's disease. *Pain* 1985;**22**:407–11.
36. Scherder E, Wolters E, Polman C, *et al.* Pain in Parkinson's disease and multiple sclerosis: its relation to the medial and lateral pain systems. *Neurosci Biobehav Rev* 2005;**29**:1047–56.
37. Schestatsky P, Kumru H, Valls-Solé J, *et al.* Neurophysiologic study of central pain in patients with Parkinson disease. *Neurology* 2007;**69**:2162–9.
38. Cleeves L, Findley L. Frozen shoulder and other shoulder disturbances in Parkinson's disease. *J Neurol Neurosurg Psychiatry* 1989;**52**:813–4.
39. Sage JI. Pain in Parkinson's disease. *Curr Treat Options Neurol* 2004;**6**:191–200.
40. Berg D, Becker G, Reiners K. Reduction of dyskinesia and induction of akinesia induced by morphine in two parkinsonian patients with severe sciatica. *J Neural Transm* 1999;**106**:725–8.
41. Ilson J, Fahn S, Cote L. Painful dystonic spasms in Parkinson's disease. *Adv Neurol*. 1984;**40**:395–8.
42. Sage JI, Kortis HI, Sommer W. Evidence for the role of spinal cord systems in Parkinson's disease-associated pain. *Clin Neuropharmacol* 1990;**13**:171–4.
43. Nausieda PA, Weiner WJ, Klawans HL. Dystonic foot response of Parkinsonism. *Arch Neurol* 1980;**37**:132–6.
44. Katzenschlager R, Costa D, Gacinovic S, Lees AJ. [^{123}I]-FP-CIT-SPECT in the early diagnosis of PD presenting as exercise-induced dystonia. *Neurology* 2002;**59**:1974–6.
45. Merskey H, Bogduk N, eds. *Classification of Chronic Pain: Descriptions of Chronic Pain Syndromes and Definitions of Pain Terms*. Prepared by the Task Force on Taxonomy of the International Association for the Study of PainASP. 2nd edn. Seattle: IASP Press, 1994.
46. Boivie J. Central pain and the role of quantitative sensory testing (QST) in research and diagnosis. *Eur J Pain* 2003;**7**:339–43.
47. Woolf CJ, Mannion RJ. Neuropathic pain: aetiology, symptoms, mechanisms, and management. *Lancet* 1999;**353**: 1959–64.
48. Attal N, Bouhassira D. Can pain be more or less neuropathic? *Pain* 2004;**110**:510–1.
49. Rasmussen PV, Sindrup SH, Jensen TS, Bach FW. Symptoms and signs in patients with suspected neuropathic pain. *Pain* 2004;**110**:461–9.
50. Cantello R, Aguggia M, Gilli M, *et al.* Analgesic action of methylphenidate on parkinsonian sensory symptoms. Mechanisms and pathophysiological implications. *Arch Neurol* 1988;**45**:973–6.
51. Pasternak GW, Inturrisi CE. Feeling pain? Who's your daddy... *Nat Med* 2006;**12**:1243–4.

52. Rainville P. Brain mechanisms of pain affect and pain modulation. *Curr Opin Neurobiol* 2002;**12**:195–204.
53. Scherder EJA, Sergeant JA, Swaab DF. Pain processing in dementia and its relation to neuropathology. *Lancet Neurol* 2003;**2**:677–86.
54. Willis WD Jr. The somatosensory system, with emphasis on structures important for pain. *Brain Res Rev* 2007;**55**:297–313.
55. Millan MJ. Descending control of pain. *Prog Neurobiol* 2002;**66**:355–474.
56. Zubieta JK, Smith YR, Bueller JA, *et al.* Regional mu opioid receptor regulation of sensory and affective dimensions of pain. *Science* 2001;**293**:311–5.
57. Becerra L, Breiter HC, Wise R, *et al.* Reward circuitry activation by noxious thermal stimuli. *Neuron* 2001;**32**:927–46.
58. Hagelberg N, Jaaskelainen SK, Martikainen IK, *et al.* Striatal dopamine D2 receptors in modulation of pain in humans: a review. *Eur J Pharmacol* 2004;**500**:187–92.
59. Cole LJ, Farrell MJ, Gibson SJ, Egan GF. Age-related differences in pain sensitivity and regional brain activity evoked by noxious pressure. *Neurobiol Aging* 2010;**31**:494–503.
60. Lindvall O, Bjorklund A, Skagerberg G. Dopamine-containing neurons in the spinal cord: anatomy and some functional aspects. *Ann Neurol* 1983;**14**:255–60.
61. Nutt JG, Carter JH. Sensory symptoms in parkinsonism related to central dopaminergic function. *Lancet* 1984;**ii**: 456–7.
62. Fleetwood-Walker SM, Hope PJ, Mitchell R. Antinociceptive actions of descending dopaminergic tracts on cat and rat dorsal horn somatosensory neurones. *J Physiol* 1988;**399**:335–48.
63. Clemens S, Rye D, Hochman S. Restless legs syndrome: revisiting the dopamine hypothesis from the spinal cord perspective. *Neurology* 2006;**67**:125–30.
64. Manning BH, Merin NM, Meng ID, Amaral DG. Reduction in opioid- and cannabinoid-induced antinociception in Rhesus monkeys after bilateral lesions of the amygdaloid complex. *J Neurosci* 2001;**21**:8238–46.
65. Helmchen C, Mohr C, Erdmann C, *et al.* Differential cerebellar activation related to perceived pain intensity during noxious thermal stimulation in humans: a functional magnetic resonance imaging study. *Neurosci Lett* 2003;**335**:202–6.
66. Altier N, Stewart J. The role of dopamine in the nucleus accumbens in analgesia. *Life Sci* 1999;**65**:2269–87.
67. Gear RW, Aley KO, Levine JD. Pain-induced analgesia mediated by mesolimbic reward circuits. *J Neurosci* 1999;**19**: 7175–81.
68. Melzack R, Casey KL. Sensory, motivational and central control determinants of pain: a new conceptual model. In: Kenshalo DR, ed. *The Skin Senses*. Springfield, IL: CC Thomas, 1968:423–39.
69. Price DD. Psychological and neural mechanisms of the affective dimension of pain. *Science* 2000;**288**:1769–1772.
70. Moisset X, Bouhassira D. Brain imaging of neuropathic pain. *NeuroImage* 2007;**37**:S80-S88.
71. George MS, Ketter TA, Parekh PI, Horwitz B, *et al.* Brain activity during transient sadness and happiness in healthy women. *Am J Psychiatry* 1995;**152**:341–51.
72. Rauch SL, Savage CR, Alpert NM, *et al.* A positron emission tomographic study of simple phobic symptom provocation. *Arch Gen Psychiatry* 1995;**52**:20–8.
73. Vogt BA, Derbyshire S, Jones AK. Pain processing in four regions of human cingulate cortex localized with co-registered PET and MR imaging. *Eur J Neurosci* 1996;**8**:1461–73.
74. Drevets WC, Price JL, Simpson JR Jr, *et al.* Subgenual prefrontal cortex abnormalities in mood disorders. *Nature* 1997;**386**:824–7.
75. Lane RD, Reiman EM, Bradley MM, *et al.* Neuroanatomical correlates of pleasant and unpleasant emotion. *Neuropsychologia* 1997;**35**:1437–44.
76. Mayberg HS, Brannan SK, Mahurin RK, *et al.* Cingulate function in depression: a potential predictor of treatment response. *NeuroReport* 1997;**8**:1057–61.
77. Blood AJ, Zatorre RJ, Bermudez P, Evans AC. Emotional responses to pleasant and unpleasant music correlate with activity in paralimbic brain regions. *Nat Neurosci* 1999;**2**:382–7.
78. Francis S, Rolls ET, Bowtell R, *et al.* The representation of pleasant touch in the brain and its relationship with taste and olfactory areas. *NeuroReport* 1999;**10**:453–9.
79. Bornhövd K, Quante M, Glauche V, *et al.* Painful stimuli evoke different stimulus–response functions in the amygdala, prefrontal, insula and somatosensory cortex: a single-trial fMRI study. *Brain* 2002;**125**:1326–36.
80. Petrovic P, Petersson KM, Hansson P, Ingvara M. Brainstem involvement in the initial response to pain. *NeuroImage* 2004;**22**:995–1005.
81. Benarroch EE. Pain–autonomic interactions. *Neurol Sci* 2006;**27**:S130–3.
82. Baron R, Levine JD, Fields HL. Causalgia and reflex sympathetic dystrophy: does the sympathetic nervous system contribute to the generation of pain? *Muscle Nerve* 1999;**22**:678–95.
83. Braak H, Sastre M, Bohl JRE, *et al.* Parkinson's disease: lesions in dorsal horn layer I, involvement of parasympathetic and sympathetic pre- and postganglionic neurons. *Acta Neuropathol* 2007;**113**:421–9.
84. Lim SY, Farrell MJ, Gibson SJ, *et al.* Do dyskinesia and pain share common pathophysiological mechanisms in Parkinson disease? *Mov Disord* 2008;**23**:1689–95.
85. Lim SY, Fox SH, Lang AE. Overview of the extranigral aspects of Parkinson's disease. *Arch Neurol* 2009;**66**:167–72.
86. Henderson JM, Carpenter K, Cartwright H, Halliday GM. Loss of thalamic intralaminar nuclei in progressive supranuclear palsy and Parkinson's disease: clinical and therapeutic implications. *Brain* 2000;**123**:1410–21.
87. Rub U, Del Tredici K, Schultz C, *et al.* Parkinson's disease: the thalamic components of the limbic loop are severely impaired by α-synuclein immunopositive inclusion body pathology. *Neurobiol Aging* 2002;**23**:245–54.
88. Braak H, Del Tredici K, Rüb U, *et al.* Staging of brain pathology related to sporadic Parkinson's disease. *Neurobiol Aging* 2003;**24**:197–211.
89. Taly AB, Muthane UB. Involvement of peripheral nervous system in juvenile Parkinson's disease. *Acta Neurol Scand* 1992;**85**:272–5.
90. Okuma Y, Hattori N, Mizuno Y. Sensory neuropathy in autosomal recessive juvenile parkinsonism (PARK2). *Parkinsonism Relat Disord* 2003;**9**:313–4.
91. Djaldetti R, Shifrin A, Rogowski Z, *et al.* Quantitative measurement of pain sensation in patients with Parkinson disease. *Neurology* 2004;**62**:2171–5.

92. Brefel-Courbon C, Payoux P, Thalamas C, *et al.* Effect of levodopa on pain threshold in Parkinson's disease: a clinical and positron emission tomography study. *Mov Disord* 2005; **20**:1557–63.
93. Urakami K, Takahashi K, Matsushima E, *et al.* The threshold of pain and neurotransmitter's change on pain in Parkinson's disease. *Jpn J Psychiatry Neurol* 1990;**44**:589–93.
94. Battista AF, Wolff BB. Levodopa and induced-pain response: a study of patients with parkinsonian and pain syndromes. *Arch Intern Med* 1973;**132**:70–4.
95. Slaoui T, Gerdelat-Mas A, Ory-Magne F, *et al.* Levodopa changes pain thresholds in Parkinson disease (PD) patients. *Mov Disord* 2006,**21**(Suppl 15):S503.
96. Vela L, Baron M, Barriga FJ, *et al.* Levodopa does not raise pain–pressure threshold in Parkinson disease. *Mov Disord* 2006;**21**(Suppl 15):S496.
97. Decina P, Mukherjee S, Caracci G, Harrison K. Painful sensory symptoms in neuroleptic-induced extrapyramidal syndromes. *Am J Psychiatry* 1992;**149**:1075–80.
98. Miley DP, Abrams AA, Atkinson JH, Janowsky DS. Successful treatment of thalamic pain with apomorphine. *Am J Psychiatry* 1978;**135**:1230–2.
99. Stuginski-Barbosa J, Rodrigues GGR, Bigal ME, Speciali JG. Burning mouth syndrome responsive to pramipexole. *J Headache Pain* 2008;**9**:43–5.
100. Trenkwalder C, Paulus W, Walters AS. The restless legs syndrome. *Lancet Neurol* 2005;**4**:465–75.
101. Ertas M, Sagduyu A, Arac N, *et al.* Use of levodopa to relieve pain from painful symmetrical diabetic polyneuropathy. *Pain* 1998;**75**:257–9.
102. Holman AJ, Myers RR. A randomized, double-blind, placebo-controlled trial of pramipexole, a dopamine agonist, in patients with fibromyalgia receiving concomitant medications. *Arthritis Rheum* 2005;**52**(8):2495–505.
103. Dickey RP, Minton JP. Levodopa relief of bone pain from breast cancer. *N Engl J Med* 1972;**286**:843.
104. Paalzow GH. L-Dopa induces opposing effects on pain in intact rats: (–)-sulpiride, SCH 23390 or α-methyl-DL-*p*-tyrosine methyle ster hydrochloride reveals profound hyperalgesia in large antinociceptive doses. *J Pharmacol Exp Ther* 1992;**263**:470–9.
105. Shyu BC, Kiritsy-Roy JA, Morrow TJ, Casey KL. Neurophysiological, pharmacological and behavioral evidence for medial thalamic mediation of cocaine-induced dopaminergic analgesia. *Brain Res* 1992;**572**:216–23.
106. Sánchez-González MA, García-Cabezas MA, Rico B, Cavada C. The primate thalamus is a key target for brain dopamine. *J Neurosci* 2005;**25**:6076–83.
107. Kupers R, Kehler H. Brain imaging of clinical pain states: a critical review and strategies for future studies. *Lancet Neurol* 2006;**5**:1033–44.
108. Guttman M, Boileau I, Warsh J, *et al.* Brain serotonin transporter binding in non-depressed patients with Parkinson's disease. *Eur J Neurol* 2007;**14**:523–8.
109. Mayeux R, Stern Y, Williams JB, *et al.* Clinical and biochemical features of depression in Parkinson's disease. *Am J Psychiatry* 1986;**143**:756–9.
110. Matsubara K, Fukushima S, Akane A, *et al.* Increased urinary morphine, codeine and tetrahydropapaveroline in parkinsonian patient undergoing L-3,4-dihydroxyphenylalanine therapy: a possible biosynthetic pathway of morphine from L-3,4-dihydroxyphenylalanine in humans. *J Pharmacol Exp Ther* 1992;**260**:974–8.
111. Mendlin A, Martín FJ, Jacobs BL. Dopaminergic input is required for increases in serotonin output produced by behavioral activation: an *in vivo* microdialysis study in rat forebrain. *Neuroscience* 1999;**93**:897–905.
112. Honey CR, Stoessl AJ, Tsui JKC, *et al.* Unilateral pallidotomy for reduction of parkinsonian pain. J Neurosurg 1999;**91**:198–201.
113. Pacchetti C, Albani G, Martignoni E, Godi L, *et al.* "Off" painful dystonia in Parkinson's disease treated with botulinum toxin. *Mov Disord* 1995;**10**:333–6.
114. Mense S. Neurobiological basis for the use of botulinum toxin in pain therapy. *J Neurol* 2004;**251**(Suppl 1):I1–7.
115. Fusina S, Conte S, Bertolasi L, *et al.* Sympathetic skin response asymmetry in early stage idiopathic Parkinson's disease. *Clin Neurophysiol* 1999;**110**:358–66.
116. Djaldetti R, Ziv I, Melamed E. The mystery of motor asymmetry in Parkinson's disease. *Lancet Neurol* 2006;**5**:796–802.
117. Lepoutre AC, Devos D, Blanchard-Dauphin A, *et al.* A specific clinical pattern of camptocormia in Parkinson's disease. *J Neurol Neurosurg Psychiatry* 2006;**77**:1229–34.
118. Lees AJ. The on-off phenomenon. *J Neurol Neurosurg Psychiatry* 1989;**52**(Suppl):29–37.
119. Nutt JG. Continuous dopaminergic stimulation: is it the answer to the motor complications of levodopa? *Mov Disord* 2007;**22**:1–9.
120. Nutt JG, Carter JH, Lea ES, Sexton GJ. Evolution of the response to levodopa during the first 4 years of therapy. *Ann Neurol* 2002;**51**:686–93.
121. Moro E, Esselink RJA, Benabid AL, Pollak P. Response to levodopa in parkinsonian patients with bilateral subthalamic nucleus stimulation. *Brain* 2002;**125**:2408–17.
122. Maricle RA, Valentine RJ, Carter J, Nutt JG. Mood response to levodopa infusion in early Parkinson's disease. *Neurology* 1998;**50**:1890–2.
123. Guigoni C, Li Q, Aubert I, *et al.* Involvement of sensorimotor, limbic, and associative basal ganglia domains in L-3,4-dihydroxyphenylalanine-induced dyskinesia. *J Neurosci* 2005;**25**:2102–7.
124. Schultz W. Dopamine neurons and their role in reward mechanisms. *Curr Opin Neurobiol* 1997;**7**:191–7.
125. Evans AH, Pavese N, Lawrence AD, *et al.* Compulsive drug use linked to sensitized ventral striatal dopamine transmission. *Ann Neurol* 2006;**59**:852–8.
126. Celerier E, Laulin J-P, Corcuff J-B, *et al.* Progressive enhancement of delayed hyperalgesia induced by repeated heroin administration: a sensitization process. *J Neurosci* 2001;**21**:4074–80.
127. Angst MS, Clark JD. Opioid-induced hyperalgesia: a qualitative systematic review. *Anesthesiology* 2006;**104**:570–87.
128. Pud D, Cohen D, Lawental E, Eisenberg E. Opioids and abnormal pain perception: new evidence from a study of chronic opioid addicts and healthy subjects. *Drug Alcohol Depend* 2006;**82**:218–23.
129. Koob GF, Le Moal M. Hedonic homeostatic dysregulation. *Science* 1997;**278**:52–8.

130. Barr AM, Markou A, Phillips AG. A 'crash' course on psychostimulant withdrawal as a model of depression. *Trends Pharmacol Sci* 2002;**23**:475–82.
131. Koob GF, Le Moal M. Plasticity of reward neurocircuitry and the 'dark side' of drug addiction. *Nat Neurosci* 2005;**8**:1442–4.
132. Nestler EJ. Is there a common molecular pathway for addiction? *Nat Neurosci* 2005;**8**:1445–9.
133. Lawrence AD, Evans AH, Lees AJ. Compulsive use of dopamine replacement therapy in Parkinson's disease: reward systems gone awry? *Lancet Neurol* 2003;**2**:595–604.
134. Funkiewiez A, Ardouin C, Krack P, *et al.* Acute psychotropic effects of bilateral subthalamic nucleus stimulation and levodopa in Parkinson's disease. *Mov Disord* 2003;**18**:524–30.
135. Poewe WH, Lees AJ, Stern GM. Dystonia in Parkinson's disease: clinical and pharmacological features. *Ann Neurol* 1988;**23**:73–8.
136. Factor SA, Brown DL, Molho ES. Subcutaneous apomorphine injections as a treatment for intractable pain in Parkinson's disease. *Mov Disord* 2000;**15**:167–9.
137. Stein WM, Read S. Chronic pain in the setting of Parkinson's disease and depression. *J Pain Symp Manage* 1997;**14**:255–8.
138. Diatchenko L, Slade GD, Nackley AG, *et al.* Genetic basis for individual variations in pain perception and the development of a chronic pain condition. *Hum Mol Genet* 2005;**14**:135–43.
139. Rakvåg TT, Klepstad P, Baar C, *et al.* The Val158Met polymorphism of the human catechol-*O*-methyltransferase (COMT) gene may influence morphine requirements in cancer pain patients. *Pain* 2005;**116**:73–8.
140. Tegeder I, Costigan M, Griffin RS, *et al.* GTP cyclohydrolase and tetrahydrobiopterin regulate pain sensitivity and persistence. *Nat Med* 2006;**12**:1269–77.
141. Gilbert GJ. Biceps pain as the presenting symptom of Parkinson disease: effective treatment with L-dopa. *South Med J* 2004;**97**:776–7.
142. O'Sullivan SS, Williams DR, Gallagher DA, *et al.* Nonmotor symptoms as presenting complaints in Parkinson's disease: a clinicopathological study. *Mov Disord* 2008;**23**:101–6.
143. Dworkin RH, Backonja M, Rowbotham MC, *et al.* Advances in neuropathic pain: diagnosis, mechanisms, and treatment recommendations. *Arch Neurol* 2003;**60**:1524–34.
144. Dworkin RH, O'Connor AB, Backonja M, *et al.* Pharmacologic management of neuropathic pain: evidence-based recommendations. *Pain* 2007;**132**:237–51.
145. Galer BS, Jensen MP. Development and preliminary validation of a pain measure specific to neuropathic pain: The Neuropathic Pain Scale. *Neurology* 1997;**48**:332–8.
146. Goy ER, Carter JH, Ganzini L. Parkinson disease at the end of life: caregiver perspectives. *Neurology* 2007;**69**:611–2.
147. Won A, Lapane K, Gambassi G, *et al.* Correlates and management of nonmalignant pain in the nursing home. SAGE Study Group – Systematic Assessment of Geriatric drug use via Epidemiology. *J Am Geriatr Soc* 1999;**47**:936–42.
148. Colloca L, Lopiano L, Lanotte M, Benedetti F. Overt versus covert treatment for pain, anxiety, and Parkinson's disease. *Lancet Neurol* 2004;**3**:679–84.
149. Shulman LM, Taback RL, Bean J, Weiner WJ. Comorbidity of the nonmotor symptoms of Parkinson's disease. *Mov Disord* 2001;**16**:507–10.
150. Weintraub D, Stern MB. Psychiatric complications in Parkinson's disease. *Am J Geriatr Psychiatry* 2005;**13**:844–51.
151. Menza M, Marin H, Kaufman K, *et al.* Citalopram treatment of depression in Parkinson's disease: the impact on anxiety, disability, and cognition. *J Neuropsychiatry Clin Neurosci* 2004;**16**:315–9.
152. Juri C, Chana P, Tapia J, *et al.* Quetiapine for insomnia in Parkinson disease: results from an open-label trial. *Clin Neuropharmacol* 2005;**28**:185–7.
153. Lim SY, Evans AH, Miyasaki JM. Impulse control and related disorders in Parkinson's disease: review. *Ann N Y Acad Sci* 2008;**1142**:85–107.
154. Drake DF, Harkins S, Qutubuddin A. Pain in Parkinson's disease: pathology to treatment, medication to deep brain stimulation. *NeuroRehabilitation* 2005;**20**:335–41.
155. Rajendran PR, Thompson RE, Reich SG. The use of alternative therapies by patients with Parkinson's disease. *Neurology* 2001;**57**:790–4.
156. Vas J, Ortega C, Olmo V, *et al.* Single-point acupuncture and physiotherapy for the treatment of painful shoulder: a multicentre randomized controlled trial. *Rheumatology* 2008;**47**:887–93.
157. Shulman LM, Wen X, Weiner WJ, *et al.* Acupuncture therapy for the symptoms of Parkinson's disease. *Mov Disord* 2002;**17**:799–802.
158. Cristian A, Katz M, Cutrone E, Walker RH. Evaluation of acupuncture in the treatment of Parkinson's disease: a double-blind pilot study. *Mov Disord* 2005;**20**:1185–8.
159. Hillen ME, Sage JI. Nonmotor fluctuations in patients with Parkinson's disease. *Neurology* 1996;**47**:1180–3.
160. Frankel JP, Lees AJ, Kempster PA, Stern GM. Subcutaneous apomorphine in the treatment of Parkinson's disease. *J Neurol Neurosurg Psychiatry* 1990;**53**:96–101.
161. Katzenschlager R, Hughes A, Evans A, *et al.* Continuous subcutaneous apomorphine therapy improves dyskinesias in Parkinson's disease: a prospective study using single-dose challenges. *Mov Disord* 2005;**20**:151–7.
162. Nyholm D, Nilsson Remahl AI, Dizdar N, *et al.* Duodenal levodopa infusion monotherapy vs oral polypharmacy in advanced Parkinson disease. *Neurology* 2005;**64**:216–23.
163. Ho B, Prakash R, Morgan JC, Sethi KD. A case of levodopa-responsive camptocormia associated with advanced Parkinson's disease. *Nat Clin Pract Neurol* 2007;**3**:526–30.
164. Kim JS, Park JW, Chung SW, *et al.* Pisa syndrome as a motor complication of Parkinson's disease. *Parkinsonism Relat Disord* 2007;**13**:126–8.
165. Friedman JH, Feinberg SS, Feldman RG. A neuroleptic malignant-like syndrome due to levodopa therapy withdrawal. *JAMA* 1985;**254**:2792–5.
166. Guindon J, Walczak JS, Beaulieu P. Recent advances in the pharmacological management of pain. *Drugs* 2007;**67**:2121–33.
167. Djaldetti R, Yust-Katz S, Kolianov V, *et al.* The effect of duloxetine on primary pain symptoms in Parkinson disease. *Clin Neuropharmacol* 2007;**30**:201–5.
168. Juncos JL. Clozapine treatment of parkinsonian pain syndromes. *Mov Disord* 1996;**11**:603–4.
169. Stoessl AJ, de la Fuente-Fernández R. Willing oneself better on placebo: effective in its own right. *Lancet* 2004;**364**:227–8.

170. Garcia-Borreguero D, Larrosa O, de la Llave Y, *et al.* Treatment of restless legs syndrome with gabapentin: a double-blind, cross-over study. *Neurology* 2002;**59**:1573–9.
171. Iranzo A, Comella CL, Santamaria J, Oertel W. Restless legs syndrome in Parkinson's disease and other neurodegenerative diseases of the central nervous system. *Mov Disord* 2007;**22**(Suppl 18):S424–30.
172. Sommer M, Bachmann CG, Liebetanz KM, *et al.* Pregabalin in restless legs syndrome with and without neuropathic pain. *Acta Neurol Scand* 2007;**115**:347–50.
173. Olson WL, Gruenthal M, Mueller ME, Olson WH. Gabapentin for parkinsonism: a double-blind, placebo-controlled, cross-over trial. *Am J Med* 1997;**102**:60–6.
174. Chaná P, de Marinis A, Barrientos N. Gabapentin and motor fluctuations in Parkinson's disease. *Mov Disord* 1997;**12**: 608.
175. Van Blercom N, Lasa A, Verger K, *et al.* Effects of gabapentin on the motor response to levodopa: a double-blind, placebo-controlled, crossover study in patients with complicated Parkinson disease. *Clin Neuropharmacol* 2004;**27**:124–8.
176. Raju PM, Walker RW, Lee MA. Dyskinesia induced by gabapentin in idiopathic Parkinson's disease. *Mov Disord* 2007;**22**:288–9.
177. Lieberman AN, Goldstein M. Reversible parkinsonism related to meperidine. *N Engl J Med* 1985;**312**:509.
178. Olivé JM, Masana L, González J. Meperidine and reversible parkinsonism. *Mov Disord* 1994;**9**:115–6.
179. Kaye J, Gage H, Kimber A, *et al.* Excess burden of constipation in Parkinson's disease: a pilot study. *Mov Disord* 2006;**21**:1270–3.
180. Klos KJ, Bower JH, Josephs KA, *et al.* Pathological hypersexuality predominantly linked to adjuvant dopamine agonist therapy in Parkinson's disease and multiple system atrophy. *Parkinsonism Relat Disord* 2005;**11**:381–6.
181. Evans AH, Lawrence AD, Potts J, *et al.* Factors influencing susceptibility to compulsive dopaminergic drug use in Parkinson disease. *Neurology* 2005;**65**:1570–4.
182. Silveira-Moriyama L, Evans AH, Katzenschlager R, Lees AJ. Punding and dyskinesias. *Mov Disord* 2006;**21**:2214–7.
183. Easterford K, Clough P, Kellett M, *et al.* Reversible parkinsonism with normal beta-CIT-SPECT in patients exposed to sodium valproate. *Neurology* 2004;**62**:1435–7.
184. Ristić AJ, Vojvodić N, Janković S, *et al.* The frequency of reversible parkinsonism and cognitive decline associated with valproate treatment: a study of 364 patients with different types of epilepsy. *Epilepsia* 2006;**47**:2183–5.
185. Svendsen KB, Jensen TS, Bach FW. Does the cannabinoid dronabinol reduce central pain in multiple sclerosis? Randomised double blind placebo controlled crossover trial. *BMJ* 2004;**329**:253.
186. Semple DM, McIntosh AM, Lawrie SM. Cannabis as a risk factor for psychosis: systematic review. *J Psychopharmacol* 2005;**19**:187–94.
187. Adler CH, Stern MB, Vernon G, Hurtig HI. Amantadine in advanced Parkinson's disease: good use of an old drug. *J Neurol* 1997;**244**:336–7.
188. Hara H, Wakayama Y, Kawase J. Clinical characteristics of painful dystonic foot response in patients with Parkinson's disease. *Rinsho Shinkeigaku* 1989;**29**:1101–5.
189. Lees AJ, Shaw KM, Stern GM. Baclofen in Parkinson's disease. *J Neurol Neurosurg Psychiatry* 1978;**41**:707–8.
190. Durif F, Debilly B, Galitzky M, *et al.* Clozapine improves dyskinesias in Parkinson disease: a double-blind, placebo-controlled study. *Neurology* 2004;**62**:381–8.
191. Cordivari C, Misra VP, Catania S, Lees AJ. Treatment of dystonic clenched fist with botulinum toxin. *Mov Disord* 2001;**16**:907–13.
192. Azher SN, Jankovic J. Camptocormia: pathogenesis, classification, and response to therapy. *Neurology* 2005;**65**:355–359.
193. Stern MB. Electroconvulsive therapy in untreated Parkinson's disease. *Mov Disord* 1991;**6**:265.
194. Moellentine C, Rummans T, Ahlskog JE, *et al.* Effectiveness of ECT in patients with parkinsonism. *J Neuropsychiatr Clin Neurosci* 1998;**10**:187–93.
195. Shulman RB. Maintenance ECT in the treatment of PD: therapy improves psychotic symptoms, physical function. *Geriatrics* 2003;**58**:43–5.
196. Abdi S, Haruo A, Bloomstone J. Electroconvulsive therapy for neuropathic pain: a case report and literature review. *Pain Physician* 2004;**7**:261–3.
197. Wasan AD, Artin K, Clark MR. A case-matching study of the analgesic properties of electroconvulsive therapy. *Pain Med* 2004;**5**:50–8.
198. Usui C, Doi N, Nishioka M, *et al.* Electroconvulsive therapy improves severe pain associated with fibromyalgia. *Pain* 2006;**121**:276–80.
199. Wolanin MW, Gulevski V, Schwartzman RJ. Treatment of CRPS with ECT. *Pain Physician* 2007;**10**:573–8.
200. Koch LD, Cofield RH, Ahlskog JE. Total shoulder arthroplasty in patients with Parkinson's disease. *J Shoulder Elbow Surg* 1997;**6**:24–8.
201. Weber M, Cabanela ME, Sim FH, *et al.* Total hip replacement in patients with Parkinson's disease. *Int Orthopaedics* 2002;**26**:66–8.
202. Shah SN, Hornyak J, Urquhart AG. Flexion contracture after total knee arthroplasty in a patient with Parkinson's disease: successful treatment with botulinum toxin type A. *J Arthroplasty* 2005;**20**:1078–80.
203. Singer C, Papapetropoulos S. Lower limb post-immobilization dystonia in Parkinson's disease. *J Neurol Sci* 2005;**239**: 111–4.
204. Idjadi JA, Aharonoff GB, Su H, *et al.* Hip fracture outcomes in patients with Parkinson's disease. *Am J Orthop* 2005;**34**: 341–6.
205. Pahwa R, Factor SA, Lyons KE, *et al.* Practice parameter: treatment of Parkinson disease with motor fluctuations and dyskinesia (an evidence-based review): Report of the Quality Standards Subcommittee of the American Academy of Neurology. *Neurology* 2006;**66**:983–95.
206. Krack P, Batir A, Van Blercom N, *et al.* Five-year follow-up of bilateral stimulation of the subthalamic nucleus in advanced Parkinson's disease. *N Engl J Med* 2003;**349**:1925–34.
207. Rodriguez-Oroz MC, Obeso JA, Lang AE, *et al.* Bilateral deep brain stimulation in Parkinson's disease: a multicentre study with 4 years follow-up. *Brain* 2005;**128**:2240–9.
208. Schupbach WMM, Chastan N, Welter ML, *et al.* Stimulation of the subthalamic nucleus in Parkinson's disease: a 5 year follow up. *J Neurol Neurosurg Psychiatry* 2005;**76**:1640–4.

209. Volkmann J, Allert N, Voges J, *et al*. Long-term results of bilateral pallidal stimulation in Parkinson's disease. *Ann Neurol* 2004;**55**:871–5.
210. Krack P, Pollak P, Limousin P, *et al*. From off-period dystonia to peak-dose chorea: the clinical spectrum of varying subthalamic nucleus activity. *Brain* 1999;**122**:1133–46.
211. Loher TJ, Burgunder JM, Weber S, *et al*. Effect of chronic pallidal deep brain stimulation on off period dystonia and sensory symptoms in advanced Parkinson's disease. *J Neurol Neurosurg Psychiatry* 2002;**73**:395–9.
212. Witjas T, Kaphan E, Régis J, *et al*. Effects of chronic subthalamic stimulation on nonmotor fluctuations in Parkinson's disease. *Mov Disord* 2007;**22**:1729–34.
213. Valldeoriola F, Pilleri M, Tolosa E, *et al*. Bilateral subthalamic stimulation monotherapy in advanced Parkinson's disease: long-term follow-up of patients. *Mov Disord* 2002;**17**:125–32.
214. Russmann H, Ghika J, Combrement P, *et al*. L-Dopa-induced dyskinesia improvement after STN-DBS depends upon medication reduction. *Neurology* 2004;**63**:153–5.
215. Tseng HM, Su PC, Liu HM, *et al*. Bilateral subthalamotomy for advanced Parkinson disease. *Surg Neurol* 2007;**68**(Suppl 1):43–51.
216. Vitek JL, Bakay RAE, Freeman A, *et al*. Randomized trial of pallidotomy versus medical therapy for Parkinson's disease. *Ann Neurol* 2003;**53**:558–69.
217. de Bie RMA, Schuurman PR, de Haan PS, *et al*. Unilateral pallidotomy in advanced Parkinson's disease: a retrospective study of 26 patients. *Mov Disord* 1999;**14**:951–7.
218. Baron MS, Vitek JL, Bakay RAE, *et al*. Treatment of advanced Parkinson's disease by posterior GPi pallidotomy: 1-year results of a pilot study. *Ann Neurol* 1996;**40**:355–66.
219. Garcia-Larrea L, Peyron R. Motor cortex stimulation for neuropathic pain: from phenomenology to mechanisms. *Neuroimage* 2007;**37**(Suppl 1):S71–9.
220. Priori A, Lefaucheur JP. Chronic epidural motor cortical stimulation for movement disorders. *Lancet Neurol* 2007;**6**:279–86.
221. Pagni CA, Zeme S, Zenga F, Maina R. Extradural motor cortex stimulation in advanced Parkinson's disease: the Turin experience: technical case report. *Operative Neurosurg* 2005; **57**.
222. Strafella AP, Lozano AM, Lang AE, *et al*. Subdural motor cortex stimulation in Parkinson's disease does not modify movement-related rCBF pattern. *Mov Disord* 2007;**22**: 2113–6.
223. Cilia R, Landi A, Vergani F, *et al*. Extradural motor cortex stimulation in Parkinson's disease. *Mov Disord* 2007:**22**: 111–4.
224. Martinez-Martin P, Schapira AHV, Stocchi F, *et al*. Prevalence of nonmotor symptoms in Parkinson's disease in an international setting: study using Nonmotor Symptoms Questionnaire in 545 patients. *Mov Disord* 2007:**22**:1623–9.
225. Iwamoto ET. Characterization of the antinociception induced by nicotine in the pedunculopontine tegmental nucleus and the nucleus raphe magnus. *J Pharmacol Exp Ther* 1991;**257**:120–33.
226. Mamede Rosa ML, Oliveira MA, Valente RB, *et al*. Pharmacological and neuroanatomical evidence for the involvement of the anterior pretectal nucleus in the antinociception induced by stimulation of the dorsal raphe nucleus in rats. *Pain* 1998;**74**:171–9.
227. Goto S, Hirano A. Catecholaminergic neurons in the parabrachial nucleus of normal individuals and patients with idiopathic Parkinson's disease. *Ann Neurol* 1991;**30**:192–6.
228. Braak H, Rüb U, Sandmann-Keil D, *et al*. Parkinson's disease: affection of brain stem nuclei controlling premotor and motor neurons of the somatomotor system. *Acta Neuropathol* 2000;**99**:489–95.

Chapter 30
Restless Legs Syndrome and Akathisia in Parkinson's Disease

Alex Iranzo[1] *& Cynthia L. Comella*[2]
[1]Neurology Service, Hospital Clinic and Institut d'Investigació Biomèdiques August Pi i Sunyer (IDIBAPS), Barcelona, Spain
[2]Department of Neurological Sciences, Rush University, Medical Center, Chicago, IL, USA

The restless legs syndrome (RLS)

Diagnosis and characteristics of RLS

Restless legs syndrome (RLS) is a chronic sensorimotor disorder characterized by an urge to move the legs, usually accompanied by unpleasant or uncomfortable sensations in the legs that begin or worsen during periods of rest or inactivity such as lying or sitting and are partially or totally relieved by movement, such as walking, stretching, or stamping [1]. RLS symptoms usually start in the evening or at night. The unpleasant sensations are usually felt deep inside the legs and most describe them as creeping and crawling. Some find it difficult to articulate the quality of the abnormal sensations and others will describe them as painful. RLS usually involves one or both lower limbs, but may sometimes involve the arms, and in severe cases the trunk, neck, and face. In the legs, the uncomfortable sensations usually involve calf muscles, but may also be described in the thighs and hips. Involvement of the feet is unusual but may occur. In the upper limbs, shoulders, arms, elbows, and forearms are more frequently affected than wrists and hands. RLS symptoms typically reach peak intensity between 11 p.m. and 3 a.m., and lessen or disappear in the morning between 6 a.m. and 10 a.m. Neurologic examination is usually normal except in those cases where RLS is secondary to another condition such as varicose veins or chronic polyneuropathy [1–3].

Periodic leg movements in sleep (PLMS) occur in about 80–90% of patients with RLS. PLMS are stereotyped repetitive movements characterized by dorsal flexion of the foot and sometimes flexion of the knee and even the hip in severe cases. The period length between two consecutive leg movements is 5–90 s. Each movement lasts between 0.5 and 10 s. PLMS appear in series of at least four movements and may occur in one or both legs [4]. In subjects with RLS, the number of PLMS is associated with RLS severity, and lessens with successful treatment of RLS. Although most RLS patients have PLMS, PLMS may occur without RLS. PLMS are also found in other disorders, such as neurodegenerative diseases, and often occur as an incidental finding in healthy individuals without motor, sensory, or sleep complaints. In healthy subjects, the prevalence of PLMS increases with age. Thus, the absence of PLMS does not exclude RLS, and the presence of PLMS is not specific for RLS. PLMS may be asymptomatic or may fragment sleep continuity, leading to a non-restorative sleep. Periodic leg movements may also be seen during wakefulness and during daytime naps when subjects are sitting or lying [4].

Differential diagnosis of RLS

The diagnosis of RLS is based on patient history, and is a clinical diagnosis [5]. The International RLS Study Group (IRLSG) has established four essential clinical criteria and three supportive criteria (Box 30.1). The differential diagnosis of RLS includes conditions related to motor restlessness, movement disorders, and leg discomfort (Box 30.2). These RLS "mimics" include akathisia, leg cramps, periodic leg movements in wakefulness, positional discomfort, leg fidgeting, chorea, athetosis, tics, myelopathy, radiculopathy, neuropathy, claudication of vascular and neurogenic origin, and painful legs and moving toes, and they may partially or fully fulfill the four essential criteria of RLS [2,3,5]. A careful history and physical examination are required to distinguish them from primary RLS.

Clinical relevance of RLS

RLS may be sporadic, familial, or secondary to several conditions, including end-stage renal disease, iron deficiency, pregnancy, some forms of peripheral neuropathy, and the use of dopamine receptor antagonists [5]. The clinical spectrum of RLS ranges from mild to severe forms [3,5], depending on the frequency and intensity of both

Parkinson's Disease: Non-Motor and Non-Dopaminergic Features, First Edition. Edited by C. Warren Olanow, Fabrizio Stocchi, and Anthony E. Lang.

Box 30.1 Diagnostic criteria of RLS [1]

Essential criteria
1 An urge to move the legs, usually accompanied or caused by uncomfortable and unpleasant sensation in the legs.
2 The urge to move or unpleasant sensations begin or worsen during periods of rest or inactivity such as lying or sitting.
3 The urge to move or unpleasant sensations are partially or totally relieved by movement such as walking or stretching, at least as the activity continues.
4 The urge to move or unpleasant sensations are worse in the evening or at night than during the day, or only occur in the evening or night.

Supportive criteria
1 Positive history of RLS.
2 Positive response to dopaminergic drugs.
3 Periodic limb movements in wakefulness or sleep as assessed with polysomnography or leg activity devices.

the urge to move and unpleasant sensations in the legs. Some cases have a progressive course, others have a stable course, and still others have unpredictable long fluctuations and remissions. In some individuals, RLS may be precipitated or aggravated by factors such as pregnancy, iron deficiency anemia, and medications such as antidepressants and dopamine receptor antagonists, including metoclopramide and risperidone [6–13]. Patients with mild RLS usually do not seek medical attention because symptoms are mild, sporadic, and not bothersome. Severe cases may be associated with impaired general quality-of-life linked either to insomnia, sleep fragmentation, daytime sleepiness, depression, anxiety, fatigue, inability to concentrate, or social limitations (e.g., inability to enjoy quiet activities at night that require sitting, such as driving for a long time, traveling by plane, dinning in a restaurant, and watching a movie) [14]. Hence, when severe RLS occurs in a patient with a disabling medical disorder such as Parkinson's disease (PD), quality-of-life may dramatically worsen.

Box 30.2 Differential diagnosis of RLS [1]

Conditions related to leg discomfort
1 Nocturnal leg cramps
2 Positional discomfort
3 Myelopathy
4 Radiculopathy
5 Sensory neuropathy
6 Claudication of vascular origin
7 Claudication of neurogenic origin
8 Painful legs and moving toes

Conditions related to movement disorders
1 Periodic leg movements in wakefulness and in sleep
2 Chorea
3 Athetosis
4 Tics

Conditions related to motor restlessness
1 Akathisia
2 Leg fidgeting
3 Foot tapping
4 Leg stretching and rolling

Demographics and epidemiology of RLS (for a review, see [5])

Although described in the medical literature in the seventeenth century by Thomas Willis, RLS has attracted scientific and medical attention only during the last 15 years. Believed for a long time to be an uncommon disorder, epidemiologic studies conducted in the USA, Canada, and Western Europe have shown prevalence rates of RLS between 3 and 15%, indicating that RLS is one of the most common movement disorders [15]. Despite using important different methodologies, the prevalence of RLS varies between 4.5 and 15% in the USA and between 8 and 11% in Canada, Germany, Spain, Sweden, Norway, Denmark, The Netherlands, France, and South Tyrol, and is 3% in Ireland, Turkey, and Greece, and less than 2% in Japan, India, and Singapore [15–25]. RLS was often first diagnosed when these studies were conducted.

Age, gender, ethnicity, and genetics influence the frequency of RLS. The disease affects both sexes and all ages. In most, but not all, studies RLS is more frequent in women than in men [23,26,27] and prevalence increases with age. One study conducted in the USA reported that experiencing RLS more than four nights per month occurred in 3% of participants aged 18–29 years, 10% of those aged 30–79 years, and 19% of those aged 80 years and older. About 20% of adults with RLS report onset of the symptoms between the ages of 10 and 20 years [28]. A population-based study performed in UK and USA showed a prevalence of 2% in children aged 8–11 years and adolescents [29]. RLS in children is common in subjects with attention deficit hyperactivity disorder (ADHD) and low serum ferritin levels, and when family members are also affected [30]. One study involving 1071 adults from east Baltimore reported that the rates of RLS were comparable between African Americans (4.7%) and Caucasian Americans (3.8%) [31]. However, studies conducted in children aged 5–7 years and in adults indicated that PLMS were more common in Caucasian Americans than in African Americans [29,32–35].

A positive family history occurs in approximately 30–60% of cases [36,37], with an autosomal dominant mode of inheritance in some. Recently, RLS and PLMS have been linked to genetic variants in the *BTBD9*, *MEIS1* and *MAP2K5-LBXCOR1* genes [38,39]. The functions of these genes are unclear, although some are thought to be involved in embryonic limb development. The worldwide distribution of the haplotypes of these three genes may account for differences in the prevalence of RLS and PLMS in different races and countries. Genetic alterations recently found in the metabolic pathways regulated by nitric oxide synthase may contribute to the origin of RLS [40].

Pathophysiology of RLS

Several lines of evidence suggest that decreased dopaminergic tone in the spinal cord and iron deficiency in the brain are involved in the pathophysiology of RLS [41–44]. Dopamine and iron share circadian rhythm variations with low levels at night, corresponding to the time when RLS symptoms usually start [45]. RLS symptom severity correlates negatively with serum ferritin levels, even in subjects without anemia [46], RLS patients have reduced CSF ferritin [47] that is relatively unrelated to serum ferritin [48], and the substantia nigra has iron metabolism abnormalities [49,50]. Iron is a cofactor necessary for dopamine synthesis in the brain and forms part of the D2 receptor, and there are iron metabolism abnormalities in subjects with idiopathic RLS which may lead to brain iron deficiency and dopaminergic dysfunction. Importantly, RLS symptoms respond to both dopaminergic agents and iron. Proposed animal models for RLS include iron-deficient diets, selective surgical lesions in the central dopaminergic systems, and dopamine receptor knockout [51–54]. There are no abnormalities in the genes coding dopamine receptors and enzymes related to dopamine synthesis [55], and there is no evidence indicating that the nigrostriatal (A8 and A9) and mesolimbic (A10) dopaminergic systems are impaired in RLS. Brain imaging studies in subjects with RLS evaluating the nigrostriatal dopaminergic system have shown variable results, although most suggest no consistent dysfunction [56–59]. It may be that RLS results from dysfunction of the diencephalospinal dopaminergic system (A11) [60], which is comprised of a very small population of neurons that originate in the hypothalamus. These neurons send processes through the dorsolateral funiculus to dorsal (sensory) and anterior (motor) horns of the spinal cord where dopaminergic receptors exist, particularly the D3 subtype. Therefore, abnormalities in the diencephalospinal dopaminergic system may account for spinal cord dysfunction (reduced supraspinal inhibitory mechanisms and facilitation of spinal flexor responses), leading to the abnormal sensations and increased motor activity (urge to move and PLMS) typically seen in RLS.

Treatment of RLS

Dopaminergic agents are considered the first-line therapy for RLS [61]. Recent large therapeutic trials have shown that small doses of dopaminergic agents such as levodopa, pergolide, pramipexole, ropinirole, cabergoline, and rotigotine are more effective than placebo. They decrease the frequency and severity of RLS-related symptoms and the number of periodic leg movements during sleep and during wakefulness [62–72]. In patients with RLS, the acute side effects of dopaminergic agents are similar to those observed in PD such as gastrointestinal (nausea, vomiting, abdominal pain, constipation) somnolence, insomnia, and even compulsive gambling [61,73]. Unlike PD, dyskinesias and motor fluctuations are not observed. This is likely related to the lack of nigrostriatal degeneration in RLS and perhaps the lower doses employed.

Long-term therapy with dopaminergic agents in RLS may lead to augmentation [74,75], a specific complication of dopaminergic treatment in RLS which includes an increase in RLS severity, earlier onset of symptoms in the afternoon, extension of symptoms to previously unaffected body parts including the upper limbs, and a shorter duration of benefit of dopaminergic medication. Augmentation is most frequent with short-acting levodopa, affecting up to 80% of patients treated [76,77]. Although augmentation also occurs with dopamine agonist therapy, it tends to be less frequent and milder [76,78,79]. Management of augmentation includes initiating therapy with or switching to dopamine agonists and reduction or discontinuation of levodopa. Non-dopaminergic medications such as gabapentin, pregabalin, opioids (e.g., oxycodone, tramadol), and iron replacement are also effective in treating RLS [43,80,80a].

The restless legs syndrome and PD

RLS in the setting of PD

With increasing evidence that RLS is linked to alterations in central dopaminergic neurotransmission, one would expect to find RLS more frequently in the setting of PD [42]. However, since RLS is a very common condition, co-occurrence with less frequent disorders such as PD, might be a matter of chance or concomitant medical problems, including iron deficiency [81]. Currently, no data suggest that patients with sporadic and familial RLS are at increased risk for developing a neurodegenerative disease [82–84]. In particular, whether RLS is associated with PD has not been established. Only a few studies have directly addressed this issue, and these have methodologic limitations yielding conflicting results.

PD affects approximately 1% of the population older than 60 years and is caused by progressive neuronal loss in many regions of the brain leading to dysfunction of several neurotransmitter systems, particularly the dopaminergic nigrostriatal and mesolimbic systems [85]. PD is characterized by motor features, but includes non-motor features such as mood, autonomic, cognitive, sleep, and sensory disturbances. Motor symptoms in PD respond dramatically to dopaminergic agents. In contrast, many of the non-motor symptoms do not. Patients with PD frequently report unpleasant sensory symptoms in the legs, such as restlessness, discomfort, stiffness, pain, tingling, burning, coldness, heat, and cramps. In many cases, the nature of these sensory symptoms is unclear and they are difficult to manage [86]. In PD, akathisia, severe ""off" states, inner tremor, and dystonic postures may be associated with sensory disturbances that occur in a temporal pattern and may resemble RLS. Patients with PD may have RLS, but it is not clear whether RLS is more frequent in PD than in the general population [81,87]. RLS has been reported both in patients with idiopathic PD and in individuals carrying *Parkin* mutations [81,88]. RLS and PD may be found in families with autosomal dominant mode of inheritance. When RLS occurs in PD, parkinsonism usually precedes the onset of RLS by several years. RLS symptoms are frequently mild in the majority of PD patients, who often do not report them spontaneously [81]. When clinically indicated, management of RLS in PD patients treated with dopaminergic agents for parkinsonism can be challenging. There are no studies addressing the issue of whether RLS in PD is pharmacologically similar to idiopathic RLS. However, in PD patients taking levodopa or dopaminergic agents, increasing the evening dose can be effective. The addition of a non-dopaminergic agent such as gabapentin can also be effective (unpublished data).

Similarities and differences between RLS and PD

Although there are some similarities between RLS and PD, especially in the response to dopaminergic drugs, there are some differences. Both PD and RLS respond dramatically to dopaminergic agents, are aggravated by dopaminergic antagonists, and are associated with the presence of PLMS, which decrease in number with the use of dopaminergic drugs [5,61,89]. However, several lines of evidence indicate that the dopaminergic impairment in PD and RLS is different. PD is characterized by neuronal loss, Lewy bodies, and increased iron deposition in the substantia nigra pars compacta [90]. In contrast, neuropathologic studies in idiopathic RLS show no cell loss in the substantia nigra pars compacta, there are no Lewy bodies, and iron staining is decreased histologically [50,91] and in neuroimaging studies [92,93]. Furthermore, neuroimaging studies show normal presynaptic nigrostriatal dopaminergic function in RLS, whereas this function is impaired in PD [59]. Moreover, there is no clinical evidence that subjects diagnosed with idiopathic RLS are at risk of developing PD [94]. Interestingly, the RLS augmentation phenomenon has not been reported in PD individuals treated with dopaminergic agents for parkinsonism. It has been suggested that in contrast to the nigrostriatal and mesolimbic dopaminergic systems involved in PD, RLS may be associated with dysfunction of the diencephalospinal area (A11), a dopaminergic system which originates in the hypothalamus and extends to the spinal cord [41,42]. One study showed that 6-hydroxydopamine lesion in the A11 nuclei of the mouse induced increased locomotor activity which could be reversed by ropinirole [54]. However, the state of the dopaminergic A11 system in humans, which contains no more than 400 neurons in rodents, has not been examined in PD. Another important difference is that RLS symptoms but not the motor features of PD may be improved with opioids, gabapentin and iron replacement [61]. Genetic variants in the *BTBD9*, *MEIS1* and *MAP2K5-LBXCOR1* genes determine a risk for developing RLS and PLMS [38,39]. The polymorphisms in these genes are not more frequent in patients with PD than age-, gender-, and ethnicity-matched controls [95]. These findings suggest that the pathogenesis of PD and RLS involves different mechanisms, and that RLS and PD have a different genetic background.

Periodic leg movements in sleep (PLMS) in PD

There are no studies addressing the issue of whether PLMS are more frequent in PD patients with RLS than without RLS. Polysomnographic studies commonly disclose PLMS in both untreated and treated patients with idiopathic PD and patients with *Parkin* mutations [96–98]. Most patients with PD who experience PLMS are unaware of the leg movements, possibly because PLMS are generally not associated with arousals (personal observations). Therefore, PLMS in PD do not appear to be a main contributing factor for sleep fragmentation and excessive daytime sleepiness. PLMS are very common in the elderly [99], and it is not clear whether they are more frequent in PD. One small study found an increase in PLMS in PD compared with MSA and controls [96]. Another small study found that in patients with parkinsonism, a reduction in dopamine transporter binding correlated with the severity of PLMS, although there were methodologic issues [100]. Finally, PLMS in patients with PD increased after bilateral subthalamic stimulation, possibly because of reduction or withdrawal of dopaminergic therapy [101].

Studies evaluating a possible relationship between RLS and PD

RLS is a common disorder that affects approximately to 8–10% of the general population over 65 years of age in Europe and North America [102], whereas the prevalence of PD in industrialized countries is about 1% in people over 60 years of age [103]. To assess whether RLS occurs more frequently in PD than in the general population would require a large prospective epidemiologic study in drug-naive PD patients compared with a

Table 30.1 Studies evaluating the frequency of restless legs syndrome in Parkinson's disease.

Study	Study design	PD patients studied (*n*)	PD patients' mean age (years)	RLS in PD (%)	RLS in controls (%)[a]
Lang and Johnson, 1987, Canada [106]	Cohort of PD	100	62	0	NA
Ondo *et al.*, 2002, USA [81]	Cohort of PD	303	67	20.8	NA
Kahn and Sahota, 2002, USA [108]	Cohort of PD	26	NA	38.4	NA
Tan *et al.*, 2002, Singapore [113]	Cohort of PD	125	65	0	NA
Krishnan *et al.*, 2003, India [111]	Case–control PD	126	57	7.9	0.8
Braga-Neto *et al.*, 2004, Brazil [107]	Cohort of PD	86	65	52.3	NA
Peralta *et al.*, 2005, Austria [109]	Cohort of PD	113	68	24.7	NA
Nomura *et al.*, 2006, Japan [112]	Case–control PD	165	68	12	2.3
Gómez-Esteban *et al.*, 2007, Spain [110]	Cohort of PD	114	68	21.9	NA
Loo and Tan, 2008, Singapore [87]	Case–control PD	400	65	3	0.5
Lee *et al.*, 2009, Korea [113a]	Cohort of PD	447	64	16	NA
Calzetti *et al.*, 2009, Italy [110a]	Cohort of PD	118	69	13	NA
Peralta *et al.*, 2009, Austria [110b]	Cohort of PD	113	67	24	NA
Verbaan *et al.*, 2010, Holland [110c]	Cohort of PD	269	61	11	NA

[a]NA, not available.

control group matched for number, age, and sex of the same geographic area without disorders known to be related to RLS. Prevalence studies in PD patients treated with dopaminergic medications may underestimate the occurrence of RLS because these drugs may mask the appearance of RLS symptoms. In support of this possibility are observations that a dose reduction of more than 70% after deep brain stimulation for PD is associated with the emergence of RLS [104] and a marked increase in the number of PLMS [101]. It should be noted, however, that a smaller decrease in levodopa equivalent dose after surgery (56%) may be associated with improvement in RLS symptoms [105]. Excluding patients taking dopaminergic agents to treat parkinsonism would not permit a determination of the prevalence of RLS in more advanced PD, where there may be a greater frequency. Few studies have addressed this complex issue, and these have had methodologic limitations and yielded different results (Table 30.1). Important methodologic limitations include different criteria for the diagnosis of RLS, referral bias, inclusion of patients only treated with dopaminergic agents, and lack of a control group. Hence the results of these studies should be interpreted with caution.

One early study published before the clinical criteria for RLS were established reported that RLS was not present in a series of 100 PD patients [106]. Although 26 PD patients experienced the need to move and inability to remain still, their symptoms could occur at any time of the day and they were diagnosed with akathisia rather than RLS. Seventeen patients reported a need to move due to rigidity, immobility, dyskinesias, and sensory complaints such as aching. Only two patients in this series experienced the inability to remain still, especially in the evening and at night, but this was not accompanied by a crawling sensation of the legs [106]. In another study, RLS symptoms were noted in 45 of 86 (52.3%) consecutive levodopa-treated PD patients seen in a movement disorders outpatient clinic [107]. RLS was diagnosed by clinical history but not the IRLSSG criteria. RLS symptoms were more frequent in patients with longer duration of parkinsonism independent of age and excessive daytime sleepiness. In a third study using mailed questionnaires and telephone interviews, 10 of 26 (38.4%) PD patients treated with dopaminergic agents reported RLS symptoms [108].

Sixty-three of 303 (20.8%) consecutively treated PD subjects had RLS using IRLSSG criteria [81]. The most predictive factor was a low serum ferritin level. In most cases, parkinsonism preceded RLS onset and severity of RLS was mild. Thus, the occurrence of RLS symptoms before parkinsonism was not common enough to suggest that RLS itself represents a risk factor for PD. Compared with patients with idiopathic RLS, those with both PD and RLS were older at RLS onset, less likely to have a family history, and had lower serum ferritin levels. No definite conclusions could be drawn because the study did not include a matched control group. The finding that RLS severity was mild could be explained, in part, by the occurrence of RLS while the patients were being treated with dopaminergic medications for parkinsonism.

In another prospective study, 28 of 113 (24.7%) patients with idiopathic PD met IRLSSG criteria. Patients with RLS were younger, had lower Hoehn and Yahr scores, and frequently experienced symptoms during the wearing-off periods. RLS was not related to PD duration, and parkinsonism preceded RLS onset in most of the patients [109].

In a recent cross-sectional study, 25 out of 114 (21.9%) consecutive PD patients without cognitive impairment were found to have mild RLS [110]. RLS was more frequent in women (68%), and five (20%) reported a positive family history for RLS. None of the patients who underwent deep brain stimulation in the subthalamic nucleus (DBS STN) had RLS. Overall quality of sleep, age, duration of parkinsonism, duration of anti-parkinsonian treatment, total levodopa equivalent dose, use of levodopa or dopamine agonists, cognitive status, parkinsonism severity, complications of dopaminergic medications, activities of daily living, overall quality-of-life, and daytime sleepiness were not different in those with and without RLS. A control group was not included and iron status was not evaluated. Three other studies conducted in Europe have found a prevalence of RLD in PD between 11 and 24% [110a,b,c].

Three studies have been conducted in Asian countries, India [111], Japan [112], and Singapore [113], where the prevalence of RLS in the general population is much lower than in Western countries. One series from India [111] using the IRLSSG criteria found RLS in 10 of 126 (7.9%) consecutive PD patients attending a movement disorder clinic and in only one of 128 (0.8%) healthy age- and sex-matched controls from the same geographic area. PD patients with RLS were older and had a higher prevalence of depression than those without RLS. Serum ferritin levels were not different in PD subjects with or without RLS. None of the subjects with RLS had a family history of RLS. In all patients RLS symptoms developed after the diagnosis of PD had been made. Of the 10 patients with RLS, nine (90%) were taking levodopa, five (50%) had mild RLS, four (40%) had moderate RLS, and one (10%) had severe RLS. Similar findings were reported in a study in Japan [112,114], where using the IRLSSG criteria RLS was found in 20 of 165 consecutive medicated PD patients (12%) and in three of 131 (2.3%) controls. Among the 20 PD patients with RLS, only two (10%) had a positive family history of RLS, and parkinsonism preceded RLS symptoms in 19 (95%). PD patients with RLS were younger and had mild discomfort. No differences between patients with or without RLS were found in serum ferritin levels, gender, PD duration, PD severity, and the use of dopaminergic agents. When compared with subjects with idiopathic RLS, PD patients with RLS had a lower prevalence of family history of RLS, similar serum ferritin and iron levels, less PLMS in polysomnographic studies, and a poorer clinical response to RLS treatment with dopamine agonists or clonazepam [49,114]. The authors of the studies in India and Japan concluded that RLS is more frequent in PD than in controls. However, given that the prevalence of RLS in PD was similar to those found in European and North American studies, and RLS prevalence in healthy controls was exceedingly low, it has been speculated that the results may be explained by ethnic differences [83]. Given that RLS is a condition that predominates in women, a limitation of the Indian study was that 90% of the subjects were male. Another study conducted in Singapore using IRLSSG criteria found that RLS did not occur in any of 125 consecutive PD outpatients, where the prevalence of RLS in the general population is 0.6%. The authors concluded that the prevalence of RLS in PD was not more common than in the general population [113]. A case–control study by the same authors involving 400 PD subjects found a higher prevalence of RLS compared with controls (3.0% versus 0.5%), although the difference was not significant [115]. Polysomnographic studies confirmed that PD subjects with RLS had an elevated PLMS index but RLS was mild and did not affect quality of sleep. None of the RLS patients reported a family history of PD or RLS. One study conducted in Korea found a prevalence of RLS in PD of 16% [113a].

Summary of the relationship between PD and RLS

Although PD and RLS are both related to central dopaminergic dysfunction, only a few studies indicate an association. Studies in general have methodologic limitations and report inconsistent results. Large long-term prospective controlled studies are warranted to assess if RLS in the setting of PD is more frequent than in the matched general population. It would not be surprising if the occurrence of RLS in the setting of PD is simply explained by a casual association between two frequent conditions in the elderly. Other conditions associated with dopaminergic deficit, such as spinocerebellar ataxia [116] and attention-deficit/hyperactivity disorder [32], are more clearly associated with RLS. Neurologists should be aware that RLS may be the underlying cause of sensory complaints in some PD patients and that they may be ameliorated with the use of appropriate medications.

Akathisia

Diagnosis and characteristics of akathisia

Akathisia (from Greek, literally "not to sit") is characterized by a subjective sensation of restlessness or an urge to move and an inability to be still [117]. Onset may be acute (acute akathisia) or chronic (tardive akathisia). Patients with any form of akathisia complain of a feeling of inner tension in the whole body, particularly the legs. They are constantly moving about, shift from one position to another when sitting, and walk incessantly in attempts to relieve their abnormal sensations. Motor manifestations are not stereotyped. They include rocking from foot to foot, shifting weight while sitting, crossing and uncrossing of the legs, toe tapping, and marching to the spot. Movements of the upper limbs, trunk twisting and rocking, and face rubbing are reported less commonly. Half of the patients experience a worsening of symptoms while standing with a tendency to move from foot to foot, and to jump or hop. Some patients report an inability to lie in bed, with a tendency to get up and walk. Typically, patients with akathisia have a little relief from the resultant movements; some patients experience some relief on lying. Family history of akathisia is usually negative and no diurnal variation of symptoms occurs. Akathisia commonly occur during the whole day, disappearing when the patient is asleep [118].

In most of the cases, patients with akathisia do not reported insomnia or other sleep disturbances despite polysomnographic studies showing PLMS. In one polysomnographic study, PLMS were present in five of nine patients with akathisia but in all 11 patients with idiopathic RLS. PLM during wakefulness were only seen in idiopathic RLS [119]. In another study, clonazepam treatment reduced PLMS in all 18 patients with RLS and four with neuroleptic-induced akathisia [120]. In a patient with schizoaffective disorder who developed neuroleptic-induced unilateral left-side akathisia, polysomnography showed right PLMS. After clonazepam treatment both akathisia and PLMS disappeared. Brain MRI findings and neurologic findings were within normal limits [121].

Diagnosis and severity can be estimated using the Barnes akathisia rating scale [122]. This clinical scale evaluates subjective (how do you feel?; do you feel you cannot sit still?; do you feel you cannot keep your legs still?) and objective features of akathisia while the patient is sitting (semi-purposeful feet movements, shifting position in chair, inability to remain seated, semi-purposeful hand and arm movements), standing (rocking from foot to foot, other normal purposeless foot movements, inability to remain standing), and lying (coarse tremor, myoclonic jerks of feet, semi-purposeful feet movements). All of these 13 items score separately as absent (0), present less than half the time (1), present more than half of the time (2), and present all of the time (3). It should be noted that patients with true RLS may exhibit high scores on this scale. The myoclonic jerks of feet and semi-purposeful feet movements when lying may represent PLM during wakefulness in subjects with RLS rather than akathisia.

The most common cause of akathisia is the recent introduction of a medication. Drugs with central anti-dopaminergic activity are the most frequently associated with akathisia [123]. Typically, akathisia develops after the use of traditional neuroleptics (e.g., phenothiazines and butyrophenones), reserpine, and anti-emetics that cross the blood–brain barrier (e.g., metoclopramide). The newer atypical anti-psychotics have a lower potential for producing akathisia than conventional neuroleptics. In half of the cases of neuroleptic-induced acute akathisia, the symptoms develop gradually within the first month of treatment and in almost 90% of cases are present by 3 months. Akathisia may also develop after long-term exposure to neuroleptics, coincident with increased dosage or change to a more potent neuroleptic. Patients with neuroleptic-induced akathisia often experience other extrapyramidal adverse effects, including dystonia, tardive dyskinesia, and parkinsonism. Akathisia has also been reported with selective serotonin reuptake inhibitor anti-depressants, tricyclic anti-depressants, lithium carbonate, methysergide, and calcium channel antagonists [118,124].

Differential diagnosis of akathisia [1–3,53]

Akathisia must be differentiated from anxiety, hyperactivity, agitation, hysteria, mannerisms, stereotyped movements including those occurring in Tourette's syndrome, dyskinesias, and exacerbation of psychosis. Symptoms that distinguish akathisia- from non-akathisia-like conditions are shifting weight from foot to foot or walking on the spot, inability to keep legs still, feelings of inner restlessness, and shifting of body position in the chair [125].

There are clinical similarities between akathisia and RLS. Patients with akathisia and RLS have subjective and objective motor manifestations. Neuroleptics and other medications that block central dopaminergic neurotransmission can cause both akathisia and RLS. Both disorders have been associated with lower serum iron or ferritin levels, and iron replacement may improve both conditions, although this is less clear for akathisia. PLMS may occur in both disorders, although less prominently in akathisia. Finally, the dopaminergic diencephalospinal system and spinal cord dysfunction are speculated to be involved in the pathophysiology of both conditions [3,126].

The following features may help to distinguish akathisia from RLS (Table 30.2). Most cases of akathisia are secondary, arising from treatment with a dopamine receptor antagonist or associated with a neurodegenerative disease, in particular PD. The majority of RLS cases are idiopathic. In RLS, the urge to move is associated with sensory discomfort, paresthesias, and dysesthesias, whereas in akathisia there is a sense of inner restlessness without more defined sensory discomfort. In contrast to akathisia, in which the unpleasant body sensation

Table 30.2 Features that distinguish restless legs syndrome from akathisia [83]

Feature	Restless legs syndrome	Akathisia
Paresthesias Dysesthesias	Common	Rare
Periodic limb movements during sleep	Common	Less frequent
Generalized restlessness	Rare	Common
Circadian pattern (worse at night)	Common	Not observed
Periodic limb movements during wakefulness	Common	Not observed
Sleep disturbance	Frequent complaint	Rare complaint

involves the whole body, RLS predominantly affects the legs. Akathisia does not have a defined circadian pattern, whereas RLS has a marked circadian pattern of symptoms with onset or a peak symptoms occurring in the evening or night. The exception to this is the augmentation of RLS induced by dopaminergic drugs, where symptoms may also occur during the daytime [74]. Symptoms of akathisia usually are not markedly relieved by movement, whereas symptoms of RLS have a partial or total improvement with activity such as walking, this being one of the core criteria for diagnosis [5]. Finally, although sleep disturbances associated with akathisia are frequent, they are generally not severe. In RLS, sleep onset delay and fragmented sleep are more pronounced, and often the presenting complaint. RLS is an autosomal dominant disorder, with a positive family history in at least 50% of patients [127]; although acute akathisia may have a genetic susceptibility [128] it is rarely an inherited disorder, and family history is infrequently positive [119].

Dopaminergic agents may be effective for both RLS and akathisia, especially in association with PD [129]. Opioids and clonazepam may also be effective in both disorders [130–134], although controlled studies are lacking. Akathisia, however, responds well to treatment with other agents, including anti-cholinergics and β-blockers, that have not been found to be effective for RLS [135,136].

Clinical relevance of akathisia

Akathisia is a common acute and tardive side effect of dopamine receptor antagonist drugs, and less frequently other psychiatric medications, including serotonergic anti-depressants [137,138], which can induce an activation syndrome [139]. Akathisia is associated with non-compliance with psychiatric medications, recurrence of psychosis, and suicide [140,141], and is considered one of the commonest and most distressing side effects of dopamine receptor antagonists. Unfortunately, it is often ignored or misdiagnosed as agitation. When correctly diagnosed, however, there are limited effective therapeutic options [118].

Demography and epidemiology of akathisia

Most studies evaluating the incidence of akathisia have been conducted in patients with schizophrenia taking conventional anti-psychotic drugs. They have diverse methodology and suffer many limitations. Incidence rates for acute akathisia with conventional anti-psychotic agents vary from 9 to 75%, with 20–30% being a conservative estimate. The newer atypical anti-psychotic drugs (e.g., clozapine, quetiapine) are much less likely to produce akathisia. Drug dose, rate of increment of dose, and drug potency seem to be important risk factors for developing akathisia. Iron status, sociodemographic factors, genetic susceptibility, and other treatment-related variables may also play a role. Drug-induced parkinsonism is significantly correlated with the occurrence of akathisia [118,125,142].

Pathophysiology of akathisia

It is surprising that although akathisia is a long-recognized and common syndrome with well-defined clinical features, very little is known regarding its pathophysiologic basis. The finding that most cases of akathisia are induced by anti-dopaminergic medications suggests that central dopaminergic dysfunction plays a key role. It has been postulated that akathisia results from a postsynaptic D2 receptor blockade in diencephalospinal and mesocortical dopaminergic systems. However, a complex interaction of dopamine with adrenergic, noradrenergic, and opioid mechanisms may play some role [143]. Abnormalities in iron metabolism have also been implicated based on the finding that patients with neuroleptic-induced akathisia have lower serum iron and ferritin levels than patients taking neuroleptics without akathisia [61–64,144–147]. Also, improvement in neuroleptic-induced akathisia has been reported with intravenous iron replacement in subjects with iron deficiency [148]. Thus, available data suggest that iron deficiency is a risk factor for akathisia, although it cannot be excluded that neuroleptics may be responsible as these drugs chelate iron [149].

Treatment of akathisia

In neuroleptic-induced akathisia, therapeutic strategies include dose reduction, changing to a lower potency neuroleptic or atypical anti-psychotic, or drug withdrawal. Akathisia may remit within days or weeks of withdrawal of the neuroleptic drug, although in some cases it may persist for several months or even be permanent. In some cases, drugs such as propranolol, gabapentin, anticholinergics, and opioids may be effective [53]. Relatively low doses of clozapine are effective for the treatment of neuroleptic-induced extrapyramidal syndromes in neuroleptic-resistant chronic schizophrenic patients. The relief of chronic akathisia in this group of patients occurs more rapidly than the reduction in psychotic symptoms [150].

Akathisia and Parkinson's disease (PD)

Akathisia in the setting of PD

If akathisia is caused by dopaminergic hypofunction in the central nervous system, one would expect a high prevalence of this disorder in patients with PD. Similarly, the now frequent use in PD of novel anti-psychotics (e.g., clozapine, quetiapine, olanzapine, and risperidone) to treat psychosis and hallucinations should be expected to be linked to an increased frequency of akathisia. However, akathisia is not a prominent feature, or at least is an under-recognized and little-studied feature, of both untreated and treated PD subjects. The introduction of classic neuroleptics in PD is more frequently associated with aggravated parkinsonism than with akathisia, although anecdotal cases of quetiapine-induced akathisia have been reported [151]. In contrast, low doses of clozapine were found to be effective in treating nocturnal akathisia in nine patients with PD. Furthermore, three patients experienced a remarkable improvement in parkinsonian rest tremor and in five the confusional state that accompanied akathisia also disappeared [152].

Studies evaluating a possible relationship between akathisia and PD

Surprisingly, there are only a few studies that have evaluated akathisia in patients with PD and no studies have evaluated subjective sleep and polysomnographic differences between patients with and without akathisia. In one study, akathisia with an inability to remain still and the need to move throughout the day was reported in 26 of 100 PD subjects [106]. Akathisia started after the initiation of levodopa in most and was not related to the presence of motor fluctuations. In some, levodopa withdrawal produced a transient elimination of symptoms. In another study, 56 consecutive PD patients completed an akathisia questionnaire [153]. Akathisia, defined as the feeling of restlessness related to an urge to move, was found in 21%. Symptoms most frequently affected the legs, and movements were suppressible for brief periods. Akathisia was most frequently related to the dosing of anti-Parkinson medications, and occurred at specific periods during the day. Furthermore, akathisia was associated with a younger age of onset and more severe parkinsonism [154]. A more recent study found that akathisia is one of the most frequent non-motor fluctuations, affecting 56% of patients with motor complications, and associated with the "off" state in 63% [129]. Following DBS STN, this symptom was markedly improved [155]. Although the underlying pathogenic mechanisms of non-motor fluctuations are not well known, the dopaminergic system is probably involved via modulation of other systems (serotonergic, adrenergic), as evidenced by the observation that non-motor fluctuations usually respond to dopaminergic treatment [129].

Summary of the relationship between akathisia and PD

Akathisia may be difficult to recognize in PD patients because they have a wide variety of motor and sensory disturbances associated with the use of dopaminergic agents. However, the occurrence of akathisia in PD has clinical importance and can be a cause of poor clinical outcome in patients chronically treated with dopaminergic agents. Indeed, akathisia may be more frequent in this population than in non-parkinsonian patients treated with dopamine receptor antagonists. It may be that neuroleptic-induced akathisia in schizophrenics and akathisia developing in PD have different pathophysiologic mechanisms and may require different therapeutic approaches. Further investigation is needed.

References

1. Allen R, Picchietti D, Hening W, *et al.* Restless legs syndrome: diagnostic criteria, special considerations, and epidemiology:a report from the restless legs syndrome diagnosis and epidemiology work shop at the National Institutes of Health. *Sleep Med* 2003;**4**:101–19.
2. Hening WA, Allen RP, Chaudhuri KR, *et al.* Clinical significance of RLS. *Mov Disord* 2007;**22**(Suppl 18):S395–400.
3. Benes H, Walters AS, Allen RP, *et al.* Definition of restless legs syndrome, how to diagnose it, and how to differentiate it from RLS mimics. *Mov Disord* 2007;**22**(Suppl 18):S401–8.
4. Hogl B, Zucconi M, Provini F. RLS, PLM, and their differential diagnosis–a video guide. *Mov Disord* 2007;**22**(Suppl 18):S414–9.
5. Garcia-Borreguero D, Egatz R, Winkelmann J. Epidemiology of restless legs syndrome: the current status. *Sleep Med Rev* 2006;**10**:153–67.
6. Allen RP, Earley CJ. The role of iron in restless legs syndrome. *Mov Disord* 2007;**22**(Suppl 18):S440–8.
7. Silber MH, Richardson JW. Multiple blood donations associated with iron deficiency in patients with restless legs syndrome. *Mayo Clin Proc* 2003;**78**(1):52–4.
8. Rottach KG, Schaner BM, Kirch MH, *et al.* Restless legs syndrome as side effect of second generation antidepressants. *J Psychiatr Res* 2008;**43**:70–5.
9. Yang C, White DP, Winkelman JW. Antidepressants and periodic leg movements of sleep. *Biol Psychiatry* 2005;**58**(6):510–4.
10. Kavanagh D, Siddiqui S, Geddes CC. Restless legs syndrome in patients on dialysis. *Am J Kidney Dis* 2004;**43**(5):763–71.
11. Merlino G, Gigli GL, Valente M. Sleep disturbances in dialysis patients. *J Nephrol* 2008;**21**(Suppl 13):S66–70.
12. Wetter TC, Stiasny K, Kohnen R, *et al.* Polysomnographic sleep measures in patients with uremic and idiopathic restless legs syndrome. *Mov Disord* 1998;**13**(5):820–4.
13. Manconi M, Govoni V, De Vito A, *et al.* Restless legs syndrome and pregnancy. *Neurology* 2004;**63**(6):1065–9.
14. Happe S, Reese JP, Stiasny-Kolster K, *et al.* Assessing health-related quality of life in patients with restless legs syndrome. *Sleep Med* 2009;**10**:295–305.
15. Wenning GK, Kiechl S, Seppi K, *et al.* Prevalence of movement disorders in men and women aged 50–89 years (Bruneck Study cohort): a population-based study. *Lancet Neurol* 2005;**4**(12):815–20.
16. Cho YW, Shin WC, Yun CH, *et al.* Epidemiology of restless legs syndrome in Korean adults. *Sleep* 2008;**31**(2):219–23.
17. Berger K, Kurth T. RLS epidemiology – frequencies, risk factors and methods in population studies. *Mov Disord* 2007;**22**(Suppl 18):S420–3.
18. Rangarajan S, Rangarajan S, D'Souza GA. Restless legs syndrome in an Indian urban population. *Sleep Med* 2007;**9**(1):88–93.

19. Hadjigeorgiou GM, Stefanidis I, Dardiotis E, *et al.* Low RLS prevalence and awareness in central Greece: an epidemiological survey. *Eur J Neurol* 2007;**14**(11):1275–80.
20. Vogl FD, Pichler I, Adel S, *et al.* Restless legs syndrome: epidemiological and clinicogenetic study in a South Tyrolean population isolate. *Mov Disord* 2006;**21**(8):1189–95.
21. Castillo PR, Kaplan J, Lin SC, *et al.* Prevalence of restless legs syndrome among native South Americans residing in coastal and mountainous areas. *Mayo Clin Proc* 2006;**81**(10):1345–7.
22. Allen RP, Walters AS, Montplaisir J, *et al.* Restless legs syndrome prevalence and impact: REST General Population Study. *Arch Intern Med* 2005;**165**(11):1286–92.
23. Hogl B, Kiechl S, Willeit J, *et al.* Restless legs syndrome: a community-based study of prevalence, severity, and risk factors. *Neurology* 2005;**64**(11):1920–4.
24. Hening W, Walters AS, Allen RP, *et al.* Impact, diagnosis and treatment of restless legs syndrome (RLS) in a primary care population: the REST (RLS epidemiology, symptoms, and treatment) primary care study. *Sleep Med* 2004;**5**(3): 237–46.
25. Sevim S, Dogu O, Camdeviren H, *et al.* Unexpectedly low prevalence and unusual characteristics of RLS in Mersin, Turkey. *Neurology* 2003;**61**(11):1562–9.
26. Winkelman JW, Finn L, Young T. Prevalence and correlates of restless legs syndrome symptoms in the Wisconsin Sleep Cohort. *Sleep Med* 2006;**7**(7):545–52.
27. Phillips B, Hening W, Britz P, Mannino D. Prevalence and correlates of restless legs syndrome: results from the 2005 National Sleep Foundation Poll. *Chest* 2006;**129**(1):76–80.
28. Phillips B, Young T, Finn L, *et al.* Epidemiology of restless legs symptoms in adults. *Arch Intern Med* 2000;**160**(14): 2137–41.
29. Picchietti D, Allen RP, Walters AS, *et al.* Restless legs syndrome: prevalence and impact in children and adolescents – the Peds REST study. *Pediatrics* 2007;**120**(2):253–66.
30. Konofal E, Cortese S, Marchand M, *et al.* Impact of restless legs syndrome and iron deficiency on attention-deficit/hyperactivity disorder in children. *Sleep Med* 2007; **8**(7–8): 711–5.
31. Lee HB, Hening WA, Allen RP, *et al.* Race and restless legs syndrome symptoms in an adult community sample in east Baltimore. *Sleep Med* 2006;**7**(8):642–5.
32. Picchietti DL, Underwood DJ, Farris WA, *et al.* Further studies on periodic limb movement disorder and restless legs syndrome in children with attention-deficit hyperactivity disorder. *Mov Disord* 1999;**14**(6):1000–7.
33. Picchietti DL, Stevens HE. Early manifestations of restless legs syndrome in childhood and adolescence. *Sleep Med* 2007;**9**(7):770–81.
34. Picchietti MA, Picchietti DL. Restless legs syndrome and periodic limb movement disorder in children and adolescents. *Semin Pediatr Neurol* 2008;**15**(2):91–9.
35. Muhle H, Neumann A, Lohmann-Hedrich K, *et al.* Childhood-onset restless legs syndrome: clinical and genetic features of 22 families. *Mov Disord* 2008;**23**(8):1113–21.
36. Winkelmann J, Polo O, Provini F, *et al.* Genetics of restless legs syndrome (RLS): state-of-the-art and future directions. *Mov Disord* 2007;**22**(Suppl 18):S449–58.
37. Winkelmann J, Muller-Myhsok B, Wittchen HU, *et al.* Complex segregation analysis of restless legs syndrome provides evidence for an autosomal dominant mode of inheritance in early age at onset families. *Ann Neurol* 2002;**52**(3):297–302.
38. Winkelmann J, Schormair B, Lichtner P, et al.Genome-wide association study of restless legs syndrome identifies common variants in three genomic regions. *Nat Genet* 2007;**39**(8):1000–6.
39. Stefansson H, Rye DB, Hicks A, *et al.* A genetic risk factor for periodic limb movements in sleep. *N Engl J Med* 2007;**357**(7):639–47.
40. Winkelmann J, Lichtner P, Schormair B, *et al.* Variants in the neuronal nitric oxide synthase (nNOS, NOS1) gene are associated with restless legs syndrome. *Mov Disord* 2008;**23**(3):350–8.
41. Clemens S, Rye D, Hochman S. Restless legs syndrome: revisiting the dopamine hypothesis from the spinal cord perspective. *Neurology* 2006;**67**(1):125–30.
42. Rye DB. Parkinson's disease and RLS: the dopaminergic bridge. *Sleep Med* 2004;**5**(3):317–28.
43. Trenkwalder C, Paulus W, Walters AS. The restless legs syndrome. *Lancet Neurol* 2005;**4**(8):465–75.
44. Paulus W, Dowling P, Rijsman R, *et al.* Pathophysiological concepts of restless legs syndrome. *Mov Disord* 2007;**22**(10):1451–6.
45. Earley CJ, Connor JR, Beard JL, *et al.* Ferritin levels in the cerebrospinal fluid and restless legs syndrome: effects of different clinical phenotypes. *Sleep* 2005;**28**(9):1069–75.
46. O'Keeffe ST, Gavin K, Lavan JN. Iron status and restless legs syndrome in the elderly. *Age Ageing* 1994;**23**(3): 200–3.
47. Earley CJ, Connor JR, Beard JL, *et al.* Abnormalities in CSF concentrations of ferritin and transferrin in restless legs syndrome. *Neurology* 2000;**54**(8):1698–700.
48. Mizuno S, Mihara T, Miyaoka T, *et al.* CSF iron, ferritin and transferrin levels in restless legs syndrome. *J Sleep Res* 2005;**14**(1):43–7.
49. Connor JR, Wang XS, Patton SM, *et al.* Decreased transferrin receptor expression by neuromelanin cells in restless legs syndrome. *Neurology* 2004;**62**(9):1563–7.
50. Connor JR, Boyer PJ, Menzies SL, *et al.* Neuropathological examination suggests impaired brain iron acquisition in restless legs syndrome. *Neurology* 2003;**61**(3):304–9.
51. Manconi M, Hutchins W, Feroah TR, *et al.* On the pathway of an animal model for restless legs syndrome. *Neurol Sci* 2007;**28**(Suppl 1):S53–60.
52. Ondo WG, He Y, Rajasekaran S, Le WD. Clinical correlates of 6-hydroxydopamine injections into A11 dopaminergic neurons in rats: a possible model for restless legs syndrome. *Mov Disord* 2000;**15**(1):154–8.
53. Qu S, Le W, Zhang X, *et al.* Locomotion is increased in a11-lesioned mice with iron deprivation: a possible animal model for restless legs syndrome. *J Neuropathol Exp Neurol* 2007;**66**(5):383–8.
54. Zhao H, Zhu W, Pan T, *et al.* Spinal cord dopamine receptor expression and function in mice with 6-OHDA lesion of the A11 nucleus and dietary iron deprivation. *J Neurosci Res* 2007;**85**(5):1065–76.

55. Desautels A, Turecki G, Montplaisir J, *et al.* Dopaminergic neurotransmission and restless legs syndrome: a genetic association analysis. *Neurology* 2001;**57**(7):1304–6.
56. Tribl GG, Asenbaum S, Klosch G, *et al.* Normal IPT and IBZM SPECT in drug naive and levodopa-treated idiopathic restless legs syndrome. *Neurology* 2002;**59**(4):649–50.
57. Eisensehr I, Wetter TC, Linke R, *et al.* Normal IPT and IBZM SPECT in drug-naive and levodopa-treated idiopathic restless legs syndrome. *Neurology* 2001;**57**(7):1307–9.
58. Trenkwalder C, Walters AS, Hening WA, *et al.* Positron emission tomographic studies in restless legs syndrome. *Mov Disord* 1999;**14**(1):141–5.
59. Linke R, Eisensehr I, Wetter TC, *et al.* Presynaptic dopaminergic function in patients with restless legs syndrome: are there common features with early Parkinson's disease? *Mov Disord* 2004;**19**(10):1158–62.
60. Ondo WG, Zhao HR, Le WD. Animal models of restless legs syndrome. *Sleep Med* 2007;**8**(4):344–8.
61. Oertel WH, Trenkwalder C, Zucconi M, *et al.* State of the art in restless legs syndrome therapy: practice recommendations for treating restless legs syndrome. *Mov Disord* 2007;**22**(Suppl 18):S466–75.
62. Oertel WH, Benes H, Garcia-Borreguero D, *et al.* Efficacy of rotigotine transdermal system in severe restless legs syndrome: a randomized, double-blind, placebo-controlled, six-week dose-finding trial in Europe. *Sleep Med* 2008;**9**(3): 228–39.
63. Trenkwalder C, Benes H, Grote L, *et al.* Cabergoline compared to levodopa in the treatment of patients with severe restless legs syndrome: results from a multi-center, randomized, active controlled trial. *Mov Disord* 2007;**22**(5):696–703.
64. Bogan RK, Fry JM, Schmidt MH, *et al.* Ropinirole in the treatment of patients with restless legs syndrome: a US-based randomized, double-blind, placebo-controlled clinical trial. *Mayo Clin Proc* 2006;**81**(1):17–27.
65. Oertel WH, Benes H, Bodenschatz R, *et al.* Efficacy of cabergoline in restless legs syndrome: a placebo-controlled study with polysomnography (CATOR). *Neurology* 2006;**67**(6):1040–6.
66. Walters AS, Ondo WG, Dreykluft T, *et al.* Ropinirole is effective in the treatment of restless legs syndrome. TREAT RLS 2: a 12-week, double-blind, randomized, parallel-group, placebo-controlled study. *Mov Disord* 2004;**19**(12):1414–23.
67. Oertel WH, Stiasny-Kolster K, Bergtholdt B, *et al.* Efficacy of pramipexole in restless legs syndrome: a six-week, multicenter, randomized, double-blind study (effect-RLS study). *Mov Disord* 2007;**22**(2):213–9.
68. Partinen M, Hirvonen K, Jama L, *et al.* Efficacy and safety of pramipexole in idiopathic restless legs syndrome: a polysomnographic dose-finding study – the PRELUDE study. *Sleep Med* 2006;**7**(5):407–17.
69. Winkelman JW, Sethi KD, Kushida CA, *et al.* Efficacy and safety of pramipexole in restless legs syndrome. *Neurology* 2006;**67**(6):1034–9.
70. Montplaisir J. Nicolas A, Denesle R, Gomez-Mancilla B. Restless legs syndrome improved by pramipexole: a double-blind randomized trial. *Neurology* 1999;**52**(5):938–43.
71. Allen R, Becker PM, Bogan R, *et al.* Ropinirole decreases periodic leg movements and improves sleep parameters in patients with restless legs syndrome. *Sleep* 2004;**27**(5): 907–14.
72. Trenkwalder C, Hundemer HP, Lledo A, *et al.* Efficacy of pergolide in treatment of restless legs syndrome: the PEARLS Study. *Neurology* 2004;**62**(8):1391–7.
73. Driver-Dunckley ED, Noble BN, Hentz JG, *et al.* Gambling and increased sexual desire with dopaminergic medications in restless legs syndrome. *Clin Neuropharmacol* 2007;**30**(5):249–55.
74. Garcia-Borreguero D, Allen RP, Kohnen R, *et al.* Diagnostic standards for dopaminergic augmentation of restless legs syndrome: report from a World Association of Sleep Medicine – International Restless Legs Syndrome Study Group consensus conference at the Max Planck Institute. *Sleep Med* 2007;**8**(5):520–30.
75. Paulus W, Trenkwalder C. Less is more: pathophysiology of dopaminergic-therapy-related augmentation in restless legs syndrome. *Lancet Neurol* 2006;**5**(10):878–86.
76. Allen RP, Earley CJ. Augmentation of the restless legs syndrome with carbidopa/levodopa. *Sleep* 1996;**19**(3):205–13.
77. Happe S, Trenkwalder C. Role of dopamine receptor agonists in the treatment of restless legs syndrome. *CNS Drugs* 2004;**18**(1):27–36.
78. Ferini-Strambi L. Restless legs syndrome augmentation and pramipexole treatment. *Sleep Med* 2002;**3**(Suppl):S23–5.
79. Silber MH, Shepard JW Jr, Wisbey JA. Pergolide in the management of restless legs syndrome: an extended study. *Sleep* 1997;**20**(10):878–82.
80. Trenkwalder C, Hogl B, Benes H, Kohnen R. Augmentation in restless legs syndrome is associated with low ferritin. *Sleep Med* 2008;**9**(5):572–4.
80a. Garcia-Borreguero D, Larrosa O, Williams AM, *et al.* Treatment of restless legs syndrome with pregabalin: a double-blind, placebo-controlled study. *Neurology* 2010;**74**:1897–904.
81. Ondo WG, Vuong KD, Jankovic J. Exploring the relationship between Parkinson disease and restless legs syndrome. *Arch Neurol* 2002;**59**(3):421–4.
82. Garcia-Borreguero D, Odin P, Serrano C. Restless legs syndrome and PD: a review of the evidence for a possible association. *Neurology* 2003;**61**(6 Suppl 3):S49–55.
83. Poewe W, Hogl B. Akathisia, restless legs and periodic limb movements in sleep in Parkinson's disease. *Neurology* 2004;**63**(8 Suppl 3):S12–6.
84. Tan EK. Restless legs syndrome and Parkinson's disease: is there an etiologic link? *J Neurol* 2006;**253**(Suppl 7):VII33–7.
85. Langston JW. The Parkinson's complex: parkinsonism is just the tip of the iceberg. *Ann Neurol* 2006;**59**(4):591–6.
86. Poewe W. Non-motor symptoms in Parkinson's disease. *Eur J Neurol* 2008;**15**(Suppl 1):14–20.
87. Loo HV, Tan EK. Case–control study of restless legs syndrome and quality of sleep in Parkinson's disease. *J Neurol Sci* 2008;**266**(1–2):145–9.
88. Adel S, Djarmati A, Kabakci K, *et al.* Co-occurrence of restless legs syndrome and *Parkin* mutations in two families. *Mov Disord* 2006;**21**(2):258–63.
89. Iranzo A, Comella CL, Santamaria J, Oertel W. Restless legs syndrome in Parkinson's disease and other neurodegenerative diseases of the central nervous system. *Mov Disord* 2007;**22**(Suppl 18):S424–30.

90. Jellinger KA. Post mortem studies in Parkinson's disease – is it possible to detect brain areas for specific symptoms? *J Neural Transm Suppl* 1999;**56**:1–29.
91. Pittock SJ, Parrett T, Adler CH, *et al.* Neuropathology of primary restless leg syndrome: absence of specific tau- and alpha-synuclein pathology. *Mov Disord* 2004;**19**(6): 695–9.
92. Allen RP, Barker PB, Wehrl F, *et al.* MRI measurement of brain iron in patients with restless legs syndrome. *Neurology* 2001;**56**(2):263–5.
93. Schmidauer C, Sojer M, Seppi K, *et al.* Transcranial ultrasound shows nigral hypoechogenicity in restless legs syndrome. *Ann Neurol* 2005;**58**(4):630–4.
94. Walters AS, LeBrocq C, Passi V, *et al.* A preliminary look at the percentage of patients with restless legs syndrome who also have Parkinson disease, essential tremor or Tourette syndrome in a single practice. J Sleep Res 2003;**12**(4):343–5.
95. Vilarino-Guell C, Soto AI, Young JE, *et al.* Susceptibility genes for restless legs syndrome are not associated with Parkinson disease. *Neurology* 2008;**71**(3):222–3.
96. Wetter TC, Collado-Seidel V, Pollmacher T, *et al.* Sleep and periodic leg movement patterns in drug-free patients with Parkinson's disease and multiple system atrophy. *Sleep* 2000;**23**(3):361–7.
97. Iranzo A, Santamaria J, Rye DB, *et al.* Characteristics of idiopathic REM sleep behavior disorder and that associated with MSA and PD. *Neurology* 2005;**65**(2):247–52.
98. Kumru H, Santamaria J, Tolosa E, *et al.* Rapid eye movement sleep behavior disorder in parkinsonism with parkin mutations. *Ann Neurol* 2004;**56**(4):599–603.
99. Hornyak M, Feige B, Riemann D, Voderholzer U. Periodic leg movements in sleep and periodic limb movement disorder: prevalence, clinical significance and treatment. *Sleep Med Rev* 2006;**10**(3):169–77.
100. Happe S, Pirker W, Klosch G, *et al.* Periodic leg movements in patients with Parkinson's disease are associated with reduced striatal dopamine transporter binding. *J Neurol* 2003;**250**(1):83–6.
101. Iranzo A, Valldeoriola F, Santamaria J, *et al.* Sleep symptoms and polysomnographic architecture in advanced Parkinson's disease after chronic bilateral subthalamic stimulation. *J Neurol Neurosurg Psychiatry* 2002;**72**(5):661–4.
102. Garcia-Borreguero D, Egatz R, Winkelmann J, Berger K. Epidemiology of restless legs syndrome: the current status. *Sleep Med Rev* 2006;**10**(3):153–67.
103. de Lau LM, Breteler MM. Epidemiology of Parkinson's disease. *Lancet Neurol* 2006;**5**(6):525–35.
104. Kedia S, Moro E, Tagliati M, *et al.* Emergence of restless legs syndrome during subthalamic stimulation for Parkinson disease. *Neurology* 2004;**63**(12):2410–2.
105. Driver-Dunckley E, Evidente VG, Adler CH, *et al.* Restless legs syndrome in Parkinson's disease patients may improve with subthalamic stimulation. *Mov Disord* 2006;**21**(8): 1287–9.
106. Lang AE, Johnson K. Akathisia in idiopathic Parkinson's disease. *Neurology* 1987;**37**(3):477–81.
107. Braga-Neto P, da Silva-Junior FP, Sueli Monte F, *et al.* Snoring and excessive daytime sleepiness in Parkinson's disease. *J Neurol Sci* 2004;**217**(1):41–5.
108. Khan SA, Sahota PK. A study to look for the incidence of restless legs sydnrome in patients with Parkinon's disease. *Sleep Med* 2002;**25**(Suppl):A378–9.
109. Peralta CM, Wolf E, Seppi K, *et al.* Restless legs in idiopathic Parkinon's disease. *Mov Disord* 2005;**20**(Suppl 10):S108.
110. Gomez-Esteban JC, Zarranz JJ, Tijero B, *et al.* Restless legs syndrome in Parkinson's disease. *Mov Disord* 2007;**22**(13):1912–6.
110a. Calzetti S, Negrotti A, Bonavina G, Angelini M, Marchesi E. Absence of comorbidity of Parkinson disease and restless legs syndrome: a case-control study in patients attending a movement disorder clinic. *Neurol Sci* 2009;**30**:119–22.
110b. Peralta CM, Frauscher B, Seppi K, *et al.* Restless legs syndrome in Parkinson's disease. *Mov Disord* 2009;**24**:2076–80.
110c. Verbaan D, Rooden SM, van Hilten J, Rijsman RM. Prevalence and clinical profile of restless legs syndrome in Parkinson's disease. *Mov Disord* 2010;**25**:2142–7.
111. Krishnan PR, Bhatia M, Behari M. Restless legs syndrome in Parkinson's disease: a case-controlled study. *Mov Disord* 2003;**18**(2):181–5.
112. Nomura T, Inoue Y, Miyake M, *et al.* Prevalence and clinical characteristics of restless legs syndrome in Japanese patients with Parkinson's disease. *Mov Disord* 2006;**21**(3):380–4.
113. Tan EK, Lum SY, Wong MC. Restless legs syndrome in Parkinson's disease. *J Neurol Sci* 2002;**196**(1–2): 33–6.
113a. Lee JE, Shin HW, Kim KS, Sohn YH. Factors contributing to the development of restless legs syndrome in patients with Parkinson's disease. *Mov Disord* 2009;**24**;579–82.
114. Nomura T, Inoue Y, Nakashima K. Clinical characteristics of Restless legs syndrome in patients with Parkinson's disease. *J Neurol Sci* 2006;**250**(1–2):39–44.
115. Look HV, Tan EK. Case-control study of restless legs syndrome and quality of sleep in Parkinon's disease. *J Neurol Sci* 2008;**266**:145–9.
116. Schols L, Haan J, Riess O, *et al.* Sleep disturbance in spinocerebellar ataxias: is the SCA3 mutation a cause of restless legs syndrome? *Neurology* 1998;**51**(6):1603–7.
117. Hodge JR. Akathisia: the syndrome of motor restlessness. *Am J Psychiatry* 1959;**116**:337–8.
118. Sachdev P, Longragan C. The present status of akathisia. *J Nerv Ment Dis* 1991;**179**(7):381–91.
119. Walters AS, Hening W, Rubinstein M, Chokroverty S. A clinical and polysomnographic comparison of neuroleptic-induced akathisia and the idiopathic restless legs syndrome. *Sleep* 1991;**14**(4):339–45.
120. Inami Y, Horiguchi J, Nishimatsu O. A polysomnographic study on periodic limb movements in patients with restless legs sydnrome and neuroleptic-induced akathisia. *Hiroshima J Med Sci* 1997;**46**:133–41.
121. Yamashita H, Horiguchi J, Mizuno S, *et al.* A case of neuroleptic-induced unilateral akathisia with periodic limb movements in the opposite side during sleep. *Psychiatr Clin Neurosci* 1999;**53**:291–3.
122. Barnes TR. A rating scale for drug-induced akathisia. *Br J Psychiatry* 1989;**154**:672–6.
123. Wirshing WC. Movement disorders associated with neuroleptic treatment. *J Clin Psychiatry* 2001;**62**(Suppl 21):15–8.
124. Jimenez-Jimenez FJ, Garcia-Ruiz PJ, Molina JA. Drug-induced movement disorders. *Drug Saf* 1997;**16**(3):180–204.

125. Sachdev P, Kruk J. Clinical characteristics and predisposing factors in acute drug-induced akathisia. *Arch Gen Psychiatry* 1994;**51**(12):963–74.
126. Sachdev PS. Neuroleptic-induced movement disorders: an overview. *Psychiatr Clin North Am* 2005;**28**(1):255–74.
127. Winkelmann J. Genetics of restless legs syndrome. *Curr Neurol Neurosci Rep* 2008;**8**(3):211–6.
128. Eichhammer P, Albus M, Borrmann-Hassenbach M, *et al.* Association of dopamine D3-receptor gene variants with neuroleptic induced akathisia in schizophrenic patients: a generalization of Steen's study on DRD3 and tardive dyskinesia. *Am J Med Genet* 2000;**96**(2):187–91.
129. Witjas T, Kaphan E, Azulay JP, *et al.* Nonmotor fluctuations in Parkinson's disease: frequent and disabling. *Neurology* 2002;**59**(3):408–13.
130. Walters A, Hening W, Chokroverty S, Fahn S. Opioid responsiveness in patients with neuroleptic-induced akathisia. *Mov Disord* 1986;**1**(2):119–27.
131. Walters AS, Hening A. Opioids a better treatment for acute than tardive akathisia: possible role for the endogenous opiate system in neuroleptic-induced akathisia. *Med Hypotheses* 1989;**28**(1):1–2.
132. Kutcher S, Williamson P, MacKenzie S, *et al.* Successful clonazepam treatment of neuroleptic-induced akathisia in older adolescents and young adults: a double-blind, placebo-controlled study. *J Clin Psychopharmacol* 1989;**9**(6):403–6.
133. Boghen D, Lamothe L, Elie R, *et al.* The treatment of the restless legs syndrome with clonazepam: a prospective controlled study. *Can J Neurol Sci* 1986;**13**(3):245–7.
134. Walters AS, Winkelmann J, Trenkwalder C, *et al.* Long-term follow-up on restless legs syndrome patients treated with opioids. *Mov Disord* 2001;**16**(6):1105–9.
135. Adler LA, Angrist B, Weinreb H, Rotrosen J. Studies on the time course and efficacy of beta-blockers in neuroleptic-induced akathisia and the akathisia of idiopathic Parkinson's disease. *Psychopharmacol Bull* 1991;**27**(2):107–11.
136. Lipinski JF Jr, Zubenko GS, Cohen BM, Barreira PJ. Propranolol in the treatment of neuroleptic-induced akathisia. *Am J Psychiatry* 1984;**141**(3):412–5.
137. Lipinski JF Jr, Mallya G, Zimmerman P, Pope HG Jr. Fluoxetine-induced akathisia: clinical and theoretical implications. *J Clin Psychiatry* 1989;**50**(9):339–42.
138. Sachdev P. The epidemiology of drug-induced akathisia: Part I. Acute akathisia. *Schizophr Bull* 1995;**21**(3):431–49.
139. Harada T, Sakamoto K, Ishigooka J. Incidence and predictors of activation syndrome induced by antidepressants. *Depress Anxiety* 2008;**25**:1014–9.
140. Gibb WR, Lees AJ. The clinical phenomenon of akathisia. *J Neurol Neurosurg Psychiatry* 1986;**49**(8):861–6.
141. Chow LY, Chung D, Leung V, *et al.* Suicide attempt due to metoclopramide-induced akathisia. *Int J Clin Pract* 1997;**51**(5):330–1.
142. Janno S, Holi M, Tuisku K, Wahlbeck K. Prevalence of neuroleptic-induced movement disorders in chronic schizophrenia inpatients. *Am J Psychiatry* 2004;**161**(1):160–3.
143. Iqbal N, Lambert T, Masand P. Akathisia: problem of history or concern of today. *CNS Spectr* 2007;**12**(9 Suppl 14):1–13.
144. Brown KW, Glen SE, White T. Low serum iron status and akathisia. *Lancet* 1987;i(8544):1234–6.
145. O'Loughlin V, Dickie AC, Ebmeier KP. Serum iron and transferrin in acute neuroleptic induced akathisia. *J Neurol Neurosurg Psychiatry* 1991;**54**(4):363–4.
146. Hofmann M, Seifritz E, Botschev C, *et al.* Serum iron and ferritin in acute neuroleptic akathisia. *Psychiatry Res* 2000;**93**(3):201–7.
147. Kuloglu M, Atmaca M, Ustundag B, *et al.* Serum iron levels in schizophrenic patients with or without akathisia. *Eur Neuropsychopharmacol* 2003;**13**(2):67–71.
148. Cotter PE, O'Keeffe ST. Improvement in neuroleptic-induced akathisia with intravenous iron treatment in a patient with iron deficiency. *J Neurol Neurosurg Psychiatry* 2007;**78**(5):548.
149. Gold R, Lenox RH. Is there a rationale for iron supplementation in the treatment of akathisia? A review of the evidence. *J Clin Psychiatry* 1995;**56**(10):476–83.
150. Spivak B, Mester R, Abesgaus J, *et al.* Clozapine treatment for neuroleptic-induced tardive dyskinesia, parkinsonism, and chronic akathisia in schizophrenic patients. *J Clin Psychiatry* 1997;**58**(7):318–22.
151. Prueter C, Habermeyer B, Norra C, Kosinski CM. Akathisia as a side effect of antipsychotic treatment with quetiapine in a patient with Parkinson's disease. *Mov Disord* 2003;**18**(6):712–3.
152. Linazasoro G, Marti Masso JF, Suarez JA. Nocturnal akathisia in Parkinson's disease: treatment with clozapine. *Mov Disord* 1993;**8**(2):171–4.
153. Braude WM, Barnes TR, Gore SM. Clinical characteristics of akathisia. A systematic investigation of acute psychiatric inpatient admissions. *Br J Psychiatry* 1983;**143**:139–50.
154. Comella CL, Goetz CG. Akathisia in Parkinson's disease. *Mov Disord* 1994;**9**(5):545–9.
155. Witjas T, Kaphan E, Regis J, *et al.* Effects of chronic subthalamic stimulation on nonmotor fluctuations in Parkinson's disease. *Mov Disord* 2007;**22**(12):1729–34.

Chapter 31 Speech and Voice Disorders in Parkinson's Disease

Lorraine Ramig[1], *Cynthia Fox*[1], *& Shimon Sapir*[2]
[1]Department of Speech, Language and Hearing Science, University of Colorado–Boulder and the National Center for Voice and Speech–Denver, CO, USA
[2]Faculty of Social Welfare and Health Sciences, University of Haifa, Haifa, Israel

Incidence and impact of speech and voice disorders in Parkinson's disease

Nearly 90% of individuals with Parkinson disease (PD) develop speech and voice disorders (dysarthria) during the course of their disease [1]. These can be among the earliest symptoms of PD [1–6] and progress throughout the course of the disease [5]. Speech and voice disorders have deleterious effects on communication, health, psychologic well-being, and quality-of-life [7–13], and are considered to be an important source of disability by many patients and their families [9,11,14,15]. Unfortunately, current pharmacologic and surgical interventions have limited effects on speech and voice disorders [16–18]. Without access to effective speech treatment, affected individuals often retire early, are forced to give up activities they enjoy, incur substantial medical costs, and have increased mortality [19–21].

Classic characteristics

Reduced vocal loudness (hypophonia), reduced pitch inflection (monotone), and breathy or hoarse voice are the main characteristics of disordered voice in PD [22–37]. Imprecise articulation may appear after the emergence of voice abnormalities and in advanced disease [1,3,5,36]; however, there is preliminary evidence for abnormal vowel articulation even at early stages of the disease [6,38]. Some patients present a tendency for speech articulation to festinate (rush), and to become hesitant and/or dysfluent [39,40]. These speech and voice disorders are collectively termed *hypokinetic dysarthria*.

Assessment

Speech and voice disorders in PD are commonly diagnosed by a speech clinician using a combination of perceptual, acoustic, and physiologic measures. These may be sensitive to disorders across all subsystems of speech production, including respiration, phonation, articulation, velopharyngeal function, and coordination of these subsystems. *Perceptual* analyses of speech are commonly used in clinical practice and research studies of PD [41,42]. Such analyses include listeners' rating of pitch, loudness, voice quality, articulation, and impact on speech intelligibility and functional communication [42,43]. An alternative, or complementary, method is *acoustic analysis* of the speech signal. Acoustic analysis can potentially provide an objective, quantitative, noninvasive, reliable, valid, and precise means to index the severity and characteristics of speech disorders in PD, and to monitor changes associated with treatment [6,44,45]. These include measures of vocal sound pressure level (vocal SPL), voice fundamental frequency, phonatory stability (jitter, shimmer, harmonics to noise ratio) and articulatory acoustics (e.g., formant frequencies) [6,38,44–48]. *Physiologic measures*, which can provide information about the movements underlying speech and voice disorders, include videostroboscopic measures of vocal fold closure [49], kinematic measures of lip, jaw, and respiratory movements [50–52], and electromyographic measures of muscle activity [53,54]. Taken together, these measures can provide a comprehensive, quantitative and qualitative description of speech and voice production of individuals with PD during the course of their disease and in response to various treatments.

Speech production in PD tends to vary according to the speaking task and environment [55–58]. Therefore, it is essential that speech and voice be evaluated across a range of tasks, including sustained vowel phonation, syllable repetition, reading aloud, and spontaneous speech. Although individuals with PD may be heard and understood in the quiet medical examination room, this situation is likely not representative of the patients' spontaneous speech production in daily living. Hence optimal

Parkinson's Disease: Non-Motor and Non-Dopaminergic Features, First Edition. Edited by C. Warren Olanow, Fabrizio Stocchi, and Anthony E. Lang.

assessment of speech functions requires testing with a variety of tasks that provide insight into both any breakdown in subsystems of speech production while simultaneously evaluating speech that is representative of functional daily communication.

Origin of speech and voice disorders in PD

Traditionally, speech disorders in PD have been attributed to dopamine deficiency and muscle rigidity. There is electromyographic evidence for hypertonicity of laryngeal muscles at rest in PD [59], and some evidence for improved respiratory function, prosodic pitch, loudness variation, and speech intelligibility with levodopa treatment [60–62]. However, other studies have failed to find a causal relationship between dopamine and speech disorders in PD [63], and it has been suggested that, in contrast to the classic motor features of PD, speech disturbances may be due to altered non-dopaminergic or special dopaminergic mechanisms, which impair internal cueing, sensorimotor gating, scaling of movement parameters, and attention to action, resulting in poor regulation of speech initiation, amplitude, and timing [5,64–68].

Currently, four pathologic mechanisms have been implicated in the speech and voice disorders in PD: (1) *motor problems* (hypokinesia/bradykinesia, deficits in scaling movement force and amplitude), (2) *sensory problems* (self-perception of voice, abnormal sensorimotor gating), (3) *cueing* (inability to cue internally), and (4) *neuropsychologic problems* (attention to action, vocal vigilance) [16,18,54,69].

Motor problems

Several studies have demonstrated a reduced range of respiratory, laryngeal, and orofacial movements during speech, with a tendency for the movements to decay (become more hypokinetic) or later in the disease to festinate (rush) during an utterance [55,57,58,70,71]. These are likely to manifest as decaying of vocal loudness, intonation, and precision of speech, resulting in reduced speech intelligibility [70,72]. When individuals with PD are asked to perform maximum duration sustained vowel phonations or a diadochokinetic speech task such as repeating a word or a syllable at a rapid rate, vocal loudness may decrease and decay and articulatory movements may become markedly smaller in amplitude [57,71]. In contrast, when individuals with PD are asked (externally cued) to speak loudly and clearly, speech is much louder and articulatory movements increase in amplitude and precision [73], prosodic pitch inflection increases and becomes more effective in imparting linguistic and emotive information, and pauses between words increase [73,74]. These phenomena suggest that under-scaling of movement amplitude, alone or in combination with timing abnormalities, underlies abnormal speech in PD. The observation that under-scaling may "disappear" with external cuing (discussed later) suggests that hypokinesia may reflect a more complex, sensorimotor, and neuropsychologic phenomenon than simply a scale-down of movement amplitude. While the pathologic mechanisms for the under-scaling of vocal and articulatory movement amplitude are not clear, they are likely to be similar to those associated with handwriting (micrographia) and gait (small, shuffling steps) [71].

Sensory problems

Numerous investigators have documented sensorimotor deficits in the orofacial system [75–78] and abnormal auditory, temporal, and perceptual processing of voice and speech [58,77–83]. These abnormalities have been implicated as important etiologic factors in the speech and voice impairment associated with PD [84]. Behavioral evidence for altered sensory processing in PD includes errors on tasks of kinesthesia [85–87], difficulties with orofacial perception, including decreased jaw proprioception, tactile localization on tongue, gums, and teeth, and targeted and tracking head movements to perioral stimulation [77], problems utilizing proprioceptive information for normal movement [77,86], and abnormal higher order processing of afferent information as demonstrated by abnormal reflex and voluntary motor responses to proprioceptive input [88]. Thus, disordered speech and voice in PD might relate to complex deficits in the utilization of specific sensory inputs to organize and guide speech movements.

The inability to scale adequately movement amplitude in speech and nonspeech functions in PD is probably linked to deficits in sensory processing and sensorimotor gating. Demirci *et al.* [89,90] have suggested that individuals with PD have problem with kinesthesia and that when they match their effort to kinesthetic feedback, they under-scale their movement, resulting in hypokinesia. It has been suggested that basal ganglia–thalamic excitatory circuits inadequately activate cortical motor centers and, as a result, motor neuron pools are not provided with adequate activation; hence movements are small and weak [91,92]. It has been proposed that the defect in motor cortex activation in PD is due to a perceptual failure to select the muscle commands to match the external force and speed requirements [93]. Collectively, these explanations implicate abnormal sensorimotor processing in hypokinetic movements secondary to basal ganglia dysfunction.

Recently, problems in sensory perception of effort have been identified as an important focus of successful voice treatment for individuals with PD [94]. Consistent with the foregoing suggestions [91–93], it has been observed that when individuals with PD are asked to produce "loud" speech (i.e., attempt large movements), they can increase their otherwise soft speech to a normal level. However, when they produce louder speech, they complain that they are talking "too loud." Individuals with PD often report that people around them "must need hearing aids" rather than recognizing that their speech is soft.

Ho, Bradshaw, and Iansek [80] contrasted the actual loudness level of speech production with perceived loudness in individuals with PD and hypophonia and in age-matched healthy individuals with normal voice and speech. To assess the ability to regulate and perceive vocal loudness, the subjects were asked to read aloud (without additional instructions) either in a loud voice or in a quiet voice using the same material, and to rate the loudness of their voice immediately after speaking, and at a later time by hearing their voice recorded on tape. These perceptual ratings were compared with the actual speech loudness (SPL) produced in reading and conversation tasks. There was less difference between patients' production and perception of speech loudness compared with those of the controls. Also, even though they spoke with a softer voice than the controls, they perceived their own speech (when it was rated immediately after speaking and later upon hearing recorded speech) to be louder than did the control subjects. PD patients also overestimated the loudness of their speech during both reading and conversation. These findings suggested that hypophonia is either the result of an abnormal perceptual mechanism, or the perceptual system is abnormal due to the generation of quiet speech.

Problems with self-perception of vocal loudness may also be related to motor-to-sensory cortical gating mechanisms. Studies have demonstrated that speech is associated with inhibitory influences on neuronal activity in the auditory cortex via cortical feed-forward, motor-to-sensory corollary efferent mechanisms [95]. Dysfunction of such feed-forward mechanisms has been documented in individuals with schizophrenia, and has been linked to inner speech and auditory hallucinations [96]. Studies using positron emission tomography (PET) and evoked response potentials (ERPs) have demonstrated the presence of abnormal (excessive) auditory cortex activity during speech in individuals with PD, suggesting abnormal collateral gating of auditory neurons [97]. This abnormality can be partially reversed (reduction in excessive auditory activity) in response to intensive voice treatment (see below) in parallel with improvements in voice and speech function and dopaminergic activity in the striatofrontal network. Importantly, this motor-to-sensory feed-forward mechanism is not specific to vocal and auditory systems, and can involve other sensory systems relevant to speech [98].

Deficits in internal cueing

The speech of individuals with PD can improve dramatically with external cueing (stimulation), such as instructing them to "speak loudly," which may compensate for deficits in internal cueing [99]. Ho and colleagues found that people with PD failed to increase or decrease vocal loudness adequately in response to implicit cues such as changes in auditory feedback from their own voice or changes in background noise [79,81]. However, when given explicit cues to increase loudness, they performed as well as healthy controls. These findings suggest an impairment with online or autophonic scaling of loudness in PD; an impairment that can be over-ridden, in the short term, with explicit (external) cueing. This hypophonic impairment is analogous to micrographic handwriting. When individuals with PD are asked to write so that the letters touch a series of dots (external cues), or when the word "big" is spoken to them (another external cue), their handwriting improves dramatically, but only during the short time that they are exposed to and/or immediately after the cue is given [100]. It is interesting to speculate on why individuals who improve speech dramatically with external cueing cannot maintain this improvement. Sensory and neuropsychologic problems are a likely explanation.

Neuropsychologic problems

The term *vocal vigilance* might be defined as the ability to pay attention to, and self-monitor, speech motor output and vocal effort as a means to ensure optimal spoken communication. Attention to action requires an intact sensorimotor mechanism, feed-back and feed-forward mechanisms, attention, working memory, adaptive responses to environmental demands, and other executive functions. The difference between a normal or near normal capacity for speech with external cuing in a PD patient versus what they produce spontaneously is most likely related to the inability of these individuals to attend to their abnormal speech output and self-correct to ensure optimal speech audibility and intelligibility. It has been demonstrated that individuals with PD, like those with Alzheimer's disease, are severely impaired in their ability to self-correct speech errors [101]. This has been attributed to attentional and frontal dysfunction [101]. Rowe *et al.* [102] compared individuals with PD with healthy controls in their ability to attend to their own motor action or to a visual distracter task. Using functional MRI, they found that in both groups, the motor task activated a distributed network that included pre-motor, motor, and parietal cortex, striatum, and cerebellum. However, in the healthy controls, but not in the individuals with PD, attention to own action, but not to the visual distractor task, increased effective connectivity between prefrontal cortex and both the lateral pre-motor cortex and the supplementary motor area. They attributed this attention to action deficit to "a context-specific functional disconnection between the prefrontal cortex and the supplementary and pre-motor cortex in Parkinson's disease" (p. 276). These findings are in line with Brown and Marsden's assertion [103] that "the basal ganglia support a basic attentional mechanism operating to bind input to output in the executive forebrain. Such focused attention provides the automatic link between voluntary effort, sensory input, and the calling up and operation of a sequence of motor programmes or thoughts" (p. 1801). There is some evidence that deficits in attention to action may be associated with non-dopaminergic mechanisms [104], which might explain why levodopa improves speech only partially, if at all, in individuals with hypophonia and hypokinetic dysarthric secondary to PD. Collectively, these findings strongly implicate the role of attention to action, supervisory, and other self-regulatory function, in addition to other executive functions, in the pathophysiology of impaired speech associated with PD. These neuropsychologic abnormalities are most likely mediated by the striatofrontal network, alone or in combination with the parietal, limbic, and thalamic network.

Although deficits in vocal vigilance may be directly related to hypokinetic dysarthria, they might be an epiphenomenon. Azulay, Mesure, and Blin [105] have argued, based on empirical evidence, that attentional processing might be part of a compensatory mechanism intended to alleviate automaticity in locomotion, bypassing the deficit of internal cueing. Obviously, if attention to action is impaired, the ability to compensate for impairment in the central motor mechanisms (e.g., scaling movement amplitude and internal cueing) must also be impaired. Importantly, deficits in attention to action and executive functions can be partially alleviated in individuals with PD by intensive training of cognitive executive function [106]. Hence it is reasonable to expect that intensive training in vocal vigilance (e.g., paying attention to the production of vocal loudness) might result in more effective control of speech output, either by restoring premorbid functions or by compensating for impairment in these functions.

As will be argued later, the LSVT® LOUD regimen may provide such a training to improve vocal loudness and speech functions. Two neural PET studies [107,108] performed before and after LSVT LOUD training show increased activity in right hemisphere networks known to mediate vigilance and attention to action. These data suggest that one therapeutic impact of the LSVT LOUD regimen may be to improve vocal vigilance. This might explain (in addition to the direct effects of motor exercise) why the therapeutic effects of the LSVT LOUD regimen are sustained over months and years [42,109]. In other words, an intensive training such as the LSVT LOUD may result in improved motor function and improved attention to motor function.

Summary of origins of speech and voice disorders in PD

The origins of the speech and voice disorders in individuals with PD are complex and only partially understood. They are likely related to *motor problems* (hypokinesia/bradykinesia reflecting reduced muscle activation, and abnormal scaling or maintenance of the gain of movement amplitude), *sensory processing problems* (abnormal gating of the somatosensory cortex, abnormal gating of the auditory cortex via feed-forward mechanisms, abnormal perception of one's own voice), *cueing problems* (reflecting deficits in internal/implicit cueing), *neuropsychologic problems* (impaired attention to action, vocal vigilance, and self-regulation of vocal output), or some combination. Additional research is needed to explore these etiologic factors and their interaction and contribution to speech impairment in PD. Given the complexity of the origins of the speech and voice disorders in PD, it is not surprising that traditional medical and behavioral treatments have had limited success in managing these problems.

Treatment of speech and voice disorders in PD

In contrast to the marked benefits of dopaminergic therapies on the classic motor features of PD, the magnitude, consistency, and long-term effects of levodopa or dopamine agonists on speech are far from satisfactory [66,110–119]. The impact of deep brain stimulation (DBS) targeting either the globus pallidus or subthalamic nucleus, on speech and voice functioning remains unclear [120,121]. A few pilot studies of non-dopaminergic agents, cranial and subdural repetitive magnetic stimulation, and laryngeal collagen augmentation injections seem to offer some positive, albeit transient, effects on voice and speech. Here we review a select number of medical treatment studies that detail these points.

Effects of dopaminergic therapy on speech

Several studies have documented improvements in various aspects of voice and speech functioning with levodopa or dopamine agonists. These studies have documented a reduction in excessive laryngeal neuromuscular activity, better laryngeal control of voice onset, and vocal fold closure during speech [122], better speech intelligibility [123], greater prosodic voice fundamental frequency (F0) inflection, greater vocal SPL, better voice quality [62,66,124], enhanced lip function during speech and non-speech tasks [125], and less voice tremor [126]. Importantly, although some of these improvements were statistically significant, they often provide limited benefits (e.g., do not improve speaker intelligibility), and were not observed in all individuals with PD. In contrast, numerous studies have failed to find significant improvement in voice and speech functions with levodopa or dopamine agonists [63,67]. These findings have led researchers to suggest that voice and speech disorders in PD might be related, at least partially if not fully, to non-dopaminergic or special dopaminergic mechanisms. In line with this suggestion, one small study documented that clonazepam at doses of 0.25–0.5 mg per day can improve some aspects of speech, such as imprecise consonants, short rushes of speech, and inappropriate silences in individuals with PD [127].

Effects of deep brain stimulation (DBS) on speech

Numerous studies have assessed the effects of DBS of the subthalamic nucleus (STN), ventral intermediate nucleus of the thalamus (Vim), and globus pallidus internus (GPi) on symptoms of PD. DBS of these neural structures has provided significant clinical benefits for individuals with PD. Specifically, stimulation of the Vim can dramatically relieve tremor, and stimulation of the STN and GPi can each reduce motor features of PD [128]. However, the effects of DBS on voice and speech have for the most part been adverse or inconclusive [120,121,129–133]. In general, left-sided stimulation seems to induce more negative effects on prosody, articulation, speech intelligibility, and language function.

In early studies, Gentil and colleagues [134–136] assessed the effects of bilateral DBS in the subthalamic nucleus (STN) on hypokinetic dysarthria in individuals with PD. Using force measurements of the articulatory organs and acoustic analysis, they reported reduced reaction and movement time of the articulatory organs, increased maximal strength and precision of these organs, and improved respiratory and phonatory functions. However, vocal intensity was not changed. In follow-up studies up to 5 years post-bilateral DBS STN [137], dysarthria worsened in spite of improvement in the articulatory forces. Other studies have documented statistically significant, although small, improvements in aspects of speech such as lip movements, voice pitch, loudness, and F0 variability with bilateral DBS STN; however, articulation was not affected and speech intelligibility was slightly reduced in the "on" stimulation condition when patients received levodopa [138,139]. DBS Vim had no effects on speech [136].

In contrast, more recent studies have reported adverse effects of bilateral DBS STN on speech, language, and executive functions [120,121,140]. These adverse effects might be related to the stereotaxic lesion or voltage spread from the stimulating electrode adversely affecting neural networks subserving speech [133,137,141,142].

Effects of transcranial/subdural stimulation on speech

The effect of repetitive transcranial magnetic stimulation (rTMS) on vocal function has been studied in individuals with PD [143]. Stimulation of the primary motor cortex (M1)–mouth area induced a significant improvement in voice F0 and intensity. Unilateral extradural motor cortex stimulation (with a quadripolar electrostimulator attached to the skull) was reported partially to relieve speech, and also tremor, akinesia, standing, anteropulsion, gait, and swallowing, in addition to dyskinesia and psychiatric complications in three individuals with severe PD [144]. Although not all such studies have had comparable results, these two studies suggest that transcortical/transdural stimulation of the motor cortex may have therapeutic effects on voice, speech, and swallowing. Further research is needed to assess the therapeutic effects of brain stimulation on speech and non-speech functions.

Collagen augmentation of the vocal folds for improved phonation

Two studies assessed the effects of collagen augmentation of the vocal folds via percutaneous injection with fiber-optic guidance on phonation in hypophonic individuals with PD [145,146]. Based on postoperative telephone interviews, the majority of the patients reported improved voicing. Poorer outcomes were found in advanced patients with aphonia, difficulty with speech initiation, dysphagia, or ambulatory difficulty. Sewall, Jiang, and Ford [147] used acoustic and perceptual methods, and also the Voice Handicap Index (VHI) questionnaire, to assess prospectively the effects of transoral vocal fold collagen injection on dysphonia in PD subjects. VHI and phonation threshold pressure improved significantly, and pitch and vocal intensity also improved, although not significantly, in five of six patients. The procedure was considered safe and well tolerated. The authors suggested that the procedure allows temporary improvement in phonatory function. Follow-up was for only 10–14 days, so the long-term efficacy of this procedure is difficult to assess [147]. Kim, Kearney, and Atkins [146] retrospectively studied 18 patients with PD who had undergone percutaneous laryngeal collagen augmentation for their hypophonia and incomplete glottic closure. All patients achieved glottic closure with this procedure, and 11 (61%) patients reported improvement in their voice for a period of at least 2 months. The patients who did not consider their voice improved had severe dysphonia, dysphagia, and/or ambulatory ability prior to surgery, and these may have been the reasons for their poor outcome. Duration of speech improvement in the 11 patients ranged from 2 to 8 months (average 3.2 months).

Behavioral speech and voice treatment for PD

In spite of high incidence of voice and speech disorders in individuals with PD, historically only a few of these individuals (3–4%) receive speech therapy [25,27]. This discrepancy might have to do with the fact that in the past treatment outcomes have been disappointing; in terms of both magnitude and long-term maintenance of any therapeutic gains [148–151]. This disappointing outcome has been observed with respect to rate control, prosody, loudness, articulation, respiration, or a combination [152,153]. Devices such as delayed auditory feedback (DAF), voice amplifiers, and pacing boards provide only transient improvement [153–155]. Evidence-based practice (EBP) for behavioral speech therapy [65] and the Academy of Neurologic Communication Disorders and Sciences guidelines [156,157] indicate that LSVT LOUD has the greatest number of positive outcome measures associated with any speech treatment examined to date in people with PD [156,158].

Intensive voice treatment (LSVT LOUD) for PD

In 1988, Ramig *et al.* [159] introduced the Lee Silverman Voice Treatment (LSVT LOUD), a Parkinson-specific approach that trains amplitude (increased vocal loudness) as a single motor control parameter, thereby targeting inadequate scaling of agonist muscle activation. LSVT LOUD also trains individuals with PD to "recalibrate" their motor and perceptual systems so that they are less inclined to under-scale (reduce amplitude) speech movement parameters. It is also geared towards overcoming or compensating for deficits in internal cueing and self-regulation of vocal effort during speech production. The LSVT LOUD trains individuals with PD to attend actively to the amount and effort and loudness required for normal voice. This directly trains vocal vigilance as a part of the sensory recalibration process. Finally, the LSVT LOUD takes advantage of the multisystemic of effects loud phonation on the entire vocal mechanism, namely simultaneous amplification of respiratory, laryngeal, and orofacial agonist muscle activity. This multisystemic upscaling of motor output manifests itself as larger amplitude of speech that more closely resembles normal speech [6,44].

Over the past 20 years, a series of studies have documented that LSVT LOUD increased movement amplitude of the respiratory–laryngeal system in individuals with PD and generated a lasting positive impact on vocal SPL [51,160,161]. These findings were consistent with perceptual data demonstrating improved loudness and voice quality [41,42]. There was no evidence of vocal hyperfunction (i.e., vocal abuse) post-treatment; on the contrary, LSVT LOUD has been shown to reduce laryngeal hyperfunction [162] and improve voice quality [41]. The target in LSVT LOUD is healthy, normal vocal loudness. Patients are not trained to yell or scream or to use pressed voice. There is also videostroboscopic evidence that the phonatory system becomes more efficient in the production of voice following LSVT LOUD, as reflected in the more adequate closure of the vocal folds and larger and more symmetrical movements of the vocal folds [160].

In addition to the direct impact on the respiratory–laryngeal systems following LSVT LOUD, studies have documented distributed effects across the speech production system. Dromey, Ramig, and Johnson [163] reported post-treatment improvements in articulation reflected in measures of transition duration, rate, and extent. Sapir *et al.* [6] compared articulatory acoustics in individuals with PD (treated and untreated) and a healthy control group. Both second formant frequency of /u/ (F2u) and the ratio of F2i and F2u (F2i/F2u) variables improved towards normalcy in participants who received LSVT LOUD and correlated with perceptual improvements in vowel ratings. No such improvement was observed in control groups. Similar findings were obtained by Sapir *et al.* [44] when they used the acoustic metric formant centralization ratio [(F2u + F2a + F1i + F1u)/(F2i + F1a)] and compared individuals with PD who received the LSVT LOUD and the two control groups (untreated patients and healthy controls): The former group, but not the latter groups, showed highly significant changes (indicative of improvement in vowel articulation) due to treatment, with a large effect size.

LSVT LOUD was also shown to improve facial expression in PD patients compared with an alternative treatment which focused on respiration [164–167]. These data underscore the relationship between face and voice in individuals with neurologic disorders [168–171] and suggest that these communicative behaviors may have overlapping neural mechanisms. LSVT LOUD was also demonstrated to improve swallowing of several bolus types using standardized radiographic studies [172]. These studies indicated that the effect of treatment extended to orofacial–swallowing musculature even though the focus of treatment was on respiratory–laryngeal movement amplitude. These studies suggest that the impact of vocal loudness training may go beyond a simple scale-up of respiratory–laryngeal movement amplitude to include the orofacial articulatory and nonspeech orofacial functions (face and swallow), even though these functions were not intentionally targeted.

Brain imaging studies using ^{15}O PET have documented changes in brain function following LSVT LOUD [97,107,108]. Specifically, while pretreatment, cued loud phonation alone activated cortical pre-motor areas, particularly the supplementary motor area (SMA), SMA activity was normalized and activity in the basal ganglia (right putamen) increased post-LSVT LOUD, suggesting a shift from abnormal cortical motor activation towards normal subcortical organization of speech–motor output. Post-LSVT LOUD changes included an increase in activity in right anterior insula and right dorsolateral prefrontal cortex, suggesting recruitment of a phylogenetically old, preverbal communication system that is involved in vocalization and emotive communication. Similarly, excess evoked potential activity in the auditory cortex of PD patients was markedly reduced to near normal levels following LSVT LOUD therapy [97]. These findings may also help to explain how a cross-system, such as swallowing, may be affected by training vocal loudness. They may also elucidate why LSVT LOUD improves voice and speech production in PD as compared with other treatments that have focused on rate or articulation, which involve primarily cortical, phylogenetically newer neural centers. Table 31.1 compares the LSVT LOUD standard protocol with traditional speech therapy.

LSVT LOUD: target, mode, and calibration

Target

The improvements in articulation, facial expression, and swallowing with LSVT LOUD are consistent with the concept of global parameters, whereby a single treatment target impacts common control mechanisms that, in turn, influence motor behaviors beyond the specific targeted function [173–175]. The neurologic bases of such global motor parameters are not known. However, several studies report evidence for neural coupling of orofacial muscles to neural systems of laryngeal and respiratory control in human studies [176–179], possibly due to efferent drive from a common brain region to motor neurons innervating orofacial, laryngeal, and respiratory muscles. Reflexogenic mechanisms may also be part of the coupling between the respiratory, laryngeal, and articulatory systems [177–179]. Another explanation for the distributed and lasting impact of LSVT LOUD is that it involves and stimulates phylogenetically old neural systems, especially the emotive brain. Speech production is a learned, highly practiced motor behavior, with many of its movements regulated in a quasi-automatic fashion [180–182]; loudness scaling is a task that both animals and humans engage in all their lives [79,80,182–185]. Hence the regulation of vocal loudness for speech may involve a phylogenetically old system that has been adapted, through learning, for speech production and comprehension.

Mode

The mode of delivery of LSVT LOUD is different from traditional forms of speech treatment. LSVT LOUD is delivered in a manner consistent with theories of motor learning [186] and skill acquisition, and also principles that drive activity-dependent neural plasticity (e.g., intensity, complexity, saliency) [187]. Therapy is administered four times per week over 4 weeks, each session lasting 50–60 min. In addition, there are daily homework and carryover assignments for the entire month of therapy. This protocol embodies many of the fundamental principles of exercise and motor training that have been shown to promote neural plasticity and brain reorganization in animal models of PD [188] and human stroke-related hemiparesis [189]. Such intensive training, especially when practiced continuously and at the onset of the disease or following brain injury, has been shown to impact molecular changes associated with cell survival, cell growth, and functional recovery which reflect neural plasticity and brain reorganization [107,188,190–192], and challenge the assumption that there is no potential for recovery of function in PD.

Calibration

LSVT LOUD includes a treatment concept called "calibration," which addresses the sensory, internal cueing, and neuropsychologic deficits that occur in PD [84]. Although intensive motor training with a single vocal loudness target is an important aspect of LSVT LOUD, the greatest barrier to generalization outside the treatment room is related to these deficits in sensory, internal cueing, and neuropsychologic functioning. During treatment, patients must be taught to self-recognize the right amount of effort and loudness needed to produce consistently a vocal loudness level that is within normal limits. Typically, this right amount of effort feels "too loud" to an individual and it requires intensive, high-effort speech exercise combined with a simple, redundant, and salient treatment target to learn to apply this loudness in functional daily living. The intensive training (four times per week for 4 weeks) is consistent with principles of motor learning, skill acquisition [193,194], and muscle training [92,93, 195,196], and is also geared to improving attention to action and vocal vigilance. This training may help maintain treatment gains over time. Table 31.2 summarizes some of the proposed principles underlying neural plasticity (column 1) to proposed deficits in Parkinson disease (column 2) and the corresponding rationale and task in LSVT LOUD (column 3).

Technology-enhanced accessibility

There are practical challenges to intensive speech therapy (four individual sessions per week for 4 weeks) necessary for promoting the principles of plasticity. There

Table 31.1 Comparison of LSVT LOUD standard protocol with traditional speech therapy.

LSVT LOUD Ramig *et al.*, 2001 [109]	Traditional speech therapy e.g., Till, Yorkston, Beukelman, 1994 [203]
Intensity: STANDARDIZED *Dosage*: 4 days per week for 4 weeks (16 sessions in 4 weeks) *Repetitions*: Minimum 15 repetitions per task **Effort*: Push for maximum patient-perceived effort each day (8 or 9 on scale of 1–10 with 10 being the most)	**Intensity**: VARIABLE *Dosage*: 2 per week for 4–16 sessions over several months *Repetitions*: Variable per task *Effort*: Moderate to low exertion; reactive to patient response in treatment
Simple focus LOUD Increased movement amplitude directed predominately to respiratory/laryngeal systems	**Complex focus** Voice, respiration, articulation, rate, posture, resonance, orofacial movement, pacing, intonation
Daily tasks first half of the treatment session (25 min) *Task 1: Maximum sustained movements* 15 reps: sustain "ah" in good quality, loud voice as long as possible *Task 2: Directional movements* 15 reps each: say "ah" in loud good quality voice going high in pitch; 15 reps each: say "ah" in loud good quality voice going low in pitch *Task 3: Functional movements* Patient self-identifies 10 phrases or sentences he/she says daily in functional living (e.g., "Good morning"), 5 reps of the list of 10 phrases. "Read phrases using same effort/loudness as you did during the long 'ah' "	**Daily tasks** **1** Variable from therapist to therapist-no standardized protocols **2** Variable from day to day (e.g., one session focus on voice loudness and intonation, next session focus on pacing, next session orofacial movements and posture
Hierarchy second half of the treatment session (25 min) • Designed to train rescaled amplitude/effort of movement achieved in CORE exercises from Daily Tasks into in context specific and variable speaking activities • Incorporate multiple repetitions with a focus on high effort (e.g., list of 20 phrases/sentences repeated 10 times for 200 repetitions) • Tasks increase complexity across weeks (words–phrases–sentences–reading–conversation) and can be tailored to each subjects goals and interests (e.g., golf versus cooking) • Tasks progress in difficulty by increasing duration (maintain LOUD for longer periods of time) amplitude (loudness – within normal limits), and complexity of tasks (dual processing, background noise and attentional distracters)	**Hierarchy** • Speech practice often does not relate back to CORE exercises focused on rescaling effort, strength or some other movement variable • Progression across treatment sessions of increasing complexity of speech tasks, often starting with speech that is more complex than single words • Diffuse focus during practice, for example, think about taking a deep breath, articulate, increase loudness, and/or slow down
Shaping techniques • Train vocal loudness that is healthy (i.e., no unwanted strain or excessive vocal fold closure) • Shape the quality and voice loudness through use of modeling ("do what I do") or tactile/visual cues • Minimal cognitive loading, behavior is not achieved through extensive instructions or explanations (which are often too complex for the patient to generalize outside the treatment room) but through modeling	**Shaping techniques** Typically use extensive verbal explanations, modeling behavior, biofeedback Complex for patient
Sensory calibration *Treatment*: Focus attention on how it feels and sounds to talk loud *Carryover activities*: start day one; daily assignments (treatment and non-treatment days); use loud voice in real-life situations; difficulty of the assignment matches the level of the hierarchy where the person is working; make patient accountable and look for comments from patient that people in their daily living have said, such as, "I can hear you better" *Homework practice*: Start day one: daily assignments to practice at home (daily tasks and hierarchy exercises); treatment days (one other time for 5–10 min); non-treatment days (two times for 10–15 min; homework book provided and patient made accountable	**Sensory calibration** No systematic approach to sensory problems associated with speech disorders in PD Carryover activities are typically used as a part of generalization. They do not typically start the very first day of treatment; rather after some period of acquisition of the trained skill Homework exercises are typically provided. Frequency and accountability for doing homework varies

Table 31.2 Translation of some of the proposed principles underlying neural plasticity (column 1) to proposed deficits in Parkinson disease (column 2), and the corresponding rationale and task in LSVT LOUD (column 3) (Data from Fox *et al.* [191]).

Principle	Deficit specific to PD	LSVT LOUD
Intensity		
Intensive practice is important for maximal plasticity. Intensity can be increased via frequency, repetitions, force/resistance, effort, and accuracy. Intensity increases activation of corticostriatal terminals inducing synaptic plasticity in striatum	Intensive, high-effort training can be difficult in PD due to sensory deficits, force control, fatigue, depression, and progressive loss of cardiac sympathetic innervation	Train intensively 1 h per day, 4 days per week, for 4 weeks; multiple repetitions (15 or more); increase resistance, amplitude (within healthy range) effort, accuracy; and daily homework exercises. Train maximum perceived effort
Complexity		
Complex movements or environmental enrichment have been shown to promote greater structural plasticity (spine density, protein expression/synapse number) in adjacent and remote interconnected regions than simple movements	As basal ganglia pathology progresses, there is a decrease in automaticity requiring greater conscious attention to task. When required to perform dual tasks, insufficient attentional resources result in a decrement in one or both of the concurrent tasks.	Train complexity of movement with single patient focus (LOUD) to multiple, motor tasks. Retrain automaticity of amplitude (LOUD) in familiar movements. Progress complexity over 4 weeks by varying contexts, adding dual cognitive/motor loads, and increasing duration and difficultly of speech tasks (progress from words to conversation)
Sailency		
Practicing rewarding tasks (success/ emotionally salient) activates basal ganglia circuitry. Rewards are associated with phasic modulation of DA levels critical to induction of striatal plasticity and learning/relearning in PD	People with early PD may experience lack of awareness of subtle motor deficits, depression, loss of motivation and a feeling of "helplessness." Hence they do not feel they need, or would not benefit from, speech therapy	We train salient familiar movements (core patterns) of speech promoting success. We provide homework tasks that reinforce success of LOUD in emotionally salient social interactions. We provide extensive positive feedback
Use it or lose it/use it and improve it		
Spared, but compromised DA neurons highly vulnerable to bouts of inactivity/activity. Inactivity may accelerate deficits Post-exercise intervention, there may be a minimum use requirement to maintain positive effects.	Deficits are subtle – not "red flag" to seek speech therapy. Persuading early PD patients to recognize the need for exercise and then convincing them to continually exercise are challenging. Decreased physical activity may be a catalyst in degenerative process	Educate people with PD on subtle deficits and improve motor function that directly impacts real life. Retrain a new way of speaking everyday life (LOUD or ENUNCIATE), thus, normal activity offers continuous exercise
Timing matters		
Early exercise has the potential to rescue DA neurons, prevent chronic disuse, promote system-wide plasticity, and halt disease progression – particularly to the asymptomatic side	People with early PD have subtle physical underactivity (small movements/soft voice). This may be coupled with a lack of awareness or self-correction, leading to further inactivity	Train people with early PD when they may not have deficits in all systems (laryngeal and orofacial). Train strategies to raise awareness/avoid neglect and increase muscle activation for normal effort/amplitude required for within normal limits vocal loudness

are not enough therapists to deliver this treatment regimen to all individuals with PD; a need which will likely increase with the aging of the "baby boomer" population. Also, many individuals with PD are not able to travel to a clinic, and some may suffer from fatigue as a result of travel, rendering treatment less effective. Furthermore, continued exercise following the conclusion of speech treatment may be needed to maintain vocal loudness as the disease progresses. Moreover, intensive treatment can be costly. Hence there is a need for expanding service delivery while containing costs and human resources. Advances in computer and web-based technology offer potential solutions. LSVT LOUD is effective when delivered online (telepractice) [197,198] and LSVT LOUD software has been developed that allows independent patient practice with documented positive outcomes similarly to previously published data both immediately post-treatment and at 6 month follow-up [199,200].

When to refer for speech treatment

It has been suggested that behavioral treatment (e.g., speech therapy, occupational therapy, physiotherapy) should be deferred until later phases of the disease [201]. However, based upon scientific evidence, it is now being suggested that these therapies should begin early in the disease process [202]. Speech and voice disorders have deleterious effects on communication, health, psychologic well-being, and quality-of-life [7–13]. Without access to effective speech treatment, affected individuals often become disabled or retire early, are forced to give up activities they enjoy, incur substantial medical costs, and have increased mortality. Treatment may be optimally efficient early in the disease when the patient has the cognitive abilities, motivation, and level of optimism necessary to learn, practice, and master the therapeutic behaviors. Factors such as depression, fatigue, and pessimism which develop as the disease progresses [199] can hinder training and therapeutic outcomes. Another reason for initiating behavioral treatment early is to maximize the potential for neural plasticity and disease modification, which are most likely to occur during the earlier stages when dopaminergic and non-domaminergic systems are not fully depleted and there is potential for recovery or development of a compensatory mechanism [190,192,201]. A third reason is that many individuals with PD are aware of their speech problems early in the course of their illness, even before other people notice these problems [6,10]. These problems can affect their ability to communicate and socialize, and also their overall psychologic wellbeing and quality-of-life [10,11,13]. Early treatment of these speech problems may prevent some of the adverse consequences of speech impairment, including social isolation and depression.

Conclusion

Speech, voice, and swallowing problems occur in nearly 90% of individuals with PD and are likely to impact negatively on communication, socialization, occupation, health, and overall quality-of-life. Although traditionally voice and speech disorders have been attributed to dopaminergic deficits and rigidity, more recent studies indicate other factors, such as deficits in scaling movement amplitude, internal cueing, sensory processing, and neuropsychologic problems (vocal vigilance). Medical and surgical treatments alone have not sufficiently alleviated speech and voice disorders for people with PD, and in some cases have exacerbated or resulted in voice and speech impairment. Behavioral speech therapy, specifically the LSVT LOUD approach, in medically managed people with PD appears at present to be the most effective type of speech intervention. There are many exciting avenues of ongoing and future speech research that it is hoped will clarify our understanding of the underlying mechanism responsible for speech disorders in PD and enhance therapy in the future.

Acknowledgment

This research was funded by National Institutes of Health (NIH) grant R01 DC1150 from the National Institutes of Deafness and Other Communication Disorders.

Disclosure

Both L. Ramig and C. Fox receive a lecturer honorarium and have ownership interest in LSVT Global, Inc.

References

1. Ho A, Iansek R, Marigliani C, *et al.* Speech impairment in a large sample of people with Parkinson's disease. *Behav Neurol* 1998;**11**:131–7.
2. Aronson AE. *Clinical Voice Disorders*. New York: Thieme-Stratton, 1990.
3. Logemann J, Fisher H, Boshes B, Blonsky E. Frequency and concurrence of vocal tract dysfunctions in the speech of a large sample of Parkinson patients. *J Speech Hear Disord* 1978;**43**:47–57.
4. Stewart C, Winfield L, Hunt A, *et al.* Speech dysfunction in early Parkinson's disease. *Mov Disord* 1995;**10**:562–5.
5. Sapir S, Pawlas AA, Ramig LO, *et al.* Voice and speech abnormalities in Parkinson disease: relation to severity of motor impairment, duration of disease, medication, depression, gender, and age. *J Med Speech Lang Pathol* 2001;**9**:213–26.
6. Sapir S, Spielman J, Ramig L, *et al.* Effects of intensive voice treatment (LSVT®) on vowel articulation in dysarthric individuals with idiopathic Parkinson disease: acoustic and perceptual findings. *J Speech Lang Hear Res* 2007;**50**:899–912.
7. Dowding CH, Shenton CL, Salek SS. A review of the health-related quality of life and economic impact of Parkinson's disease. *Drugs Aging* 2006;**23**:693–721.
8. Findley LJ. The economic impact of Parkinson's disease. *Parkinsonism Relat Disord* 2007;**13**(Suppl): S8–12.
9. Miller N, Noble E, Jones D, Burn D. Hard to swallow: dysphagia in Parkinson's disease. *Age Ageing* 2006;**35**:614–8.
10. Miller N, Noble E, Jones D, Burn D. Life with communication changes in Parkinson's disease. *Age Ageing* 2006;**35**:235–9.
11. Miller N, Allcock L, Jones D, *et al.* Prevalence and pattern of perceived intelligibility changes in Parkinson's disease. *J Neurol Neurosurg Psychiatry* 2007;**78**:1188–90.
12. Pell MD, Cheang HS, Leonard CL. The impact of Parkinson's disease on vocal-prosodic communication from the perspective of listeners. *Brain Lang* 2006;**97**:123–34.
13. Pitcairn TK, Clemie S, Gray JM, Pentland B. Non-verbal cues in the self-presentation of parkinsonian patients. *Br J Clin Psychol* 1990;**29**:177–84.
14. Fox C, Ramig L. Vocal sound pressure level and self-perception of speech and voice in men and women with idiopathic Parkinson disease. *Am J Speech Lang Pathol* 1997;**2**:29–42.
15. Miller N, Noble E, Jones D, *et al.* How do I sound to me? Perceived changes in communication in Parkinson's disease. *Clin Rehabil* 2008;**22**:14–22.

16. Ramig L, Fox C, Sapir S. Speech treatment for Parkinson disease. *Expert Rev Neurother* 2008;**8**:299–311.
17. Sapir S, Ramig L, Fox C. Voice, speech and swallowing disorders. In: Factor S, Weiner W, eds. *Parkinson Disease: Diagnosis and Clinical Management*. New York: Demos Medical Publishing, 2008: 77–97.
18. Sapir S, Ramig L, Fox C. The Lee Silverman Voice Treatment for voice, speech and other orofacial disorders in patients with Parkinson's disease. *Fut Neurol* 2006;**1**:563–70.
19. D'Amelio M, Ragonese P, Morgante L, *et al.* Long-term survival of Parkinson's disease: a population-based study. *J Neurol* 2006;**253**:33–7.
20. Schenkman M, Zhu CW, Cutson TM, Whetten-Goldstein K. Longitudinal evaluation of economic and physical impact of Parkinson's disease. *Parkinsonism Relat Disord* 2001;**2**:41–50.
21. Wermuth L, Stenager EN, Stenager E, Boldsen J. Mortality in patients with Parkinson's disease. *Acta Neurol Scand* 1995;**92**:55–8.
22. Atarashi J, Uchida E. A clinical study of parkinsonism. *Rec Adv Res Nerv Syst* 1959;**3**:871–82.
23. Canter GJ. Speech characteristics of patients with Parkinson's disease: III. Articulation, diadochokinesis and overall speech adequacy. *J Speech Hear Disord* 1965;**30**:217–24.
24. Canter GJ. Speech characteristics of patients with Parkinson's disease: II. Physiological support for speech. *J Speech Hear Disord* 1965;**30**:44–9.
25. Hartelius L, Svensson P. Speech and swallowing symptoms associated with Parkinson's disease and multiple sclerosis: a survey. *Folia Phoniatr* 1994;**46**:9–17.
26. Hoberman SG. Speech techniques in aphasia and parkinsonism. *J Mich State Med Soc* 1958;**57**:1720–3.
27. Mutch R, Strucwick A, Roy S, *et al.* Parkinson's disease: disability review and management. *Br Med J* 1986;**293**:675–7.
28. Oxtoby M. *Parkinson's Disease Patients and Their Social Needs*. London: Parkinson's Disease Society, 1982.
29. Scott S, Caird FI, Williams BO. *Communication in Parkinson's Disease*. Rockville, MD: Aspen, 1985.
30. Selby G. Parkinson's disease. In: Vinken PJ, Bruyn GW, eds. *Handbook of Clinical Neurology*. North-Holland: Amsterdam, 1968:173–211.
31. Streifler M, Hofman S. Disorders of verbal expression in parkinsonism. In: Hassler RG, Christ JF. eds. *Advances in Neurology*. New York: Raven Press, 1984:385–93.
32. Uziel A, Bohe M, Cadilhac J, *et al.* Les troubles de la voix et de la parole dans les syndromes parkinsoniens. *Folia Phoniatr* 1975;**27**:166–76.
33. Darley FL, Aronson AE, Brown JR Clusters of deviant speech dimensions in the dysarthrias. *J Speech Hear Res* 1969;**12**:462–9.
34. Darley FL, Aronson A, Brown J. Differential diagnostic patterns of dysarthria. *J Speech Hear Res* 1969;**12**:246–69.
35. Darley FL, Aronson AE, Brown JR. *Motor Speech Disorders*. Philadelphia: Saunders, 1975.
36. Logemann J, Boshes B, Fisher H. The steps in the degeneration of speech and voice control in Parkinson's disease. In: Siegfried J, ed. *Parkinson's Diseases: Rigidity, Akinesia, Behavior*. Vienna: Hans Huber, 1973:101–12.
37. Ludlow CL, Bassich CJ. Relationships between perceptual ratings and acoustic measures of hypokinetic speech. In: McNeil MR, Rosenbek JC, Aronson AE, eds. *The Dysarthrias: Physiology, Acoustics, Perception, Management*. San Diego, CA: College-Hill Press, 1984:163–95.
38. Skodda S, Visser W, Schlegel U. Vowel articulation in Parkinson's disease. *J Voice* 2010; Apr 30 [Epub ahead of print].
39. Moreau C, Ozsancak C, Blatt JL, *et al.* Oral festination in Parkinson's disease: biomechanical analysis and correlation with festination and freezing of gait. *Mov Disord* 2007;**22**:1503–1506.
40. Skodda S, Schlegel U. Speech rate and rhythm in Parkinson's disease. *Mov Disord* 2008;**23**:985–92.
41. Baumgartner CA, Sapir S, Ramig LO. Voice quality changes following phonatory–respiratory effort treatment (LSVT®) versus respiratory effort treatment for individuals with Parkinson disease. *J Voice* 2001;**15**:105–14.
42. Sapir S, Ramig L, Hoyt P, *et al.* Speech loudness and quality 12 months after intensive voice treatment (LSVT) for Parkinson's disease: a comparison with an alternative speech treatment. *Folia Phoniatr* 2002;**54**:296–303.
43. Ramig L. The role of phonation in speech intelligibility: a review and preliminary data from patients with Parkinson's disease. In: Kent RD, ed. *Intelligibility in Speech Disorders: Theory, Measurement, and Management*. Amsterdam: John Benjamin, 1992: 119–56.
44. Sapir S, Ramig LO, Spielman JL, Fox C. Formant centralization ratio: a proposal for a new acoustic measure of dysarthric speech. *J Speech Lang Hear Res* 2010;**53**:114–25.
45. Fox C, Ramig L. Vocal sound pressure level and self-perception of speech and voice in men and women with idiopathic Parkinson disease. *Am J Speech Lang Pathol* 1997;**6**: 85–94.
46. King J, Ramig L, Lemke JH, Horii Y. Parkinson disease: longitudinal changes in acoustic parameters of phonation. *J Med Speech Lang Pathol* 1994;**2**:29–42.
47. Winholtz W, Ramig L. The vocal demodulator for analysis of vocal tremor. *J Speech Hear Res* 1992;**35**:562–73.
48. Ramig L, Scherer R, Titze I, Ringel S. Acoustic characteristics of voice of patients with neurological disease: a preliminary report. *Ann Otol Rhinol Laryngol* 1988;**97**:164–72.
49. Smith M, Ramig LO, Dromey C, *et al.* Intensive voice treatment in Parkinson's disease: laryngostroboscopic findings. *J Voice* 1995;**9**:453–9.
50. Kleinow J, Smith A, Ramig, L. Speech stability in idiopathic Parkinson disease: effects of rate and loudness manipulations. *J Speech Lang Hear Res* 2001;**44**:1041–51.
51. Huber J, Stathopoulos E, Ramig L, Lancaster S. Respiratory function and variability in individuals with Parkinson disease: pre and post Lee Silverman Voice Treatment (LSVT®). *J Med Speech Lang Pathol* 2003;**11**:185–201.
52. Solomon NP, Hixon TJ. Speech breathing in Parkinson's disease. *J Speech Lang Hear Res* 1993;**36**:294–310.
53. Baker K, Ramig LO, Luschei E, Smith M. Thyroarytenoid muscle activity associated with hypophonia in Parkinson disease and aging. *Neurology* 1998;**51**(6): 1592–8.
54. Luschei ES, Ramig LO, Baker KL, *et al.* Discharge characteristics of laryngeal single motor units during phonation in young and older adults and in persons with Parkinson disease. *J Neurophys* 1999;**81**:2131–9.
55. Caligiuri M. The influence of speaking rate on articulatory hypokinesia in parkinsonian dysarthria. *Brain Lang* 1989;**36**:493–502.

56. Kempler D, Van Lancker D. Effect of speech task on intelligibility in dysarthria: a case study of Parkinson's disease. *Brain Lang* 2002;**80**:449–64.
57. Rosen KM, Kent RD, Duffy JR. Task-based profile of vocal intensity decline in Parkinson's disease. *Folia Phoniatr* 2005;**57**:28–37.
58. Ackermann H, Ziegler W. Articulatory deficits in parkinsonian dysarthria: an acoustic analysis. *J Neurol Neurosurg Psychiatry* 1991;**54**:1093–8.
59. Zarzur AP, Duprat AC, Shinzato G, Eckley CA. Laryngeal electromyography in adults with Parkinson's disease and voice complaints. *Laryngoscope* 2007;**117**:831–4.
60. De Letter M, Santens P, De Bodt M, *et al.* The effect of levodopa on respiration and word intelligibility in people with advanced Parkinson's disease. *Clin Neurol Neurosurg* 2007;**109**:495–500.
61. De Letter M, Santens P, Estercam I, *et al.* Levodopa-induced modifications of prosody and comprehensibility in advanced Parkinson's disease as perceived by professional listeners. *Clin Linguist Phon* 2007;**21**:783–91.
62. Ho AK, Bradshaw JL, Iansek FR. For better or worse: the effect of levodopa on speech in Parkinson's disease. *Mov Disord* 2008;**23**:574–80.
63. Larson K, Ramig LO, Scherer RC. Acoustic and glottographic voice analysis during drug-related fluctuations in Parkinson's disease. *J Med Speech Lang Pathol* 1994;**2**:211–26.
64. Goberman A. Correlation between acoustic speech characteristics and non-speech motor performance in Parkinson disease. *Med Sci Monit* 2005;**11**:CR109–16.
65. Trail M, Fox C, Ramig LO, *et al.* Speech treatment for Parkinson's disease. *NeuroRehabilitation* 2005;**20**:205–21.
66. Goberman A, Coelho C, Robb M. Phonatory characteristics of parkinsonian speech before and after morning medication: the ON and OFF states. *J Commun Disord* 2002;**35**:217–39.
67. Kompoliti K, Wang QE, Goetz CG, *et al.* Effects of central dopaminergic stimulation by apomorphine on speech in Parkinson's disease. *Neurology* 2000;**54**:458–62.
68. Netsell R, Daniel B, Celesia GG. Acceleration and weakness in parkinsonian dysarthria. *J Speech Hear Disord* 1975;**40**:170–8.
69. Fox C, Ramig L, Ciucci M, *et al.* The science and practice of LSVT/LOUD: neural plasticity-principled approach to treating individuals with Parkinson disease and other neurological disorders. *Semin Speech Lang* 2006;**27**:283–99.
70. Forrest K, Weismer G, Turner GS. Kinematic, acoustic, and perceptual analyses of connected speech produced by Parkinsonian and normal geriatric adults. *J Acoust Soc Am* 1989;**85**:2608–22.
71. Ho AK, Iansek R, Bradshaw JL. Motor instability in parkinsonian speech intensity. *Neuropsychiatry Neuropsychol Behav Neurol* 2001;**14**:109–16.
72. Liss JM, Spitzer SM, Caviness JN, Adler C. The effects of familiarization on intelligibility and lexical segmentation in hypokinetic and ataxic dysarthria. *J Acoust Soc Am* 2002;**112**:3022–30.
73. Dromey C, Ramig L. Intentional changes in sound pressure level and rate: Their impact on measures of respiration, phonation, and articulation. *J Speech Lang Hear Res* 1998;**41**:1003–18.
74. Goberman AM, Elmer LW. Acoustic analysis of clear versus conversational speech in individuals with Parkinson disease. *J Commun Disord* 2005;**38**:215–30.
75. Caligiuri M, Abbs JH. Response properties of the perioral reflex in Parkinson's disease. *Exp Neurol* 1987;**98**:563–72.
76. Diamond SG, Schneider JS, Markham CH. Oral sensorimotor defects in people with Parkinson's disease. *Adv Neurol* 1987;**45**:335–8.
77. Schneider JS, Diamond SG, Markham CH. Deficits in orofacial sensorimotor function in Parkinson's disease. *Ann Neurol* 1986;**19**:275–82.
78. Schneider JS, Lidsky TI. *Basal Ganglia and Behavior: Sensory Aspects of Motor Functioning*. Toronto: Hans Huber, 1987.
79. Ho AK, Iansek R, Bradshaw JL. Regulations of parkinsonian speech volume: the effect of interlocuter distance. *J Neurol Neurosurg Psychiatry* 1999;**67**:199–202.
80. Ho AK, Bradshaw JL, Iansek T. Volume perception in parkinsonian speech. *Mov Disord* 2000;**15**:1125–31.
81. Ho AK, Bradshaw JL, Iansek R, Alfredson R. Speech volume regulation in Parkinson's disease: effects of implicit cues and explicit instructions. *Neuropsychologia* 1999;**37**:1453–60.
82. Graber S, Hertrich I, Daum I, *et al.* Speech perception deficits in Parkinson's disease: Underestimation of time intervals compromises identification of durational phonetic contrasts. *Brain Lang* 2002;**82**:65–74.
83. Solomon NP, Robin DA, Lorell DM, *et al.* Tongue function testing in Parkinson's disease: indicators of fatigue. In: Till JA, Yorkston KM, Beukelman R, eds. *Motor Speech Disorders: Advances in Assessment and Treatment*. Baltimore, MD: Paul H. Brooks, 1994: 147–60.
84. Fox CM, Morrison CE, Ramig LO, Sapir S. Current perspectives on the Lee Silverman Voice Treatment (LSVT) for people with idiopathic Parkinson's disease. *Am J Speech Lang Pathol* 2002;**11**:111–23.
85. Demirci M, Grill S, McShane L, Hallett M. A mismatch between kinesthetic and visual perception in Parkinson's disease. *Ann Neurol* 1997;**41**:781–8.
86. Jobst EE, Melnick ME, Byl NN, *et al.* Sensory perception in Parkinson's disease. *Arch Neurol* 1997;**54**:450–4.
87. Klockgether T, Borutta M, Rapp H., *et al.* A defect of kinesthesia in Parkinson's disease. *Brain* 1997;**120**:460–5.
88. Rickards C, Cody FW. Proprioceptive control of wrist movements in Parkinson's disease. *Brain* 1997;**120**:977–90.
89. Demirci M, Grill S, McShane L, Hallett M. A mismatch between kinesthetic and visual perception in Parkinson's disease. *Ann Neurol* 1997;**41**:781–8.
90. Demirci M, Grill S, McShane L, Hallet M. Impairment of kinesthesia in Parkinson's disease. *Neurology* 1995;**45**:A218.
91. Albin RL, Young AB, Penny JB. The functional anatomy of basal ganglia disorders. *Trends Neurosci* 1989;**12**:366–75.
92. Penny JB, Young AB. Speculations on the functional anatomy of basal ganglia disorders. *Annu Rev Neurosci* 1983;**6**:73–94.
93. Berardelli A, Dick JP, Rothwell JC, *et al.* Scaling of the size of the first agonist EMG burst during rapid wrist movements in patients with Parkinson's disease. *J Neurol Neurosurg Psychiatry* 1986;**49** 1273–9.
94. Ramig LO, Fox CM. *LSVT LOUD Training and Certification Workshop Manual*. Tucson, AZ: LSVT Global, 2009.

95. Curio G, Neuloh G, Numminen J, *et al.* Speaking modifies voice-evoked activity in the human auditory cortex. *Hum Brain Mapp* 2000;**9**:183–91.
96. Ford JM, Mathalon DH. Electrophysiological evidence of corollary discharge dysfunction in schizophrenia during talking and thinking. *J Psychiatr Res* 2004;**38**:37–46.
97. Liotti M, Vogel D, Sapir S, *et al.* Abnormal auditory gating in Parkinson's disease before and after LSVT®. *Paper presented at the Annual Meeting of the American Speech, Language and Hearing Association*, Washington, DC, 2000.
98. Boecker H, Ceballos-Baumann A, Bartenstein P, *et al.* Sensory processing in Parkinson's and Huntington's disease: investigations with 3D $H_2{}^{15}O$-PET. *Brain* 1999;**122**:1651–65.
99. Cunnington R, Iansek R, Bradshaw JL, Phillips JG. Movement-related potentials in Parkinson's disease. Presence and predictability of temporal and spatial cues. *Brain* 1995; **118**:935–50.
100. Oliveira RM, Gurd JM, Nixon P, *et al.* Micrographia in Parkinson's disease: the effect of providing external cues. *J Neurol Neurosurg Psychiatry* 1997;**63**:429–33.
101. McNamara P, Obler LK, Au R, *et al.* Speech monitoring skills in Alzheimer's disease, Parkinson's disease, and normal aging. *Brain Lang* 1992;**42**:38–51.
102. Rowe J, Stephan KE, Friston K, *et al.* Attention to action in Parkinson's disease: impaired effective connectivity among frontal cortical regions. *Brain* 2002;**125**:276–8.
103. Brown P, Marsden CD. What do the basal ganglia do? *Lancet* 1999;**351**:1801–4.
104. Bohnen NI, Kaufer DI, Hendrickson R, *et al.* (2006) Cognitive correlates of cortical cholinergic denervation in Parkinson's disease and parkinsonian dementia. *J Neurol.* **253**, 242–7.
105. Azulay JP, Mesure S, Blin O. Influence of visual cues on gait in Parkinson's disease: contribution to attention or sensory dependence? *J Neurol Sci* 2006;**248**:192–5.
106. Sammer G, Reuter I, Hullmann K, *et al.* Training of executive functions in Parkinson's disease. *J Neurol Sci.* 2006;**248**:115–9.
107. Liotti M, Ramig LO, Vogel D, *et al.* Hypophonia in Parkinson's disease. neural correlates of voice treatment revealed by PET. *Neurology* 2003;**60**:432–40.
108. Narayana S, Fox PT, Zhang W, *et al.* Neural correlates of efficacy of voice therapy in Parkinson's disease identified by performance-correlation analysis. *Hum Brain Mapp* 2010;**31**, 222–36.
109. Ramig LO, Sapir S, Countryman S, *et al.* Intensive voice treatment (LSVT®) for patients with Parkinson's disease: a 2 year follow up. *J Neurol Neurosurg Psychiatry* 2001;**71**:493–8.
110. Radad K, Gille G, Rausch W. Short review on dopamine agonists: insight into clinical and research studies relevant to Parkinson's disease. *Pharmacol. Rep* 2005;**57**:701–12.
111. Critchley EMR. Speech disorders of parkinsonism: a review. *J Neurol Neurosurg Psychiatry* 1981;**44**:751–8.
112. Mawdsley C. Speech and levodopa. *Adv Neurol* 1973;**3**:33–47.
113. Mawdsley C, Gamsu CV. Periodicity of speech in parkinsonism. *Nature* 1971;**231**:315–6.
114. Nakano KK, Zubick H, Tyley HR Speech defects of parkinsonian patients. *Neurology* 1973;**23**:865–70.
115. Rigrodsky S, Morrison EB. Speech changes in parkinsonism during L-dopa therapy: preliminary findings. *J Am Geriatr Soc* 1970;**18**:142–51.
116. Wolfe VI, Garvin J, Bacon M, Waldrop W. Speech changes in Parkinson's disease during treatment with L-dopa. *J Commun Disord* 1975;**8**:271–9.
117. Yaryura-Tobias JA, Diamond B, Merlis S. Verbal communication with L-dopa treatment. *Nature* 1971;**234**:224–5.
118. Hunter PC, Crameri J, Austin S, *et al.* Response of parkinsonian swallowing dysfunction to dopaminergic stimulation. *J Neurol Neurosurg Psychiatry* 1997;**63**:579–83.
119. Tison F, Wiart L, Guatterie M, *et al.* Effects of central dopaminergic stimulation by apomorphine on swallowing disorders in Parkinson's disease. *Mov Disord* 1996;**11**:729–32.
120. Klosterman F, Ehlen F, Vesper J, *et al.* Effects of subthalamic deep brain stimulation on dysarthrophonia in Parkinson's disease. *J Neurol Neurosurg Psychiatry* 2008;**79**:522–9.
121. Tripoliti E, Zrinzo L, Martinez-Torres I, *et al.* Effects of contact location and voltage amplitude on speech and movement in bilateral subthalamic nucleus deep brain stimulation. *Mov Disord* 2008;**23**(16):2377–83.
122. Gallena S, Smith PJ, Zeffiro T, Ludlow CL. Effects of levodopa on laryngeal muscle activity for voice onset and offset in Parkinson disease. *J Speech Lang Hear Res* 2001;**44**: 1284–99.
123. De Letter M, Santens P, Van Borsel J. The effects of levodopa on word intelligibility in Parkinson's disease. *J Commun Disord* 2005;**38**:187–96.
124. Sanabria J, Ruiz PG, Gutierrez R, *et al.* The effect of levodopa on vocal function in Parkinson's disease. *Clin Neuropharmacol* 2001;**24**:99–102.
125. Cahill L, Murdoch BE, Theodoros DG, *et al.* Effect of oral levodopa treatment on articulatory function in Parkinson's disease: preliminary results. *Motor Control* 1998;**2**:161–72.
126. Jiang J, Lin E, Wang J, Hanson DG. Glottographic measures before and after levodopa treatment in Parkinson's disease. *Laryngoscope* 1999;**109**:1287–94.
127. Biary N, Pimental PA, Langenberg PW. A double-blind trial of clonazepan in the treatment of parkinsonian dysarthria. *Neurology* 1988;**38**:255–8.
128. Perlmutter JS, Mink JW. Deep brain stimulation. *Annu Rev Neurosci* 2006;**29**:229–57.
129. Pahwa R, Lyons KE, Wilkinson SB, *et al.* Long-term evaluation of deep brain stimulation of the thalamus. *J Neurosurg* 2006;**104**:506–12.
130. Rodriguez-Oroz MC, Obeso JA, Lang AE, *et al.* Bilateral deep brain stimulation in Parkinson's disease: a multicentre study with 4 years follow-up. *Brain* 2005;**128**:2240–9.
131. Krack P, Batir A, Van Blercom N, *et al.* Five-year follow-up of bilateral stimulation of the subthalamic nucleus in advanced Parkinson's disease. *N Engl J Med* 2003;**349**:1925–34.
132. Santens P, De Letter M, Van Borsel J, *et al.* Lateralized effects of subthalamic nucleus stimulation on different aspects of speech in Parkinson's disease. *Brain Lang* 2003;**87**: 253–8.
133. Wang E, Verhagen Metman L, Bakay R, *et al.* The effect of unilateral electrostimulation of the subthalamic nucleus on respiratory/phonatory subsystems of speech production in Parkinson's disease-a preliminary report. *Clin Linguist Phonet* 2003;**17**:283–9.
134. Gentil M, Pinto S, Pollak P, Benabid AL. Effect of bilateral stimulation of the subthalamic nucleus on parkinsonian dysarthria. *Brain Lang* 2003;**85**:190–6.

135. Gentil M, Garcia-Ruiz P, Pollak P, Benabid AL Effect of bilateral deep-brain stimulation on oral control of patients with parkinsonism. *Eur Neurol* 2000;**44**:147–52.
136. Gentil M, Chauvin P, Pinto S, *et al.* Effect of bilateral stimulation of the subthalamic nucleus on parkinsonian voice. *Brain Lang* 2001;**78**:233–40.
137. Pinto S, Gentil M, Fraix V, *et al.* Bilateral subthalamic stimulation effects on oral force control in Parkinson's disease. *J Neurology* 2003;**250**:179–87.
138. Dromey C, Kumar R, Lang AE, Lozano AM. An investigation of the effects of subthalamic nucleus stimulation on acoustic measures of voice. *Mov Disord* 2000;**15**:1132–8.
139. Rousseaux M, Krystkowiak P, Kozlowski O, *et al.* Effects of subthalamic nucleus stimulation on parkinsonian dysarthria and speech intelligibility. *J Neurol* 2000;**251**:327–34.
140. Saint-Cyr JA, Trepanier LL, Kumar R, *et al.* Neuropsychological consequences of chronic bilateral stimulation of the subthalamic nucleus in Parkinson's disease. *Brain* 2000;**123**:2091–108.
141. McIntyre CC, Mori S, Sherman DL, *et al.* Electric field and stimulating influence generated by deep brain stimulation of the subthalamic nucleus. *Clin Neurophysiol* 2004;**115**:589–95.
142. Tornqvist AL, Schalen, L, Rehncrona S. Effects of different electrical parameter settings on the intelligibility of speech in patients with Parkinson's disease treated with subthalamic deep brain stimulation. *Mov Disord* 2005;**20**:416–23.
143. Dias AE, Barbosa ER, Coracini K, *et al.* Effects of repetitive transcranial magnetic stimulation on voice and speech in Parkinson's disease. *Acta Neurol Scand* 2006;**113**:92–9.
144. Pagni CA, Zeme S, Zenga F. Further experience with extradural motor cortex stimulation for treatment of advanced Parkinson's disease. Report of 3 new cases. *J Neurosurg Sci* 2003;**47**:189–93.
145. Berke GS, Gerratt B, Kreiman J, Jackson K. Treatment of parkinson hypophonia with percutaneous collagen augmentation. *Laryngoscope* 1999;**109**:1295–9.
146. Kim SH, Kearney JJ, Atkins JP. Percutaneous laryngeal collagen augmentation for treatment of parkinsonian hypophonia. *Otolaryngol Head Neck Surg* 2002;**126**:653–6.
147. Sewall GK, Lang J, Ford CN. Clinical evaluation of Parkinson's-related dysphonia. *Laryngoscope* 2006;**116**:1740–4.
148. Allan CM. Treatment of non-fluent speech resulting from neurological disease: treatment of dysarthria. *Br J Disord Commun* 1970;**5**:3–5
149. Greene HCL. *The Voice and Its Disorders*. London: Pitman Medical, 1980.
150. Weiner WJ, Lang AE. *Movement Disorders; a Comprehensive Survey*. Mount Kisco, NY: Futura, 1989.
151. Sarno MT. Speech impairment in Parkinson's disease. *Arch Phys Med Rehabil* 1968;**49**:269–75.
152. Yorkston KM. Treatment efficacy: dysarthria. *J Speech Hear Res* 1996;**39**:S46–57.
153. Adams SG. Hypokinetic dysarthria in Parkinson's disease. In: McNeil MR, ed. *Clinical Management of Sensorimotor Speech Disorders*. New York: Thieme, 1997.
154. Helm N. Management of palilalia with a pacing board. *J Speech Hear Disord* 1979;**44**:350–3.
155. Downie AW, Low JM, Lindsay DD. Speech disorders in parkinsonism: usefulness of delayed auditory feedback in selected cases. *Br J Disord Commun* 1981;**16**:135–9.
156. Yorkston KM, Spencer KA, Duffy JR. Behavioral management of respiratory/phonatory dysfunction from dysarthria: a systematic review of the evidence. *J Med Speech Lang Pathol* 2003;**11**:xiii–xxxviii.
157. Yorkston KM, Hakel, M, Beukelman DR, Fager S. Evidence for effectiveness of treatment of loudness, rate, or prosody in dysarthria: a systematic review. *J Med Speech Lang Pathol* 2007;**15**:xi–xxxvi.
158. Pinto S, Ozsancak C, Tripoliti E, Thobois S, *et al.* Treatments for dysarthria in Parkinson's disease. *Lancet Neurol* 2004;**3**:547–56.
159. Ramig L, Mead C, Scherer R, *et al.* Voice therapy and Parkinson's disease: a longitudinal study of efficacy. Paper presented at the Clinical Dysarthria Conference, San Diego, CA, February 1988.
160. Smith M, Ramig LO, Dromey C, *et al.* Intensive voice treatment in Parkinson's disease: laryngostroboscopic findings. *J Voice* 1995;**9**:453–9.
161. Ramig LO, Dromey C. Aerodynamic mechanisms underlying treatment-related changes in SPL in patients with Parkinson disease. *J Speech Hear Res* 1996;**39**:798–807.
162. Countryman S, Hicks J, Ramig L. Supraglottic hyperadduction in an individual with Parkinson disease: treatment outcome. *Am J Speech Lang Pathol* 1997;**6**:85–94.
163. Dromey C, Ramig LO, Johnson A. Phonatory and articulatory changes associated with increased vocal intensity in Parkinson disease: a case study. *J Speech Hear Res* 1995;**38**:751–63.
164. Borod JC, Pick LH, Hall S, *et al.* Relationships among facial, prosodic, and lexical channels of emotional perceptual processing. *Cogn Emotion* 2000;**14**:193–211.
165. Spielman J, Borod J, Ramig L. The effects of intensive voice treatment on facial expressiveness in Parkinson disease: preliminary data. *Cogn Behav Neurol* 2003;**16**:177–88.
166. Borod JC, Koff E, Lorch MP, Nicholas M. Channels of emotional expression in patients with unilateral brain damage. *Arch Neurol* 1985;**42**:345–8.
167. Borod JC, Welkowitz J, Alpert M, *et al.* Parameters of emotional processing in neuropsychiatric disorders: conceptual issues and a battery of tests. *J Commun Disord* 1990;**23**:247–71.
168. Canino E, Borod JC, Madigan N, *et al.* Development of procedures for rating posed emotional expressions across facial, prosodic, and lexical channels. *Percept Mot Skills* 1999;**89**:57–71.
169. Ross ED, Mesulam MM. Dominant language functions of the right hemisphere? Prosody and emotional gesturing. *Arch Neurol* 1979;**36**:144–8.
170. Porges SW. Orienting in a defensive world: mammalian modifications of our evolutionary heritage. A polyvagal theory. *Psychophysiology* 1995;**32**:301–18.
171. Porges SW. Emotion: an evolutionary by-product of the neural regulation of the autonomic nervous system. *Ann N Y Acad Sci* 1997;**807**:62–77.
172. Sharkawi AE, Ramig L, Logemann JA, *et al.* swallowing and voice effects of Lee Silverman Voice Treatment (LSVT®): a pilot study. *J Neurol Neurosurg Psychiatry* 2002;**72**:31–6.
173. Dromey C, Ramig L. Intentional changes in sound pressure level and rate: their impact on measures of respiration, phonation, and articulation. *J Speech Lang Hear Res* 1998;**41**:1003–18.

174. Allen G. Segmental timing control in speech production. *J Phonet* 1973;**1**:219–37.
175. Gandour J, Dechongkit S, Ponglorpisit S, Khunadorn F. Speech timing at the sentence level in Thai after unilateral brain damage. *Brain Lang* 1994;**46**:419–38.
176. McClean MD, Tasko SM. Association of orofacial with laryngeal and respiratory motor output during speech. *Exp Brain Res* 2002;**146**:481–9.
177. Higgins MB, Netsell R, Schulte L. Vowel-related differences in laryngeal articulatory and phonatory function. *J Speech Lang Hear Res* 1998;**41**:712–24.
178. Larson KK, Sapir S. Orolaryngeal reflex responses to changes in affective state. *J Speech Lang Hear Res* 1995;**38**:990–1000.
179. Sapir S. The intrinsic pitch of vowels: theoretical, physiological, and clinical considerations. *J Voice* 1989;**3**:44–51.
180. Ackermann H, Wildgruber D, Daum I, Grodd W. Does the cerebellum contribute to cognitive aspects of speech production? A functional magnetic resonance imaging (fMRI) study in humans. *Neurosci Lett* 1998;**247**:187–90.
181. Hirano S, Kojima H, Naito Y, *et al.* Cortical speech processing mechanisms while vocalizing visually presented languages. *NeuroReport* 1996;**8**:363–7.
182. Jurgens U, Kirzinger A, von Cramon D. The effects of deep-reaching lesions in the cortical face area on phonation. A combined case report and experimental monkey study. *Cortex* 1982;**18**:125–30.
183. Kitchen DM, Cheney DL, Seyfarth RM. Male chacma baboons (*Papio hamadryas ursinus*) discriminate loud call contests between rivals of different relative ranks. *Anim Cogn* 2005;**8**:1–6.
184. Leinonen L, Laakso ML, Carlson S, Linnankoski I. Shared means and meanings in vocal expression of man and macaque. *Logoped. Phoniatr Vocol* 2003;**28**:53–61.
185. Tecumseh W. The phonetic potential of nonhuman vocal tracts: comparative cineradiographic observations of vocalizing animals. *Phonetica* 2000;**57**:205–18.
186. Ofer-Noy N, Dudai Y, Karni A. Skill learning in mirror reading: how repetition determines acquisition. *Cogn Brain Res* 2003;**17**:507–21.
187. Tillerson J, Miller G. Forced limb-use and recovery following brain injury. *Neuroscientist* 2002;**8**:574–85.
188. Fisher B, Petzinger G, Nixon K, *et al.* Exercise-induced behavioral recovery and neuroplasticity in the 1-methyl-4-phenyl-1,2,3,6-tetrahydropyridine-lesioned mouse basal ganglia. *J Neurosci Res* 2004;**77**:378–90.
189. Liepert J, Miltner W, Bauder H, *et al.* Motor cortex plasticity during constraint-induced movement therapy in stroke patients. *Neurosci Lett* 1998;**250**:5–8.
190. Kleim J, Jones T, Schallert T. Motor enrichment and the induction of plasticity before or after brain injury, *Neurochem Res* 2003;**11**:1757–69.
191. Fox C, Ramig L, Ciucci M, *et al.* The science and practice of LSVT/LOUD: neural plasticity-principled approach to treating individuals with Parkinson disease and other neurological disorders. *Semin Speech Lang* 2006;**27**(4):283–99.
192. Taub E. Harnessing brain plasticity through behavioral techniques to produce new treatments in neurorehabilitation. *Am. Psychol* 2004;**59**:692–704.
193. Schmidt RA. A schema theory of discrete motor skill learning. *Psychol Rev* 1975;**82**:225–60.
194. Schmidt RA. *Motor Control and Learning*. Champaign, IL: Human Kinetic Publishers, 1988.
195. Astrand PO, Rodahl K. *Textbook of Work Physiology*. New York: McGraw-Hill.
196. Stelmach GE. (1991) Basal ganglia impairment and force control. In: Requin J, Stelmach GE, eds. *Tutorial in Motor Neuroscience*. Dordrecht: Kluwer, 1970.
197. Theodoros DG, Constantinescu G, Russell TG, *et al.* Treating the speech disorder in Parkinson's disease online. *J Telemed Telecare* 2006;**12**:88–91.
198. Howell S, Tripoliti E, Pring T. Delivering the Lee Silverman Voice Treatment (LSVT) by web camera: a feasibility study. *J Lang Commun Disord* 2009;**44**:287–300.
199. Halpern AE, Matos C, Ramig L, *et al.* LSVTC – a PDA supported speech treatment for Parkinson's disease. Presented at the Annual American Speech–Language–Hearing Association Meeting, Philadelphia, PA, 2004.
200. Halpern A, Matos C, Ramig L, *et al.* LSVTC – a PDA supported speech treatment for Parkinson's disease. Presented at the 9th International Congress of Parkinson's Disease and Movement Disorders, New Orleans, LA, 2005.
201. Rajput A, Rajput AH. Parkinson's disease management strategies. *Expert Rev Neurother* 2006;**6**:91–9.
202. Zigmond MJ, Cameron JL, Leak RK, *et al.* Triggering endogenous neuroprotective processes through exercise in models of dopamine deficiency. *Parkinsonism Relat Disord* 2009;**15**(Suppl 3): S42–45.
203. Till JA, Yorkston KM, Beukelman R. *Motor Speech Disorders: Advances in Assessment and Treatment*. Baltimore, MD: Paul H Brooks, 1994.

Chapter 32
Gait, Postural Instability, and Freezing

Yvette A.M. Grimbergen[1], *Arlène D. Speelman*[2], *Marjolein A. van der Marck*[2], *Yvonne Schoon*[3], *& Bastiaan R. Bloem*[2]

[1]Department of Neurology, Leiden University Medical Centre, Leiden, and Department of Neurology, Sint Franciscus Gasthuis, Rotterdam, The Netherlands

[2]Department of Neurology and Parkinson Centre Nijmegen, Donders Institute for Brain Cognition and Behaviour, Radboud University Nijmegen Medical Centre, Nijmegen, The Netherlands

[3]Department of Geriatrics, Radboud University Nijmegen Medical Centre, Nijmegen, The Netherlands

Introduction

A chapter on gait and balance impairment is inevitable in a book on non-motor and non-dopaminergic features of Parkinson's disease (PD), for several reasons. First, even though gait impairment and postural instability (jointly referred to as "axial motor disability") are traditionally regarded as "motor" features of PD, evidence is accumulating that the ability to walk and maintain balance are governed, at least in part, by cognitive processes. For example, many PD patients find it difficult to walk and talk at the same time and, when they nevertheless try to combine these two seemingly easily tasks, falls result [1]. Also, the appearance of axial motor disability typically coincides with cognitive decline, as is obvious in patients with the PIGD (postural instability and gait disability) subtype of PD [2–4]. This co-occurrence could be a chance finding reflecting more widespread disease pathology in this subtype of PD. An interesting alternative explanation is that patients may only begin to fall when they fail to compensate consciously for axial motor deficits. In its most striking form, this is seen in patients with progressive supranuclear palsy (PSP), who have an unusually high risk of falling, not only because their balance is poor, but also because they fail to adjust their behavior due to lack of insight – a feature sometimes referred to as "motor recklessness" [5]. Taken together, these observations suggest that difficulties with gait or balance are perhaps more "non-motor" than initially considered.

Second, axial disability can rightly be included among the non-dopaminergic features of PD. Gait impairment and postural instability are typically "late" features of PD, appearing at a time when the disease extends beyond the dopaminergic substantia nigra [6,7]. Several observations support a non-dopaminergic basis for axial motor disability in PD. Axial motor features are typically inadequately controlled with dopaminergic medication [8–10]. This is particularly the case for postural instability and, to a lesser extent, for gait abnormalities. Indeed, most falls in PD occur when patients are in the ON state [11]. Such clinical observations have been tested with dynamic posturography: evaluating balance quantitatively while standing subjects are perturbed by sudden movements of a support surface [12]. The results suggest that several balance problems (mainly the reactive automatic postural responses) in PD are not primarily dopamine dependent [10,13–15]. In fact, dopaminergic medication can paradoxically increase the frequency of falls by inducing ON period freezing, orthostatic hypotension leading to syncopal falls, or violent dyskinesias that can literally throw the patients off their feet [16–19].

Third, neuropathologic and biochemical studies suggest that non-dopaminergic lesions emerge at about the same time that gait and balance problems develop [20]. Specifically, postmortem brain studies in patients with gait and balance impairment demonstrate substantial cell loss within the locus coeruleus, particularly the caudal part that projects mainly to the spinal cord and cerebellum [21,22]. Consistent with this cell loss in the locus coeruleus, CSF analyses and postmortem brain studies have shown reduced norepinephrine levels in PD. Further, there is a correlation between the reduced concentration of norepinephrine and the severity of gait and postural disturbances, and levels of norepinephrine are significantly reduced in patients with freezing of gait [23]. Gait impairment, especially freezing (and possibly also balance abnormalities), may further be linked to dysfunction of the mixed cholinergic–glutamatergic pedunculopontine nucleus (PPN) in the dorsal brainstem [24–26]. The PPN normally governs step initiation and step maintenance. PPN dysfunction in PD is partially caused by excessive inhibition from the internal globus pallidus

Parkinson's Disease: Non-Motor and Non-Dopaminergic Features, First Edition. Edited by C. Warren Olanow, Fabrizio Stocchi, and Anthony E. Lang.

and substantia nigra pars reticulata. In addition, cell loss occurs within the cholinergic portion of the PPN, and this neurodegeneration likely further aggravates the gait problems [26].

Observations in patients with atypical parkinsonism provide a final argument to support a non-dopaminergic basis for axial motor disability in PD. Generally, gait and balance problems emerge earlier and are more prominent in patients with atypical parkinsonism; this includes patients with PSP, multiple system atrophy (MSA), corticobasal degeneration (CBD), dementia with Lewy bodies (DLB), and vascular parkinsonism [5,27,28]. These atypical parkinsonian syndromes are all typically characterized by more widespread pathology compared with PD, including abundant extranigral and non-dopaminergic lesions.

This is not to say, of course, that gait and balance problems can be ascribed entirely to the presence of non-dopaminergic lesions. For many patients, dopamine replacement therapy can provide partial benefit, particularly in early stages of the disease, more so for gait than posture or balance. The bradykinetic gait in early disease stages – characterized by a reduced walking velocity and small, shuffling steps – usually improves with dopaminergic treatment. Also, freezing of gait – which usually appears later in the course of the disease – may also improve when dopaminergic therapy is started or augmented [17,29]. Freezing may become more resistant in later stages of the disease, but the issue here may be related to inadequate dosing because of adverse effects of treatment such as motor complications or hallucinations. Indeed, it has been our impression that the threshold for obtaining a therapeutic response may be higher for freezing than for other motor signs (Figure 32.1). This could partially explain the presence of ON period freezing of gait: at certain doses most motor signs will have improved, but freezing persists, falsely creating the impression that medication actually induced the freezing symptoms. Future research will need to substantiate this assumption, for example by carefully monitoring the response of freezing and other disease signs to a levadopa challenge, using controlled increases in dosage. A link to dopaminergic lesions was made in a large prospective aging study, where postmortem examination of 50 subjects without PD detected an association between cell loss in the dorsolateral quadrant of the substantia nigra and UPDRS scores for postural instability, stooped posture, and gait disturbances [30].

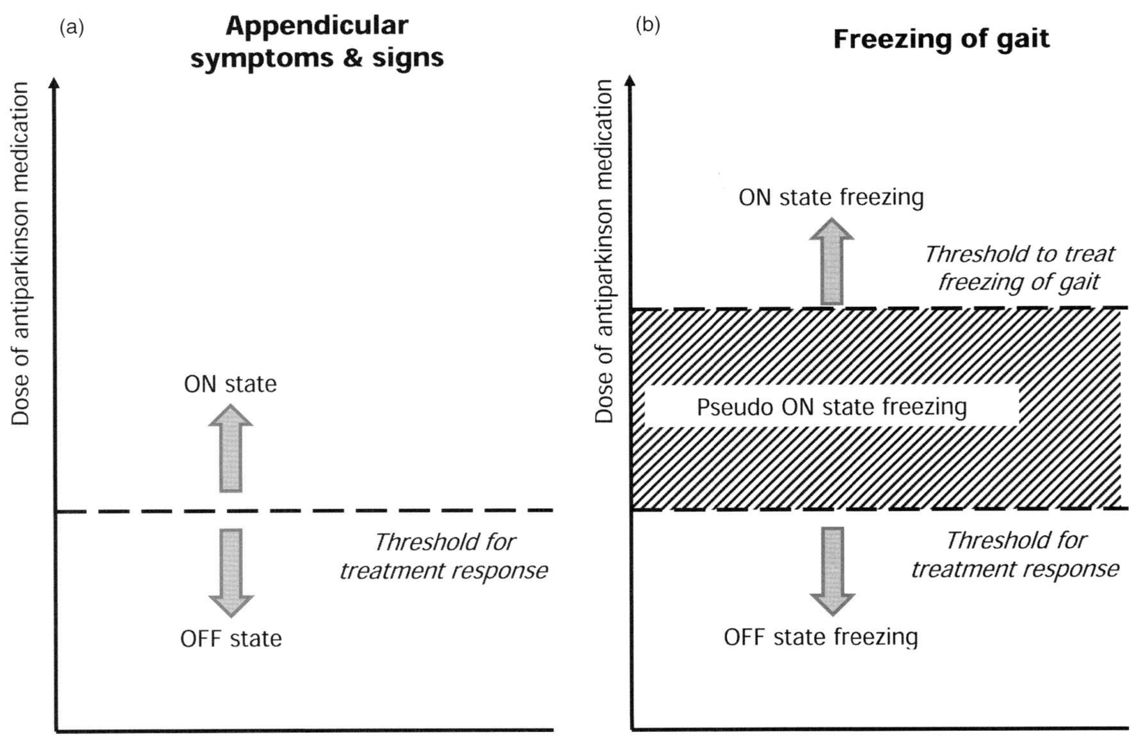

Figure 32.1 Treatment of freezing of gait, in relation to other motor symptoms and signs. The threshold for symptoms and signs to improve may be lower for appendicular manifestations of PD (a), compared with the threshold for freezing of gait to improve (b). This creates an intermediate level, occurring at doses where patients generally appear to respond well to medication, but nevertheless experience freezing of gait. Although counterintuitive, we recommend first increasing the dose of anti-parkinson medication in these patients, provided that they do not experience dose-limiting side effects. If freezing improves, the patient actually has "pseudo ON" freezing. If freezing worsens, the patient has true ON period freezing, and the dose should be reduced.

The most devastating consequence of gait and balance impairment is falling. In this chapter, we summarize the dominant clinical features of axial motor disability in PD, provide a pathophysiologic framework for falls in PD, and consider how to develop an individually tailored and multifactorial falls prevention program. We propose a battery of measures that are based on published observations in PD, personal experience, and knowledge obtained with falls prevention in the elderly. The protocol proposed here may serve both as a guide for current clinical use and also as a basis for future formal evaluation in adequately designed randomized clinical trials.

Clinical assessment of balance and gait

Importance

Careful recognition of gait and balance abnormalities is crucial, for several reasons (Box 32.1). First, axial features can often assist clinicians in refining their differential diagnosis in patients presenting with a hypokinetic–rigid syndrome. It is not rare for the specific gait or balance features to provide the clue to correct diagnosis. Examples include the occurrence of seemingly spontaneous backward falls in the first year of the disease – suggesting a diagnosis of PSP – or the presence of dominant lower-body parkinsonism with early and levodopa-resistant freezing of gait – suggesting a diagnosis of vascular parkinsonism.

Box 32.1 Importance of gait and balance assessment in clinical practice

- Support for the differential diagnosis
- Basis for individually tailored treatment
- Prevention of complications
  - Falls
  - Injuries
  - Constipation
  - Pressure sores
  - Insomnia
  - Osteoporosis
  - Physical inactivity
  - Loss of independence
  - Social isolation
  - Fear of falling
  - Reduced quality-of-life
  - Caregiver stress
- Marker of poor prognosis/greater disease severity and associated symptoms
  - Depression
  - Anxiety
  - Rapid disease progression
  - Urinary incontinence
  - Cognitive decline
  - Nursing home admission
  - Reduced survival
- Marker for underlying abnormalities
  - Frontal executive deficits
  - Underlying cerebrovascular disease
- Socio-economic impact
  - Loss of productivity
  - Costs related to injuries

Second, as indicated earlier, careful clinical assessment provides the basis for subsequent treatment, aimed at improving gait and balance, reducing or preventing falls, and minimizing their consequences. Indeed, falls in PD often have devastating consequences, leading to a poor overall prognosis. Hip fractures occur in about 25% of patients within 10 years of diagnosis [31] and are associated with high morbidity, admission to a nursing home, and mortality [32–34]. Fractures of the wrist are less common, perhaps because the hands are not stretched out fast enough after a fall [35]. "Minor" injuries such as bruises or lacerations are even more common than fractures. Furthermore, reduced mobility is associated with other incapacitating complications, including constipation, pressure sores, insomnia, and osteoporosis, which increase fracture risk in the future. Immobility also deprives patients of their independence and social contacts. These problems are aggravated by a commonly present and incapacitating fear of renewed falls [11]. When this fear of falling becomes excessive, patients become unnecessarily immobilized, with consequences for their social interactions and physical fitness.

Third, the presence of gait and balance abnormalities serves as a marker for other signs that are perhaps less obvious during routine clinical examination, such as frontal executive deficits [36–39] or underlying cerebrovascular disease [40]. This is discussed in more detail in the section on clinical manifestations.

Fourth, gait and balance abnormalities have considerable prognostic importance. In a group of 362 patients who were originally enrolled as part of the DATATOP study and who were carefully followed for disease progression, the current level of gait dysfunction did not predict future changes in health-related quality-of-life [41]. However, worsening gait and balance over time were accompanied by worsening mental and physical health-related quality-of-life, underscoring the need to preserve balance in order to prevent a worsening of health-related quality-of-life. Furthermore, a prior fall is the best predictor of future falls [42], and postural instability and falls are associated with reduced survival [27,43,44]. This increased mortality is explained by the occurrence of lethal falls and by secondary immobilization, which reduces general fitness and increases the risk of cardiovascular disease. Importantly, the disease also appears to progress at a faster rate once falls are present [28].

Finally, gait and balance abnormalities have implications for society at large. Falls and fall-related injuries are extremely costly and contribute to the overall costs of PD [45,46]. Falls are also a major reason for caregiver stress [47,48], and healthcare costs rise considerably when the caregiver support collapses.

In the light of these considerations, it should be appreciated that the clinical examination of parkinsonian patients is incomplete without a proper gait and balance assessment. Whenever possible, patients should be examined during both the OFF state (preferably following withdrawal of anti-parkinson medication for at least 12 h) and the "best ON" state. It is recommended to have a sufficiently large examination room, or else to take the patients to the corridor to examine their gait. At the same time, gait and balance need to be challenged using a series of tests, in order to bring about the full range of abnormalities. Note that performance is usually much better in the hospital, where lighting is optimal and gait is rarely complicated by obstacles in the pathway. Hospital examination is also obscured by a phenomenon termed "kinesia paradoxica," namely the ability of poorly mobile patients with advanced disease to move unexpectedly well under emotional circumstances (such as a doctor's visit). In contrast, at home patients are more at ease, and they need to walk in crowded living rooms (forcing them to make narrow turns), with poor lighting or loose rugs on the floor. Some of these domestic factors can be copied in the examination room, for example by forcing patients to turn around in tight quarters to provoke freezing [49]. Nevertheless, it is often informative to have a physiotherapist or occupational therapist pay a home visit to witness the patient's performance in their own habitat.

Gait

For most patients, walking changes can already be detected in early stages of the disease, and can even be the presenting symptom, for example, an asymmetrically reduced or absent arm swing [50]. Other early features include difficulties turning around in a standing or recumbent position. As the disease progresses, gait becomes slower and the typical parkinsonian gait emerges with shuffling and short steps, bilaterally reduced arm swing, and slow turns which are executed *en bloc*. In contrast to most other gait disorders, gait is typically not wide-based [51]. The presence of a broad-based gait generally suggests an atypical parkinsonism. A simple test is to ask patients to take 10 consecutive tandem steps; patients with idiopathic PD can usually perform this without difficulty, even when moderately severely affected [52]. Hence, taking even a single corrective side step is suggestive of atypical parkinsonism, particularly in early stages of the disease. Note that patients may compensate for their "automatic" gait problems by paying conscious attention to the act of walking. Distraction or asking the patient to perform a double or secondary task (answering questions, carrying an object) interferes with this compensatory strategy and often aggravates the gait disorder, causing patients to slow down or completely stop walking.

Freezing of gait

The features described above represent a form of "continuous" gait abnormality that are more or less continuously present. In addition, PD patients can also experience "episodic" gait disorders, that is, walking problems that are only irregularly present, intermingled with periods when gait is much better [53]. The prime example of these episodic gait disorders is freezing of gait, when patients experience sudden and usually brief moments where the feet subjectively seem to become "glued to the floor" [17]. For practical purposes, freezing of gait was recently defined as "a brief episode during which patients find it impossible to generate effective forward stepping movements, in the absence of another cause than parkinsonism or higher cortical deficits" [54]. The prevalence of freezing increases with disease duration and progression of disease severity, although it can be present in early stages of PD, and occasionally even at disease onset. However, early freezing episodes should alert the clinician to the presence of a form of atypical parkinsonism, or a disorder called primary progressive freezing of gait [55]. In patients with PD, freezing is more common after prolonged dopaminergic treatment, but this does not necessarily imply that the drugs are causally related (because more severe symptoms also require more medication). Indeed, freezing can occur in drug-naïve patients, and most forms of freezing in PD improve with dopaminergic medication. Note that freezing may also occur in other parkinsonian disorders (e.g., PSP, MSA, vascular parkinsonism, and normal pressure hydrocephalus) [56,57]. However, freezing is rare in drug-induced parkinsonism.

Freezing most commonly appears when patients are making turns, especially in tight quarters. Other circumstances that commonly provoke freezing include negotiating a narrow passage such as a door, trying to initiate gait ("start hesitation"), executing a double task (such as talking while walking), or upon reaching a target. It is less common for freezing to occur during straight, undisturbed walking. Although the name suggests otherwise, freezing is usually not an "immobile" blockade of walking movements (complete akinesia), but is a more dynamic phenomenon. The most common presentation is with shuffling small steps, or a characteristic "trembling" of the legs, with the frozen foot in plantar flexion and the forefoot stuck to the floor [58]. Freezing of just one leg may occur, particularly when turning. Most freezing episodes are brief, usually lasting only a few seconds or less, although in more advanced stages of the disease freezing may persist for minutes. Freezing episodes are also much briefer during the ON than the OFF phase.

Detection of freezing often depends on a careful history taking, with attention to the provoking circumstances. It can be difficult to assess freezing reliably during physical examination, because the anxiety associated with the doctor's visit may suppress the phenomenon. A freezing of gait questionnaire has been developed for this purpose. There is now an updated version where patients and their immediate carers are shown video clips of characteristic freezing events, in order to facilitate recognition of the phenomenon [59]. This updated questionnaire also addresses the impact of freezing on daily life, for example, fear of falling.

Physical examination should include a dedicated "freezing of gait trajectory" that features specific triggers to elicit freezing: gait initiation, undisturbed walking in an open space, and walking under challenging situations (crossing a door or other narrow space, turning around, negotiating obstacles and performing a dual task) (Figure 32.2). Interestingly, many patients only experience freezing during full turns (360–540°) and not during partial turns (180°), so a standardized gait trajectory should include full turns (in both directions, because freezing often shows a directional sensitivity, being much worse and sometimes even exclusively present for turns in one direction). In addition to attempts to *provoke* freezing, it is useful to evaluate the response to external cues. This may have diagnostic importance, because freezing will improve in PD patients, but generally not in patients with higher level gait disorders [53]. Evaluating the effect of cues may also help to determine possible therapeutic interventions. Finally, various quantitative gait assessments have been proposed, but these methods do not yet have a proven value for clinical practice.

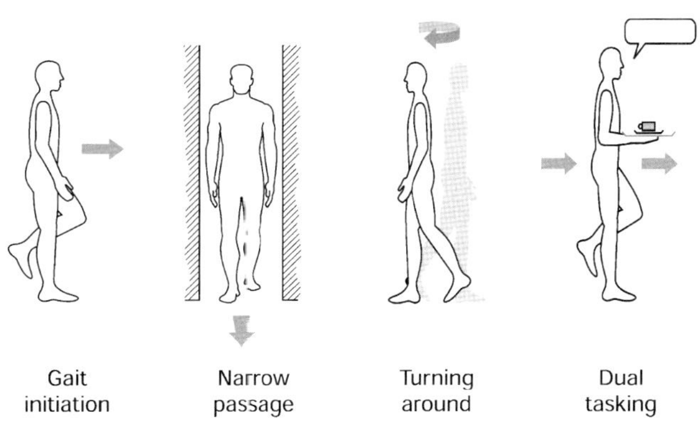

Figure 32.2 Essential elements of a dedicated "freezing of gait trajectory". Reproduced from Snijders *et al.* [49] with permission from John Wiley & Sons, Inc.

Postural abnormalities

Changes in posture can provide important diagnostic information. A gently stooped posture can be seen in early stages of PD, becoming more pronounced in later stages of the disease, usually with some lateral leaning of the trunk. However, severe and persistent lateroflexion – the so-called "Pisa syndrome" or pleurothotonus – often (but not always) suggests neuroleptic-induced dystonia, MSA, or post-encephalitic parkinsonism [60–62]. Camptocormia refers to a marked anteflexion of the thoracolumbar spine (between 30 and 90°), but without forward flexion of the neck [63]. This can occur in both PD (where it may occasionally improve with dopaminergic medication or deep brain surgery) and forms of atypical parkinsonism. Camptocormia is apparent on standing, worsens while walking, but decreases while sitting and even disappears when lying down. This last feature separates camptocormia from the fixed kyphoscoliosis seen in patients with degenerative changes of the spine. An extreme degree of antecollis relative to other body parts, with the neck held in a relatively fixed and severely flexed position, or when the chin touches the chest, is unusual and suggests a diagnosis of MSA [64,65]. Antecollis develops in about half of pathologically proven MSA patients, usually in the middle or late stages of the disease [65]. In contrast, retroflexion of the neck (retrocollis) suggests a diagnosis of PSP [66], but is usually not an early feature [66]. In PSP, axial rigidity of the neck is greater than in the trunk, whereas the opposite pattern occurs in PD [67].

Balance impairment

Postural stability is preserved early in the course of PD, and falls never occur at onset or within the first 2 years of the disease in pathologically confirmed cases of idiopathic PD [28]. Balance impairment can gradually develop as the disease progresses [68], appearing later (and in less prominent form) in patients with the tremor-dominant type of PD. Being unable to stand on one leg, for example while getting dressed, is one of the earliest signs of postural instability.

A battery of clinical tests is needed to capture the complex nature of balance problems in patients with basal ganglia disorders. Functional "every day" tests should be performed whenever possible. These include rising from a chair, sitting down, and getting in and out of a bed. It is particularly important to test the so-called defensive balance reactions, which are evoked by imminent falls. Examples include the ability to take corrective steps or to make protective arm movements (to grasp for support, or to cushion the impact of an impending fall). Evaluation of these defensive reactions is often difficult in a clinical setting because patients must be brought close to (or even beyond) their limits of stability. Quantified assessment following standardized balance perturbations – using dynamic posturography – is perhaps more suited for this purpose, although the clinical utility for the management of individual patients remains unclear [69]. In clinical practice, the retropulsion test is typically used to test defensive reactions, but this test is not without problems. There is great variability in test performance across clinicians (depending on subjective preferences, but also on the height or weight of both the patient and investigator), scoring of the response is subjective, and its interpretation is not straightforward. For example, it is unclear how many corrective steps can still be regarded as "normal." Interestingly, taking more steps is usually equated with greater balance impairment, but this may not be correct because corrective steps are important defensive reactions. Indeed, the most abnormal reaction is not taking any corrective step at all, leading to a fall "like a pushed toy soldier" (note that freezing can be a "confounder" here, interfering with the ability to step backward and leading to a fall "like a log" into the arms of the investigator, even when balance itself is otherwise preserved). We recommend taking the speed and quality of balance reactions into account (rather than merely counting the number of corrective steps), and to regard a slow response as abnormal even if only one or two steps are taken. A particular problem is the inconsistency in the strength of the shoulder pull, within and between raters (depending on experience or physical strength), and also within and between patients who may have different degrees of instability. Consequently, the retropulsion test has an only moderate intra- and inter-rater consistency, correlates poorly with objective measures of postural instability (as quantitatively ascertained in a balance laboratory), and is a poor predictor of actual falls in daily life [70]. We usually deliver one shoulder pull without specific prior warning, as this may best mimic daily life circumstances where falls are usually unexpected events. We then repeat the test several times and regard failure to "habituate" to the test as another sign of balance impairment. As such, the retropulsion test indexes the degree of postural instability. However, the test fails to predict falls, at least in PD [11], probably because falling is the net result of a complex interplay between gait, balance, and protective mechanisms.

The "push and release" test was recently proposed as a more consistent and sensitive alternative to the pull test (or retropulsion test) [71]. The essence is to eliminate the inconsistency of the stimulus by instructing subjects actively to push backwards against the palms of the examiner's hands (placed on the subject's scapulae), allowing the trunk to move backwards while the examiner supports the subject's weight. Balance is then perturbed when the examiner suddenly removes the external support, forcing the patient to take a backward step to regain balance. Initial experience suggests that the "push and release" test correlates better with self-reported prior falls than the retropulsion test, and that it could be used in both the ON and the OFF states [71,72]. A drawback of the "push and release" test is that patients may have difficulty following the instructions, and some are hesitant to push back adequately into the examiner's hands due to lack of confidence.

Falls

Falls are a devastating consequence of postural and gait disturbances. Prospective surveys in PD note high rates of falls that exceed those of community-dwelling elderly subjects [42]. The incidence of falls is even higher when near-falls are included [73], and these near-falls typically precede the onset of actual falling [74]. The risk of falling is highest when patients reach Hoehn and Yahr stage 2.5–3, when balance becomes impaired but patients are still sufficiently mobile to be at risk of falling. In these moderately affected PD patients, the risk of sustaining a single fall was six times higher than in healthy age-matched peers, and the risk of recurrent falls was nine times higher. The falling rate may level off in the later stages due to disease progression and increasing immobility [42]. Indeed, patients in Hoehn and Yahr stage 5 who are bound to their bed or wheelchair are for this reason unlikely to fall. Furthermore, patients may compensate for their worsening balance by moving more safely and purposely restricting their activities.

It is important to realize that most falls occur when patients are in the ON state, possibly reflecting their increased mobility. This observation underscores that dopaminergic medication usually provides little or no improvement of postural instability. In fact, dopaminergic medication can cause dyskinesias that may perturb patients and increase falls. In addition, medication may cause or aggravate cognitive dysfunction, causing delirium and risky wandering behavior, leading to more falls. Most falls involve movements of the trunk, in particular sudden turning movements, presumably because this provokes freezing. Changes in posture ("transfers"), such as rising from a chair, are also commonly responsible. Orthostatic hypotension has been mentioned as an independent risk factor for falls in PD [75]. However, falls due to preceding loss of consciousness are rare, and when this occurs clinicians should consider MSA, where syncope due to autonomic dysfunction is common [76].

Cognitive deficits

PD patients with gait and balance problems should always receive a cognitive examination, especially testing frontal executive functions and attention. This may seem unnecessary, because gait and balance control are traditionally considered to be a largely automatic process, governed mainly at a subconscious level by spinal and perhaps brainstem neural structures. However, recent studies have shown that neuropsychologic processes such as attention are necessary for maintaining balance. Walking is an even more complex process than standing, involving a range of cognitive systems [77]. This role of cognition is obvious during many activities of daily living, when people need to perform multiple actions simultaneously or quickly shift attention and control from one task to another. To perform such actions, cognitive abilities are needed effectively to monitor the environment, choose flexible response patterns to appearing threats, and to make appropriate motor responses necessary for completing goals – and this is precisely where patients PD experience great difficulties, perhaps explaining why gait and balance deficits are such prominent features of PD. Indeed, cognitive dysfunction is particularly prominent in patients with the PIGD subtype of PD [2,3,78]. It may also explain why falls seem to be particularly prominent in disorders that are characterized by a combination of both motor deficits (gait impairment, postural instability) plus a concurrent decline in cognitive functions. PD itself is one good example, but there are many other such disorders, including various forms of atypical parkinsonism (PSP, Lewy body dementia, vascular parkinsonism), and Alzheimer's disease [79]. Patients with PD have difficulty executing two different motor tasks simultaneously, such as walking and carrying an object [80–88], and these dual task problems are associated with the risk of falling [1]. Various studies have shown that frontal executive dysfunction is related to gait impairment in PD patients [89] and is associated with an increased risk of falls [90]. Moreover, frontal executive dysfunction and freezing frequently co-occur, but there is as yet no proof of a direct causal interrelationship [36]. Recklessness, decreased ability to learn cues, and an increased sensitivity to cognitive overload (for example, when dual tasking) may explain why patients with frontal executive dysfunction are more prone to falls. Moreover, the presence of frontal executive dysfunction may give a clue to the underlying etiology, as it is more prominent in atypical parkinsonism than idiopathic PD. A clear example is provided by patients with PSP, where "motor recklessness" combined with progressive balance deficits are jointly responsible for the high rates of falls [5]. Emotional problems should also be considered. Depression is associated with falls [91], and possibly increased freezing [58], and freezing is also associated with anxiety and panic attacks [92].

Treatment

A multifactorial falls prevention program

Adequate treatment of gait and balance impairment is crucial in view of their potentially devastating consequences. The key goals should be prevention, preservation of safe mobility, and independence. We have recently reviewed the specific medical and non-medical treatment options for specific gait and balance problems in PD [93]. Rather than reiterating these treatment recommendations, we focus here on a newly developed protocol for a multidisciplinary falls prevention program. To achieve this, it is important to consider the pathophysiology of falls, as this offers a rationale for preventive strategies. Falls in PD patients are usually not caused by a single factor – such as a reduced step height – but are typically the net result of a complex and multifactorial pathophysiology. This includes both "extrinsic" or environmental factors (e.g., loose rugs on the floor) and "intrinsic" or patient-related factors (e.g., balance impairment, gait disability, and freezing of gait). Many of these factors are specific for PD, but patients may also fall due to generic risk factors for falls that apply to any elderly person ("generic risk factors").

It is therefore unlikely that, by themselves, single interventions will be able to prevent patients from falling. Instead, we anticipate that a multifactorial falls prevention program is needed, including PD-specific therapeutic measures plus a set of generic strategies. The merits of such a comprehensive falls prevention program have never been evaluated in PD, and in fact, there is no accepted menu of interventions. Here we propose such a program, based on (a) determination of previously identified risk factors for falls in PD and (b) to distil all relevant risk factors, defined as those factors that were consistently present in the literature, that conveyed a substantial risk of falling (i.e. were either commonly present, or associated with a high relative risk of falling, or both) and that appeared potentially amenable to therapeutic intervention. We subsequently tailored a menu of therapeutic interventions to address risk factors, including not only disease-specific strategies, but also a selection of "generic" falls prevention strategies derived from the literature and from published national and international falls prevention guidelines (Table 32.1). A challenge here was to identify therapeutic strategies that would be both relevant and feasible for PD patients. For example, standing with both legs crossed is an accepted intervention to reduce falls caused by orthostatic hypotension, but is unlikely to be an acceptable treatment for PD patients given their postural instability. Also, each falls prevention strategy needs to strike a balance between being both comprehensive (covering every single potential risk factor) and tolerable (not too demanding for PD patients, given their fatigue and at times limited learning abilities). Based on these considerations, we have constructed a concept for a Multifactorial Parkinson Falls Prevention Strategy that accomodates the above factors. This protocol is summarized in Table 32.1. Below we briefly discuss a few elements of the multifactorial strategy.

Table 32.1 Selected generic and disease-specific risk factors for falls, and tailored interventions.

Risk factor for falls	Tailored intervention
PD specific	
Gait impairment (e.g., reduced step height)	• Increase anti-parkinson medication • Physiotherapy (cueing strategies) [94,95]
Freezing of gait	• Optimize anti-parkinson medication – ON phase freezing: decrease levodopa (after excluding pseudo-ON-freezing) – OFF increase freezing: increase levodopa; MAO-blocker • Physiotherapy (cueing strategies) [94,95] • Eliminate domestic hazards [96]
Postural instability	• Optimize anti-parkinson medication (usually ineffective) • Physiotherapy (balance training) [94] • Lower limb strength training [97]
Bradykinesia (e.g., slow protective arm movements)	• Increase dopaminergic medication
Dyskinesias	• Optimize anti-parkinson medication
Inability to handle dual tasks	• Avoiding dual tasks (physiotherapy, occupational therapy) [1,89] • Cognitive movement strategies (chaining) [94]
Transfers	• Increase anti-parkinson medication • Cognitive movement strategies [94]
Generic	
Polypharmacy	• Reduction of medication (consult a geriatrician)
Sedative drugs (benzodiazepines)	• Stop when possible
Daily use of alcohol	• Minimize alcohol intake
Fear of falling	• Increase balance confidence [94]
Impaired ADL	• Occupational therapist [96]
Physical inactivity	• Physiotherapy: improve physical capacity, muscle power, mobility, muscle length [94]
Improper use of assistive device	• Train use of assistive devices (physical therapist; occupational therapist)
Visual impairment	• Consult eye specialist • Restrict use of multifocal glasses • Cataract surgery [98]
Cognitive impairment	• Medication (no evidence for PD to reduce falls) – Cholinesterase inhibitor • Physiotherapy – Avoid multitasking – Minimize hazardous behavior
Behavioral disturbances	• Atypical neuroleptics • Restriction of activities (only if all other measures fail)
Muscle weakness	• Muscle strength training [94,97,99]
Postural hypotension	• Decrease anti-parkinson medication • Decrease other hypotensive medication [100] • Increase dietary salt and fluid intake • Anti-orthostatic maneuvers (if balance is good) • Pressure stockings • Small meals • Raising cranial end of the bed • Symptomatic medication: – Fludrocortisone – Midrodine
Urinary incontinence and nocturia	• Reduce coffee and alcohol in the evening • Adequate night-time lighting • Incontinence materials
Environmental risk factors	• Occupational therapy at home

Medication

As outlined at the outset of this chapter, dopaminergic medication has mixed effects on gait, balance, and falls. On the one hand, some axial motor features can improve following treatment with dopaminergic medication. For example, freezing is usually seen during the OFF state, and such OFF-state freezing of gait may improve when dopaminergic medication is increased. However, other gait and balance problems are more resistant to treatment [8–10] or are even aggravated by dopaminergic medication [16–19]. It is therefore important to review carefully the relation between falls and the timing of intake of dopaminergic medication. When freezing appears to occur during the ON state [101,102] – which is the case in only a small proportion of PD patients – the first step is nevertheless to increase further the dose of dopaminergic therapy, as some patients actually have "pseudo-ON freezing" (see Figure 32.1). In a few patients, freezing will worsen further, suggesting that it is a true ON period sign, and this necessitates a dose reduction. Benzodiazepines and other sedative medication need to be avoided whenever possible, as they may further increase the risk of falling [11].

Pharmacotherapy of gait and balance problems should ideally aim at correction of both dopaminergic and non-dopaminergic deficits. Attention is now shifting towards the development of "non-dopaminergic" drugs directed at other neurotransmitter systems [20,103]. Unfortunately, such drugs are not yet available for treatment of axial disability.

Physiotherapy

There is increasing evidence to support the use of physiotherapy as part of a comprehensive falls prevention program [94,104–108]. Patients who have difficulties with initiating or maintaining gait often report that simple tricks can promote walking; these include cues that are environmental (e.g., stepping over an object on the floor) or self-generated (e.g., counting). This technique of using internal or external cueing can be exploited to train patients to use auditory cues (such as listening to rhythmic sounds of a metronome), visual cues (such as stepping over lines pasted on to the floor), tactile cues (such as tapping on the leg), or mental cues (such as simple arithmetic, or generating a mental image of the appropriate step length). Physiotherapists can also teach patients how to handle their freezing episodes. The risk of falling appears highest in patients who actively try to "overcome" their gait blockade, so patients should be instructed simply to wait for the freezing to disappear. Physiotherapists can also address the cognitive aspects of falling, by teaching patients to avoid multitasking in daily life, and to split complex tasks into several less complex sub-movements (a technique called "chaining"). Such cognitive strategies have been shown to improve transfers or rolling over in bed in PD patients [94]. Another approach is to restore confidence and diminish the fear of falling. This may help to restore mobility and promote independence. There is no specific evidence in PD, but studies in the elderly suggest that group treatment using a behavioral–cognitive approach to change attitudes, in addition to training with a physiotherapist, can help [109]. The use of an assistive device and gait training can enhance self-confidence. Instructions on how to stand up may also decrease fear of falling. An entirely different approach is required for cognitively impaired patients, who can be overly confident and inappropriately "over-rate" their own balance, resulting in risky behavior and falls. For them, restriction of hazardous activities might be the best solution to prevent recurrent falls. It is also important to inform the caregiver about activities that should be avoided.

Prevention of complications

Despite all efforts, most patients will continue to sustain at least occasional falls, and for patients with advanced PD the problem may become treatment resistant. For this group, attention should increasingly be focused on preventing the complications of falls. For example, patients with PD can have a coexisting osteoporosis (caused by immobilization and perhaps endocrine disorders) [110], that increase the risk of fracture. In PD patients presenting with a fracture, one should consider performing DEXA bone densitometry to establish whether osteoporosis is present. Treatment of osteoporosis may then reduce the risk of new fractures.

Who should be candidates?

It is necessary to identify patients who are most at risk of falling. Various factors are related to falling, but many are interrelated. Prior falls, disease severity (Hoehn and Yahr stage 3 being most prominently associated with falls), and disease duration appear to be the most consistent predictors of falls. In a meta-analysis, the only independent predictor of falling was earlier falls [42], and this is not a satisfactory predictor because patients have already begun falling. Less robust, but potentially interesting, predictors of falls were fear of falling, avoiding activities because of this fear, and presence of prior near-falls. This may offer a way to identify eligible candidates for fall prevention, even before the first real fall has occurred.

One size fits all?

For clinicians, this is a familiar problem in clinical practice. The good part of the falls prevention approach, as described above, is its comprehensive character: this minimizes the risk of "missing" relevant risk factors, and theoretically provides the most aggressive and complete "gunshot" approach to the falling problem. However, there are less attractive sides of the coin. Being comprehensive, the program is costly and, importantly, it may be excessive for patients where a single factor is obviously responsible for the falling problem. For example, when patients only fall because they trip over a rug in the living room, simply removing this rug may treat the problem and obviate the need for the remainder of the comprehensive falls prevention program. Alternatively, when patients fall because of syncope, is it necessary to pay a home visit and eliminate domestic risk factors for tripping? There is no evidence to support any particular strategy, but a practical compromise may be the following. When patients consistently display a specific type of fall, where one obvious risk factor is consistently responsible for the falls, then simply tackling this single factor may suffice. Figure 32.3 shows the most common fall types,

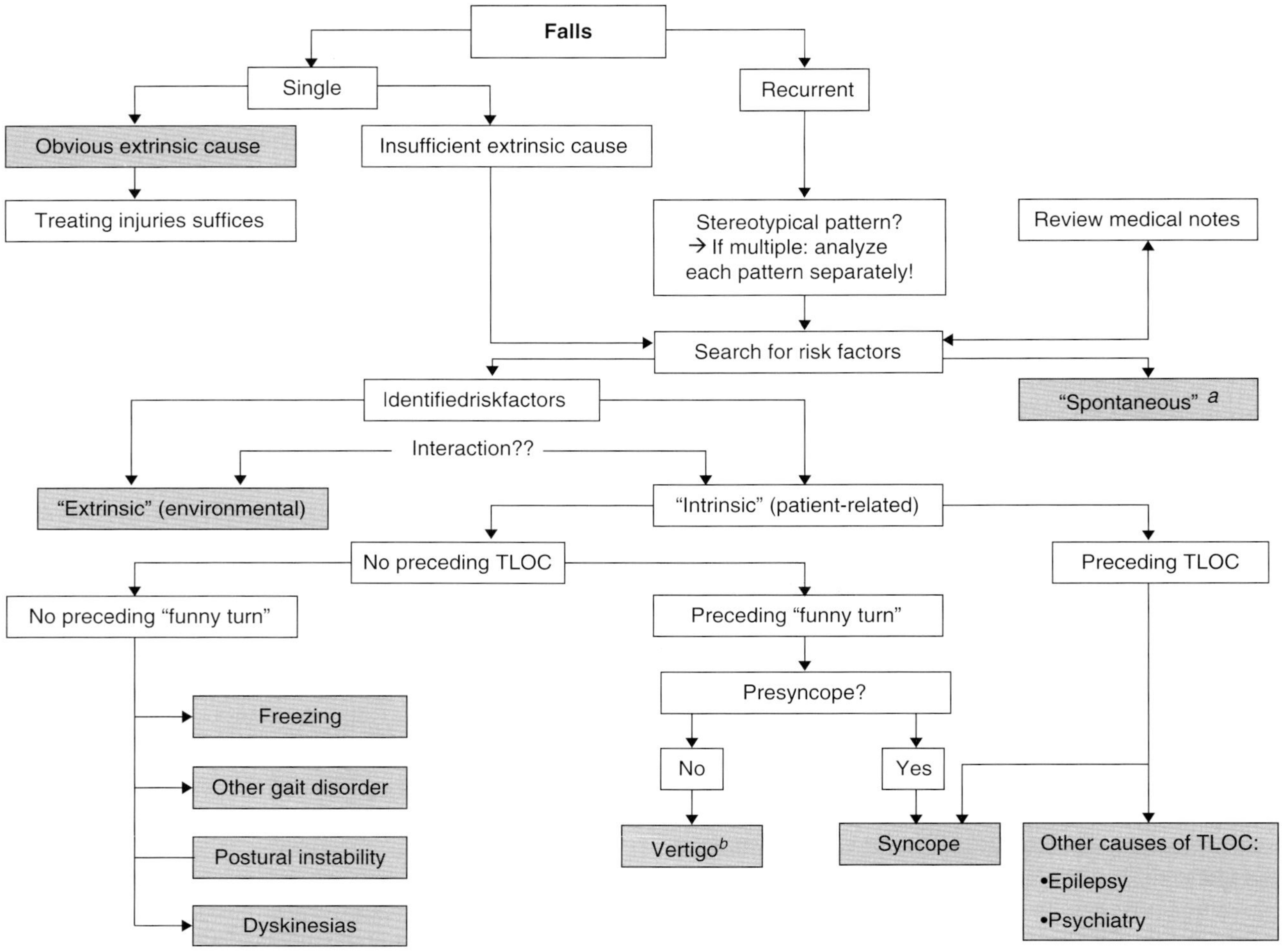

Figure 32.3 Diagnostic algorithm to classify the main types of falls in patients with a hypokinetic–rigid syndrome, modified after Voermans *et al.* [111]. The main categories of falls are shown in gray boxes. TLOC = transient loss of consciousness. [a]When patients claim to fall spontaneously, this is usually caused by either freezing of gait (that is not recognized as such by the patient), or transient loss of consciousness (which is often incorrectly denied by elderly patients). [b]Although there is only little supportive literature [112], it has been our impression that vertigo – in particular that caused by benign position-dependent vertigo – is not rare in patients with PD, perhaps because their relative immobility promotes development of debris in the semicircular canals.

and also a pragmatic approach to ascertain which specific type of fall is present. In other patients, a comprehensive multifactorial approach is recommended.

Conclusion

This chapter underscores that gait disability, postural instability, and falls are common and frequently devastating features of PD. We have reviewed the clinical features, briefly reviewed therapy, and considered a rational basis for a multifactorial falls prevention program. This approach includes identifying both generic and PD-specific risk factors, in order to define a program that is tailored to each individual patient. This program includes: optimizing dopaminergic medication; reducing the use of sedative drugs; physiotherapy to improve transfers, gait (including freezing), balance and balance confidence, physical activity, and the use of assistive devices; occupational therapy (home visits to eliminate domestic hazards); and treatment of orthostatic hypotension, urinary incontinence, and visual impairment. More research is needed to underpin the merits of the proposed multidisciplinary falls prevention program and to evaluate its cost-effectiveness. We also need to develop better ways of finding those patients who are most at risk for falling.

Acknowledgment

This work was supported by a ZonMw VIDI research grant (No. 016.076.352] to B.R.B.

References

1. Bloem BR, Grimbergen YA, van Dijk JG, Munneke M. The "posture second" strategy: a review of wrong priorities in Parkinson's disease. *J Neurol Sci* 2006;**248**:196–204.
2. Alves G, Larsen JP, Emre M, *et al*. Changes in motor subtype and risk for incident dementia in Parkinson's disease. *Mov Disord* 2006;**21**:1123–30.
3. Burn DJ, Rowan EN, Allan LM, *et al*. Motor subtype and cognitive decline in Parkinson's disease, Parkinson's disease with dementia, and dementia with Lewy bodies. *J Neurol Neurosurg Psychiatry* 2006;**77**:585–9.
4. Post B, Merkus MP, De Haan RJ, Speelman JD. Prognostic factors for the progression of Parkinson's disease: a systematic review. *Mov Disord* 2007;**22**:1839–51.
5. Bloem BR, Bhatia KP. Gait and balance in basal ganglia disorders. In: Bronstein AM, Brandt T, Nutt JG, Woollacott MH, eds. *Clinical Disorders of Balance, Posture and Gait*, 2nd edn. Arnold: London, 2004: 173–206.
6. Schrag A, Dodel R, Spottke A, *et al*. Rate of clinical progression in Parkinson's disease. A prospective study. *Mov Disord* 2007;**22**:938–45.
7. Ahlskog JE. Beating a dead horse: dopamine and Parkinson disease. *Neurology* 2007;**69**:1701–11.
8. Lakke JPWF. Axial apraxia in Parkinson's disease. *J Neurol Sci* 1985;**69**:37–46.
9. Bonnet AM, Loria Y, Saint-Hilaire MH, *et al*. Does long-term aggravation of Parkinson's disease result from nondopaminergic lesions? *Neurology* 1987;**37**:1539–42.
10. Bloem BR, Beckley DJ, van Dijk JG, *et al*. Influence of dopaminergic medication on automatic postural responses and balance impairment in Parkinson's disease. *Mov Disord* 1996;**11**:509–21.
11. Bloem BR, Grimbergen YA, Cramer M, *et al*. Prospective assessment of falls in Parkinson's disease. *J Neurol* 2001;**248**:950–8.
12. Bloem BR, Visser JE, Allum JH. Posturography. In: Hallett M, ed. *Handbook of Clinical Neurophysiology*. Amsterdam: Elsevier Science, 2003: 295–336.
13. Dietz V, Berger W, Horstmann GA. Posture in Parkinson's disease: impairment of reflexes and programming. *Ann Neurol* 1988;**24**:660–9.
14. Horak FB, Frank JS, Nutt JG. Effects of dopamine on postural control in parkinsonian subjects: scaling, set, and tone. *J Neurophysiol* 1996;**75**:2380–96.
15. Bloem BR, Beckley DJ, van Dijk JG, *et al*. Medium latency stretch reflexes in young-onset Parkinson's disease and MPTP-induced parkinsonism. *J Neurol Sci* 1994;**123**:52–8.
16. Bloem BR. Postural instability in Parkinson's disease. *Clin Neurol Neurosurg* 1992;**94** (Suppl.):S41–5.
17. Bloem BR, Hausdorff JM, Visser JE, Giladi N. Falls and freezing in Parkinson's disease: a review of two interconnected, episodic phenomena. *Mov Disord* 2004;**19**:871–84.
18. Bloem BR, van Vugt JP, Beckley DJ. Postural instability and falls in Parkinson's disease. *Adv Neurol* 2001;**87**:209–23.
19. Giladi N, Kao R, Fahn S. Freezing phenomenon in patients with parkinsonian syndromes. *Mov Disord* 1997;**12**:302–5.
20. Grimbergen YA, Langston JW, Roos RA, Bloem BR. Postural instability in Parkinson's disease: the adrenergic hypothesis and the role played by the locus coeruleus. *Exp Rev Neurother* 2009;**9**:279–90.
21. Hoogendijk WJ, Pool CW, Troost D, *et al*. Image analyser-assisted morphometry of the locus coeruleus in Alzheimer's disease, Parkinson's disease and amyotrophic lateral sclerosis. *Brain* 1995;**118**:131–43.
22. Braak H, Rub U, Sandmann-Keil D, *et al*. Parkinson's disease: affection of brain stem nuclei controlling premotor and motor neurons of the somatomotor system. *Acta Neuropathol (Berl)* 2000;**99**:489–95.
23. Tohgi H, Abe T, Saheki M, *et al*. Concentration of catecholamines and indoleamines in the cerebrospinal fluid of patients with vascular parkinsonism compared to Parkinson's disease patients. *J Neural Transm* 1997;**104**:441–9.
24. Jellinger KA. Pathology of Parkinson's disease. Changes other than the nigrostriatal pathway. *Mol Chem Neuropathol* 1991;**14**:153–97.
25. Pahapill PA, Lozano AM. The pedunculopontine nucleus and Parkinson's disease. *Brain* 2000;**123**:1767–83.
26. Zweig RM, Jankel WR, Hedreen JC, *et al*. The pedunculopontine nucleus in Parkinson's disease. *Ann Neurol* 1989;**26**: 41–6.
27. Wenning GK, Bosch S, Verny M, *et al*. Time course of severe gait disturbance in parkinsonian disorders: a clinicopathological study. *Mov Disord* 1999;**13**(Suppl.2): 127.
28. Wenning GK, Ebersbach G, Verny M, *et al*. Progression of falls in postmortem-confined parkinsonian disorders. *Mov Disord* 1999;**14**:947–50.
29. Schaafsma JD, Balash Y, Gurevich T, *et al*. Characterization of freezing of gait subtypes and the response of each to levodopa in Parkinson's disease. *Eur J Neurol* 2003;**10**:391–8.
30. Ross GW, Petrovitch H, Abbott RD, *et al*. Parkinsonian signs and substantia nigra neuron density in decendents elders without PD. *Ann Neurol* 2004;**56**:532–9.
31. Johnell O, Melton ILJ, Atkinson EJ, *et al*. Fracture risk in patients with parkinsonism: a population based study in Olmsted County, Minnesota. *Age Ageing* 1992;**21**:32–8.
32. Nutt JG, Hammerstad JP, Gancher ST. *Parkinson's Disease: 100 Maxims*. London: Edward Arnold, 1992.
33. Temlett JA, Thompson PD. Reasons for admission to hospital for Parkinson's disease. *Intern Med J* 2006;**36**:524–6.
34. Hely MA, Morris JGL, Traficante R, *et al*. The Sydney multicentre study of Parkinson's disease: progression and mortality at 10 years. *J Neurol Neurosurg Psychiatry* 1999;**67**: 300–7.
35. Bloem BR, Carpenter MG, Allum JH, Honegger F. Trunk control and protective arm responses to multidirectional postural perturbations in Parkinson's disease. In: Duysens JE, Smits-Engelsman BCM, Kingma H, eds. *Control of Posture and Gait. Maastricht: Symposium of the International Society for Postural and Gait Research*, 2001: 916–9.
36. Giladi N, Huber-Mahlin V, Herman T, Hausdorff JM. Freezing of gait in older adults with high level gait disorders: association with impaired executive function. *J Neural Transm* 2007;**114**:1349–53.
37. Hausdorff JM, Doniger GM, Springer S, *et al*. A common cognitive profile in elderly fallers and in patients with Parkinson's disease: the prominence of impaired executive function and attention. *Exp Aging Res* 2006;**32**:411–29.

38. Snijders AH, Verstappen CC, Munneke M, Bloem BR. Assessing the interplay between cognition and gait in the clinical setting. *J Neural Transm* 2007;**114**:1315–21.
39. Yogev-Seligmann G, Hausdorff JM, Giladi N. The role of executive function and attention in gait. *Mov Disord* 2008;**23**:329–42.
40. Ebersbach G, Sojer M, Muller J, *et al.* Dysequilibrium in idiopathic Parkinson disease. The effect of cerebrovascular comorbidity. *Nervenarzt* 2002;**73**:162–5 (in German).
41. Marras C, Mcdermott MP, Rochon PA, *et al.* Predictors of deterioration in health-related quality of life in Parkinson's disease: results from the DATATOP trial. *Mov Disord* 2008;**23**:653–9.
42. Pickering RM, Grimbergen YA, Rigney U, *et al.* A meta-analysis of six prospective studies of falling in Parkinson's disease. *Mov Disord* 2007;**22**:1892–900.
43. Bennett DA, Beckett LA, Murray AM, Shannon KM, *et al.* Prevalence of parkinsonian signs and associated mortality in a community population of older people. *N Engl J Med* 1996;**334**:71–6.
44. Ebmeier KP, Calder SA, Crawford JR, *et al.* Mortality and causes of death in idiopathic Parkinson's disease: results from the Aberdeen whole population study. *Scott Med J* 1990;**35**(6): 173–5.
45. Chrischilles EA, Rubenstein LM, Voelker MD, *et al.* The health burdens of Parkinson's disease. *Mov Disord* 1998;**13**: 406–13.
46. Pressley JC, Louis ED, Tang MX, *et al.* The impact of comorbid disease and injuries on resource use and expenditures in parkinsonism. *Neurology* 2003;**60**:87–93.
47. Schrag A, Hovris A, Morley D, *et al.* Caregiver-burden in parkinson's disease is closely associated with psychiatric symptoms, falls, and disability. *Parkinsonism Relat Disord* 2006;**12**:35–41.
48. Balash Y, Peretz C, Leibovich G, *et al.* Falls in outpatients with Parkinson's disease. Frequency, impact and identifying factors. *J Neurol* 2005;**252**:1310–5.
49. Snijders AH, Nijkrake MJ, Bakker M, *et al.* Clinimetrics of freezing of gait. *Mov Disord* 2008;**23**(Suppl 2): S468–74.
50. Lees AJ. When did Ray Kennedy's Parkinson's disease begin? *Mov Disord* 1992;**7**:110–6.
51. Charlett A, Weller C, Purkiss AG, *et al.* Breadth of base whilst walking: effect of ageing and parkinsonism. *Age Ageing* 1998;**27**:49–54.
52. Abdo WF, Borm GF, Munneke M, *et al.* Ten steps to identify atypical parkinsonism. *J Neurol Neurosurg Psychiatry* 2006;**77**:1367–9.
53. Snijders AH, van de Warrenburg BP, Giladi N, Bloem BR. Neurological gait disorders in elderly people: clinical approach and classification. *Lancet Neurol* 2007;**6**:63–74.
54. Giladi N, Nieuwboer A. Understanding and treating freezing of gait in parkinsonism, proposed working definition, and setting the stage. *Mov Disord* 2008;**23**(Suppl 2): S423–5.
55. Factor SA, Higgins DS, Qian J. Primary progressive freezing gait: a syndrome with many causes. *Neurology* 2006;**66**:411–4.
56. Giladi N. Freezing of gait. Clinical overview. *Adv Neurol* 2001;**87**:191–7.
57. Stolze H, Kuhtz-Buschbeck JP, Drucke H, *et al.* Comparative analysis of the gait disorder of normal pressure hydrocephalus and Parkinson's disease. *J Neurol Neurosurg Psychiatry* 2001;**70**:289–97.
58. Giladi N, Mcdermott MP, Fahn S, *et al.* Freezing of gait in PD: prospective assessment in the DATATOP cohort. *Neurology* 2001;**56**:1712–21.
59. Nieuwboer A, Herman T, Rochester L, Giladi N. Evaluation of freezing of gait severity in patients with Parkinson's disease: the perception of caregivers. *Mov Disord* 2006;**21**(Suppl. 15):S493.
60. Martin JP. Curvature of the spine in post-encephalitic parkinsonism. *J Neurol Neurosurg Psychiatry* 1965;**28**:395–400.
61. Colosimo C. Pisa syndrome in a patient with multiple system atrophy. *Mov Disord* 1998;**13**:607–9.
62. Yassa R, Nastase C, Cvejic J, Laberge G. The Pisa syndrome (or pleurothotonus): prevalence in a psychogeriatric population. *Biol Psychiatry* 1991;**29**:942–5.
63. Djaldetti R, Mosberg-Galili R, Sroka H, *et al.* Camptocormia (bent spine) in patients with Parkinson's disease – characterization and possible pathogenesis of an unusual phenomenon. *Mov Disord* 1999;**14**:443–7.
64. Wenning GK, Ben-Shlomo Y, Magalhaes M, *et al.* Clinical features and natural history of multiple system atrophy. An analysis of 100 cases. *Brain* 1994;**117**:835–45.
65. Quinn NP. Disproportionate antecollis in multiple system atrophy. *Lancet* 1989;**i**:844.
66. Litvan I, Mangone CA, Mckee A, *et al.* Natural history of progressive supranuclear palsy (Steele–Richardson–Olszewski syndrome) and clinical predictors of survival: a clinicopathological study. *J Neurol Neurosurg Psychiatry* 1996;**61**:615–20.
67. Tanigawa A, Komiyama A, Hasegawa O. Truncal muscle tonus in progressive supranuclear palsy. *J Neurol Neurosurg Psychiatry* 1998;**64**:190–6.
68. Muller J, Wenning GK, Jellinger K, *et al.* Progression of Hoehn and Yahr stages in Parkinsonian disorders: a clinicopathologic study. *Neurology* 2000;**55**:888–91.
69. Visser JE, Carpenter MG, van der KH, Bloem BR. The clinical utility of posturography. *Clin Neurophysiol* 2008;**119**(11): 2424–36.
70. Hass CJ, Bloem BR, Okun MS. Pushing or pulling to predict falls in Parkinson disease? *Nat Clin Pract Neurol* 2008;**4**:530–1.
71. Jacobs JV, Horak FB, Van TK, Nutt JG. An alternative clinical postural stability test for patients with Parkinson's disease. *J Neurol* 2006;**253**:1404–13.
72. Valkovic P, Brozova H, Botzel K, *et al.* Push and release test predicts better Parkinson fallers and nonfallers than the pull test: comparison in OFF and ON medication states. *Mov Disord* 2008;**23**:1453–7.
73. Gray P, Hildebrand K. Fall risk factors in Parkinson's disease. *J Neurosci Nursing* 2000;**32**:222–8.
74. Stack E, Ashburn A. Fall events described by people with Parkinson's disease: implications for clinical interviewing and the research agenda. *Physiother Res Int* 1999;**4**:190–200.
75. Dennison AC, Noorigian JV, Robinson KM, *et al.* Falling in Parkinson disease: identifying and prioritizing risk factors in recurrent fallers. *Am J Phys Med Rehabil* 2007;**86**:621–32.
76. Bloem BR, Overeem S, van Dijk JG. Syncopal falls, drop attacks and their mimics. In: Bronstein AM, Brandt T, Nutt JG, Woollacott MH, eds. *Clinical Disorders of Balance, Posture and Gait*, 2 edn. London: Arnold, 2004: 286–316.

77. Hausdorff JM, Yogev G, Springer S, *et al.* Walking is more like catching than tapping: gait in the elderly as a complex cognitive task. *Exp Brain Res* 2005;**164**(4):541–8.
78. Post B, Merkus MP, De Haan RJ, Speelman JD. Prognostic factors for the progression of Parkinson's disease: a systematic review. *Mov Disord* 2007;**22**:1839–51.
79. Buchner DM, Larson EB. Falls and fractures in patients with Alzheimer-type dementia. *JAMA* 1987;**257**:1492–5.
80. Ashburn A, Stack E, Pickering RM, Ward C. A community-dwelling sample of people with Parkinson's disease: characteristics of fallers and non-fallers. *Age Ageing* 2001;**30**:47–52.
81. Baker K, Rochester L, Nieuwboer A. The immediate effect of attentional, auditory, and a combined cue strategy on gait during single and dual tasks in Parkinson's disease. *Arch Phys Med Rehabil* 2007;**88**:1593–600.
82. Bloem BR, Valkenburg VV, Slabbekoorn M, van Dijk JG. The Multiple Tasks Test. Strategies in Parkinson's disease. *Exp Brain Res* 2001;**137**:478–86.
83. Bond JM, Morris ME. Goal-directed secondary motor tasks: their effects on gait in subjects with Parkinson disease. *Arch Phys Med Rehabil* 2000;**81**:110–6.
84. Camicioli RM, Oken BS, Sexton G, *et al.* Verbal fluency task affects gait in Parkinson's disease with motor freezing. *J Geriatr Psychiatry Neurol* 1998;**11**:181–5.
85. Canning CG. The effect of directing attention during walking under dual-task conditions in Parkinson's disease. *Parkinsonism Relat Disord* 2005;**11**(2):95–9.
86. Hausdorff JM, Balash J, Giladi N. Effects of cognitive challenge on gait variability in patients with Parkinson's disease. *J Geriatr Psychiatry Neurol* 2003;**16**:53–8.
87. Morris ME, Iansek R, Smithson F, Huxham F. Postural instability in Parkinson's disease: a comparison with and without a concurrent task. *Gait Posture* 2000;**12**:205–16.
88. Rochester L, Hetherington V, Jones D, *et al.* Attending to the task: interference effects of functional tasks on walking in Parkinson's disease and the roles of cognition, depression, fatigue, and balance. *Arch Phys Med Rehabil* 2004;**85**:1578–85.
89. Yogev G, Giladi N, Peretz C, *et al.* Dual tasking, gait rhythmicity, and Parkinson's disease: which aspects of gait are attention demanding? *Eur J Neurosci* 2005;**22**:1248–56.
90. Hausdorff JM, Doniger GM, Springer S, *et al.* A common cognitive profile in elderly fallers and in patients with Parkinson's disease: the prominence of impaired executive function and attention. *Exp Aging Res* 2006;**32**(4):411–29.
91. Schrag A, Jahanshahi M, Quinn NP. What contributes to depression in Parkinson's disease? *Psychol Med* 2001;**31**:65–73.
92. Lieberman A. Are freezing of gait (FOG) and panic related? *J Neurol Sci* 2006;**248**(1–2):219–22.
93. Bloem BR, Geurts AC, Hassin-Baer S, Giladi N. Treatment of gait and balance disorders. In: Hallett M, Poewe WH, eds. *Therapeutics of Parkinson's Disease and Other Movement Disorders*. Chichester: John Wiley & Sons, Ltd., 2008: 417–43.
94. Keus SH, Bloem BR, Hendriks EJ, *et al.* Evidence-based analysis of physical therapy in Parkinson's disease with recommendations for practice and research. *Mov Disord* 2007;**22**:451–60.
95. Nieuwboer A, Kwakkel G, Rochester L, *et al.* Cueing training in the home improves gait-related mobility in Parkinson's disease: the RESCUE trial. *J Neurol Neurosurg Psychiatry* 2007;**78**:134–40.
96. Sturkenboom IH, Thijssen MC, Gons-van de Elsacker JJ, *et al. Ergotherapie bij de Ziekte van Parkinson. Een Richtlijn van Ergotherapie Nederland*. Utrecht/Den Haag: Uitgeverij Lemma, 2008.
97. Pessiglione M, Guehl D, Agid Y, *et al.* Impairment of context-adapted movement selection in a primate model of presymptomatic Parkinson's disease. *Brain* 2003;**126**(Pt 6): 1392–408.
98. Lord SR. Visual risk factors for falls in older people. *Age Ageing* 2006;**35**(Suppl **2**):ii42–5.
99. Horlings CG, van Engelen BG, Allum JH, Bloem BR. A weak balance: the contribution of muscle weakness to postural instability and falls. *Nat Clin Pract Neurol* 2008;**4**:504–15.
100. Finelli PF, Gupta F, Zeevi N. Neuroimaging of bilateral caudate infarction manifesting as Parkinsonian gait disorder. *Conn Med* 2007;**71**(3):149–50.
101. Ambani LM, Van Woert MH. Start hesitation – a side effect of long-term levodopa therapy. *N Engl J Med* 1973;**288**:1113–5.
102. Ahlskog JE, Muenter MD, Bailey PA, Stevens PM. Dopamine agonist treatment of fluctuating parkinsonism. D-2 (controlled-release MK-458) vs combined D-1 and D-2 (pergolide). *Arch Neurol* 1992;**49**:560–8.
103. Fox SH, Brotchie JM, Lang AE. Non-dopaminergic treatments in development for Parkinson's disease. Lancet Neurol 2008;**7**:927–38.
104. Falvo MJ, Schilling BK, Earhart GM. Parkinson's disease and resistive exercise: rationale, review, and recommendations. *Mov Disord* 2008;**23**:1–11.
105. Jobges EM, Spittler-Schneiders H, Renner CI, Hummelsheim H. Clinical relevance of rehabilitation programs for patients with idiopathic Parkinson syndrome. II: Symptom-specific therapeutic approaches. *Parkinsonism Relat Disord* 2007;**13**:203–13.
106. Kwakkel G, de Goede CJ, van Wegen EE. Impact of physical therapy for Parkinson's disease: a critical review of the literature. *Parkinsonism Relat Disord* 2007;**13**(Suppl 3): S478–87.
107. Giladi N, Balash Y. The clinical approach to gait disturbances in Parkinson's disease; maintaining independent mobility. *J Neural Transm Suppl* 2006;(70): 327–32.
108. Lim I, van Wegen E, de Goede C, *et al.* Effects of external rhythmical cueing on gait in patients with Parkinson's disease: a systematic review. *Clin Rehabil* 2005;**19**(7):695–713.
109. Rucker D, Rowe BH, Johnson JA, *et al.* Educational intervention to reduce falls and fear of falling in patients after fragility fracture: results of a controlled pilot study. *Prev Med* 2006;**42**(4): 316–9.
110. Sato Y, Manabe S, Kuno H, Oizumi K. Amelioration of osteopenia and hypovitaminosis D by 1α-hydroxyvitamin D3 in elderly patients with Parkinson's disease. *J Neurol Neurosurg Psychiatry* 1999;**66**(1):64–8.
111. Voermans NC, Snijders AH, Schoon Y, Bloem BR. Why old people fall (and how to stop them). *Pract Neurol* 2007;**7**: 158–71.
112. Aranke SV, Sethi KD. Benign paroxysmal positional vertigo in Parkinson's disease. *Neurology* 2003;**61**:1156.

Chapter 33
Orthopedic Complications of Parkinson's Disease

Joseph Rudolph[1] *& Michele Tagliati*[2]
[1]Department of Neurology, Mount Sinai School of Medicine, New York, NY, USA
[2]Department of Neurology, Cedars-Sinai Medical Center, Los Angeles, CA, USA

Introduction

The orthopedic complications of Parkinson's disease (PD) represent an area that is often overlooked, but often as important as the primary neurological aspects of the disease, particularly in the advanced stages of the illness. In his seminal early description of the disease, Charcot notably pointed to skeletal deformities that occur in PD patients, which he noted to be similar to those seen in rheumatoid arthritis [1]. Fractures, osteoporosis, scoliosis, surgical interventions, and other orthopedic issues are all seen in PD patients with greater frequency than in the general population [2]. Unfortunately, these patients are often denied surgical intervention, as orthopedic surgeons have historically been hesitant to bring a PD patient to the operating table, fearing a postoperative course that might have higher morbidity and mortality than in the general population.

Orthopedic complications of PD can be classified under several headings. First, there are the direct effects of the disease, including dyskinetic movement, on the musculoskeletal system of the patient. Also important are the secondary effects (usually bone fractures) due to the higher frequency of falls and trauma that occur as a consequence of postural instability and altered cognition typical of the late stages of the disease. Finally, PD may lead to postoperative complicating factors. Indeed, unique complications and morbidities have been reported in the PD population following a variety of orthopedic procedures, including hip, knee, shoulder, and spine surgeries [3–8]. This chapter considers the orthopedic problems associated with PD.

Primary orthopedic complications

Primary orthopedic problems in PD patients are essentially comprised of joint abnormalities or skeletal deformities secondary to rigidity and dystonia, a condition characterized by involuntary muscle contractions that produce abnormal postures or repetitive movements [9]. Dystonia is more common in young-onset PD and may predate the more typical signs of PD, such as tremor, bradykinesia, and rigidity. Positive family history and rapidly progressive disease generally correlate with the development of dystonic spasms in PD, which tend to affect the side of the body where motor symptoms first occur. Dystonia can present both as features of untreated PD and as a complication of treatment with levodopa. Over the long term, some dystonias can result in fixed muscle contractures and abnormal wearing of the bones or joints. Ultimately, dystonia may induce skeletal deformities such as striatal hand and toe, severe torticollis, camptocormia, and other spinal abnormalities [10]. Over one-third of PD patients have been reported to develop axial, limb, or truncal deformities, a level that can approach 70% in patients with atypical parkinsonism [2]. PD patients who develop deformities are more likely to be on levodopa therapy, which may indicate a more advanced stage of the disease rather than a causative relationship [11]. Table 33.1 summarizes the principal features of limb and axial deformities in PD.

Limb deformities

Striatal hand and foot

The most common type of skeletal deformity in PD is the so-called "striatal" hand or foot. A striatal hand has been described in 8.4% and striatal foot occurred in 5.9% of advanced-stage PD patients in one series [2]. The incidence of hand deformity in the pre-levodopa era was probably much higher, reaching 24% in one study [12]. Striatal abnormalities are more frequent in multiple system atrophy, where they have been described in 26.3% of individuals [2]. Historically, the occurrence of

Parkinson's Disease: Non-Motor and Non-Dopaminergic Features, First Edition. Edited by C. Warren Olanow, Fabrizio Stocchi, and Anthony E. Lang.

Table 33.1 Limb and axial deformities in PD.

	Deformity	Characteristics[a]
Limb	Striatal hand	MCP flexion PIP extension DIP flexion Ulnar deviation (not required)
	Striatal foot	Great toe extension or flexion Plantarflexion of remaining toes Ankle inversion (not required)
	Frozen shoulder	Slow onset Shoulder stiffness Pain Decreased range of motion, active and passive No obvious joint abnormality
Axial	Camptocorm a	Marked flexion (>45°) of thoracolumbar spine when standing or sitting Until advanced stages, improves in recumbent position
	Lateral flexion	Lateral deviation of spine with tendency to lean Flexes away from (usually) side of initial PD symptoms
	Pisa syndrome	Lateral deviation of spine Subacute onset Usually secondary to anti-psychotic medication
	Anterocollis	Marked neck flexion (>45°) • Neck flexor overactivity (dystonia) • Weakness of neck extensors (myopathy)

[a]MCP, metacarpophalangeal joints; PIP, proximal interphalangeal joints; DIP, distal interphalangeal joints

striatal hand was particularly high in post-encephalitic parkinsonism, where 71% of patients developed such deformities in one series [12].

Striatal hand is characterized by flexion of the distal interphalangeal (DIP) joints, extension of the proximal interphalangeal (PIP) joints with flexion of the metacarpophalangeal (MCP) joints, fifth digit abduction, ulnar wrist deviation, and occasionally tight fist clenching [2,12,13]. The positioning mimics that of rheumatoid arthritis, but there are no signs of local joint involvement, such as tenderness, heat, and swelling (Figure 33.1). Further, rheumatoid arthritis is usually bilateral, while the striatal hand in PD tends to be asymmetric [14]. Hand deformity significantly correlates with rigidity, as 72% of those with deformity have severe rigidity [12].

Striatal foot is characterized by the extension of the great toe with flexion of the remaining toes, often with equinovarus foot dystonia (Figure 33.2). Whereas striatal hand is a finding that may go unnoticed, foot deformities are frequently symptomatic and disabling. Patients who develop such deformities tend to be younger and to have a genetic form of PD [2]. Similarly to axial skeletal deformities, the side of the hand or foot deformity tends to coincide with the side of initial symptoms and worse PD-related disability [2]. Thalamotomy has been reported to improve hand deformities [14,15], but it is not yet clear whether deep brain stimulation (DBS) has a consistent effect on striatal hand or foot.

Frozen shoulder

Adhesive capsulitis or periarthritis, also known as *"frozen shoulder,"* occurs at higher rates in PD patients, with an incidence approaching 13% in some series [16]. This syndrome is characterized by the insidious development of shoulder stiffness, pain, and loss of active and passive external rotation in the absence of an obvious intrinsic

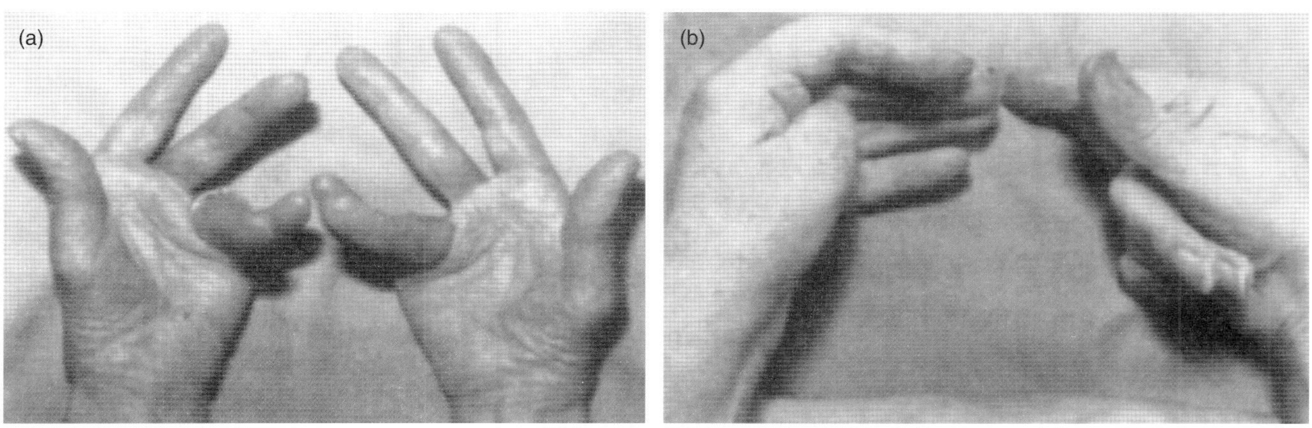

Figure 33.1 Striatal hands. Typical abnormalities resembling rheumatoid arthritis, with ulnar deviation of the fingers (a), flexion of the metacarpophalangeal joints (MCP) and extension of interphalangeal joints (a, b). Reproduced from Reynolds and Petropoulos [12]. Copyright (1965), with permission from Elsevier.

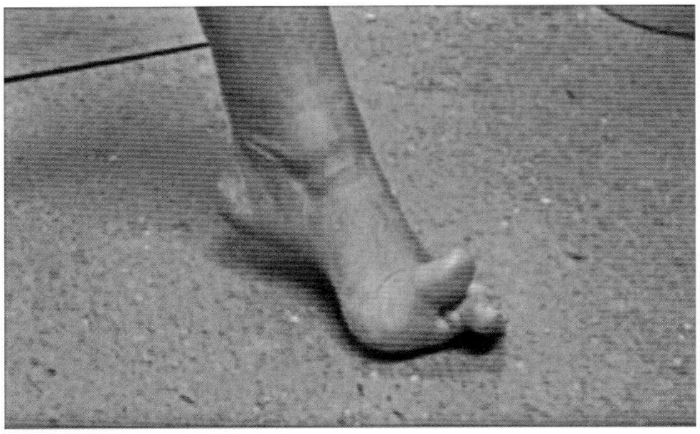

Figure 33.2 Striatal foot in a patient with multiple system atrophy (MSA).

joint abnormality [14]. The condition usually improves without intervention, but the immobility may last weeks to months longer than the pain. Often an account of undiagnosed shoulder symptoms is elicited from PD patients in retrospect. In fact, most patients who developed PD after the episode of frozen shoulder show the initial parkinsonian symptoms on the same side as the periarthritis and are generally more likely to develop an akinetic-rigid form of PD [16]. These features raise the possibility that "frozen shoulder" may be an early and presenting symptom of PD, that reflects restricted movement of the arm that was unappreciated by the patient.

Axial deformities

Several axial deformities can complicate the progression of PD, with stooped posture being the most common and most frequently recognized. In his original monograph, James Parkinson described a "propensity to bend the trunk forward" that became one of the clinical hallmarks of the disease [17]. About 8.4% of PD patients develop spinal deformities, a prevalence that is higher than in the general population [14]. In general, spinal deformities occur in patients who are receiving levodopa, most likely because they have advanced disease rather than because of any direct causal relationship.

Axial deformities that are commonly recognized in patients with PD and atypical parkinsonism include camptocormia (bent spine), lateral flexion (scoliosis), Pisa syndrome (leaning to one side), and anterocollis (flexion of the head on to the chest). These manifestations may ultimately represent different expressions of the same motor disorder, affecting different spinal levels. In most cases, the abnormal postures in PD patients are complex, and include elements of lateral and forward flexion [18].

Differential diagnosis of spinal deformities in PD is summarized in Table 33.2 and therapies for skeletal deformities are outlined in Table 33.3.

Table 33.2 Differential diagnosis of spinal deformities in PD.

Camptocormia
- Idiopathic
- Parkinsonism
  - Idiopathic Parkinson disease
  - Multiple system atrophy
  - Autosomal recessive juvenile parkinsonism (parkin mutation)
  - Postencephalitic parkinsonism
  - Atypical parkinsonism
- Dystonia
  - Primary
  - Secondary associated with parkinsonism
  - Secondary dystonia associated with structural lesions in the brain or spinal cord
- Spine deformities
- Stroke
- Neuromuscular
  - Focal myopathy
  - Amyotrophic lateral sclerosis
  - Inclusion body myositis
  - Nemaline myopathy
- Psychogenic
- Miscellaneous
  - Drug-induced
  - Grave's disease
  - Paraneoplastic
  - Tourette's syndrome

Lateral flexion and Pisa syndrome
- Parkinsonism
  - Idiopathic Parkinson disease
  - Multiple system atrophy
- Drugs
  - Typical neuroleptics
  - Atypical neuroleptics
  - Cholinesterase inhibitors
  - Tricyclic antidepressants
  - Selective serotonin reuptake inhibitors
  - Anti-emetics
  - Lithium
  - Dopaminergic agonists

Anterocollis
- Parkinsonism
  - Idiopathic Parkinson's disease
  - Multiple system atrophy
- Drugs
  - Dopaminergic agonists

Camptocormia (bent spine)

One of the most typical forms of dystonia affecting PD patients is camptocormia, or the "bent-spine" syndrome, which has an incidence of 12.9% [14]. Camptocormia is defined by marked trunk anteroflexion, which subsides in the recumbent position or when leaning against a wall or other type of support (Figure 33.3). It usually shows no or minimal response to levodopa [20,21]. PD patients with camptocormia are typically older, predominantly male, and have long disease duration with early axial

Table 33.3 Therapies for skeletal deformities.

Type	Treatment	Therapy
Medications	Muscle relaxants (centrally acting)	Cyclobenzaprine
		Tizanadine
		Baclofen
		Benzodiazepines
	Locally active	Botulinum toxin injection
Neurosurgical	Medication delivery	Baclofen pump
	Stereotactic surgery	Ablation
		DBS
Orthopedic	Nonsurgical	Casting/bracing
		Physical therapy
	Surgical	Joint reconstruction
		Tendon release

involvement, motor fluctuations, and autonomic symptoms [19,22], although it has been reported as the presenting symptom of PD [23]. Spondyloarthritic changes are very frequent and may be a risk factor for developing camptocormia [19,24]. Lumbar or thoracolumbar scoliosis coexist with camptocormia in 61% of patients and a mild to moderate low-back pain is present in 77% of patients [25]. Although the most frequent etiology is PD, camptocormia may be associated with other parkinsonian syndromes, primary dystonia, vascular lesions, and muscular and rheumatologic disorders [25].

The pathogenesis of camptocormia in PD is poorly explained. There are two schools of thought regarding the underlying mechanism [24]. The first speculates that camptocormia represents a focal action dystonia of the spine and reflects a central disorder [20,21]. This theory is supported by electromyographic findings of dystonic discharges from paraspinal muscles and anecdotal reports of clinical improvement after DBS [26]. In addition, acute onset dystonic camptocormia has been associated with lenticular lesions, suggesting that the basal ganglia play an important role in the maintenance of axial posture [27]. The second theory hypothesizes that camptocormia is primarily a muscle problem affecting trunk extension, and therefore a peripheral disorder [28]. Imaging evidence of muscle hypodensity, myopathic changes in biopsy specimens and electromyograms of the paraspinal muscles, and positive effects of steroid treatment support this alternative hypothesis. These two theories are probably not mutually exclusive and might even be linked, as atrophy of the paraspinal muscles might be secondary to a primary action dystonia of the spine [19].

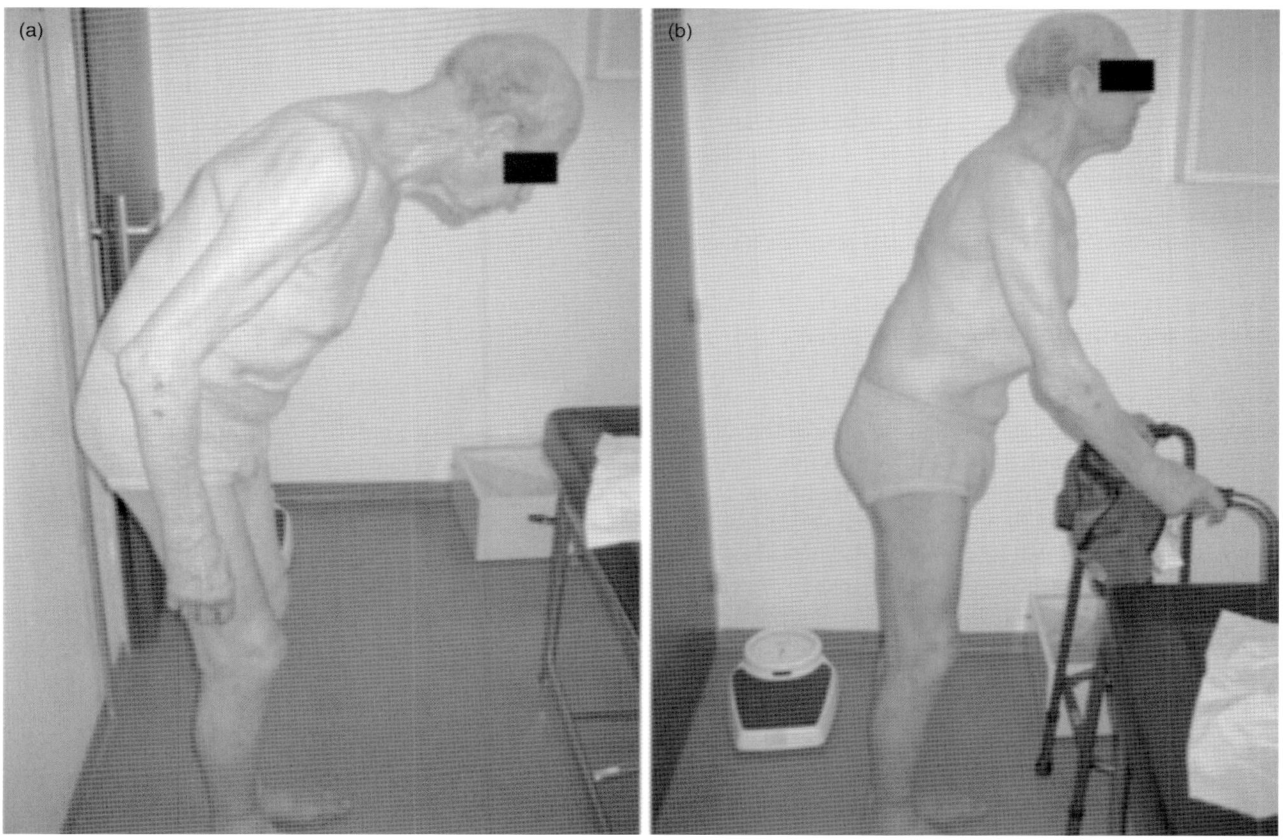

Figure 33.3 Camptocormia. Severe forward flexion of the trunk (a), which appears reducible (b) when leaning over a walker. Reproduced from Lepoutre *et al.* [19] with permission from the BMJ.

Various pharmacologic treatments had been tried in PD patients with camptocormia, including levodopa, anti-cholinergics, amantadine, dopamine agonists, muscle relaxants, tetrabenazine, and intrathecal baclofen infusion, but none has provided consistent postural improvement [10,20]. Moderate to marked improvement was observed in some patients after injecting 300–600 units of botulinum toxin into their abdominal muscles [20]. Pallidal DBS can provide substantial relief of the postural abnormality in patients with idiopathic camptocormia [29,30] and there is anecdotal evidence that DBS can also effectively treat abnormal postures in PD, provided that it is performed before the onset of fixed spinal deformities [18,31]. In evaluating patients with camptocormia, it is important to rule out treatable underling causes such as disc disease with root compression, with spine flexion occurring in an attempt to relieve pain.

Lateral flexion and Pisa syndrome

Lateral flexion in PD is characterized by a lateral deviation of the spine and a corresponding tendency to lean to one side, usually away from the side of initial parkinsonian symptoms [32]. This abnormality is frequent seen in advanced stages of PD, with an observed incidence of 80–95% in some series [19,32]. There is some disagreement in the literature regarding gender frequency: some studies have shown that women have a higher propensity to develop limb and spinal abnormalities [11], whereas others demonstrate a more even distribution between men and women [2]. Interestingly, a positive family history of PD is associated with a greater likelihood of developing axial skeletal deformities, possibly indicating a different underlying genetic disorder [2].

Lateral flexion in PD can have a chronic or subacute presentation, which is very similar to the so-called Pisa syndrome (Figure 33.4), a rare form of axial dystonia, commonly related to anti-psychotic therapy [33]. The chronic type of lateral flexion in PD has a subtle onset and worsens gradually, following the progression of the disease. The evolution of the subacute type of lateral flexion is more rapid and may lead to severely abnormal posture and balance instability as a consequence [18]. A prominent asymmetry of the paraspinal muscles can be observed, with a pathological enlargement of those contralateral to the lateral flexion, which is interpreted as a sign of dystonia (Figure 33.5). Therapy with a number of dopamine agonists has been associated with subacute truncal dystonia in PD [34,35]. Spontaneous occurrence of Pisa syndrome has also been reported rarely in MSA patients [36,37].

Interestingly, PD patients are often unaware of their abnormal postures, suggesting an underlying disturbance of the ability to determine body position in space [18]. Classical observations of the inability of PD patients to judge the visual vertical and horizontal both with the

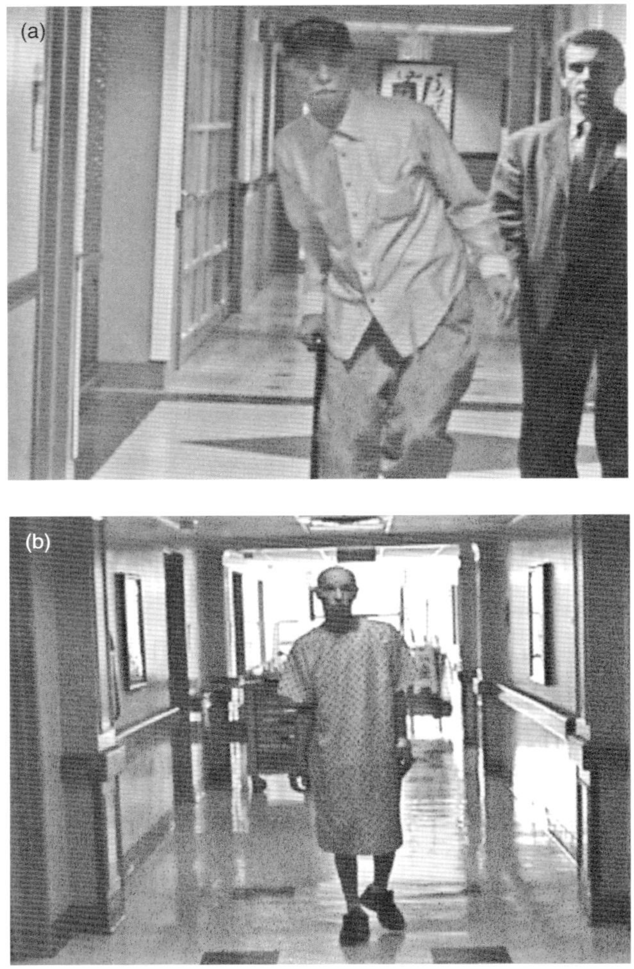

Figure 33.4 Pisa syndrome in a patient with advanced PD on clozapine (a), with resolution of abnormal posture after discontinuation of the atypical neuroleptic (b).

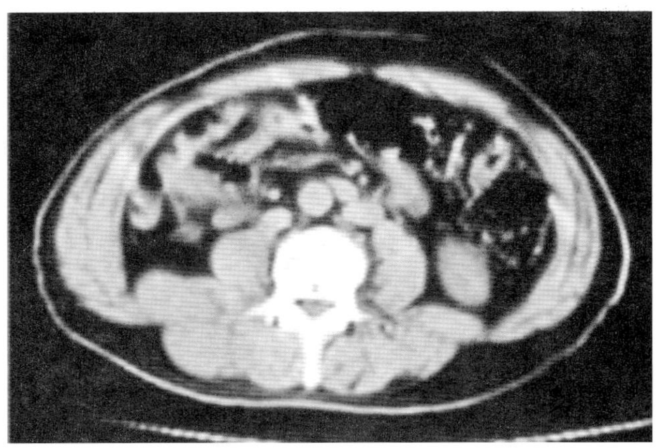

Figure 33.5 Computed tomographic scan showing hypertrophy of the left paraspinal muscles in a PD patient with right lateral flexion of the spine. Reproduced from Yocochi [18] with permission from Dietrich/Steinkopff Verlag.

body tilted and in the upright position point to a specific basal ganglia deficit [38,39] and may explain the progressive disturbance in posture. The curvature of the spine occurs as the paraspinal muscles on the affected side become more hypertonic. This rigidity is reversed by administration of levodopa or dopamine agonists unless the curvature has affected the vertebrae or is very severe. Although the exact pathogenesis of PD scoliosis has not been elucidated, a dopaminergic–cholinergic imbalance has been speculated. In a rat model of PD, 6-hydroxydopamine injections caused ipsilateral deviation and a scoliosis-like skeletal deformity, the severity of which correlated with a decrease in extracellular striatal dopamine level [40]. The occurrence of Pisa syndrome after neuroleptic therapy and its resolution with anticholinergic medications further suggest a neurochemical imbalance in the basal ganglia as the possible cause of the postural deformity [33].

Lateral flexion in PD is poorly responsive to treatment with anti-parkinsonian drugs, although some success with levodopa was anecdotally reported [41]. If there is suspicion that dopamine agonists lead to the development of lateral flexion, this should be discontinued. Ultimately, the best treatment of lateral flexion in PD would be the prevention of the abnormal paraspinal hypertonic contractions, although this may be very difficult to accomplish. Similarly to what is observed with camptocormia, DBS can effectively treat abnormal lateral flexion before it induces an irreversible spine deformity [18]. Corrective surgery is usually not an option for PD scoliosis as the asymmetric paraspinal dystonia may ultimately lead to failure. In the only successful case reported in the literature, a 73-year-old woman with advanced PD and right-leaning kyphoscoliosis improved dramatically after a two-step spine procedure including anterior decompression and fusion and posterior placement of Isola rods [42]. Orthopedic surgery is not indicated in Pisa syndrome, which normally responds to withdrawal of the causative medications (Figure 33.4).

Anterocollis (dropped head)

The first account of anterocollis in PD was provided by James Parkinson, who described a case in whom "the chin is now almost immovably bent down upon the sternum." In reality, anterocollis or "dropped head" (Figure 33.6) is more commonly observed in patients with MSA [44], whereas neck extension or retrocollis is more frequently found in PSP and tardive syndromes [2]. The incidence of dropped head in PD has not been extensively investigated, but it is probably around 5–6% [45,46]. When present, anterocollis in PD may progress either slowly or subacutely over a period of several days, causing important disability [45].

The pathogenesis of anterocollis is heterogeneous and includes either neck flexor overactivity (dystonia) or

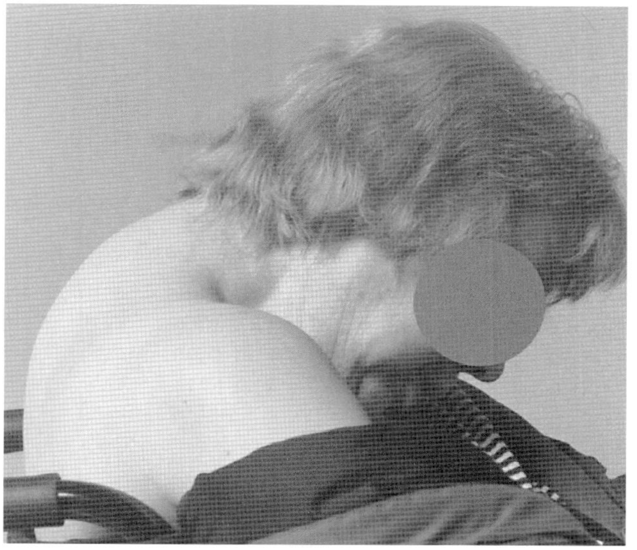

Figure 33.6 Anterocollis caused by neck extensor myopathy in a patient with advanced parkinsonism. Reproduced from Askmark *et al.* [43] with permission.

weakness of neck extensors (myopathy). When dystonia is the causative factor, the sternocleidomastoid muscles are hypertonic and prevent neck extension. Typical agonist/antagonist co-contraction can be documented by EMG, which shows simultaneous contraction of the anterior and posterior neck muscles [45,47]. When myopathic mechanisms prevail, the dropped head is caused primarily by weakness of the extensor neck muscles [43,48,49]. Similarly to what has been proposed for camptocormia, the two theories may not be mutually exclusive and a neck extensor inflammatory myopathy may be secondary to the mechanical overstretching caused by dystonia and rigidity [48]. This hypothesis is exemplified by a case in which pallidal DBS resolved the abnormal dystonic contraction of anterior neck muscles, only to leave the patient still unable to lift the head up [45].

Anterocollis with a clear dystonic component should initially be treated with levodopa, or a dose increase if already in use [50,51]. Dopamine agonists should not be used or tapered if already part of the therapeutic regimen, as these agents may worsen anterocollis in PD [45,52]. Alternative treatments for dystonic anterocollis include muscle block of the sternocleidomastoid muscles with either lidocaine or ethanol [47]; botulinum toxin injections are usually not effective and can result in dysphagia and dysphasia [53]. Pallidal DBS has been reported to treat anterocollis successfully in one PD patient [45].

Other skeletal deformities

It is unclear whether other skeletal deformities that occur in the general population, such as Dupuytryen's contracture, hammertoes, and trigger finger, appear with a higher frequency among PD patients, as this has not been formally studied [2].

Secondary orthopedic complications

Although bone fractures are not a primary symptom of PD, trauma is not uncommon in the late stages of the disease. Trauma, usually due to a fall, is the most frequent acute co-morbidity in emergency room visits among PD patients. In one study, 12 out of 49 (24%) PD patients admitted to the hospital for non-neurological reasons had a fall or other trauma; of 48 PD patients seen in the emergency department, nine had fractures, three had head trauma, and one had a hip prosthesis displacement. In total, 25 out of 90 (30.5%) PD patients presented to the hospital with an orthopedic issue [54]. In addition, PD patients have a high rate of in-hospital orthopedic complications: eight out of 50 inpatient consultations in one study were to orthopedists [54]. Levodopa treatment may paradoxically exacerbate the issue, as it improves mobility with less effect on postural stability, resulting in increased risk of falls even among those who are well managed medically [55].

PD patients have a significant increase in fracture risk, which is about double that for age-matched controls [56–59]. Ten years after diagnosis, 27% of PD patients experienced a hip fracture in one study, with fracture patterns suggesting that the increased risk was due more to specific types of falls than to osteoporosis [56]. There is also a disproportionate frequency of hip fractures in PD patients when compared with age-matched controls, where fractures of the forearm are predominant [56,58,59]. Falls are primarily related to gait disturbances and postural instability, which are generally manifestations of the later stages of the disease, and usually occur after the onset of non-motor symptoms [25,60]. Several other factors contribute to postural instability with falling in PD patients, including orthostatic hypotension, age-related sensory changes, and their ability to integrate visual, vestibular, and proprioceptive inputs and cognitive impairment ([25], and elsewhere in this book).

PD patients have a tendency to fall backwards or to the side, without adequately directed arm movements to attenuate falling impact [56,61,62]. Kinematic studies have shown that PD patients have a decreased arm flexion in the forward-afterward direction, and an increased adduction in the medial-lateral direction [63]. These abnormally directed arm responses prevent proper grasping for support and performing a "counterbalance" function [64]. This peculiar deficit, typical of parkinsonian syndromes, could explain why upper extremity injuries are relatively rare in PD, whereas hip fractures are frequent due to the trauma to the unprotected trochanter (Figure 33.7).

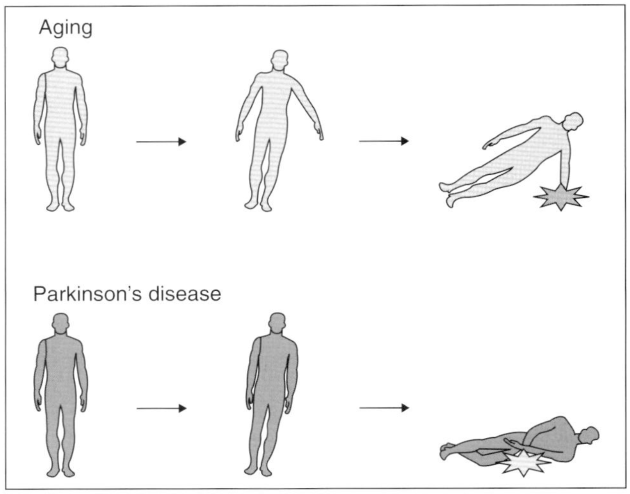

Figure 33.7 PD fall mechanisms. Healthy elderly individuals stretch out their arms in the direction of the impending fall, whereas PD patients adduct their arms against the trunk, thereby exposing the unprotected hip. Reproduced from Grimbergen *et al.* [61] with permission from Lippincott Williams & Wilkins.

The increase in hip fracture risk in PD is also attributed to a variety of other factors, including low bone mineral density (BMD). As parkinsonian patients stand and walk less, their bones lose mass and structural density and, as a consequence, the occurrence of osteoporosis in PD is higher than in the general population [65]. Low body mass index (BMI), low BMD, serum 25-OHD concentrations $\leq 5\,\text{ng ml}^{-1}$ with secondary hyperparathyroidism also contribute to increased risk of hip fracture, particularly in female PD patients with long postmenopausal intervals [57,66].

A diagnosis of PD may influence the type of hip fracture that occurs secondary to a fall. There are two primary anatomic locations of a hip fracture, the femoral neck (also referred to as the cervical or subcapsular region) and the intertrochanteric area, which has a higher proportion of trabecular bone than the femoral neck (Figure 33.8). There is a general tendency to develop femoral neck fractures secondary to poor functional ability, while risk factors for intertrochanteric fractures include aging, lower BMI, and osteoporosis [59,67–69]. PD patients appear to suffer more femoral neck than intertrochanteric fractures [5,59,70], but it is controversial whether the type of hip fracture affects outcome and mortality in PD patients [5,71,72]. PD patients, overall, do not seem to have increased mortality with fracture of the femoral neck, although individual factors, such as age or treatment option, may have an effect. For example, patients more than 80 years old also had significantly worse mortality than those younger than 80 years, independent of fracture type or method of repair [72].

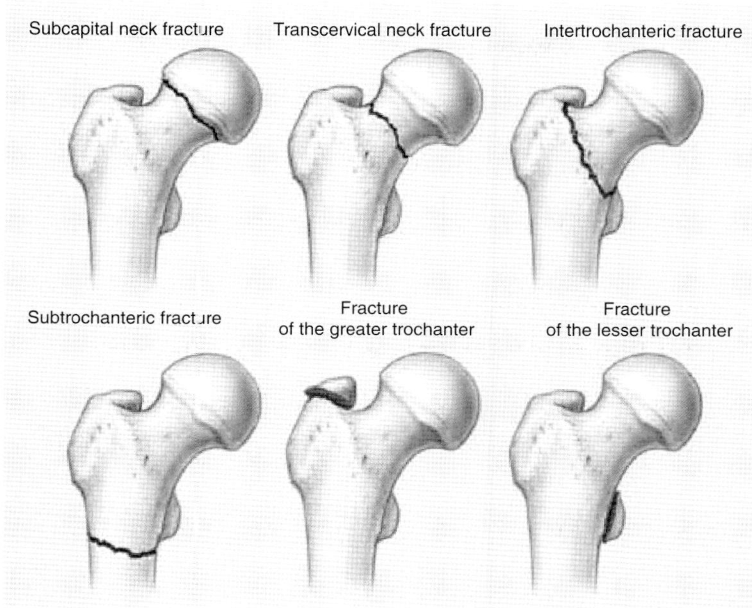

Figure 33.8 Types of femoral fractures.

Fall prevention is obviously the most important therapeutic approach to traumatic fractures in PD, but none of the existing strategies, ranging from optimized pharmacologic treatment to functional neurosurgery, physiotherapy, and multidisciplinary interventions, have provided consistent benefits [25,61]. The treatment of osteoporosis plays a pivotal role in hip fracture prevention in PD patients. Two recent randomized controlled trials showed a reduction of hip fracture incidence in PD patients over a 2-year follow-up with the administration of vitamin D and oral alendronate [73] or oral risedronate [74], although statistical significance was not achieved in the latter study. Vitamin D supplementation may reduce fracture incidence independent of its trophic actions on bone because vitamin D deficiency is common in PD [75] and it exerts extra-skeletal effects that reduce fall risk and ameliorate ability to function [59].

Given the higher postoperative morbidity and mortality rates, there is little consensus on whether and how to perform hip repair surgery in PD patients after a fracture [72]. Several studies did not find increased mortality in PD patients with femoral neck fractures treated with internal fixation, with rates between 15 and 28% at 2 years follow-up [76,77]. However, mortality increased significantly in those treated with endoprosthesis, possibly related to the prolonged postoperative immobilization compared with internal fixation patients [71]. It was therefore suggested that endoprosthesis may be contraindicated in PD [77] or that an anterior approach might be preferable, as this would allow earlier mobilization, reducing the risk of dislocation and mortality [71]. Yet others found that mortality and dislocation rates were not related to type, severity, or treatment of the fracture, which included non-operative, internal fixation for trochanteric fractures and endoprosthesis, via a posterolateral approach, for subcapital fractures [5,78].

A final orthopedic complication of PD worth mentioning is patellar insufficiency fracture (Figure 33.9), an otherwise rare event. In a published case, osteoporosis and osteoarthritis were PD co-morbidities likely leading to bilateral patellar fractures without a direct trauma, which recovered well with conservative management [79]. Therefore, pre-patellar pain in PD patients should not be underestimated.

Parkinsonism complicating orthopedic surgery

PD is generally associated with a higher risk of technical complications and need for re-operation following orthopedic procedures, which stems from a combination of poor bone quality and a severe neuromuscular disorder [8]. Early mobilization, intense rehabilitation, and proper postoperative reinstitution of levodopa therapy have all been suggested as strategies to prevent surgery failures in PD [5,55]. However, delivery of oral PD medications may be difficult in the perioperative period and a parenteral form of levodopa is not clinically available [7]. The particular challenges presented by PD patients have been studied in the settings of various orthopedic surgeries.

Hip replacement

As noted, parkinsonian patients are particularly prone to suffer hip fractures, which are further complicated by high rates of postoperative complications, unsatisfactory

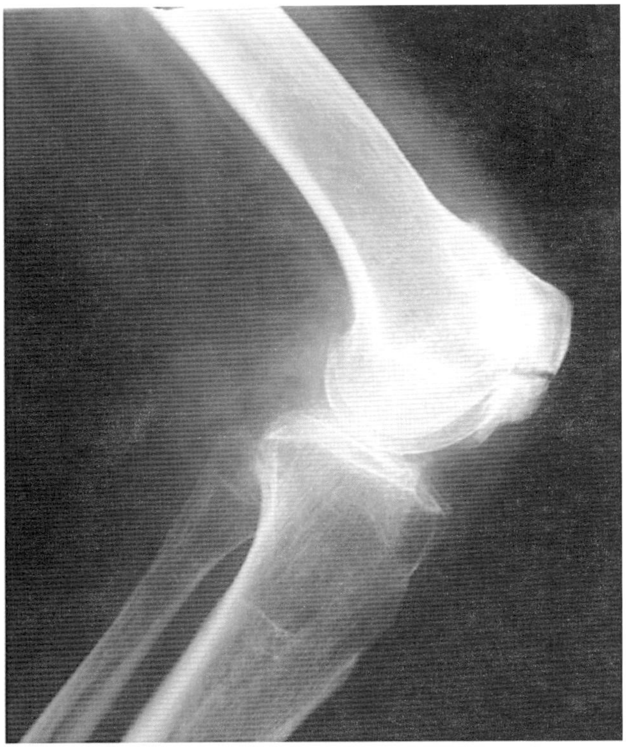

Figure 33.9 Radiograph of insufficiency patellar fracture in a PD patient. Reproduced from Moretti *et al.* [79] with permission from Wiley-Blackwell.

results, and death after hip replacement surgery. Six-month mortality rates for PD patients ranged from 20 to 49% in the earlier literature [4,5,71]; although mortality rates after hip replacement in PD are currently as low as 5.6%, they are still higher than those in the general population [4]. Although PD patients with a hip fracture have a high mortality in general, those undergoing surgery usually have better function after several months than those who do not [4,5]. Interestingly, although long-term mortality rates of PD patients approach the rates for the general population, PD patients are more likely than other patients to have a longer hospital course and to need transfer to a "skilled nursing facility" rather than progressing to short-term rehabilitation [80].

Among specific postoperative morbidities, prosthesis dislocations are a frequent problem in PD patients undergoing hip replacement [5,71]. Dislocations occur more often in PD patients with more severe disease, and possibly in those who have received hip surgery before [4]. Opinions differ as to whether the type of surgical approach can affect the outcome and likelihood of dislocation [5].

Another important postoperative morbidity is infections, including urinary tract infections and pneumonia, which tend to be more common than in the general population [4,78,81]. Prophylactic antibiotic treatment for 5–7 days postoperatively has been used to try to reduce the frequency of urinary tract infections and pneumonia. A unique issue that arises among patients with neuromuscular disease, including PD, is adduction contracture; tendon releases were necessary on 7–10% of patients in one series [78]. Regardless of surgical outcome, however, most PD patients continue to decline neurologically, often dying or becoming severely disabled within a few years after surgical repair. Nonetheless, as these patients often return to ambulation prior to their ultimate deterioration, there appears to be a clear benefit to be gained from operating on this population [4,5].

Spine surgery

Many of the issues mentioned for hip surgery come into play during recuperation from spine surgery, as parkinsonian patients tend to have greater postoperative difficulty and more frequent failures, often necessitating re-operation. The literature regarding surgery for spinal pathology in PD patients is sparse, but there is evidence that they experience spinal problems of a different nature and degree than patients without PD. In one retrospective study, 86% of PD patients required additional surgery, with 79% undergoing additional procedures at the same or adjacent level for instability [8]. Multiple re-operations for hardware failure or pullout (Figure 33.10) were necessary in almost one-third of patients [8]. Even in those with a successful procedure and postoperative course, instability at a remote spinal segment may occur. In this series, two patients (14%) developed wound infections during the course of treatment. Other spinal problems that could contribute to failure are spondylolisthesis, pseudoarthrosis, and most frequently kyphosis. Indeed, the "relentless kyphosis" occurring at levels adjacent to the surgical sites is considered the most important cause of instrument failure after spinal surgery in PD [8]. Decreased bone mass is another important factor, as osteoporosis has a high prevalence among this population [82,83].

Knee replacement

There is very little discussion in the literature about total knee arthroplasty (TKA) in PD patients. PD was originally considered a contraindication to knee surgery, because of the extremely high risk of complications, such as implant failure or tendon contractures, preventing rehabilitation [6], However, larger series have since shown more optimistic outcomes in PD patients undergoing TKA. In a review of nine patients with 12 TKAs, 75% of outcomes were rated as excellent and 25% as good at the time of the final follow-up examination [84]. A retrospective review of 24 consecutive PD patients who underwent primary cemented condylar TKA showed equally encouraging results: no mortality at an average follow-up of 33 months, generally good pain relief and functional recovery at least in those patients who did not show

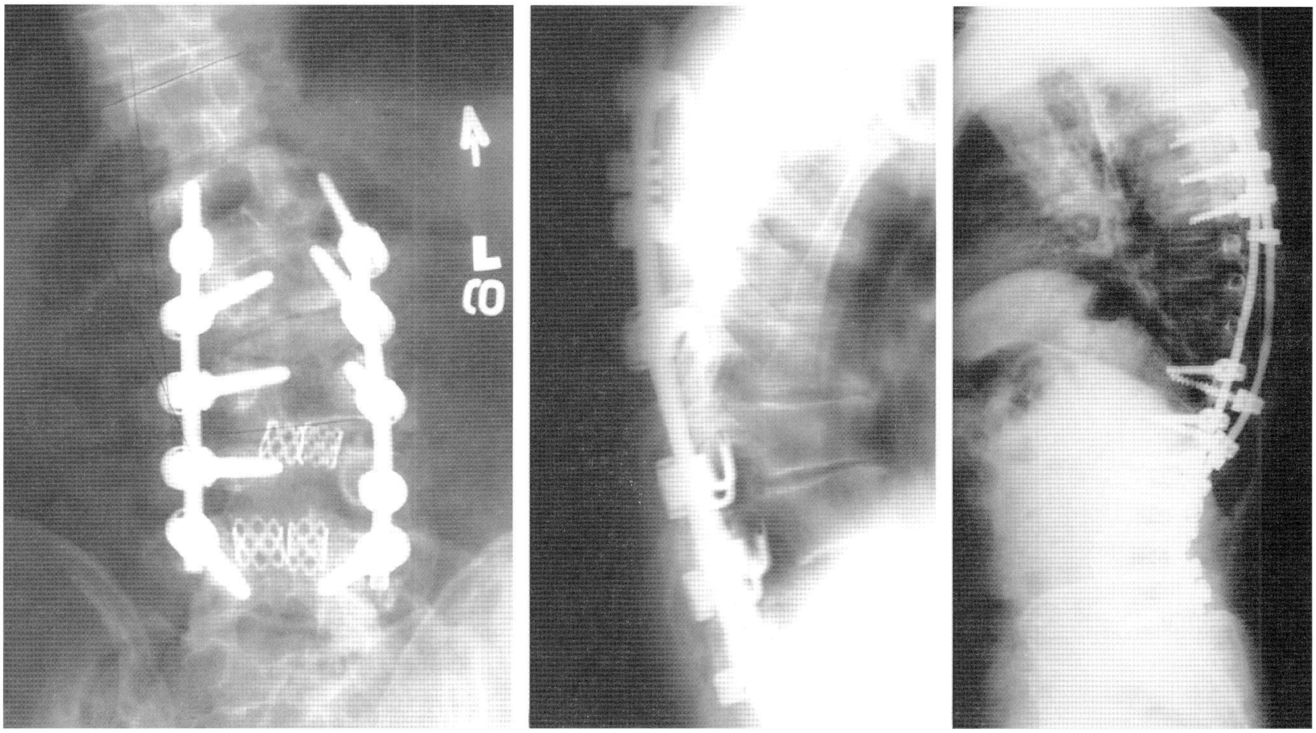

(a) (b) (c)

Figure 33.10 Multiple radiographs of lumbar (a) and thoracic (b, c) pull-out failures of spine instrumentation with acute kyphoscoliosis due to progressive kyphoscoliosis in PD patients. Reproduced from Babat *et al.* [8] with permission from Lippincott Williams & Wilkins.

subsequent progression of PD, and no hamstring rigidity or extensor mechanism problems [85].

With careful consideration of age and severity of disease, TKA appears to improve the function of PD patients, in particular those with intact ambulatory and cognitive function prior to surgery [86]. However, the rehabilitation process may be significantly prolonged and more difficult even in patients suffering from mild PD. Botulinum toxin injections have been reported to be useful in conjunction with limb manipulation under anesthesia and a static brace, to help ease contractures that inhibit full range of motion, allowing the joint to respond better to rehabilitation [87]. Finally, early neurologic consultation and reinstitution of medications can significantly decrease length of stay and improve early outcomes after TKA. [88].

Shoulder surgery

Similarly to what has been observed for knee and hip surgery, PD patients may benefit less than members of the general population from shoulder arthroplasty. In a small report of 15 PD patients who underwent total shoulder arthroplasty (TSA), successful pain relief was mitigated by poor overall functional results, which were attributed to increased muscle tone, severity of tremor, and an increased mortality rate [7]. A larger series of TSAs performed in PD patients for osteoarthritis of the shoulder also found marginal results, with 20/49 (47%) achieving unsatisfactory results [89]. The authors found significant improvements in pain, external rotation, and active abduction, but no significant improvement in internal rotation. In addition, there was a higher rate of postoperative joint instability [89]. Specific complications of TSA in PD may include subluxation of the humerus and equipment loosening. It is more common to see complications in older patients (more than 65 years old), although age is not by itself a strict predictive factor.

Good outcome predictors for TSA in PD patients include well-controlled neurological symptoms before surgery, minimal shoulder rigidity, and absence of cognitive deterioration. Muscle rigidity of the rotator cuff, typical of PD, may prevent proper rehabilitation and therefore adaptation of the repaired joint. Better outcomes are also associated with the absence of clinical or radiographic evidence of significant rotator cuff tearing, a limited amount of asymmetric glenoid wear, and only a mild amount of humeral subluxation. If there is moderate or severe subluxation preoperatively, it is unlikely that shoulder arthroplasty will satisfactorily control it [89]. Similarly to what has been suggested for other orthopedic surgeries, anti-parkinsonian drugs should be reinstituted as soon as feasible, aggressive and early mobilization and rehabilitation of the operated limb should be performed, and aggressive pulmonary care and antibiotic prophylaxis introduced [7]. Finally, adequate caregiver assistance and support are crucial in the postoperative period.

Conclusion

PD is a prime example of how a neuromuscular disorder can be associated with and complicate orthopedic conditions. There are numerous complications that may arise as a primary effect of parkinsonian muscle rigidity, and also conditions that are complicated by the co-morbid presence of PD. Parkinsonian dystonia can affect posture and head control and also cause limb deformities. Surgical correction may be possible in some cases, but not in all. Postural instability and the related propensity to fall are also a complicating factor in PD patients, with a potential for devastating trauma. Certain types of fractures, including hip injuries, may be more common in PD patients given the higher frequency of osteoporosis and falling patterns. In the postoperative setting, PD patients have historically demonstrated a higher rate of complication and implant failure. However, with careful consideration of age and severity of disease, several arthroplasty procedures appear to improve the function of PD patients. Complications can be minimized with early utilization of levodopa therapy and also early mobilization and physical therapy. Also of vital importance in this population are the prevention and careful management of medical perioperative issues, such as respiratory toilet and infection.

References

1. Charcot JM. *Lectures on the Diseases of the Nervous System, Lecture V*. London: New Sydenham Society, 1877:140–7.
2. Ashour R, Jankovic J. Joint and skeletal deformities in Parkinson's disease, multiple system atrophy, and progressive supranuclear palsy. *Mov Disord* 2006;**21**:1856–63.
3. Segatore M. Managing the surgical orthopaedic patient with Parkinson's disease. *Orthop Nurs* 1998;**17**:13–20.
4. Weber M, Cabanela ME, Sim FH, *et al*. Total hip replacement in patients with Parkinson's disease. *Int Orthop* 2002;**26**:66–8.
5. Eventov I, Moreno M, Geller E, *et al*. Hip fractures in patients with Parkinson's syndrome. *J Trauma* 1983;**23**:98–101.
6. Oni OOA, MacKenney RP. Total knee replacement in patients with Parkinson's disease. *J Bone Joint Surg* 1985:**67B**(3), 424–5.
7. Koch LD, Cofield RH, Ahlskog JE. Total shoulder arthroplasty in patients with Parkinson's disease. *J Shoulder Elbow Surg* 1997;**6**:24–8.
8. Babat LB, McLain RF, Bingaman W, *et al*. Spinal surgery in patients with Parkinson's disease: construct failure and progressive deformity. *Spine* 2004;**29**:2006–12.
9. Fahn S, Bressman S, Marsden CD. Classification of dystonia. *Adv Neurol* 1998;**78**:1–10.
10. Jankovic J, Tintner R. Dystonia and parkinsonism. *Parkinsonism Relat Disord* 2001;**8**:109–21.
11. Hu MT, Bland J, Clough C, *et al*. Limb contractures in levodopa-responsive parkinsonism: a clinical and investigational study of seven new cases. *J Neurol* 1999;**246**:671–6.
12. Reynolds FW, Petropoulos GC. Hand Deformities in Parkinsonism. *J Chron Dis* 1965;**18**:593–595.
13. Dorwart BD, Schumacher HR. Hand deformities resembling rheumatoid arthritis. *Semin Arthritis Rheum* 1974;**4**:53–71.
14. Ashour R, Tintner R, Jankovic J. Striatal deformities of the hand and foot in Parkinson's disease. *Lancet Neurol* 2005;**4**:423–31.
15. Gortvai P. Deformities of the hands and feet in Parkinsonism and their reversibility by operation. *J Neurol Neurosurg Psychiatry* 1963;**26**:33–6.
16. Riley D, Lang AE, Blair RD, *et al*. Frozen shoulder and other shoulder disturbances in Parkinson's disease. *J Neurol Neurosurg Psychiatry* 1989;**52**(1):63–6.
17. Parkinson J. *An Essay on the Shaking Palsy*. London: Whittingham and Rowland, 1817.
18. Yokochi F. Lateral flexion in Parkinson's disease and Pisa syndrome. *J Neurol* 2006;**253**(Suppl 7):vii17–20.
19. Lepoutre AC, Devos D, Blanchard-Dauphin A, *et al*. A specific clinical pattern of camptocormia in Parkinson's disease. *J Neurol Neurosurg Psychiatry* 2006;**77**:1229–34.
20. Azher SN, Jankovic J. Camptocormia: pathogenesis, classification, and response to therapy. *Neurology* 2005;**65**:355–9.
21. Bloch F, Houeto JL, Tezenas du Montcel S, *et al*. Parkinson's disease with camptocormia. *J Neurol Neurosurg Psychiatry* 2006;**77**:1223–8.
22. Djaldetti R, Mosberg-Galili R, Sroka H, *et al*. Camptocormia (bent spine) in patients with Parkinson's disease – characterization and possible pathogenesis of an unusual phenomenon. *Mov Disord* 1999;**14**:443–7.
23. Bouzgarou E, Dupeyron A, Castelnovo G, *et al*. Camptocormia disclosing Parkinson's disease. *Ann Readapt Med Phys* 2007;**50**:55–9 (in French).
24. Djaldetti R, Melamed E. Camptocormia in Parkinson's disease: new insights. *J Neurol Neurosurg Psychiatry* 2006;**77**:1205.
25. Benatru I, Vaugoyeau M, Azulay JP. Postural disorders in Parkinson's disease. *Neurophysiol Clin/Clin Neurophysiol* 2008;**38**:459–65.
26. Micheli F, Cersosimo MG, Piedimonte F. Camptocormia in a patient with Parkinson disease: beneficial effects of pallidal deep brain stimulation. Case report. *J Neurosurg* 2005;**103**:1081–3.
27. Nieves AV, Miyasaki JM, Lang AE. Acute onset dystonic camptocormia caused by lenticular lesions. *Mov Disord* 2001;**16**:177–80.
28. Schäbitz WR, Glatz K, Schuhan C, *et al*. Severe forward flexion of the trunk in Parkinson's disease: focal myopathy of the paraspinal muscles mimicking camptocormia. *Mov Disord* 2003;**18**:408–14.
29. Nandi D, Parkin S, Scott R, *et al*. Camptocormia treated with bilateral pallidal stimulation. *J Neurosurg* 2002;**97**:461–6.
30. Fukaya C, Otaka T, Obuchi T, *et al*. Pallidal high-frequency deep brain stimulation for camptocormia: an experience of three cases. *Acta Neurochir Suppl* 2006;**99**:25–8.
31. Yamada K, Goto S, Matsuzaki K, *et al*. Alleviation of camptocormia by bilateral subthalamic nucleus stimulation in a patient with Parkinson's disease. *Parkinsonism Relat Disord* 2006;**12**:372–5.

32. Duvoisin RC, Marsden CD. Note on the scoliosis of Parkinsonism. *J Neurol Neurosurg Psychiatry* 1975;**38**:787–93.
33. Suzuki M, Hirai T, Ito Y, *et al.* Pramipexole-induced antecollis in Parkinson's disease. *J Neurol Sci* 2008;**264**:195–7.
34. Cannas A, Solla P, Floris G, *et al.* Reversible Pisa syndrome in Parkinson's disease during treatment with pergolide: a case report. *Clin Neuropharm* 2005;**28**:252.
35. Gambarin M, Antonini A, Moretto G, *et al.* Pisa syndrome without neuroleptic exposure in a patient with Parkinson's disease: case report. *Mov Disord* 2006;**21**:270–3.
36. Hozumi I, Piao YS, Inuzuka T, *et al.* Marked asymmetry of putaminal pathology in an MSA-P patient with Pisa syndrome. *Mov Disord* 2004;**19**:470–2.
37. Colosimo C. Pisa syndrome in a patient with multiple system atrophy. *Mov Disord* 1998;**13**:607–9.
38. Proctor F, Riklan M, Cooper IS, *et al.* Judgment of visual and postural vertical by parkinsonian patients. *Neurology* 1964; **14**:287–93.
39. Danta G, Hilton RC. Judgment of the visual vertical and horizontal in patients with parkinsonism. *Neurology* 1975;**25**: 43–7.
40. Herrera-Marschitz M, Utsumi H, Ungerstedt U. Scoliosis in rats with experimentally-induced hemiparkinsonism: dependence upon striatal dopamine denervation. *J Neurol Neurosurg Psychiatry* 1990;**53**:39–43.
41. Kim JS, Park JW, Chung SW, *et al.* Pisa syndrome as a motor complication of Parkinson's disease. *Parkinsonism Relat Disord* 2007;**13**:126–8.
42. Tabamo RE, Fernandez HH, Friedman JH, Lucas PR. Spinal surgery for severe scoliosis in Parkinson's disease. *Med Health R I* 2000;**83**:114–5.
43. Askmark H, Eeg-Olofsson KE, Johansson A, *et al.* Parkinsonism and neck extensor myopathy: a new syndrome or coincidental findings? *Arch Neurol* 2001;**58**:232–7.
44. Quinn NP. Disproportionate antecollis in multiple system atrophy. *Lancet* 1989;**333**:844.
45. Fujimoto K. Dropped head in Parkinson's disease. *J Neurol* 2006;**253**(Suppl 7):vii21–6.
46. Kashihara K, Ohno M, Tomita S. Dropped head syndrome in Parkinson's disease. *Mov Disord* 2006;**21**:1213–6.
47. Yoshiyama Y, Takama J, Hattori T. The dropped head sign in parkinsonism. *J Neurol Sci* 1999;**167**:22–5.
48. Katz JS, Wolfe GI, Burns DK, *et al.* Isolated neck extensor myopathy: a common cause of dropped head syndrome. *Neurology* 1996;**46**:917–21.
49. Okamiya S, Ito H, Saito T, *et al.* A case of isolated neck extensor myopathy with parkinsonism. *Rinsho Shinkeigaku* 1997;**37**:393–6.
50. Jorens PG, Eycken MP, Parizel GA, Martin JJ. Antecollis in parkinsonism. *Lancet* 1989;**333**:1320–1.
51. Horiuchi M, Uehara K, Kamo T, *et al.* A case of elderly onset Parkinson's disease complicated by dropped head syndrome. *Jpn J Geriat* 2001;**38**:693–5.
52. Suzuki T, Matsuzaka H. Drug-induced Pisa syndrome (pleurothotonus): epidemiology and management. *CNS Drugs* 2002;**16**:165–74.
53. Quinn NP. Parkinsonism and dystonia, pseudoparkinsonism and pseudodystonia. *Adv Neurol* 1993;**60**:540–3.
54. Martignoni E, Godi L, Citterio A, *et al.* Parkinson's Disease Comorbidity Study Group. Comorbid disorders and hospitalisation in Parkinson's disease: a prospective study. *Neurol Sci* 2004;**25**:66–71.
55. Rothermel JE, Garcia A. Treatment of hip fractures in patients with Parkinson's syndrome on levodopa therapy. *J Bone Joint Surg Am* 1972;**54**:1251–4.
56. Johnell O, Melton LJ III, Atkinson EJ, *et al.* Fracture risk in patients with parkinsonism: a population-based study in Olmsted County, Minnesota. *Age Ageing* 1992;**21**:32–8.
57. Sato Y, Kaji M, Tsuru T, Oizumi K. Risk factors for hip fracture among elderly patients with Parkinson's disease. *J Neurol Sci* 2001;**82**:89–93.
58. Genever RW, Downes TW, Medcalf P. Fracture rates in Parkinson's disease compared with age- and gender-matched controls: a retrospective cohort study. *Age Ageing* 2005;**34**: 21–4.
59. Di Monaco M, Vallero F, Di Monaco R, *et al.* Type of hip fracture in patients with Parkinson disease is associated with femoral bone mineral density. *Arch Phys Med Rehabil* 2008;**89**:2297–301.
60. Jankovic J. Parkinson's disease: clinical features and diagnosis. *J Neurol Neurosurg Psychiatry* 2008;**79**:368–76.
61. Grimbergen YA, Munneke M, Bloem BR. Falls in Parkinson's disease. *Curr Opin Neurol* 2004;**17**:405–15.
62. Winogrodzka A, Wagenaar RC, Booij J, Wolters EC. Rigidity and bradykinesia reduce interlimb coordination in Parkinsonian gait. *Arch Phys Med Rehabil* 2005;**86**:183–9.
63. Carpenter MG, Allum JH, Honegger F, *et al.* Postural abnormalities to multidirectional stance perturbations in Parkinson's disease. *J Neurol Neurosurg Psychiatry* 2004;**75**: 1245–54.
64. Allum JH, Carpenter MG, Honegger F, *et al.* Age-dependent variations in the directional sensitivity of balance corrections and compensatory arm movements in man. *J Physiol (Lond)* 2002;**542**:643–63.
65. Yamada T, Kachi T, Ando K. Osteoporosis and fractures in Parkinson's disease. *Nippon Ronen Igakkai Zasshi* 1995;**32**: 637–40 (in Japanese).
66. Vaserman N. Parkinson's disease and osteoporosis. *Joint Bone Spine* 2005;**72**:484–8.
67. Vega E, Mautalen C, Gómez H, *et al.* Bone mineral density in patients with cervical and trochanteric fractures of the proximal femur. *Osteoporos Int* 1991;**1**:81–6.
68. Stewart A, Porter RW, Primrose WR, *et al.* Cervical and trochanteric hip fractures: bone mass and other parameters. *Clin Rheumatol* 1999;**18**:201–6.
69. Fox KM, Cummings SR, Williams E, Stone K. Femoral neck and intertrochanteric fractures have different risk factors:a prospective study. *Osteoporosis Int* 2000;**11**:1018–23.
70. Christodoulou NA, Dretakis EK. Significance of muscular disturbances in the localization of fractures of the proximal femur. *Clin Orthop Relat Res* 1984;**187**:215–7.
71. Coughlin L, Templeton J. Hip fractures in patients with Parkinson's disease. *Clin Orthop Relat Res* 1980;**148**:192–5.
72. Clubb VJ, Clubb SE, Buckley S. Parkinson's disease patients who fracture their neck of femur: a review of outcome data. *Injury* 2006;**37**:929–34.
73. Sato Y, Iwamoto J, Kanoko T, Satoh K. Alendronate and vitamin D_2 for prevention of hip fracture in Parkinson's disease: a randomized controlled trial. *Mov Disord* 2006;**21**: 924–9.

74. Sato Y, Honda Y, Iwamoto J. Risedronate and ergocalciferol prevent hip fracture in elderly men with Parkinson disease. *Neurology* 2007;**68**:911–5.
75. Sato Y, Kaji M, Tsuru T, *et al.* Vitamin K deficiency and osteopenia in vitamin D-deficient elderly women with Parkinson's disease. *Arch Phys Med Rehabil* 2002;**83**:86–91.
76. Londos E, Nilsson LT, Stromqvist B. Internal fixation of femoral neck fractures in Parkinson's disease. 32 patients followed for 2 years. *Acta Orthop Scand* 1989;**60**: 682–5.
77. Turcotte R, Godin C, Duchesne R, Jodoin A. Hip fractures and Parkinson's disease. A clinical review of 94 fractures treated surgically. *Clin Orthop* 1990;**256**:132–6.
78. Staeheli JW, Frassica FJ, Franklin H. Prosthetic replacement of the femoral head for fracture of the femoral neck in patients who have Parkinson disease. *J Bone Joint Surg Am* 1988;**704**:565–8.
79. Moretti B, Speciale D, Garofalo R, *et al.* Spontaneous bilateral fracture of patella. *Geriatr Gerontol Int* 2008;**8**:55–8.
80. Idjadi JA, Aharonoff GB, Su H, *et al.* Hip fracture outcomes in patients with Parkinson's disease. *Am J Orthop* 2005;**34**(7):341–6.
81. Hammer AJ. Intertrochanteric and femoral neck fractures in patients with parkinsonism. *S Afr Med J* 1991;**79**:200–2.
82. Ishizaki F, Harada T, Katayama S, *et al.* Relationship between osteopenia and clinical characteristics of Parkinson's disease. *Mov Disord* 1993;**8**:507–11.
83. Kao CH, Chen CC, Wang SJ, *et al.* Bone mineral density in patients with Parkinson's disease measured by dual photon absorptiometry. *Nucl Med Commun* 1994;**15**:173–7.
84. Vince KG, Insall JN, Bannerman CE. Total knee arthroplasty in the patient with Parkinson's disease. *J Bone Joint Surg* 1989;**71** B:51.
85. Duffy GP, Trousdale RT. Total knee arthroplasty in patients with Parkinson's disease. *J Arthroplasty* 1996;**11**:899.
86. Fast A, Mendelsohn E, Sosner J. Total knee arthroplasty in Parkinson's disease. *Arch Phys Med Rehabil* 1994;**75**:1269.
87. Shah SN, Hornyak J, Urquhart AG. Flexion contracture after total knee arthroplasty in a patient with Parkinson's disease: successful treatment with botulinum toxin type A. *J Arthroplasty* 2005;**20**:1078–80.
88. Mehta S, Vankleunen JP, Booth RE, *et al.* Total knee arthroplasty in patients with Parkinson's disease: impact of early postoperative neurologic intervention. *Am J Orthop* 2008;**37**: 513–6.
89. Kryzak TJ, Sperling JW, Schleck CD, Cofield RH. Total shoulder arthroplasty in patients with Parkinson's disease. *J Shoulder Elbow Surg* 2009;**18**:96–9.

Chapter 34
Other Non-Motor Symptoms of Parkinson's Disease

Mark J. Edwards & Kailash P. Bhatia
Sobell Department of Motor Neuroscience and Movement Disorders, Institute of Neurology, University College London, Queen Square, London, UK

Visual disturbances

A variety of visual disturbances occur in patients with Parkinson's disease (PD), although there are no epidemiologic data on their prevalence. Typical complaints from patients are of blurred vision, particularly problems with vision in low light conditions, double vision, and more generally just complaints of "I can't see properly." Despite these complaints, visual examinations are often normal.

A number of different problems may contribute to poor vision in patients with PD. Patients often have a relatively flexed neck and body posture, and this, combined with age-related restriction of up gaze and lid dehiscence, can lead to a markedly restricted ability to view objects in the upper part of the visual field [1]. Patients with PD also often have poor contrast sensitivity [2–8], a factor that impairs vision in low-light conditions. Deficits in contrast sensitivity can be reversed to a certain extent with levodopa or apomorphine [9,10], but become more prominent as the disease progresses [6,11]. The cause of contrast sensitivity deficits is not clear, but may result from a combination of retinal dopaminergic cell degeneration (as indicated by delayed visual evoked potentials and abnormal electroretinograms in PD [12–15]), specific problems in color perception [16,17] (again likely to be mainly due to retinal degeneration), and cortical abnormalities in visual processing [18–21].

Patients with PD may complain of double vision or blurring of vision during reading or other tasks that involve focusing on near objects. The exact origin of these difficulties is not clear, but there is some evidence that the mechanism may represent "convergence insufficiency" [22]. This failure of convergence might be helped by exercises that are generally recommended for convergence problems (e.g. "pencil push-ups," computer based vergence training [23]), but evidence for the effectiveness of these techniques in PD specifically is lacking.

Bedside testing of eye movements and saccades is typically normal in PD, but subtle deficits in eye movement, often only detectable by electro-oculography, are common [24]. Saccades are often hypometric and slower than controls (although with significant overlap between the groups) [25]. Patients with PD may have specific problems with self-paced saccades or saccades towards a remembered target [26–30]. Repeated pursuit eye movements may also be abnormal, tending to decrease in magnitude with repetition (similar to bradykinesia seen with other repetitive movements) [31,32]. This abnormality can be present early in the course of the disease and is responsive to dopaminergic therapy [33]. The clinical consequences of these subtle eye movement abnormalities are not known.

Pupil size is typically normal in normal light conditions, but patients with PD may show a delayed and incomplete pupilary light reflex in response to increases in light, with no particular abnormalities seen in response to reduction in ambient light intensity [34–36]. The origin of this deficit has been proposed as a central one involving the Edinger–Westphal nucleus, although an additional peripheral parasympathetic deficit has also been reported [35].

Drugs used to treat PD may contribute to visual problems. Anti-cholinergic drugs can cause dry eyes and blurred vision and can precipitate closed angle glaucoma. Pramipexole has been associated with dry eyes, conjunctivitis, and glaucoma. All dopamine agonists (and to a lesser extent other dopaminergic drugs) have been associated with the precipitation or worsening of visual hallucinations. Amantadine has been associated with superficial keratitis, mydriasis, and reduced ability to perform accommodation.

In PD patients who complain of visual problems, a routine ophthalmologic assessment is helpful to rule out correctable problems such as cataracts and glaucoma.

Parkinson's Disease: Non-Motor and Non-Dopaminergic Features, First Edition. Edited by C. Warren Olanow, Fabrizio Stocchi, and Anthony E. Lang.

Consideration should be given as to whether drugs (those prescribed for PD or for other illnesses) might be contributing to the visual problems. Visual hallucinations are often managed by reducing the number, type, and/or dose of dopaminergic medications. Visual hallucinations may also respond to cholinesterase inhibitor and dopamine receptor blocking medications (especially atypical neuroleptics).

Other practical steps to help with visual problems include increasing ambient light in the home (installing higher wattage bulbs, increasing the number or lights), avoiding placement of visual information high in the visual field, ensuring that flooring and surfaces have high contrast between them, particularly around changes in floor level, removing clutter from walkways, and reducing/stopping driving in low-light conditions [1].

Salivation

Sialorrhea is a common complaint of patients with PD, with a prevalence reported at between 49 and 78% [37–39], in contrast to a prevalence of 6% in a control population [37]. The severity of drooling is reported as mild to moderate in 73% of affected patients (only lips wet, or lips and chin wet) and severe in the remainder (clothing soiled or clothing hands, etc., moist or wet) [39]. Drooling is most often reported during relaxation or when tired, and less often during eating [39]. Sialorrhea can have an adverse impact on the quality-of-life of patients with PD. Using a non-standard questionnaire, Kalf *et al.* reported sialorrhea to be associated with restriction of social contact and a lack of self-confidence [39].

There is clear evidence that the pathophysiology of sialorrhea in PD is primarily related to a reduction in spontaneous swallowing (and a flexed head posture), rather than an excessive production of saliva [40]. In fact, a number of studies have found a reduction in the rate of saliva production in PD. Using either spit collection or weighing a cotton pad before and after it had been placed under the tongue for 2 min, saliva flow rates in PD (both *de novo* and treated) appear lower than those in a control age-matched population [41–44]. Saliva flow rates also seem to decrease with increasing disease severity [45].

There is an association between drooling and dysphagia, with 86% of those with dysphagia complaining of drooling compared with 44% of those without [38]. In addition, impaired swallow even in the absence of specific symptoms is common in PD, even in those with early disease [46,47]. Levodopa was found to increase salivation in one study [45], but this was not replicated in a second study [43]. Deep brain stimulation of the sub-thalamic nucleus increased sialorrhea in one patient [48], but there have been no other reports of this association.

Both anti-cholinergic medications and the central adrenergic agonist clonidine have been tested for PD patients with sialorrhea. Atropine drops given sublingually reduced sialorrhea in an open-label study of six patients, but side effects included hallucinations [49]. Ipratropium bromide spray was evaluated in a double-blind, placebo-controlled trial in 17 patients with PD and sialorrhea [50]. Two sprays (total dose 42 μg) were given sublingually up to a maximum of four times daily. Response was assessed by weighing a cotton roll before and after it had been placed under the tongue for 5 min, an also by patient-completed subjective measures of saliva production. No significant difference was found between ipratropium and placebo in terms of weight of cotton pad, but there was a trend towards improvement on subjective measures of salivation for patients on active treatment. No significant side effects were reported. Clonidine at a dose of 0.15 mg per day has been reported to have a beneficial effect on saliva production in a double-blind, placebo-controlled trial in a total of 32 patients with PD [51]. In a 3-month study, there was a significant improvement in subjective reports of hypersalivation in the active treatment group, and no significant side effects were reported.

Botulinum toxin injection into the salivary glands has been extensively assessed in patients with sialorrhea and PD [52–63]. In summary, botulinum toxin serotypes A and B have both been demonstrated to be effective for patients with PD and sialorrhea. Improvement is maintained for at least 1 month, and in most studies has returned to baseline by 3 months. Injections (given with or without ultrasound guidance) have most commonly been given into the parotid glands bilaterally, although some studies have injected the submandibular gland (using ultrasound guidance) [59,60]. Similar results have been reported for the two injection sites. Side effects reported in these studies have been limited to transient mild swallowing difficulties, and in one study using botulinum toxin type B, mild and transient dry mouth, worsened gait, diarrhea, and neck pain [59]. There have been no trials directly comparing botulinum serotypes A and B. In studies of patients with cranio-cervical dystonia, botulinum toxin type B injections are more commonly associated with the side effect of dry mouth compared with injections of type A toxin [64], which could suggest a theoretical advantage for the use of botulinum toxin type B for sialorrhea.

Other treatments that have been tried include behavioral modification using a cue (a beeping watch) to prompt swallowing. This was shown to be effective in the short term, but long-term results were poor, probably due to a decline in motivation [65]. Radiotherapy (radiation of the salivary glands) has been tried with some benefit in groups of patients with chronic neurologic conditions causing sialorrhea, including six patients with PD [66]. The treatment was of benefit, but side effects, including the long-term risk of inducing a neoplasm, make this treatment less attractive.

Fatigue

Fatigue in PD is a complex problem to study. Fatigue is a very common phenomenon in the normal population, and particularly common in patients with chronic diseases. There are numerous potentially confounding associations with fatigue, such as depression, poor sleep, cognitive deficits, and reduced physical exercise, and all of these are common symptoms of PD. The prevalence of fatigue in PD patients has been estimated to range between 33 and 81% [67–75]. The methods of assessment and the patient characteristics varied in all these studies, but some important points can be gleaned from reviewing the data. First, fatigue appears to be an early, even premotor, symptom of PD. For example, in a group of 50 non-depressed men with PD who complained of fatigue, half reported that their fatigue preceded the onset of motor symptoms of PD [74]. Second, fatigue in PD is probably as common and as severe as that reported in multiple sclerosis [68]. Third, the prevalence of fatigue in PD patients may increase with disease duration [76], although a separate (smaller) cohort study did not replicate this finding [68].

The experience of fatigue for patients with PD is a personal, subjective one. Brown *et al.* [77] found that patients with PD often did not spontaneously use the word "fatigue" to describe their symptoms, preferring such words as "tiredness," "lack of energy," or "exhaustion." There are indications that fatigue is an important symptom for many PD patients. For example, 15% of patients in one study rated fatigue as their worst symptom, with 54% rating it as equally severe as their other PD symptoms [74]. Quality-of-life studies in patients with PD and fatigue have found a poorer quality-of-life in patients with fatigue than in those without, with the main domains affected being "bodily discomfort," "emotional well-being," and "mobility" [75,78]. As indicated above, it is very difficult to disentangle the relative contributions of other common non-motor symptoms in PD (e.g., depression, sleep disturbance, cognitive deficits, physical inactivity) to fatigue [76]. Certainly, fatigue is reported early in PD in patients who do not score in the abnormal range on scales assessing mood and cognitive function [75]. However, fatigue may be secondary to the effect of mild disturbances in mood, cognition, and sleep that are not picked up by standard scales. Multiple non-motor symptoms, including fatigue, commonly cluster together, making the task of disentangling the pathophysiology of fatigue in PD even harder.

Treatment of fatigue in PD depends on the presence of other identifiable associated factors. Most important amongst these are depression and sleep disturbance. There have been general benefits reported for physical exercise programs in PD [79], although their specific impact on fatigue is not known. There has been one small, randomized controlled trial of methylphenidate in patients with PD and fatigue [80]. Thirty-six non-depressed PD patients were randomized to receive either methylphenidate [10 mg t.i.d.) or placebo for 6 weeks, and the response was assessed using two self-completed fatigue questionnaires. No formal screening for the co-occurrence of depression or sleep disturbance was performed. There was a significant reduction in fatigue scores in the active treatment group and side effects slightly favored those in the methylphenidate group.

Sweating

Disordered sweating (dyshidrosis) was recognized many years ago as a potential feature of PD, appearing, for example, in descriptions of patients with PD by Gowers in his *Manual of Disease of the Nervous System*, published in 1893. The prevalence of dyshidrosis in PD has been the subject of a number of studies, with estimates ranging widely. Taking those studies with the largest number of PD patients, estimates of prevalence of dyshidrosis vary between 46 and 64% of patients [81–83]. In one of these studies, the prevalence of dyshidrosis in PD patients was significantly different from that in a healthy control population surveyed using the same questionnaire (12.5%) [83].

The main clinical features of dyshidrosis in PD patients are hyperhidrosis (including focal/asymmetric excessive sweating and generalized drenching sweats) and hypohidrosis (including heat intolerance and excessive fatigue brought on by hot weather). In the epidemiology studies mentioned above, the prevalence of hypohidrosis was slightly less than that of hyperhidrosis. There is no clear correlation between duration of disease, disease severity, medication used to treat PD, and presence of dyshidrosis. However, there is a correlation between the presence of severe dyskinesia or motor fluctuations and dyshidrosis [81,83–85]. Hyperhidrosis tends to be most prominent when patients are "off" or when severe dyskinesias are occurring. In one study [85] in which the presence of sweating was measured serially every hour in two groups of PD patients with and without "on"/"off" fluctuations, excessive sweating was present only in the fluctuating group, and was most prominent when the Unified Parkinson's Disease Rating Scale (UPDRS) was at its highest level (i.e., patients were in their most severe parkinsonian state). There are also correlations between the presence of dyshidrosis and other autonomic symptoms, notably urinary frequency and sialorrhea.

Both central and peripheral factors have been proposed to cause dyshidrosis in PD. Although skin biopsies have not found abnormal cholinergic fibers, tests examining the post-ganglionic component of sweating (local pilocarpine test, local acetylcholine test) are abnormal in late-stage PD [82,86]. A decrease in the number of sweat glands has also been reported in some PD patients. Sympathetic skin responses have, in some studies, been found to be absent or suppressed whereas other studies have found normal results. Centrally, the pathways from the medial hypothalamus thought to be involved in control of sweating are degenerate in postmortem studies of PD brains. It is possible that one component of excessive sweating seen in PD is a compensatory response to centrally and peripherally driven hypohidrosis [87]. Excessive sweating during severe dyskinesia could be explained simply by the physical exertion of such movements. However, the "off" period emergence of excessive sweating cannot be simply explained by this mechanism, and therefore a hypodopaminergic state (or at least fluctuation from a hyper- to a hypo-dopaminergic state) may cause particular problems in control of sweating for some patients with PD [84,85]. Although its relevance to disorders of sweating and skin appearance is unknown, immunoreactivity to phosphorylated α-synuclein has recently been described in 70% of skin biopsy samples in a retrospective cohort of patients with pathologically proven PD [88].

Assessments of activities of daily living with current scales are unimpaired by the presence of dyshidrosis. However, quality-of-life can be affected by dyshidrosis, in particular for those with drenching sweats. A correlation has been found between the pain subscore of the PDQ-39 and the presence of dyshidrosis and also with the visual analog scale component of the EQ-5D quality-of-life scale [83]. This reflects the anecdotal reports of patients who experience social embarrassment and restriction of activities from dyshidrosis, disturbed sleep from drenching night sweats, and even a requirement for extra care due to excessive sweating.

Treatment is difficult. For those who experience hyperhidrosis in response to severe dyskinesia or "off" periods, successful medical or surgical management of these aspects of their motor symptoms may improve their excessive sweating. Indeed, there is evidence that the effects of subthalamic nucleus (STN) deep brain stimulation may extend to modification of some non-motor symptoms, including excessive sweating [89]. Some patients with focal excessive sweating may benefit from local treatments, such as powerful anti-perspirants or botulinum toxin injections. Anti-cholinergic drugs can reduce sweating, but commonly cause side effects in older patients such as hallucinations, confusion, drowsiness, and dry mouth, which may limit their usefulness.

Skin disorders

Seborrhea

Seborrhea has been noted since the 1920s as an additional component of Parkinson's disease, and its prevalence has been reported to be as high as 52% [90]. This prevalence may, however, depend on the treatment status of the patients, as levodopa has been reported to increase sebum production [91] (although this is not a universal finding [92]). In line with this, rates of seborrhea in an untreated cohort of PD patients have been reported to be lower at 19% [90]. Apart from levodopa treatment itself, no clear additional cause of the high prevalence of seborrhea in PD has been identified. It has been suggested that central drivers of sebum production (α-melanocyte stimulating hormone, androgens) may play a role [92], but there is no clear evidence to support this hypothesis [90]. Patients may complain of a rather waxy, greasy appearance of the skin, but no studies to date have focused on the impact of this symptom on patients. There is no evidence regarding how commonly treatment is required, or the most satisfactory methods of treatment.

Malignant melanoma and other skin cancers

There has been a long-running debate regarding the possibility of an increased risk of malignant melanoma in patients with PD, and in particular if that risk might be attributable to levodopa or other dopaminergic therapy. Recent large epidemiologic studies have provided some welcome clarity to this debate. In a large follow-up study using a health database in Denmark, which included over 14 000 people with PD, a twofold increase in the incidence of malignant melanoma was found [93]. This study was complemented by two further studies in the Danish population. One, which included over 8000 PD patients, found that there was an increased prevalence of malignant melanoma and other skin cancers (squamous cell carcinoma, basal cell carcimoma) before the diagnosis of PD [94]. The second study, a case–control study, again found an excess of cases of malignant melanoma in patients with PD, but no association between the presence of this cancer and the cumulative levodopa dose [95].

It is currently unclear what causes the increased risk of malignant melanoma in patients with PD. There is a positive correlation between social class and melanoma, as there is between social class and not smoking. Given that non-smokers are at higher risk of developing PD, it may be that social class could be a confounding factor in the association between melanoma and PD [96]. However, in the large Danish epidemiologic study [94], the authors dismissed this argument as an association between smoking and social class is not a significant one in Denmark. This large Danish study found a reduction in cancers at sites usually associated with smoking-related cancers (lung, larynx, mouth, bladder), even when data were corrected for smoking history [94]. This may indicate an interaction between genetic risk factors for the development of PD and the development of certain cancers, but protection against the development of others. A possible mechanism for the association of PD with certain specific types of cancer is that dysfunction in the ubiquitin–proteasome system, clearly implicated in the development of PD, is also associated with the promotion of certain oncogenes and therefore the development of cancer [97].

References

1. Hutton JT, Morris JL. Vision in Parkinson's disease. *Adv Neurol* 2001;**86**:279–88.
2. Bodis-Wollner I, Marx MS, Mitra S, *et al*. Visual dysfunction in Parkinson's disease. Loss in spatiotemporal contrast sensitivity. *Brain* 1987;**110**(Pt 6):1675–98.
3. Bulens C, Meerwaldt JD, Van der Wildt GJ, Keemink CJ. Contrast sensitivity in Parkinson's disease. *Neurology* 1986;**36**(8):1121–5.
4. Harris JP, Calvert JE, Phillipson OT. Processing of spatial contrast in peripheral vision in Parkinson's disease. *Brain* 1992;**115**(Pt 5):1447–57.
5. Haug BA, Trenkwalder C, Arden GB, *et al*. Visual thresholds to low-contrast pattern displacement, color contrast, and luminance contrast stimuli in Parkinson's disease. *Mov Disord* 1994;**9**(5):563–70.
6. Hutton JT, Morris JL, Elias JW, *et al*. Spatial contrast sensitivity is reduced in bilateral Parkinson's disease. *Neurology* 1991;**41**(8):1200–2.
7. Mestre D, Blin O. Serratrice G, Pailhous J. Spatiotemporal contrast sensitivity differs in normal aging and Parkinson's disease. *Neurology* 1990;**40**(11):1710–4.
8. van Tebartz EL, Greenlee MW, Foley JM, Lucking CH. Contrast detection, discrimination and adaptation in patients with Parkinson's disease and multiple system atrophy. *Brain* 1997;**120**(Pt 12):2219–28.
9. Bulens C, Meerwaldt JD, Van der Wildt GJ, Van Deursen JB. Effect of levodopa treatment on contrast sensitivity in Parkinson's disease. *Ann Neurol* 1987;**22**(3):365–9.
10. Buttner T, Muller T, Kuhn W. Effects of apomorphine on visual functions in Parkinson's disease. *J Neural Transm* 2000;**107**(1):87–94.
11. Diederich NJ, Raman R, Leurgans S, Goetz CG. Progressive worsening of spatial and chromatic processing deficits in Parkinson disease. *Arch Neurol* 2002;**59**(8):1249–52.
12. Langheinrich T, van Tebartz EL, Lagreze WA, *et al*. Visual contrast response functions in Parkinson's disease: evidence from electroretinograms, visually evoked potentials and psychophysics. *Clin Neurophysiol* 2000;**111**(1):66–74.
13. Sartucci F, Orlandi G, Lucetti C, *et al*. Changes in pattern electroretinograms to equiluminant red–green and blue–yellow gratings in patients with early Parkinson's disease. *J Clin Neurophysiol* 2003;**20**(5):375–81.
14. Sartucci F, Orlandi G, Bonuccelli U, *et al*. Chromatic pattern-reversal electroretinograms (ChPERGs) are spared in multiple system atrophy compared with Parkinson's disease. *Neurol Sci* 2006;**26**(6):395–401.
15. Sartucci F, Porciatti V. Visual-evoked potentials to onset of chromatic red–green and blue–yellow gratings in Parkinson's disease never treated with L-dopa. *J Clin Neurophysiol* 2006;**23**(5):431–5.
16. Pieri V, Diederich NJ, Raman R, Goetz CG. Decreased color discrimination and contrast sensitivity in Parkinson's disease. *J Neurol Sci* 2000;**172**(1):7–11.
17. Price MJ, Feldman RG, Adelberg D, Kayne H. Abnormalities in color vision and contrast sensitivity in Parkinson's disease. *Neurology* 1992;**42**(4):887–90.
18. Lieb K, Brucker S, Bach M, *et al*. Impairment in preattentive visual processing in patients with Parkinson's disease. *Brain* 1999;**122**(Pt 2):303–13.
19. Abe Y, Kachi T, Kato T, *et al*. Occipital hypoperfusion in Parkinson's disease without dementia: correlation to impaired cortical visual processing. *J Neurol Neurosurg Psychiatry* 2003;**74**(4):419–22.
20. Bulens C, Meerwaldt JD, Van der Wildt GJ. Effect of stimulus orientation on contrast sensitivity in Parkinson's disease. *Neurology* 1988;**38**(1):76–81.
21. Crevits L. Abnormal psychophysical visual perception in Parkinson's disease patients. *Acta Neurol Belg* 2003;**103**(2): 83–7.
22. Corin MS, Elizan TS, Bender MB. Oculomotor function in patients with Parkinson's disease. *J Neurol Sci* 1972;**15**(3): 251–65.
23. Randomized clinical trial of treatments for symptomatic convergence insufficiency in children. *Arch Ophthalmol* 2008; **126**(10):1336–49.
24. Shibasaki H, Tsuji S, Kuroiwa Y. Oculomotor abnormalities in Parkinson's disease. *Arch Neurol* 1979;**36**(6):360–4.
25. White OB, Saint-Cyr JA, Tomlinson RD, Sharpe JA. Ocular motor deficits in Parkinson's disease. II. Control of the saccadic and smooth pursuit systems. *Brain* 1983;**106**(Pt 3):571–87.
26. Bronstein AM, Kennard C. Predictive ocular motor control in Parkinson's disease. *Brain* 1985;**108**(Pt 4):925–40.
27. O'Sullivan EP, Shaunak S, Henderson L, *et al*. Abnormalities of predictive saccades in Parkinson's disease. *Neuroreport* 1997;**8**(5):1209–13.
28. Shaunak S, O'Sullivan E, Blunt S, *et al*. Remembered saccades with variable delay in Parkinson's disease. *Mov Disord* 1999;**14**(1):80–6.
29. Ventre J, Zee DS, Papageorgiou H, Reich S. Abnormalities of predictive saccades in hemi-Parkinson's disease. *Brain* 1992;**115**(Pt 4):1147–65.
30. Vermersch AI, Rivaud S, Vidailhet M, *et al*. Sequences of memory-guided saccades in Parkinson's disease. *Ann Neurol* 1994;**35**(4):487–90.
31. Sharpe JA, Fletcher WA, Lang AE, Zackon DH. Smooth pursuit during dose-related on–off fluctuations in Parkinson's disease. *Neurology* 1987;**37**(8):1389–92.
32. White OB, Saint-Cyr JA, Tomlinson RD, Sharpe JA. Ocular motor deficits in Parkinson's disease. II. Control of the saccadic and smooth pursuit systems. *Brain* 1983;**106**(Pt 3):571–87.
33. Bares M, Brazdil M, Kanovsky P, *et al*. The effect of apomorphine administration on smooth pursuit ocular movements

in early Parkinsonian patients. *Parkinsonism Relat Disord* 2003;**9**(3):139–44.
34. Hori N, Takamori M, Hirayama M, *et al.* Pupillary supersensitivity and visual disturbance in Parkinson's disease. *Clin Auton Res* 2008;**18**(1):20–7.
35. Knopp W, Rotenberg M, Boye R. L-Dopa, Parkinson's disease and pupillary reaction to light. *Monogr Hum Genet* 1972;**6**: 198.
36. Micieli G, Tassorelli C, Martignoni E, *et al.* Disordered pupil reactivity in Parkinson's disease. *Clin Auton Res* 1991;**1**(1):55–8.
37. Edwards LL, Pfeiffer RF, Quigley EM, *et al.* Gastrointestinal symptoms in Parkinson's disease. *Mov Disord* 1991;**6**(2):151–6.
38. Eadie MJ, Tyrer JH. Alimentary disorder in Parkinsonism. *Australas Ann Med* 1965;**14**: 13–22.
39. Kalf JG, Smit AM, Bloem BR, *et al.* Impact of drooling in Parkinson's disease. *J Neurol* 2007;**254**(9):1227–32.
40. Chou KL, Evatt M, Hinson V, Kompoliti K. Sialorrhea in Parkinson's disease: a review. *Mov Disord* 2007;**22**(16):2306–13.
41. Bagheri H, Damase-Michel C, Lapeyre-Mestre M, *et al.* A study of salivary secretion in Parkinson's disease. *Clin Neuropharmacol* 1999;**22**(4):213–5.
42. Nicaretta DH, de Rosso AL, Maliska C, Costa MM. Scintigraphic analysis of the parotid glands in patients with sialorrhea and Parkinson's disease. *Parkinsonism Relat Disord* 2008;**14**(4):338–41.
43. Proulx M, de Courval FP, Wiseman MA, Panisset M. Salivary production in Parkinson's disease. *Mov Disord* 2005;**20**(2):204–7.
44. Tumilasci OR, Cersosimo MG, Belforte JE, *et al.* Quantitative study of salivary secretion in Parkinson's disease. *Mov Disord* 2006;**21**(5):660–7.
45. Persson M, Osterberg T, Granerus AK, Karlsson S. Influence of Parkinson's disease on oral health. *Acta Odontol Scand* 1992;**50**(1):37–42.
46. Bushmann M, Dobmeyer SM, Leeker L, Perlmutter JS. Swallowing abnormalities and their response to treatment in Parkinson's disease. *Neurology* 1989;**39**(10):1309–14.
47. Fuh JL, Lee RC, Wang SJ, *et al.* Swallowing difficulty in Parkinson's disease. *Clin Neurol Neurosurg* 1997;**99**(2):106–12.
48. Thobois S, Mertens P, Guenot M, *et al.* Subthalamic nucleus stimulation in Parkinson's disease: clinical evaluation of 18 patients. *J Neurol* 2002;**249**(5):529–34.
49. Hyson HC, Johnson AM, Jog MS. Sublingual atropine for sialorrhea secondary to parkinsonism: a pilot study. *Mov Disord* 2002;**17**(6):1318–20.
50. Thomsen TR, Galpern WR, Asante A, *et al.* Ipratropium bromide spray as treatment for sialorrhea in Parkinson's disease. *Mov Disord* 2007;**22**(15):2268–73.
51. Serrano-Duenas M. Treatment of sialorrhea in Parkinson's disease patients with clonidine. Double-blind, comparative study with placebo. *Neurologia* 2003;**18**(1):2–6 (in Spanish).
52. Santamato A, Ianieri G, Ranieri M, *et al.* Botulinum toxin type A in the treatment of sialorrhea in Parkinson's disease. *J Am Geriatr Soc* 2008;**56**(4):765–7.
53. Fuster Torres MA, Berini AL, Gay EC. Salivary gland application of botulinum toxin for the treatment of sialorrhea. *Med Oral Patol Oral Cir Bucal* 2007;**12**(7):E511–7.
54. Kalf JG, Smit AM, Bloem BR, *et al.* Botulinum toxin A for drooling in Parkinson's disease: a pilot study to compare submandibular to parotid gland injections. *Parkinsonism Relat Disord* 2007;**13**(8):532–4.
55. Nobrega AC, Rodrigues B, Torres AC, *et al.* Does botulinum toxin decrease frequency and severity of sialorrhea in Parkinson's disease? *J Neurol Sci* 2007;**253**(1–2): 85–7.
56. Contarino MF, Pompili M, Tittoto P, *et al.* Botulinum toxin B ultrasound-guided injections for sialorrhea in amyotrophic lateral sclerosis and Parkinson's disease. *Parkinsonism Relat Disord* 2007;**13**(5):299–303.
57. Lagalla G, Millevolte M, Capecci M, *et al.* Botulinum toxin type A for drooling in Parkinson's disease: a double-blind, randomized, placebo-controlled study. *Mov Disord* 2006;**21**(5):704–7.
58. Tan EK. Botulinum toxin treatment of sialorrhea: comparing different therapeutic preparations. *Eur J Neurol* 2006;**13**(Suppl 1):60–4.
59. Ondo WG, Hunter C, Moore W. A double-blind placebo-controlled trial of botulinum toxin B for sialorrhea in Parkinson's disease. *Neurology* 2004;**62**(1):37–40.
60. Mancini F, Zangaglia R, Cristina S, *et al.* Double-blind, placebo-controlled study to evaluate the efficacy and safety of botulinum toxin type A in the treatment of drooling in parkinsonism. *Mov Disord* 2003;**18**(6):685–8.
61. Friedman A, Potulska A. Botulinum toxin for treatment of parkinsonian sialorrhea. *Neurol Neurochir Pol* 2001;**35**(Suppl 3):23–7.
62. Friedman A, Potulska A. Quantitative assessment of parkinsonian sialorrhea and results of treatment with botulinum toxin. *Parkinsonism Relat Disord* 2001;**7**(4):329–32.
63. Jost WH. Treatment of drooling in Parkinson's disease with botulinum toxin. *Mov Disord* 1999;**14**(6):1057.
64. Comella CL, Jankovic J, Shannon KM, *et al.* Comparison of botulinum toxin serotypes A and B for the treatment of cervical dystonia. *Neurology* 2005;**65**(9):1423–9.
65. Marks L, Turner K, O'Sullivan J, *et al.* Drooling in Parkinson's disease: a novel speech and language therapy intervention. *Int J Lang Commun Disord* 2001;**36**(Suppl):282–7.
66. Borg M, Hirst F. The role of radiation therapy in the management of sialorrhea. *Int J Radiat Oncol Biol Phys* 1998;**41**(5): 1113–9.
67. Abe K, Takanashi M, Yanagihara T. Fatigue in patients with Parkinson's disease. *Behav Neurol* 2000;**12**(3):103–6.
68. Friedman J, Friedman H. Fatigue in Parkinson's disease. *Neurology* 1993;**43**(10):2016–8.
69. Havlikova E, Rosenberger J, Nagyova I, *et al.* Impact of fatigue on quality of life in patients with Parkinson's disease. *Eur J Neurol* 2008;**15**(5):475–80.
70. Karlsen K, Larsen JP, Tandberg E, Jorgensen K. Fatigue in patients with Parkinson's disease. *Mov Disord* 1999;**14**(2): 237–41.
71. Larsen JP, Karlsen K, Tandberg E. Clinical problems in non-fluctuating patients with Parkinson's disease: a community-based study. *Mov Disord* 2000;**15**(5):826–9.
72. Shulman LM, Taback RL, Rabinstein AA, Weiner WJ. Non-recognition of depression and other non-motor symptoms in Parkinson's disease. *Parkinsonism Relat Disord* 2002;**8**(3): 193–7.
73. van Hilten JJ, Hoogland G, van der Velde EA, *et al.* Diurnal effects of motor activity and fatigue in Parkinson's disease. *J Neurol Neurosurg Psychiatry* 1993;**56**(8):874–7.

74. van Hilten JJ, Weggeman M, van der Velde EA, *et al.* Sleep, excessive daytime sleepiness and fatigue in Parkinson's disease. *J Neural Transm Park Dis Dement Sect* 1993;**5**(3):235–44.
75. Havlikova E, Rosenberger J, Nagyova I, *et al.* Clinical and psychosocial factors associated with fatigue in patients with Parkinson's disease. *Parkinsonism Relat Disord* 2008;**14**(3): 187–92.
76. Alves G, Wentzel-Larsen T, Larsen JP. Is fatigue an independent and persistent symptom in patients with Parkinson disease? *Neurology* 2004;**63**(10):1908–11.
77. Brown RG, Dittner A, Findley L, Wessely SC. The Parkinson fatigue scale. *Parkinsonism Relat Disord* 2005;**11**(1):49–55.
78. Herlofson K, Larsen JP. The influence of fatigue on health-related quality of life in patients with Parkinson's disease. *Acta Neurol Scand* 2003;**107**(1):1–6.
79. Crizzle AM, Newhouse IJ. Is physical exercise beneficial for persons with Parkinson's disease? *Clin J Sport Med* 2006;**16**(5): 422–5.
80. Mendonca DA, Menezes K, Jog MS. Methylphenidate improves fatigue scores in Parkinson disease: a randomized controlled trial. *Mov Disord* 2007;**22**(14):2070–6.
81. Hirayama M. Sweating dysfunctions in Parkinson's disease. *J Neurol* 2006;**253**(Suppl 7):VII42–7.
82. Saito H, Kogure K. Thermal sudomotor deficits in Parkinson's disease. *Rinsho Shinkeigaku* 1989;**29**(6):734–40 (in Japanese).
83. Swinn L, Schrag A, Viswanathan R, *et al.* Sweating dysfunction in Parkinson's disease. *Mov Disord* 2003;**18**(12):1459–63.
84. Pursiainen V, Haapaniemi TH, Korpelainen JT, *et al.* Sweating in parkinsonian patients with wearing-off. *Mov Disord* 2007;**22**(6):828–32.
85. Sage JI, Mark MH. Drenching sweats as an off phenomenon in Parkinson's disease: treatment and relation to plasma levodopa profile. *Ann Neurol* 1995;**37**(1):120–2.
86. Hirashima F, Yokota T, Hayashi M. Sympathetic skin response in Parkinson's disease. *Acta Neurol Scand* 1996;**93**(2–3):127–32.
87. Turkka JT, Myllyla VV. Sweating dysfunction in Parkinson's disease. *Eur Neurol* 1987;**26**(1):1–7.
88. Ikemura M, Saito Y, Sengoku R, *et al.* Lewy body pathology involves cutaneous nerves. *J Neuropathol Exp Neurol* 2008;**67**(10):945–53.
89. Witjas T, Kaphan E, Regis J, *et al.* Effects of chronic subthalamic stimulation on nonmotor fluctuations in Parkinson's disease. *Mov Disord* 2007;**22**(12):1729–34.
90. Fischer M, Gemende I, Marsch WC, Fischer PA. Skin function and skin disorders in Parkinson's disease. *J Neural Transm* 2001;**108**(2):205–13.
91. Kohn SR, Pochi PE, Strauss JS, *et al.* Sebaceous gland secretion in Parkinson's disease during L-dopa treatment. *J Invest Dermatol* 1973;**60**(3):134–6.
92. Villares JC, Carlini EA. Sebum secretion in idiopathic Parkinson's disease: effect of anticholinergic and dopaminergic drugs. *Acta Neurol Scand* 1989;**80**(1):57–63.
93. Olsen JH, Friis S, Frederiksen K, *et al.* Atypical cancer pattern in patients with Parkinson's disease. *Br J Cancer* 2005;**92**(1):201–5.
94. Olsen JH, Friis S, Frederiksen K. Malignant melanoma and other types of cancer preceding Parkinson disease. *Epidemiology* 2006;**17**(5):582–7.
95. Olsen JH, Tangerud K, Wermuth L, *et al.* Treatment with levodopa and risk for malignant melanoma. *Mov Disord* 2007;**22**(9):1252–7.
96. Zanetti R, Loria D, Rosso S. Melanoma, Parkinson's disease and levodopa: causal or spurious link? A review of the literature. *Melanoma Res* 2006;**16**(3):201–6.
97. Paul S. Dysfunction of the ubiquitin–proteasome system in multiple disease conditions: therapeutic approaches. *Bioessays* 2008;**30**(11–12):1172–84.

Chapter 35
Overview of the Medical Treatment of the Non-Motor and Non-Dopaminergic Features of Parkinson's Disease

Mark Stacy[1] *& Joseph Jankovic*[2]
[1]Division of Neurology, Duke University Medical School, Durham, NC, USA
[2]Parkinson's Disease Center and Movement Disorders Clinic, Department of Neurology, Baylor College of Medicine,, Houston, TX, USA

Introduction

Non-motor symptoms in Parkinson's disease (PD) patients have become the focus of care in tertiary movement disorder centers. These include behavioral, cognitive, sensory, autonomic, and sleep disturbances [1]. Patients often develop depression, passive attitude and apathy, and cognitive decline leading to dementia. Frontal release or "cortical disinhibition" signs, such as the glabellar signs [2] or the applause sign [3], accompany other mental and motor symptoms of PD, but are not specific. Neuro-ophthalmologic abnormalities include decreased blink rate, ocular surface irritation, altered tear film, blepharospasm, apraxia of eyelid opening, limitation of upward gaze, ocular saccade impairment, and convergence abnormalities [4]. Gastrointestinal symptoms encompass delayed gastric emptying, constipation and anismus, while urogenital symptoms include incontinence and sexual dysfunction [5]. Sensory symptoms such as pain, burning, coldness, or numbness are reported by about half of PD patients [6]. Seborrhea, seen in some patients, may represent systemic involvement in PD [1,7]. This chapter provides an overview of the management of these non-motor, poorly dopa-responsive symptoms.

Neuropsychiatric disorders

Cognitive disorders

Dementia occurs in more than 30% of PD patients, particularly in those older than 70 years [8,9], with frequency depending on the assessment tool. A long-term follow-up of 233 subjects in Norway found that dementia was present in 60.1% of PD subjects by 12 years into their disease [10]. Others report significant cognitive symptoms in more than 80% of end-stage patients [11]. A review of 873 PD outpatients in Germany found that 28.6% of subjects met DSM-IV criteria for dementia; age and disease severity increased the risk of cognitive decline [12]. The Movement Disorders Society recently reviewed the criteria for cognitive assessment in PD (Box 35.1) [13]. PD with dementia (PDD) is characterized by a subcortical dementia dominated by distractibility, passivity, and slow thinking, typically affecting visuospatial, attentional, and executive functions. This contrasts with the cortical type of dementia found in Alzheimer's disease (AD) and dementia with Lewy bodies (DLB), which primarily affects storage processing (memory and language) [14]. Cognitive changes associated with PDD usually begin more than 10 years after motor symptoms, but can begin much earlier, and even precede the development of parkinsonian features (typically referred to as DLB). Patients can also develop a mixed picture of PD and AD, in which patients experience cognitive and language abnormalities early in the course of the illness [15].

Cognitive symptoms seen in PD are associated with dysfunction of the basal forebrain cholinergic system. Cholinergic neuronal loss and depletion of choline acetyltransferase are found early in the course of PD and DLB [14]. Furthermore, positron emission tomography (PET) measuring cortical acetylcholinesterase (AChE) activity demonstrates a greater reduction in PDD (21%) than PD without dementia (13%) [16]. Treatment with cholinesterase inhibitors can improve cognition [17], whereas anti-cholinergics may further disturb attention and precipitate hallucinations and should be avoided, even in the setting of mild cognitive deficits. Other possible causes of dementia should be excluded in PD patients, including subdural hematoma, multiple brain infarctions,

Parkinson's Disease: Non-Motor and Non-Dopaminergic Features, First Edition. Edited by C. Warren Olanow, Fabrizio Stocchi, and Anthony E. Lang.

Box 35.1 Algorithm for diagnosing PDD [2007]

- A diagnosis of Parkinson's disease based on the UK Brain Bank criteria for PD
- PD developed prior to the onset of dementia
- MMSE <26
- Cognitive deficits severe enough to impact daily living
- Impairment in at least two of the following tests:
  - Months reversed or seven backward
  - Lexical fluency or clock drawing
  - MMSE pentagons
  - Three-word recall

normal pressure hydrocephalus, nonconvulsive seizures, metabolic disturbances, thyroid abnormalities, pernicious anemia, and subacute meningitis [18].

Treatment of cognitive disorders in PD

Cholinesterase inhibitors such as donepezil, rivastigmine, and galantamine can provide meaningful improvement of cognitive impairment and other behavioral problems in PD. A double-blind, randomized, placebo-controlled, 10-week study of 14 patients with PD and cognitive impairment showed that donepezil (5 or 10 mg per day) was associated with a 2.1-point increase in the mean MMSE score compared with a 0.3 point increase on placebo. This benefit was not associated with worsening of parkinsonism [19]. However, other studies suggest that cholinergic side effects and worsening parkinsonism may be limiting factors [20,21]. Rivastigmine inhibits both acetyl and butyryl cholinesterase, molecules accounting for 40% of cholinergic activity in the cortex and 60% in the hippocampus in AD brains. A study of 541 PD patients with symptoms of dementia randomized to rivastigmine or placebo [17] demonstrated significant benefit in the mean ADAS-Cog score (2.1 versus 0.7 points in the rivastigmine and placebo groups respectively; $p < 0.001$) and in the MMSE (0.8 points versus 0.2; $p = 0.03$). Nausea, vomiting, dizziness, and tremor were significantly more frequent in the rivastigmine group. Although the maximum suggested dose for rivastigmine is 24 mg per day, 55.5% of subjects were receiving 9–12 mg per day at final visit. A follow-up report demonstrated sustained benefit in a 48-week extension study [22]. Rivastigmine also significantly improved attention in a study of 487 PD patients with dementia [23], but caused slight worsening of tremor in PDD patients [24]. In a 12-week study comparing donepezil and rivastigmine, both drugs improved cognition comparably, but donepezil was better tolerated [25]. In general, it can be concluded that cholinesterase inhibitors are effective treatments for dementia in PD, but improvement is modest and motor side effects may occur [25]. Memantine is reported to improve symptoms in moderate to advanced cases of AD and PD, but is also known to trigger psychosis in PD patients. Memantine effects likely reflect activities at both NMDA and dopamine D2 receptors [26]. The AAN Quality Standards Subcommittee has summarized current practice parameters for depression, psychosis, and dementia [27]. As dementia is such an important problem in PD and a major cause of disability and nursing home placement for advanced patients, more effective treatments are required.

Psychiatric disorders

Psychosis in PD is often linked to cognitive decline and the use of anti-PD drugs. The presence of psychosis is a strong predictor of institutionalization and dementia. PD patients living in Nursing Care Facilities have a 16-fold higher likelihood of hallucinations than those living at home [28]. A review of PD patients with psychosis found that hallucinations were linked to dementia (68%), nursing home placement (42%), and death (25%) [29]. An NIH working group proposed criteria for defining psychosis in PD (Box 35.2) [30]. Psychosis in PD typically begins 10 years after the diagnosis; early-onset psychosis suggests DLB, AD, or a pre-existing psychiatric disorder [31]. Using the administrative healthcare databases of Ontario, Canada, 10 347 individuals aged 66 years or older newly treated with dopaminergic agents were

Box 35.2 Proposed diagnostic criteria for PD associated psychosis [2007]

- Presence of at least one of the following symptoms
  - Illusions
  - False sense of presence
  - Hallucinations
  - Delusions
- UK brain bank criteria for PD
- The symptoms of psychosis occur after the onset of PD
- The symptoms of psychosis are recurrent or continuous for 1 month
- The symptoms of psychosis are not better accounted for by
  - Diffuse Lewy body disease
  - Schizophrenia
  - Schizoaffective disorder
  - Delusional disorder
  - Mood disorder with psychotic features
  - General medical condition including delirium
- Associated features
  - With/without insight
  - With/without dementia
  - With/without treatment for PD

identified. The estimated cumulative probability of requiring an anti-psychotic at 7 years was 35%; 499 individuals (4.8%; 5.2/100 person-years) were prescribed an anti-psychotic within 1 year of starting dopaminergic therapy. With the introduction of atypical neuroleptics, the proportion of initial prescriptions for typical anti-psychotics decreased from 56% (42 of 75) in 1998 to 9% (8 of 88) in 2002 [32]. Although anti-PD therapy can trigger psychosis, a relationship to levodopa-equivalent doses cannot always be established [33]. Indeed, symptoms of psychosis were well recognized in the pre-levodopa era [34], indicating that drug therapy alone is not the definitive etiologic factor. Autopsy series report high concentrations of Lewy bodies in the parahippocampus, amygdala, and frontal, temporal, and parietal lobes in parkinsonian patients with psychosis.

Symptoms of psychosis include hallucinations and delusional thought. Traditionally, benign hallucinations are not usually bothersome to patients, and the patient retains insight that these are not real experiences. Malignant hallucinations are associated with a loss of this insight. The distinction between benign and malignant hallucinations is somewhat arbitrary, and should not imply progression of disease. More recent categorization divides these phenomena into transient and persistent phenomena. Presence or passing (vague images in the peripheral vision) hallucinations and visual illusions are early symptoms, and persistent images are superimposed on a normal environment [35]. Visual hallucinations are by far the most common type of hallucinatory experience. These are usually well-formed people, animals, or inanimate objects, and appear and vanish suddenly [7]. Caregivers report that alerting stimuli will usually improve symptoms. Auditory hallucinations are less common and may range from simple sounds (such as ringing or knocking) to indistinct whispers. Some patients, particularly with hearing loss, may report hearing music. Unlike schizophrenia, auditory hallucinations in PD are rarely threatening or disturbing, and usually accompany visual hallucinations. Tactile, olfactory, and gustatory hallucinations are uncommon, and almost always accompany visual experiences. Delusions are usually paranoid in nature and typically include suspicions of spousal infidelity or abandonment. Grandiose, somatic, and religious delusions are relatively infrequent [36].

Delirium is common in PD patients due to co-morbid medical problems and multiple medications. Distinguishing delirium from drug-induced psychosis may be difficult, especially in a demented patient [18]. Fluctuating levels of consciousness, marked declines in cognitive performance, increased confusion, and disorientation from baseline are hallmark signs of delirium. In psychotic patients, baseline memory, orientation, and cognition are usually unimpaired, but the presence of psychosis can be a harbinger of dementia.

Treatment of psychotic disorders

Treatment of psychosis in PD is typically accomplished with atypical anti-psychotic agents that do not affect striatal dopamine receptors [36,37], although there is little supporting evidence in double-blind trials. Two trials did show significantly better outcomes for low-dose clozapine versus placebo with respect to both psychosis and motor function. In contrast, two double-blind trials failed to show efficacy of quetiapine over placebo [38]. A trial comparing clozapine with quetiapine showed relatively equivalent efficacy and tolerability, although benefits favored clozapine. In this study, 27 patients with PD and recent-onset psychosis were randomly allocated to 22 weeks of treatment with quetiapine or clozapine. Clozapine had a trend over quetiapine in controlling the frequency of hallucinations ($p = 0.097$) and a significant advantage in reducing delusions ($p = 0.011$). In two placebo-controlled trials, the atypical neuroleptic olanzapine did not improve psychotic symptoms and caused extrapyramidal side effects [39]. A more recent 3-month study randomized age- and disease duration-matched subjects ($n = 30$) to quetiapine or placebo [28]. The study did not show a beneficial effect for quetiapine in the treatment of psychosis in PD [39], although the withdrawal rates were high. Another randomized, double-blind, placebo-controlled trial in 40 patients with dementia and parkinsonism also found no significant benefit of quetiapine versus placebo. Large placebo effects, inadequate dosages (mean 120 mg per day), and inadequate power may have contributed to the inability to detect benefit. Quetiapine was generally well tolerated and did not worsen parkinsonism [40]. In another study, 35 PD patients with dementia were treated with quetiapine and followed for 24 months. At the end of the study, 31% of patients were still on quetiapine [41]. Fifteen non-responding patients were switched to clozapine, and 12 (80%) had a positive result. An open-label pilot study evaluated the effect of the atypical anti-psychotic aripiprazole on psychosis in PD. Fourteen patients were started on 1 mg per day and titrated up to a maximum dose of 5 mg per day. Although some had a favorable response, aripiprazole was associated with exacerbation of motor symptoms, and therefore does not appear promising as a treatment for psychosis in PD [42].

Overall, psychosis is an important problem in PD and can limit adequate utilization of dopaminergic therapy. Clozapine is considered to be the most effective treatment, but is associated with hematologic side effects and periodic monitoring must be employed. Quetiapine has not been convincingly shown to be effective in double-blind trials, but anecdotal experience suggests that many patients respond well, it permits an increase in levodopa dose, and it is well tolerated. For this reason, many physicians will initially try quetiapine before going on to a trial of clozapine. Occasional anti-psychotic benefits have been observed with anti-cholinesterase agents.

Depression

Depression is reported to occur in 30–90% of PD patients, increases with cognitive decline, and may present as "pseudo-dementia," [43]. In 537 patients with PDD, 58% had associated depression [44]. A systematic review of depression in PD has found the average prevalence of major depression to be 17%, dysthymia occurring in 13% and minor depression in 22% [45]. Vegetative symptoms of depression (slowness, lack of energy, poor concentration, and sleep disturbance) are correlated with duration of illness and changes in activities of daily living, and may reflect parkinsonism. Therefore, if depression is suspected, the clinician must inquire about early-morning awakening, low mood with diurnal variation, apathy, crying, withdrawal, and suicidal tendencies [7]. Unique features attributed to depression in PD include increased dysphoria, irritability, sadness, anxiety, brooding, cognitive deficits, pessimism, and suicidal ideation without action. PD patients appear to have less guilt and self-blame than other populations [28].

Treatment of depression

A survey of 22 827 parkinsonian patients showed that 20% were taking anti-depressant medications [46]. A cross-sectional study in Italy (PRIAMO) found that 169 of 1072 (15.8%) PD patients were treated for depression [47]. Tricyclic anti-depressants such as amitriptyline or nortriptyline may be helpful and may improve sialorrhea because of their anti-cholinergic side effects, but may compromise cognitive function. Selective serotonin reuptake inhibitors (SSRIs) are also helpful in treating depression in PD patients and seem to be well tolerated, although they may exacerbate tremors [48], and there is a theoretical risk of a serotonin reaction if combined with MAO-B inhibitors. Sertraline has relatively low selectivity for serotonin relative to dopamine reuptake and has been suggested to have the most favorable profile. Compared with tricyclics, sertraline improves quality-of-life, activities of daily living (ADL), mobility, and stigma [47] and may even improve motor symptoms [49].

Some have investigated whether symptoms such as depression, anxiety, lack of energy, and sexual dysfunction in PD are related to co-morbid testosterone deficiency (found in 35% of patients) and suggested that testosterone treatment may be appropriate [50]. However, in a controlled clinical trial, testosterone was not found to be beneficial [51]. Cognitive training interventions have been reported to improve cognitive ability in PD patients [52]. Active musical therapy has been reported to improve affective and behavioral functions and possibly bradykinesia in PD [53].

Behavioral disorders – anxiety, apathy and fatigue

Approximately 40% of PD patients experience clinically significant anxiety, including panic disorder, generalized anxiety, and phobic disorders [7]. This rate is higher than that in the general population and in groups of patients with similar disabilities. Anxiety may appear prior to motor symptoms or occur as a psychologic reaction to having PD. Concerns about and fear of institutionalization, going insane, or dying contribute to anxiety among patients with PD. Symptoms of anxiety may be difficult to differentiate from and wrongly attributed to PD, including tremor, numbness, tingling, breathlessness, chest discomfort, sweating, abdominal discomfort, restlessness, and dizziness [54]. Typically the "off" state is more distressing, and because of this patients prefer to be "on" with dyskinesia [55].

Variable degrees of apathy have been found in about half of patients with PD [56], and may be noted prior to motor symptoms. Apathy is characterized by an isolated lack of motivation, hopelessness, and low mood, but not necessarily anhedonia. Rarely, apathy progresses to abulia (severe apathy and lack of initiative and spontaneity) and even akinetic mutism and catatonia. Apathy is believed to be a prefrontal lobe dysfunction and has no known treatment [7].

Fatigue is reported by 42% of PD patients, and is defined as an overwhelming sense of tiredness, lack of energy, or feeling of exhaustion [7]. Differentiating fatigue syndromes from depression can be difficult. The underlying pathophysiology of apathy and fatigue remains poorly understood. Fatigue can be multifactorial and result from sleepiness, hypotension, drug effect, and co-morbid illness.

Treatment of behavioral disorders

Leentjens *et al.* have reviewed pooled data from seven registry trials of pramipexole in the treatment of motor symptoms of PD [56]. *Post hoc* comparison of placebo versus active therapy groups for question four (motivation) of the UPDRS found benefit in 64.7% of pramipexole-treated patients and 43.4% of those receiving placebo ($n = 480$; $p < 0.001$). A randomized controlled trial of paroxetine CR, nortriptyline, and placebo in 52 patients with PD and depression found nortriptyline, but not paroxetine CR, to be superior to placebo for change in HAM-D ($p < 0.002$). Response rates favored nortriptyline ($p = 0.024$): nortriptyline 53%, paroxetine CR 11%, placebo 24%. Nortriptyline was also superior to placebo in sleep, anxiety, and social functioning, whereas paroxetine CR was not.

Impulse control disorders

Behavioral disturbances in PD associated with dopaminergic therapy have been recognized for over 30 years.

Hypersexuality (HS), hyperlibidinous behavior, and hypomania were emphasized in the early levodopa literature. More recently, pathologic gambling (PG), compulsive shopping (CS), and binge eating (BE) have also been recognized to be relatively common and socially damaging complications of anti-PD treatment [57–61]. In addition, some PD patients develop compulsive motor behaviors, which they may deny but are obvious to the physician or family. Dopamine dysregulation syndrome describes patients who take high doses of dopamine replacement therapy and exhibit severe dyskinesias, cyclical mood disorder with hypomania or manic psychosis, and impaired social and occupational function. To describe the constellation of symptoms and maladaptive behaviors that emerge with PD progression and anti-parkinsonian medications, the term "impulse control disorder" (ICD) has been used. This includes disruptive behaviors (e.g., punding), destructive behaviors (e.g., compulsive spending, gambling, binge eating, or hypersexuality), and addictive behaviors (e.g. excessive use and abuse of anti-parkinsonian medications) (Box 35.3) [58].

Box 35.3 Proposed diagnostic criteria for impulse control disorder: risk factors for ICD; possible ICD; definite ICD

Diagnosis prior to 50 years of age
Diagnosis >5 years
Male gender
Reported change in personality or behavior, increased secrecy

Compulsive behavior (punding) greater than 1 h per day
H/O depression, anxiety or bipolar disorder

Increased time at hobbies or work
Addictive behavior
Gambling
Shopping
Prior drug/alcohol abuse
Decreasing need for sleep or complaints of insomnia
Increased libido
Hypersexual behavior
Bing eating
Prior gambling or other behavioral addiction
Increased medication intake

Family history of mental illness
Hoarding medications

Family history of drug/alcohol addiction

Dyskinesias

Levodopa or equivalent DA dosages >1000 mg per day

Dopamine agonist therapy

Punding refers to aimless, repetitive activity, often involving seemingly endless manipulations of a familiar object [62]. The term is borrowed from the vernacular of Swedish intravenous amphetamine addicts, meaning "blockhead." Examples include inordinate writing, doodling, painting, walkabouts, assembly/disassembly, collecting things, shuffling through papers, blogging, excessive cleaning or gardening or sorting household objects, humming or singing, and reciting meaningless soliloquies without an audience [63]. Interestingly, performance of these behaviors may be linked to increased synaptic dopamine, since amphetamine, cocaine, and levodopa share a presynaptic mechanism. In addition, these activities seem to be more prominent during "on time" and "on time with dyskinesias" [64]. PG, CS, BE and HS have been reported predominantly in PD patients using dopamine agonists used as monotherapy or in addition to levodopa, rather than with levodopa alone [65–68]. Features associated with these behaviors include early age of onset, duration of disease, family history of psychiatric disorders, depression, and prior history of gambling. Patients with binge eating usually have other behavioral addictions, punding, and a history of weight control issues.

The anatomic substrate for ICDs is not fully elucidated [58]. The D2 dopamine receptor mediates neuronal activity in the indirect pathway, and is thought to have a prominent role in ICDs in PD and in addiction disorders. Within the D2-type receptor family attention has particularly focused on D3 receptors, which reside within the ventral striatum/nucleus accumbens and modulate non-motor circuits. These non-motor circuits include the dorsolateral prefrontal cortex, regulating executive function; the lateral orbito-frontal cortex, modulating socially appropriate behavior and mood; and the anterior cingulate cortex, initiating activity and maintaining interest. Involvement of these pathways has been postulated to play a role in the development of ICDs.

Treatment of ICDs

At present, there are no prospective studies evaluating treatment strategies for ICDs in patients with PD [71] and treatment approaches are largely anecdotal. In general, each case should be evaluated for the presence of other ICDs and psychiatric conditions, such as substance abuse or mood disorders, and also for the overuse of dopaminergic therapies and features consistent with DDS. Symptoms of ICD most often respond to reduction or withdrawal of dopaminergic therapy, particularly dopamine agonists (Box 35.4). The addition of SSRIs, quetiapine, valproic acid, naltrexone, or topiramate may be helpful [71]. Successful treatment has also been reported with accomprosate, donezepil, and clozapine [72–75]. There are also reports of improvement after deep brain stimulation surgery, in the context of dopaminergic therapy

Box 35.4 Treatment of non-dopaminergic symptoms associated with PD

Cognitive impairment, tip-of-the- tongue phenomenon, bradyphrenia
  Rivastigmine, donepezil, galantamine, memantine
Depression, apathy, anhedonia, fatigue, other behavioral and psychiatric problems
  SSRIs, tricyclics, modafinil, armodafinil, quetiapine, clozapine
Sensory symptoms: anosmia, ageusia, pain (shoulder, back), paresthesias
  Gabapentin, pregabalin, duloxetine
Dysautonomia (orthostatic hypotension, constipation, urinary and sexual dysfunction, abnormal sweating, seborrhea), weight loss
  Fludrocortisone, midodrine, poly(ethylene glycol), lubiprostone, botulinum toxin, tolterodine, solifenacin, darifenacin, sildenafil
Sleep disorders (RBD, vivid dreams, daytime drowsiness, sleep fragmentation, RLS)
  Modafinil, armodafinil, CNS stimulants, clonazepam, melatonin, zolpidem, quetiapine, dopamine agonists

reduction [76]. However, some report worsening or emergence of ICD behaviors after surgery [77].

Several case reports and series indicate improvement of ICDs subsequent to a decrease in dosage or discontinuation of dopaminergic therapy. Dodd *et al.* reported that seven of 18 patients with an ICD had resolution of the behavior with discontinuation ($n = 4$) or dosage reduction ($n = 2$) of a dopamine agonist [68]. In a series of 13 patients with HS, all cases resolved following discontinuation of dopaminergic medications [77]; similar results were observed in a retrospective chart review [78]. Similarly, a decrease in agonist dosage improved punding behavior [64], and food cravings in those with binge eating [79].

Pharmacologic approaches may be useful. Resolution of symptoms in individuals has been reported after decreasing dopamine agonist therapy and adding quetiapine/valproate or olanzapine/lithium [80]. However, there are reports of patients who did not respond to decreases in DRT or to trials of quetiapine or citalopram [72]. In patients with DDS and punding, quetiapine was found to abort or improve punding behavior [24]. Clozapine 50 mg per day was effective in treating paraphilia in one patient [75], and risperidone 1 mg per day was associated with resolution of PG in another [81]. Two patients with hyperlibidinous behavior and depression benefited from anti-depressant monotherapy [82]. However, citalopram 40 mg per day was reported to improve depression but not PG in one case [61]. The anti-androgen cyproterone has been used for HS in patients with DDS, sometimes in conjunction with decreases in DRT [62], and clomipramine reduced punding in a patient with DDS [62]. Recently, amantadine has been shown to be effective in treating PG in a prospective, blinded setting [69]. However, others report that subjects taking amantadine showed no greater decrease in frequency of ICD behaviors than subjects not taking this agent [70]. Other treatment approaches remain largely anecdotal.

Counseling has not been formally studied in the management of ICDs but may be of benefit. Several reports note beneficial effects of counseling in some patients [5,8,9]. Counseling in conjunction with anti-depressants has been considered [67], and a combination of decreased DRT, psychotherapy, and treatment with sertraline reportedly allowed one patient to overcome gambling behavior [83]. Limiting access to money and restricting medications have been advocated for those with PG [9], and treatment of punding with DDS [62]. In one patient with PD and PG, cognitive–behavioral therapy, monitoring of spending, SSRIs, and attending a self-help group were not effective, whereas a reduction in DRT improved gambling behaviors [28]. Acamprosate was approved for the treatment of alcohol dependence in 2004. Because acamprosate is an mGluR5 antagonist and appears to modify D2 receptor density in the nucleus acumbans, it may modify impulsive behavior without significant adverse motor effects [73,74], but it has not yet been formally tested.

Several recent reports have addressed the use of deep brain stimulation (DBS) of the subthalamic nucleus (STN) for the treatment of ICDs and DDS [84–86], particularly for the subset of patients receiving high dosages of DRT. Two patients with motor fluctuations, dyskinesias, DDS, and HS underwent bilateral STN DBS [84]. One had a history of alcohol abuse, hypersexuality, and walkabouts. Postoperatively he was able to stop all DRT and HS behavior resolved. Following bilateral STN DBS, a second patient was able to decrease DRT by 75% with improvement in his disruptive behaviors [85]. When considering DBS STN for PG, it must be noted that post-operatively new onset PG has been reported in five of thirty-nine patients, some in the absence of dopamine agonist use [87]. A recent multicenter retrospective review of 598 patients with PD and DBS STN identified seven subjects with PG at the time of surgery [86]. Prior interventions had not been successful, including behavioral therapy in four patients and clozapine in one. Four of the patients also met criteria for DDS. Postoperatively, dopamine agonist therapy was stopped in three patients with an average reduction in DRT of 74%; PG was improved postoperatively, although some still gambled to a mild degree. Three patients had postoperative depression that triggered gambling which reportedly was less pleasurable than preoperatively. Several other ICDs resolved subsequent to DBS. HS was reported in five of seven preoperatively, one of six at 3 months postoperatively, and in none of the seven followed for 2–6 years after surgery. CS was present in three of seven preoperatively, one of six at 3 months, and one of seven at 2–6 years after surgery. BE was present in two subjects prior to surgery, three of six at 3 months, and one of seven at 2–6 years. There was transient worsening of PG in two patients immediately postoperation due to mania. In two patients whose medications could not be reduced, PG persisted.

Sleep disorders

Sleep difficulties are estimated to occur in 60–98% of PD patients, and night-time awakenings are three times more frequent than in healthy age-matched controls (38.9% versus 12%) [88]. Polysomnography found that PD patients not taking medication had less total sleep time, less sleep efficiency, more frequent awakenings, and greater overall waking time compared with controls [89]. Stimulation of dopaminergic neurons is associated with arousal and suppression of rapid eye movement (REM) sleep. Levodopa or use of a dopamine agonist was the strongest predictor of sleep disturbance [90].

Excessive daytime sleepiness (EDS) is more common in PD than controls, and is associated with advancing disease, increasing dopaminergic therapy, disease duration, and male gender [91]. Contributing factors include disease severity, concurrent illness, sedating medication, and additional sleep disorders. In a survey of more than 200 patients, sleep benefit was reported in 42% of respondents, and this was associated with years of levodopa therapy, motor fluctuations, and dyskinesias [92]. When PD patients were compared with normal controls and patients with a chronic disease (diabetes mellitus), similar frequencies of mild daytime sleepiness were found, but PD respondents had significantly higher EDS (15.5% in PD versus 4% in diabetics). Although EDS in PD may relate to neuropathologic changes, it also may be a function of anti-PD therapy [88]. With the possible exception of selegiline, all anti-parkinsonian medications have some potential to induce EDS. Polysomnograms in patients complaining of an irresistible desire to sleep demonstrate transition into stage 1–2 sleep within 30–60 min of a levodopa dose. Follow-up studies while off medication revealed normal multiple sleep latency tests [90]. In addition, REM suppression has been documented in patients receiving levodopa infusion [93].

Circadian rhythm disruption is common in advancing PD, and patients often nap frequently during the day, with resulting night-time wakefulness. The advanced sleep phase syndrome in which the patent retires early in the evening is also common in PD. Environmental factors such as noise, frequent awakenings by a bed partner, and nocturia are common causes of insomnia in both the normal and PD populations. Sleep may further be affected in PD because of delayed gastric emptying and potential protein competition for levodopa absorption producing poor mobility. Bradykinesia, rigidity, and other PD symptoms increase nocturnal immobility [96]. Rarely, a low-amplitude tremor occurs in stage 1 or 2 sleep, after arousals, and during sleep stage transitions [92]. These arousals are more likely to delay return to sleep. Choreiform dyskinesias are rarely associated with increased awakenings, but correlate with delay in sleep return.

Parasomnias associated with sleep disorders include confusional arousals, sleep terrors, sleep talking, nocturnal leg cramps, nightmares, REM sleep behavior disorder (RBD), sleep bruxism, and nocturnal paroxysmal dystonia [94]. In RBD there is failure of the normal suppression of EMG activity during REM sleep and an absence of atonia. Affected individuals physically act out their dreams, sometimes causing injury to themselves or their bed-partners. In one study, 50% of PD patients undergoing screening polysomnography were found to have RBD [93]. Another study found a 38% increase in risk of developing PD in patients diagnosed with RBD followed for a mean of 13 years [95]. In a review of 93 consecutive patients with RBD, 49 carried the additional diagnosis of PD, dementia, or multiple system atrophy, and in more than half of PD patients with RBD the sleep behavior disorder occurred prior to onset of other features of parkinsonism [96].

Sleep attacks have been described in PD patients receiving dopamine agonists who fell asleep while driving [97]. Similar case histories for apomorphine, bromocriptine, cabergoline, pergolide, lisuride, and other dopamine agonists have been reported [88]. A retrospective review noted daytime somnolence in 22 of 45 subjects participating in three double-blind, randomized, placebo-controlled pramipexole clinical trials [98] and 21 of 37 subjects reported somnolence in the open-label extension studies, with 14 subjects having EDS. In a follow-up structured interview completed in 12 of these subjects, seven reported feeling drowsy all the time and would fall asleep during periods of inactivity, and three reported discrete episodes of irresistible sleepiness. Sleep apnea, common in multiple system atrophy and other parkinsonism-plus syndromes, has not been shown to be more common in patients with PD than controls.

Treatment of sleep disorders

Physicians should be aware of the frequency of sleep disorders in PD and seek out these problems. History alone may not reveal the magnitude of the problem and more objective evaluation scales such as the Epworth Sleepiness Scale should be employed. In general, PD patients should be encouraged to have good sleep hygiene, sleep disorders should be ruled out as appropriate, and dose reductions, particularly of dopamine agonists, should be considered for patients with sleepiness. Patients should also be counseled against driving if they are tired. REM RBD generally responds to night-time treatment with low doses of clonazepam or melatonin [99] (Box 35.4). Modafinil 200–400 mg per day may be effective in reversing EDS and the sedative effects of anti-PD medications [100]. However, no objective benefit on Multiple Sleep Latency Test, Epworth Sleepiness Scale (ESS), Fatigue Severity Scale, or Hamilton Depression Scale were demonstrated in a double-blind, placebo-controlled study [101]. Nocturnal administration of sodium oxybate improved EDS and fatigue in an open-label polysomnographic study of 38 subjects [102].

Autonomic dysfunction

A wide range of autonomic symptoms, such as orthostatic hypotension, sphincter dysfunction, and sexual impotence occur in PD. Some of these may respond to specific treatments (Box 35.4). A recent comparison 420 patients and 150 controls found that PD patients reported more gastrointestinal and urologic symptoms [103]. Higher age, greater disease severity, and higher doses of dopaminergic medication were related to more autonomic problems. In turn, autonomic symptom severity was associated with motor dysfunction, depressive symptoms, cognitive dysfunction, psychiatric complications, night-time sleep disturbances, and excessive daytime sleepiness ($p \leq 0.01$) [103].

Gastrointestinal disturbances

Nausea and loss of appetite are commonly associated with anti-parkinsonian medications. Most often these begin with the initiation of levodopa, but may occur with any anti-parkinsonian agent. This usually results from stimulation of the area postrema, the emesis center of the brain, which is not protected by the blood–brain barrier [104]. Loss of appetite may occur even without associated nausea. Swallowing difficulties increase with progression of PD, and increase risk for developing aspiration pneumonia. A videofluroscopic study of 71 PD patients found multiple abnormalities in mastication and oral-lingual delivery and normal bolus transport in only two patients [105]. Constipation, associated with prolonged gastrointestinal transit time, is seen in most PD patients, and represents one of the most common complaints among such patients [105]. Paralytic ileus affects 7.1% of PD patients; symptoms include abdominal bloating, pain, nausea, vomiting, and abdominal distension [106]. Anismus, or an inability to relax the external anal sphincter for defecation, is seen in "off" periods [107].

Treatment

Nausea and vomiting associated with dopaminergic drugs frequently disappear over time (tachyphylaxis). Levodopa is routinely administered with a decarboxylase inhibitor, which reduces peripheral dopamine accumulation and dramatically reduces nausea and vomiting. Persistent nausea and vomiting can be treated by giving levodopa with food, increasing the dose of carbidopa in order to block the decarboxylase enzyme more completely, or co-administration of a peripheral dopamine receptor blocker such as domperidone. Only rarely do nausea and vomiting limit the use of dopaminergic agents.

Constipation should be approached prophylactically, ensuring that patients drink sufficient fluids and eat leafy green vegetables and diets rich in bran, with laxatives being used only after ensuring proper diet. Agents that increase gastrointestinal motility such as cisapride have been useful, but have been removed from the market because of cardiac toxicity. Persistent constipation can be treated with psyllium, poly(ethylene glycol), bisacodyl, and magnesium sulfate [108]. Other drugs for constipation include lubiprostone, which locally activates intestinal ClC-2 chloride channels and increases intestinal fluid secretion without altering serum electrolyte levels, and tegaserod maleate, a novel selective serotonin receptor type-4 [5-HT(4)] partial agonist that stimulates upper gastrointestinal motility [109,110]. Another agent, macrogol, an isosomotic electrolyte, has been found to increase significantly the frequency of bowel movements and to improve stool consistency [111]. Prucalopride, a selective, high-affinity 5-hydroxytryptamine 4 receptor agonist, at 4 mg per day increased bowel frequency in about half of patients with severe chronic constipation, but this agent has not been specifically tested in patients with PD [112]. Other strategies used in the management of recalcitrant constipation include neostigmine, symbiotic yogurt-containing components, such as *Bifidobacterium* and fructoligosaccharide, subcutaneous methylnaltrexone in opioid-related constipation, botulinum toxin injections, and sacral nerve stimulation [113].

Urologic dysfunction

Lower urinary tract symptoms in PD range from 38 to 71%, of patients and are attributed to the loss of the dopaminergic inhibitory effect on micturition [114]. Bladder detrusor overactivity causes urgency, frequency, and incontinence. In one study, urge episodes and urge incontinence were observed in 53 and 27% of the patients with PD, respectively, and detrusor overactivity in 46% of the patients with PD, which was less prevalent than in patients with DLB and AD, whereas mean voided volume, free flow, cystometric bladder capacity, and detrusor pressor were similar in the groups [115].

Bladder contraction is mediated through the cholinergic, parasympathetic (muscarinic) pelvic nerve, whereas relaxation results from noradrenergic sympathetic receptors at the hypogastric nerve [115]. Urethral contraction is linked to noradrenergic, sympathetic hypogastric nerve and cholinergic (nicotinic), somatic pudendal nerve activity. Urinary storage depends on autonomic sacral spinal cord segments. The pontine storage center is influenced by the hypothalamus, cerebellum, basal ganglia, and frontal cortex [5]. Micturition is dependent on the spino-bulbo-spinal reflex, involving midbrain periaqueductal gray and the pontine micturition center, which facilitates sacral bladder preganglionics by glutamate, and inhibits the motor nucleus by GABA and glycine. Voiding is initiated by the hypothalamus and prefrontal cortex. Detrussor overactivity is increased by glutamatergic and D2 dopaminergic activity, although the bladder wall contains predominantly D1 receptors. Functional neuroimaging during bladder filling activates the globus pallidus in normal volunteers and in the putamen in patients with PD. Stimulation of the SNpc inhibits micturition, and striatal dopamine increases urinary storage [5].

Increased urinary frequency due to overactive bladder often improves not only with levodopa treatment [116], but also with anti-muscarinic oxybutynin 5 mg three or four times per day, oxybutynin transdermal patch, one patch twice per week, tolterodine 2 mg three times per day, solifenacin 5–10 mg per day, or darifenacin 7.5–15 mg per day [117]. More recently, botulinum toxin injections into the bladder wall have been reported to be beneficial [118,119].

Sexual dysfunction

Sexual dysfunction ranges from 12 to 60% in men with PD [120]. In a review of sexual functioning of 32 women and 43 men with PD, women reported difficulties with arousal (87.5%) and reaching orgasm (75.0%), and sexual dissatisfaction (37.5%) [96]. Men reported erectile dysfunction (68.4%), sexual dissatisfaction (65.1%), premature ejaculation (40.6%), and difficulties reaching orgasm (39.5%). Pre-morbid sexual dysfunction may contribute to cessation of sexual activity during the course of the disease (among 23.3% of men and 21.9% of women). Associated illnesses, use of medications, motor difficulties, depression, anxiety, and advanced stage of PD contributed to sexual dysfunction. Sildenafil citrate has been found to be safe and effective in the treatment of erectile dysfunction associated with PD, but may unmask orthostatic hypotension [121]. This side effect may be prevented with a new formulation of phosphodiesterase type 5 inhibitors, which can be applied topically with a novel delivery system utilizing nanoparticles [122].

Excessive sweating

Excessive sweating appears to be related to plasma levodopa fluctuations with peak dose dyskinesias associated with mild increased sweating, and the more bothersome, drenching sweats being associated with an end-of-dose, "off" period [97]. Skin changes, such as seborrheic dermatitis, occur with increasing oiliness of the skin and a fungal infection, typically located on the forehead, malar, and chin regions of the face [1,7]. The skin may also become erythematous and scaly, and dandruff is common. Treatment of sweating hinges on achieving stable plasma levodopa levels, while the skin rash often responds to treatment with dandruff shampoo [123].

Orthostatic hypotension

Orthostatic hypotension is reported in 10–20% of patients, and increases with age and severity of PD; if unrecognized, it may lead to unnecessary evaluations for dizziness [124]. Symptoms include lightheadedness, initial dizziness when standing, fatigue, and pain across the back of the shoulders and neck. Frequent monitoring with standing and sitting blood pressure measurements are helpful in following this problem, and may often be done by caregivers [36].

Orthostatic hypotension can be treated with salt, fludrocortisone and midodrine [125,126]. DOPS (Droxidopa) (Chelsea Therapeutics) is currently being investigated for the treatment of orthostatic hypotension [127]. Droxidopa (L-*threo*-3,4-dihydroxyphenylserine or L-DOPS) is a synthetic amino acid precursor of norepinephrine that has been marketed in Japan since 1989 for the treatment of orthostatic hypotension.

Sensory disturbances

Visual disturbances

Visual acuity, contrast sensitivity, color discrimination, temporal sensitivity, motion perception, peripheral visual field sensitivity, and visual processing speed have been reported in PD [128,129]. An ophthalmologic study comparing 31 early untreated PD and 31 control subjects found ocular surface irritation, altered tear film, visual hallucinations, blepharospasm, decreased blink rate, and decreased convergence amplitudes to be more common in PD [130]. Electrophysiologic testing suggests that retinal ganglion cell impairment plays a role in the loss of acuity in PD subjects. Indirect evidence for this includes prolonged visual evoked potential latencies and abnormal electroretinographic patterns noted in these subjects [131]. Interestingly, both of these neurophysiologic assessments respond to levodopa [132,133]. Abnormalities of color perception, especially in the blue–green axis, and of visual contrast sensitivity (VCS) are also seen. Finally, a review of 81 patients found that non-motor tasks were affected by visual or visuospatial impairment [134]. Motor disturbances were directly attributed to visual hallucinations, double vision, and estimating spatial relations, and most often produced freezing of gait.

Olfactory dysfunction

Loss of olfactory sense and discrimination is seen in up to 90% of PD patients and increases with disease progression. The olfactory system has been suggested as the original site of Lewy pathology, but this has not been confirmed [4]. There are no known treatments.

Pain and paresthesia

Shoulder pain is recognized as an early, and sometimes initial, symptom of PD [135]. Two recent studies have determined that pain may be much more common in people with PD, and may be subdivided into dystonic or non-dystonic varieties. In a report of 402 PD patients (mean age 67 years, mean disease duration 7.5 years) versus 317 healthy age-matched controls, the rates of non-dystonic pain (arthralgia and neuropathic) were similar, whereas dystonic and cramping pain occurred only in PD subjects [136]. In the PD group, dystonic pain occurred in 7% of patients, with symptoms distributed to the leg or foot (5.5%), neck or shoulder (2.2%), and arm (1%). In addition, more PD patients experienced pain for at least 3 months (69% versus 63%, $p = 0.04$). A review of 450 consecutive PD patients at 25 centers found chronic pain, attributed to PD, to be present in 167 patients (37%) [137]. Patients with pain had younger onset, higher depression, and more motor complications.

Although the mechanism of central or peripheral pain symptoms in PD is unknown, recently some authors have suggested a pain threshold difference in patients in the "on" or "off" states [138]. In the "off" condition, patients with PD had lower heat pain and laser pinprick thresholds, and less habituation than both PD patients without pain and control subjects. In addition, these abnormalities lateralized to the more affected parkinsonian side of the body. Because the abnormalities attenuated with levodopa, there may be dopamine-dependent centers regulating both autonomic function and inhibitory modulation of pain inputs.

Other sensory disorders

Restless legs syndrome (RLS) and PD overlap in some features, including response to dopaminergic drugs, but whether the two disorders are pathogenically linked is controversial [139,140]. Akathisia is an inability to sit still, and unlike RLS, involves the entire body. This symptom is most often associated with dopamine receptor blocking drugs, such as metoclopramide and haloperidol, and is characterized by stereotyped and repetitive crossing of the legs or pacing in place, and inner feelings of restlessness.

Bulbar disorders

Dysarthria

Dysarthria in PD results from a combination of functional disorders, including impaired vocal cord adduction and diminished diaphragmatic excursion, producing hypophonia, breathiness, poor articulation, and loss of speech prosody [141]. Dysarthria also results from poor lingual, labial, and guttural coordination and is present in both dyskinetic and "off" periods. Hypophonia occurs in approximately 70% of PD patients, and results from both rigidity and fatigability of the thyroarytenoid muscles during vocalization. Although the neurologic substrate of hypophonia has not been defined, it is well accepted that lesions within the basal ganglia may adversely affect speech volume, supporting a central cause [142].

Salivary disturbances

Sialorrhea is has been reported in as many as 78% of parkinsonian patients [143]. Although the exact mechanism of sialorrhea remains poorly understood, this symptoms probably result from a combination of excessive saliva production and difficulties in clearing saliva from the mouth, due to infrequent and impaired swallowing. Three major pairs of salivary glands (parotid, submandibular, and sublingual) produce over 90% of the saliva. At rest, the submandibular gland produces most of the saliva, but the parotid gland appears to be more active during eating.

Treatment of bulbar disorders

Drooling (sialorrhea), one of the most embarrassing symptoms of PD, caused by impaired swallowing, has been successfully treated with botulinum toxin injections [144–146]. Speech therapy designed to stimulate increased vocal fold adduction with instructions to "increase loudness," the Lee Silverman Voice Treatment (LSVT) [147], may improve the volume and quality of the speech.

Respiratory disturbances

Respiratory difficulties experienced by patients with PD result from a variety of mechanisms, including a restrictive component due to rigid respiratory muscles and levodopa-induced respiratory dyskinesias [148,149]. Two main types of upper airway obstruction have been described in patients with PD [150]. The first is termed respiratory flutter and is characterized by a pattern of airway obstruction with superimposed rapid oscillations of the supraglottic structures and vocal cords. These rhythmic oscillations are time-locked to the 4–8 Hz resting tremor in PD patients and can be verified by endoscopy or flow-volume loops. The second pattern of upper airway obstruction is characterized by irregular, abrupt changes in the flow-volume loop, at times indicating complete obstruction. Rigidity and hypokinesia of both the upper airway and the chest wall are thought to contribute to this second pattern. Upper airway obstruction is thought to be a direct result of the pathology within the basal ganglia causing irregularities in agonist and antagonist respiratory muscles. When PD patients were compared with healthy controls, those with PD were found to swallow significantly more often during inhalation, at low tidal volumes, and exhibited significantly more post-swallow inhalation [150]. Impaired coordination of breathing and swallowing may contribute to the high frequency of aspiration pneumonia in PD. Sleep apnea, which appears to occur more frequently in patients with PD than controls, has already been discussed in the section on sleep disorders. Treatment of chest wall rigidity and disordered breathing associated with dyskinesias relies individualization of dopaminergic therapy. Sleep apnea is treated with continuous positive airway pressure after proper titration and mask fitting in a sleep laboratory.

Pleuropulmonary fibrosis is induced by ergot-derived dopamine agonists and, because it is not seen with agents such as pramipexole and ropinirole, it is increasingly rare [151]. Clinical symptoms include dyspnea, pleuritic pain, and nonproductive cough, with pulmonary infiltrates and pleural effusions present on chest radiograph. The sedimentation rate may be elevated and the pleural fluid may show inflammatory cells with a predominance of eosinophils. The inflammatory response may reflect serotonergic activation from the ergotaminergic mechanisms.

Orthopedic problems

Joint and axial deformities in PD are common and may manifest as "striatal" hand and foot deformities, kyphoscoliosis, bent spine or dropped head syndrome, Pisa syndrome (a marked leaning to the right or left side), and camptocormia (marked truncal flexion) [152–154]. Camptocormia in PD is defined by marked anteroflexion of the trunk that improves in the recumbent position or when a patient is asked to stand straight by pushing up from a tabletop or bench. Neither condition responds to levodopa. Although thought primarily an action dystonia of the spine producing an active change in posture, some have suggested it may be a myopathic disorder, and is associated with weakness [155]. There are no known treatments for these axial changes in posture.

Conclusion

Non-motor symptoms in PD are increasingly recognized as a significant cause of disability, and may involve almost any aspect of the nervous system. Autonomic nervous system dysfunction includes gastrointestinal disturbances, urogenital dysfunction, orthostatic hypotension, and thermoregulatory difficulties. Peripheral nervous system involvement is seen with changes in olfactory, vision, and sensory decline. Higher cortical dysfunction results in symptoms of cortical or subcortical dementia, while basal ganglia disturbances may result in impulsive or compulsive behaviors. Brainstem involvement may result in fatigue, bulbar, respiratory, and sleep dysfunction. Symptoms attributed to non-nervous system dysfunction include nausea, postural changes, and dermatitis.

Although many of these symptoms do not respond to therapy, some may improve with a reduction of antiparkinsonian medications. These include panic attacks, excessive sweating, impulse control disorders, orthostatic hypotension, and nausea. In addition, anismus and bladder urgency and hesitancy may respond to dopaminergic therapy. Other symptoms, such as dementia, orthostatic hypotension, urinary frequency, and erectile dysfunction, respond to non-dopaminergic interventions.

An increasing number of reports draw attention to the importance of non-motor symptoms and their impact on quality of life [156,157]. The American Academy of Neurology Quality Measurement and Reporting Subcommittee proposed 10 quality measures for PD, largely focusing on non-motor symptoms, such as an annual PD review, assessments of psychiatric and cognitive impairment, querying about autonomic dysfunction, sleep disturbances, falls, and medication-related motor complications, discussing rehabilitative and surgical options, and counseling regarding safety issues [158].

References

1. Jankovic J. Parkinson's disease: clinical features and diagnosis. *J Neurol Neurosurg Psychiatry* 2008;**79**:368–76.
2. Brodsky H, Dat Vuong K, Thomas M, Jankovic J. Glabellar and palmomental reflexes in parkinsonian disorders. *Neurology* 2004;**63**:1096–8.
3. Wu LJC, Sitburana O, Davidson A, Jankovic J. Applause sign in parkinsonian disorders and Huntington's disease. *Mov Disord* 2008;**23**(16):2307–11.
4. Biousse V, Skibell BC, Watts RL, *et al.* Ophthalmologic features of Parkinson's disease. *Neurology* 2004;**62**:177–80.
5. Sakakibara R, Uchiyama T, Yamanishi T, *et al.* Bladder and bowel dysfunction in Parkinson's disease. *J Neural Transm* 2008;**115**:443–60.
6. Tinazzi M, Del Vesco C, Fincati E, *et al.* Pain and motor complications in Parkinson's disease. *J Neurol Neurosurg Psychiatry* 2006;**77**:822–5.
7. Borek LL, Amick MM, Friedman JH, Non-motor aspects of Parkinson's disease. *CNS Spectr* 2006;**11**:541–54.
8. Aarsland D, Tandberg E, Largsen JP, Cummings JL. Frequency of dementia in Parkinson disease. *Arch Neurol* 1996;**53**:538–42.
9. Biggins CA, Boyd JL, Harrop FA, *et al.* A controlled, longitudinal study of dementia in Parkinson's disease. *J Neurol Neurosurg Psychiatry* 1992;**55**:566–72.
10. Buter TC, van den Hout A, Matthews FE, *et al.* Dementia and survival in Parkinson disease: a 12-year population study. *Neurology* 2008;**70**:1017–22.

11. Riedel O, Klotsche J, Spottke A, *et al.* Cognitive impairment in 873 patients with idiopathic Parkinson's disease. Results from the German Study on Epidemiology of Parkinson's Disease with Dementia (GEPAD). *J Neurol* 2008;**255**:255–64.
12. Hely MA, Reid WGJ, Adena MA, *et al.* The Sydney multicenter study of Parkinson's disease: the inevitability of dementia at 20 years. *Mov Disord* 2008;**23**:837–44.
13. Dubois B, Burn D, Goetz C, *et al.* Diagnostic procedures for Parkinson's disease dementia: recommendations from the Movement Disorder Society Task Force. *Mov Disord* 2007;**22**:2314–24.
14. Tröster AI. Neuropsychological characteristics of dementia with Lewy bodies and Parkinson's disease with dementia: differentiation, early detection, and implications for "mild cognitive impairment" and biomarkers. *Neuropsychol Rev* 2008;**18**:103–19.
15. Halliday G, Hely M, Reid W, Morris J. The progression of pathology in longitudinally followed patients with Parkinson's disease *Acta Neuropathol* 2008;**115**:409–15.
16. Hilker R, Thomas AV, Klein JC, *et al.* Dementia in Parkinson disease: functional imaging of cholinergic and dopaminergic pathways. *Neurology* 2005;**65**:1716–22.
17. Emre M, Aarsland D, Albanese A, *et al.* Rivastigmine for dementia associated with Parkinson's disease. *N Engl J Med* 2004;**351**:2509–18.
18. Stacy M. Recognizing and treating nonmotor symptoms in Parkinson's disease. *CNS Spectr* 1998;**3**:415.
19. Aarsland D, Laake K, Larsen JP, Janvin C. Donepezil for cognitive impairment in Parkinson's disease: a randomized controlled study. *J Neurol Neurosurg Psychiatry* 2002;**72**: 708–12.
20. Leroi I, Brandt J, Reich SG, *et al.* Randomized placebo-controlled trial of donepezil in cognitive impairment in Parkinson's disease. *Int J Geriatr Psychiatry* 2004;**19**:1–8.
21. Ravina B, Putt M, Siderowf A, *et al.* Donepezil for dementia in Parkinson's disease: a randomised, double blind, placebo controlled, crossover study. *J Neurol Neurosurg Psychiatry* 2005;**76**:934–9.
22. Poewe W, Wolters E, Emre M, *et al.*; EXPRESS Investigators. Long-term benefits of rivastigmine in dementia associated with Parkinson's disease: an active treatment extension study. *Mov Disord* 2006;**21**:456–61.
23. Wesnes KA, McKeith I, Edgar C, *et al.* Benefits of rivastigmine on attention in dementia associated with Parkinson disease. *Neurology* 2005;**65**:1654–6.
24. Gurevich TY, Shabtai H, Korczyn AD, *et al.* Effect of rivastigmine on tremor in patients with Parkinson's disease and dementia. *Mov Disord* 2006;**21**:1663–6.
25. Wilkinson DG, Passmore AP, Bullock R, *et al.* A multinational, randomised, 12-week, comparative study of donepezil and rivastigmine in patients with mild to moderate Alzheimer's disease. *Int J Clin Pract* 2002;**56**:441–6.
26. Seeman P, Caruso C, Lasaga M. Memantine agonist action at dopamine D2High receptors. *Synapse* 2008;**62**(2):149–53.
27. Miyasaki JM, Shannon K, Voon V, *et al.*; Quality Standards Subcommittee of the American Academy of Neurology Practice Parameter: evaluation and treatment of depression, psychosis, and dementia in Parkinson disease (an evidence-based review): report of the Quality Standards Subcommittee of the American Academy of Neurology *Neurology* 2006;**66**:996–1002.
28. Goetz CG, Stebbins GT. Risk factors for nursing home placement in advanced Parkinson's disease. *Neurology* 1993;**43**: 2227–9.
29. Goetz CG, Stebbins GT. Mortality and hallucinations in nursing home patients with advanced Parkinson's disease. *Neurology* 1995;**45**:669–71.
30. Ravina B, Marder K, Fernandez H, *et al.* Diagnostic criteria for psychosis in Parkinson's disease: report of an NINDS/NIMH Work Group. *Mov Disord* 2007;**22**:1061–8.
31. Goetz CG, Vogel C, Tanner CM, Stebbins GT. Early dopaminergic drug-induced hallucinations in parkinsonian patients. *Neurology* 1998;**51**:811–4.
32. Marras C, Kopp A, Qiu F, *et al.* Antipsychotic use in older adults with Parkinson's disease. *Mov Disord* 2007;**22**:319–23.
33. Fénelon G, Goetz CG, Karenberg A. Hallucinations in Parkinson disease in the pre-levodopa era. *Neurology* 2006;**66**: 93–8.
34. Fénelon G. Psychosis in Parkinson's disease: phenomenology, frequency, risk factors, and current understanding of pathophysiologic mechanisms. *CNS Spectr* 2008;**13**(3 Suppl 4):18–25.
35. Goetz CG, Pappert EJ, Blasucci LM, *et al.* Intravenous levodopa infusions in hallucinating Parkinson's disease patients: high-dose challenge does not precipitate hallucinations. *Neurology* 1998;**50**:515–7.
36. Stacy M. Managing late complications of Parkinson's disease. *Med Clin North Am* 1999;**83**:469–81.
37. Frieling H, Hillemacher T, Ziegenbein M, *et al.* Treating dopamimetic psychosis in Parkinson's disease: structured review and meta-analysis. *Eur Neuropsychopharmacol* 2007;**17**:165–71.
38. Rabey JM, Prokhorov T, Miniovitz A, *et al.* Effect of quetiapine in psychotic Parkinson's disease patients: a double-blind labeled study of 3 months' duration. *Mov Disord* 2007;**22**:313–8.
39. Merims D, Balas M, Peretz C, *et al.* Rater-blinded, prospective comparison: quetiapine versus clozapine for Parkinson's disease psychosis. *Clin Neuropharmacol* 2006;**29**:331–7.
40. Kurlan R, Cummings J, Raman R, Thal L; Alzheimer's Disease Cooperative Study Group. Quetiapine for agitation or psychosis in patients with dementia and parkinsonism. *Neurology* 2007;**68**(17):1356–63.
41. Klein C, Prokhorov T, Miniovich A, *et al.* Long-term follow-up (24 months) of quetiapine treatment in drug-induced Parkinson disease psychosis. *Clin Neuropharmacol* 2006;**29**(4):215–9.
42. Friedman JH, Berman RM, Goetz CG, F, *et al.* Open-label flexible-dose pilot study to evaluate the safety and tolerability of aripiprazole in patients with psychosis associated with Parkinson's disease. *Mov Disord* 2006;**21**:2078–81.
43. Ravina B, Camicioli R, Como PG, *et al.* The impact of depressive symptoms in early Parkinson's disease. *Neurology* 2007;**69**:342–7.
44. Aarsland D, Bronnick K, Ehrt U, *et al.* Neuropsychiatric symptoms in patients with Parkinson's disease and dementia: frequency, profile and associated care giver stress. *J Neurol Neurosurg Psychiatry* 2007;**78**:36–42.

45. Reijnders JSAM, Ehrt U, Weber WEJ, *et al.* A systematic review of prevalence studies of depression in Parkinson's disease. *Mov Disord* 2008;**23**:183–9.
46. Brandt-Christensen M, Kvist K, Nilsson FM, *et al.* Treatment with antiparkinson and antidepressant drugs: a register-based, pharmaco-epidemiological study. *Mov Disord* 2007;**22**: 2037–42.
47. Antonini A, Colosimo C, Marconi R, *et al.*; PRIAMO study group. The PRIAMO study: background, methods and recruitment. *Neurol Sci* 2008;**29**(2):61–5.
48. Dell'Angnello G, Ceravalo R, Nuti A, *et al.* SSRIs do not worsen Parkinson's disease: evidence from an open-label, prospective study. *Clin Neuropharmacol* 2001;**24**:221–7.
49. Kulisevsky J, Pagonabarraga J, Pascual-Sedano B, *et al.* Motor changes during sertraline treatment in depressed patients with Parkinson's disease. *Eur J Neurol* 2008;**15**:953–9.
50. Okun MS, Walter BL, McDonald WM, *et al.* Beneficial effects of testosterone replacement for the nonmotor symptoms of Parkinson disease. *Arch Neurol* 2002;**59**:1750–3.
51. Okun MS, Fernandez HH, Rodriguez RL, *et al.* Testosterone therapy in men with Parkinson disease: results of the TEST-PD Study. *Arch Neurol* 2006;**63**:729–35.
52. Press DZ, Mechanic DJ, Tarsy D, Manoach DS. Cognitive slowing in Parkinson's disease resolves after practice. *J Neurol Neurosurg Psychiatry* 2002;**73**:524–8.
53. Pacchetti C, Mancini F, Aglieri R, *et al.* Active music therapy in Parkinson's disease: an integrative method for motor and emotional rehabilitation. *Psychosom Med* 2000;**62**: 386–93.
54. Stacy M, Bowron A, Guttman M, *et al.* Identification of motor and non-motor wearing-off in Parkinson's disease: comparison of a patient questionnaire versus a clinician assessment. *Mov Disord* 2005;**20**:726–33.
55. Stacy M, Hauser R; Wearing Off Study Group. Development of a Wearing-Off Patient Questionnaire to facilitate recognition of the motor and non-motor symptoms of wearing-off in Parkinson's disease. *J Neural Transm* 2007;**114**:211–7.
56. Leentjens AF, Koester J, Fruh B, *et al.* The effect of pramipexole on mood and motivational symptoms in Parkinson's disease: a meta-analysis of placebo-controlled studies. *Clin Ther* 2009;**31**(1):89–98.
57. Menza M, Dobkin RD, Marin H, *et al.* A controlled trial of antidepressants in patients with Parkinson disease and depression. *Neurology* 2009;**72**(10):886–92.
58. Ferrara JM, Stacy M. Impulse control disorders and Parkinson's disease. *CNS Spectr* 2008;**13**:690–8.
59. Mamikonyan E, Siderowf AD, Duda JE, *et al.* Long-term follow-up of impulse control disorders in Parkinson's disease. *Mov Disord* 2008;**23**:75–80.
60. Stamey W, Jankovic J. Impulse control disorders and pathological gambling in patients with Parkinson disease. *Neurologist* 2008;**14**:89–99.
61. Kurlan R. Disabling repetitive behaviors in Parkinson's disease. *Mov Disord* 2004;**19**:433–7.
62. Evans AH, Katzenschlager R, Paviour D, *et al.* Punding in Parkinson's disease: its relation to the dopamine dysregulation syndrome, *Mov Disord* 2004;**19**:397–405.
63. Silveira-Moriyama L, Evans AH, Katzenschlager R, Lees AJ. Punding and dyskinesias. *Mov Disord* 2006;**21**:2214–7.
64. Friedman JH. Punding on levodopa. *Biol Psychiatry* 1994; **36**(5):350–1.
65. Weintraub D, Siderowf AD, Potenza MN, *et al.* Association of dopamine agonist use with impulse control disorders in Parkinson disease. *Arch Neurol* 2006;**63**(7):969–73.
66. Wingo TS, Evatt M, Scott B, *et al.* Impulse control disorders arising in three patients treated with rotigotine. *Clin Neuropharmacol* 2009;**32**(2):59–62.
67. Driver-Dunckley E, Samanta J, Stacy M. Pathological gambling associated with dopamine agonist therapy in Parkinson's disease. *Neurology* 2003;**61**:422–3.
68. Dodd ML, Klos KJ, Bower JH, *et al.* Pathological gambling caused by drugs used to treat Parkinson disease. *Arch Neurol* 2005;**62**(9):1377–81.
69. Thomas A, Bonnani L, Gambi F, *et al.* Pathological gambling in Parkinson's disease is reduced by amantadine. *Ann Neurol* 2010;**68**:400–4.
70. Weintraub D, Sohr M, Potenza MN, *et al.* Amantadine use associated with impulse control disorders in Parkinson disease in cross-sectional study. *Ann Neurol* 2010;**68**:963–8.
71. Galpern WR, Stacy M. Management of impulse control disorders in Parkinson's disease. *Curr Treat Options Neurol* 2007;**9**:189–97.
72. Ivanco LS, Bohnen NI. Effects of donepezil on compulsive hypersexual behavior in Parkinson disease: a single case study. *Am J Ther* 2005;**12**:467–8.
73. De Witte P, Littleton J, Parot P, Koob G. Neuroprotective and abstinence-promoting effects of acamprosate: elucidating the mechanism of action. *CNS Drugs* 2005;**19**:517–37.
74. Cowen MS, Adams C, Kraehenbuehl T, *et al.* The acute anticraving effect of acamprosate in alcohol-preferring rats is associated with modulation of the mesolimbic dopamine system. *Addict Biol.* 2005;**10**:233–42.
75. Fernandez HH, Durso R. Clozapine for dopaminergic-induced paraphilias in Parkinson's disease. *Mov Disord* 1998;**13**(3):597–8.
76. Ardouin C, Voon V, Worbe Y, *et al.* Pathological gambling in Parkinson's disease improves on chronic subthalamic nucleus stimulation. *Mov Disord* 2006;**21**(11):1941–6.
77. Uitti RJ, Tanner CM, Rajput AH, *et al.* Hypersexuality with antiparkinsonian therapy. *Clin Neuropharmacol* 1989;**12**(5): 375–83.
78. Klos KJ, Bower JH, Josephs KA, *et al.* Pathological hypersexuality predominantly linked to adjuvant dopamine agonist therapy in Parkinson's disease and multiple system atrophy. *Parkinsonism Relat Disord* 2005;**11**(6):381–6.
79. Nirenberg MJ, Waters C. Compulsive eating and weight gain related to dopamine agonist use. *Mov Disord* 2006;**21**(4):524–9.
80. Klos KJ, Bower JH, Josephs KA, *et al.* Pathological hypersexuality predominantly linked to adjuvant dopamine agonist therapy in Parkinson's disease and multiple system atrophy. *Parkinsonism Relat Disord* 2005;**11**(6):381–6.
81. Seedat S, Kesler S, Niehaus DJ, Stein DJ. Pathological gambling behaviour: emergence secondary to treatment of Parkinson's disease with dopaminergic agents. *Depress Anxiety* 2000;**11**(4):185–6.
82. Voon V, Hassan K, Zurowski M, *et al.* Prevalence of repetitive and reward-seeking behaviors in Parkinson disease. *Neurology* 2006;**67**(7):1254–7.

83. Avanzi M, Uber E, Bonfa F. Pathological gambling in two patients on dopamine replacement therapy for Parkinson's disease. *Neurol Sci* 2004;**25**(2):98–101.
84. Witjas T, Baunez C, Henry JM, *et al.* Addiction in Parkinson's disease: impact of subthalamic nucleus deep brain stimulation. *Mov Disord* 2005;**20**(8):1052–5.
85. Bandini F, Primavera A, Pizzorno M, Cocito L. Using STN DBS and medication reduction as a strategy to treat pathological gambling in Parkinson's disease. *Parkinsonism Relat Disord* 2007;**13**:369–71.
86. Ardouin C, Voon V, Worbe Y, *et al.* Pathological gambling in Parkinson's disease improves on chronic subthalamic nucleus stimulation. *Mov Disord* 2006;**21**(11):1941–6.
87. Klos KJ, Bower JH, Josephs KA, *et al.* Pathological hypersexuality predominantly linked to adjuvant dopamine agonist therapy in Parkinson's disease and multiple system atrophy. *Parkinsonism Relat Disord* 2005;**11**(6):381–6.
88. Stacy, M. Sleep disorders in Parkinson's disease: epidemiology and management. *Drugs Aging* 2002;**19**:733–9.
89. Van Hilten B, Hoff JI, Huub AM. Sleep disruption in Parkinson's disease. *Arch Neurol* 1995;**51**:922–8.
90. Nausieda PA, Weiner WJ, Kaplan LR, *et al.* Sleep disruption in the course of chronic levodopa therapy: an early feature of the levodopa psychosis. *Clin Neuropharmacol* 1982;**5**: 183–94.
91. Verban D, van Rooden SM, Visser M, *et al.* Nighttime sleep problems and daytime sleepiness in Parkinson's disease. *Mov Disord* 2008;**23** 35–41.
92. Tandberg E, Larsen JP, Karlsen K. Excessive daytime sleepiness and sleep benefit in Parkinson's disease: a community-based study. *Mov Dis* 1999;**14**:922–7.
93. Comella CL, Tanner CM, Ristanovic RL. Polysomnographic sleep measures in Parkinson's disease patients with treatment induced hallucinations. *Ann Neurol* 1993;**34**:710–4.
94. Currie LJ, Bennett JP, Harrison MB, *et al.* Clinical correlates of sleep benefit in Parkinson's disease. *Neurology* 1997;**47**:1115–7.
95. Schenck CH, Bundlie SR, Mahowald MW. Delayed emergence of a Parkinsonian disorder in 38% of 29 older men initially diagnosed with idiopathic rapid eye movement sleep behavior disorder. *Neurology* 1996;**46**:388–93.
96. Olson EJ, Boeve BF, Silber MH. Rapid eye movement sleep behavior disorder: demographic, clinical and laboratory findings in 93 cases. *Brain* 2000;**123**:331–9.
97. Frucht S, Rogers JD, Greene PE, *et al.* Falling asleep at the wheel: motor vehicle mishaps in persons taking pramipexole and ropinirole. *Neurology* 1999;**52**:1908–10.
98. Hauser RA, Gauger L, Anderson WM, Zesiewicz TA. Pramipexole induced somnolence and sleep episodes of daytime sleep. *Mov Disord* 2000;**15**:658–63.
99. Gagnon JF, Postuma RB, Montplaisir J. Update on the pharmacology of REM sleep behavior disorder. *Neurology* 2006;**67**:742–7.
100. Adler CH, Caviness JN, Hentz JG, *et al.* Randomized trial of modafinil for treating subjective daytime sleepiness in patients with Parkinson's disease. *Mov Disord* 2003;**18**:287–93.
101. Ondo WG, Fayle R, Atassi F, Jankovic J. Modafinil for daytime somnolence in Parkinson's disease: double blind, placebo controlled parallel trial. *J Neurol Neurosurg Psychiatry* 2005;**76**:1636–9.
102. Ondo WG, Perkins T, Swick T, *et al.* Sodium oxybate for excessive daytime sleepiness in Parkinson disease: an open-label polysomnographic study. *Arch Neurol* 2008;**65**: 1337–40.
103. Verbaan D, Marinus J, Visser M, *et al.* Patient-reported autonomic symptoms in Parkinson disease. *Neurology* 2007;**69**:333–41.
104. Edwards LL, Quigley EMM, Hofman R, *et al.* Gastrointestinal symptoms in Parkinson's disease: an 18-month follow-up study. *Mov Disord* 1993;**8**:83–6.
105. Cersosimo MG, Benarroch EE. Neural control of the gastrointestinal tract: implications for Parkinson disease. *Mov Disord* 2008;**23**:1065–75.
106. Wullner U, Schmitz-Hubsch T, Antony G, *et al.*, on behalf of the KNP. Autonomic dysfunction in 3414 Parkinson's disease patients enrolled in the German Network on Parkinson's disease: the effect of aging. *Eur J Neurol* 2007;**14**:1405–8.
107. Mathers SE, Kempster PA, Law PJ, *et al.* Anal sphincter dysfunction in Parkinson's disease. *Arch Neurol* 1989;**46**:1061–4.
108. Eichhorn TE, Oertel WH. Macrogol 3350/electrolyte improves constipation in Parkinson's disease and multiple system atrophy. *Mov Disord* 2001;**16**:1176–7.
109. Degen L, Petrig C, Studer D, *et al.* Effect of tegaserod on gut transit in male and female subjects. *Neurogastroenterol Motil* 2005;**17**:821–6.
110. Sullivan KL, Staffetti JF, Hauser RA, *et al.* Tegaserod (Zelnorm) for the treatment of constipation in Parkinson's disease. *Mov Disord* 2006;**21**:115–6.
111. Zangaglia R, Martignoni E, Glorioso M, *et al.* Macrogol for the treatment of constipation in Parkinson's disease. A randomized placebo-controlled study. *Mov Disord* 2007;**22**:1239–44.
112. Camilleri M, Kerstens R, Rykx A, Vandeplassche L. A placebo-controlled trial of prucalopride for severe chronic constipation. *N Engl J Med* 2008;**358**(22):2344–54.
113. Kapoor S. Management of constipation in the elderly: emerging therapeutic strategies. *World J Gastroenterol* 2008;**14**(33): 5226–7.
114. Fitzmaurice H, Fowler CJ, Rickards D, *et al.* Micturition disturbance in Parkinson's disease. *Br J Urol* 1985;**57**:652–6.
115. Ransmayr GN, Holliger S, Schletterer K, *et al.* Lower urinary tract symptoms in dementia with Lewy bodies, Parkinson's disease and Alzheimer disease. *Neurology* 2008;**70**;299–303.
116. Brusa L, Petta F, Pisani A, *et al.* Acute vs chronic effects of *l*-dopa on bladder function in patients with mild Parkinson disease. *Neurology* 2007;**68**:1455–9.
117. Brunton S, Kuritzky L. Recent developments in the management of overactive bladder: focus on the efficacy and tolerability of once daily solifenacin succinate 5 mg. *Curr Med Res Opin* 2005;**21**:71–80.
118. Ouslander JG. Management of overactive bladder. *N Engl J Med* 2004;**350**:786–99.
119. Sahai A, Khan MS, Arya M, *et al.* The overactive bladder: review of current pharmacotherapy in adults. Part 2: treatment options in cases refractory to anticholinergics. *Expert Opin Pharmacother* 2006;**7**:529–38.
120. Bronner G, Royter V, Korczyn AD, Giladi N. Sexual dysfunction in Parkinson's disease. *J Sex Marital Ther* 2004;**30**:95–105.
121. Hussain IF, Brady CM, Swinn MJ, *et al.* Treatment of erectile dysfunction with sildenafil citrate (Viagra) in parkinsonism

due to Parkinson's disease or multiple system atrophy with observations on orthostatic hypotension. *J Neurol Neurosurg Psychiatry* 2001;**71**:371–4.

122. Han G, Tar M, Dwaraka S. *et al.* Nanoparticles as a novel delivery vehicle for therapeutics targeting erectile dysfunction. *J Sexual Med* 2010;**7**(1 Pt 1):224–33.
123. Pursiainen V, Haapaniemi TH, Korpelainen JT, *et al.* Sweating in Parkinsonian patients with wearing-off. *Mov Disord* 2007;**22**:828–32.
124. Hillen ME, Wagner ML, Sage JI. "Subclinical" orthostatic hypotension is associated with dizziness in elderly patients with Parkinson's disease. *Arch Phys Med Rehab* 1996;**77**:710–2.
125. Jankovic J, Gilden JL, Hiner BC, *et al.* Neurogenic orthostatic hypotension: a double-blind placebo-controlled study with midodrine. *Am J Med* 1993;**95**:38–48.
126. Low PA, Gilden JL, Freeman R, *et al.* Efficacy of midodrine vs placebo in neurogenic orthostatic hypotension. A randomized, double-blind multicenter study. *JAMA* 1997;**277**: 1046–51.
127. Mostile G, Jankovic J. Treatment of dysautonomia associated with Parkinson's disease. *Parkinsonism Relat Disord* 2009;**15**(Suppl 3):S224–32.
128. Uc EY, Rizzo M, Anderson SW, *et al.* Visual dysfunction in Parkinson disease without dementia. *Neurology* 2005;**65**: 1907–13.
129. Diederich NJ, Raman R, Leurgans S, Goetz CG. Progressive worsening of spatial and chromatic processing deficits in Parkinson's disease. *Arch Neurol* 2002;**59**:1249–52.
130. Biousse V, Skibell BC, Watts RL, *et al.* Ophthalmologic features of Parkinson's disease. *Neurology* 2004;**62**:177–80.
131. Sartucci F, Orlandi G, Lucetti C, *et al.* Changes in pattern electroretinograms to equiluminant red–green and blue–yellow gratings in patients with early Parkinson's disease. *J Clin Neurophysiol* 2003;**20**:375–81.
132. Rascol O, Clanet M, Montastruc JL, *et al.* Abnormal ocular movements in Parkinson's disease: evidence for involvement of dopaminergic systems. *Brain* 1989;**112**:1193–214.
133. Hood AJ, Amador SC, Cain AE, *et al.* Levodopa slows prosaccades and improves antisaccades: an eye movement study in Parkinson's disease. *J Neurol Neurosurg Psychiatry* 2007;**78**:565–70.
134. Davidsdottir S, Cronin-Golomb A, Lee A. Visual and spatial symptoms in Parkinson's disease. *Vision Res* 2005;**45**:1285–96.
135. Stamey W, Davidson A, Jankovic J. Shoulder pain: a presenting symptom of Parkinson disease. *J Clin Rheumatol* 2008;**14**:253–4.
136. Defazio G, Berardelli A, Fabbrini G, *et al.* Pain as a nonmotor symptom of Parkinson disease: evidence from a case–control study. *Arch Neurol* 2008;**65**:1191–4.
137. Nègre-Pagès L, Regragui W, Bouhassira D, *et al.*; DoPaMiP Study Group. Chronic pain in Parkinson's disease: the cross-sectional French DoPaMiP survey. *Mov Disord* 2008;**23**:1361–9.
138. Schestatsky P, Kumru H, Valls-Solé J, *et al.* Neurophysiologic study of central pain in patients with Parkinson disease. *Neurology* 2007;**69**:2162–9.
139. Ondo WG, Vuong DK, Jankovic J. Exploring the relationship between Parkinson's disease and restless legs syndrome. *Arch Neurol* 2002;**59**:421–4.
140. Gomez-Esteban JC, Zarranz JJ, Tijero B, *et al.* Restless legs syndrome in Parkinson's disease. *Mov Disord* 2007;**22**:1912–6.
141. Skodda S, Schlegel U. Speech rate and rhythm in Parkinson's disease. *Mov Disord* 2008;**23**:985–92.
142. Shill HA, Stacy M. Respiratory complications of Parkinson's disease. *Semin Respir Crit Care Med* 2002;**23**:261–6.
143. Chou KL, Evatt M, Hinson V, Kompoliti K. Sialorrhea in Parkinson's disease: a review. *Mov Disord* 2007;**22**:2306–13.
144. Sheffield JK, Jankovic J. Botulinum toxin in the treatment of tremors, dystonias, sialorrhea and other symptoms associated with Parkinson's disease. *Expert Rev Neurother* 2007;**7**:637–47.
145. Jankovic J. Disease-oriented approach to botulinum toxin use. *Toxicon* 2009;**54**:614–23.
146. Capaccio P, Torretta S, Osio M, *et al.* Botulinum toxin therapy: a tempting tool in the management of salivary secretory disorders. *Am J Otolaryngol* 2008;**29**:333–8.
147. Sharkawi AE, Logemann JA, Pauloski BR, *et al.* Swallowing and voice effects of Lee Silverman Voice Treatment (LSVT): a pilot study. *J Neurol Neurosurg Psychiatry* 2002;**72**:31–6.
148. Rice JE, Antic R, Thompson PD. Disordered respiration as a levodopa-induced dyskinesia in Parkinson's disease. *Mov Disord* 2002;**17**:524–7.
149. Mehanna R, Jankovic J. Respiratory problems in neurologic movement disorders. *Parkinsonism Relat Disord* 2010;**16**: 628–38.
150. Gross RD, Atwood CW Jr, Ross SB, *et al.* The coordination of breathing and swallowing in Parkinson's disease. *Dysphagia* 2008;**23**:136–45.
151. Tintner R, Manian P, Gauthier P, Jankovic J. Pleuropulmonary fibrosis after long-term treatment with the dopamine agonist pergolide for Parkinson disease. *Arch Neurol* 2005;**62**: 1290–5.
152. Ashour R, Tintner R, Jankovic J. "Striatal" hand and foot deformities in Parkinson's disease. *Lancet Neurol* 2005;**4**: 423–31.
153. Ashour R, Jankovic J. Joint and skeletal deformities in Parkinson's sisease, multiple system atrophy, and progressive supranuclear palsy. *Mov Disord* 2006;**21**:1856–63.
154. Azher SN, Jankovic J. Camptocormia: pathogenesis, classification, and response to therapy. *Neurology* 2005;**65**: 353–9.
155. Djaldetti R, Melamed E. Camptocormia in Parkinson's disease: new insights. *J Neurol Neurosurg Psychiatry* 2006;**77**: 1205.
156. Politis M, Wu K, Molloy S, *et al.* Parkinson's disease symptoms: the patient's perspective. *Mov Disord* 2010;**25**: 1646–51.
157. Gallagher DA, Lees AJ, Schrag A. What are the most important nonmotor symptoms in patients with Parkinson's disease and are we missing them? *Mov Disord* 2010;**25**: 2493–500.
158. Cheng EM, Tonn S, Swain-Eng R, *et al.* American Academy of Neurology Parkinson Disease Measure Development Panel. Quality improvement in neurology: AAN Parkinson disease quality measures: report of the Quality Measurement and Reporting Subcommittee of the American Academy of Neurology. *Neurology* 2010;**75**:2021–7.

Chapter 36
Surgery for Non-Dopaminergic and Non-Motor Features of Parkinson's Disease

Brian J. Snyder[1] *& Andres M. Lozano*[2]
[1]Division of Neurosurgery, Toronto Western Hospital, University of Toronto, Toronto, ON, Canada
[2]Division of Neurosurgery, University of Toronto and Toronto Western Research Institute, Toronto, ON, Canada

Introduction

With over 80 000 patients treated to date, deep brain stimulation (DBS) has become a mainstay for the treatment of patients with advanced Parkinson's disease (PD). Similarly to levodopa, DBS surgery is highly effective for the treatment of some aspects of PD, but ineffective for the management of others. Motor signs including tremor, rigidity, and akinesia are improved significantly with stimulation or lesions of either the globus pallidus pars internus (GPi) or the subthalamic nucleus (STN). Further, surgical stimulation or ablation of STN or GPi produces striking improvements in the motor complications induced by levodopa treatment, including motor fluctuations and dyskinesias. Despite these significant advances, however, it is very apparent that with disease progression and involvement of non-dopaminergic and non-motor systems, patients develop increasing disability that cannot be adequately controlled with available therapies. These disturbances in the non-motor and non-dopaminergic systems occur with increasing frequency and severity as the disease progresses. In fact, for a large number of patients, these non-motor and non-dopaminergic problems lead to greater disability than the classic motor features which are typically well controlled with dopaminergic medications [1]. Although certain non-motor components may be alleviated to a limited extent with dopaminergic therapy, the majority are not adequately managed with either current medical therapy or conventional surgical approaches [2]. These therapeutic shortcomings are responsible for ongoing disability and reduced quality-of-life [3].

This chapter focuses on the effects of current DBS-based neurosurgical interventions on certain non-motor and non-dopaminergic features of PD, including psychiatric conditions such as depression, cognitive dysfunction, and sensory dysfunction (pain and paresthesias). We also briefly evaluate emerging surgical treatments that are more specifically directed at these problems [3].

Challenges in the non-motor and non-dopaminergic aspects of PD

There are a number of limitations that must be considered in a discussion of neurosurgery as a possible therapy for the non-motor and non-dopaminergic features of PD. These include the issue of how to ascertain these impairments and the availability and implementation of appropriate scales to assess their severity and the impact of a surgical intervention. Much discussion in the literature outlines the benefits of pallidotomy and subsequently DBS of the GPi and STN for the treatment of motor dysfunction. Less well studied are the effects of DBS on non-motor and non-dopaminergic dysfunction in PD. The commonly used outcome instruments in surgical trials such as the Unified Parkinson's Disease Rating Scale (UPDRS) are predominantly weighted towards motor dysfunction. Interventions that have effects on non-motor systems may not be identified because their impact in these instruments is dwarfed by the weighted contribution of the motor components to the overall score.

Psychiatric symptoms

Depression

The prevalence rates of depression in PD patients range widely, from 2.7% to greater than 90%, depending on the source being consulted. A recent review of the literature calculated the prevalence of the disease to be approximately 17% [4].

STN-DBS has been reported to improve depression in some instances, but it has more frequently been described as having a negative impact on mood, depression, anxiety,

Parkinson's Disease: Non-Motor and Non-Dopaminergic Features, First Edition. Edited by C. Warren Olanow, Fabrizio Stocchi, and Anthony E. Lang.

and mania [5,6]. Transient or chronic depression has been observed in as many as 25% of patients following STN-DBS and yet others have reported small but significant improvements in depression associated with STN stimulation [7].

In addition to risk factors such as a history of mood disorders and difficulties adjusting to familial or psychosocial problems associated with PD, poor tolerance to the adverse effects of DBS has been shown to correlate with depression following STN-DBS surgery [8]. It has also been suggested that the reduction in levodopa dosage or other dopaminergic agents that often accompanies DBS surgery may cause or contribute to the development or worsening of depression and other psychiatric symptoms following this procedure [9]. Furthermore, DBS has been shown specifically to induce depressive symptoms when the electrode is thought to be located within the zona incerta or the substantia nigra pars reticulata (SNr) [10]. It is therefore incumbent on the physician evaluating a patient with new onset depression following DBS to ensure that the electrode is positioned in the appropriate location. In one series, 25% of patients suffered significant worsening of their mood state following surgery despite improvement in motor function. Indeed, half of these patients were reported to have become transiently suicidal [11–13]. Further, the appearance of frontal behavioral changes has been reported by family members to be observed in 30–50% of patients who have undergone STN stimulation [6,14]. It is interesting that the incidence of suicide in patients with PD has been reported to be both the same as [15] and 10 times lower than [16] that in an aged-matched population. However, in a series of patients who underwent STN-DBS there was a very high incidence of suicidality, with 2% of patients having attempted and 1% having committed suicide during a mean of 12 months postoperatively, despite "successful" surgical results [9]. In a larger review of patients having undergone STN-DBS, 0.4 and 0.9% of patients were found to have completed/attempted suicide. It is therefore now well accepted that depression after STN-DBS occurs, and is a major risk factor for committing suicide [17]. The relationship between STN-DBS and suicide, however, remains incompletely understood and is likely multifactorial.

Although depression is obviously an important risk factor for suicide, a loss of impulse control associated with stimulation has also been suggested [18]. STN-DBS has been reported to be associated with a decrease in impulse control disorders such as pathologic gambling, likely due to decreases in dopaminergic medication made possible after DBS [19,20]. More frequently, however, are observations suggesting that there is an increase in impulse control disorders following surgery such as gambling [21], compulsive behaviors, punding, and hypersexual behavior [22,23].

The origins of changes in impulsivity are hypothesized to be due to effects of stimulation on the limbic component of the STN. The STN has been functionally divided into three territories with the sensorimotor circuit occupying the dorsolateral STN, the ventral STN being connected to associative areas and the medial STN related to the limbic circuit [24]. It is currently hypothesized that stimulation within the "wrong" portion of the STN may be associated with decreased efficacy on motor symptoms and an increased likelihood of inducing mood dysfunction. Although electrode location is known to correlate with efficacy in general, due to the small size of the STN, if an electrode is placed correctly enough to produce beneficial motor effects with stimulation, the potential that current might spread and spill over to affect the associative and limbic portions of the STN would seem to be inevitable, perhaps leading to adverse effects in the respective associative and limbic domains in some patients. Electrode locations were evaluated in a series of STN-DBS patients whose cognitive and or psychiatric function declined after surgery [25]. No correlation was found between motor, cognitive, or behavioral effects and active location of the electrode with the STN. Further studies to determine better how and why STN-DBS leads to depression with suicidality are clearly warranted.

Other psychiatric disturbances

Dopamine dysregulation syndrome (DDS) is closely related to the dysfunctions that occur in impulsivity in many patients with PD. DDS is a disorder that is characterized by dopamine addiction, whereby PD patients tend to take escalating doses of the drug as a psychostimulant, independent of a need to control motor symptoms better [26]. This in turn may result in hypomanic behavior, mood swings, and gambling. The effects of STN-DBS on this behavior remain disputed. Postoperatively, patients frequently *need* less dopamine, which may, therefore, help to decrease the desire for the euphorigenic effect of the medication. Furthermore, there is some evidence that suggests that STN lesions may have a direct effect that limits some of the reward associated with cocaine [27]. Witjas *et al.* described two patients who noted significant improvement in their behavioral dysfunction following STN stimulation [20].

Patients with PD may also have other, more complex, psychiatric disturbances. Some are dopamine dependent whereas others are not. A study reported a patient with severe disturbances consisting of panic, bradyphrenia, headache, and back pain associated with being in the "off" state; these symptoms were in addition to motor fluctuations and dyskinesias. The patient underwent uneventful STN-DBS, which successfully treated the motor features and complications, but the patient was unable to be tapered off of levodopa because this led to worsening of the non-motor symptoms [28]. These types of "non-motor" off symptoms are said to occur in as many as 60% of PD patients [29]. Although response to levodopa has been demonstrated to be a good predictor of motor response to STN-DBS [30], cases such as this highlight the fact that levodopa responsiveness to non-motor dysfunction may not respond reliably to stimulation.

Future therapy in psychiatric aspects of PD

Increasing attention is now being directed towards depression and other psychiatric disturbances in patients with PD. The relationship between STN stimulation and psychiatric illness in PD patients remains incompletely understood. Advances in the understanding of the pathophysiology and circuitry of depression have led to consideration of novel surgical interventions. For example, surgery for depression is now being studied using DBS in the subgenual cingulate gyrus, and other potential targets have been proposed.

Our group has published results on DBS of the subgenual cingulate gyrus in the treatment of major depressive disorder (MDD). Our early results demonstrated that four out of six patients (66%) met the criteria of disease response [a 50% or greater reduction in the patient's score on the Hamilton Depression Rating Scale (HDRS-17)] [31]. We have also maintained a similar disease remission rate in our more recent patients. It should be noted that many patients who do not meet the criteria for a full response still achieve some degree of clinical improvement following DBS. The rationale for our having moved forwards with this intervention was the finding that pretreatment PET scans in our severely depressed patients revealed increased activity in the subgenual area at baseline.

So far, there have been very limited studies involving functional imaging in patients with PD-associated depression. One group found changes in fractional anisotropy values in the region thought to correspond to the anterior cingulate gyrus in patients with depression and PD. These changes were not observed in those patients with PD who did not have depression [32]. Confirmation that these same structural regions of the brain that are being targeted in patients with MDD are also present in PD patients with depression suggests that there could be possible benefit with DBS in these regions in PD patients with severe depressive symptoms in whom more conventional therapy has failed. Whether these targets will be useful in a treatment-resistant PD depression state is unknown.

It is noteworthy that DBS is also being applied to treat Tourette's syndrome and obsessive compulsive disorder (OCD) [33–38]. Knowledge gained from these studies might also have an impact in treating psychiatric manifestations in patients with PD.

Cognitive dysfunction

Cognitive deterioration is a prominent feature associated with PD [39]. The origins of dementia in PD are multifactorial. The degree of degeneration of the basal forebrain cholinergic pathway and the loss of neurons within the nucleus basalis of Meynert have been shown to correlate with the severity of cognitive deficits in PD patients [40]. Similarly, the evolution of cortical Lewy body pathology has been shown to correlate with the development of dementia. As patients develop progressive histopathologic changes and presence of Lewy bodies within a greater number of central nervous system structures, there is an increasing rate of dementia [41], such that by Braak stage 6 every patient would be expected to have diffuse cortical Lewy bodies and clinical evidence of dementia.

MR imaging of PD patients, when compared when controls, demonstrates greater volume loss in the temporal lobe, hippocampus, and parahippocampal gyrus, and also in the occipital lobe, right frontal lobe, and left parietal lobe [42]. Similar loss of volume in frontal and temporal lobes was found by voxel-based morphometry analysis in another study [43], although these changes were less than found in patients with Alzheimer's disease.

The effects of STN-DBS on cognition remain somewhat in dispute. Various studies have found that STN-DBS is associated with improvements in executive function following surgery [44,45], whereas others have reported cognitive decline following STN-DBS[14,25,46]. Still others have noted that there was a general preservation of cognitive performance without significant improvement or deterioration associated with the surgery [5,47]. In a systematic review of the literature, one group found that 41% of patients experienced cognitive problems following surgery [48,49].

"Slowness of thinking" as a particular complaint was examined in one study. In this series, 41% of patients had this particular complaint on preoperative assessment, usually most pronounced during the "off" state. Following STN-DBS, only 7% of patients continued to complain of slowness of thinking [50]. Others studies have found a worsening in verbal fluency following stimulation [51], and an association between age at surgery and a potential decline in executive function with surgery [6,7].

At present there is no surgical therapy that can be directed towards the cognitive and memory declines in PD. Recent work suggests that enhancing cognitive function with DBS may not be very far off. A recent report suggests that cognitive function may be enhanced in PD with DBS in the basal nucleus of Meynert [48]. In addition, our group has reported enhancement in memory function in a patient with fornix/hypothalamic DBS [52]. Standardized low-resolution electromagnetic tomography (sLORETA) conducted 11 months following implantation revealed that fornix/hypothalamic stimulation significantly increased activity in the ipsilateral mesial temporal structures. These observations point to the possibility that in the future, surgical therapies directed at this or other regions may become available and may be useful for treating cognitive dysfunction in PD.

Gait

STN stimulation produces variable but often unsustained improvements in gait function. STN DBS has been shown to increase walking speed [53,54] and to improve gait initiation in patients with PD [55]. These effects, however, have been shown to be relatively short lived. By 1 year postoperatively, improvements in gait as assessed by the UPDRS are lost and after 5 years of follow-up there is significant worsening in gait [8]. Long-term follow-up of patients with STN-DBS reveals that despite continued good motor control, patients develop increased disability secondary to gait dysfunction and freezing, which occur in 5–20% of patients [56].

Recent work suggests that patients with existing STN-DBS may obtain "new benefit" in gait and freezing if the stimulations settings are switched from a high-frequency (130 Hz) paradigm to a lower frequency (60 Hz). It has been hypothesized that the possible improvement is not related to stimulation of the STN in this situation, but is due to effects on neighboring structures including the pedunculopontine nucleus (PPN) [56].

Understanding the pathophysiology of gait disturbances in PD and identifying its neuroanatomic substrates have been challenging. In 1966, Sterman and Fairchild noted that in experimental animals there were a number of brainstem regions where stimulation produced locomotor activity [57]. In the 1980s, it was found that focal injections of neuroactive substances into the brainstem of rodents could drive locomotor activity. Observations in MPTP-treated non-human primates have shown that there is very pronounced synaptic metabolic activity in the vicinity of the PPN, an observation consistent with the enhanced activity of the descending GABAergic projections from basal ganglia outflow nuclei in parkinsonian states [58]. Further experiments by the group at Oxford have shown that it is possible to reverse experimental parkinsonism in MPTP treated non-human primates by microinjections of the excitatory agent bicuculline within the PPN area [59].

Based of these preclinical data, we initiated studies testing the effect of implanting DBS electrodes within the PPN in PD patients with gait disturbances [60]. We found that this region is populated with movement-responsive neurons in patients with PD [61]. Low-frequency PPN-DBS (25–75 Hz) has now been reported to improve axial symptoms such as rising from a chair, posture, gait, and postural stability, even in patients who have previously undergone STN-DBS. Interestingly, high-frequency stimulation does not appear to replicate these beneficial effects on gait [62–64].

In patients who were not candidates for STN-DBS due to prominent axial difficulties and falls, we have recently shown that PPN-DBS improves falls [65]. PPN-DBS appears to be well tolerated. A consistent but reversible stimulation-related adverse effect is paresthesia, likely due to the proximity of the target to the medial lemniscus [64]. This is controlled by reducing the current and frequency settings of the DBS stimulation.

Autonomic dysfunction

Autonomic dysfunction is commonly described to occur in patients with PD. Orthostatic hypotension in particular is prone to be exacerbated by the tendency for levodopa to lower blood pressure and heart rate at rest and thereby to increase orthostatic hypotension [66]. There are reports of transient ipsilateral increases in sweating and mydriasis associated with STN-DBS. This is hypothesized to be due to stimulation of descending sympathetic fibers located within the zona incerta and has been described to disappear with hours to days after initiation of stimulation.

Many PD patents experience drenching sweats during the "off" period. In fact, this has been found to be the most frequent non-motor complaint in one series of PD patients. In a series investigating the benefits of STN-DBS, an 87% improvement was found in complaints relating to sweating and other dysautonomic symptoms following surgery [50]. In another study, STN-DBS was found to have little direct effect on the autonomic system but, due to the decreased dose of levodopa permitted by the DBS procedure, patients experienced a relative improvement in their autonomic state following surgery. There are currently no surgical therapies that directly address autonomic dysfunction in PD. One could speculate, however, that stimulation of the hypothalamus or peripheral ganglia might one day prove useful.

Pain and fatigue

Little is known about how surgery affects PD-related pain and fatigue. Pain in PD is complex and frequently associated with motor fluctuations [67] or "off" dystonia [68]. In one study, pain related to "off" dystonia was found to be the most successfully treated non-motor symptom in a cohort of patients undergoing STN-DBS surgery [68]. Fatigue is a also a very common complaint in patients with advanced PD. The origin of fatigue in PD is not known and is likely to be multifactorial. Fatigue can be difficult to assess and does not necessarily correlate with physiologic fatigue associated with performing a motor task [69]. In one particular study that examined fatigue, it was found to have a trend towards improvement following surgery, but with less obvious benefit than the effects of DBS on motor or other non-motor functions [50]. Furthermore, this may be countered by apathy, which may appear as patients are weaned off dopaminergic medications following surgery [70]. Patients may misinterpret their feelings of apathy and loss of motivation as fatigue. There are no current direct surgical treatments for fatigue.

Conclusion

Although an important first step, it is obviously not adequate merely to treat PD symptoms with dopaminergic therapy in an attempt to restore balance to the nigrostriatal dopaminergic motor circuitry. Treatments for the motor component have improved significantly, but the course of PD is relentless and, even with complete control of dopaminergic features, patients continue to suffer disability due to the development of non-motor and non-dopaminergic features. The current surgical therapies of GPi-DBS and STN-DBS were developed and popularized because of their dramatic effects on the motor fluctuations and dyskinesia in patients with advanced PD. It is time now to turn our attention to the development of novel strategies aimed at treating the non-motor and non-dopaminergic symptoms. The association of STN-DBS with depression and possibly cognitive dysfunction offers the potential for providing a new form of therapy, or at least better understanding the pathophysiology of these problems. The early work on PPN-DBS for gait dysfunction is encouraging, and further studies are under way to understand better the possible benefits of this intervention. We are encouraged that there may be utility in applying DBS to other regions of the brain to treat other non-motor features of PD. There certainly may come a time when the movement disorders team has a variety of different targets proven beneficial such that an individual patient can have a tailored surgical approach to treat the symptoms that are most disabling to them.

References

1. Witjas T, *et al.* Nonmotor fluctuations in Parkinson's disease: frequent and disabling. *Neurology* 2002;**59**(3):408–13.
2. Gunal DI, *et al.* The clinical profile of nonmotor fluctuations in Parkinson's disease patients. *Can J Neurol Sci* 2002;**29**(1):61–4.
3. Adler CH. Nonmotor complications in Parkinson's disease. *Mov Disord* 2005;**20**(Suppl 11):S23–9.
4. Reijnders JS, *et al.* A systematic review of prevalence studies of depression in Parkinson's disease. *Mov Disord* 2008;**23**(2):183–9; quiz 313.
5. Ardouin C, *et al.* Bilateral subthalamic or pallidal stimulation for Parkinson's disease affects neither memory nor executive functions: a consecutive series of 62 patients. *Ann Neurol* 1999;**46**(2):217–23.
6. Saint-Cyr JA, *et al.* Neuropsychologic consequences of chronic bilateral stimulation of the subthalamic nucleus in Parkinson's disease. *Brain* 2000;**123**(Pt 10):2091–108.
7. Funkiewiez A, *et al.* Long term effects of bilateral subthalamic nucleus stimulation on cognitive function, mood, and behaviour in Parkinson's disease. *J Neurol Neurosurg Psychiatry* 2004;**75**(6):834–9.
8. Krack P, *et al.* Five-year follow-up of bilateral stimulation of the subthalamic nucleus in advanced Parkinson's disease. *N Engl J Med* 2003;**349**(20):1925–34.
9. Soulas T, *et al.* Attempted and completed suicides after subthalamic nucleus stimulation for Parkinson's disease. *J Neurol Neurosurg Psychiatry* 2008;**79**(8):952–4.
10. Bejjani BP, *et al.* Transient acute depression induced by high-frequency deep-brain stimulation. *N Engl J Med* 1999; **340**(19):1476–80.
11. Berney A, *et al.* Effect on mood of subthalamic DBS for Parkinson's disease: a consecutive series of 24 patients. *Neurology* 2002;**59**(9):1427–9.
12. Kulisevsky J, *et al.* Mania following deep brain stimulation for Parkinson's disease. *Neurology* 2002;**59**(9):1421–4.
13. Houeto JL, *et al.* Behavioural disorders, Parkinson's disease and subthalamic stimulation. *J Neurol Neurosurg Psychiatry* 2002;**72**(6):701–7.
14. Dujardin K, *et al.* Influence of chronic bilateral stimulation of the subthalamic nucleus on cognitive function in Parkinson's disease. *J Neurol* 2001;**248**(7):603–11.
15. Stenager EN, *et al.* Suicide in patients with Parkinson's disease. An epidemiologic study. *Acta Psychiatr Scand* 1994;**90**(1):70–2.
16. Myslobodsky M, Lalonde FM, Hicks L. Are patients with Parkinson's disease suicidal? *J Geriatr Psychiatry Neurol* 2001; **14**(3):120–4.
17. Voon V, Krack P, Lang AE. Factors associated with suicide risk following STN DBS for Parkinson's disease. *Mov Disord* 2006; **21**(Suppl 15):S691.
18. Frank MJ, *et al.* Hold your horses: impulsivity, deep brain stimulation, and medication in parkinsonism. *Science* 2007; **318**(5854):1309–12.
19. Ardouin C, *et al.* Pathologic gambling in Parkinson's disease improves on chronic subthalamic nucleus stimulation. *Mov Disord* 2006;**21**(11):1941–6.
20. Witjas T, *et al.* Addiction in Parkinson's disease: impact of subthalamic nucleus deep brain stimulation. *Mov Disord* 2005; **20**(8):1052–5.
21. Smeding HM, *et al.* Pathologic gambling after bilateral subthalamic nucleus stimulation in Parkinson disease. *J Neurol Neurosurg Psychiatry* 2007;**78**(5):517–9.
22. Visser-Vandewalle V, *et al.* Long-term effects of bilateral subthalamic nucleus stimulation in advanced Parkinson disease: a four year follow-up study. *Parkinsonism Relat Disord* 2005; **11**(3):157–65.
23. Albanese A, *et al.* Suicide after successful deep brain stimulation for movement disorders. *Neurology* 2005;**65**(3):499–500; author reply 499–500.
24. Parent A, Smith Y. Organization of efferent projections of the subthalamic nucleus in the squirrel monkey as revealed by retrograde labeling methods. *Brain Res* 1987;**436**(2):296–310.
25. Perriol MP, *et al.* Stimulation of the subthalamic nucleus in Parkinson's disease: cognitive and affective changes are not linked to the motor outcome. *Parkinsonism Relat Disord* 2006; **12**(4):205–10.

26. Giovannoni G, *et al.* Hedonistic homeostatic dysregulation in patients with Parkinson's disease on dopamine replacement therapies. *J Neurol Neurosurg Psychiatry* 2000;**68**(4): 423–8.
27. Baunez C, *et al.* Opposite effects of subthalamic nucleus lesions on motivation for natural reward versus drugs of abuse in rats. *Soc Neurosci Abstr* 2003;**29**:724.2.
28. Cersosimo MG, *et al.* Bilateral STN-DBS fails to improve nonmotor fluctuations in a PD patient. *Parkinsonism Relat Disord* 2007;**13**(8):537–8.
29. Raudino F. Non-motor off in Parkinson's disease. *Acta Neurol Scand* 2001;**104**(5):312–5.
30. Charles PD, *et al.* Predictors of effective bilateral subthalamic nucleus stimulation for PD. *Neurology* 2002;**59**(6):932–4.
31. Mayberg HS, *et al.* Deep brain stimulation for treatment-resistant depression. *Neuron* 2005;**45**(5):651–60.
32. Matsui H, *et al.* Depression in Parkinson's disease. Diffusion tensor imaging study. *J Neurol* 2007;**254**(9):1170–3.
33. Aouizerate B, *et al.* Deep brain stimulation of the ventral caudate nucleus in the treatment of obsessive-compulsive disorder and major depression. Case report. *J Neurosurg* 2004; **101**(4):682–6.
34. Greenberg BD, *et al.* Three-year outcomes in deep brain stimulation for highly resistant obsessive-compulsive disorder. *Neuropsychopharmacology* 2006;**31**(11):2384–93.
35. Lipsman N, Neimat JS, Lozano AM. Deep brain stimulation for treatment-refractory obsessive-compulsive disorder: the search for a valid target. *Neurosurgery* 2007;**61**(1):1–11; discussion 11–3.
36. Diederich NJ, *et al.* Efficient internal pallidal stimulation in Gilles de la Tourette syndrome: a case report. *Mov Disord* 2005; **20**(11):1496–9.
37. Maciunas RJ, *et al.* Prospective randomized double-blind trial of bilateral thalamic deep brain stimulation in adults with Tourette syndrome. *J Neurosurg* 2007;**107**(5):1004–14.
38. Servello D, *et al.* Deep brain stimulation in 18 patients with severe Gilles de la Tourette syndrome refractory to treatment: the surgery and stimulation. *J Neurol Neurosurg Psychiatry* 2008;**79**(2):136–42.
39. Agid Y, *et al.* Parkinson's disease is a neuropsychiatric disorder. *Adv Neurol* 2003;**91**: 365–70.
40. Whitehouse PJ, *et al.* Basal forebrain neurons in the dementia of Parkinson disease. *Ann Neurol* 1983;**13**(3):243–8.
41. Braak H, *et al.* Cognitive status correlates with neuropathologic stage in Parkinson disease. *Neurology* 2005;**64**(8):1404–10.
42. Burton EJ, *et al.* Cerebral atrophy in Parkinson's disease with and without dementia: a comparison with Alzheimer's disease, dementia with Lewy bodies and controls. *Brain* 2004; **127**(Pt 4):791–800.
43. Beyer MK, *et al.* A magnetic resonance imaging study of patients with Parkinson's disease with mild cognitive impairment and dementia using voxel-based morphometry. *J Neurol Neurosurg Psychiatry* 2007;**78**(3):254–9.
44. Benabid AL, *et al.* Deep brain stimulation of the subthalamic nucleus for Parkinson's disease: methodologic aspects and clinical criteria. *Neurology* 2000;**55**(12 Suppl 6):S40–4.
45. Jahanshahi M, *et al.* The impact of deep brain stimulation on executive function in Parkinson's disease. *Brain* 2000;**123**(Pt 6): 1142–54.
46. Trepanier LL, *et al.* Neuropsychologic outcome of GPi pallidotomy and GPi or STN deep brain stimulation in Parkinson's disease. *Brain Cogn* 2000;**42**(3):324–47.
47. Pillon B, *et al.* Neuropsychologic changes between "off" and "on" STN or GPi stimulation in Parkinson's disease. *Neurology* 2000;**55**(3):411–8.
48. Temel Y, *et al.* Behavioural changes after bilateral subthalamic stimulation in advanced Parkinson disease: a systematic review. *Parkinsonism Relat Disord* 2006;**12**(5):265–72.
49. Freund HJ, *et al.* Cognitive functions in a patient with Parkinson-dementia syndrome undergoing deep brain stimulation. *Arch Neurol* 2009;**66**(6):781–5.
50. Witjas T, *et al.* Effects of chronic subthalamic stimulation on nonmotor fluctuations in Parkinson's disease. *Mov Disord* 2007;**22**(12):1729–34.
51. York MK, *et al.* Cognitive declines following bilateral subthalamic nucleus deep brain stimulation for the treatment of Parkinson's disease. *J Neurol Neurosurg Psychiatry* 2008;**79**(7): 789–95.
52. Hamani C, *et al.* Memory enhancement induced by hypothalamic/fornix deep brain stimulation. *Ann Neurol* 2008; **63**(1):119–23.
53. Bejjani BP, *et al.* Axial parkinsonian symptoms can be improved: the role of levodopa and bilateral subthalamic stimulation. *J Neurol Neurosurg Psychiatry* 2000;**68**(5):595–600.
54. Stolze H, *et al.* Effects of bilateral subthalamic nucleus stimulation on parkinsonian gait. *Neurology* 2001;**57**(1):144–6.
55. Liu W, *et al.* Bilateral subthalamic stimulation improves gait initiation in patients with Parkinson's disease. *Gait Posture* 2006;**23**(4):492–8.
56. Moreau C, *et al.* STN-DBS frequency effects on freezing of gait in advanced Parkinson disease. *Neurology* 2008;**71**(2): 80–4.
57. Sterman MB, Fairchild MD. Modification of locomotor performance by reticular formation and basal forebrain stimulation in the cat: evidence for reciprocal systems. *Brain Res* 1966;**2**(3):205–17.
58. Mitchell IJ, *et al.* Neural mechanisms underlying parkinsonian symptoms based upon regional uptake of 2-deoxyglucose in monkeys exposed to 1-methyl-4-phenyl-1,2,3,6-tetrahydropyridine. *Neuroscience* 1989;**32**(1):213–26.
59. Nandi D, *et al.* Reversal of akinesia in experimental parkinsonism by GABA antagonist microinjections in the pedunculopontine nucleus. *Brain* 2002;**125**(Pt 11):2418–30.
60. Pahapill PA, Lozano AM. The pedunculopontine nucleus and Parkinson's disease. *Brain* 2000;**123**(Pt 9):1767–83.
61. Weinberger M, *et al.* Pedunculopontine nucleus microelectrode recordings in movement disorder patients. *Exp Brain* Res 2008;**188**(2):165–74.
62. Plaha P, Gill SS. Bilateral deep brain stimulation of the pedunculopontine nucleus for Parkinson's disease. *Neuroreport* 2005;**16**(17):1883–7.
63. Mazzone P, *et al.* Implantation of human pedunculopontine nucleus: a safe and clinically relevant target in Parkinson's disease. *Neuroreport* 2005;**16**(17):1877–81.
64. Stefani A, *et al.* Bilateral deep brain stimulation of the pedunculopontine and subthalamic nuclei in severe Parkinson's disease. *Brain* 2007;**130**(Pt 6):1596–607.

65. Moro E, *et al.* Unilateral pedunculopontine stimulation improves falls in Parkinson's disease. *Brain* 2010;**133**(Pt 1): 215–24.
66. Ludwig J, *et al.* Effects of subthalamic nucleus stimulation and levodopa on the autonomic nervous system in Parkinson's disease. *J Neurol Neurosurg Psychiatry* 2007;**78**(7):742–5.
67. Goetz CG, *et al.* Pain in Parkinson's disease. *Mov Disord* 1986;**1**(1):45–9.
68. Tinazzi M, *et al.* Pain and motor complications in Parkinson's disease. *J Neurol Neurosurg Psychiatry* 2006;**77**(7):822–5.
69. Lou JS, *et al.* Levodopa improves physical fatigue in Parkinson's disease: a double-blind, placebo-controlled, crossover study. *Mov Disord* 2003;**18**(10):1108–14.
70. Krack P, *et al.* Subthalamic nucleus or internal pallidal stimulation in young onset Parkinson's disease. *Brain* 1998;**121**(Pt 3): 451–7.

Chapter 37
Effects of Exercise on Basal Ganglia Function in Parkinson's Disease and Its Animal Models

Giselle M. Petzinger[1,2], *Beth E. Fisher*[1,2], *Charlie K. Meshul*[3], *John P. Walsh*[4], *Garnik Akopian*[4], *& Michael W. Jakowec*[1,2]

[1]Department of Neurology, Keck School of Medicine, University of Sothern California, Los Angeles, CA, USA
[2]Division of Biokinesiology and Physical Therapy, University of Southern California, Los Angeles, CA, USA
[3]Department of Behavioral Neurosciences, Oregon Health Sciences University, Portland, OR, USA
[4]Andrus Gerontology Center, University of Southern California, Los Angeles, CA, USA

Introduction

The beneficial effects of physical therapy and general forms of exercise in individuals with Parkinson's disease (PD) have been reported in numerous studies [1–8]. Epidemiologic studies have also revealed that increased physical activity, particularly strenuous exercise, throughout life has been associated with a lower risk of developing neurodegenerative disorders such as PD [9–11]. These studies have served as a catalyst to determine whether exercise may represent a critical therapeutic intervention in PD and, more importantly, to investigate whether exercise leads to central nervous system (CNS) compensatory or neuroprotective changes with the potential to alter disease progression. Over the past few decades, studies have demonstrated that the brain is altered by experience, including exercise. This phenomenon termed experience-dependent neuroplasticity is defined as modifications within the CNS in response to physical activity that promotes a skill acquisition process. As such, (i) intensity, (ii) specificity, and (iii) complexity of practice appear to be important parameters for driving neuroplasticity with potential lasting effects on both brain and behavior. While the importance of these parameters have been primarily established in both the healthy brain and brain injury secondary to stroke, this framework has more recently been adopted to study experience-dependent neuroplasticity and particularly the effects of exercise on neurodegenerative diseases, such as PD, and to examine its potential to modify disease progression. The aim of this chapter is to highlight findings from exercise studies in normal brain and toxin-induce animal models and in individuals with PD, focusing on aspects important to basal ganglia circuitry and motor control.

The traditional approach to physical therapy for individuals with PD has focused on teaching patients compensatory strategies to bypass symptoms associated with basal ganglia pathology and also to prevent secondary strength and mobility impairments that may arise from disuse. The use of external cues and cognitive strategies has been considered the main training option. Thus, individuals with PD are instructed consciously to process movement information such as thinking about swinging the arms or taking large steps. In addition, the physical demands of many of the exercise protocols have been at low to moderate levels of intensity. The goal of traditional therapy has been largely to help people maintain what motor capability they have for as long as possible and to help them adjust as their function inevitably declines. This traditional approach to physical therapy stems from the assumption that in the case of a neurodegenerative process such as that seen in PD, there is no potential for neurologic recovery.

This assumption has been challenged by (i) the recognition that the adult brain has capacity for recovery from injury and, importantly, (ii) the demonstration that exercise can promote brain plasticity and increase neuroprotective and neuroregenerative processes. In addition, in the last few decades there has been accumulating evidence that brain injury and progressive degeneration may support an environment by which experience can facilitate neuroplasticity through molecular, eletrophysiological, or structural events that could enhance functional outcome [12,13].

Parkinson's Disease: Non-Motor and Non-Dopaminergic Features, First Edition. Edited by C. Warren Olanow, Fabrizio Stocchi, and Anthony E. Lang.

Effects of exercise on the normal brain

Studies in normal (non-injured) animals have been extremely valuable in elucidating the neurobiological basis for the beneficial effects of exercise. These studies support the concept that exercise effects on the brain may be related to up-regulated mechanisms of neuroprotection, neuroplasticity, neurogenesis, and/or angiogenesis. Although we classify these exercise effects as being categorically distinct, there is tremendous overlap with respect to their potential role in modulating behavior and function. The following sections examine some of these features.

Neurotrophic factors

Animal studies examining effects of exercise have shown that physical activity, primarily running, can increase brain neurotrophic factors including brain-derived neurotrophic factor (BDNF), glia-derived neurotrophic factor (GDNF), neuronal growth factor (NGF), fibroblast growth factor (FGF), and insulin-like growth factor 1 (IGF-1). Exercise-induced up-regulation of neurotrophic factors has been documented in a number of brain regions involved in learning, memory, mental processing, mood, and motor control, including the hippocampus, cerebellum, cerebral cortex, and striatum [14–17]. Neurotrophic factors in the CNS are expressed at different levels in a number of various cell types, including neurons, microglia, and astrocytes. The precise mechanism that may trigger neurotrophic expression with exercise is not fully elucidated. Metabolic demand, neurotransmitter release, and other released factors may serve as intrinsic local agents that induce neurotrophic factor activation. In addition, the peripheral immune system may contribute to exercise-induced alterations in neurotrophic factor levels and may complement CNS-derived sources.

BDNF up-regulation has been closely linked to exercise and may be an important factor in exercise-derived benefits [17–20]. BDNF is a neurotrophin widely distributed throughout different regions of the brain. It provides both neurotrophic and neuroprotective support to many subpopulations of neurons throughout both development and adulthood. BDNF is a key mediator of synaptic efficacy and experience-dependent neuroplasticity and is associated with both learning and memory processes within the hippocampus. Exercise modulates the induction of BDNF in a time-dependent manner within the hippocampus and cerebral cortex contributing to brain plasticity and functional maintenance [21]. BDNF mRNA and its protein appear quickly within days in rodents undergoing voluntary running wheel exercise, and induced levels are sustained for several weeks after completion of an exercise regimen. Exercise also primes the molecular memory for BDNF induction where a brief second session of exercise can more rapidly re-induce BDNF protein expression. The induction of the major receptors for BDNF through exercise, including the tyrosine kinases TrkB and p75, are also important for experience-dependent neuroplasticity since the balance between these two receptors can dictate the preferences for long-term potentiation (LTP) or long-term depression (LTD) within the hippocampus and striatum [22,23]. The molecular details underlying the beneficial effects of exercise mediated through BNDF are not yet fully elucidated. However, it is believed that neurotrophic factors may promote neurogenesis, angiogenesis, and synaptogenesis at dendritic sites (local effects) or cell bodies of neurons and glia (global effects) through (i) activation of kinases, including the mitogen-activated kinase (MAPK) cascades, (ii) induction of local protein translation within dendrites, thus modifying synaptic morphology and synaptic strength, (iii) induction of gene expression at the level of the cell nucleus, or (iv) the regulation of presynaptic neurotransmitter release. These mechanisms play a key role in lowering the threshold for potentiating activation of processes involved in neuroplasticity and repair.

Neurogenesis and exercise

Physical activity may have neuroregenerative and/or neuroprotective influences by stimulating neurogenesis, the birth and development of new cells. Within the normal adult brain, it has been well documented that specific anatomic regions can display robust neurogenesis, including within the dentate gyrus of the hippocampus, the subventricular zone, and the olfactory bulb [24–27]. Newborn neurons are thought to replace dying or defective neurons directly through neurogenesis within these anatomic sites. Alternatively, they may be translocated to specific regions via routes such as the rostral–caudal migratory pathway [28,29]. Experience is thought to enhance neurogenesis. For example, the initial identification of enhanced neurogenesis within the hippocampal dentate gyrus was reported in rats housed under conditions of environmental enrichment with objects to promote social interactions, reduce stress, and provide voluntary exercise with running wheels [30,31]. Interestingly, when the individual components used in environmental enrichment were separated it was revealed that the running wheel itself was predominantly associated with enhancing neurogenesis [32,33] and that neurogenesis in the context of voluntary exercise, in contrast to enriched housing, has a potentially distinct pathway [34]. Subsequent studies using a variety of techniques have shown that normal rodents subjected to treadmill running have potentiated neurogenesis within the dentate gyrus of the hippocampus associated with changes in blood flow [35], neurotrophic factors [36], and glutamate neurotransmission [37]. Neurogenesis within the basal ganglia circuitry, either within the substantia nigra pars compacta, where midbrain dopaminergic neurons reside, or within the striatum has not yet been demonstrated in the context of exercise. However, two studies in 6-OHDA lesioned rats subjected to environmental enrichment have demonstrated enhanced neurogenesis within the striatum based on doublecortin immunoreactivity [38] and within the substantia nigra based on labeling for BrdU incorporation [39]. The precise role of neurogenesis within the brain is far from complete. Newborn neurons could replace dying neurons, expand the neuronal population, or act as protection from insult or injury. Interestingly, the fact that behavioral benefits of environmental enrichment may not necessarily require hippocampal neurogenesis [40] raises questions regarding the role of neurogenesis in this region and also its role at sites of injury. Since voluntary running wheel exercise has been shown to elevate neurotrophic factor expression within the hippocampus, it is thought that factors such as BDNF, IGF-1, and other neurotrophic factors have a major effect on promoting neurogenesis and also synaptogenesis and cell survival [16,41–43].

Blood flow and angiogenesis

Physical activity, including running and endurance training, has been shown to increase blood flow and angiogenesis, and to alter factors involved in maintaining the integrity of the blood-brain barrier. Exercise has specifically been shown to induce angiogenesis and blood flow within the cerebellar and motor cortices [44–47]. The cerebrovascular changes that occur in response to exercise are likely due to changes in metabolic demand of underlying neural circuits. While the precise mechanisms involved in exercise-induced increase of blood flow and angiogenesis are not clearly elucidated, some basic understanding is beginning to emerge. Potentially important factors include angiopoietin and vascular epithelial growth factor (VEGF). VEGF, initially termed vascular permeability factor, is constitutively expressed to maintain vessel integrity, and increased expression of the protein in conjunction with its receptor results in increased angiogenesis and increased permeability of the blood–brain barrier. Angiopoietin also increases local angiogenesis but, unlike VEGF, does not have as pronounced an effect on blood–brain barrier permeability. Mechanisms underlying VEGF elevation by exercise are not clear, but one possible process may involve changes in oxygen demand whereby a state of hypoxia may trigger VEGF expression. Alternatively, both local CNS and peripheral sources of IGF-1 could elevate transcription factors such as hypoxia-inducible factor 1 (HIF-1), leading to induction of VEGF. The role of VEGF in disrupting the blood–brain barrier may be important for recruiting factors from the periphery such as activated macrophages, cytokines, or other molecules which may participate in exercise-induced angiogenesis. Physical activity has also been shown to increase astrocytic and epidermal cell proliferation in both the motor cortex and striatum, which may reflect alterations in the blood–brain barrier and contribute to both angiogenesis and passage of factors from the peripheral to central nervous system [16,36,48]. Interestingly, different forms of exercise may mediate various degrees of angiogenesis. For example, endurance training creates a local metabolic demand leading to increased angiogenesis whereas skilled motor training might not [44,49].

Synaptogenesis and dendritic morphology

Changes in dendritic spine density and morphology can be induced by physical exercise through skilled motor training in several regions of the normal adult rat brain, including the motor cortex, hippocampus, and cerebellum. For example, long-term voluntary running increases the density of dendritic spines in the entorhinal cortex and hippocampus [50], and also in the granule cells of the dentate gyrus in adult rats [51]. A study involving rats trained to navigate successfully through a complex obstacle course showed that after 5–10 days of motor skill training there was a significant increase in synaptic connectivity as measured by synapse-to-neuron ratio within the motor cortex [52]. In addition, similar training of adult rats induced an increase in dendritic arborization of stellate interneurons within the cerebellar cortex [53]. Finally, adult rats undergoing a motor skill learning task for 30 days showed a significant increase in the number of synaptic connections in the cerebellum between parallel-fiber and climbing-fiber inputs to Purkinje neurons [54].

Whereas exercise-related mechanisms in the normal brain have been well documented, the effects of exercise as an intervention on the injured brain, including the role of neurotrophic factors, neurogenesis, synaptogenesis, and angiogenesis on experience-dependent neuroplasticity, have only recently begun to be explored. In addition, it is unclear to what extent these exercise-related processes observed in the normal brain may modify disease progression in PD and other neurodegenerative disorders.

Exercise in animal models of Parkinson's disease

PD is characterized by loss of nigrostriatal dopaminergic neurons and the depletion of striatal dopamine. These features can be replicated in the 1-methyl-4-phenyl-1,2,3,6-tetrahydopyridine (MPTP)- and 6-hydroxydopamine (6-OHDA)-lesioned animal models. The focus of exercise studies in PD models has been to examine for neuroprotective or neurorestorative effects on the dopaminergic system and its downstream targets. These are relevant to the major goals in PD research of preventing dopaminergic neuronal loss, promoting survival of remaining neurons, and enhancing compensatory mechanisms important for basal ganglia function and motor performance. Table 37.1 summarizes published animal studies

Table 37.1 List of published studies examining the effects of exercise or skilled training on basal ganglia circuitry and motor control[a,b].

Study	Species	Lesioning regimen	Exercise regimen	Outcome measurements	Results/notes/conclusions
MacRae *et al.* 1987 [113]	Rats SD, 3 or 18 months old	None	Treadmill running, screen 2 weeks at 5–10 min per day. Controls: 5 min per day at 5–10 m min^{-1} for 2 days per week. Trained group: 12 weeks ramping to 20 m min^{-1} for 1 h, 5 days per week	DA, DOPAC, HVA by HPLC DA-D2R (spiperone) binding	Showed 27% enhancement of citrate synthase activity in older exercised rats. Older runners had higher striatal DOPAC levels. No changes in DA levels. Higher HVA/DA ratio with older runners. Elevated D2-R binding in older runners
MacRae *et al.* 1987 [74]	Rats SD, 3 months old	None	Same as MacRae *et al.* [113] except used 6 months of treadmill Compared young control with young runner	DA, DOPAC, HVA by HPLC DA-D2R (spiperone) binding	Exercise increases D2-R binding and stabilizes DA metabolism. The beneficial effects of exercise may be enhanced in aging
Dishman *et al.* 1997 [114]	Rats SD, 1 month old	None	Activity wheel (motorized)	Escape latency from foot-shock DA, 5HT, and their metabolites by HPLC	Exercised rats had 34% reduction in latency to escape foot-shock. Changes in NE and 5HT suggest that exercise reduced anxiety and depression. No changes in DA
Bland *et al.* 1999 [116]	Rats LE	None Casting	Spontaneous movement in cylinder	Glutamate by microdialysis	Spontaneous movement increased extracellular levels of Glu. Casted animals showed reduced Glu on contralateral side. Use-dependent arborization may involve Glu
Meeusen *et al.* 1997 [115]	Rats Wistar	None	Exercise 5 days per week for 6 weeks from 19 m min^{-1} for 30 min to 26 m min^{-1} for 80 min	Microdialysis after 1 h exercise in trained and control rats	Trained rats increased extracellular Glu levels in striatum, reduced basal activity of striatum, levels of DA and Glu reduced. Propose a functional link between Glu and DA
Humm *et al.* 1999 [117]	Rats LE	Lesion of sensorimotor cortex (FL-SMC)	In some lesioned rats the affected limb was cast and some received MK-801. Sham controls were included	Behavior with forelimb placing and cylinder tests Microdialysis in CPu for glutamate TH-ir of SN to sample cell number	Blocking glutamate spared SN neuron loss, and blocked use-dependent exaggeration of cortical injury. Forelimb placing ability recovered by blocking glutamate but not landing from rearing position
Tillerson *et al.* 2001 [58]	Rats LE	6-OHDA MFB	Forced use of impaired limb by casting for 1–7, 3–9, or 7–13 days after lesioning	Behavioral testing for limb akinesia, wall exploration, limb placement, Apo rotation DA and metabolites, DAT, TH, VMAT2 protein	Early cast showed no difference in limb asymmetry compared with control in a range of measures. Reduced or no benefit to casting at later time points. Early casting protected DA levels from depletion. Partial benefit seen in day 3–9 casting
Tumer *et al.* 2001 [118]	Rats Fisher SD	None	Motorized treadmill, gradual increase in speed and duration over 2 weeks reaching 1 h per day running	Analysis of mRNA expression for TH, NPY, DBH Mobility shift assay for AP-1 and CREB	Increased TH mRNA in old but not young rats after exercise in SN. Increased TH mRNA in VTA and LC of young rats

(*continued*)

Table 37.1 (*Cont.*)

Study	Species	Lesioning regimen	Exercise regimen	Outcome measurements	Results/notes/conclusions
Tillerson *et al.* 2002 [119]	Rats Fisher Mice C57BL/6 (retired breeders)	6-OHDA to MFB; MPTP 2 × 15 mg, 12 h apart	Treadmill 1 day prior to lesion at 15 m min^{-1} for 10 min. Baseline analysis 2 h after lesion. Rats run day 1–9, 15 m min^{-1} for 2 × 15 min. Mice on treadmill 1 day before lesion at 5 m min^{-1} and then from day of last lesion to 9 days at 5 m min^{-1} for 2 × 5 min	Behavioral testing for limb asymmetry, limb placement, stride length, grid-walking (length and faults), HPLC of DA, WIB for TH, DAT, VMAT2	Treadmill running resulted in recovery from limb asymmetry and akinesia, protected from behavioral deficits seen in MPTP lesion mice, resulted in normalization of DA levels and sparing of TH, DAT, and VMAT2 depletion. Suggest exercise-induced sprouting. Neuroprotective effect leaving more surviving cells. No assessment of degree of lesioning
Tillerson *et al.* 2002 [120]	Rats LE	6-OHDA MFB Mild, severe	Casted unaffected forelimb days 1–7 after lesioning for forced-use followed by period of non-use	Behavioral testing limb asymmetry, akinesia, placing. Apo-rotation, HPLC of DA, and WIB for TH, DAT, VMAT2	Casting the unimpaired forelimb in first 7 days resulted in enhanced injury
Bezard *et al.* 2003 [66]	Mice C57BL/6	MPTP 4 × 20 mg	Weaned at 21 days then in EE for 2 months EE large cage, toys, running wheel SE standard cage	Cocaine behavior in activity cages MPP+ levels D1-R, D2-R, Enk, BDNF, TrkB, DAT mRNA	EE mice less responsive to cocaine, altered c-fos pattern, and reduced novel locomotor reactivity, fewer SNpc neurons, resistant to MPTP, with same levels of MPP+ in EE and SE mice. DAT binding and mRNA reduced in EE. BDNF increased but trkA/B unchanged. D1-R, D2-R, PPE, PPT mRNA unchanged
Cohen *et al.* 2003 [59]	Rats LE and SD	6-OHDA MFB and limb casting	None; casting of one limb for disuse Fore limb was cast for 7 days prior to lesion in the ipsilateral side	Behavior in forelimb asymmetry and akinesia. Apo-induced rotation. DA by HPLC. Striatal GDNF levels	Cast rats prior to lesioning showed reduced forelimb asymmetry and akinesia with lesioning, attenuated both contralateral turning and loss of DA. Elevated GDNF in striatum corresponding to cast limb that returned to baseline
Dobrossy and Dunnett 2003 [112]	Rats SD	6-OHDA 10 weeks post-transplant	EE with visual stimulus and more intense training than deprived groups	Apo-induced rotation Paw reaching and Skinner box Striatal TH-ir to assess graft survival	Rats in EE showed increased graft survival with improved behavior and reduced rotations
Verara-Aragon *et al.* 2003 [122]	Rats LE	6-OHDA MFB	Skilled reaching task taught to rats for 14 days 3 weeks after lesioning	Behavioral testing included skilled reaching, cylinder test, Apo-induced rotation. TH-ir	Results suggest improved reaching due to development of compensatory movements ipsilateral to the lesion through training
Fisher *et al.* 2004 [88]	Mice C57BL/6, 10 weeks old	MPTP 4 × 20 mg kg^{-1} free-base	Treadmill exercise started 4 days after MPTP for 30 days (6 days per week) Ramping 10–25 m min^{-1}, 1 h per day	Analysis after 30 days. Behavior (velocity and duration), TH and DAT striatal protein, D1 and D2 striatal mRNA. Immuno-EM for glutamate	Enhanced velocity and endurance in MPTP+E. Exercise suppressed DAT and TH protein, elevated D2 but not D1 mRNA, and normalized immunogold labeling in striatum

Mabandla *et al.* 2004 [123]	Rats LE	6-OHDA MFB	Running wheels 7 days before lesioning and then 14 days after lesioning	Apo-induced rotation	Exercised rats did not rotate, suggesting protection
Faherty *et al.* 2005 [67]	Mice C57BL/6	MPTP 4 × 20 mg	Housed in EE, exercise, or standard cages. Running wheels provided but not monitored	WIB for TH for cell counting PCR for BDNF, GDNF, DAT, VMAT2 MPP+ in subset of mice	EE in adult mice provides protection from MPTP. Elevated striatal BDNF in EE. No change in GDNF in striatum but elevated in SN. Reduced DAT and VMAT2 in EE and exercise
Jadavji *et al.* 2006 [128]	Rats LE	6-OHDA MFB	EE and SE before lesioning. Skilled reaching and skilled walking	Behavior test skilled walking and reaching, open field, forelimb asymmetry, Apo-induced rotation, TH-ir, CORT	More SN TH-ir neuron in EE rats. Improved behavior and lower CORT levels in EE rats
Howells *et al.* 2005 [124]	Rats LE	6-OHDA MFB	Voluntary running wheel in home cage Groups runners, runners + stress, sedentary. Running started 1 week before lesion, continued for 3 weeks, 2 weeks sedentary	Behavior with Apo-induced contralateral rotation Sample SNpc TH-ir neurons	Running was neuroprotective. Stress reduced the benefits of running
Li *et al.*, 2005 [48]	Rats SD	None	Motorized treadmill, 15 m min^{-1}, 30 min per day, 6 weeks	Astrocyte proliferation by GFAP-ir in dorsolateral striatum and cortex	Elevated astrocyte activation in exercise groups that persisted after exercise completion.
Poulton and Muir 2005 [125]	Rats LE, 9–10 months old	6-OHDA MFB	All 2-week runway training. Treadmill 3 × 20 min 2 weeks prior to lesioning at 0 or 13 m min^{-1}. Treadmill started 24 h or 7 days after lesioning for 6 days per week for a 30-day period at 13 m min^{-1}	Extent of DA depletion evaluated 2 weeks after lesion. Behavioral testing at 3 and 6 weeks post-lesion for forelimb akinesia, ladder walking (stride, speed, errors). Ground reaction force, DA	Treadmill caused attenuation of DA loss. Treadmill training did not ameliorate behavioral deficits. No return of symmetrical presurgical gait. Used ratio of L and R hemispheres for DA by HPLC. Suggest that studies that start intervention too early are in fact providing protection from lesion event
Steiner *et al.* 2006 [39]	Rats SD	6-OHDA Striatum	EE with rotarod and SE	AMPH-induced rotation. BrdU labeling, ICC for TH-ir	EE rats had increased numbers of BrdU-labeled TH-ir cells and glia in the SN. EE rats improved rotation
Al-Jarrah *et al.* 2007 [126]	Mice C57BL/6, 10–12 weeks old	MPTP + probenacid 2 × 25 mg kg^{-1} per week for 5 weeks	Motorized treadmill 18 m min^{-1}, 40 min per day, 5 days per week, for 4 weeks	Behavior open field with AMPH challenge. ECG. VO2, VCO2, HR. Citrate synthase. HPLC of DA, DOPAC. TH-ir CPu, SN	In lesioned mice, exercise led to reduced heart rate, restoration of R-wave amplitude, decline in VO2, increased AMPH-induced locomotor activity. Slight elevation of TH. No change in DA or DOPAC
Anstrom *et al.*, 2007 [129]	Rats SD	6-OHDA MFB	Focused sensorimotor training by vibrissae-elicited forelimb placing before/after 6-OHDA	Behavior placing test, spontaneous limb use, TH-ir in SN and striatum	Intervention showed behavioral benefits and protection from DA depletion and cell loss

(continued)

Table 37.1 (*Cont.*)

Study	Species	Lesioning regimen	Exercise regimen	Outcome measurements	Results/notes/conclusions
O'Dell *et al.* 2007 [68]	Rats SD	6-OHDA striatum	Voluntary or forced running or running wheel starting 2.5 weeks before lesioning and continuing for additional 4 weeks	Behavioral stepping test, cylinder test, elevated grid. DAT autoradiography. TH-ir in midbrain to count SNpc neurons	Running resulted in recovery of motor deficits without recovery of DAT or TH-ir neurons
Yoon *et al.* 2007 [127]	Rats SD	6-OHDA striatum	Treadmill exercise was started 1 day after lesioning at 2–3 m min^{-1} for 14 days	Apo rotation. Striatal TH-ir. SN cell TH-ir counts by sampling	Treadmill exercise lesioned rat had 33% less rotation, 30% more TH-ir cell, and 10% greater striatal TH-ir than 6-OHDA non-exercise rats
Petzinger *et al.*, 2007 [69]	Mice C57BL/6	MPTP 4 × 20 mg kg^{-1} (free base)	10-week-old mice, treadmill exercise started 5 days after MPTP. Treadmill exercise for 30 days (5 days per week). Ramping 10–25 m min^{-1}, 1 h per day	Analysis after 30 days of exercise. Behavior (velocity and duration), TH and DAT striatal protein, midbrain DA cell counts, HPLC analysis of striatal DA DA release by voltammetry	Motor behavioral recovery not accompanied by increased DA or change in midbrain DA cell number. Increased evoked release of DA in dorsolateral striatum
Urakawa *et al.* 2007 [38]	Rats Wistar	6-OHDA Striatum or SN	EE with running wheels and SE	Beam walking, cylinder test, BrdU-labeling, TH-ir	EE rats showed improved behavior, no cell loss protection with EE, more migrating cells in EE, different response in SN compared with striatal injury

[a] These studies were carried in rodents without dopamine lesioning or with subjects lesioned with 6-OHDA or MPTP. This table serves as a synopsis of the variations in rodent models used and outcome measures evaluating either neuroprotection or neurorestoration.

[b] Abbreviations: AMPH, amphetamine; Apo, apomorphine; BDNF, brain-derived neurotrophic factor; BrdU, bromodeoxyuridine; CORT, corticosterone; CPu, caudate putamen; DA, dopamine; DA-D1R; dopamine D1 receptor; DA-D2R, dopamine D2 receptor; DAT, dopamine transporter; DBH, dopamine β-hydroxylase; EE, environment enrichment; GDNF, glia-derived neurotrophic factor; Glu, glutamate; HPLC high-performance liquid chromatography; 5-HT, serotonin; HVA, homovanillic acid; LE, Long Evans; MFB, medial forebrain bundle; NE, norepinephrine; NPY, neuropeptide Y; PPE, preproenkephalin; PPT, preprotachykinin; SD, Sprague–Dawley; SE, standard environment; SN, substantia nigra; TH-ir, tyrosine hydroxylase immunoreactivity; VTA, ventral tegmental area.

examining the effects of exercise on the basal ganglia and its circuitry in normal and dopamine-depleted rodent models. In the following sections we highlight some of these findings.

Exercise and neuroprotection

The administration of either 6-OHDA or MPTP to rodents leads to midbrain dopaminergic cell death and depletion of striatal dopamine, and provides two important animal models to study the effects of exercise on basal ganglia injury [55,56]. Studies examining the effects of motor enrichment or exercise exposure prior to 6-OHDA or MPTP administration show attenuation of motor deficits and protection of dopaminergic neurons. Exercise-induced neuroprotection is demonstrated with respect to (i) the neuronal integrity of dopamine production and handling through gene and protein expression of tyrosine hydroxylase (TH), dopamine transporter (DAT), and vesicular transporter type 2 (VMAT-2); (ii) the survivability of midbrain dopaminergic cells through comparative cell counts; and/or (iii) the maintenance of dopaminergic neuronal integrity through analysis of striatal dopamine levels and its metabolites. Specifically, exercise initiated 1 day prior to 6-OHDA or MPTP lesioning and continued for 1 week post-injury showed improved motor behavior, attenuation of striatal dopamine depletion, and a reduction in the loss of the dopaminergic markers TH, DAT, and VMAT-2 when measured at completion of the exercise regimen [57]. The application of intense motor training (forced use) on the impaired limb in the unilateral 6-OHDA-lesioned rat also provides protection of dopamine integrity and motor behavior when used either pre-lesioning or within the first week post-lesioning [58,59]. However, starting forced use at time points greater than 7 days post-lesioning showed no benefit, indicating that the phases of neuroprotection and lack of efficacy may be distinct. One hypothesis accounting for neuroprotection in these exercise studies is through the elevation of neurotrophic factors such as BDNF, GDNF, or IGF-1, which could provide protection by activating downstream signaling cascades, including second messenger systems and protein kinases that may enhance neuronal function [60]. An alternative hypothesis accounting for exercise-induced neuroprotection from both 6-OHDA and MPTP is a reduction in the bioavailability of the neurotoxin. For example, dopaminergic neurons may be protected due to exercise-induced alterations in the expression of DAT or VMAT-2, transporters important for neurotoxin uptake at the dopaminergic neuronal terminal or vesicular uptake from the cell cytoplasm, respectively [61–63]. Exercise-induced alterations in the blood–brain barrier or xenobiotic detoxification in the liver may also affect brain levels of neurotoxin. The time course of exercise intervention relative to the neurotoxicant administration/exposure is also important, since both MPTP and 6-OHDA have prolonged periods of toxin-induced cell death ranging from 3 to 28 days, respectively, and an exercise-induced suppression of DAT and/or VMAT-2 during this time frame could result in reduced bioavailability of the toxin and subsequent cell death [64,65]. Indeed, two studies using environmental enrichment that included an exercise component in the form of a voluntary running wheel showed that protection from MPTP lesioning was likely due to suppression of DAT and VMAT-2 protein expression in midbrain dopaminergic neurons [66,67]. Studies by O'Dell *et al.* using pre-lesioning voluntary exercise with a forced-exercise component post-lesioning for 4 weeks showed improvement in motor performance but without protection against 6-OHDA-induced injury of midbrain dopaminergic neurons. This suggests alternative mechanisms for exercise benefits including compensatory changes in remaining dopaminergic neurons and/or increased function of other striatal pathways [68].

Exercise and neurorestoration – effects on the DA and glutamate systems

After injury, there exists an opportunity to enhance neuroplasticity through exercise, including skilled or voluntary running. Our studies have focused on exercise-induced compensatory changes of the dopaminergic and glutamatergic systems, two systems important for normal basal ganglia function and motor control. Intensive treadmill exercise in the post-injury state leads to improved motor performance and dopaminergic signaling within the basal ganglia. Specifically, intensive treadmill training initiated 5 days after MPTP administration (when cell death is complete) and continued for 30 days (5 days per week, 1 hour per day) leads to task-specific benefits in both running velocity and endurance and also improved balance using an accelerating rotarod [69]. The MPTP model for these studies consisted of the administration of four intraperitoneal injections of $20\,mg\,kg^{-1}$ (free base) at 2 h intervals for a total administration of $80\,mg\,kg^{-1}$, which results in 60–70% destruction of nigrostriatal dopaminergic neurons and >95% depletion of striatal dopamine levels. Similarly to what is seen in patients with PD, this lesioning regimen spares a subset of surviving neurons, which may subsequently act as a template for experience-dependent neuroplasticity [65,70]. In our exercise paradigm, behavioral benefits from treadmill exercise were accompanied by an increase in evoked dopamine release within the striatum and a decrease in extracellular decay as measured using fast-scan cyclic voltammetry. Enhanced dopamine release was most significant in the dorsolateral region of the striatum, a region involved in motor control [69,71]. Additionally, treadmill exercise led to down-regulation of the DAT (measuring both mRNA transcript and protein) within the striatum. The elevated evoked release of striatal dopamine from surviving nigrostriatal dopaminergic terminals, in conjunction with reduced levels of DAT (the primary route for presynaptic removal of dopamine), leads to an increased synaptic occupancy of dopamine and hence increased dopamine neurotransmission [72,73]. Analysis of the pattern of expression of the dopamine receptors also showed an exercise-induced elevation of dopamine D2 receptor (DA-D2R), but no change in the expression of the dopamine D1 receptor (DA-D1R) in striatal MSNs. Studies using [^{18}F]fallypride with PET imaging have also shown an exercise-induced increase in the DA-D2R. [^{18}F]Fallypride is a high-affinity D2/D3 receptor radioligand that can be used to detect changes in DA-D2R expression within the basal ganglia after exercise. Interestingly there were no exercise-induced changes in either the total level of striatal dopamine, as measure by HPLC homogenates, or the number of substantia nigra neurons, supporting the role of high-intensity exercise in modulating compensatory changes in dopamine handling and neurotransmission in surviving dopaminergic neurons. In support of the exercise-induced changes of the DA-D2R, a similar effect has been observed using *in vitro* receptor autoradiography in the striatum of normal rats after chronic exercise [74]. DA-D2R activation is important for normal function of the basal ganglia, establishing LTD and motor learning and may be a key factor for compensation after injury [75,76]. Some of the effects of dopamine neurotransmission may be mediated thorough its effects on glutamate. When DA-D2R are activated or blocked, glutamate release decreases or increases, respectively [77–79], indicating that alterations in the level of DA-R expression and/or dopamine levels can have profound effects on nearby glutamate neurotransmission. Taken together, these findings suggest that increased dopamine neurotransmission through the DA-D2R pathway may represent an important mechanism for experience-dependent neuroplasticity and the functional benefits of exercise.

In addition to the dopaminergic system, studies in our laboratory and others support the notion that the beneficial effects of exercise may be due to alterations in glutamatergic neurotransmission within the basal ganglia and its circuitry. Glutamatergic projections from either the corticostriatal or thalamostriatal pathways on to striatal medium spiny neurons (MSNs) play a major role in mediating basal ganglia function and motor control [80–83]. There is compelling evidence that the loss of nigral dopaminergic neurons and the depletion of striatal dopamine are responsible for an increase in glutamatergic corticostriatal drive leading to hyperexcitability of MSNs, contributing to the motor deficits in PD [84–87]. A possible mechanism by which exercise may lead to beneficial effects in PD is through the attenuation of corticostriatal hyperexcitability. Studies in our laboratory suggest that exercise-induced neuroplasticity of the glutamatergic system may diminish corticostriatal hyperexcitability and underlie the motor improvement observed in exercised mice. Specifically, using immuno-electron microscopy we observed that 30 days of treadmill exercise initiated 5 days after MPTP lesioning reversed the MPTP-induced increase in *presynaptic* glutamate immunolabeling within striatal terminals, suggesting that exercise reduces the amount of glutamate available for release [88]. In addition, recent studies demonstrate that treadmill exercise also modulates *postsynaptic* glutamate receptors, including the α-amino-3-hydroxy-5-methyl-4-isoxazolepropionic acid receptor (AMPA-R) subtype, in the MPTP-lesioned mouse model. The AMPA-R subtype of glutamate receptors is responsible for the majority of fast excitatory neurotransmission in the CNS and regulates activation of *N*-methyl-D-aspartate receptors (NMDA-Rs) [89,90]. AMPA-Rs are located on the postsynaptic MSN and act as ionotropic channels that convert the chemical signal of presynaptically released glutamate into a postsynaptic electrical signal through the mobilization of cations such as Na^+ and Ca^{2+} [91]. Pathologic elevation of AMPA-R function in PD could act to depolarize striatal MSNs into a region of instability, through the recruitment of NMDA-Rs and voltage-dependent Ca^{2+} channels, which could lead to oscillatory bursts of activity. Indeed, modeling studies have shown that changing AMPA/NMDA receptor ratios by itself changes the oscillatory behavior of ventral striatal MSNs [92]. We found that the AMPA/NMDA receptor ratio increased in MPTP mice and that high-intensity treadmill exercise reduced the receptor ratio back towards the level seen in saline mice (unpublished observation). These data add support not only to exercise as a modality for restoring normal corticostriatal drive, but also for reducing pathologic oscillations in the basal ganglia seen with dopamine depletion. In addition to the exercise-induced changes in glutamate receptor expression, we also observed changes in AMPA-R subunit composition after treadmill running. The electrophysiologic properties of AMPA-R channels are influenced by its subunit composition. The AMPA-R is a heteromeric tetramer consisting of four subunits (GluR1 through GluR4) with the most abundant in the striatum being GluR1 and GluR2 [89,93]. Studies in our laboratory have revealed that treadmill exercise leads to increased expression of the GluR2 subunit in MPTP-lesioned mice. AMPA-R channels with predominant GluR2 subunit composition have been shown to reduce the unitary conductance of AMPA receptors and to reduce the Ca^{2+} permeability of AMPA-R, thus serving as an important mechanism for diminishing postsynaptic hyperexcitability due to dopamine depletion [94,95].

A fundamentally important correlate to these molecular findings is the relationship between AMPA-R expression and the electrophysiologic properties of striatal MSNs. Using organotypic slice cultures, we examined the effects of treadmill exercise on excess excitation and/or

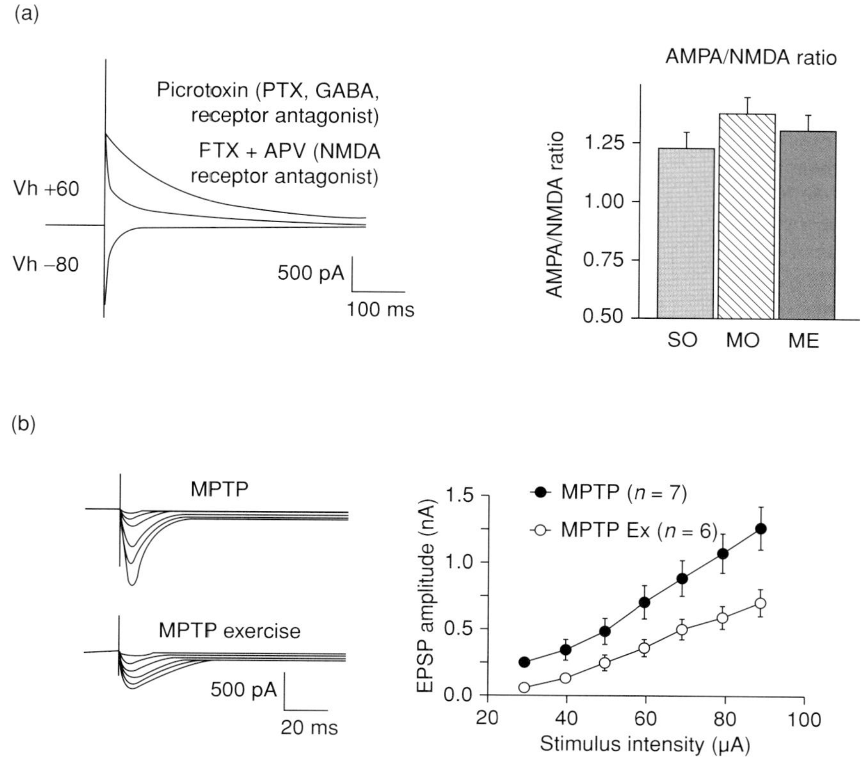

Figure 37.1 Electrophysiological measures of corticostriatal excitation. (a) AMPA receptor participation is reduced with exercise in the MPTP-lesioned mouse. The voltage clamp traces on the left illustrate the experimental approach for measuring AMPA and NMDA receptor-mediated synaptic responses. The bar graph on the right indicates that MPTP lesioning increased the AMPA/NMDA ratio, whereas exercise in the MPTP-lesioned mouse reduced the AMPA/NMDA ratio. Saline only (SO, $n = 11$), MPTP only (MO, $n = 7$), and MPTP + exercise (ME, $n = 10$). (b) Corticostriatal afferents were stimulated *in vitro* at the same stimulus intensity in all brain slices. The examples to the left illustrate the reduction in the size of AMPA receptor-mediated synaptic responses with exercise in the MPTP-lesioned mouse. The graph to the right illustrates the input (stimulus intensity)–output (excitatory postsynaptic current or EPSC) relationship for MPTP alone ($n = 7$) and MPTP + exercise ($n = 6$) groups.

alteration in the frequency of discharge in striatal MSNs in MPTP-lesioned mice. Stimulation of corticostriatal afferents in these *in vitro* brain slice preparations produced large AMPA-R-mediated synaptic events [in the form of excitatory postsynaptic currents (EPSCs)] in MPTP-lesioned mice that were reduced back to normal after exercise (see the comparison of input/output relationship in Figure 37.1). These molecular and electrophysiologic results suggest that exercise-mediated reduction in the size of corticostriatal synaptic events could be due, at least in part, to an increase in the expression and thus influence of GluR2 subunits [91,96,97].

In summary, the findings suggest that alterations in both dopaminergic and glutamatergic neurotransmission through experience-dependent processes modulate cortical hyperexcitability of the basal ganglia, and may underlie exercise-induced behavioral improvement. An important next step is to investigate whether high-intensity exercise has similar benefits in patients with PD.

Exercise-induced neuroplasticity in brain injury

An exciting advance in neuroscience over the last two decades has been the recognition that the capacity for recovery from injury in the human adult brain is far greater than previously thought. It is now recognized that the brain has the ability to reorganize and undergo neuroplastic changes after disease or injury, and that this phenomenon can be facilitated through experience-dependent processes, including forced use, complex skills training, and exercise. Most of our understanding of this experience-dependent neuroplasticity is derived from studies of brain injury related to stroke and spinal cord injury. Lesions in the cortex of rodents and nonhuman primates have permitted investigation of neuroplasticity by studying the effect of forced active use on body segment(s) impaired by brain injury. In addition, basic science research has provided substantial evidence that functional locomotor recovery occurs in animal models of stroke and spinal cord injury when intense, locomotor training is employed.

Noninvasive imaging and stimulation techniques now offer evidence that experience-dependent reorganization occurs in the human brain in response to exercise, locomotor training, and motor skill learning. This experience-dependent neuroplasticity has been shown to play a major role in the recovery of function after stroke. An important example of this is preliminary work using functional magnetic resonance imaging (fMRI) before and after treadmill training with body weight support (BWSTT) that involves an overhead harness that can ease the transition into ambulation [98,99]. Because patients are protected from falling, BWSTT allows them to train safely at greater walking speeds. It is proposed that task-specific BWSTT promotes neural recovery rather than compensation because of significant improvements in velocity of locomotion, motor control of the hemiparetic limbs, and alterations in fMRI activation patterns [98,99].

Physical therapy and exercise in Parkinson's disease

Historically, the goal of exercise programs for PD has not been to examine whether we can induce neuroplasticity, since the general belief has been that the potential for experience-dependent neuroplasticity would be limited in a neurodegenerative process. Rather, the goal has been to maintain the highest possible level of function as people inevitably decline. Exercise studies in mild to moderate states of PD have focused on avoiding secondary impairments from disuse such as weakness and limitations in mobility. Some approaches have been to teach the patient with PD to rely on external cues (visual, auditory) to compensate for impaired internal generation of behavior normally derived from activity in cortico-basal ganglia loops [100].

Over the last 50 years, there have been numerous studies demonstrating the beneficial effects of exercise in individuals with PD [1–8,101–103]. An analysis of exercise studies in PD over this period shows that overall the physical demands of the exercise protocols for the most part were low to moderate in intensity. The activities could be grouped into six categories: (i) passive range of motion (ROM) and stretching; (ii) active ROM; (iii) balance activities; (iv) gait; (v) resistance training; and (vi) practicing functional activities and transitional movements (i.e., sit-to-stand). These studies have shown that exercise is an important adjunct to pharmacologic treatment and helps walking ability and activities of daily living, in addition to slowness, stiffness, and balance dysfunction [104,105].

More recently, a number of studies examining the effects of treadmill training have shown that individuals with PD can benefit from treadmill exercise in which gait behavior is driven more automatically. Improved motor performance has been reported and treadmill speeds have gradually increased from studies in which subjects trained at self-selected velocities for comfort to speeds above over-ground walking velocity. For example, Pohl *et al.* examined the short-term effects of unsupported, speed-dependent treadmill training on patients with early PD [106]. Significant, immediate differences were observed following a single treadmill training intervention versus conventional gait therapy in both walking speed and stride length [106]. In two separate randomized, controlled trials, Miyai and colleagues [107,108] compared immediate and long-term effects of two interventions for individuals with PD: BWSTT and a standard physical therapy regimen involving general conditioning, range of motion, and gait training exercises. After 12 treatment sessions, the BWSTT group exhibited significantly greater improvement on the Unified Parkinson's Disease Rating Scale (UPDRS), whereas the conventional therapy group showed negligible change. Furthermore, both velocity and cadence over a distance of 10 m improved in the BWSTT group and benefits persisted after a 4-week period of no training. A similar report from Toole *et al.* using BWSTT demonstrated functional benefits after six weeks that were sustained 4 weeks later [109]. The intensity of this training was greater than in previous studies but still relatively modest. A recent trend has demonstrated that patients with PD can participate in and benefit from more intensive exercise. In a study by Hirsch *et al.* subjects with PD participated in 10 weeks (three times per week) of high-intensity lower extremity resistance *and* balance training and were assessed before, immediately after training, and 4 weeks later. Muscle strength and balance increased substantially and this effect persisted for at least 4 weeks [8]. Additionally, Dibble *et al.* examined changes in quadriceps muscle volume, muscle force production, and mobility as a result of a 12-week high-force eccentric resistance training program in PD. Eccentric resistance training led to muscle hypertrophy, improved strength, and mobility in persons with PD [110].

Although exercise interventions are gradually becoming more intense, an important next step is to examine if, similarly to what has been seen in the animal models described above, intensive exercise in PD leads to neuroplastic changes and disease modification. Human epidemiologic studies support this hypothesis by demonstrating a neuroprotective role of strenuous exercise [9,111]. Borrowing from our treadmill studies in MPTP-lesioned mice, we are currently using intensive exercise with BWSTT to explore the potential for brain changes and concomitant behavioral improvement in PD. In order to examine the potential disease-modifying role of exercise, our studies have focused on earlier stages of disease where the chances of detecting significant exercise effects may be optimized. We recently completed a randomized, controlled trial to examine the effects of high-intensity exercise using BWSTT on functional performance in people with early-stage PD (Hoehn and Yahr stage 1 or 2) relative to exercise at low (physical therapy) and no intensity. An important part of the study was to determine whether improved performance was accompanied by changes in the brain (neuroplasticity) as measured with transcranial magnetic stimulation (TMS). TMS is a noninvasive neuro-imaging technique that assesses the responsiveness (excitability) of the corticomotor system, Subjects in the two exercise groups completed 24 exercise sessions over 8 weeks, whereas subjects in the zero-intensity group completed six education classes over 8 weeks. Subjects in the high-intensity exercise group worked on an average metabolic equivalent level (MET) of 4.3 with a range between 2.5 and 13.3 METs and speeds ranging from 8.0 to 12.8 km h^{-1} (5.0–8.0 mph). Proper gait kinematics for stance and swing (upright posture, extending and flexing the hip, knee, and ankle, and coordinating limb movements to achieve symmetric limb cadence and equal step length) were maintained during the treadmill training. Subjects in the PT group participated in individualized exercise sessions, which included active and passive range of motion, strengthening, gait, and balance activities. In this study, we found that people with PD participating in high-intensity BWSTT improved in kinematic measures of gait performance (i.e., step length, stride length, hip extension excursion), and lower extremity symmetry of ground reaction forces during a sit-to-stand task. This improvement was not observed consistently in the other groups. In addition, using TMS we observed lengthening of maximal cortical silent period (CSP) duration in all subjects in the high-intensity exercise group. Changes in CSP duration were not observed in subjects in the low-intensity and no exercise groups. Among TMS studies examining corticomotor excitability in patients with PD, CSP durations are among the most consistent abnormalities reported in PD, with shorter duration reflecting increased corticomotor excitability and greater parkinsonian symptoms. Similarly to the observed effects of high-intensity exercise, CSP durations are increased in PD patients after taking levodopa, apomorphine, and pergolide, drugs known to provide effective symptomatic relief of motor symptoms. The findings from our study demonstrate the capability of individuals with PD to engage in intensive exercise and suggest a potential role of intense exercise in driving experience-dependent neuroplasticity and functional improvement in people with PD, and this warrants further investigation.

Conclusion

Although the benefits of exercise and physical therapy in PD are recognized, only recently has there been interest in examining the effects of exercise on brain function and disease modification. To this end, studies have utilized challenging and complex interventions designed to retrain and re-educate normal motor function. Animal models provide an opportunity to test specific hypotheses regarding the mechanisms by which exercise leads to experience-dependent neuroplasticity. In addition, neurotoxin-induced animal models, including rodents and potentially nonhuman primates, and also some of the recently developed transgenic mouse models of PD, can be used to explore fundamentally important aspects of exercise, including the role of the central and peripheral immune systems, the effects of exercise on non-motor features including affective behavior (anxiety and depression), learning, and other cortical functions such as attention and executive function. In the light of the potential application of progenitor and stem cells, and also various virus-based vector construct approaches as treatments for disorders such as PD, studies testing if the survival and integration of these agents can be influenced by the target environment including brains undergoing exercise are warranted [112]. Overall, studies in both healthy and PD animal models provide evidence for exercise-induced neuroplasticity and have ignited interest in further testing of the effects of exercise in patients with PD.

Acknowledgments

We would like to thank our colleagues for helpful discussions and contributions, including Daniel Holschneider, Marta Vuckovic, Breyda Ortega, Jon VanLeeuwen, Wendy Gilmore, Brett Lund, Ruth Wood, and Michael Zigmond. Studies discussed in this chapter were supported from the US Army NETRP, NIH, Team Parkinson, The Parkinson Alliance, Whittier PD Support Group, Department of Veterans Affairs Merit Review Program, and the Kinetics Foundation. This chapter is dedicated to the memory of Dr George Boone, whose vision and support inspired many of the studies in our laboratories.

References

1. Hurwitz A. The benefit of a home exercise regimen for ambulatory Parkinson's disease patients. *J Neurosci Nurs* 1989;**21**:180–4.
2. Reuben DB, Siu AL. An objective measure of physical function of elderly outpatients. The Physical Performance Test. *J Am Geriatr Soc* 1990;**38**:1105–12.
3. Formisano R, Pratesi L, Modarelli FT, *et al.* Rehabilitation and Parkinson's disease. *Scand J Rehabil Med* 1992;**24**:157–60.
4. Comella CL, Stebbins GT, Brown-Toms N, *et al.* Physical therapy and Parkinson's disease: a controlled clinical trial. *Neurology* 1994;**44**:376–8.
5. Sunvisson H, Lokk J, Ericson K, *et al.* Changes in motor performance in persons with Parkinson's disease after exercise in a mountain area. *J Neurosci Nurs* 1997;**29**:255–60.
6. de Goede CJ, Keus SH, Kwakkel G, *et al.* The effects of physical therapy in Parkinson's disease: a research synthesis. *Arch Phys Med Rehabil* 2001;**82**:509–15.
7. Bergen JL, Toole T, Elliott RG III, *et al.* Aerobic exercise intervention improves aerobic capacity and movement initiation in Parkinson's disease patients. *NeuroRehabilitation* 2002;**17**:161–8.
8. Hirsch MA, Toole T, Maitland CG, *et al.* The effects of balance training and high-intensity resistance training on persons with idiopathic Parkinson's disease. *Arch Phys Med Rehabil* 2003;**84**:1109–17.
9. Sasco AJ, Paffenbarger RSJ, Gendre I, *et al.* The role of physical exercise in the occurrence of Parkinson's disease. *Arch Neurol* 1992;**49**:360–5.
10. Tsai CH, Lo SK, See LC, *et al.* Environmental risk factors of young onset Parkinson's disease: a case–control study. *Clin Neurol Neurosurg* 2002;**104**:328–33.
11. Chen X, Li Y, Kline AE, *et al.* Gender and environmental effects on regional brain-derived neurotrophic factor expression after experimental traumatic brain injury. *Neuroscience* 2005;**135**:11–7.

12. Kleim JA, Jones TA, Schallert T. Motor enrichment and the induction of plasticity before or after brain injury. *Neurochem Res* 2003;**28**:1757–69.
13. Kleim JA, Jones TA. Principles of experience-dependent neural plasticity: implications for rehabilitation after brain damage. *J Speech Lang Hear Res* 2008;**51**:S225–39.
14. Neeper SA, Gomez-Pinilla F, Choi J, *et al.* Physical activity increases mRNA for brain-derived neurotrophic factor and nerve growth factor in rat brain. *Brain Res* 1996;**726**:49–56.
15. Gomez-Pinilla F, Dao L, So V. Physical exercise induces FGF-2 and its mRNA in the hippocampus. *Brain Res* 1997;**764**:1–8.
16. Carro E, Trejo JL, Busiguina S, *et al.* Circulating insulin-like growth factor I mediates the protective effects of physical exercise against brain insults of different etiology and anatomy. *J Neurosci* 2001;**21**:5678–84.
17. Berchtold NC, Chinn G, Chou M, *et al.* Exercise primes a molecular memory for brain-derived neurotrophic factor protein induction in the rat hippocampus. *Neuroscience* 2005;**133**:853–61.
18. Cotman CW, Berchtoldb NC. Exercise: a behavioral intervention to enhance brain health and plasticity. *Trends Neurosci* 2002;**25**:295–301.
19. Gomez-Pinilla F, Ying Z, Roy RR, *et al.* Voluntary exercise induces a BDNF-mediated mechanism that promotes neuroplasticity. *Neurophysiology* 2002;**88**:2187–95.
20. Vaynman S, Gomez-Pinilla F. License to run: exercise impacts functional plasticity in the intact and injured central nervous system by using neurotrophins. *Neurorehabil Neural Repair* 2005;**19**:283–95.
21. Adlard PA, Perreau VM, Engesser-Cesar C, *et al.* The time-course of induction of brain-derived neurotrophic factor mRNA and protein in the rat hippocampus following voluntary exercise. *Neurosci Lett* 2004;**363**:43–8.
22. Klintsova AY, Dickson E, Yoshida R, *et al.* Altered expression of BDNF and its high-affinity receptor TrkB in response to complex motor learning and moderate exercise. *Brain Res* 2004;**1028**:92–104.
23. Liu YF, Chen HI, Yu L, *et al.* Upregulation of hippocampal TrkB and synaptotagmin is involved in treadmill exercise-enhanced aversive memory in mice. *Neurobiol Learn Mem* 2008;**90**:81–9.
24. Alvarez-Buylla A, Garcia-Verdugo JM. Neurogenesis in adult subventricular zone. *J Neurosci* 2002;**22**:629–34.
25. Lledo PM, Alonso M, Grubb MS. Adult neurogenesis and functional plasticity in neuronal circuits. *Nat Rev Neurosci* 2006;**7**:179–93.
26. Taupin P. Adult neurogenesis in mammals. *Curr Opin Mol Ther* 2006;**8**:345–51.
27. Ehninger D, Kempermann G. Neurogenesis in the adult hippocampus. *Cell Tissue Res* 2008;**331**:243–50.
28. Alvarez-Buylla A, Herrera DG, Wichterle H. The subventricular zone: source of neuronal precursors for brain repair. *Prog Brain Res* 2000;**127**:1–11.
29. Yamashima T, Tonchev AB, Yukie M. Adult hippocampal neurogenesis in rodents and primates: endogenous, enhanced, and engrafted. *Rev Neurosci* 2007;**18**:67–82.
30. Kempermann G, Kuhn HG, Gage FH. More hippocampal neurons in adult mice living in an enriched environment. *Nature* 1997;**386**:493–5.
31. Kempermann G, Kuhn HG, Gage FH. Experience-induced neurogenesis in the senescent dentate gyrus. *J Neurosci* 1998;**18**:3206–12.
32. van Praag H, Christie BR, Sejnowski TJ, *et al.* Running enhances neurogenesis, learning, and long-term potentiation in mice. *Proc Natl Acad Sci USA* 1999;**96**:13427–31.
33. van Praag H, Kempermann G, Gage FH. Running increases cell proliferation and neurogenesis in the adult mouse dentate gyrus. *Nat Neurosci* 1999;**2**:266–70.
34. Olson AK, Eadie BD, Ernst C, *et al.* Environmental enrichment and voluntary exercise massively increase neurogenesis in the adult hippocampus via dissociable pathways. *Hippocampus* 2006;**16**:250–60.
35. Pereira AC, Huddleston DE, Brickman AM, *et al.* An *in vivo* correlate of exercise-induced neurogenesis in the adult dentate gyrus. *Proc Natl Acad Sci USA* 2007;**104**:5638–43.
36. Trejo JL, Carro E, Torres-Aleman I. Circulating insulin-like growth factor I mediates exercise-induced increases in the number of new neurons in the adult hippocampus. *J Neurosci* 2001;**21**:1628–34.
37. Kitamura T, Mishina M, Sugiyama H. Enhancement of neurogenesis by running wheel exercises is suppressed in mice lacking NMDA receptor epsilon 1 subunit. *Neurosci Res* 2003;**47**:55–63.
38. Urakawa S, Hida H, Masuda T, *et al.* Environmental enrichment brings a beneficial effect on beam walking and enhances the migration of doublecortin-positive cells following striatal lesions in rats. *Neuroscience* 2007;**144**:920–33.
39. Steiner B, Winter C, Hosman K, *et al.* Enriched environment induces cellular plasticity in the adult substantia nigra and improves motor behavior function in the 6-OHDA rat model of Parkinson's disease. *Exp Neurol* 2006;**199**:291–300.
40. Meshi D, Drew MR, Saxe M, *et al.* Hippocampal neurogenesis is not required for behavioral effects of environmental enrichment. *Nat Neurosci* 2006;**9**:729–31.
41. Carro E, Nunez A, Busiguina S, *et al.* Circulating insulin-like growth factor I mediates effects of exercise on the brain. *J Neurosci* 2000;**20**:2926–33.
42. Ang ET, Wong PT, Moochhala S, *et al.* Neuroprotection associated with running: is it a result of increased endogenous neurotrophic factors? *Neuroscience* 2003;**118**:335–45.
43. Adlard PA, Cotman CW. Voluntary exercise protects against stress-induced decreases in brain-derived neurotrophic factor protein expression. *Neuroscience* 2004;**124**:985–92.
44. Black JE, Isaacs KR, Anderson BJ, *et al.* Learning causes synaptogenesis, whereas motor activity causes angiogenesis, in cerebellar cortex of adult rats. *Proc Natl Acad Sci USA* 1990;**87**:5568–72.
45. Kleim JA, Cooper NR, VandenBerg PM. Exercise induces angiogenesis but does not alter movement representations within rat motor cortex. *Brain Res* 2002;**934**:1–6.
46. Holschneider DP, Yang J, Guo Y, *et al.* Reorganization of functional brain maps after exercise training: importance of cerebellar–thalamic–cortical pathway. *Brain Res.* 2007;**1184**: 96–107
47. Yang J, Sadler TR, Givrad TK, *et al.* Changes in brain functional activation during resting and locomotor states after unilateral nigrostriatal damage in rats. *Neuroimage* 2007;**36**: 755–73.

48. Li J, Ding YH, Rafols JA, *et al.* Increased astrocyte proliferation in rats after running exercise. *Neurosci Lett* 2005;**386**:160–4.
49. Isaacs KR, Anderson BJ, Alcantara AA, *et al.* Exercise and the brain: angiogenesis in the adult rat cerebellum after vigorous physical activity and motor skill learning. *J Cereb Blood Flow Metab* 1992;**12**:110–9.
50. Stranahan AM, Khalil D, Gould E. Running induces widespread structural alterations in the hippocampus and entorhinal cortex. *Hippocampus* 2007;**17**:1017–22.
51. Eadie BD, Redila VA, Christie BR. Voluntary exercise alters the cytoarchitecture of the adult dentate gyrus by increasing cellular proliferation, dendritic complexity, and spine density. *J Comp Neurol* 2005;**486**:39–47.
52. Kleim JA, Lussnig E, Schwarz ER, *et al.* Synaptogenesis and Fos expression in the motor cortex of the adult rat after motor skill learning. *J Neurosci* 1996;**16**:4529–35.
53. Kleim JA, Swain RA, Czerlanis CM, *et al.* Learning-dependent dendritic hypertrophy of cerebellar stellate cells: plasticity of local circuit neurons. *Neurobiol Learn Mem* 1997;**67**:29–33.
54. Kleim JA, Swain RA, Armstrong KA, *et al.* Selective synaptic plasticity within the cerebellar cortex following complex motor skill learning. *Neurobiol Learn Mem* 1998;**69**:274–89.
55. Dauer W, Przedborski S. Parkinson's disease: mechanisms and models. *Neuron* 2003;**39**:889–909.
56. Petzinger GM, Jakowec MW. The MPTP-lesioned model of Parkinson's disease with emphasis on mice and nonhuman primates. *CompMed* 2004;**54**:497–513.
57. Tillerson JL, Caudle WM, Reveron ME, *et al.* Exercise induces behavioral recovery and attenuates neurochemical deficits in rodent models of Parkinson's disease. *Neuroscience* 2003;**119**:899–911.
58. Tillerson JL, Cohen AD, Philhower J, *et al.* Forced limb-use effects on the behavioral and neurochemical effects of 6-hydroxydopamine. *J Neurosci* 2001;**21**:4427–35.
59. Cohen AD, Tillerson JL, Smith AD, *et al.* Neuroprotective effects of prior limb use in 6-hydroxydopamine-treated rats: possible role of GDNF. *J Neurochem* 2003;**85**:299–305.
60. Shen H, Tong L, Balazs R, *et al.* Physical activity elicits sustained activation of the cyclic AMP response element-binding protein and mitogen-activated protein kinase in the rat hippocampus. *Neuroscience* 2001;**107**:219–29.
61. Pifl C, Giros B, Caron MG. Dopamine transporter expression confers cytotoxicity to low doses of the parkinsonism-inducing neurotoxin 1-methyl-4-phenylpyridinium. *J Neurosci* 1993;**13**:4246–53.
62. Gainetdinov RR, Fumagalli F, Jones SR, *et al.* Dopamine transporter is required for *in vivo* MPTP neurotoxicity: evidence from mice lacking the transporter. *J Neurochem* 1997;**69**:1322–25.
63. Takahashi N, Miner LL, Sora I, *et al.* VMAT2 knockout mice: heterozygotes display reduced amphetamine-conditioned reward, enhanced amphetamine locomotion, and enhanced MPTP toxicity. *Proc Natl Acad Sci USA* 1997;**94**:9938–43.
64. Sauer H, Oertel W. Progressive degeneration of nigrostriatal dopamine neurons following intrastriatal terminal lesions with 6-hydroxydopamine: a combined retrograde tracing and immunocytochemical study in the rat. *Neuroscience* 1994;**59**:401–15.
65. Jackson-Lewis V, Jakowec M, Burke RE, *et al.* Time course and morphology of dopaminergic neuronal death caused by the neurotoxin 1-methyl-4-phenyl-1,2,3,6-tetrahydropyridine. *Neurodegeneration* 1995;**4**:257–69.
66. Bezard E, Dovero S, Belin D, *et al.* Enriched environment confers resistance to 1-methyl-4-phenyl-1,2,3,6-tetrahydropyridine and cocaine: involvement of dopamine transporter and trophic factors. *J Neurosci* 2003;**23**:10999–1007.
67. Faherty CJ, Raviie Shepherd K, Herasimtschuk A, *et al.* Environmental enrichment in adulthood eliminates neuronal death in experimental parkinsonism. *Brain Res Mol Brain Res* 2005;**134**:170–9.
68. O'Dell SJ, Gross NB, Fricks AN, *et al.* Running wheel exercise enhances recovery from nigrostriatal dopamine injury without inducing neuroprotection. *Neuroscience* 2007;**144**:1141–51.
69. Petzinger GM, Walsh JP, Akopian G, *et al.* Effects of treadmill exercise on dopaminergic transmission in the 1-methyl-4-phenyl-1,2,3,6-tetrahydropyridine-lesioned mouse model of basal ganglia injury. *J Neurosci* 2007;**27**:5291–300.
70. Tatton WG, M. M. Kwan, M. C. Verrier, N. A. Seniuk, and E. Theriault. MPTP produces reversible disapperance of tyrosine hydroxylase-containing retinal amacrine cells. *Brain Res* 1990;**527**:21–31.
71. Holschneider DP, Maarek JM. Mapping brain function in freely moving subjects. *Neurosci Biobehav Rev* 2004;**28**:449–61.
72. Mortensen OV, Amara SG. Dynamic regulation of the dopamine transporter. *Eur J Pharmacol* 2003;**479**:159–70.
73. Cragg SJ, Rice ME. DAncing past the DAT at a DA synapse. *Trends Neurosci* 2004;**27**:270–7.
74. MacRae PG, Spirduso WW, Walters TJ, *et al.* Endurance training effects on striatal D2 dopamine receptor binding and striatal dopamine metabolites in presenescent older rats. *Psychopharmacology (Berl)* 1987;**92**:236–40.
75. Wise RA. Dopamine, learning and motivation. *Nat Rev Neurosci* 2004;**5**:483–94.
76. Pisani A, Centonze D, Bernardi G, *et al.* Striatal synaptic plasticity: implications for motor learning and Parkinson's disease. *Mov Disord* 2005;**20**:395–402.
77. Calabresi P, Maj R, Pisani A, *et al.* Long-term synaptic depression in the striatum: physiological and pharmacological characterization. *J Neurosci* 1992;**12**:4224–33.
78. Yamamoto B, Davy,S. Dopaminergic modulation of glutamate release in striatum as measured by microdialysis. *J Neurochem* 1992;**58**:1736–42.
79. Bamford NS, Robinson S, Palmiter RD, *et al.* Dopamine modulates release from corticostriatal terminals. *J Neurosci* 2004;**24**:9541–52.
80. Bouyer JJ, Park DH, Joh TH, *et al.* Chemical and structural analysis of the relation between cortical inputs and tyrosine hydroxylase-containing terminals in rat neostriatum. *Brain Res* 1984;**302**:267–75.
81. Meshul CK, Stallbaumer RK, Taylor B, *et al.* Haloperidol-induced synaptic changes in striatum are associated with glutamate synapses. *Brain Res* 1994;**648**:181–95.
82. Gundersen V, Ottersen OP, Storm-Mathisen J. Selective excitatory amino acid uptake in glutamatergic nerve terminals and in glia in the rat striatum: quantitative electron microscopic immunocytochemistry of exogenous (D)-aspartate and

endogenous glutamate and GABA. *Eur J Neurosci* 1996;**8**: 758–65.

83. Lacey CJ, Boyes J, Gerlach O, *et al.* GABA(B) receptors at glutamatergic synapses in the rat striatum. *Neuroscience* 2005;**136**:1083–95.
84. Schwarting RK, Huston JP. The unilateral 6-hydroxydopamine lesion model in behavioral brain research. Analysis of functional deficits, recovery and treatments. *Prog Neurobiol* 1996;**20**:275–331.
85. Meshul CK, Emre N, Nakamura CM, *et al.* Time-dependent changes in striatal glutamate synapses following a 6-hydroxydopamine lesion. *Neuroscience* 1999;**88**:1–16.
86. Cepeda C, Hurst RS, Altemuis KL, *et al.* Facilitated glutamatergic transmission in the striatum of D2 dopamine receptor-deficient mice. *J Neurophysiol* 2001;**85**:659–70.
87. Neely MD, Schmidt DE, Deutch AY. Cortical regulation of dopamine depletion-induced dendritic spine loss in striatal medium spiny neurons. *Neuroscience* 2007;**149**:457–64.
88. Fisher BE, Petzinger GM, Nixon K, *et al.* Exercise-induced behavioral recovery and neuroplasticity in the 1-methyl-4-phenyl-1,2,3,6-tetrahydropyridine-lesioned mouse basal ganglia. *J Neurosci Res* 2004;**77**:378–90.
89. Isaac JT, Ashby M, McBain CJ. The role of the GluR2 subunit in AMPA Receptor function and synaptic plasticity. *Neuron* 2007;**54**:859–71.
90. Esteban JA. Intracellular machinery for the transport of AMPA receptors. *Br J Pharmacol* 2008;**153**(Suppl 1):S35–43.
91. Hollmann M, M. Hartley, and S. Heinemann. Ca^{2+} permeability of KA-AMPA-gated glutamate receptor channels depends on subunit composition. *Science* 1991;**252**:851–3.
92. Wolf JA, Moyer JT, Lazarewicz MT, *et al.* NMDA/AMPA ratio impacts state transitions and entrainment to oscillations in a computational model of the nucleus accumbens medium spiny projection neuron. *J Neurosci* 2005;**25**:9080–95.
93. Bernard V, P. Somogyi, and J. P. Bolam. Cellular, subcellular, and subsynaptic distribution of AMPA-type glutamate receptor subunits in the neostriatum of the rat. *J Neurosci* 1997;**17**:819–33.
94. Bowie D, Mayer ML. Inward rectification of both AMPA and kainate subtype glutamate receptors generated by polyamine-mediated ion channel block. *Neuron* 1995;**15**:453–62.
95. Swanson GT, Kamboj SK, Cull-Candy SG. Single-channel properties of recombinant AMPA receptor depend on RNA editing, splice variation, and subunit composition. *J Neurosci* 1997;**17**:58–69.
96. Pellegrini-Giampietro DE, Bennett ML, Zukin RS. Are Ca^{2+}-permeable kainate/AMPA receptors more abundant in immature brain? *Neurosci Lett* 1992;**144**:65–9.
97. Geiger JR, Melcher T, Koh DS, *et al.* Relative abundance of subunit mRNAs determines gating and Ca^{2+} permeability of AMPA receptors in principal neurons and interneurons in rat CNS. *Neuron* 1995;**15**:193–204.
98. Fisher B, Sullivan KJ. Activity-dependent factors affecting post-stroke functional outcomes. *Top Stroke Rehabil* 2001;**8**:31–44.
99. Dobkin BH, Firestine A, West M, *et al.* Ankle dorsiflexion as an fMRI paradigm to assay motor control for walking during rehabilitation. *Neuroimage* 2004;**23**:370–81.
100. Romo R, Schultz W. Role of primate basal ganglia and frontal cortex in the internal generation of movements. III. Neuronal activity in the supplementary motor area. *Exp Brain Res* 1992;**91**:396–407.
101. Watkins AL. Physical medicine and rehabilitation for the elderly neurologic patient. *Geriatrics* 1954;**9**:227–229.
102. Bilowit DS. Establishing physical objectives in the rehabilitation of patients with Parkinson's disease; gymnasium activities. *Phys Ther Rev* 1956;**36**:176–8.
103. Clark EC, Clements BG, Erickson DJ, *et al.* Therapeutic exercises in management of paralysis agitans. *J Am Med Assoc* 1956;**162**:1041–3.
104. Hass CJ, Waddell DE, Fleming RP, *et al.* Gait initiation and dynamic balance control in Parkinson's disease. *Arch Phys Med Rehabil* 2005;**86**:2172–6.
105. Hackney ME, Earhart GM. Tai Chi improves balance and mobility in people with Parkinson disease. *Gait Posture* 2008;**28**:456–60.
106. Pohl M, Rockstroh G, Ruckriem S, *et al.* Immediate effects of speed-dependent treadmill training on gait parameters in early Parkinson's disease. *Arch Phys Med Rehabil* 2003;**84**:1760–6.
107. Miyai I, Fujimoto Y, Ueda Y, *et al.* Treadmill training with body weight support: its effect on Parkinson's disease. *Arch Phys Med Rehabil* 2000;**1**:849–52.
108. Miyai I, Fujimoto Y, Yamamoto H, *et al.* Long-term effect of body weight-supported treadmill training in Parkinson's disease: a randomized controlled trial. *Arch Phys Med Rehabil* 2002;**83**:1370–3.
109. Toole T, Maitland CG, Warren E, *et al.* The effects of loading and unloading treadmill walking on balance, gait, fall risk, and daily function in Parkinsonism. *NeuroRehabilitation* 2005;**20**:307–22.
110. Dibble LE, Hale TF, Marcus RL, *et al.* High-intensity resistance training amplifies muscle hypertrophy and functional gains in persons with Parkinson's disease. *Mov Disord* 2006;**21**:1444–52.
111. Chen H, Zhang SM, Schwarzschild MA, *et al.* Physical activity and the risk of Parkinson disease. *Neurology* 2005;**64**: 664–9.
112. Dobrossy MD, Dunnett SB. Motor training effects on recovery of function after striatal lesions and striatal grafts. *Exp Neurol* 2003;**184**:274–84.
113. MacRae PG, Spirduso WW, Cartee GD, *et al.* Endurance training effects on striatal D2 dopamine receptor binding and striatal dopamine metabolite levels. *Neurosci Lett* 1987;**79**: 138–44.
114. Dishman RK, Renner KJ, Youngstedt SD, *et al.* Activity wheel running reduces escape latency and alters brain monoamine levels after footshock. *Brain Res Bull* 1997;**42**:399–406.
115. Meeusen R, Smolders I, Sarre S, *et al.* Endurance training effects on neurotransmitter release in rat striatum: an *in vivo* microdialysis study. *Acta Physiol Scand* 1997;**159**:335–41.
116. Bland ST, Gonzale RA, Schallert T. Movement-related glutamate levels in rat hippocampus, striatum, and sensorimotor cortex. *Neurosci Lett* 1999;**277**:119–22.
117. Humm JL, Kozlowski DA, Bland ST, *et al.* Use-dependent exaggeration of brain injury: is glutamate involved? *Exp Neurol* 1999;**157**:349–59.

118. Tumer N, Demirel HA, Serova L, *et al.* Gene expression of catecholamine biosynthetic enzymes following exercise: modulation by age. *Neuroscience* 2001;**103**:703–11.
119. Tillerson JL, Caudle WM, Reveron ME, *et al.* Detection of behavioral impairments correlated to neurochemical deficits in mice treated with moderate doses of 1-methyl-4-phenyl-1,2,3,6-tetrahydropyridine. *Exp Neurol* 2002;**178**:80–90.
120. Tillerson JL, Cohen AD, Caudle WM, *et al.* Forced nonuse in unilateral parkinsonian rats exacerbates injury. *J Neurosci* 2002;**22**:6790–9.
121. Tillerson JL, Miller GW. Forced limb-use and recovery following brain injury. *Neuroscientist* 2002;**8**:574–85.
122. Vergara-Aragon P, Gonzalez CL, Whishaw IQ. A novel skilled-reaching impairment in paw supination on the "good" side of the hemi-Parkinson rat improved with rehabilitation. *J Neurosci* 2003;**23**:579–86.
123. Mabandla M, Kellaway L, St Clair Gibson A, *et al.* Voluntary running provides neuroprotection in rats after 6-hydroxydopamine injection into the medial forebrain bundle. *Metab Brain Dis* 2004;**19**:43–50.
124. Howells FM, Russell VA, Mabandla MV, *et al.* Stress reduces the neuroprotective effect of exercise in a rat model for Parkinson's disease. *Behav Brain Res* 2005;**165**:210–20.
125. Poulton NP, Muir GD. Treadmill training ameliorates dopamine loss but not behavioral deficits in hemi-parkinsonian rats. *Exp Neurol* 2005;**193**:181–97.
126. Al-Jarrah M, Pothakos K, Novikova L, *et al.* Endurance exercise promotes cardiorespiratory rehabilitation without neurorestoration in the chronic mouse model of Parkinsonism with severe neurodegeneration. *Neuroscience* 2007;**149**:28–37.
127. Yoon MC, Shin MS, Kim TS, *et al.* Treadmill exercise suppresses nigrostriatal dopaminergic neuronal loss in 6-hydroxydopamine-induced Parkinson's rats. *Neurosci Lett* 2007;**423**:12–7.
128. Jadavji NM, Kolb B, Metz GA. Enriched environment improves motor function in intact and unilateral dopamine-depleted rats. *Neuroscience* 2006;**140**:1127–38.
129. Anstrom KK, Schallert T, Woodlee MT, *et al.* Repetitive vibrissae-elicited forelimb placing before and immediately after unilateral 6-hydroxydopamine improves outcome in a model of Parkinson's disease. *Behav Brain Res* 2007;**179**:183–91.

Chapter 38
Non-Dopaminergic Approaches to the Treatment of Parkinson's Disease

Susan H. Fox[1] *& Jonathan M. Brotchie*[2]
[1]Movement Disorders Clinic, Division of Neurology, University of Toronto, Toronto, ON, Canada
[2]Toronto Western Research Institute, Toronto Western Hospital, Toronto, ON, USA

Introduction

The pathology of Parkinson's disease (PD) primarily involves degeneration of the nigrostriatal dopaminergic pathway resulting in bradykinesia, tremor, and rigidity. As such, the primary treatment for the motor symptoms of PD involves dopamine replacement therapy with dopamine receptor agonists or the dopamine precursor, levodopa. However, over time, PD patients experience motor fluctuations and levodopa-induced dyskinesia (LID). These motor complications result in increased disability and impaired quality-of-life. One potential treatment approach maybe to target non-dopaminergic systems.

The basal ganglia circuitry controlling movement utilizes a range of non-dopaminergic neurotransmitters and neuromodulators. In PD and LID, abnormal dopamine receptor stimulation alters the activity of GABAergic striatal efferents of the "direct" dopamine D_1 and "indirect" dopamine D_2 pathways. Abnormal striatal output, in turn, alters the firing rate, patterning and, most likely, synchronization of neuronal firing, the substantia nigra pars reticulata (SNpr) and internal segment of the globus pallidus (GPi), the output regions of the basal ganglia,. Subsequently, inhibition of motor cortex results in parkinsonian symptoms or excess activation results in LID [1–3]. In addition, the activity of these striatal output pathways is regulated by cortical and subthalamic glutamatergic inputs, striatal cholinergic interneurons, and a range of receptors for neuromodulators, including adenosine, cannabinoids, histamine, opioids, and serotonin.

It is clear that non-dopaminergic systems contribute to the pathophysiology of parkinsonism and several non-dopaminergic approaches have been suggested by preclinical studies. However, to date, no non-dopaminergic drug has shown comparable clinical efficacy to dopaminergic agents in alleviating PD motor symptoms in early or advanced disease. Several preclinical studies have suggested that non-dopaminergic therapies can be used as part of a "levodopa-sparing" strategy to prevent the development of levodopa-induced motor complications. However, clinical studies have generally investigated the effects of non-dopaminergic agents in advanced PD patients receiving large doses of dopaminergic drugs. Not surprisingly, such studies have shown either mild or no benefit in alleviating PD motor symptoms, although several have been demonstrated to reduce wearing-off. Non-dopaminergic approaches have also been studied to try to treat LID directly, potentially to *prevent* the onset of levodopa-induced motor complications, and to address "non-levodopa-responsive" elements of the disease. This chapter discusses how several non-dopaminergic transmitter systems have been investigated as means to address these problems (Table 38.1).

Anti-cholinergics

Acetylcholine receptor antagonists (anti-cholinergics) are the best known, non-dopaminergic agents used in the treatment of PD. The non-selective anti-cholinergics, scopolamine and atropine, were first used in the nineteenth century, and synthetic anti-cholinergics were widely used in the treatment of PD in the pre-levodopa era. In recent years, anti-cholinergics have still occasionally been used for the treatment of parkinsonian tremor [4]. However, side effects related cholinergic blockade, such as dry mouth, sphincter dysfunction, impaired memory, and confusion, often limit the use of these agents. In addition, double-blind, randomized controlled trials (RCTs) using benzhexol, orphenadrine, benztropine, bornaprine, benapryzine, and methixine report variable improvement in PD symptoms, including tremor [5].

Parkinson's Disease: Non-Motor and Non-Dopaminergic Features, First Edition. Edited by C. Warren Olanow, Fabrizio Stocchi, and Anthony E. Lang.

Table 38.1 Neurotransmitter and neuromodulatory systems that have been investigated in animal models and in clinical trials as potential treatments for PD motor symptoms and levodopa-induced dyskinesia[a].

Neurotransmitter	Receptor class	Receptor subtype	Preclinical efficacy			Clinical applicability
			Parkinsonism	Wearing-off	LID	
Acetylcholine	Muscarinic (mAChR)	M_1, M_4, possibly M_3 antagonist	+ (tremor)		+ May reduce levodopa-induced dystonia	Non-selective subtype or M_1-selective mAChR antagonists are in clinical use but have poor tolerability
	Nicotinic (nAChR)	Nonselective agonists			+	
		$\alpha 4\beta 2$ nAChR agonists	+			Not known; SIB-1508Y had poor tolerability
Adenosine	Adenosine antagonist	A_{2A} antagonist	+	+	No LID in primed animals	Istradefylline, as add-on to optimal levodopa, reported variable effects on reducing wearing-off. Good tolerability. BIIB0014, preladenant ongoing studies
Glutamate	NMDA	Nonselective receptor antagonist	– Can worsen at high doses		+ Can reduce chorea but also worsen dystonia	Amantadine in clinical use for LID; may cause side effects and benefit may wane Amantadine also has mild effect on motor symptoms in early PD Memantine, remacemide had no benefit on LID; dextromethorphan reduced LID
		NR2A-NMDA antagonist			– Worsens LID	
		NR2B-NMDA antagonist	+		+/– Can also exacerbate LID	Ifenprodil had no effect on LID or PD disability. CP101,606 and eliprodil – ongoing
	AMPA	AMPA receptor antagonists			+	Talampanel RCT not reported. Perampanel ineffective on LID
	Metabotropic glutamate receptor (mGLuR)	$mGluR_4$ agonist	+			
		$mGluR_5$ antagonist			+	AFQ056 – ongoing
	Glutamate release inhibition			+		Riluzole was ineffective on PD or LID. Safinamide had mild effect on motor symptoms. Zonisamide reduced "off" time but a low dose of levodopa was used. FP0011 improved PD symptoms
Noradrenaline	α_2 adrenoceptors	α_2 agonist			+	Clonidine – ineffective on motor symptoms
		$\alpha_{2A/2C}$ antagonist	+	+	+	Idazoxan: variable effect on LID with poor tolerability. Fipamezole – ongoing

Table 38.1 (*Cont.*)

Neurotransmitter	Receptor class	Receptor subtype	Preclinical efficacy: Parkinsonism	Preclinical efficacy: Wearing-off	Preclinical efficacy: LID	Clinical applicability
Serotonin		5-HT_{1A} agonists	– Or can worsen parkinsonism		+	Mirtazapine can reduce LID and PD tremor. Buspirone and tandospirone reduced LID and worsened PD. Sarizotan reduced LID but worsened PD motor symptoms. Piclozotan and pardoprunox under development
		5-HT_{1B} agonists	–		+	
		5-HT_{2A} antagonists	May worsen parkinsonism		+	ACP 103 – under development Clozapine reduces PD tremor; does not worsen other PD motor symptoms; can reduce LID. Requires regular blood monitoring. Quetiapine – no effect
		5-HT_{2C} receptor antagonists	+		+	
Endocannabinoids	Exogenous cannabinoids	CB_1 agonist	– Worsens parkinsonism		+	Nabilone reduced LID. Cannabidiol/Δ^9-THC extract no effect. No worsening of PD; mild sedative and postural hypotension side effects
		CB_1 antagonist	+		+	Rimonabant – no effect on PD or LID. No adverse effects
	Enhances endocannabinoid levels	FAAH inhibitor	+ (in combination with D2 agonists)			
Opioids		δ-Opioid agonist	+		+	
		κ-Opioid agonist	+/–		+	
		ORL-1 antagonist	+		– Worsens LID with high-dose levodopa	
		Nonselective antagonist			+/– Variable effects	Naloxone (i.v.): variable effects, reduced LID or had no effect; increased "on" time Naltrexone: mild effect at high dose only. No effect on PD; good tolerability
		μ-Opioid antagonist			+	
		δ-Opioid antagonist			+	
Histamine		Histamine H_3 agonist			+	

[a]Key: +, significant positive effect; –, significant negative effect; LID, levodopa-induced dyskinesia; FAAH, fatty-acid amide hydrolase; ORL-1, opioid-like receptor.

Despite their many years of use, the mechanism of action in potentially reducing tremor remains unclear [6].

Muscarinic acetylcholine receptor antagonists

Muscarinic acetylcholine receptors (mAChRs) are widely distributed in the brain; to date, five subtypes of receptor, M_1–M_5, have been described. M_1, M_3, and M_5 are excitatory, whereas M_2 and M_4 are generally inhibitory. The M_1, M_2, and M_4 subtypes are found in the highest levels within the striatum; M_1 and M_4 are located on medium spiny neurons and M_2 is the principal autoreceptor on aspiny cholinergic interneurons [7]. Within the striatum, acetylcholine plays a key role in synaptic function and controls the activity of both the dopamine D_1- and D_2-mediated striatopallidal pathways [8]. In general, when dopamine levels are reduced in the striatum, acetylcholine is released, whereas dopamine D_2 receptor stimulation reduces acetylcholine release [9,10]. Thus increased acetylcholine release and stimulation of M_1 mAChR subtype may contribute to overactivation of the D_2-mediated striatopallidal pathway associated with parkinsonian symptoms [11]. Hence M_1 receptor antagonists would potentially have an anti-parkinsonian action. Trihexyphendyl is a putative M_1 antagonist, but in preclinical studies had only a mild effect on reversing parkinsonism [12] and is rarely useful in treating PD symptoms. On the other hand, activation of inhibitory M_4 receptors on the direct pathway which exert an inhibitory control over D_1 receptor-mediated locomotion may contribute to parkinsonism [13,14]. This suggests that M_4-selective mAChR antagonists might reduce PD symptoms by increasing activity in the D_1-mediated direct pathway [15]. In preclinical studies, an animal model of jaw tremor using pilocarpine has been used to investigate the role of mAChRs in PD tremor [16]. In this model, the M_4 antagonists appear to be the most effective at reducing tremor [17]. Studies in the clinic, however, are limited owing to a lack of highly selective M_4 antagonists that penetrate the blood–brain barrier.

Alternatively, acetylcholine may contribute to the generation of parkinsonian symptoms, in particular PD tremor, via an action in the subthalamic nucleus (STN). Part of the drive for STN overactivity in PD may relate to increased cholinergic input from the pedunculopontine (PPN) [18] that is excitatory [19,20]. Increased stimulation of cholinergic receptors may drive STN activity in PD [21] and possibly tremor. Although there is loss of acetylcholine neurons within the PPN in PD [22], the functional activity of the cholinergic input to the STN and other basal ganglia regions remains unclear. More specifically, cholinergic drive to the STN may facilitate tremor by generating synchronized oscillatory burst discharges at low frequencies. Such oscillatory bursts correlate with tremor; and are controlled by an STN–GPe feedback system that synchronizes the bursting [23]. Activity from this STN–GPe central oscillator is transmitted via trans-cortical pathways to the periphery and is modulated by cholinergic transmission from the PPN to GPi [24]. Anticholinergics which act via the M_3 receptor reduce STN overactivity and thus may have potential anti-parkinsonian actions [25]. Injection of subtype-selective M_3 antagonists into the STN in reserpine-treated rats improves muscle rigidity [26]. To date, no M_3 subtype-selective mAChR antagonists have been investigated in PD. However, as M_3 receptors are widely distributed in both the periphery and CNS, side effects may limit the use of M_3 subtype-selective antagonists in PD.

Muscarinic cholinergic antagonists and levodopa-induced dystonia

Anti-cholinergics are also useful in the treatment of idiopathic dystonia and have been proposed to help levodopa-induced dystonia [27], but may increase chorea [28]. This may occur via an action within the striatum but also possibly within the GPi. Thus, M_1 mAChRs are found within the GPi and in postmortem studies there is an increase in binding of $[^3H]$QNB, a marker of M_1, in the GPi in levodopa-treated PD patients and in MPTP-lesioned primates with dyskinesia [29]. Thus, anticholinergics could induce or worsen chorea or reduce levodopa-induced dystonia [30].

In conclusion, despite some clinical evidence and theoretical rationale for the involvement of enhanced mAChR transmission in the generation of parkinsonian symptoms, at present the precise anatomic or receptor subtype substrates for those actions remain unclear. The development of clinically applicable subtype-selective agents may be required to resolve these issues.

Nicotinic acetylcholine receptor agonists

Although much focus has been placed upon mAChRs, nicotinic acetylcholine receptors (nAChRs) have also been investigated as potential targets for PD treatment. Neuronal nAChRs are composed of multiple subtypes with α and β subunits [31]. To date, several subtypes have been linked to striatal function and are located on GABAergic interneurons, cholinergic interneurons, and dopaminergic terminals, where their activation enhances dopamine release [32]. Given a location on dopaminergic terminals, it is not surprising that reduced levels of nAChRs have been reported in the striatum in animal models of parkinsonism and in postmortem PD studies [33,34]. In preclinical studies, the nonselective nAChR agonist nicotine reduced LID in MPTP-lesioned primates without adversely affecting the anti-parkinsonian actions of levodopa [35]. The mechanism by which this occurs remains to be resolved. Identification of the subtype(s) of nAChRs involved may, in due course, allow this finding to be translated to the clinic. The $\alpha6(^*)$ subtype of nAChRs has shown a relatively selective localization to the nigrostriatal pathway and activation results in striatal dopamine release [36]. Thus, $\alpha 6(*)$ nAChR agonists may enhance dopaminergic effects and provide symptomatic benefits. However, this subtype-selective nicotinic agonist has not yet been investigated in PD [37]. The $\alpha 4\beta 2$ subtype may also be a target for anti-parkinsonian agents. SIB-1508Y, an agonist at $\alpha 4\beta 2$ nAChRs, when combined with a subtherapeutic dose of levodopa, had significant therapeutic benefit in MPTP-lesioned monkeys [38]. However, clinical studies using SIB-1508Y monotherapy in PD patients had poor tolerability [39].

Adenosine A_{2A} antagonists

Adenosine is an endogenous nucleoside found extracellularly in the CNS. Levels of adenosine rise in response to ischemia, hypoxia, neurotoxicity, and inflammation and adenosine receptor antagonists are being investigated as neuroprotective agents [40,41]. Adenosine is also an important neuromodulator within the basal ganglia. Adenosine A_{2A} receptors are selectively located on cell bodies and terminals of GABAergic indirect striatal output pathway neurons and are functionally linked to dopamine D_2 receptor function [42]. Adenosine, via the A_{2A} receptor, may contribute to the overactivity of the indirect pathway in PD by enhancing GABA release in the GPe [43]. Corticostriatal glutamatergic activity via *N*-methyl D-aspartate (NMDA) receptor stimulation is increased in PD and results in adenosine release and stimulation of A_{2A} receptors, an action that may further increase activity of the indirect GABAergic pathway [44].

Changes in adenosine A_{2A} receptors have been reported in PD. In postmortem studies, adenosine A_{2A} mRNA is increased by 60% in the putamen and by 24% in the GPe in PD patients with LID, compared with PD patients without dyskinesia and age-matched controls; perhaps suggesting increased adenosine A_{2A} signaling in the indirect pathway [45]. Studies in MPTP-lesioned primates also showed increased adenosine A_{2A} mRNA in the striatum of animals with LID, an effect reversed by co-treatment with selective NMDA receptor antagonists [46], further linking adenosine A_{2A} receptors with expression of LID.

Several adenosine A_{2A} antagonists are under development as treatments for PD. Preclinical studies have shown that adenosine A_{2A} antagonist monotherapy can alleviate parkinsonism in the 6-hydroxydopamine (6-OHDA)-lesioned rodent model [47–49] and in the MPTP-lesioned primate without inducing LID, even in "primed" animals (i.e., animals that exhibit dyskinesia if treated with levodopa) [50,51]. In combination with a low dose of levodopa, adenosine A_{2A} antagonists can enhance anti-parkinsonian actions without exacerbating LID. Furthermore, if administered in combination with dopaminergic therapy *de novo*, A_{2A} antagonists can prevent the development of dyskinesia.

Istradefylline is a selective A_{2A} antagonist which has anti-parkinsonian actions as monotherapy in MPTP-lesioned primates and does not induce dyskinesia, even in primed animals [52]. Co-treatment of low-dose levodopa with istradefylline potentiated the peak anti-parkinsonian action of levodopa with no significant effect on dyskinesia [53], but it has not been tested in combination with optimal doses of levodopa in MPTP-lesioned primates. Phase IIa clinical studies testing istradefylline (80 mg) monotherapy were ineffective,. In PD patients, istradefylline potentiated the anti-parkinsonian action of low-dose i.v. levodopa and extended its duration of action without affecting LID [54]. However, when given in combination with optimal i.v. doses of levodopa, there was no beneficial effect of istradefylline on dyskinesia or parkinsonism. In a Phase IIb placebo-controlled study in levodopa-treated patients with motor fluctuations, istradefylline [20 and 40 mg per day) significantly reduced "off" time but increased "on" time with dyskinesia [55]. However, in-office assessments of LID showed no significant difference compared with placebo. Phase III studies have reported either modest or no benefit compared with placebo when used as an add-on to optimized dopaminergic therapy [56–60]. Based on these equivocal results, istradefylline did not receive FDA approval for PD and further development has been halted in the USA, but is ongoing in Japan.

Other adenosine A_{2A} antagonists are in earlier stages of development, for example, BIIB0014 [61] and preladenant (SCH 420814) [62]. However, no preclinical data have been published to evaluate the potential efficacy of these agents. Overall, preclinical studies support further testing of adenosine A_{2A} antagonists in PD as monotherapy in an attempt to prevent dyskinesia, and in combination with a low dose of levodopa, to enhance the anti-parkinsonian action without exacerbating LID. This is supported by a single Phase II study. It is important to appreciate that Phase III trials performed to date have not been designed to replicate benefits seen in monkey studies, so it remains unresolved as to whether these agents will be effective in the clinic.

Glutamate antagonists

The neural mechanisms underlying both PD and LID involve enhanced corticostriatal glutamatergic activity [3,63]. In PD, this may result in increased activity of the dopamine D_2-mediated indirect GABAergic pathway, possibly via an interaction with adenosine A_{2A} receptors (see above). In contrast, in LID, enhanced glutamatergic activity may drive increased activity of the dopamine

D_1-mediated direct pathway, with resultant inhibition of basal ganglia outputs [3]. Enhanced corticostriatal activity is thought to be mediated by phosphorylation of subunits of the NMDA and AMPA receptors, involving changes in the subcellular distribution of subunits between the synapse and cytoplasm and/or alterations in the adaptor proteins to which these receptors bind and which regulate their function [64,65]. In addition, glutamate receptors are critical to synaptic plasticity, and in parkinsonism and LID, abnormal synaptic plasticity similar to long-term depression (LTD) and long-term potentiation (LTP) seen in the hippocampus likely contribute to symptom generation. Thus, in the striatum in PD, loss of LTD in the indirect pathway may lead to enhanced glutamatergic signaling and overactivity of that pathway. In contrast, abnormal LTP may contribute to the development of dyskinesia and motor fluctuations [66,67]. Hence modulating glutamate activity may reduce PD motor symptoms and LID.

NMDA receptor antagonists

Preclinical studies in the MPTP-lesioned primate demonstrate that NMDA-selective glutamate antagonists, for example, MK801 and LY235959, reduce levodopa-induced dyskinesia but may exacerbate levodopa-induced dystonia and worsen parkinsonism [68–70]. The NMDA receptor antagonist amantadine has been shown in preclinical studies to reduce levodopa-induced dyskinesia (by 95%) but to worsen motor features when combined with low-dose, but not high-dose, levodopa [71,72]. Amantadine is now a well-established therapy for LID in PD [73,74]. Clinical trials in relatively small numbers of PD patients [75] have demonstrated a dyskinesia reduction of 24–60% [76–78] without worsening of PD motor symptoms, probably reflecting its use with relatively high doses of levodopa [79]. In clinical practice, only a proportion of PD patients respond well to amantadine and many experience tachyphylaxis [80]. Follow-up studies report maintained benefit after 1 year [81], but longer-term follow up studies have not been reported. Some PD patients experience side effects, including hallucinations, confusion, livedo reticularis, and edema, which limit its use. Hyperpyrexia with sudden withdrawal of amantadine has been reported [82], and slow taper is advised. There are isolated reports of amantadine benefit for fatigue [83], prevention of cognitive problems [84], as a predictor of survival in PD [85], possibly via GDNF-mediated action [86], and as a treatment for punding [87]. The related uncompetitive NMDA receptor antagonist memantine, in contrast to amantadine, had no significant effect on dyskinesia in 12 PD patients assessed in a cross-over design [88]. This agent, however, is effective in the treatment of cognitive problems in Alzheimer's disease [89] and may also be helpful in treating PD dementia.

Other NMDA receptor antagonists have shown variable efficacy for dyskinesia. Remacemide did not show any significant benefit compared with placebo in 39 PD patients [90], whereas dextromethorphan (which also activates sigma receptors) improved dyskinesia in a rat model of PD [91] and in a small clinical study (six patients), without affecting parkinsonism [92]

Theoretically, NMDA antagonists should reduce overactivity of the indirect pathway and alleviate parkinsonian symptoms, although this has not been demonstrated with the compounds discussed above, presumably because any benefit afforded by reducing activity of the indirect pathway would be countered by reducing activity of the direct pathway (amantadine can have a mild symptomatic effect in early PD, but this may be via a dopaminergic action). Given these issues, the next development would be to identify a selective agonist that targets the subtype of NMDA receptor specifically involved in the generation of parkinsonism and LID.

NMDA receptors are composed of subunits belonging to two major families, termed NR1 and NR2, the latter existing in four major forms, NR2A–D. The differential combination of these subunits produces subtypes of NMDA receptors with different functional and pharmacologic properties. Thus, NMDA receptor antagonists with selectivity for NR2B-containing receptors can improve parkinsonian symptoms as monotherapy (e.g., ifenprodil [93]), potentiate the anti-parkinsonian effects of levodopa (e.g., CP-101,606 [94,95]), reduce LID (e.g., Co 101244 [96]), and prevent the development of dyskinesia in *de novo* levodopa-treated animals (e.g., CI 1041 [97]). There is some inconsistency with respect to the ability of NR2B antagonists to reduce established dyskinesia. Thus, Co 101244 reduces LID whereas CP101,606 exacerbates dyskinesia. This discrepancy may relate to the molecular mechanism of action of these different drugs [94], and reduction of LID may not be a general property of all NR2B antagonists. In MPTP-lesioned monkeys, a selective NR2A receptor antagonist, MDL 100,453, exacerbated established dyskinesia by 25% [96]. Overall subtype-selective NMDA antagonists with actions at NR2B-containing NMDA receptors appear the most promising for clinical development.

There are currently only a few available agents in these categories and to date clinical studies have reported no benefit in reducing LID or on parkinsonism (e.g., ifenprodil [96], CP 101,606 [98], and eliprodil [99]), although the one compound shown to be effective in the monkey, Co 101244, has not been evaluated in the clinic [96].

AMPA receptor antagonists

Selective AMPA receptor antagonists have demonstrated efficacy in preclinical studies but clinical benefit is unclear. The selective AMPA receptor antagonist talampanel significantly reduced LID by up to 40%, with no effect on parkinsonism [100], but results from a large clinical trial have not been reported [101]. The selective non-competitive AMPA-receptor antagonist parampanel reduced LID in MPTP-lesioned primates but was ineffective in clinical trials and development has been discontinued [102]. Sub-therapeutic doses of the AMPA antagonist GYKI-47261 combined with amantadine were reported to reduce dyskinesia by 51%; the effect on parkinsonism was not reported [103].

Metabotropic glutamate receptor agonists and antagonists

Targeting metabotropic glutamate receptors (mGluRs) has been investigated in PD and may be a better option than NMDA or AMPA antagonists due to a wider therapeutic index [104]. $mGluR_4$ agonists reduce GABA release from terminals of the indirect pathway [105] and alleviate parkinsonian symptoms in rodents [106,107], but have not been tested in primates or patients. Levels of $mGluR_5$ are enhanced in the striatum of MPTP-lesioned primates with LID [108] and $mGluR_5$ antagonists reduce LID in rodents [109,1110]. No demonstration of anti-dyskinetic effects with $mGluR_5$ antagonists have been reported in PD patients; however, AFQ056, a presumed $mGluR_5$ receptor antagonist, is under development for LID [111].

Glutamate release inhibition

Other agents that may potentially reduce overactive glutamate neurotransmission in PD include riluzole, which acts to inhibit glutamate release by blocking activated Na^+ channels. However, this agent had no significant effect on parkinsonism or LID in a small trial in 15 PD patients [112]. The anti-epileptic agents safinamide and zonisamide both have multiple modes of action, including MAO-B inhibition and glutamate release inhibition. Safinamide, as an adjunct to dopamine agonists, benefits motor symptoms in early PD and delays the need for levodopa at doses thought to inhibit glutamate release rather than MAO-B [113–115]. In advanced PD, safinamide decreased motor fluctuations in 13 patients [116]. Further studies are ongoing [117]. Zonisamide was efficacious in small studies in advanced PD patients with motor fluctuations [118]. A large Phase III trial reported a significant reduction in "off" time [–1.3 h (50 mg) and –1.63 h (100 mg) compared with –0.2 h (placebo)] [118]. There was also a significant improvement in "on" period motor UPDRS scores and there was no significant effect on dyskinesia. Further studies are required to evaluate fully the mechanism of action and effects in PD patients with motor fluctuations taking higher doses of levodopa. FP00011 is a novel glutamate release inhibitor that improved motor symptoms in MPTP-lesioned primates [119] and in a small clinical trial in PD patients [120].

Noradrenaline

The role of noradrenaline (NA) and adrenergic receptors in PD remains unclear, but topical and potentially therapeutically relevant. Indeed, the differences in antiparkinsonian action between levodopa and dopamine receptor agonists may relate to the former's ability to act as a precursor for noradrenaline as well as dopamine. The locus coeruleus contains noradrenergic cell bodies and sends projections to the cerebral cortex, hypothalamus, and the basal ganglia [121]. Noradrenergic terminals, uptake sites, and receptors are located within the striatum, STN, and substantia nigra [122,123]. The neurodegenerative processes in PD involve Lewy body pathology within the locus coeruleus [124,125] with noradrenergic cell loss between 50 and 80% compared with 40% loss in normal age-matched controls [126]. Of interest, a *parkin* null (exon 7) mouse model has a selective loss of catecholamine cells in the locus coeruleus, and deficiency of NA, although no impairment of nigrostriatal dopamine [127]. In limited postmortem studies in PD patients with *parkin* mutations, there is loss of dopamine SNpc cells and also locus coeruleus neurons [128,129]. Thus, loss of LC neurons is characteristic of both idiopathic PD and monogenic parkinsonism. Loss of LC neurons results in reduced NA in the striatum, particularly caudate and nucleus accumbens and cortex in animal models of parkinsonism and PD patients [130–134]. Platelet levels of α_2 adrenoceptors are reduced in untreated PD, but this is reversed with levodopa [135]. Within the brain, α_{2A} receptor levels are reduced in the prefrontal cortex of PD patients[136], suggesting that loss of noradrenergic neurotransmission is linked to non-motor symptoms such as dementia [137], depression [138,139], and alertness [140]. Loss of noradrenaline in PD is also associated with orthostatic hypotension [141] and gait and balance dysfunction [142].

Noradrenergic system and motor symptoms of PD

Despite the evidence for NA having a role in non-motor symptoms, its role in motor symptoms is less well defined. There is little evidence to suggest that NA replacement has any therapeutic effect in PD. Clonidine, an α_2 adrenoceptor agonist, was ineffective in alleviating symptoms in PD when administered both with and without levodopa [143,144]. This may not be surprising as clonidine can reduce NA release due to an inhibitory effect on LC firing [145] with reduced stimulation of adrenoceptors. The use of α_2 adrenoceptor antagonists that enhance NA release may be a better approach.

In animal models of PD, α_2 adrenergic receptor antagonists reverse reserpine-induced parkinsonism [146], increase locomotor activity in 6-OHDA-lesioned rats

[147], and potentiate the effect of apomorphine [148, 149]. In MPTP-lesioned primates, monotherapy with the α_{2A} adrenoceptor antagonist idazoxan improved motor symptoms, although to only a moderate extent [150]. Moreover, idazoxan and fipamezole enhanced the anti-parkinsonian actions of levodopa [151,152]. The site of action mediating these effects remains unclear, however, but may involve reduced activation of the STN [147] and increased dopamine release as lesioning the locus coeruleus in normal rats decreases striatal dopamine release [153].

α_2 Adrenoceptor antagonists and dyskinesia

Clinical investigation of α_2 antagonists in PD has focused primarily on their potential to reduce LID. Within the striatum, the α_{2C} adrenoceptors are located on GABAergic spiny neurons [154] and appear to modulate activity of the direct striatopallidal pathway, possibly by regulating GABA release [155]. Thus, reducing activity of the overactive direct striatopallidal pathway via α_{2C} receptor antagonism may reduce LID, as highlighted in a seminal study in MPTP macaques [69]. Thus, the α_2 adrenoceptor antagonist yohimbine reduced LID without affecting the anti-parkinsonian actions of L-dopa. Subsequent studies using selective α_2 adrenoceptor antagonists idazoxan, rauwolscine, and fipamezole in MPTP-lesioned primates confirmed these findings and showed a significant increase in "on" time [152,156,157]. α_2 Adrenoceptor antagonism may reduce LID by enhancing the release of NA, produced from metabolic conversion of levodopa into NA [158]. Thus, in MPTP-lesioned primates, idazoxan significantly reduces LID, but not dyskinesia induced by the direct-acting dopamine receptor agonist apomorphine [151].

In Phase IIa studies, idazoxan reduced LID following an acute levodopa challenge in 20 PD patients, although at higher doses a paradoxical increase in LID was noted [159]. Another study in eight advanced PD patients with LID showed no significant effect of idazoxan on apomorphine-induced dyskinesia [160], confirming the findings in monkeys and suggesting that the anti-dyskinesia effect of α_2 antagonists is due to blocking NA effects resulting from levodopa metabolism. A Phase III study of idazoxan in LID has not been reported and it is currently not being further developed for PD. Fipamezole, another selective $\alpha_{2A/2C}$ adrenoceptor, showed a significant reduction in LID and prolonged levodopa duration of action in 21 PD patients [161]. A larger multicenter study is ongoing [162].

Serotonin

The serotonergic system is a widely distributed neurotransmitters system, innervating virtually all regions of the CNS. Serotonin participates in many basic physiologic functions, such as sleep, arousal, feeding, and satiety, in addition to more complex activities such as emotion and cognition. The diverse functions of the serotonergic system are exemplified by the 14 distinct subtypes of 5-HT receptors. The dense serotonergic innervation of the basal ganglia, particularly the striatum and the output regions of the basal ganglia (SNpr and GPi) [163], from the dorsal raphe nuclei (DRN) suggest a role in movement also [164]. In advanced PD, there is approximately 30–60% depletion of serotonin in the caudate, hypothalamus, and frontal cortex [130,165], which may be secondary to neurodegeneration within the raphe nuclei [166,167]. Imaging studies demonstrated decreased serotonin transporter binding in thee striatum in PD, further suggesting depletion of serotonergic innervation [168,169].

5-HT receptors and PD motor symptoms

Most studies of 5-HT in PD have focused on LID, as serotonergic agents appear to have no benefit on motor features [170,171]. Further, serotonergic agents such as SSRIs have been reported to worsen PD [172], although epidemiologic studies suggest that this is not a significant problem [173]. However, clinical studies suggest that 5-HT may be involved in PD tremor, as mirtazapine, a 5-HT_{1A} agonist and 5-HT_2 and 5-HT_3 antagonist, reduces parkinsonian tremors [174]. Several studies have reported that clozapine, which binds to $5\text{-HT}_{2A/2C}$ receptors, also suppresses PD tremor [175–177], although this may relate to its anti-cholinergic properties. A PET study in advanced PD patients showed a 27% reduction in midbrain raphe 5-HT_{1A} binding that correlated with tremor, but not bradykinesia or rigidity [178].

5-HT_{2C} receptor antagonists

5-HT_{2C} receptors are a potentially useful therapeutic target. In the brain, 5-HT_{2C} receptors are selectively located within the output regions of the basal ganglia, SNpr and GPi, with moderate expression in the STN and caudate [179]. 5-HT_{2C} receptor binding is increased in the SNpr in advanced PD [180]. Serotonin binding to $5\ \text{HT}_{2C}$ receptors is excitatory in the SNpr and GPi [181,182] and stimulation may contribute to increased activity of these structures in PD. Systemic administration of selective 5-HT_{2C} antagonists to 6-OHDA-lesioned rodents potentiates the anti-parkinsonian action of dopamine D_1 and D_2 agonists [183–185]. 5-HT_{2C} receptor antagonism may therefore be the mechanism whereby the atypical neuroleptics clozapine and quetiapine, which have dopamine D_2 antagonist effects, can be used in PD without worsening motor symptoms. Subtype-selective 5-HT_{2C} receptor antagonists have not been further investigated in PD.

5-HT$_{1B}$ agonists

5-HT$_{1B}$ receptors are selectively located within the basal ganglia on terminals of 5-HT neurons in the striatum and on GABAergic striatopallidal output neurons in the SNpr and globus pallidus, suggesting a potential role in movement [186,187]. A postmortem study demonstrated no change in 5-HT$_{1B}$ receptors levels within the stratum and substantia nigra in six PD patients compared with age-matched controls [188]. However, opportunities for targeting 5-HT$_{1B}$ receptors in parkinsonism may exist. Thus, 5-HT activation of 5-HT$_{1B}$ receptors suppresses GABA release in the GPe in normal awake monkeys [189] and in the homologous structure, the globus pallidus, in brain slices prepared from normal rats [190]. This action would reduce inhibition of the indirect pathway and have an anti-parkinsonian action. The 5-HT$_{1B}$ agonist CP-93129, when injected into the globus pallidus in reserpine-lesioned rats, improved akinesia [191]. Systemic administration of a 5-HT$_{1B}$ agonist in the MPTP-lesioned primate, however, had no anti-parkinsonism effect [192]. Studies of 5-HT$_{1B}$ agonists have focused more on a potential effect on LID.

5-HT receptors and dyskinesia

5-HT$_{1A}$ receptors in the DRN and striatum, 5-HT$_{1B}$ receptors on striatopallidal pathways, and 5-HT$_{2A/2C}$ receptors within the SNpr and GPi modulate dopamine, GABA, and glutamate release and have attracted interest as possible therapies for LID.

5-HT$_{1A}$ agonists

5-HT$_{1A}$ receptors are located on cell bodies of the DRN, where they inhibit cell firing, [193]. Neurodegeneration in PD results in a loss of 5-HT input from DRN to the striatum, albeit to a lesser extent than the loss of dopamine. Levodopa can be converted to dopamine in remaining serotonergic neurons, and its non-physiologic release from striatal serotonergic terminals may result in abnormal stimulation of dopamine receptors in striatopallidal pathways leading to dyskinesia [194]. Presynaptic 5-HT$_{1A}$ agonists might reduce dyskinesia by suppressing levodopa-derived dopamine release from 5-HT striatal inputs, but possibly with worsening parkinsonism. 5-HT$_{1A}$ agonists might also reduce LID through postsynaptic reduction of glutamatergic activity in the striatum [195], or pallidum [189], although effects on GPe might exacerbate parkinsonism whereas effects on GPi might alleviate parkinsonism but exacerbate LID. Therefore, depending on relative actions in different regions, 5HT$_{1A}$ agonists could have different effects on motor function.

In the 6-OHDA-lesioned rat, selective 5-HT$_{1A}$ agonists can reduce LID [194,196–198]. In MPTP-lesioned primates, selective 5-HT$_{1A}$ agonists reduced LID by 50%, but worsened parkinsonism [199]. In MPTP-lesioned monkeys, the 5-HT$_{1A}$ receptor agonist sarizotan reduced LID by >90% and had no adverse effect on parkinsonism, and these effects were blocked by the selective 5-HT$_{1A}$ antagonist WAY 100635 [200]. These contrasting results suggest that there may be differences between doses of drug, species, or the detailed pharmacology of individual agonists that define the relative distribution of actions of systemically administered drugs in different basal ganglia regions.

Clinical studies have been performed with 5-HT$_{1A}$ agonists. A small Phase II trial reported that buspirone reduced LID without worsening parkinsonian disability [201]. A buspirone-like drug, tandospirone citrate, improved dyskinesia in five of 10 PD patients, but with worsening parkinsonism [202]. Sarizotan (10 mg) reduced LID by 40% in 18 advanced PD patients, without affecting the anti-parkinsonian action of optimal levodopa infusion [203], and reduced LID in 64 PD patients, but doses had to be reduced in 50% because of worsening parkinsonism [204]. However, in a large double-blind trial (398 PD patients), sarizotan [2, 4, 10 mg per d) failed to reduce "on" time without dyskinesia, compared with placebo [205]. The lower dose improved activities of daily living without worsening parkinsonism, but higher doses were associated with increased "off" time and no effect on LID. Two additional double-blind trials [206,207] of 2 mg sarizotan showed no significant improvement in LID [208]. These studies suggest that either 5-HT$_{1A}$ agonists have to be used at a critical dose due to their potential to reduce dopamine release or glutamate activity, or, in the case of sarizotan, PD worsening may be related to its actions as a dopamine D_2/D_3 receptor antagonist [209]. In any case, it appears that it may be difficult in the clinic to define a window for 5-HT$_{1A}$ agonists that can provide anti-dyskinetic benefit without compromising anti-parkinsonian efficacy.

The non-selective anti-depressant mirtazapine, which acts as a 5-HT$_{1A}$ agonist and 5-HT$_2$ and 5-HT$_3$ antagonist, and has noradrenergic and anti-cholinergic actions, has also been reported to improve LID without worsening parkinsonism in open-label studies [210,211]. Other agents under development include piclozotan, a highly selective 5-HT$_{1A}$ agonist with 1000-fold selectivity over dopamine D_2 receptors [212]. Pardoprunox (SLV308) is a 5-HT$_{1A}$ agonist and also a partial dopamine $D_{2/3}$ agonist that is also under development for PD, but the effects on dyskinesia are unknown [213].

5-HT$_{1B}$ agonists

5-HT$_{1B}$ agonists have also been investigated in LID. In the 6-OHDA-lesioned rat, chronic levodopa induces an increase in 5-HT$_{1B}$ receptors and p11 (a protein involved in the functional expression of 5-HT$_{1B}$ receptors) on the D1-mediated striatonigral pathway [214]. Stimulation of striatal 5-HT$_{1B}$ receptors can reduce 5-HT release [215] and dopamine release from serotonergic neurons analogous to that proposed for 5-HT_{1A} receptors [194]. Stimulation of 5-HT_{1B} receptors in SNpr also reduces GABA release [216]. These mechanisms might be expected to reduce LID, but with potential to exacerbate parkinsonian features.

Preclinical studies have shown that selective 5-HT_{1B} agonists can reduce LID in 6-OHDA-lesioned rats [194,214]. In the MPTP-lesioned primate, the non-selective 5-HT_{1B} agonist SKF-99101 reduced LID but worsened parkinsonism [192]. The non-selective serotonergic drug MDMA also reduced LID in MPTP-lesioned primates by stimulation of 5-HT_{1B} receptors [199]. Hence 5-HT_{1B} agonists are plausible candidates for development as anti-dyskinetic agents, although these drugs may depend on selective basal ganglia activity and have a narrow therapeutic window. Despite the widespread clinical availability of agents of this class, no clinical trials have evaluated selective 5-HT_{1B} agonists in PD.

5-HT_{2A} antagonists

5-HT_{2A} receptors are the most widely distributed subtype of 5-HT receptor in the brain, found predominantly in the multiple areas of cortex, basal ganglia, and claustrum. In PD, a postmortem study showed an increase in 5-HT_{2A} receptors in the neocortex of PD patients[217]. In the 6-OHDA-lesioned rat, there was increased 5-HT_{2A} mRNA in the striatum but not cortex or STN [218,219]. Following long-term levodopa therapy, this increase was reversed [219], suggesting that striatal 5-HT_{2A} receptors are modulated by nigrostriatal dopamine function [220].

In preclinical studies, a selective 5-HT_{2A} receptor antagonist, M100907, failed to reduce LID in the 6-OHDA-lesioned rat but reduced dyskinesia induced by the dopamine D_1 agonist SKF82958 [221]. Studies in the MPTP-lesioned primate have shown that methysergide, a nonselective 5-HT_2 antagonist, can reduce LID, but with adverse effects on parkinsonism [69]. Low-dose clozapine (which binds to both 5-HT_{2A} and 5-HT_{2C} receptors) ($0.1\,mg\,kg^{-1}$) significantly reduced LID in the MPTP-lesioned primate, without exacerbating parkinsonism. However, higher doses ($1.0\,mg\,kg^{-1}$) worsened parkinsonism [222]. In contrast, in another study using the same dose of clozapine ($1.0\,mg\,kg^{-1}$), there was a significant reduction in LID in MPTP-lesioned primates without worsening parkinsonism [223]. Quetiapine, which also has $5HT_{2A/2C}$ antagonist properties, significantly reduced LID in MPTP-lesioned primates, without affecting parkinsonism [223,224].

In clinical studies, a single RCT, using low-dose clozapine (average dose 39 mg per day) demonstrated a significant effect on LID without worsening PD [225]. The reduction was only in LID when measured at rest and not when the patient was performing activities, hence the clinical applicability is unclear. In addition, clozapine requires regular monitoring for the risk of agranulcytosis. In a Phase IIa study, quetiapine did not have an anti-dyskinetic effect compared with placebo, although a very low dose (25 mg) was used [226]. A selective 5-HT_{2A} receptor inverse agonist, ACP-103, is under development for LID. A double-blind, RCT Phase II trial of ACP-103 in 12 PD patients with LID and motor complications demonstrated good tolerability and reduced dyskinesia, without worsening of parkinsonian symptoms [227].

Endocannabinoid system

The medicinal properties of naturally occurring cannabinoids, derived from the plant, *Cannabis sativa* (marijuana), have been known for millennia. Anecdotal reports have suggested benefit in muscle spasms, pain, and seizures. However, concerns regarding the cognitive and psychotropic effects of cannabinoids have limited the clinical development of these drugs. Currently, the oral cannabinoid drugs nabilone and dronabinol are licensed in some territories for clinical use in nausea and anorexia, and the mixed cannabinoid preparation spray Δ^9-tetrahydrocannabinol + cannabinol is licensed for pain.

The role of cannabinoids in locomotion is well known; indeed, a classical cannabinomimetic effect in animals is parkinsonian symptoms with reduced locomotion and rigidity [228,229]. The discovery in the 1990s of receptors for exogenous cannabinoids including *Cannabis sativa*, namely the cannabinoid CB_1 and CB_2 receptors (CB_2 receptors are principally located and function in the immune system and are not considered here), and the endogenous ligands (endocannabinoids) anandamide and 2-arachidonylglycerol (2-AG) has led to an explosion of research in this field.

A role for the endocannabinoid system in movement is suggested by high concentrations of CB_1 receptors within the basal ganglia. Within the striatum, CB_1 receptors are located on dendrites, cell bodies, and terminals of the GABAergic medium spiny neurons, paravalbumin positive interneurons, and glutamatergic terminals [230,231]. Striatal endocannabinoid synthesis and release are under dopaminergic control [232] and receptor stimulation can modulate GABA [233–235] and glutamate transmission [236–238]. In GPe, GPi, and SNpr, CB_1 receptor stimulation enhances GABA levels either by increasing release or decreasing reuptake. Within the output regions of the basal ganglia, CB_1 stimulation reduces glutamate release from STN afferents. Thus cannabinoid receptor stimulation modulates multiple neurotransmitter systems within the basal ganglia circuitry and, depending on the site of action, may play a role in the pathophysiology of parkinsonism and LID.

The cannabinoid system is an attractive target in PD, as opportunities exist for both anti-parkinsonian and anti-dyskinetic actions, and several means to obtain these effects are apparent. To date, studies of CB_1 receptor ligands have focused on LID because of their effect on locomotion [233,239], whereas in untreated PD, endogenous cannabinoids have been evaluated. As with other neurotransmitters/modulators discussed in this chapter, the multiplicity of actions makes translation to clinical efficacy a challenge. Beneficial actions in one region of the basal ganglia circuit may be compromised by adverse actions elsewhere. Similarly, opposing manipulations of endocannabinoid function may have the same clinical outcome depending on which brain region is preferentially targeted.

Cannabinoid modulation and PD

In untreated PD patients, increased endocannabinoids are found in cerebrospinal fluid [240], and enhanced endocannabinoid levels have been reported in the striatum of animal models [241–243]. Because of their potential to reduce glutamate, this enhancement of endocannabinoids may represent a compensation for dopamine loss and an attempt to reduce excitation in the indirect pathway that leads to parkinsonian symptoms. On one level, stimulation of CB_1 receptors decreases corticostriatal glutamatergic transmission by promoting the reuptake mechanism and indirect stimulation of presynaptic mGluRs [237]. In addition, an increase in endogenous cannabinoids may induce plasticity of glutamatergic corticostriatal synapses. Thus in parkinsonism, overactivity of the indirect striatopallidal pathway may be due in part to reduced ability to undergo long-term depression (LTD), an effect dependent upon not only stimulation of D_2 dopamine receptors but also endocannabinoids [244].

Given these actions, enhancing endocannabinoids may result in enhanced compensation and suppression of PD motor symptoms. Fatty acid amide hydrolase (FAAH) is involved in the breakdown of endocannabinoids and inhibition of FAAH reduces excitatory striatal glutamate activity in 6-OHDA-lesioned rats [242]. Combined treatment of 6-OHDA-lesioned or reserpinized rats with dopamine D_2 agonists and URB597, a selective inhibitor of endocannabinoid degradation, reversed parkinsonism [244]. However, no anti-parkinsonian action of monotherapy with FAAH inhibitors has yet been described. Alternatively, enhanced extra-striatal endocannabinoids may contribute to the generation, rather than suppression, of parkinsonian symptoms. Thus, in reserpinized rats and untreated MPTP-lesioned primates, there are increased levels of endocannabinoids in the GPe [241,243]. By stimulating CB_1 receptors within the GPe, and reducing GABA reuptake [245], endocannabinoids may reduce GPe activity, a key abnormality in PD. Indeed, the CB_1-selective antagonist rimonabant has a mild effect on reversal of motor symptoms in the 6-OHDA-lesioned rat [246] and the MPTP-lesioned primate [243]. In addition, the selective CB_1 antagonist carboxylic acid amide benzenesulfonate (CE) enhanced the anti-parkinsonian actions of levodopa in MPTP-lesioned primates [247]. That these agents do not completely alleviate parkinsonian symptoms may reflect a balance between anti-parkinsonian actions and suppression of striatal compensatory mechanisms, thus exacerbating parkinsonism. It is likely that there may be only a narrow window of therapeutic doses for the anti-parkinsonian action of CB_1 antagonists or that a means of selectively targeting GPe may be required to appreciate these actions fully. Indeed, a small trial of rimonabant as add-on therapy in four advanced PD patients reported no effect on PD motor symptoms, although there were no adverse effects [248]. To date, no further clinical studies have been performed.

Cannabinoid modulation and LID

Cannabinoid CB_1 receptor agonists or enhancement of endocannabinoid levels might treat LID by reducing overactive corticostriatal glutamate activity (see above). Stimulation of CB_1 receptors on striatopallidal terminals of indirect pathway GABAergic neurons also reduces GABA reuptake [249,250] and thus GPe activity. In preclinical studies, the cannabinoid agonist WIN55,212 reduced levodopa-induced hyperkinesias in reserpinized rats [251], whereas WIN55,212 and the FAAH inhibitor UEB597 reduced abnormal involuntary movements in the 6-OHDA-lesioned rat model of LID [252,253], and the cannabinoid agonist nabilone reduced LID in MPTP-treated monkeys without affecting the anti-parkinsonian action of levodopa [254]. In an acute challenge cross-over study in seven PD patients, nabilone significantly reduced "on"-period dyskinesia and "off"-period dystonia [250]. There was no effect on parkinsonian disability but all patients experienced side effects, including mild sedation and dizziness. Another trial using an oral extract of *Cannabis sativa* containing Δ^9-tetrahydrocannabinol and cannabidiol showed no significant effect on LID [255]. No further studies have yet been performed to assess the effects of cannabinoid receptor stimulation in LID. However, several case reports have suggested a potential use for cannabinoids in focal dystonia [256–258], but a randomized trial failed to show benefit in idiopathic generalized dystonia [259].

In apparent contradiction to the above, studies in rodents suggest that the CB_1 cannabinoid receptor antagonist rimonabant may potentially reduce LID [251]. In the MPTP-lesioned marmoset, rimonabant significantly reduced LID, without affecting parkinsonian disability [243]. The mechanism of action is not clear, although likely different from that of CB_1 agonists. Hence endocannabinoid-mediated enhancement of GABA transmission from terminals of the direct pathway is suggested as being a component of the mechanism leading to enhanced direct pathway signaling in LID. CB1 receptor antagonists, by reversing this, would have anti-dyskinetic properties. However, despite the strong preclinical data, rimonabant had no significant effect on LID as assessed by UPDRS IV and an acute levodopa challenge using a modified AIMS scale [248].

The ability of both cannabinoid receptor stimulation and blockade to alleviate parkinsonism and LID highlights the fact that cannabinoid neurotransmission is differentially altered in basal ganglia pathways, under different conditions. Depending on the site of action, and possibly dose administered, CB_1 receptor modulation could lead to a range of clinical effects. Future development of cannabinoids in PD also needs to focus on safety and development of tolerance with long-term use of cannabinoids.

Opioid system

Opioid peptides and their precursors are located within the basal ganglia and act as modulators of GABA, dopamine, and glutamate neurotransmission. The effects of opioid peptides are mediated via δ, μ, and κ receptor subtypes, all of which are found in high concentration within the striatum, co-localized on GABAergic neurons, and throughout the basal ganglia in regions receiving input from the striatum. The striatopallidal GABAergic projection neurons are segregated with respect to the opioid peptides used as co-transmitters. Thus, indirect striatopallidal projection neurons express enkephalins derived from the precursor pre-proenkephalin A (PPE-A), whereas striatonigral neurons of the direct pathway express opioids derived from pre-proenkephalin B (PPE-B) [260], [261]. PPE-A is the precursor for leu- and met-enkephalins, which predominantly activate δ-opioid receptors. The opioid peptides derived from PPE-B include dynorphin A and B, α-neoendorphin, and β-neoendorphin and activate δ, μ, and κ subtypes of opioid receptors with varying levels of selectivity [262,263]. Other endogenous opioids found within the basal ganglia are endomorphin 1 and 2, the precursor for which is unknown; these predominantly activate μ-opioid receptors. Another opioid peptide system found in the striatum, SNpc, and SNpr is nociceptin/orphanin FQ and its receptor the opioid-like receptor (ORL1) or N/OFQ peptide (NOP) receptor.

Opioids and PD motor symptoms

Regulation of levels of basal ganglia opioid peptides is closely linked to dopamine levels and dopamine receptor stimulation. However, the role of opioids in PD remains unclear. In particular, it remains unknown if opioid peptides play a role in mediating motor dysfunction or are simply a compensatory effect consequent to altered firing patterns based on the pathologic abnormality, or a plastic mechanism attempting to compensate for breakdown in dopaminergic function. Thus, in the dopamine-depleted striatum, PPEA mRNA and enkephalin protein levels are elevated and striatal PPE-B mRNA and dynorphin levels are decreased [261,264–266]. Given the localization of PPE-A to the indirect pathway and the understanding that increased activity of the indirect striatopallidal GABAergic pathway is critical to the development of parkinsonian symptoms, a role for enkephalin in parkinsonism has long been proposed.

Enkephalin activation of δ-opioid receptors in the GPe reduces GABA release from the indirect pathway, hence elevated levels may be a compensatory attempt to reduce activity of the indirect striaopallidal pathway [245,267]. In MPTP-treated macaques, elevation of PPE-A mRNA has been demonstrated prior to the onset of motor symptoms, suggesting a compensatory role for loss of dopamine, rather than a mediator of, or response to, symptoms [268]. Enhancement of this compensatory mechanism provides an attractive means to try to alleviate parkinsonian symptoms. Indeed, in rodent and primate models of PD, δ-opioid agonists have anti-parkinsonian actions [269,270] that are of the same magnitude as dopaminergic replacement.

Given the reduction in PPE-B and dynorphin in neurons of the direct pathway in parkinsonism, dynorphin replacement therapy might seem attractive. Moreover, reduced stimulation of κ-opioid receptors in the striatum and GPi would enhance glutamate release in these regions [271,272], which could contribute to the generation of parkinsonian symptoms. Indeed, the κ-opioid agonist enadoline enhanced locomotion in reserpine-treated rats and reversed parkinsonism in MPTP-lesioned primates [271,273]. However, another κ-opioid agonist, U50,488, worsened PD [274]. To date, no subtype-selective opioid agonists have been assessed in PD.

Nociceptin/orphanin FQ, via ORL1 activation, reduces dopamine neurotransmission and increases GABA and glutamate release. In rodent studies, the selective ORL1 antagonist J113397 reduced parkinsonism [275,276] and potentiated the effects of sub-therapeutic doses of levodopa [277]. In MPTP-lesioned primates, J113397 enhances the actions of high dose levodopa by reducing glutamate release in the SNpr and enhancing nigrostriatal dopaminergic neurotransmission, but with increased LID [278]. Further research is required to define how, and whether, it is possible to combine ORL1 antagonists with levodopa to alleviate parkinsonism without worsening LID.

Opioids and dyskinesia

Following long-term levodopa therapy and the development of LID, there is enhanced production of mRNA for PPE-A (even above that seen after dopamine depletion alone) and PPE-B (reversing the reduction induced by lesioning to above normal), and corresponding opioid peptides [279–282]. These increases are correlated with LID expression, as no enhancement of opioid peptides is seen with dopamine agonists that do not induce dyskinesia [282–284], although one study reported no elevation of PPE-A in squirrel monkeys with LID [285]. Elevation in PPE-A and PPE-B have also been reported in postmortem studies of patients with PD [266,286,287]. In addition, positron emission tomography (PET) studies show abnormalities in opioid receptor function, consistent with enhanced opioid transmission in the striatum of PD patients with dyskinesia compared with non-dyskinetic patients [288].

These findings suggest that increased opioid neuropeptide neurotransmission at least accompanies, and may be involved in, the pathophysiology of dyskinesia. However, in preclinical studies, non-subtype-selective opioid receptor antagonists have various effects; thus naloxone and naltrexone had no effect on LID [69], significantly reduced dyskinesia [289,290], or increased LID [291]. In clinical studies, the non-subtype-selective opioid receptor antagonist naloxone has been reported to reduce LID [292,293] in small numbers of patients. In a double-blind trial, naltrexone $1\,mg\,kg^{-1}$ failed to show any effect [294] and $5\,mg\,kg^{-1}$ had a minimal effect [295]; neither dose exacerbated dyskinesia or affected parkinsonian disability. Intravenous infusion of naloxone, at a dose known to block central opioid receptors, also failed to reduce dyskinesia, but did extend the duration of action of levodopa [296].

This disparity makes it uncertain whether elevated opioids represent a compensatory/protective mechanism or cause dyskinesia [297]. Alternatively, the non-selective nature of these agents may result in effects on multiple opioid receptors, some of which may be pro- and others anti-dyskinetic. Different doses, agents, and species of animal used may affect the balance between these effects. Subtype-selective antagonists may therefore be necessary to provide anti-dyskinetic actions.

In the MPTP-lesioned primate model of LID, there is enhanced striatal μ-opioid receptor, with less κ- and δ-opioid-mediated transmission, suggesting that μ-opioid receptor antagonists may treat LID [298,299]. Indeed, the μ-opioid receptor antagonist cyprodime alleviated LID in MPTP-lesioned primates [289]. The same study demonstrated that δ-subtype-selective opioid antagonists may also reduce LID. Potential mechanisms whereby μ- and δ-opioid receptor stimulation might contribute to LID expression include enhanced enkephalin release in the GPe causing reduce GABA release via activation of δ-opioid receptors [245] and opioid released from the terminals of the direct pathway may active μ-opioid receptors to increase GABA release [289,300]. Both actions would reduce firing in the output regions of the basal ganglia and result in LID. To date, no subtype-selective opioid receptor antagonists are available for clinical study

Histamine

The central histaminergic system is a subcortical aminergic system involved in several regulatory functions, including thermoregulation, eating, sexual activity, sleep–wakefulness cycle, and hormonal regulation through activation of three receptor subtypes, H_1, H_2, and H_3. Its role in motor activity is less clear and little studied, although there is strong histaminergic innervation of the basal ganglia arising from the tuberomammillary nucleus of the posterior hypothalamus. Histamine levels are increased in the putamen, SNpc, GPe, and GPi in PD [301], and the density of histaminergic fibers is increased in the SNpc and SNpr in PD, suggestive of compensatory up-regulation of input [302]. Histamine H_2 receptors are located in the caudate, putamen, and accumbens, particularly on GABAergic striatopallidal pathways [303,304]. Histamine has excitatory effects and increases striatopallidal activity [305]. However, no changes have been reported in striatal H_2 receptors in PD [303]. Stimulation of H_2 receptors on striatal cholinergic interneurons increases acetylcholine release [306], reminiscent of the effects of dopamine D_1-mediated activation [8]. Thus H_2 antagonists might reduce activity in the direct striatopallidal pathway and potentially reduce LID. To date, no subtype-selective H_2 antagonists have been investigated in PD though an open-label study using the H_2 antagonist famotidine induced mild anti-parkinsonian actions in seven PD patients [307].

Histamine H_3 receptors are principally located within the CNS, and striatal H_3 binding is unchanged in PD [308], although increases in the SNpc and increased mRNA in the GPe have been proposed compared with age-matched controls [309]. Histamine H3 receptors are presynaptic and are either heteroceptors located on corticostriatal terminals in the striatum, on direct and indirect pathway projection terminals in SNpc, GPe, and GPi, and serotonergic terminals in GPi and SNpr [308,310]. Hence histamine H_3 receptors thus potentially can modulate neurotransmission by reducing striatal glutamate transmission [311], GABA in GPe and GPi/SNpr, and 5-HT in SNpr [312,313]. In addition, histamine H_3 receptors are autoreceptors on histaminergic inputs throughout the basal ganglia that reduce histamine release. Histamine H_3 agonists could potentially reverse enhanced striatal glutamatergic and GPi/SNpr GABAergic transmission observed in LID. Histamine H_3 agonists could also indirectly reduce striatal H_2-mediated transmission (see above) by reducing histamine release.

In preclinical studies, histamine H_3 agonists reduce levodopa- and apomorphine-induced contralateral turning in the 6-OHDA-lesioned rat via an action in the SNpr [313,314]. In MPTP-lesioned primates, H_3 agonists reduce levodopa-induced chorea but not dystonia, and worsen parkinsonism [315]. This effect may be due to an indirect effect on acetylcholine release in the striatum, as increasing acetylcholine may worsen or induce dystonia but reduce chorea [28,30]. To date, no subtype-selective histamine H_3 agonists have been evaluated for treatment of LID in PD patients.

Conclusions

The neural mechanisms underlying the motor symptoms of PD and complications of long-term levodopa involve several non-dopaminergic neurotransmitters and neuromodulators. Drugs that act on these systems have been, and will continue to be, investigated as potential therapies for these symptoms at a preclinical level and some are now under clinical development. Future developments need to focus on understanding how to deliver treatments that target only those regions of the basal ganglia involved in PD.

References

1. Obeso JA, Rodriguez-Oroz MC, Rodriguez M, *et al.* Pathophysiology of levodopa-induced dyskinesias in Parkinson's disease: problems with the current model. *Ann Neurol* 2000;**47**(4 Suppl 1):S22–32; discussion S32–4.
2. Bezard E, Brotchie JM, Gross CE. Pathophysiology of levodopa-induced dyskinesia: potential for new therapies. *Nat Rev Neurosci* 2001;**2**(8):577–88.
3. Brotchie JM, Lee J, Venderova K. Levodopa-induced dyskinesia in Parkinson's disease. *J Neural Transm* 2005;**112**(3): 359–91.
4. Fishman PS. Paradoxical aspects of parkinsonian tremor. *Mov Disord* 2008;**23**(2):168–73.
5. Katzenschlager R, Sampaio C, Costa J, Lees A. Anticholinergics for symptomatic management of Parkinson's disease. *Cochrane Database Syst Rev* 2003;(2):CD003735.
6. Deuschl G, Raethjen J, Lindemann M, Krack P. The pathophysiology of tremor. *Muscle Nerve* 2001;**24**(6):716–35.
7. Hersch SM, Gutekunst CA, Rees HD, *et al.* Distribution of m1–m4 muscarinic receptor proteins in the rat striatum: light and electron microscopic immunocytochemistry using subtype-specific antibodies. *J Neurosci* 1994;**14**(5 Pt 2): 3351–63.
8. Pisani A, Bernardi G, Ding J, Surmeier DJ. Re-emergence of striatal cholinergic interneurons in movement disorders. *Trends Neurosci* 2007;**30**(10):545–53.
9. Stoof JC, Drukarch B, de Boer P, Westerink BH, Groenewegen HJ. Regulation of the activity of striatal cholinergic neurons by dopamine. *Neuroscience* 1992;**47**(4):755–70.
10. Gerber DJ, Sotnikova TD, Gainetdinov RR, *et al.* Hyperactivity, elevated dopaminergic transmission, and response to amphetamine in M1 muscarinic acetylcholine receptor-deficient mice. *Proc Natl Acad Sci USA* 2001;**98**(26):15312–7.
11. Shen W, Tian X, Day M, *et al.* Cholinergic modulation of Kir2 channels selectively elevates dendritic excitability in striatopallidal neurons. *Nat Neurosci* 2007;**10**(11):1458–66.
12. Domino EF, Ni L. Trihexyphenidyl potentiation of L-DOPA: reduced effectiveness three years later in MPTP-induced chronic hemiparkinsonian monkeys. *Exp Neurol* 1998;**152**(2):238–42.
13. Di Chiara G, Morelli M, Consolo S. Modulatory functions of neurotransmitters in the striatum: ACh/dopamine/NMDA interactions. *Trends Neurosci* 1994;**17**(6):228–33.
14. Gomeza J, Zhang L, Kostenis E, *et al.* Enhancement of D1 dopamine receptor-mediated locomotor stimulation in M(4) muscarinic acetylcholine receptor knockout mice. *Proc Natl Acad Sci USA* 1999;**96**(18):10483–8.
15. Tzavara ET, Bymaster FP, Davis RJ, *et al.* M4 muscarinic receptors regulate the dynamics of cholinergic and dopaminergic neurotransmission: relevance to the pathophysiology and treatment of related CNS pathologies. *FASEB J* 2004;**18**(12):1410–2.
16. Salamone JD, Correa M, Carlson BB, *et al.* Neostriatal muscarinic receptor subtypes involved in the generation of tremulous jaw movements in rodents implications for cholinergic involvement in parkinsonism. *Life Sci* 2001;**68**(22–23):2579–84.
17. Betz AJ, McLaughlin PJ, Burgos M, *et al.* The muscarinic receptor antagonist tropicamide suppresses tremulous jaw movements in a rodent model of parkinsonian tremor: possible role of M4 receptors. *Psychopharmacology (Berl)* 2007; **194**(3):347–59.
18. Bevan MD, Bolam JP. Cholinergic, GABAergic, and glutamate-enriched inputs from the mesopontine tegmentum to the subthalamic nucleus in the rat. *J Neurosci* 1995; **15**(11):7105–20.
19. Feger J, Hammond C, Rouzaire-Dubois B. Pharmacological properties of acetylcholine-induced excitation of subthalamic nucleus neurones. *Br J Pharmacol* 1979;**65**(3):511–5.
20. Weinberger M, Hamani C, Hutchison WD, *et al.* Pedunculopontine nucleus microelectrode recordings in movement disorder patients. *Exp Brain Res* 2008;**188**(2):165–74.
21. Breit S, Lessmann L, Benazzouz A, Schulz JB. Unilateral lesion of the pedunculopontine nucleus induces hyperactivity in the subthalamic nucleus and substantia nigra in the rat. *Eur J Neurosci* 2005;**22**(9):2283–94.
22. Rinne JO, Ma SY, Lee MS, *et al.* Loss of cholinergic neurons in the pedunculopontine nucleus in Parkinson's disease is related to disability of the patients. *Parkinsonism Relat Disord* 2008;**14**(7):553–7.
23. Plenz D, Kital ST. A basal ganglia pacemaker formed by the subthalamic nucleus and external globus pallidus. *Nature* 1999;**400**(6745):677–82.
24. Niktarash AH, Shahidi GA. Effects of the activity of the internal globus pallidus-pedunculopontine loop on the transmission of the subthalamic nucleus–external globus pallidus–pacemaker oscillatory activities to the cortex. *J Comput Neurosci* 2004;**16**(2):113–27.
25. Shen KZ, Johnson SW. Presynaptic dopamine D2 and muscarine M3 receptors inhibit excitatory and inhibitory

transmission to rat subthalamic neurones *in vitro*. *J Physiol* 2000;**525**(Pt 2):331–41.
26. Hernandez-Lopez S, Flores G, Rosales MG, *et al*. Muscarinic antagonists microinjected into the subthalamic nucleus decrease muscular rigidity in reserpinized rats. *Neurosci Lett* 1996;**213**(3):157–60.
27. Fahn S, Burke R, Stern Y. Antimuscarinic drugs in the treatment of movement disorders. *Prog Brain Res* 1990;**84**: 389–97.
28. Nomoto M, Thompson PD, Sheehy MP, *et al*. Anticholinergic-induced chorea in the treatment of focal dystonia. *Mov Disord* 1987;**2**(1):53–6.
29. Griffiths PD, Sambrook MA, Perry R, Crossman AR. Changes in benzodiazepine and acetylcholine receptors in the globus pallidus in Parkinson's disease. *J Neurol Sci* 1990;**100**(1–2): 131–6.
30. Pearce RKB, Banerji T, Jackson M, *et al*. Cholinergic manipulation of L-DOPA-induced chorea and dystonia in the MPTP-lesioned common marmoset. *Mov Disord* 1999;**11**(Suppl 1):60.
31. Lukas RJ, Changeux JP, Le Novere N, *et al*. International Union of Pharmacology. XX. Current status of the nomenclature for nicotinic acetylcholine receptors and their subunits. *Pharmacol Rev* 1999;**51**(2):397–401.
32. Zhou FM, Liang Y, Dani JA. Endogenous nicotinic cholinergic activity regulates dopamine release in the striatum. *Nat Neurosci* 2001;**4**(12):1224–9.
33. Clarke PB, Pert A. Autoradiographic evidence for nicotine receptors on nigrostriatal and mesolimbic dopaminergic neurons. *Brain Res* 1985;**348**(2):355–8.
34. Kulak JM, McIntosh JM, Quik M. Loss of nicotinic receptors in monkey striatum after 1-methyl-4-phenyl-1,2,3,6-tetrahydropyridine treatment is due to a decline in alpha-conotoxin MII sites. *Mol Pharmacol* 2002;**61**(1):230–8.
35. Quik M, Cox H, Parameswaran N, *et al*. Nicotine reduces levodopa-induced dyskinesias in lesioned monkeys. *Ann Neurol* 2007;**62**(6):588–96.
36. Bordia T, Grady SR, McIntosh JM, Quik M. Nigrostriatal damage preferentially decreases a subpopulation of $\alpha6\beta2^*$ nAChRs in mouse, monkey, and Parkinson's disease striatum. *Mol Pharmacol* 2007;**72**(1):52–61.
37. Quik M, McIntosh JM. Striatal $\alpha6^*$ nicotinic acetylcholine receptors: potential targets for Parkinson's disease therapy. *J Pharmacol Exp Ther* 2006;**316**(2):481–9.
38. Schneider JS, Pope-Coleman A, Van Velson M, *et al*. Effects of SIB-1508Y, a novel neuronal nicotinic acetylcholine receptor agonist, on motor behavior in parkinsonian monkeys. *Mov Disord* 1998;**13**(4):637–42.
39. Parkinson Study Group. Randomized placebo-controlled study of the nicotinic agonist SIB-1508Y in Parkinson disease. *Neurology* 2006;**66**:408–10.
40. Pedata F, Corsi C, Melani A, *et al*. Adenosine extracellular brain concentrations and role of A2A receptors in ischemia. *Ann N Y Acad Sci* 2001;**939**:74–84.
41. Schwarzschild MA, Chen JF, Ascherio A. Caffeinated clues and the promise of adenosine A(2A) antagonists in PD. *Neurology* 2002;**58**(8):1154–60.
42. Hillion J, Canals M, Torvinen M, *et al*. Coaggregation, cointernalization, and codesensitization of adenosine A2A receptors and dopamine D2 receptors. *J Biol Chem* 2002;**277**(20):18091–7.
43. Schwarzschild MA, Agnati L, Fuxe K, *et al*. Targeting adenosine A2A receptors in Parkinson's disease. *Trends Neurosci* 2006;**29**(11):647–54.
44. Nash JE, Brotchie JM. A common signaling pathway for striatal NMDA and adenosine A2a receptors: implications for the treatment of Parkinson's disease. *J Neurosci* 2000; **20**(20):7782–9.
45. Calon F, Dridi M, Hornykiewicz O, *et al*. Increased adenosine A2A receptors in the brain of Parkinson's disease patients with dyskinesias. *Brain* 2004;**127**(Pt 5):1075–84.
46. Morissette M, Dridi M, Calon F, *et al*. Prevention of dyskinesia by an NMDA receptor antagonist in MPTP monkeys: effect on adenosine A2A receptors. *Synapse* 2006;**60**(3):239–50.
47. Morelli M, Pinna A. Interaction between dopamine and adenosine A2A receptors as a basis for the treatment of Parkinson's disease. *Neurol Sci* 2001;**22**(1):71–2.
48. Bove J, Marin C, Bonastre M, Tolosa E. Adenosine A2A antagonism reverses levodopa-induced motor alterations in hemiparkinsonian rats. *Synapse* 2002;**46**(4):251–7.
49. Lundblad M, Vaudano E, Cenci MA. Cellular and behavioural effects of the adenosine A2a receptor antagonist KW-6002 in a rat model of l-DOPA-induced dyskinesia. *J Neurochem* 2003;**84**(6):1398–410.
50. Grondin R, Bedard PJ, Hadj Tahar A, *et al*. Antiparkinsonian effect of a new selective adenosine A2A receptor antagonist in MPTP-treated monkeys. *Neurology* 1999;**52**(8):1673–7.
51. Bibbiani F, Oh JD, Petzer JP, *et al*. A2A antagonist prevents dopamine agonist-induced motor complications in animal models of Parkinson's disease. *Exp Neurol* 2003;**184**(1):285–94.
52. Kanda T, Jackson MJ, Smith LA, *et al*. Adenosine A2A antagonist: a novel antiparkinsonian agent that does not provoke dyskinesia in parkinsonian monkeys. *Ann Neurol* 1998;**43**(4):507–13.
53. Kanda T, Jackson MJ, Smith LA, *et al*. Combined use of the adenosine A(2A) antagonist KW-6002 with L-DOPA or with selective D1 or D2 dopamine agonists increases antiparkinsonian activity but not dyskinesia in MPTP-treated monkeys. *Exp Neurol* 2000;**162**(2):321–7.
54. Bara-Jimenez W, Sherzai A, Dimitrova T, *et al*. Adenosine A(2A) receptor antagonist treatment of Parkinson's disease. *Neurology* 2003;**61**(3):293–6.
55. Hauser RA, Hubble JP, Truong DD. Randomized trial of the adenosine A(2A) receptor antagonist istradefylline in advanced PD. *Neurology* 2003;**61**(3):297–303.
56. LeWitt PA, Guttman M, Tetrud JW, *et al*. Adenosine A2A receptor antagonist istradefylline (KW-6002) reduces "off" time in Parkinson's disease: a double-blind, randomized, multicenter clinical trial (6002-US-005). *Ann Neurol* 2008;**63**(3):295–302.
57. Stacy M, Silver D, Mendis T, *et al*. A 12-week, placebo-controlled study (6002-US-006) of istradefylline in Parkinson disease. *Neurology* 2008;**70**(23):2233–40.
58. Trugman JM, 6002-US-013 Clinical Investigator Group. Efficacy of istradefylline (KW-6002) in levodopa-treated Parkinson's disease patients with motor response complications: primary efficacy results of the KW-6002–US-013 study. *Mov Disord* 2006;**21**(Suppl 15):682.
59. Guttman M, 6002-US-018 Clinical Investigator Group. Efficacy of istradefylline in Parkinson's disease patients treated

with levodopa with motor response complications; results of the KW-6002–US-018 study focusing on functional and motor improvements. *Mov Disord* 2006;**21**(Suppl 15):934.

60. Fernandez H, 6002-US-018 Clinical Investigator Group. Istradefylline for the treatment of motor response complications on levodopa in PD patients; results of the KW-6002–US-018 study focusing on functional and motor improvements. *Mov Disord* 2006;**21**(Suppl 15):1136.
61. Biogen Idec. Dose-Finding Safety Study of BIIB014 in Combination with Levodopa in Moderate to Late Stage Parkinson's Disease. http://clinicaltrials.gov/ct2/show/NCT00438607, 2008.
62. Schering-Plough. Dyskinesia in Parkinson's Disease (Study P04501AM3). http://clinicaltrials.gov/ct2/show/NCT00406029, 2008.
63. Chase TN, Oh JD, Konitsiotis S. Antiparkinsonian and antidyskinetic activity of drugs targeting central glutamatergic mechanisms. *J Neurol* 2000;**247**(Suppl 2):II36–42.
64. Chase TN, Bibbiani F, Oh JD. Striatal glutamatergic mechanisms and extrapyramidal movement disorders. *Neurotox Res* 2003;**5**(1–2): 139–46.
65. Ravenscroft P, Brotchie J. NMDA receptors in the basal ganglia. *J Anat* 2000;**196**(Pt 4):577–85.
66. Calabresi P, Giacomini P, Centonze D, Bernardi G. Levodopa-induced dyskinesia: a pathological form of striatal synaptic plasticity? *Ann Neurol* 2000;**47**(4 Suppl 1):S60–8; discussion S68–9.
67. Picconi B, Centonze D, Hakansson K, *et al.* Loss of bidirectional striatal synaptic plasticity in L-DOPA-induced dyskinesia. *Nat Neurosci* 2003;**6**(5):501–6.
68. Rupniak NM, Boyce S, Steventon MJ, *et al.* Dystonia induced by combined treatment with L-dopa and MK-801 in parkinsonian monkeys. *Ann Neurol* 1992;**32**(1):103–5.
69. Gomez-Mancilla B, Bedard PJ. Effect of nondopaminergic drugs on L-dopa-induced dyskinesias in MPTP-treated monkeys. *Clin Neuropharmacol* 1993;**16**(5):418–27.
70. Papa SM, Chase TN. Levodopa-induced dyskinesias improved by a glutamate antagonist in Parkinsonian monkeys. *Ann Neurol* 1996;**39**(5):574–8.
71. Blanchet PJ, Konitsiotis S, Chase TN. Amantadine reduces levodopa-induced dyskinesias in parkinsonian monkeys. *Mov Disord* 1998;**13**(5):798–802.
72. Hill MP, Ravenscroft P, Bezard E, *et al.* Levetiracetam potentiates the antidyskinetic action of amantadine in the 1-methyl-4-phenyl-1,2,3,6-tetrahydropyridine (MPTP)-lesioned primate model of Parkinson's disease. *J Pharmacol Exp Ther* 2004;**310**(1):386–94.
73. Goetz CG, Poewe W, Rascol O, Sampaio C. Evidence-based medical review update: pharmacological and surgical treatments of Parkinson's disease: 2001 to 2004. *Mov Disord* 2005;**20**(5):523–39.
74. Pahwa R, Factor SA, Lyons KE, *et al.* Practice Parameter: treatment of Parkinson disease with motor fluctuations and dyskinesia (an evidence-based review): report of the Quality Standards Subcommittee of the American Academy of Neurology. *Neurology* 2006;**66**(7):983–95.
75. Crosby NJ, Deane KH, Clarke CE. Amantadine for dyskinesia in Parkinson's disease. *Cochrane Database Syst Rev* 2003;(2):CD003467.
76. Luginger E, Wenning GK, Bosch S, Poewe W. Beneficial effects of amantadine on L-dopa-induced dyskinesias in Parkinson's disease. *Mov Disord* 2000;**15**(5):873–8.
77. Verhagen Metman L, Del Dotto P, van den Munckhof P, *et al.* Amantadine as treatment for dyskinesias and motor fluctuations in Parkinson's disease. *Neurology* 1998;**50**(5):1323–6.
78. Snow BJ, Macdonald L, McAuley D, Wallis W. The effect of amantadine on levodopa-induced dyskinesias in Parkinson's disease: a double-blind, placebo-controlled study. *Clin Neuropharmacol* 2000;**23**(2):82–5.
79. Moresco RM, Volonte MA, Messa C, *et al.* New perspectives on neurochemical effects of amantadine in the brain of parkinsonian patients: a PET – [^{11}C]raclopride study. *J Neural Transm* 2002;**109**(10):1265–74.
80. Thomas A, Iacono D, Luciano AL, *et al.* Duration of amantadine benefit on dyskinesia of severe Parkinson's disease. *J Neurol Neurosurg Psychiatry* 2004;**75**(1):141–3.
81. Metman LV, Del Dotto P, LePoole K, *et al.* Amantadine for levodopa-induced dyskinesias: a 1-year follow-up study. *Arch Neurol* 1999;**56**(11):1383–6.
82. Paci C, Thomas A, Onofrj M. Amantadine for dyskinesia in patients affected by severe Parkinson's disease. *Neurol Sci* 2001;**22**(1):75–6.
83. Martinez-Martin P, Catalan MJ, Benito-Leon J, *et al.* Impact of fatigue in Parkinson's disease: the Fatigue Impact Scale for Daily Use (D-FIS). *Qual Life Res* 2006;**15**(4):597–606.
84. Inzelberg R, Bonuccelli U, Schechtman E, *et al.* Association between amantadine and the onset of dementia in Parkinson's disease. *Mov Disord* 2006;**21**(9):1375–9.
85. Uitti RJ, Rajput AH, Ahlskog JE, *et al.* Amantadine treatment is an independent predictor of improved survival in Parkinson's disease. *Neurology* 1996;**46**(6):1551–6.
86. Caumont AS, Octave JN, Hermans E. Amantadine and memantine induce the expression of the glial cell line-derived neurotrophic factor in C6 glioma cells. *Neurosci Lett* 2006;**394**(3):196–201.
87. Kashihara K, Imamura T. Amantadine may reverse punding in Parkinson's disease – observation in a patient. *Mov Disord* 2008;**23**(1):129–30.
88. Merello M, Nouzeilles MI, Cammarota A, Leiguarda R. Effect of memantine (NMDA antagonist) on Parkinson's disease: a double-blind crossover randomized study. *Clin Neuropharmacol* 1999;**22**(5):273–6.
89. Reisberg B, Doody R, Stoffler A, *et al.* Memantine in moderate-to-severe Alzheimer's disease. *N Engl J Med* 2003;**348**(14):1333–41.
90. Parkinson Study Group. Evaluation of dyskinesias in a pilot, randomized, placebo-controlled trial of remacemide in advanced Parkinson disease. *Arch Neurol* 2001;**58**(10): 1660–8.
91. Paquette MA, Brudney EG, Putterman DB, *et al.* Sigma ligands, but not *N*-methyl-D-aspartate antagonists, reduce levodopa-induced dyskinesias. *Neuroreport* 2008;**19**(1):111–5.
92. Verhagen Metman L, Del Dotto P, Natte R, *et al.* Dextromethorphan improves levodopa-induced dyskinesias in Parkinson's disease. *Neurology* 1998;**51**(1):203–6.
93. Nash JE, Fox SH, Henry B, *et al.* Antiparkinsonian actions of ifenprodil in the MPTP-lesioned marmoset model of Parkinson's disease. *Exp Neurol* 2000;**165**(1):136–42.

94. Nash JE, Ravenscroft P, McGuire S, *et al.* The NR2B-selective NMDA receptor antagonist CP-101,606 exacerbates L-DOPA-induced dyskinesia and provides mild potentiation of anti-parkinsonian effects of L-DOPA in the MPTP-lesioned marmoset model of Parkinson's disease. *Exp Neurol* 2004;**188**(2):471–9.
95. Steece-Collier K, Chambers LK, Jaw-Tsai SS, *et al.* Antiparkinsonian actions of CP-101,606, an antagonist of NR2B subunit-containing N-methyl-D-aspartate receptors. *Exp Neurol* 2000;**163**(1):239–43.
96. Blanchet PJ, Konitsiotis S, Whittemore ER, *et al.* Differing effects of *N*-methyl-D-aspartate receptor subtype selective antagonists on dyskinesias in levodopa-treated 1-methyl-4-phenyl-tetrahydropyridine monkeys. *J Pharmacol Exp Ther* 1999;**290**(3):1034–40.
97. Hadj Tahar A, Gregoire L, Darre A, *et al.* Effect of a selective glutamate antagonist on l-dopa-induced dyskinesias in drug-naive parkinsonian monkeys. *Neurobiol Dis* 2004;**15**(2):171–6.
98. Pfizer. The Effects of an NR2B NMDA Antagonist, CP-101,606, in Patients with Parkinson's Disease. http://clinicaltrials.gov/ct2/show/NCT00163085, 2008.
99. National Institute of Neurological Disorders and Stroke (NINDS). Treatment of Parkinson's Disease with Eliprodil. http://clinicaltrials.gov/ct2/show/NCT00001929, 2008.
100. Konitsiotis S, Blanchet PJ, Verhagen L, *et al.* AMPA receptor blockade improves levodopa-induced dyskinesia in MPTP monkeys. *Neurology* 2000;**54**(8):1589–95.
101. Teva *Neuroscience*. Effects of Talampanel on Patients with Advanced Parkinson's Disease. http://clinicaltrials.gov/ct2/show/NCT00036296, 2008.
102. Eisei. Evaluation of the Long-Term Safety, Tolerability, and Efficacy of Perampanel (E2007) as an Adjunctive Therapy in Levodopa Treated Parkinson's Disease Subjects with Motor Fluctuations. http://clinicaltrials.gov/ct2/show/NCT00505622, 2008.
103. Bibbiani F, Oh JD, Kielaite A, *et al.* Combined blockade of AMPA and NMDA glutamate receptors reduces levodopa-induced motor complications in animal models of PD. *Exp Neurol* 2005;**196**(2):422–9.
104. Conn PJ, Battaglia G, Marino MJ, Nicoletti F. Metabotropic glutamate receptors in the basal ganglia motor circuit. *Nat Rev Neurosci* 2005;**6**(10):787–98.
105. Ossowska K, Konieczny J, Wardas J, *et al.* An influence of ligands of metabotropic glutamate receptor subtypes on parkinsonian-like symptoms and the striatopallidal pathway in rats. *Amino Acids* 2007;**32**(2):179–88.
106. Dawson L, Chadha A, Megalou M, Duty S. The group II metabotropic glutamate receptor agonist, DCG-IV, alleviates akinesia following intranigral or intraventricular administration in the reserpine-treated rat. *Br J Pharmacol* 2000;**129**(3):541–6.
107. Bradley SR, Marino MJ, Wittmann M, *et al.* Activation of group II metabotropic glutamate receptors inhibits synaptic excitation of the substantia nigra pars reticulata. *J Neurosci* 2000;**20**(9):3085–94.
108. Samadi P, Gregoire L, Morissette M, *et al.* Basal ganglia group II metabotropic glutamate receptors specific binding in non-human primate model of L-Dopa-induced dyskinesias. *Neuropharmacology* 2008;**54**(2):258–68.
109. Dekundy A, Pietraszek M, Schaefer D, *et al.* Effects of group I metabotropic glutamate receptors blockade in experimental models of Parkinson's disease. *Brain Res Bull* 2006;**69**(3):318–26.
110. Mela F, Marti M, Dekundy A, *et al.* Antagonism of metabotropic glutamate receptor type 5 attenuates l-DOPA-induced dyskinesia and its molecular and neurochemical correlates in a rat model of Parkinson's disease. *J Neurochem* 2007;**101**(2):483–97.
111. Novartis. Efficacy and Safety of AFQ056 in Reducing L-Dopa Induced Dyskinesias in Parkinson's Disease Patients, and Safety in Combination with L-Dopa. http://clinicaltrials.gov/ct2/show/NCT00888004, 2008.
112. Bara-Jimenez W, Dimitrova TD, Sherzai A, *et al.* Glutamate release inhibition ineffective in levodopa-induced motor complications. *Mov Disord* 2006;**21**(9):1380–3.
113. Stocchi F, Arnold G, Onofrj M, *et al.* Improvement of motor function in early Parkinson disease by safinamide. *Neurology* 2004;**63**(4):746–8.
114. Anand R OM, Schapira AH, 015 Study Group. Safinamide potentiates the effects of DA-agonists in early stage Parkinson's disease patients. *Mov Disord* 2007;**22**(Suppl 16):797.
115. Shapira AH BR, Stoccchi F, *et al.* Long term safety and efficacy of safinamide added to dopamine agonists in early Parkinson's disease. *Neurology* 2008;**70**(Suppl 1):424.
116. Stocchi F, Vacca L, Grassini P, *et al.* Symptom relief in Parkinson disease by safinamide: biochemical and clinical evidence of efficacy beyond MAO-B inhibition. *Neurology* 2006;**67**(7 Suppl 2):S24–9.
117. MOTION, Safinamide in Early IPD, as Add-On to Dopamine Agonist. http://clinicaltrials.gov/ct2/show/NCT00605683, 2010.
118. Murata M, Horiuchi E, Kanazawa I. Zonisamide has beneficial effects on Parkinson's disease patients. *Neurosci Res* 2001;**41**(4):397–9.
119. Brotchie JM, Johnston TH, Fox SH *et al.* FP0011 extends the duration of the anti-parkinsonian actions of L-DOPA and reduces L-DOPA-induced dyskinesia in the MPTP-lesioned macaque model of Parkinson's disease. *Mov Disord* 2007;**22**(Suppl 16):310.
120. Rascol O, Lacomblez L, Ferreira J, Negre-Pages L. A $N = 1$ randomised placebo controlled multiple cross-over pilot study of FP0011, a novel antiglutamate agent in advanced PD. *Mov Disord* 2007;**22**(Suppl 16):912.
121. Ungerstedt U. Stereotaxic mapping of the monoamine pathways in the rat brain. *Acta Physiol Scand Suppl* 1971;**367**: 1–48.
122. Scheinin M, Lomasney JW, Hayden-Hixson DM, *et al.* Distribution of alpha 2-adrenergic receptor subtype gene expression in rat brain. *Brain Res Mol Brain Res* 1994;**21**(1–2): 133–49.
123. Rosin DL, Talley EM, Lee A, Stornetta RL, *et al.* Distribution of alpha 2C-adrenergic receptor-like immunoreactivity in the rat central nervous system. *J Comp Neurol* 1996;**372**(1):135–65.
124. Chan-Palay V. Locus coeruleus and norepinephrine in Parkinson's disease. *Jpn J Psychiatry Neurol* 1991;**45**(2):519–21.
125. Braak H, Del TrediciK, Rub U, *et al.* Staging of brain pathology related to sporadic Parkinson's disease. *Neurobiol Aging* 2003;**24**(2):197–211.

126. Mann DM, Yates PO. Pathological basis for neurotransmitter changes in Parkinson's disease. *Neuropathol Appl Neurobiol* 1983;**9**(1):3–19.
127. Von Coelln R, Thomas B, Savitt JM, *et al.* Loss of locus coeruleus neurons and reduced startle in parkin null mice. *Proc Natl Acad Sci USA* 2004;**101**(29):10744–9.
128. Hayashi S, Wakabayashi K, Ishikawa A, *et al.* An autopsy case of autosomal-recessive juvenile parkinsonism with a homozygous exon 4 deletion in the parkin gene. *Mov Disord* 2000;**15**(5):884–8.
129. Gouider-Khouja N, Larnaout A, Amouri R, *et al.* Autosomal recessive parkinsonism linked to parkin gene in a Tunisian family. Clinical, genetic and pathological study. *Parkinsonism Relat Disord* 2003;**9**(5):247–51.
130. Fahn S, Libsch LR, Cutler RW. Monoamines in the human neostriatum: topographic distribution in normals and in Parkinson's disease and their role in akinesia, rigidity, chorea, and tremor. *J Neurol Sci* 1971;**14**(4):427–55.
131. Jenner P, Sheehy M, Marsden CD. Noradrenaline and 5-hydroxytryptamine modulation of brain dopamine function: implications for the treatment of Parkinson's disease. *Br J Clin Pharmacol* 1983;**15**(Suppl 2):277S–289S.
132. Russ H, Mihatsch W, Gerlach M, *et al.* Neurochemical and behavioural features induced by chronic low dose treatment with 1-methyl-4-phenyl-1,2,3,6-tetrahydropyridine (MPTP) in the common marmoset: implications for Parkinson's disease? *Neurosci Lett* 1991;**123**(1):115–8.
133. Hornykiewicz O. Biochemical aspects of Parkinson's disease. *Neurology* 1998;**51**(2 Suppl 2):S2–9.
134. Scatton B, Javoy-Agid F, Rouquier L, *et al.* Reduction of cortical dopamine, noradrenaline, serotonin and their metabolites in Parkinson's disease. *Brain Res* 1983;**275**(2):321–8.
135. Villeneuve A, Berlan M, Lafontan M, *et al.* Platelet alpha 2 adrenoceptors in Parkinson's disease: decreased number in untreated patients and recovery after treatment. *Eur J Clin Invest* 1985;**15**(6):403–7.
136. Cash R, Ruberg M, Raisman R, Agid Y. Adrenergic receptors in Parkinson's disease. *Brain Res* 1984;**322**(2):269–75.
137. D'Amato RJ, Zweig RM, Whitehouse PJ, *et al.* Aminergic systems in Alzheimer's disease and Parkinson's disease. *Ann Neurol* 1987;**22**(2):229–36.
138. Chan-Palay V, Asan E. Quantitation of catecholamine neurons in the locus coeruleus in human brains of normal young and older adults and in depression. *J Comp Neurol* 1989;**287**(3):357–72.
139. Remy P, Doder M, Lees A, *et al.* Depression in Parkinson's disease: loss of dopamine and noradrenaline innervation in the limbic system. *Brain* 2005;**128**(Pt 6):1314–22.
140. Stern Y, Mayeux R, Cote L. Reaction time and vigilance in Parkinson's disease. Possible role of altered norepinephrine metabolism. *Arch Neurol* 1984;**41**(10):1086–9.
141. Goldstein DS, Holmes C, Sharabi Y, *et al.* Plasma levels of catechols and metanephrines in neurogenic orthostatic hypotension. *Neurology* 2003;**60**(8):1327–32.
142. Tohgi H, Abe T, Takahashi S, *et al.* Monoamine metabolism in the cerebrospinal fluid in Parkinson's disease: relationship to clinical symptoms and subsequent therapeutic outcomes. *J Neural Transm Park Dis Dement Sect* 1993;**5**(1):17–26.
143. Tarsy D, Parkes JD, Marsden CD. Clonidine in Parkinson disease. *Arch Neurol* 1975;**32**(2):134–6.
144. Shoulson I, Chase TN. Clonidine and the anti-parkinsonian response to L-DOPA or piribedil. *Neuropharmacology* 1976;**15**(1):25–7.
145. Norenberg W, Schoffel E, Szabo B, Starke K. Subtype determination of soma-dendritic alpha2-autoreceptors in slices of rat locus coeruleus. *Naunyn Schmiedebergs Arch Pharmacol* 1997;**356**(2):159–65.
146. Colpaert FC. Pharmacological characteristics of tremor, rigidity and hypokinesia induced by reserpine in rat. *Neuropharmacology* 1987;**26**(9):1431–40.
147. Belujon P, Bezard E, Taupignon A, *et al.* Noradrenergic modulation of subthalamic nucleus activity: behavioral and electrophysiological evidence in intact and 6-hydroxydopamine-lesioned rats. *J Neurosci* 2007;**27**(36):9595–606.
148. Mavridis M, Colpaert FC, Millan MJ. Differential modulation of (+)-amphetamine-induced rotation in unilateral substantia nigra-lesioned rats by alpha 1 as compared to alpha 2 agonists and antagonists. *Brain Res* 1991;**562**(2):216–24.
149. Haapalinna A, Leino T, Heinonen E. The alpha 2-adrenoceptor antagonist atipamezole potentiates anti-Parkinsonian effects and can reduce the adverse cardiovascular effects of dopaminergic drugs in rats. *Naunyn Schmiedebergs Arch Pharmacol* 2003;**368**(5):342–51.
150. Bezard E, Brefel C, Tison F, *et al.* Effect of the alpha 2 adrenoreceptor antagonist, idazoxan, on motor disabilities in MPTP-treated monkey. *Prog Neuropsychopharmacol Biol Psychiatry* 1999;**23**(7):1237–46.
151. Fox SH, Henry B, Hill MP, *et al.* Neural mechanisms underlying peak-dose dyskinesia induced by levodopa and apomorphine are distinct: evidence from the effects of the alpha(2) adrenoceptor antagonist idazoxan. *Mov Disord* 2001;**16**(4):642–50.
152. Savola JM, Hill M, Engstrom M, *et al.* Fipamezole (JP-1730) is a potent alpha2 adrenergic receptor antagonist that reduces levodopa-induced dyskinesia in the MPTP-lesioned primate model of Parkinson's disease. *Mov Disord* 2003;**18**(8):872–83.
153. Srinivasan J, Schmidt WJ. Potentiation of parkinsonian symptoms by depletion of locus coeruleus noradrenaline in 6-hydroxydopamine-induced partial degeneration of substantia nigra in rats. *Eur J Neurosci* 2003;**17**(12):2586–92.
154. Holmberg M, Scheinin M, Kurose H, Miettinen R. Adrenergic alpha2C-receptors reside in rat striatal GABAergic projection neurons: comparison of radioligand binding and immunohistochemistry. *Neuroscience* 1999;**93**(4):1323–33.
155. Hill MP, Brotchie JM. The adrenergic receptor agonist, clonidine, potentiates the anti-parkinsonian action of the selective kappa-opioid receptor agonist, enadoline, in the monoamine-depleted rat. *Br J Pharmacol* 1999;**128**(7):1577–85.
156. Henry B, Fox SH, Peggs D, *et al.* The alpha2-adrenergic receptor antagonist idazoxan reduces dyskinesia and enhances anti-parkinsonian actions of L-dopa in the MPTP-lesioned primate model of Parkinson's disease. *Mov Disord* 1999;**14**(5):744–53.
157. Domino EF, Ni L, Colpaert F, Marien M. Effects of (±)-idazoxan alone and in combination with L-DOPA methyl

ester in MPTP-induced hemiparkinsonian monkeys. *Receptors Channels* 2003;**9**(5):335–8.

158. Alachkar A, Brotchie J, Jones OT. alpha2-Adrenoceptor-mediated modulation of the release of GABA and noradrenaline in the rat substantia nigra pars reticulata. *Neurosci Lett* 2006;**395**(2):138–42.
159. Rascol O, Arnulf I, Peyro-Saint Paul H, *et al.* Idazoxan, an alpha-2 antagonist, and L-DOPA-induced dyskinesias in patients with Parkinson's disease. *Mov Disord* 2001;**16**(4):708–13.
160. Manson AJ, Iakovidou E, Lees AJ. Idazoxan is ineffective for levodopa-induced dyskinesias in Parkinson's disease. *Mov Disord* 2000;**15**(2):336–7.
161. Bara-Jimenez W, Morris M, Dimitrova T, *et al.* Alpha-2A adrenergic antagonistic effects in advanced Parkinson's disease. *Mov Disord* 2004;**19**(Suppl 9):37.
162. Juvantia Pharma. Safety and Efficacy Study of Fipamezole in Treatment of Motor Dysfunctions in Parkinson's Disease (Fjord). http://clinicaltrials.gov/ct2/show/NCT00559871, 2008.
163. Lavoie B, Parent A. Immunohistochemical study of the serotoninergic innervation of the basal ganglia in the squirrel monkey. J Comp Neurol 1990;**299**(1):1–16.
164. van der Kooy D, Hattori T. Dorsal raphe cells with collateral projections to the caudate-putamen and substantia nigra: a fluorescent retrograde double labeling study in the rat. *Brain Res* 1980;**186**(1):1–7.
165. Kish SJ, Tong J, Hornykiewicz O, *et al.* Preferential loss of serotonin markers in caudate versus putamen in Parkinson's disease. *Brain* 2008;**131**(Pt 1):120–31.
166. Halliday GM, Blumbergs PC, Cotton RG, *et al.* Loss of brainstem serotonin- and substance P-containing neurons in Parkinson's disease. *Brain Res* 1990;**510**(1):104–7.
167. Jellinger KA. Pathology of Parkinson's disease. Changes other than the nigrostriatal pathway. *Mol Chem Neuropathol* 1991;**14**(3):153–97.
168. Guttman M, Boileau I, Warsh J, *et al. Brain* serotonin transporter binding in non-depressed patients with Parkinson's disease. *Eur J Neurol* 2007;**14**(5):523–8.
169. Albin RL, Koeppe RA, Bohnen NI, *et al.* Spared caudal brainstem SERT binding in early Parkinson's disease. *J Cereb Blood Flow Metab* 2008;**28**(3):441–4.
170. Hall CD, Weiss EA, Morris CE, Prange AJ Jr. Rapid deterioration in patients with parkinsonism following tryptophan–pyridoxine administration. *Neurology* 1972;**22**(3):231–7.
171. Beasley BL, Davenport RW, Chase TN. Fenfluramine hydrochloride treatment of parkinsonism. *Arch Neurol* 1977;**34**(4):255–6.
172. Richard IH, Maughn A, Kurlan R. Do serotonin reuptake inhibitor antidepressants worsen Parkinson's disease? A retrospective case series. *Mov Disord* 1999;**14**(1):155–7.
173. Arbouw ME, Movig KL, Neef C, *et al.* Influence of initial use of serotonergic antidepressants on antiparkinsonian drug use in levodopa-using patients. *Eur J Clin Pharmacol* 2007;**63**(2):181–7.
174. Gordon PH, Pullman SL, Louis ED, *et al.* Mirtazapine in Parkinsonian tremor. *Parkinsonism Relat Disord* 2002;**9**(2):125–6.
175. Friedman JH, Koller WC, Lannon MC, *et al.* Benztropine versus clozapine for the treatment of tremor in Parkinson's disease. *Neurology* 1997;**48**(4):1077–81.
176. Jansen EN. Clozapine in the treatment of tremor in Parkinson's disease. *Acta Neurol Scand* 1994;**89**(4):262–5.
177. Bonuccelli U, Ceravolo R, Salvetti S, *et al.* Clozapine in Parkinson's disease tremor. Effects of acute and chronic administration. *Neurology* 1997;**49**(6):1587–90.
178. Doder M, Rabiner EA, Turjanski N, *et al.* Tremor in Parkinson's disease and serotonergic dysfunction: an ^{11}C-WAY 100635 PET study. *Neurology* 2003;**60**(4):601–5.
179. Hoyer D, Pazos A, Probst A, Palacios JM. Serotonin receptors in the human brain. II. Characterization and autoradiographic localization of 5-HT1C and 5-HT2 recognition sites. *Brain Res* 1986;**376**(1):97–107.
180. Fox SH, Brotchie JM. 5-HT2C receptor binding is increased in the substantia nigra pars reticulata in Parkinson's disease. *Mov Disord* 2000;**15**(6):1064–9.
181. Rick CE, Stanford IM, Lacey MG. Excitation of rat substantia nigra pars reticulata neurons by 5-hydroxytryptamine *in vitro*: evidence for a direct action mediated by 5-hydroxytryptamine 2C receptors. *Neuroscience* 1995;**69**(3):903–13.
182. Invernizzi RW, Pierucci M, Calcagno E, *et al.* Selective activation of 5-HT(2C) receptors stimulates GABA-ergic function in the rat substantia nigra pars reticulata: a combined *in vivo* electrophysiological and neurochemical study. *Neuroscience* 2007;**144**(4):1523–35.
183. Fox S, Brotchie J. Normethylclozapine potentiates the action of quinpirole in the 6-hydroxydopamine lesioned rat. *Eur J Pharmacol* 1996;**301**(1–3):27–30.
184. Fox SH, Brotchie JM. 5-HT(2C) receptor antagonists enhance the behavioural response to dopamine D(1) receptor agonists in the 6-hydroxydopamine-lesioned rat. *Eur J Pharmacol* 2000;**398**(1):59–64.
185. Fox SH, Moser B, Brotchie JM. Behavioral effects of 5-HT2C receptor antagonism in the substantia nigra zona reticulata of the 6-hydroxydopamine-lesioned rat model of Parkinson's disease. *Exp Neurol* 1998;**151**(1):35–49.
186. Pazos A, Palacios JM. Quantitative autoradiographic mapping of serotonin receptors in the rat brain. I. Serotonin-1 receptors. *Brain Res* 1985;**346**(2):205–30.
187. Barnes NM, Sharp T. A review of central 5-HT receptors and their function. *Neuropharmacology* 1999;**38**(8):1083–152.
188. Castro ME, Pascual J, Romon T, *et al.* 5-HT1B receptor binding in degenerative movement disorders. *Brain Res* 1998;**790**(1–2):323–8.
189. Kita H, Chiken S, Tachibana Y, Nambu A. Serotonin modulates pallidal neuronal activity in the awake monkey. *J Neurosci* 2007;**27**(1):75–83.
190. Rav-Acha M, Bergman H, Yarom Y. Pre and post synaptic serotoninergic excitation of globus pallidus neurons. *J Neurophysiol* 2008;**100**:1053–66.
191. Chadha A, Sur C, Atack J, Duty S. The 5HT(1B) receptor agonist, CP-93129, inhibits [^{3}H]-GABA release from rat globus pallidus slices and reverses akinesia following intrapallidal injection in the reserpine-treated rat. *Br J Pharmacol* 2000;**130**(8):1927–32.

192. Jackson MJ, Al-Barghouthy G, Pearce RK, *et al.* Effect of 5-HT1B/D receptor agonist and antagonist administration on motor function in haloperidol and MPTP-treated common marmosets. *Pharmacol Biochem Behav* 2004;**79**(3):391–400.

193. Pompeiano M, Palacios JM, Mengod G. Distribution and cellular localization of mRNA coding for 5-HT1A receptor in the rat brain: correlation with receptor binding. *J Neurosci* 1992;**12**(2):440–53.

194. Carta M, Carlsson T, Kirik D, Bjorklund A. Dopamine released from 5-HT terminals is the cause of L-DOPA-induced dyskinesia in parkinsonian rats. *Brain* 2007;**130**(Pt 7): 1819–33

195. Antonelli T, Fuxe K, Tomasini MC, *et al.* Effects of sarizotan on the corticostriatal glutamate pathways. *Synapse* 2005;**58**(3):193–9.

196. Tomiyama M, Kimura T, Maeda T, *et al.* A serotonin 5-HT1A receptor agonist prevents behavioral sensitization to L-DOPA in a rodent model of Parkinson's disease. *Neurosci Res* 2005;**52**(2):185–94.

197. Dupre KB, Eskow KL, Negron G, Bishop C. The differential effects of 5-HT(1A) receptor stimulation on dopamine receptor-mediated abnormal involuntary movements and rotations in the primed hemiparkinsonian rat. *Brain Res* 2007;**1158**:135–43.

198. Eskow KL, Gupta V, Alam S, *et al.* The partial 5-HT(1A) agonist buspirone reduces the expression and development of l-DOPA-induced dyskinesia in rats and improves l-DOPA efficacy. *Pharmacol Biochem Behav* 2007;**87**(3):306–14.

199. Iravani MM, Tayarani-Binazir K, Chu WB, *et al.* In 1-methyl-4-phenyl-1,2,3,6-tetrahydropyridine-treated primates, the selective 5-hydroxytryptamine 1a agonist (*R*)-(+)-8-OHDPAT inhibits levodopa-induced dyskinesia but only with increased motor disability. *J Pharmacol Exp Ther* 2006;**319**(3):1225–34.

200. Bibbiani F, Oh JD, Chase TN. Serotonin 5-HT1A agonist improves motor complications in rodent and primate parkinsonian models. *Neurology* 2001;**57**(10):1829–34.

201. Bonifati V, Fabrizio E, Cipriani R, *et al.* Buspirone in levodopa-induced dyskinesias. *Clin Neuropharmacol* 1994; **17**(1):73–82.

202. Kannari K, Kurahashi K, Tomiyama M, *et al.* Tandospirone citrate, a selective 5-HT1A agonist, alleviates L-DOPA-induced dyskinesia in patients with Parkinson's disease. *No To Shinkei* 2002;**54**(2):133–7 (in Japanese).

203. Bara-Jimenez W, Bibbiani F, Morris MJ, *et al.* Effects of serotonin 5-HT1A agonist in advanced Parkinson's disease. *Mov Disord* 2005;**20**(8):932–6.

204. Olanow CW, Damier P, Goetz CG, *et al.* Multicenter, open-label, trial of sarizotan in Parkinson disease patients with levodopa-induced dyskinesias (the SPLENDID Study). *Clin Neuropharmacol* 2004;**27**(2):58–62.

205. Goetz CG, Damier P, Hicking C, *et al.* Sarizotan as a treatment for dyskinesias in Parkinson's disease: a double-blind placebo-controlled trial. *Mov Disord* 2007;**22**(2):179–86.

206. Rascol O, Damier P, Goetz CG, *et al.* A large phase III study to evaluate the safety and efficacy of sarizotan in the treatment of L-dopa-induced-dyskinesia associated with PD: the Paddy-1 study. *Mov Disord* 2006;**21**(Suppl 15):492–493.

207. Müller T, Olanow CW, Nutt J, *et al.* The Paddy-2 study: the evaluation of sarizotan for treatment-associated for dyskinesia in PD patients. *Mov Disord* 2006;**21**(Suppl 15):591.

208. Goetz CG, Laska E, Hicking C, *et al.* Placebo influences on dyskinesia in Parkinson's disease. *Mov Disord* 2008;**23**:700–7.

209. Bartoszyk GD, Van Amsterdam C, Greiner HE, *et al.* Sarizotan, a serotonin 5-HT1A receptor agonist and dopamine receptor ligand. 1. Neurochemical profile. *J Neural Transm* 2004;**111**(2):113–26.

210. Pact V, Giduz T. Mirtazapine treats resting tremor, essential tremor, and levodopa-induced dyskinesias. *Neurology* 1999;**53**(5):1154.

211. Meco G, Fabrizio E, Di Rezze S, *et al.* Mirtazapine in L-dopa-induced dyskinesias. *Clin Neuropharmacol* 2003;**26**(4):179–81.

212. Asubio Pharmaceuticals. Preliminary Study of Piclozotan in Patients with Motor Complications Associated with Parkinson's Disease. http://clinicaltrials.gov/ct2/show/NCT00623363, 2008.

213. Bronzova J, Sampiano C, Hauser RA, *et al.* Pardoprunox (SLV308) improves motor symptoms in patients with early stage Parkinson's disease – a double-blind placebo controlled multi centre study. *Neurology* 2008;**70**(Suppl 1):2.028.

214. Zhang X, Andren PE, Greengard P, Svenningsson P. Evidence for a role of the 5-HT1B receptor and its adaptor protein. p11, in L-DOPA treatment of an animal model of Parkinsonism. *Proc Natl Acad Sci USA* 2008;**105**(6):2163–8.

215. Knobelman DA, Kung HF, Lucki I. Regulation of extracellular concentrations of 5-hydroxytryptamine (5-HT) in mouse striatum by 5-HT(1A) and 5-HT(1B) receptors. *J Pharmacol Exp Ther* 2000;**292**(3):1111–7.

216. Stanford IM, Lacey MG. Differential actions of serotonin, mediated by 5-HT1B and 5-HT2C receptors, on GABA-mediated synaptic input to rat substantia nigra pars reticulata neurons *in vitro*. *J Neurosci* 1996;**16**(23):7566–73.

217. Chen CP, Alder JT, Bray L, *et al.* Post-synaptic 5-HT1A and 5-HT2A receptors are increased in Parkinson's disease neocortex. *Ann N Y Acad Sci* 1998;**861**:288–9.

218. Numan S, Lundgren KH, Wright DE, *et al.* Increased expression of 5HT2 receptor mRNA in rat striatum following 6-OHDA lesions of the adult nigrostriatal pathway. *Brain Res Mol Brain Res* 1995;**29**(2):391–6.

219. Zhang X, Andren PE, Svenningsson P. Changes on 5-HT2 receptor mRNAs in striatum and subthalamic nucleus in Parkinson's disease model. *Physiol Behav* 2007;**92**(1–2):29–33.

220. Di Matteo V, De Blasi A, Di Giulio C, Esposito E. Role of 5-HT(2C) receptors in the control of central dopamine function. *Trends Pharmacol Sci* 2001;**22**(5):229–32.

221. Taylor JL, Bishop C, Ullrich T, *et al.* Serotonin 2A receptor antagonist treatment reduces dopamine D1 receptor-mediated rotational behavior but not L-DOPA-induced abnormal involuntary movements in the unilateral dopamine-depleted rat. *Neuropharmacology* 2006;**50**(6):761–8.

222. Grondin R, Doan VD, Gregoire L, Bedard PJ. D1 receptor blockade improves L-dopa-induced dyskinesia but worsens parkinsonism in MPTP monkeys. *Neurology* 1999;**52**(4):771–6.

223. Visanji NP, Gomez-Ramirez J, Johnston TH, *et al.* Pharmacological characterization of psychosis-like behavior in the MPTP-lesioned nonhuman primate model of Parkinson's disease. *Mov Disord* 2006;**21**(11):1879–91.

224. Oh JD, Bibbiani F, Chase TN. Quetiapine attenuates levodopa-induced motor complications in rodent and primate parkinsonian models. *Exp Neurol* 2002;**177**(2):557–64.
225. Durif F, Debilly B, Galitzky M, *et al.* Clozapine improves dyskinesias in Parkinson disease: a double-blind, placebo-controlled study. *Neurology* 2004;**62**(3):381–8.
226. Katzenschlager R, Manson AJ, Evans A, *et al.* Low dose quetiapine for drug induced dyskinesias in Parkinson's disease: a double blind cross over study. *J Neurol Neurosurg Psychiatry* 2004;**75**(2):295–7.
227. Roberts C. ACP-103, a 5-HT2A receptor inverse agonist. *Curr Opin Investig Drugs* 2006;**7**(7):653–60.
228. Pertwee RG, Greentree SG. Delta-9-tetrahydrocannabinol-induced catalepsy in mice is enhanced by pretreatment with flurazepam or chlordiazepoxide. *Neuropharmacology* 1988;**27**(5):485–91.
229. Cravatt BF, Demarest K, Patricelli MP, *et al.* Supersensitivity to anandamide and enhanced endogenous cannabinoid signaling in mice lacking fatty acid amide hydrolase. *Proc Natl Acad Sci USA* 2001;**98**(16):9371–6.
230. Di Marzo V, Bifulco M, De Petrocellis L. The endocannabinoid system and its therapeutic exploitation. *Nat Rev Drug Discov* 2004;**3**(9):771–84.
231. Uchigashima M, Narushima M, Fukaya M, *et al.* Subcellular arrangement of molecules for 2-arachidonoyl-glycerol-mediated retrograde signaling and its physiological contribution to synaptic modulation in the striatum. *J Neurosci* 2007;**27**(14):3663–76.
232. Giuffrida A, Parsons LH, Kerr TM, *et al.* Dopamine activation of endogenous cannabinoid signaling in dorsal striatum. *Nat Neurosci* 1999;**2**(4):358–63.
233. Pertwee RG, Wickens AP. Enhancement by chlordiazepoxide of catalepsy induced in rats by intravenous or intrapallidal injections of enantiomeric cannabinoids. *Neuropharmacology* 1991;**30**(3):237–44.
234. Glass M, Brotchie JM, Maneuf YP. Modulation of neurotransmission by cannabinoids in the basal ganglia. *Eur J Neurosci* 1997;**9**(2):199–203.
235. Wallmichrath I, Szabo B. Analysis of the effect of cannabinoids on GABAergic neurotransmission in the substantia nigra pars reticulata. *Naunyn Schmiedebergs Arch Pharmacol* 2002;**365**(4):326–34.
236. Gerdeman G, Lovinger DM. CB1 cannabinoid receptor inhibits synaptic release of glutamate in rat dorsolateral striatum. *J Neurophysiol* 2001;**85**(1):468–71.
237. Brown TM, Brotchie JM, Fitzjohn SM. Cannabinoids decrease corticostriatal synaptic transmission via an effect on glutamate uptake. *J Neurosci* 2003;**23**(35):11073–7.
238. Kofalvi A, Rodrigues RJ, Ledent C, *et al.* Involvement of cannabinoid receptors in the regulation of neurotransmitter release in the rodent striatum: a combined immunochemical and pharmacological analysis. *J Neurosci* 2005;**25**(11):2874–84.
239. Maneuf YP, Crossman AR, Brotchie JM. The cannabinoid receptor agonist WIN 55,212-2 reduces D2, but not D1, dopamine receptor-mediated alleviation of akinesia in the reserpine-treated rat model of Parkinson's disease. *Exp Neurol* 1997;**148**(1):265–70.
240. Pisani A, Fezza F, Galati S, *et al.* High endogenous cannabinoid levels in the cerebrospinal fluid of untreated Parkinson's disease patients. *Ann Neurol* 2005;**57**(5):777–9.
241. Di Marzo V, Hill MP, Bisogno T, *et al.* Enhanced levels of endogenous cannabinoids in the globus pallidus are associated with a reduction in movement in an animal model of Parkinson's disease. *FASEB J* 2000;**14**(10):1432–8.
242. Maccarrone M, Gubellini P, Bari M, *et al.* Levodopa treatment reverses endocannabinoid system abnormalities in experimental parkinsonism. *J Neurochem* 2003;**85**(4):1018–25.
243. van der Stelt M, Fox SH, Hill M, *et al.* A role for endocannabinoids in the generation of parkinsonism and levodopa-induced dyskinesia in MPTP-lesioned non-human primate models of Parkinson's disease. *FASEB J* 2005;**19**(9):1140–2.
244. Kreitzer AC, Malenka RC. Endocannabinoid-mediated rescue of striatal LTD and motor deficits in Parkinson's disease models. *Nature* 2007;**445**(7128):643–7.
245. Maneuf YP, Mitchell IJ, Crossman AR, Brotchie JM. On the role of enkephalin cotransmission in the GABAergic striatal efferents to the globus pallidus. *Exp Neurol* 1994;**125**(1):65–71.
246. Gonzalez S, Scorticati C, Garcia-Arencibia M, *et al.* Effects of rimonabant, a selective cannabinoid CB1 receptor antagonist, in a rat model of Parkinson's disease. *Brain Res* 2006;**1073–1074**:209–19.
247. Cao X, Liang L, Hadcock JR, *et al.* Blockade of cannabinoid type 1 receptors augments the antiparkinsonian action of levodopa without affecting dyskinesias in 1-methyl-4-phenyl-1,2,3,6-tetrahydropyridine-treated rhesus monkeys. *J Pharmacol Exp Ther* 2007;**323**(1):318–26.
248. Mesnage V, Houeto JL, Bonnet AM, *et al.* Neurokinin B, neurotensin, and cannabinoid receptor antagonists and Parkinson disease. *Clin Neuropharmacol* 2004;**27**(3):108–10.
249. Maneuf YP, Duty S, Hille CJ, *et al.* Modulation of GABA transmission by diazoxide and cromakalim in the globus pallidus: implications for the treatment of Parkinson's disease. *Exp Neurol* 1996;**139**(1):12–6.
250. Sieradzan KA, Fox SH, Hill M, *et al.* Cannabinoids reduce levodopa-induced dyskinesia in Parkinson's disease: a pilot study. *Neurology* 2001;**57**(11):2108–11.
251. Segovia G, Mora F, Crossman AR, Brotchie JM. Effects of CB1 cannabinoid receptor modulating compounds on the hyperkinesia induced by high-dose levodopa in the reserpine-treated rat model of Parkinson's disease. *Mov Disord* 2003;**18**(2):138–49.
252. Ferrer B, Asbrock N, Kathuria S, *et al.* Effects of levodopa on endocannabinoid levels in rat basal ganglia: implications for the treatment of levodopa-induced dyskinesias. *Eur J Neurosci* 2003;**18**(6):1607–14.
253. Morgese MG, Cassano T, Cuomo V, Giuffrida A. Anti-dyskinetic effects of cannabinoids in a rat model of Parkinson's disease: role of CB(1) and TRPV1 receptors. *Exp Neurol* 2007;**208**(1):110–9.
254. Fox SH, Henry B, Hill M, *et al.* Stimulation of cannabinoid receptors reduces levodopa-induced dyskinesia in the MPTP-lesioned nonhuman primate model of Parkinson's disease. *Mov Disord* 2002;**17**(6):1180–7.
255. Carroll CB, Bain PG, Teare L, *et al.* Cannabis for dyskinesia in Parkinson disease: a randomized double-blind crossover study. *Neurology* 2004;**63**(7):1245–50.

256. Consroe P, Sandyk R, Snider SR. Open label evaluation of cannabidiol in dystonic movement disorders. *Int J Neurosci* 1986;**30**(4):277–82.
257. Jabusch HC, Schneider U, Altenmuller E. Delta9-tetrahydrocannabinol improves motor control in a patient with musician's dystonia. *Mov Disord* 2004;**19**(8):990–1.
258. Gauter B, Rukwied R, Konrad C. Cannabinoid agonists in the treatment of blepharospasm – a case report study. *Neuro Endocrinol Lett* 2004;**25**(1–2):45–8.
259. Fox SH, Kellett M, Moore AP, *et al.* Randomised, double-blind, placebo-controlled trial to assess the potential of cannabinoid receptor stimulation in the treatment of dystonia. *Mov Disord* 2002;**17**(1):145–9.
260. Cuello AC. Endogenous opioid peptides in neurons of the human brain. *Lancet* 1978;**ii**(8084):291–3.
261. Gerfen CR, Engber TM, Mahan LC, *et al.* D1 and D2 dopamine receptor-regulated gene expression of striatonigral and striatopallidal neurons. *Science* 1990;**250**(4986):1429–32.
262. Seizinger BR, Grimm C, Hollt V, Herz A. Evidence for a selective processing of proenkephalin B into different opioid peptide forms in particular regions of rat brain and pituitary. *J Neurochem* 1984;**42**(2):447–57.
263. Breslin MB, Lindberg I, Benjannet S, *et al.* Differential processing of proenkephalin by prohormone convertases 1(3) and 2 and furin. *J Biol Chem* 1993;**268**(36):27084–93.
264. Jiang HK, McGinty JF, Hong JS. Differential modulation of striatonigral dynorphin and enkephalin by dopamine receptor subtypes. *Brain Res* 1990;**507**(1):57–64.
265. Herrero MT, Augood SJ, Hirsch EC, *et al.* Effects of L-DOPA on preproenkephalin and preprotachykinin gene expression in the MPTP-treated monkey striatum. *Neuroscience* 1995;**68**(4):1189–98.
266. Nisbet AP, Foster OJ, Kingsbury A, *et al.* Preproenkephalin and preprotachykinin messenger RNA expression in normal human basal ganglia and in Parkinson's disease. *Neuroscience* 1995;**66**(2):361–76.
267. Brotchie J, Crossman A, Mitchell I, *et al.* Chemical signalling in the globus pallidus in parkinsonism. *Prog Brain Res* 1993;**99**:125–39.
268. Bezard E, Crossman AR, Gross CE, Brotchie JM. Structures outside the basal ganglia may compensate for dopamine loss in the presymptomatic stages of Parkinson's disease. *FASEB J* 2001;**15**(6):1092–4.
269. Hille CJ, Fox SH, Maneuf YP, *et al.* Antiparkinsonian action of a delta opioid agonist in rodent and primate models of Parkinson's disease. *Exp Neurol* 2001;**172**(1):189–98.
270. Hudzik TJ, Howell A, Payza K, Cross AJ. Antiparkinson potential of delta-opioid receptor agonists. *Eur J Pharmacol* 2000;**396**(2–3):101–7.
271. Maneuf YP, Mitchell IJ, Crossman AR, *et al.* Functional implications of kappa opioid receptor-mediated modulation of glutamate transmission in the output regions of the basal ganglia in rodent and primate models of Parkinson's disease. *Brain Res* 1995;**683**(1):102–8.
272. Hill MP, Brotchie JM. Modulation of glutamate release by a kappa-opioid receptor agonist in rodent and primate striatum. *Eur J Pharmacol* 1995;**281**(1):R1–2.
273. Hughes NR, McKnight AT, Woodruff GN, *et al.* Kappa-opioid receptor agonists increase locomotor activity in the monoamine-depleted rat model of parkinsonism. *Mov Disord* 1998;**13**(2):228–33.
274. Cox H, Togasaki DM, Chen L, *et al.* The selective kappa-opioid receptor agonist U50,488 reduces L-dopa-induced dyskinesias but worsens parkinsonism in MPTP-treated primates. *Exp Neurol* 2007;**205**(1):101–7.
275. Marti M, Mela F, Guerrini R, *et al.* Blockade of nociceptin/orphanin FQ transmission in rat substantia nigra reverses haloperidol-induced akinesia and normalizes nigral glutamate release. *J Neurochem* 2004;**91**(6):1501–4.
276. Marti M, Mela F, Veronesi C, *et al.* Blockade of nociceptin/orphanin FQ receptor signaling in rat substantia nigra pars reticulata stimulates nigrostriatal dopaminergic transmission and motor behavior. *J Neurosci* 2004;**24**(30):6659–66.
277. Marti M, Trapella C, Viaro R, Morari M. The nociceptin/orphanin FQ receptor antagonist J-113397 and L-DOPA additively attenuate experimental parkinsonism through overinhibition of the nigrothalamic pathway. *J Neurosci* 2007;**27**(6):1297–307.
278. Visanji N, de Bie RM, Johnston TH, *et al.* The nociceptin/orphanin FQ receptor antagonist J-113397 enhances the effects of levodopa in the MPTP-lesioned non-human primate model of Parkinson's disease. *Mov Disord* 2008;**23**(13):1922–5.
279. Engber TM, Boldry RC, Chase TN. The kappa-opioid receptor agonist spiradoline differentially alters the rotational response to dopamine D1 and D2 agonists. *Eur J Pharmacol* 1991;**200**(1):171–3.
280. Duty S, Brotchie JM. Enhancement of the behavioral response to apomorphine administration following repeated treatment in the 6-hydroxydopamine-lesioned rat is temporally correlated with a rise in striatal preproenkephalin-B, but not preproenkephalin-A, gene expression. *Exp Neurol* 1997;**144**(2):423–32.
281. Cenci MA, Lee CS, Bjorklund A. L-DOPA-induced dyskinesia in the rat is associated with striatal overexpression of prodynorphin- and glutamic acid decarboxylase mRNA. *Eur J Neurosci* 1998;**10**(8):2694–706.
282. Henry B, Crossman AR, Brotchie JM. Effect of repeated L-DOPA, bromocriptine, or lisuride administration on preproenkephalin-A and preproenkephalin-B mRNA levels in the striatum of the 6-hydroxydopamine-lesioned rat. *Exp Neurol* 1999;**155**(2):204–20.
283. Morissette M, Goulet M, Soghomonian JJ, *et al.* Preproenkephalin mRNA expression in the caudate-putamen of MPTP monkeys after chronic treatment with the D2 agonist U91356A in continuous or intermittent mode of administration: comparison with L-DOPA therapy. *Brain Res Mol Brain Res* 1997;**49**(1–2):55–62.
284. Ravenscroft P, Chalon S, Brotchie JM, Crossman AR. Ropinirole versus L-DOPA effects on striatal opioid peptide precursors in a rodent model of Parkinson's disease: implications for dyskinesia. *Exp Neurol* 2004;**185**(1):36–46.
285. Quik M, Police S, Langston JW, Di Monte DA. Increases in striatal preproenkephalin gene expression are associated with nigrostriatal damage but not L-DOPA-induced dyskinesias in the squirrel monkey. *Neuroscience* 2002;**113**(1):213–20.

286. Henry B, Duty S, Fox SH, *et al.* Increased striatal pre-proenkephalin B expression is associated with dyskinesia in Parkinson's disease. *Exp Neurol* 2003;**183**(2):458–68.
287. Calon F, Birdi S, Rajput AH, *et al.* Increase of pre-proenkephalin mRNA levels in the putamen of Parkinson disease patients with levodopa-induced dyskinesias. J Neuropathol *Exp Neurol* 2002;**61**(2):186–96.
288. Piccini P, Weeks RA, Brooks DJ. Alterations in opioid receptor binding in Parkinson's disease patients with levodopa-induced dyskinesias. *Ann Neurol* 1997;**42**(5):720–6.
289. Henry B, Fox SH, Crossman AR, Brotchie JM. Mu- and delta-opioid receptor antagonists reduce levodopa-induced dyskinesia in the MPTP-lesioned primate model of Parkinson's disease. *Exp Neurol* 2001;**171**(1):139–46.
290. Klintenberg R, Svenningsson P, Gunne L, Andren PE. Naloxone reduces levodopa-induced dyskinesias and apomorphine-induced rotations in primate models of parkinsonism. *J Neural Transm* 2002;**109**(10):1295–307.
291. Samadi P, Gregoire L, Bedard PJ. Opioid antagonists increase the dyskinetic response to dopaminergic agents in parkinsonian monkeys: interaction between dopamine and opioid systems. *Neuropharmacology* 2003;**45**(7):954–63.
292. Sandyk R, Snider SR. Naloxone treatment of L-dopa-induced dyskinesias in Parkinson's disease. *Am J Psychiatry* 1986;**143**(1):118.
293. Trabucchi M, Bassi S, Frattola L. Effect of naloxone on the "on–off' syndrome in patients receiving long-term levodopa therapy. *Arch Neurol* 1982;**39**(2):120–1.
294. Rascol O, Fabre N, Blin O, *et al.* Naltrexone, an opiate antagonist, fails to modify motor symptoms in patients with Parkinson's disease. *Mov Disord* 1994;**9**(4):437–40.
295. Manson AJ, Katzenschlager R, Hobart J, Lees AJ. High dose naltrexone for dyskinesias induced by levodopa. *J Neurol Neurosurg Psychiatry* 2001;**70**(4):554–6.
296. Fox S, Silverdale M, Kellett M, *et al.* Non-subtype-selective opioid receptor antagonism in treatment of levodopa-induced motor complications in Parkinson's disease. *Mov Disord* 2004;**19**(5):554–60.
297. Samadi P, Bedard PJ, Rouillard C. Opioids and motor complications in Parkinson's disease. *Trends Pharmacol Sci* 2006;**27**(10):512–7.
298. Chen L, Togasaki DM, Langston JW, *et al.* Enhanced striatal opioid receptor-mediated G-protein activation in L-DOPA-treated dyskinetic monkeys. *Neuroscience* 2005;**132**(2):409–20.
299. Hallett PJ, Brotchie JM. Striatal delta opioid receptor binding in experimental models of Parkinson's disease and dyskinesia. *Mov Disord* 2007;**22**(1):28–40.
300. You ZB, Herrera-Marschitz M, *et al.* Effect of morphine on dynorphin B and GABA release in the basal ganglia of rats. *Brain Res* 1996;**710**(1–2):241–8.
301. Rinne JO, Anichtchik OV, Eriksson KS, *et al.* Increased brain histamine levels in Parkinson's disease but not in multiple system atrophy. *J Neurochem* 2002;**81**(5):954–60.
302. Anichtchik OV, Rinne JO, Kalimo H, Panula P. An altered histaminergic innervation of the substantia nigra in Parkinson's disease. *Exp Neurol* 2000;**163**(1):20–30.
303. Martinez-Mir MI, Pollard H, Moreau J, *et al.* Loss of striatal histamine H2 receptors in Huntington's chorea but not in Parkinson's disease: comparison with animal models. *Synapse* 1993;**15**(3):209–20.
304. Honrubia MA, Vilaro MT, Palacios JM, Mengod G. Distribution of the histamine H(2) receptor in monkey brain and its mRNA localization in monkey and human brain. *Synapse* 2000;**38**(3):343–54.
305. Chen K, Wang JJ, Yung WH, *et al.* Excitatory effect of histamine on neuronal activity of rat globus pallidus by activation of H2 receptors *in vitro*. *Neurosci Res* 2005;**53**(3): 288–97.
306. Prast H, Tran MH, Lamberti C, *et al.* Histaminergic neurons modulate acetylcholine release in the ventral striatum: role of H1 and H2 histamine receptors. *Naunyn Schmiedebergs Arch Pharmacol* 1999;**360**(5):552–7.
307. Molinari SP, Kaminski R, Di Rocco A, Yahr MD. The use of famotidine in the treatment of Parkinson's disease: a pilot study. *J Neural Transm Park Dis Dement Sect* 1995;**9**(2–3):243–7.
308. Goodchild RE, Court JA, Hobson I, *et al.* Distribution of histamine H3-receptor binding in the normal human basal ganglia: comparison with Huntington's and Parkinson's disease cases. *Eur J Neurosci* 1999;**11**(2):449–56.
309. Anichtchik OV, Peitsaro N, Rinne JO, *et al.* Distribution and modulation of histamine H(3) receptors in basal ganglia and frontal cortex of healthy controls and patients with Parkinson's disease. *Neurobiol Dis* 2001;**8**(4):707–16.
310. Prast H, Tran MH, Fischer H, *et al.* Histaminergic neurons modulate acetylcholine release in the ventral striatum: role of H3 histamine receptors. *Naunyn Schmiedebergs Arch Pharmacol* 1999;**360**(5):558–64.
311. Doreulee N, Yanovsky Y, Flagmeyer I, *et al.* Histamine H(3) receptors depress synaptic transmission in the corticostriatal pathway. *Neuropharmacology* 2001;**40**(1):106–13.
312. Threlfell S, Cragg SJ, Kallo I, *et al.* Histamine H3 receptors inhibit serotonin release in substantia nigra pars reticulata. *J Neurosci* 2004;**24**(40):8704–10.
313. Garcia-Ramirez M, Aceves J, Arias-Montano JA. Intranigral injection of the H3 agonist immepip and systemic apomorphine elicit ipsilateral turning behaviour in naive rats, but reduce contralateral turning in hemiparkinsonian rats. *Behav Brain Res* 2004;**154**(2):409–15.
314. Huotari M, Kukkonen K, Liikka N, *et al.* Effects of histamine H(3)-ligands on the levodopa-induced turning behavior of hemiparkinsonian rats. *Parkinsonism Relat Disord* 2000;**6**(3):159–164.
315. Gomez-Ramirez J, Johnston TH, Visanji NP, *et al.* Histamine H3 receptor agonists reduce L-dopa-induced chorea, but not dystonia, in the MPTP-lesioned nonhuman primate model of Parkinson's disease. *Mov Disord* 2006;**21**(6):839–46.

Chapter 39
Prospects for Neuroprotective Therapies That Can Modulate Non-Dopaminergic Features in Parkinson's Disease

C. Warren Olanow[1] *& Anthony E. Lang*[2]

[1]Departments of Neurology and Neuroscience, Mount Sinai School of Medicine, New York, NY, USA
[2]Department of Neurology, University of Toronto, Toronto, ON, Canada

Introduction

The clinical significance of the non-motor and non-dopaminergic features of Parkinson's disease (PD) described throughout this book highlight the need for more effective therapies. Current anti-parkinsonian treatments are primarily dopaminergic, and as such they do not satisfactorily control the non-motor and non-dopaminergic features of the illness which currently constitute the primary source of disability for patients with advanced PD. Moderately effective treatments exist for some of these features, such as mood disorders, autonomic dysfunction, and sleep problems, but effective treatments are basically lacking for the more disabling features such as freezing of gait, postural disturbances, falling, cognitive impairment, and dementia. Indeed, these are the major reasons for nursing home placement for PD patients. A disease-modifying or neuroprotective therapy that could be instituted in the early stages of the illness and delay or prevent the emergence of these non-dopaminergic and non-motor features therefore represents an urgent priority.

Although there are many promising candidate targets and several putative neuroprotective agents have been identified, none has been definitively established to have a disease-modifying effect [1]. Selegiline, coenzyme Q10, and the dopamine agonists ropinirole and pramipexole have been shown to protect dopamine neurons in animal models and to have positive results in clinical trials, but could not be definitively determined to be disease-modifying because of potential confounding symptomatic or pharmacologic effects [2–5]. Rasagiline 1 mg per day had positive effects in a delayed-start study consistent with a disease-modifying effect, and showed benefits on some measures of non-motor features, but rasagiline 2 mg per day failed to provide benefit in this same trial [6]. The basis of this dissociation remains unresolved and leaves the question of whether rasagiline has true disease modification effects unanswered. Cell-based and gene delivery of trophic factors have attracted considerable attention, but have not yet shown benefit in double-blind, controlled trials. Further, to date these therapies have focused on restoring the nigrostriatal dopamine system, and it is hard to envision how these strategies as they are currently employed will meaningfully benefit non-dopaminergic pathology [7]. This chapter briefly reviews some of the obstacles that have limited the development of a neuroprotective therapy that might benefit the non-motor and non-dopaminergic features of PD, and the progress that has been made in attempting to overcome these problems.

Etiopathogenesis of PD

A major obstacle to the development of a neuroprotective or disease-modifying therapy for PD has been uncertainty as to the precise etiology and pathogenesis of the disorder. Putative neuroprotective agents studied to date have largely aimed at interfering with pathogenic processes implicated in the cell death process primarily based on postmortem studies. These factors include oxidative stress, mitochondrial dysfunction, calcium-mediated cytotoxicity, inflammation, proteolytic stress, and signal-mediated apoptosis. However, clinical trials to date testing agents that interfere with these processes have failed to detect an effect on disease progression. Indeed, after more than two decades of study, it remains unknown which, if any, of these mechanisms represent the primary driver of the cell death process, which play only a

Parkinson's Disease: Non-Motor and Non-Dopaminergic Features, First Edition. Edited by C. Warren Olanow, Fabrizio Stocchi, and Anthony E. Lang.

secondary role, and whether any or all are merely unrelated epiphenomena. It remains possible that cell death in PD develops in response to an as yet unidentified etiopathogenic process that differs from all of the mechanisms implicated to date. It may also be that initiating therapies in even the early stages of PD may be too late to interfere effectively with the disease process. Further, treating single mechanisms may not be sufficient and cocktails of agents that interfere with multiple mechanisms may be required.

Treating the fundamental cause of the disease is desirable, but there is now evidence that multiple factors may be involved in the etiology of PD, and they may well differ in different individuals. Twin studies suggest that in individuals older than 50 years, PD is likely to be predominantly environmental in origin [8]. MPTP and rotenone are toxic to mitochondria and cause dopaminergic lesions in laboratory models, but do not precisely replicate PD pathology and have not been shown to cause PD. Epidemiologic studies have implicated rural living, exposure to pesticides, and drinking well water as risk factors, but no specific toxin has yet been established to cause the disease. Genetic causes have attracted more recent attention, as several mutations have been identified in familial and even some sporadic cases of PD. These include α-synuclein, UCH-L1, parkin, DJ-1, PINK1, LRRK2, OMI/HTRA2, ATP13A2, and mutations in GBA in Gaucher's disease [9]. Although these affect relatively small numbers of individuals, and most cases occur sporadically, these mutations provide an opportunity to study the mechanism by which the mutant protein can induce cell death in at least one form of PD, with the hope that this is relevant to the more common sporadic form of the disease. Towards this end, gene mutations identified to date primarily point towards defects in mitochondrial function and protein misfolding and accumulation as being central to the development of PD.

Mitochondrial dysfunction

PD is known to be associated with reduced staining and activity of complex I of the mitochondrial respiratory chain in the substantia nigra pars compacta (SNc) [10,11], and toxins such as MPTP and rotenone that specifically affect complex I induce a model of PD [12,13]. Several of the gene mutations identified in PD also point to mitochondrial dysfunction as an important factor in the disease. PINK1 (PTEN-induced putative kinase) has a mitochondrial targeting sequence [14] and acts to sense mitochondrial stress and to protect against apoptosis [15,16]. Knockout of PINK1 causes mitochondrial dysfunction with enlargement and fragmentation of christae [17,18]. Parkin mutations also lead to alterations in mitochondrial morphology and enhance damage caused by PINK1 mutations [18]. Interestingly, overexpression of parkin protects against PINK1 mutations, but PINK1 does not protect against parkin mutations [19,20], suggesting that PINK1 and parkin are linked via a common pathway with parkin being downstream. DJ-1 acts as a sensor of oxidative stress in mitochondria and mutations cause a form of PD [21]. Overexpression of the protein protects dopamine neurons from oxidative stress [22], and mutation or knockout of the protein leads to oxidative stress [23,24]. Alterations in mitochondrial function due to any of these causes could lead to reduced ATP production critical for normal cell function. Hence the mitochondrion and related proteins such as parkin, PINK1 and DJ-1 are candidate targets for a putative neuroprotective therapy aimed at restoring or enhancing mitochondrial function. Agents that are thought to enhance mitochondrial function such as coenzyme Q10 and creatine are currently being tested in double-blind trials.

Protein accumulation

Protein accumulation has been implicated in the etiology of PD, as Lewy bodies and Lewy neurites which contain misfolded and aggregated proteins are the pathologic hallmark of the disease. The role of proteins has attracted even more attention with the appreciation that neurodegeneration with protein accumulation is widespread in PD and appears to involve the olfactory system, lower brainstem, and peripheral autonomic nervous system prior to the SNc [25]. Protein accumulation could result from increased production or impaired clearance of proteins, and is thought to lead to the formation of toxic oligomers and cell death. Gene mutations associated with familial PD could cause protein accumulation through either of these mechanisms. Mutations in α-synuclein are associated with familial PD [26], and the mutant protein is prone to misfold and generate potentially toxic oligomers and aggregates [27], suggesting that increased levels of abnormal proteins can drive the PD process. Importantly, duplication or triplication of wild-type α-synuclein [28,29] also causes familial PD, indicating that even increased production of normal proteins can cause the disorder. This concept is supported by studies showing that gene delivery of α-synuclein to the region of the SNc can replicate many of the behavioral and pathologic features of PD in rodents and primates [30,31].

Other gene mutations associated with familial PD could interfere with protein clearance. Parkin is a ubiquitin ligase which attaches ubiquitin to unwanted proteins to signal for their transport to, and degradation by, the proteasome [32]. Mutations associated with PD can interfere with this process and prevent clearance of substrate proteins. UCH-L1 de-ubiquitinates ubiquitinated proteins to permit their entry into the proteasome [33]. Mutations in UCH-L1 can inhibit this function. In further support of this concept, postmortem studies demonstrate defects in proteasomal and lysosomal function in the SNc of patients with sporadic PD [34], and proteasome and

UCH inhibition in the laboratory induce degeneration of dopamine neurons with Lewy body-like inclusions [35].

Regardless of the cause of accumulation, proteins can damage UPS and lysosomal functions, thereby further impairing protein clearance. Thus, a vicious cycle might occur whereby increased production of mutant or wild-type proteins could interfere with clearance mechanisms, while impaired clearance could result in further protein accumulation. Continued protein accumulation resulting from this vicious cycle could eventually exceed the capacity of the cell to degrade the unwanted proteins, thereby leading to a state of proteolytic stress with consequent protein accumulation, oligomer formation, aggregation, and cell death.

The possibility that proteolytic stress may be a key factor in the cell death process in PD provides several novel candidate targets for a putative neuroprotective therapy. Such therapies could be designed to prevent the production of misfolded proteins, facilitate refolding, enhance proteasomal or lysosomal degradation, and promote the dissolution or prevent the formation of toxic oligomers or polymers. Preliminary studies in the laboratory have focused on upregulation of heat shock proteins [36–38], vaccination-induced production of antibodies directed against oligomeric α-synuclein [39], rifampicin which inhibits oligomerization and disaggregates α-synuclein [40], and the sirtuin family of proteins (SIRTs) that are involved in histone deacetylation and autophagy [41]. Although these various approaches are interesting, none has yet been tested in PD patients, and safety issues remain to be more fully evaluated before clinical trials can be considered.

The role of proteins in the cell death process has been further supported by the recent finding that embryonic dopamine neurons implanted into the striatum of advanced PD patients developed α-synuclein-positive inclusions identical with Lewy bodies [42,43]. While the mechanism responsible for these pathologic changes is not known, the fact that genetically unrelated embryonic dopamine neurons can develop PD pathology raises the possibility that α-synuclein can act like a prion and be transmitted from host to implanted dopamine neurons [44]. Indeed, there is evidence that neurons can release and take up α-synuclein *in vitro* [45,46] and *in vivo* [47]. One might therefore envision that transmission of α-synuclein from affected to unaffected cells could account for the sequential evolution of α-synuclein pathology described by Braak *et al.* [25]. Studies are currently under way to determine whether inoculates derived from α-synuclein aggregates in PD patients can be transmitted to other species and cause the disease. This concept provides a rationale for targets that could interfere with a prion-like process in PD.

It is noteworthy that proteasomal and mitochondria functions are interdependent and that damage to one system can lead to dysfunction in the other. Adenosine triphosphate (ATP) generated by mitochondria is essential for normal proteasomal function, and mitochondrial toxins lead to proteasomal impairment, whereas proteasome inhibitors result in mitochondrial dysfunction. Indeed, α-synuclein overexpression induces both mitochondrial and proteasomal dysfunction [48,49], suggesting that the two mechanisms may be linked.

LRRK2 has received particular attention as a possible target for a neuroprotective therapy because mutations have been described in patients with both familial and "sporadic" PD [50], and because this mutation accounts for as many as 40% of PD cases in Ashkenazi Jews and some North African populations [51,52]. LRRK2 is linked to the outer mitochondrial membrane and has kinase [53] and guanosine triphosphatase (GTPase) [54] activities. Mutations found in PD are associated with reduced guanosine triphosphate (GTP) hydrolysis and alterations that reduce kinase activity in mutant LRRK2 reduce neuronal toxicity [55]. These observations suggest that cell death may relate to altered phosphorylation of target proteins, possibly as a result of an increase in levels of misfolded substrate proteins. LRRK2 may therefore be a novel target for neuroprotective drugs, and agents that alter or inhibit its kinase activity are currently being actively explored.

Although the large majority of PD cases occur sporadically and are of unknown etiology, the identification of mutations associated with some forms of PD potentially permits elucidation of the precise mechanism and signaling pathways that are associated with the cell death process in one form of PD and provides an opportunity to identify candidate targets for novel neuroprotective agents. Although the causes of genetic forms of PD may differ from each other and from sporadic cases, it is not unreasonable to anticipate that they might share a common pathogenic pathway, and that interventions that are protective against one of these forms might also be applicable to others.

This brief sample of experimental studies illustrates the many possible candidate targets that are currently being pursued, and it is likely that many more will be identified as new gene mutations associated with PD continue to be identified and explored.

Animal models of PD

Most preclinical studies evaluating potential new therapies for the treatment of PD have relied primarily on the 6-OHDA and MPTP models. These models, and particularly the MPTP monkey, provide excellent models of dopamine depletion and have facilitated the development of anti-parkinsonian and anti-dyskinesia drugs and treatment strategies. They do not, however, provide a good

Box 39.1 Desired feature in an animal model of PD

- Etiopathogenesis is relevant to PD
- Models the dopaminergic pathology of PD – including Lewy body formation
- Models the non-dopaminergic pathology of PD – including Lewy body formation
- Progressive, levodopa-responsive, behavioral syndrome
- Can be induced in small animals (e.g., *Drosophila*, *Caenorhabditis elegans*) to permit high-throughput testing
- Can be induced in large animals (e.g., non-human primates) to permit behavioral testing

model of PD for purposes of developing neuroprotective therapies as illustrated in Box 39.1. There is no evidence to suggest that MPTP or 6-OHDA is involved in the etiology of the disease or that cell death induced by these toxins is in any way associated with the pathogenesis of cell death in PD. Importantly, especially from the perspective of the non-dopaminergic features of the disease, they do not induce the full spectrum of non-dopaminergic pathology that characterizes the illness and are not associated with Lewy body pathology. Finally, although MPTP induces a good phenotype of the motor dysfunction of PD, it does not produce a progressive behavioral disorder in which to test the value of putative neuroprotective agents on disease progression as they would be employed in PD. It is therefore not surprising that positive results found in MPTP models have not consistently translated into positive results in clinical trials in PD. By contrast, it is possible that an agent that provides no benefits in the MPTP or 6-OHDA model might still prove effective in PD. Efforts to develop models of PD based on pathogenic factors such as iron infusion and buthionine sulfoxamine (oxidative stress), LPS (inflammation), and rotenone (mitochondrial damage) induce neurodegenerative changes, but similarly do not fully recapitulate the pathology or behavior of PD and have not been widely used for assessing potential new therapies.

More hope has been placed on transgenic models generated from mutations that are specifically associated with PD and therefore have an etiopathogenesis that is relevant to at least one form of the disease. To date, transgenic models have been developed based on the α-synuclein, parkin, and more recently LRRK2 mutations [56]. Although these models are promising, and alterations in dopamine synthesis, release, inclusions, and altered morphology of dopamine terminals have been described, none of the models developed to date adequately replicates the behavioral or pathologic (dopamine and non-dopamine) features of PD. Another methodology that has been employed involves gene delivery of α-synuclein to the region of the substantia nigra [30,31,34]. This methodology induces a model with progressive behavioral change, dopamine neuronal degeneration with inclusion bodies, and changes to the proteasome and lysosome systems that more closely model what is found in PD. As such, this may prove to be a valuable model, particularly as overexpression of even wild-type α-synuclein can cause a form of PD. However, this model as it is currently generated does not result in non-dopaminergic pathology, which, as outlined in great detail in this book, represents a major source of disability for many patients. An agent that blocks degeneration of dopamine neurons will not necessarily prevent non-dopaminergic neurodegeneration.

It is possible that a complete model of PD may not be achievable as spontaneously occurring PD has not been described in animal species, and it may be that the neurodegenerative process that occurs in PD is relatively specific to the human and cannot be fully modeled because of differences in metabolism, vulnerability factors, or compensatory mechanisms. Genetic models may nonetheless be of great importance for the development of neuroprotective agents as the changes that are induced likely occur through a similar pathway as the neurodegeneration of PD. Agents that interfere with this mechanism may therefore be more likely to have protective effects in PD than agents that protect against MPTP or 6-OHDA, which likely cause cell death through a different process. To date, few putative disease-modifying agents have been tested in genetic animal models as a prelude to clinical trials, but this is likely to change in the near future. It is also possible that with further modifications and new genetic models, we will develop a model that more closely replicates the pathologic and behavioral phenotype of PD.

Outcome measures and study designs to detect disease-modification

A study design or endpoint that accurately delineates disease modification is another important obstacle to defining a neuroprotective therapy. Study designs used to date have not been able to differentiate a disease-modifying effect from confounding symptomatic or pharmacologic effects of the study intervention [1]. To try to overcome this problem, the delayed-start design has been proposed [57]. This is a two-period study: in the first period, subjects are randomized to active treatment or placebo, and in the second period, subjects in both groups receive active treatment. Benefits seen at the end of the first period could be due to symptomatic or disease-modifying effects, or both. If the change from baseline at the end of the second period is no different in the early versus delayed-start groups when both groups are receiving the same treatment, this would argue that the drug has only symptomatic effects. However, if the benefits of early start persist at the end of the second period, then the results are not readily explained by a symptomatic effect and are consistent with the drug having a disease-modifying effect [58]. The ADAGIO study was the first prospective study to employ a delayed-start design [59]. In this study, rasagiline 1 mg per day met all three primary endpoints, consistent with the drug having a disease-modifying effect. Indeed, benefits were detected in both dopaminergic and non-dopaminergic features of the disease. Rasagiline 2 mg per day failed. The basis for these discrepant results remains unknown, although it has been proposed that the symptomatic effects of the higher dose may have masked the ability to detect a disease-modifying effect in this very mild population of patients [59].

The delayed-start study is designed primarily to determine if a study intervention provides benefits that cannot be explained by symptomatic effects alone, and is consistent with disease modification. It does not, however, necessarily provide information on the clinical significance of this benefit. To accomplish this, long-term studies such as the "long-term simple study" are required. These studies assess the impact of the drug on cumulative disability using an endpoint that incorporates measures of gait, cognitive function, and quality-of-life in addition to the standard UPDRS [60]. The delayed-start study thus provides information regarding mechanism, but not on clinical relevance, whereas the long-term simple study provides information on clinical significance but does not address mechanism. It is anticipated that the combination of a delayed-start study and a long-term simple study will provide the necessary information for regulatory authorities and clinicians to define a disease-modifying drug and its clinical significance [60].

Optimal population to study in disease-modifying trials

The population to study in a neuroprotection trial is potentially important and perhaps has not received sufficient attention. Most studies accept "all comers," which has the advantage of providing generalizable results, but may fail to detect benefits in sub-populations. For example, agents that enhance mitochondrial function might best be studied in patients with reduced mitochondrial complex I activity in platelets. Neuroprotective therapies may be more effective in early patients where more neurons are available to protect, whereas outcome measures that assess cumulative disability due to gait impairment and dementia may be more useful in a more advanced patient population where these events are more likely to occur.

There is increasing evidence suggesting that PD might be detected prior to the emergence of the classic motor features of the disease. Braak and others have proposed that α-synuclein pathology can be detected in olfactory, lower brainstem, and peripheral autonomic neurons prior to the appearance of neurodegeneration in the SNc. Correspondingly, anosmia, REM behavior disorder, and constipation frequently precede the clinical diagnosis of PD. Indeed, it has been proposed that these features are not just risk factors for the development of PD but in fact represent an early stage of the disease that precedes tremor, rigidity, and bradykinesia [61]. Identification of such a population might be valuable for testing putative disease-modifying agents that might be most effective in the earliest stages of the illness. Importantly, the introduction of an agent that has disease-modifying effects at such an early stage might prevent the emergence of the classic motor features entirely.

Conclusions

A disease-modifying therapy that slows or stops disease progression, and particularly has a positive impact on the emergence of disabling non-dopaminergic features, is a major unmet need in PD. Although no agent has as yet been unequivocally demonstrated to provide disease-modifying effects, much progress has occurred. Genetic studies have defined factors that are possibly central to the etiopathogenesis of PD, and suggest many new candidate targets for disease-modifying drugs. Similarly, animal models based on gene mutations associated with at least some forms of PD are likely to be more predictive of the potential value of a disease-modifying agent in PD patients than currently used models. Finally, new study designs such as the delayed-start and the long-term simple study offer promise for detecting agents that have disease-modifying effects and providing information that will be of value to both regulatory authorities and treating physicians.

References

1. Schapira AHV, Olanow CW. Neuroprotection in Parkinson's disease: myths, mysteries, and misconceptions. *JAMA* 2004; **291**:358–64.
2. Parkinson's Study Group. Effects of tocopherol and deprenyl on the progression of disability in early Parkinson's disease. *N Engl J Med* 1993;**328**:176–83.
3. Shults CW, Oakes D, Kieburtz K, *et al*. Effects of coenzyme Q10 in early Parkinson disease: evidence of slowing of the functional decline. *Arch Neurol* 2002;**59**:1541–50.
4. Whone AL, Watts RL, Stoessl AJ, *et al*. Slower progression of Parkinson's disease with ropinirole versus levodopa: the REAL-PET Study. *Ann Neurol* 2003;**54**:93–101.

5. Parkinson Study Group. Dopamine transporter brain imaging to assess the effects of pramipexole vs levodopa on Parkinson disease progression. *JAMA* 2002;**287**:1653–61.
6. Olanow CW, Rascol O, Hauser R, *et al.* A double-blind delayed-start study of rasagiline in early Parkinson's disease. *N Engl J Med* 2009;**361**:1268–78.
7. Olanow CW, Kordower JH, Lang AE, Obeso JA. Dopaminergic transplantation for Parkinson's disease: current status and future prospects. *Ann Neurol* 2009;**66**:591–6.
8. Tanner CM, Ottman R, Goldman SM, *et al.* Parkinson disease in twins: an etiologic study. *JAMA* 1999;**281**:341–6.
9. Hardy J, Cai H, Cookson MR, *et al.* Genetics of Parkinson's disease and parkinsonism. *Ann Neurol* 2006;**60**:389–98.
10. Schapira AHV, Cooper JM, Dexter D, *et al.* Mitochondrial complex I deficiency in Parkinson's disease. *J Neurochem* 1990; **54**:823–7.
11. Mizuno Y, Ohta S, Tanaka M, *et al.* Deficiencies in complex I subunits of the respiratory chain in Parkinson's disease. *Biochem Biophys Res Commun* 1989;**163**:1450–5.
12. Langston JW, Ballard P, Tetrud JW, Irwin I. Chronic parkinsonism in humans due to a product of meperidine-analog synthesis. *Science* 1983;**219**:979–80.
13. Betarbet R, Sherer TB, MacKenzie G, *et al.* Chronic systemic pesticide exposure reproduces features of Parkinson's disease. *Nat Neurosci* 2000;**3**:1301–6.
14. Valente EM, Abou-Sleiman PM, Caputo V, *et al.* Hereditary early-onset Parkinson's disease caused by mutations in PINK1. *Science* 2004;**304**:1158–60.
15. Pridgeon JW, Olzmann JA, Chin LS, Li L. PINK1 protects against oxidative stress by phosphorylating mitochondrial chaperone TRAP1. *PLoS Biol* 2007;**5**:e172.
16. Alnemri ES. HtrA2 and Parkinson's disease: think PINK? *Nat Cell Biol* 2007;**9**:1227–9.
17. Clark IE, Dodson MW, Jiang C, *et al.* *Drosophila* pink1 is required for mitochondrial function and interacts genetically with parkin. *Nature* 2006;**441**:1162–6.
18. Park J, Lee SB, Lee S, *et al.* Mitochondrial dysfunction in *Drosophila* PINK1 mutants is complemented by parkin. *Nature* 2006;**441**:1157–61.
19. Yang Y, Gehrke S, Imai Y, *et al.* Mitochondrial pathology and muscle and dopaminergic neuron degeneration caused by inactivation of *Drosophila* Pink1 is rescued by Parkin. *Proc Natl Acad Sci USA* 2006;**103**:10793–8.
20. Exner N, Treske B, Paquet D, *et al.* Loss-of-function of human PINK1 results in mitochondrial pathology and can be rescued by parkin. *J Neurosci* 2007;**27**:12413–8.
21. Bonifati V, Rizzu P, van Baren MJ, *et al.* Mutations in the DJ-1 gene associated with autosomal recessive early-onset parkinsonism. *Science* 2003;**299**:256–9.
22. Inden M, Taira T, Kitamura Y, *et al.* PARK7 DJ-1 protects against degeneration of nigral dopaminergic neurons in Parkinson's disease rat model. *Neurobiol Dis* 2006;**24**:144–58.
23. Yang Y, Gehrke S, Haque ME, Iet al. Inactivation of *Drosophila* DJ-1 leads to impairments of oxidative stress response and phosphatidylinositol 3-kinase/Akt signaling. *Proc Natl Acad Sci USA* 2005;**102**:13670–5.
24. Yokota T, Sugawara K, Ito K, *et al.* Down regulation of DJ-1 enhances cell death by oxidative stress, ER stress, and proteasome inhibition. *Biochem Biophys Res Commun* 2003;**312**:1342–8.
25. Braak H, Del Tredici K, Rub U, *et al.* Staging of brain pathology related to sporadic Parkinson's disease. *Neurobiol Aging* 2003; **24**:197–211.
26. Polymeropoulos MH, Lavedan C, Leroy E, *et al.* Mutation in the alpha-synuclein gene identified in families with Parkinson's disease. *Science* 1997;**276**:2045–7.
27. Conway KA, Lee SJ, Rochet JC, *et al.* Acceleration of oligomerization, not fibrillization, is a shared property of both alpha-synuclein mutations linked to early-onset Parkinson's disease: implications for pathogenesis and therapy. *Proc Natl Acad Sci USA* 2000;**97**:571–6.
28. Chartier-Harlin MC, Kachergus J, Roumier C, *et al.* Alpha-synuclein locus duplication as a cause of familial Parkinson's disease. *Lancet* 2004;**364**:1167–9.
29. Singleton AB, Farrer M, Johnson J. Alpha-synuclein locus triplication causes Parkinson's disease. *Science* 2003;302: 841.
30. St Martin JL, Klucken J, Outeiro TF, *et al.* Dopaminergic neuron loss and up-regulation of chaperone protein mRNA induced by targeted over-expression of alpha-synuclein in mouse substantia nigra. *J Neurochem* 2007;**100**:1449–57.
31. Kirik D, Annett LE, Burger C, *et al.* Nigrostriatal alpha-synucleinopathy induced by viral vectormediated overexpression of human alpha-synuclein: a new primate model of Parkinson's disease. *Proc Natl Acad Sci USA* 2003;**100**:2884–9.
32. Kitada T, Asakawa S, Hattori N, *et al.* Mutations in the parkin gene cause autosomal recessive juvenile parkinsonism. *Nature* 1998;**392**:605–8.
33. Leroy E, Boyer R, Auburger G, *et al.* The ubiquitin pathway in Parkinson's disease. *Nature* 1998;**395**:451–2.
34. Chu Y, Dodiya1 H, Aebischer P, *et al.* Alterations in lysosomal and proteasomal markers in Parkinsons disease: relationship to alpha synuclein inclusions. *Neurobiol Dis* 2009;**35**:385–98.
35. McNaught KSP, Mytilineou C, JnoBaptiste R, *et al.* Impairment of the ubiquitin–proteasome system causes dopaminergic cell death and inclusion body formation in ventral mesencephalic cultures. *J Neurochem* 2002;**81**:301–6.
36. Klucken J, Shin Y, Masliah E, *et al.* Hsp70 reduces alpha-synuclein aggregation and toxicity. *J Biol Chem* 2004;**279**:25497–502.
37. Auluck PK, Chan E, Trojanowski JQ, *et al.* Chaperone suppression of alpha-synuclein toxicity in a *Drosophila* model of Parkinson's disease. *Science* 2002;**295**:865–8.
38. McLean PJ, Klucken J, Shin Y, Hyman BT. Geldanamycin induces Hsp70 and prevents alpha-synuclein aggregation and toxicity *in vitro*. *Biochem Biophys Res Commun* 2004;**321**: 665–9.
39. Masliah E, Rockenstein E, Adame A, *et al.* Effects of alpha-synuclein immunization in a mouse model of Parkinson's disease. *Neuron* 2005;**46**:857–68.
40. Li J, Zhu M, Rajamani S, *et al.* Rifampicin inhibits alpha-synuclein fibrillation and disaggregates fibrils. *Chem Biol* 2004; **11**:1513–21.
41. Outeiro TF, Kontopoulos E, Altmann SM, *et al.* Sirtuin 2 inhibitors rescue alpha-synuclein-mediated toxicity in models of Parkinson's disease. *Science* 2007;**317**:516–9.
42. Kordower JH, Chu Y, Hauser RA, *et al.* Parkinson's disease pathology in long-term embryonic nigral transplants in Parkinson's disease. *Nat Med* 2008;**14**:504–6.

43. Li JY, Englund E, Holton JL, *et al.* Lewy bodies in grafted neurons in subjects with Parkinson's disease suggest host-to-graft disease propagation. *Nat Med* 2008;**14**:501–3.
44. Olanow CW, Prusiner SB. Is Parkinson's disease a prion disorder? *Proc Natl Acad Sci USA* 2009;**106**:12571–2.
45. Lee H-J, Patel S, Lee S-J. Intravesicular localization and exocytosis of alpha-synuclein and its aggregates. *J Neurosci* 2005;**25**:6016–24.
46. Lee H-J, Suk JE, Bae EJ, *et al.* Assembly-dependent endocytosis and clearance of extracellular alpha-synuclein. *Int J Biochem Cell Biol* 2008;**40**:1835–49.
47. Desplats P, Lee HJ, Bae EJ, *et al.* Inclusion formation and neuronal cell death through neuron-to-neuron transmission of alpha-synuclein. *Proc Natl Acad Sci USA* 2009;**106**:13010–5.
48. Chen L, Thiruchelvam MJ, Madura K, Richfield EK. Proteasome dysfunction in aged human alpha-synuclein transgenic mice. *Neurobiol Dis* 2006;**23**:120–6.
49. Martin LJ, Pan Y, Price AC, *et al.* Parkinson's disease alpha-synuclein transgenic mice develop neuronal mitochondrial degeneration and cell death. *J Neurosci* 2006;**26**:41–50.
50. Gilks WP, Abou-Sleiman PM, Gandhi S, *et al.* A common LRRK2 mutation in idiopathic Parkinson's disease. *Lancet* 2005;**365**:415–6.
51. Ozelius LJ, Senthil G, Saunders-Pullman R, *et al.* LRRK2 G2019S as a cause of Parkinson's disease in Ashkenazi Jews. *N Engl J Med* 2006;**354**:424–5.
52. Lesage S, Dürr A, Tazir M, *et al.* LRRK2 G2019S as a cause of Parkinson's disease in North African Arabs. *N Engl J Med* 2006;**354**:422–3.
53. West AB, Moore DJ, Biskup S, *et al.* Parkinson's disease-associated mutations in leucine-rich repeat kinase 2 augment kinase activity. *Proc Natl Acad Sci USA* 2005;**102**:16842–7.
54. Li X, Tan Y, Poulose S, *et al.* Leucine-rich repeat kinase 2/PARK8 possesses GTPase activity that is altered in familial Parkinson's disease R1441C/G mutant. *J Neurochem* 2007;**103**:238–47.
55. Smith WW, Pei Z, Jiang H, *et al.* Kinase activity of mutant LRRK2 mediates neuronal toxicity. *Nat Neurosci* 2006;**9**:1231–3.
56. Olanow CW, Kordower J. Modeling Parkinson's disease. *Ann Neurol* 2009;**66**:432–6.
57. Leber P. Slowing the progression of Alzheimer disease: methodologic issues. *Alzheimer Dis Assoc Disord* 1997;**11**(Suppl 5):S10–21; discussion S37–9.
58. Olanow CW, Hauser R, Jankovic J, *et al.* A randomized, double-blind, placebo-controlled, delayed start study to assess rasagiline as a disease modifying therapy in Parkinson's disease (the ADAGIO Study): rationale, design, and baseline characteristics. *Mov Disord* 2008;**23**:2194–201.
59. Olanow CW, Rascol O, Hauser R, *et al.* A double-blind delayed-start study of rasagiline in early Parkinson's disease. *N Engl J Med* 2009;**361**:1268–78.
60. Olanow CW, Kieburtz K. Prospects for defining disease-modifying therapies in PD – a step forward. *Mov Disord* 2010;**25**:1774–9.
61. Langston JW. The Parkinson's complex: parkinsonism is just the tip of the iceberg. *Ann Neurol* 2006;**59**:591–6.

Index

Page numbers in *italics* denote figures, those in **bold** denote tables.

Parkinson's Disease: Non-Motor and Non-Dopaminergic Features, First Edition. Edited by C. Warren Olanow, Fabrizio Stocchi, and Anthony E. Lang.